IMMUNOPATHOLOGY OF THE SKIN

IMMUNOPATHOLOGY OF THE SKIN

THIRD EDITION

Edited by

ERNST H. BEUTNER, Ph.D.
Professor of Microbiology and Dermatology
Schools of Medicine and Dentistry
State University of New York at Buffalo
Buffalo, New York

TADEUSZ P. CHORZELSKI, M.D.
Professor of Dermatology
Warsaw Academy of Medicine
Warsaw, Poland

VIJAY KUMAR, Ph.D.
Associate Research Professor
Department of Microbiology and Dermatology
Schools of Medicine and Dentistry
State University of New York at Buffalo
Buffalo, New York

A WILEY MEDICAL PUBLICATION
JOHN WILEY & SONS
New York • Chichester • Brisbane • Toronto • Singapore

Library of Congress Cataloging in Publication Data:

Immunopathology of the skin.

(A Wiley medical publication)
Bibliography: p.
Includes index.
1. Skin—Diseases—Immunopathological aspects.
2. Immunopathology. 3. Skin—Diseases—Diagnosis.
4. Fluorescent antibody technique. I. Beutner, Ernst H., 1923– . II. Chorzelski, Tadeusz P.
III. Kumar, Vijay, 1945– IV. Series.
RL96.I45 1987 616.5′079 86-28081
ISBN 0-471-84074-2

Printed in the United States of America

10 9 8 7 6 5 4 3 2 1

Contributor List

Boris Albini, M.D.
Professor of Microbiology, State University of New York at Buffalo, Buffalo, New York

Elaine L. Alexander, M.D., Ph.D.
Assistant Professor of Medicine, Johns Hopkins Medical Institutions, Baltimore, Maryland

Grant J. Anhalt, M.D.
Assistant Professor of Dermatology, Johns Hopkins Medical Institutions, Baltimore, Maryland

Samuel F. Bean, M.D.
Clinical Professor of Dermatology, University of Texas Medical School, Houston, Texas, Clinical Associate Professor of Dermatology, Baylor College of Medicine, Houston, Texas

Wilma Fowler Bergfeld, M.D.
Head, Dermatopathology, Department of Pathology, Cleveland Clinic Foundation, Cleveland, Ohio

Ernst H. Beutner, Ph.D.
Professor of Microbiology and Dermatology, Schools of Medicine and Dentistry, State University of New York at Buffalo, Buffalo, New York

Maria Blaszczyk, M.D.
Associate Professor, Department of Dermatology, Warsaw Academy of Medicine, Warsaw, Poland

Robert A. Briggaman, M.D.
Professor of Dermatology, University of North Carolina School of Medicine, Chapel Hill, North Carolina

Thomas K. Burnham, M.B., B.S.
Staff Physician, Department of Dermatology, Henry Ford Hospital, Detroit, Michigan

Tadeusz P. Chorzelski, M.D.
Professor of Dermatology, Warsaw Academy of Medicine, Warsaw, Poland

Roger C. Cornell, M.D.
Head, Division of Dermatology, Scripps Clinic and Research Foundation, La Jolla, California

Roger K. Cunningham, Ph.D.
Associate Professor, Department of Microbiology, State University of New York at Buffalo, Buffalo, New York

Mark V. Dahl, M.D.
Professor of Dermatology, University of Minnesota Medical School, Minneapolis, Minnesota

Jau-Shyong Deng, M.D.
Assistant Professor, Department of Dermatology, University of Pittsburgh, Chief of Dermatology, Veteran's Administration Medical Center, Pittsburgh, Pennsylvania

Luis A. Diaz, M.D.
Associate Professor of Dermatology, Johns Hopkins Medical Institutions, Baltimore, Maryland

Liliane Didierjean, Ph.D.
Clinique de Dermatologie, Hôpital Cantonal Universitaire, Geneva, Switzerland

N. Fred Eaglstein, D.O.
Postdoctoral Research Fellow, Department of Dermatology, Johns Hopkins Medical Institutions, Baltimore, Maryland

Jo-David Fine, M.D.
Associate Professor of Dermatology, University of Alabama School of Medicine, Birmingham, Alabama

Lionel Fry, B.Sc., M.D., F.R.C.P.
Consultant Dermatologist, St. Mary's Hospital, London, England

Nancy L. Furey, M.D.
Department of Dermatology, Northwestern University Medical School, Chicago, Illinois

W. Ray Gammon, M.D.
Associate Professor of Dermatology, University of North Carolina School of Medicine, Chapel Hill, North Carolina

James N. Gilliam, M.D. (Deceased)
Professor and Chairman, Division of Dermatology, Department of Internal Medicine, University of Texas, Southwestern Medical School, Dallas, Texas

Gerald P. Haffenden, F.I.M.L.S.
Senior Chief MLSO, Department of Histopathology, St. Mary's Hospital, London, England

John B. Harley, M.D., Ph.D.
Assistant Professor, Oklahoma Medical Research Foundation, Oklahoma City, Oklahoma

Peter Hebborn, Ph.D.
Director, Research and Development, Owen Laboratories, Fort Worth, Texas

Frederick Helm, M.D.
Professor and Chairman, Department of Dermatology, State University of New York at Buffalo, Buffalo, New York

Helmut Hintner, M.D.
Associate Professor of Dermatology, University of Innsbruck, Innsbruck, Austria

Karl Holubar, M.D.
Professor and Chairman, Department of Dermatology, Hadassah University Hospital, Jerusalem, Israel

Stefania Jablonska, M.D.
Professor and Chairman, Department of Dermatology, Warsaw Academy of Medicine, Warsaw, Poland

Naresh Jain, Ph.D.
Research Associate, Department of Microbiology, State University of New York at Buffalo, Buffalo, New York

Jerzy Januszkiewicz, M.D.
Professor and Chief, Department of Infectious Diseases, Pomerian Medical Academy, Institute of Internal Diseases, Szczecin, Poland

Maria Jarzabek-Chorzelska, Ph.D.
Assistant Professor, Department of Dermatology, Warsaw Academy of Medicine, Warsaw, Poland

Pamela C. Jones, Ph.D.
Postdoctoral Research Associate, State University of New York at Buffalo, Buffalo, New York

Stephen I. Katz, M.D., Ph.D.
Chief, Dermatology Branch, National Cancer Institute, National Institutes of Health, Bethesda, Maryland

Teresa Krainska, Ph.D.
Assistant Professor, Department of Dermatology, Warsaw Academy of Medicine, Warsaw, Poland

Susan A. Krasny, Ph.D.
Clinical Instructor, Department of Microbiology, State University of New York at Buffalo, Buffalo, New York

Vijay Kumar, Ph.D.
Clinical Professor, Department of Microbiology and Dermatology, State University of New York at Buffalo, Schools of Medicine and Dentistry, Buffalo, New York

Thomas J. Lawley, M.D.
Senior Investigator, Dermatology Branch, National Institutes of Health, Bethesda, Maryland

Jonathan N. Leonard, B.Sc., M.D., M.R.C.P.
Senior Registrar, Dermatology Department, St. Mary's Hospital, London, England

Aaron Lerner, M.D.
Lecturer, Department of Pediatrics, Technion-Israel Institute of Technology, Lady Davis Carmel Hospital, Haifa, Israel

Robert M. Lewis, D.V.M.
Professor and Chairman, Department of Pathology, New York State College of Veterinary Medicine, Cornell University, Ithaca, New York

Rona M. Mackie, M.D.
Department of Dermatology, University of Glasgow, Glasgow, Scotland

Beno Michel, M.D.
Clinical Professor of Dermatology, Case Western Reserve University, Cleveland, Ohio

Rodolfo Molina, M.D.
Department of Medicine, Good Samaritan Hospital, Baltimore, Maryland, Present address: Major, U.S. Air Force, Chief of Rheumatology, U.S. Air Force Medical Center, Andrews Air Force Base, Maryland

Patricia L. Myskowski, M.D.
Assistant Attending, Dermatology Service, Memorial Sloan-Kettering Cancer Center, New York, New York

Russell J. Nisengard, D.D.S. Ph.D.
Professor of Periodontology and Microbiology, State University of New York at Buffalo, Buffalo, New York

Harish P. Patel, M.D.
Assistant Professor of Dermatology, Johns Hopkins Medical Institutions, Baltimore, Maryland

Thomas T. Provost, M.D.
Professor and Chairman, Department of Dermatology, Johns Hopkins Medical Institutions, Baltimore, Maryland

Morris Reichlin, M.D.
Head, Arthritis and Immunology Lab, Professor of Medicine, Chief Immunology Section, Oklahoma Medical Research Foundation, Oklahoma City, Oklahoma

Georg Reimer, M.D.
Research Associate, Scripps Clinic and Research Foundation, La Jolla, California

Nicola P. Ring, F.I.M.L.S.
Chief, MLSO, Department of Histopathology, Brompton Hospital, London, England

Roy S. Rogers III, M.D.
Professor of Dermatology, Mayo Medical School, Rochester, Minnesota

Tomasz Rogozinski, M.D.
Assistant Professor, Department of Dermatology, Warsaw Academy of Medicine, Warsaw, Poland

Justin T. Roscoe, M.D.
Postdoctoral Research Fellow, Department of Dermatology, Johns Hopkins Medical Institutions, Baltimore, Maryland

Bijan Safai, M.D. D.Sc.
Chief, Dermatology Service, Memorial Sloan-Kettering Cancer Center, New York, New York, Professor of Medicine, Cornell University Medical Center, Ithaca, New York

W. Mitchell Sams, M.D.
Professor and Chairman, Department of Dermatology, University of Alabama School of Medicine, Birmingham, Alabama

Jean Hilaire Saurat, M.D.
Professor and Chairman, Clinique de Dermatologie, Hôpital Cantonal Universitaire, Geneva, Switzerland

Daniel Schmitt, Ph.D.
Directeur de Recherche, INSERM, Lyon, France

Danny W. Scott, D.V.M.
Associate Professor of Medicine, Department of Clinical Sciences, Chief, Dermatology Service, New York State College of Veterinary Medicine, Cornell University, Ithaca, New York

Robert J. Seiler, B.V.Sc., Ph.D.
Regional Veterinary Laboratory, Victoria, Australia

Suyh Shu, Ph.D.
Associate Professor of Pathology, University of Pittsburgh, Senior Investigator, Pittsburgh Cancer Institute, Pittsburgh, Pennsylvania

Philip S. Spencer, M.D.
Clinical Assistant Instructor of Dermatology, State University of New York at Buffalo, Buffalo, New York

Jadwiga Sulej, Ph.D.
Assistant Professor, Department of Dermatology, Warsaw Academy of Medicine, Warsaw, Poland

Eng M. Tan, M.D.
Director, W. M. Keck Autoimmune Disease Center, Scripps Clinic and Research Foundation, La Jolla, California

Jean Thivolet, M.D.
Professor of Dermatology, Université Claude Bernard, Lyon, France

Denny L. Tuffanelli, M.D.
Clinical Professor, Department of Dermatology, University of California, San Francisco, California

Mitchell S. Turner, M.D.
Assistant Clinical Instructor, Department of Dermatology, State University of New York at Buffalo, Buffalo, New York

Hiroaki Ueki, M.D.
Professor and Chairman, Department of Dermatology, Kawasaki Medical School, Kurashiki-shi, Japan

D. J. Unsworth, B.Sc., Ph.D.
Bone and Joint Research Unit, The London Hospital Medical College, London, England, Present address: St. Bartholomew's Hospital, London, England

Rafael Valenzuela, M.D.
Head, General Immunology Section, Department of Immunopathology, Cleveland Clinic Foundation, Cleveland, Ohio

Rosemarie M. Watson, M.D., M.R.C.P.I.
Postdoctoral Research Fellow, Department of Dermatology, Johns Hopkins Medical Institutions, Baltimore, Maryland

B. Dale Wilson, M.D.
Associate Professor of Dermatology, State University of New York at Buffalo, Buffalo, New York

Klaus Wolff, M.D.
Professor and Chairman, Department of Dermatology, University of Vienna, Vienna, Austria

Kim B. Yancey, M.D.
Assistant Professor, Dermatology Department, Uniformed Services University of the Health Sciences, Bethesda, Maryland

Hideo Yaoita, M.D.
Department of Dermatology, University of Tsukuba, Ibaraki-Ken, Japan

Preface to Third Edition

The function of this third edition, as of the first two editions of *Immunopathology of the Skin,* is to focus primarily on the clinical and laboratory findings in bullous and connective tissue diseases and other skin diseases in which immunofluorescence and other relevant laboratory methods can provide useful diagnostic and prognostic information. The large volume of literature on skin immunopathology that has appeared since publication of the first two editions has, in effect, converted this field into a viable subdiscipline of medicine. In this edition, the connective tissue diseases, vesiculo-bullous diseases, and other diseases with immunopathologically recognizable changes are considered in terms of concepts and clinical findings, the actual methods of performing test procedures, and the evaluation of their reproducibility or validity.

This book is written primarily for immunopathologists, dermatopathologists (i.e., for dermatologists who want to specialize through the certification program of the American Dermatologic Society for Allergy and Immunology), immunologists who specialize through a certification program of the American Board of Medical Laboratory Immunology, and manufacturers of reagents for these specialties. Importantly, the third edition is intended as a reference book not only for larger dermatology clinics, but also for general dermatologists and pathologists to help them deal with bullous and connective tissue diseases with present-day methods.

Significant progress toward the establishment of a subdiscipline of immunodermatology has been made since the publication of the first edition in 1973 and the second edition in 1979. This was the basic goal set forth in the preface of the first edition. Recent advances are notably in the training of specialists, further evolution of methods, and the number and quality of publications. As evidence of the growth in this discipline, this edition contains about twice as much material as in the second edition. While everything has been rewritten, the material in this edition is self-sufficient. That is, relevant information from the second edition is condensed and modified for this edition. It is organized into four sections: 1) basic concepts and methods, 2) vesiculo-bullous diseases, 3) connective tissue diseases, and 4) other dermatoses with significant immunohistologic findings. The new material includes chapters on standardization of immunofluorescence, monoclonal antibodies for lymphocyte subsets, immune complexes, the major advances relating to dermatitis herpetiformis and other forms of gluten-sensitive enteropathy, the identification of antigens to which systemic lupus patients develop autoimmunity, wart viruses, and other clinically relevant advances.

Ernst H. Beutner, Ph.D.
Tadeusz P. Chorzelski, M.D.
Vijay Kumar, Ph.D.

Buffalo, New York
Warsaw, Poland
Buffalo, New York
February 1987

Preface to Second Edition

The goals of studies in the field of immunopathology of the skin as set forth in the preface of the first edition remain unchanged. Some significant steps towards the achievement of these goals are set forth in this second edition, using the same basic methodology of defined immunofluorescence described in the first edition. Importantly, the wider use of the transport medium for skin biopsies now serves to make the immunofluorescence studies of tissues available to practitioners in all parts of the world.

This second edition deals with extensions of and refinements in the utilization of immunofluorescence and other immunologic studies of the skin diseases. These now include not only the bullous and connective tissue diseases, the vasculitides and conditions such as lichen planus but also the scaling dermatoses, most notably psoriasis. From the point of view of research valuable contributions now come from ultrastructural studies by immunoelectron microscopy. From a practical standpoint other serologic methods such as precipitation and agglutination tests for extractable nuclear antigens now play a more prominent role in immunodermatologic diagnosis.

Serodiagnostic studies of syphilis have been deleted from this second edition, in part, to accommodate the expanding body of knowledge in immunodermatology and in part because most dermatologists throughout the world now no longer deal with venereology.

All of the editors are deeply indebted to the wise guidance and thoughtful advice of Dr. Stefania Jablonska. Without her help this book would not have come into being.

ERNST H. BEUTNER, Ph.D.

Buffalo, New York, January 1979

Preface to First Edition

This book represents a first attempt to organize into a subdiscipline the clinically relevant research, methodologies and clinical experience with studies of immunodermatology. At present this subdiscipline deals primarily with immunopathologic and immunohistologic studies of the skin. It centers on the use of defined immunofluorescent staining for studies of bullous diseases and certain collagen diseases. The reproducibility of findings and more specifically the use of defined immunofluorescent methods necessary for achieving reproducible results constitute a prerequisite for the meaningful studies of the diseases under consideration.

It took half a century to elaborate the subdiscipline of the histopathology of the skin. The immunohistology and immunopathology of the skin will probably prove to be even more difficult to elaborate to a comparable degree of sophistication since the quantitative serology, immunochemistry and the defined immunofluorescence which is derived from them are rather demanding disciplines in and of themselves. However, the efforts required to establish reproducibly defined test systems seem justified since they already appear to be fruitful in terms of diagnosis and management of bullous diseases and collagen diseases.

It must be kept in mind that immunofluorescent tests of the type described in this book when performed by inexperienced workers frequently lead to misinterpretations and thus *can do more harm than good for the patients* whose specimens are examined. To use these methods successfully the laboratory worker should have about a half year of training in immunology and immunodermatology. Since the number of cases of the diseases in which the methods described in this book are limited, and the prerequisites for the proper performance of the indicated immunodermatologic studies are rather demanding, these studies should be performed at large institutions that have the necessary trained personnel, resources and experience to do the work properly.

To elaborate and evaluate even a single fully documented set of immunodermatologic test procedures may require the better part of a decade. The aim of the editors and contributors to this book is to strike a middle ground between the rigorous discipline of laboratory work required to lay a firm foundation for each test system and the less rigorously controlled exploratory work necessary to discover new potential uses of immunofluorescence and other immunologic methods for the diagnosis. The book is organized in such a way as to stress which procedures are of proven value and which findings are of an exploratory nature. The hope of the editors is to lay a firm but not a restrictive foundation for the subdiscipline of immunodermatology. The objective is to try to maintain and increase the value of immunodermatology in the diagnosis and management of dermatoses with immunologic hallmarks.

ERNST H. BEUTNER. Ph.D.

Buffalo, New York, October 1973

Acknowledgments

The preparation of this book would not have been possible without the outstanding and devoted secretarial and editorial work of Mrs. Gloria Griffin.

The support of the Summerhill Foundation was of vital importance in the preparation of this monograph.

Contents

Abbreviations

A	absorbance
AA	anti-antibody
Ab	antibodies or autoantibodies
AbP	Antibody concentration or antibody protein
A-B	avidin biotin
ABC	avidin biotin peroxidase complex
ABMZA	antibasement membrane zone antibodies
Ab/P	Antibody protein to total protein ratio
ABS	avidin biotin system
ACA	anticentromere antibodies (a type of ANA)
AEC	aminoethyl carbozol
Ag	antigens or autoantigens
AGA	antigliadin antibodies
AHG	aggregated human gamma globulin
AMA	antimitochondrial antibodies
ANA	antinuclear antibodies
ARA	American Rheumatism Association
ARM	autoimmune repair mechanism
AV	atrioventricular
A self	accessible self-antigens (or type antibodies to them)
A self-Ab	autoantibodies to A self-Ag
ASMA	antismooth muscle antibodies
BCBDC	benign chronic bullous disease of childhood
BCC	basal cell cytoplasm
BCyt (BCL)	basal cytoplasmic
BESLE	bullous eruption of systemic lupus erythematosus
BF	blister fluid
BMMP	benign mucous membrane pemphigoid (referred to elsewhere in this book as cicatricial pemphigoid)

BMT	bone marrow transplantation
BMZ	basement membrane zone
BP	bullous pemphigoid
BPF	Brazilian pemphigus foliaceus
BPV	bovine fibropapilloma
BPab(s)	BP antibody(ies)
BV	blood vessels
C	complement
C3	complement component C3
CAH	chronic active hepatitis
CBDC	chronic bullous disease of childhood
CD	celiac disease
CF	complement fixation
CHB	congenital heart block
CIC	circulating immune complexes
CIF	complement immunofluorescence
CIN	cervical in situ neoplasia
CMI	cell-mediated immunity
CMV	cytomegalovirus
CNS	central nervous system
CPK	creatinine phosphokinase
CSF	cerebrospinal fluid
CREST	Calcinosis, Raynauds, esophageal immotility, sclerodactyly, and telangiectasia
CTD	connective tissue disease
DAB	3,3 diaminobenzidene, (diaminobenzidene) tetrahydrochloride
DABCO	1,4-diazobicyclo-(2,2,2)-octane (an antifading agent)
DACM	N-(7-dimethylamino-4-methylcoumarinyl)-maleimide
DDLE	disseminated discoid lupus erythematosus
dDNA or nDNA	double-stranded DNA or native DNA
DEJ	dermal-epidermal junction
DH	dermatitis herpetiformis
DIF	direct immunofluorescence
DLE	discoid lupus erythematosus
DM	dermatomyositis
DNCB	2,4, dinitrochlorobenzene
DNase	deoxribonuclease
DSS	desired specific staining
EA	erythrocyte antibody complexes
EB	epidermolysis bullosa
EBA	epidermolysis bullosa acquisita
EBER	Epstein-Barr virus associated RNA

EBNA	Epstein-Barr virus nuclear antigen
EBV	Epstein-Barr virus
EC	epidermal cells
ECG	electrocardiogram, electrocardiographic
EDAC	1-ethyl-3-(3-dimethylaminopropyl) carbodiimide
EDTA	ethylenediamine tetracetic acid
ELISA	enzyme-linked immunosorbent assay
EM	electron microscopy
ENA	extractable nuclear antigens
ESR	electron spin resonance (Chap. 13)
ESR	erythrocyte sedimentation rate (Chap. 44, Part 1)
EV	epidermodysplasia verruciformis
EmA	endomysial antibodies
F	fibrin (Chap. 44, Part 2)
F	fluorescein (Chap. 1)
F/P	fluorescein-to-protein ratios
FCS	fetal calf serum
FDA	fluorescein diacetate
FITC	fluorescein isothiocyanate
FLAC	fluorescein-labeled affinity chromatography
FTA	fluorescent tneponemal antibody
Fab_2, Fab, FC	fragments of immunoglobulins
GCyt (GEC)	general cytoplasmic
GE	gluten-sensitive enteropathy
GEC	generalized epidermal cytoplasmic
GFD	gluten-free diet
GP	glycoprotein
GVH, GVHR	graft-versus-host reaction
GVHD	graft-versus-host disease
H self	hidden self-antigens
H self-Ab	autoantibodies to H self-Ag
H&E	hematoxylin and eosin
HB	hepatitis B
HBsAg	hepatitis B surface antigen
HETE	hydroxyeicosatetraenoic acid
HG	herpes gestationis
HLA	human leukocyte antigens
HLA, Dr, Dw loci	genetic loci within major histocompatibility complex
HPV	human papilloma virus
HRP	horseradish peroxidase
HS	human skin
HSV	herpes simplex virus

HTLA	human T-lymphocyte surface antigens
HX cells	histiocytosis X cells
IC	intercellular
ICS	intercellular cement substance
ID	intradermal
IEM	immunoelectron microscopy
IEP	immunoelectrophoresis
IF	immunofluorescent or immunofluorescence
Ig	immunoglobulin
IHC	immunohistochemistry
IIF	indirect immunofluorescence
IP	intraperitoneal (Chap. 12)
IP	immunoperoxidase (Chap. 6)
IPO	indirect peroxidase
IR	immune response (Chap. 19)
IV	intravenous
IVD	inflammatory vascular disease
IgA-EmA	IgA endomysial antibody (Chap. 27)
IgA-EmA	IgA-class antiendomysial antibodies (Chap. 8)
IgG	immunoglobulin G
KC	keratinocyte cytoplasm
KCAbs	keratinocyte cytoplasmic antibodies
KCAg/Ab	keratinocyte cytoplasm antigen/antibodies
KCS	keratoconjunctivitis sicca
KCAgs	keratinocyte cytoplasmic antigens
kd	kilodalton
KIF	keratin intermediate filaments
LABD	linear IgA bullous dermatosis
LATS	long-acting thyroid stimulator
LC	Langerhans cells
LCA	leukocytoclastic vasculitis
LDL	low-density lipoproteins
LE	lupus erythematosus
LIA	lymphocyte-induced angiogenesis
LP	lichen planus
LPSA	lichen planus-specific antigen
LSANA	leukocyte-specific antinuclear antibodies
LTB_4	leucotriene B4
La (SS-B, Ha)	RNA protein complex localized predominantly in the nucleus
M	mucosa
M_w	molecular weight
MCA	monoclonal antibodies

MCTD	mixed connective tissue disease
MEM	minimal essential medium
MF	mycosis fungoides
mg P/ml	mg protein/ml
MHC	major histocompatibility complex
MIVD	mononuclear inflammatory vascular disease
MLC	mixed leukocyte culture assay
MT_2	an additional loci located near DR loci, also referred to as secondary DR loci
Mrs PAH	mixed reverse solid-phase hemagglutination assay
NCCLS	National Committee for Clinical Laboratory Standards
NHS	normal human serum
NIVD	neutrophilic inflammatory vascular disease
NK	natural killer
NLE	neonatal lupus erythematosus
NSS	nonspecific staining
NYSCVM	New York State College of Veterinary Medicine
OK	orthokeratosis
OPD	O-phenylene diamine
OS	optical standard
P	protein
P-IgG	pemphigus IgG
PA	plasminogen activator
PAF	pemphigus acantholysis factor
PAHO	Pan American Health Organization
PAP	peroxidase-antiperoxidase
PAS	periodic acid Schiff (stain)
PB cells	peripheral blood cells
PBC	primary biliary cirrhosis
PBS	phosphate-buffered saline
PCNA	proliferating cell nuclear antigen
PCT	porphyria cutanea tarda
PECC	primary epidermal cell cultures
PEG	polyethylene glycol
PEP	plateau endpoint (of a conjugate)
PK	parakeratosis
PLA	pemphigus-like antibodies
PM	polymyositis
PMN	polymorphonuclear leukocytes
PMSF	Phenylmethyl sulfonylfluorid
POPA	protein A peroxidase
PPD	purified protein derivative

PPP	prepinpoint papule
PSS	progressive systemic sclerosis
PT	plateau titer (of a serum)
PUVA	psoralen ultraviolet A
PV	pemphigus vulgaris (Chap. 12)
PV	papilloma virus (Chap. 38)
Pab (s)	pemphigus antibody (ies)
Pag (s)	pemphigus antigen (s)
Po	peroxidase
r	coefficient of correlation
R (H) self	reactive form of H-self
RA	rheumatoid arthritis
RAP	rheumatoid arthritis precipitin
RANA	rheumatoid arthritis-associated nuclear antigen
RBC	red blood cells
RE	rabbit esophagus
RES	reticuloendothelial system
RF	rheumatoid factor
RNP	ribonucleoprotein
RNase	ribonuclease
Ro	one of the ENA
Ro/SS-A (SS-A/Ro), La/SS-B(SS-B/La), PM-1, Jo-1, Ku, Sm, nRNP	RNA protein cytoplasmic macromolecule See Tables 1–3, Chap. 32
RRID	reverse radial immunodiffusion
rRNA	ribosomal RNA
r_s	Spearman rank coefficient of correlation
RZ	Reaktionszahl (reaction number)
s	secretory (chap. 41)
S_G	standard deviation of geometric mean titer
SC	stratum corneum or SC antibodies
SCAb	SC autoantibodies
SCAg	SC autoantigens
SCLE	subacute cutaneous lupus erythematosus
SDS	sodium dodecyl sulfate
SDS-PAGE	sodium dodecyl sulfate polyacrylamide gel electrophoresis
SHB	subepidermal hyaline bodies
SLE	systemic lupus erythematosus
SLT	speckle-like thready
Sm	an acidic glycoprotein
SPA	staphyloccocal protein A

SRB, SRBC	sheep red blood cells
SS	Sjögren's syndrome (Chap. 34)
SS	systemic sclerosis (Chap. 3)
SS_A	Sjögren's syndrome with active central nervous system disease
SS_{IA}	Sjögren's syndrome with inactive central nervous system disease
SS-A/Ro, SS-B/La, Ma, Pm-1, Mi-1, Jo-1, Ku	See Table 3
ssDNA	single-stranded DNA
T- cell	T lymphocyte
TAg	T antigens of red blood cells (RBC) (after Thomsen)
TR	trypsin resistant (i.e., TR-type SCAg)
TS	trypsin sensitive (i.e., TS-type SCAg)
Tk	a variant of TAg of RBC
Tn	another variant of TAg of RBC
Ts_1, Ts_2, Ts_3	forms of Ts cells
Ts cells	T-suppressor cells (lymphocytes)
TsF	Ts cell factor
TsF_1, TsF_2, TsF_3	forms of TsF
UCyt (UEC)	upper cytoplasmic
UEC	upper epidermal cytoplasmic
μm	micrometer
USS	undesired specific staining
UV	ultraviolet
VARNA	adenovirus-associated RNA
WHO	World Health Organization
X or X_G	geometric mean titer
w/w	weight/weight

Section I

1
Defined Immunofluorescence in Immunodermatology

Ernest H. Beutner

Vijay Kumar

Susan A. Krasny

Tadeusz P. Chorzelski

INTRODUCTION

Background information on the basic techniques of immunofluorescence is reviewed in detail in a number of books (16,18,27,28,33–36,50) and symposia (2,7,21,22,29) on the subject.

Since the second edition of this book was published, significant improvements in optical equipment, commercially available conjugates, mounting media plus stabilizing agents, and methodologies have made it possible to attain more reproducible results, at least in some systems. On the basis of past work on defined methods, the basic methods employed in a standardization of immunofluorescence have evolved significantly as indicated in Chapter 2. In the future, industry should assume more responsibility for standardization of diagnostic, labeled antibody methods. The definition of methods of immunofluorescence is still needed, however, in research and for skin immunopathology. This chapter affords a review of the established methods for defining immunofluorescence and provides more detailed reports on the newer developments related to the uses of defined methods in clinical immunodermatology and research. Appendix Section G affords a detailed description of procedures indicated for detection of antiepithelial antibodies, including intercellular antibodies and the basement membrane zone (BMZ) antibodies. In brief, this chapter (together with other selected chapters in this volume) affords a comprehensive review of those aspects of immunofluorescence that are relevant to studies of immunopathology of the skin.

Readers interested in establishing clinical immunodermatology services are well advised to focus first on direct immunofluorescence studies of skin biopsy specimens, using

The preparation of this chapter is supported by a grant from the Summerhill Foundation.

conjugates that are specifically pretested and prepared for clinical immunopathologic studies. It is also recommended that immunofluorescence staining of skin biopsies be performed by technicians who are qualified in this field, and that the cryostat sections used for immunofluorescence be checked by people who have some expertise in the field before diagnostic studies are undertaken. For laboratories closely affiliated with dermatologic clinics, which perform small numbers of serum studies for autoantibodies associated with bullous and/or connective tissue diseases, it is recommended that small numbers of sera (less than 10 to 20 per week) be sent to major reference laboratories that do a volume necessary to maintain high levels of competence.

NATURE OF IMMUNOFLUORESCENCE STUDIES USED IN IMMUNODERMATOLOGY

In clinical immunodermatology, the two basic test systems are direct immunofluorescence (DIF) studies of biopsy specimens and indirect immunofluorescence (IIF) tests of patient sera, as described below. Both DIF and IIF entail the use of fluorescein-labeled antibodies to the human immunoglobulin or complement components. For DIF, antibodies to immunoglobulins and other human serum proteins are labeled. Specifically, fluorescein in the form of fluorescein isothiocyanate (FITC) (see Fig. 1) is coupled to these antibodies via a thiocarbamido linkage. (The technique for conjugation is detailed in Section A of the Appendix.) Fluorescein affords a uniquely sensitive labeling component because of its high degree of resonance (Fig. 1). The fact that the diacetate derivative of fluorescein, which cannot undergo such resonant configurational changes, is nonfluorescent and colorless points to the role of resonance in the uniquely high level of fluorescence of this molecule.

Method for the Performance of Immunofluorescence Studies

As indicated above, the best hopes for standardization of diagnostic immunofluorescence procedures lies in the commercial production of all components of test kits for well-standardized procedures. For antinuclear antibody (ANA) tests, this standardization is in the process of developing as indicated in Chapter 2, but this has not as yet evolved effectively for antiepithelial antibodies. Thus, the reproducibility of the latter between laboratories is still poor, as revealed by a survey in 1983 by the American Academy of Dermatology. Until some industrial standardization is achieved, the only recourse is to use the defined methods described in Section G of the Appendix. Discussion of some of the factors contributing to the reproducibility of immunofluorescence tests follows.

Direct Immunofluorescence

Briefly, the direct immunofluorescence (DIF) staining of skin biopsy specimens entails the following steps:

1. Collection of specimens—almost all studies are now performed with skin biopsy specimens collected in a transport medium described by Michel et al. (32). (See Appendix Section B for details on this medium.) Earlier controversies over the use of the transport medium (32,45) seem to have been resolved by careful maintenance of a neutral pH. This transport medium can now be purchased commercially, and is supplied free of charge by some laboratories that perform immunopathologic studies of skin. A recent report describes a simplified transport medium composed only of ammonium sulfate (38; Appendix Section B). This merits independent evaluation.

2. After washing the biopsy specimens in the transport medium (without the ammonium sulfate) according to standard methods and snap-freezing them, frozen sections

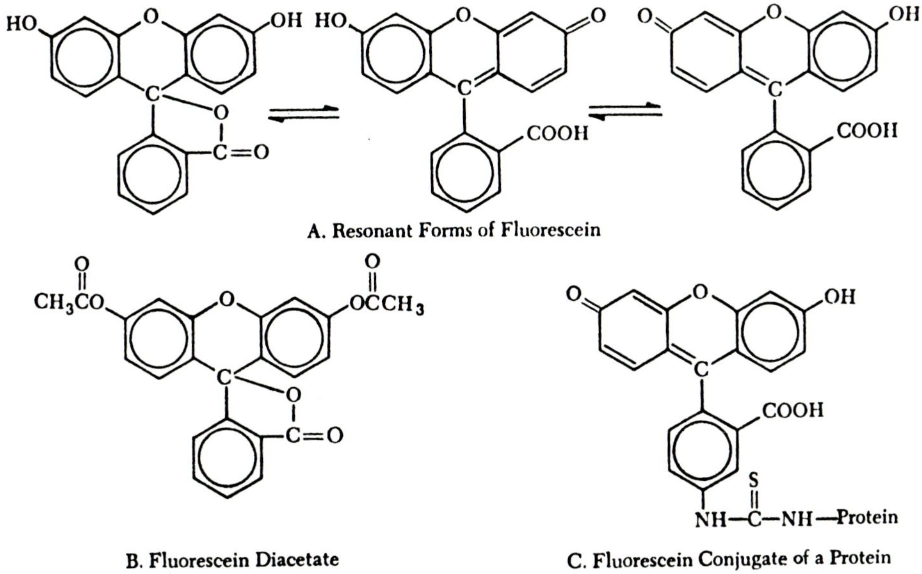

Figure 1. A. Three of the many resonant forms of fluorescein. The high degree of resonance of this molecule, particularly in its ionized form as a sodium salt (at a pH of 8.0 or more), accounts for its unusually high level of fluorescence. B. The diacetate form of fluorescein. This molecule cannot resonate to the carbonile form. It is a nonfluorescent colorless compound. C. Fluorescein conjugated to a free amino group (e.g., epsilon amino group of lysine) via a thiocarbamido linkage. This linkage is formed by allowing the protein to react with FITC in an alkaline solution. (Reprinted with permission from Beutner EH, et al.: Immunofluorescence and immunoenzyme staining. In Rose NR, Milgrom F, van Oss CJ (Eds): ed. 2. Macmillan, New York, 1979.

are cut at 4 μm. These must be of a good quality to perform reliable studies. To obtain good morphologic characteristics, the sections could be placed on albumin-coated slides (see below). A "mapping" technique (described in the next subsection) is recommended to obtain comparable sections for each of the reagents tested.

3. Preferably, two or more sections should be treated with carefully defined reagents (see below) with the following specificities: anti-IgG, anti-IgM, anti-IgA, anticomplement C3, and antifibrin. Each reagent should be tested on a separate slide. Tests for other complement and serum components may be added.

For "mapping," the sequence of sections should be of the following type:

Slide 1,	section 1,	11 & 21	anti-IgG
Slide 2,	section 2,	12 & 22	anti-IgA
Slide 3,	section 3.	13 & 23	anti-IgM
Slide 4,	section 4,	14 & 24	antifibrin
Slide 5,	section 5,	15 & 25	anti-C3
Slide 6,	section 6,	16 & 26	Extra slides for other tests and repeat tests
Slide 7,	section 7,	17 & 27	
Slide 8,	section 8,	18 & 28	
Slide 9,	section 9,	19 & 29	
Slide 10,	section 10,	20 & 30	

The criteria for defining conjugates used for these studies are given below (see conjugate characteristics). Well-defined, pretested, and prediluted reagents are now available commercially. Comparative studies of the commercially available reagents remain to be done.

4. Following 30 minutes of incubation for skin biopsy sections with the selected defined conjugates, they are rinsed quickly to remove the bulk of the conjugate from each slide (only one conjugate should be used per slide) and are washed in phosphate-buffered saline (PBS) for 10 minutes. Slides should be mounted in a semipermanent mounting medium, so that they can be stored in a freezer if desired. Stabilizers of fluorescence (which are reviewed in the section of this chapter on "Mounting Media") should be added (see Appendix Section C).

Quick freezing affords somewhat better clarity of morphologic characteristics especially of certain dermal structures; blood vessels notably have more "natural" morphologic characteristics than the structures seen after handling in transport medium. However, with modern cryostats and a bit of experience with specimens handled in transport medium, these problems can be overcome. Multiple sections from different areas of the biopsy specimens obtained by "mapping" should be tested with each conjugate to provide a reasonable sampling of the tissues examined. The selection of biopsy sites for DIF studies of bullous connective tissue and vascular diseases are of critical importance (see Chaps. 8, 9, 15, 21, and 30).

Indirect Immunofluorescence

In principle, indirect immunofluorescence (IIF) is used in immunodermatology principally for serologic studies; that is, for the detection of antibodies in a patient's serum. The most reliable serologic tests are performed with commercially standardized test systems (see Chap. 2). Details of the basic procedures are given in the Appendix Section D. In essence, the steps are, with minor variations among manufacturers, as follows: 1) substrate is treated with selected dilutions of patients or control sera for 30 minutes in a moist chamber; 2) following a rinse in PBS to remove unbound serum proteins, sections are treated with an anti-IgG or other antibody conjugates of defined specificity and sensitivity (see the section in this chapter on conjugate characteristics for details on criteria for defining these reagents); 3) following a rinse of at least 10 minutes in PBS to remove unbound conjugate and mounting of the slides with glycerine, they are examined under a fluorescence microscope (see the section in this chapter on microscopy).

Albumin Coating of Slides

Tissue sections are usually placed directly on slides as obtained from the manufacturer. However, these sections sometimes either wash off or are folded during processing of the specimen for IF staining. There are various reasons the sections might not adhere adequately; notably: 1) slides are dirty or oily, 2) sections are too thick, 3) inadequate drying, and 4) rough handling during the staining and washing period of the slides. These can be prevented or at least minimized, to a large extent, if the slides are precleaned and coated with albumin. In some problem cases, the elimination of cover-glasses aids in minimizing distortion.

The slides can be coated with egg albumin as follows:

1. Clean the slides in 1% HCl, and in 70% ethanol by immersion and agitation for 10 minutes. Remove the slides from acid alcohol, and then dip the slides in acetone and air dry.

2. Prepare an egg albumin solution by blending egg white from one egg in 500 ml of distilled water containing 1 ml of concentrated ammonium hydroxide. Filter the egg albumin solution through a filter paper just before use. This solution should be made fresh.
3. Dip the clear slides in the egg albumin solution for 1 minute. Remove the slides from the solution, drain excess solution on a paper towel, and dry them overnight at 60°C.

Many slides can be prepared at one time and can be kept for long periods of time (up to 1 year). Up to 500 slides can be prepared from 500 ml of the solution.

Type of Fluorescence

Immunofluorescence methods yield not only desired specific staining, but also undesired specific staining due to unwanted antibodies present either in the conjugates or the sera, and nonspecific staining due to the fluorochroming activity of fluorescein (F) conjugates. These three types of staining, DSS, NSS, and USS need to be distinguished not only from each other, but also from the autofluorescence of the tissue. These may be distinguished as follows:

1. Desired specific staining (DSS) is true immunofluorescence. It is due to the labeled specific antibodies selected for study, and is a function of the amount of reactive antigen, the labeled antibody concentration, and the labeling ratio of conjugate. The latter is expressed as a molar fluorescein-to-protein (F/P) ratio.
2. Autofluorescence occurs naturally in untreated tissues and other substrates, as seen by exposure to the light of the optical system. Since the emission wavelength of autofluorescence differs from that of F, its appearance varies with the filter system (as indicated in Table 1), and with the nature of the antigenic substrate. It is distinguished from other types of fluorescence by its occurrence in untreated ("saline") control sections.
3. Nonspecific staining (NSS) is fluorochroming due to the staining capacity of FITC-labeled conjugates. It is a function of the concentration of bound (and sometimes also free) F in the diluted conjugate, its F/P ratio, and the nature of the antigenic substrate.
4. Undesired specific staining (USS) is due to unwanted antibodies present in the labeled or unlabeled globulins. For example, anti-immunoglobulin conjugates used in fluorescent treponemal antibody or FTA tests should be free of "natural" antibodies to saprophytic treponemata, as well as to cross-reactive antibodies to rabbit immunoglobulin (14). Both of these can cause USS. Cross-reactive antibodies to rabbit immunoglobulin need to be removed, because the treponemata, grown in rabbit testes and used as antigens in the FTA test, may contain surface-bound rabbit antibodies to the treponemata. Also, the animal sera from which conjugates are prepared may contain "natural" antibodies to treponemata that cross-react with the *Treponema pallidum* used as antigen in the FTA test. Thus, conjugates may need to be absorbed with rabbit immunoglobulin and with suspensions of treponemata before use in the FTA test. In practice, the use of equal parts of "FTA sorbent" (a sonicated suspension of *T. reiter* used in the standard FTA-ABS test) and normal rabbit serum (or Cohn fraction II of rabbit serum) as a diluent for the first 1:2 dilution of conjugate, followed by centrifugation, may suffice to remove these types of USS.

MICROSCOPY

Fluorescent microscopy has become a powerful tool in immunodermatology, cell biology, and many other areas. This has been partially due to the development of new and better microscopes, better filters, and availability of high-intensity light sources (44,46). The availability of epi-illumination microscopy (40,41) is replacing substage-transmitted light microscopy. The intensity as well as the sensitivity of a microscope can be increased by increasing the excitation intensity. This has resulted in the development and marketing of new and better microscopes. The various aspects of the microscope that affect the specificity and sensitivity are: 1) light sources, 2) filters, and 3) lenses (objective and ocular).

1. Light sources: High-pressure mercury bulbs (HBO 100 and 200) and halogen lamps have been employed for many years as the light energy source. Even though they are suitable in routine diagnostic testing, other systems such as xenon arc and lasers have been found to be of significant value in increasing the sensitivity of the system, especially in areas of cell biology and receptor-binding studies. Thomson and Hageage (46) found xenon arc 450 XBO to be of sufficient energy to produce at least twice as much fluorescence compared to HBO 200 mercury lamps. Another light source used on an experimental basis and routinely in fluorescent cell sorters is the laser. Lasers emit high-energy (44), monochromic, and highly constant waves of light at 488 and 514 nm. Their high cost, however, has prevented their use in routine diagnostic laboratories. The intensity of fluorescence emitted by the use of lasers is 10^3-fold higher compared to mercury lamps.

2. Filters: The type of filters used in immunofluorescence are indicated in Table 1. For epi-illumination systems, both exciter and barrier filters are provided as filter cubes. Cubes that afford "narrow band" excitation (i.e., that eliminate light below about 450 nm) are preferable.

3. Optics: With substage illumination, there is a decrease in light intensity with an increase in magnification of the objective lens. Hence, in general, low-to-moderate power dry objectives are preferred in substage illumination. The reverse, however, is true in incident illumination or epi-illumination. In addition, with epi-illumination, the light collection is proportional to the fourth power of the numerical aperture (41). Thus, it is important in epi-illumination to have objectives of moderate magnification with maximal numerical aperture. However, with higher intensities of illumination, there is an increased risk of fluorescence intensity fading.

Optical sensitivity of systems can be estimated roughly with optical standard (OS) slides, which have beads of varying intensities of fluorescence* referred to as 100%, 50%, 25%, 12.5%, 2%, and 0% bright. (A 6.25% bright was added in 1985.) The microfluorospectrophotometric readings of these beads in arbitrary units with three types of illumination systems are summarized on page 10.

The illumination systems used were as follows:

Epi-tungsten: A.O.[a] equipped with 100 W Tungsten-halogen lamp and read with 40× objective.

Epi-mercury: A.O. equipped with HBO 50 W mercury vapor lamp.

Sub-mercury: A.O. substage equipped with HBO 100 W mercury vapor lamp.

[a]A.O.—American Optical Co., Buffalo, NY

*OS slides are available from Behring Diagnostics, La Jolla, CA.

Table 1. Light Sources and Filters Available for Immunofluorescence

Types, light source (Indications for use)	*Role*	*Color of filter in daylight (Transmission wavelength)*	*Common examples*
Substage illumination			
UV, Mercury (Hg) vapor light	Exciter	Black or faint blue or purple (under 400 nm)	Corning C 5970, C 5860 Schott UGI, UG2, UG5
	Barrier	Colorless or pale yellow (over 400 nm)	Wratten W2A, W2B, W2E Schott I 103, I 102, I 805
BV, Hg vapor light	Exciter	Blue (400 to 450 nm)	Corning C 5850, C 5113 Schott BG k2m BG 25
(DNA antibodies, FTA)	Barrier	Yellow or yellow green (over 500 nm)	Corning CP-OY4, CP-OY3 Schott SOG-4, SOG-1 Wratten W-12, W-15
Interference Hg vapor or quartz halogen	Barrier	Silver mirror (over nm of KP no. and under K no. of filters)	KP 490 or KP 500 (+ K 450 or K 480 for narrow band illumination)
	Exciter	Yellow green (over nm of filter no.)	510 or 520
Incident illumination			
Dichroic mirror	Exciter Barrier	Silver mirror	(As for interference filters)

	Percent Brightness (as per Coulter Electronics)				
Illumination	*100%*	*50%*	*25%*	*12.5%*	*2%*
Epi-tungsten	248.30 ± 16.3	107.70 ± 12.3	43.1 ± 4.2	20.90 ± 7.9	2.70 ± 0.8
Epi-mercury	168.25 ± 31.3	82.95 ± 10.2	35.9 ± 3.9	17.70 ± 4.0	2.28 ± 1.0
Sub-mercury	120.19 ± 15.8	47.44 ± 9.1	21.8 ± 6.3	13.43 ± 4.7	2.40 ± 0.9
	Expected Results in Immunofluorescent Studies				
"Strong" light sources	positive	positive	positive	positive	weak
"Weak" light sources	positive	positive	positive	weak	trace

These OS slides are of practical value in estimating the relative sensitivity of fluorescence microscopes. For routine immunopathologic studies, a "strong" light source should be used.

CRITERIA FOR CHARACTERIZATION, SELECTION, AND DILUTION OF ANTI-Ig ANTIBODIES CONJUGATED WITH FLUORESCEIN ISOTHIOCYANATE (FITC)

The criteria used are of two types: 1) those used by manufacturers, and 2) those employed by immunopathology laboratories.

Manufacturers' Responsibilities for Conjugate Characterization: Writers' Views

Table 2 summarizes the key factors in the characterization of FITC conjugates of immunoglobulin fractions of hyperimmune sera with anti-Ig antibodies by manufacturers. The basic methods for performing assays for fluorescein (F) and protein (P) and calculating F/P ratios are given in Appendix Section E. Also, a new method for assaying the concen-

Table 2. Characterization of FITC-labeled Anti-Ig Conjugates

Characteristics	*Assay methods*
Specificity	IEP, gel precipitation, IIF (with Ig class-restricted Ab)
Sensitivity	
F and P conc.	NCCLS methods
F/P ratios	NCCLS methods
Ab concentration (≥10%)	a Reverse radial immunodiffusion, and/or b. Unitage assay, and c. Chessboard titration[a]
Use dilution	a. 50 μg Ab/ml (25–100 μg/ml), and/or b. ¼ U/ml (⅛ to ½ U/ml) check for PEP and NSS

[a]See Table 3.

tration of labeled antibodies in anti-Ig conjugates are given in Appendix Section F. The key factors in characterizing conjugates are their specificity and sensitivity for the conjugates. The relationship of the biochemical and immunochemical characteristics to their performance in immunofluorescent tests is determined by two-dimensional or chessboard titration. Table 3 affords an example of such a titration with a serum containing ANA. The relationships of the characteristics of conjugates to their performance may be summarized briefly as follows:

1. Tests of the Ig class specificity of conjugates by chessboard titrations of the type shown in Tables 4 and 5 reveal not only the presence or absence of but also the degree of cross-reactivity.
2. The F/P ratio or optical sensitivity ratio governs primarily: a) The titer and intensity of specific or DSS reactions. b) The degree of NSS.
3. The concentration of specific antibody governs primarily the dilution of the conjugate at which routine tests should be performed at its use dilution.

Manufacturers' Responsibilities for Conjugate Characterization: Views of Others

Similar views are now being expressed by others. Chantler and Batty (10) state that the major quality control factors for the manufacturer of FITC-labeled reagents are: 1) the selection of antisera for conjugation, 2) the specificity assessment, 3) the control of the degree of labeling, and 4) the potency assessment of such conjugates.

Table 3. Chessboard Titration of a Serum Containing ANA on Mouse Kidney Sections with Serial Dilutions of an Antihuman IgG Conjugate

Human sera tested	*Dilutions tested*		*Strength of ANA obtained with dilutions of conjugate containing the following antibody concentrations in U/ml (1/2 to 1/64) and in antibody protein (100 to 3.1 mg/ml)*					
		U/ml: *Mg/ml:*	*1/2* *100*	*1/4* *50*	*1/8* *25*	*1/16* *12.5*	*1/32* *6.3*	*1/64* *3.1*
Saline	—		—	—	—	—	—	—
Normal	1:10		NSS	—	—	—	—	—
ANA pos	1:80		++	++	++	++	+	+
"	1:160		++	++	++	++	+	Weak
"	1:320		+	+	+	+	Weak	±
"	1:640		+	+	+	Weak	±	±
"	1:1280		Weak	Weak	Weak	±	±	±
"	1:2560		±	±	±	±	±	–
	Titers		1280	1280	1280	640	320	160
		Comments:	Trace of NSS	Use dilution	Conj. PEP			
				Plateau titer range				

Table 4. Chessboard Titrations of IgG and IgM Class ANA with Three Types of Conjugates

Anti-IgG conjugate[b]

			Use dil.[a]		(PEP)	
		640	—	—	—	—
	(PT)	320	w+	w+/±	±	—
		160	+	+	w+/±	—
		80	++	+/w+	+/w+	—
		40	++	++	+/w+	—
IgG ANA		1/20	+++	++	+/w+	—
NHS[a]		1/10	—	—	—	—
U/ml[a] anti-IgG			1/4	1/8	1/16	1/32
g/ml anti-IgG			56	28	14	7
U/ml anti-IgM			—	—	—	—
Dilution			1/16	1/32	1/64	1/128

	320	—	—	—
	160	—	—	—
	80	—	—	—
	40	—	—	—
	1/20	—	—	—
IgM ANA	1/10	—	—	—
NHS	1/10	—	—	—
		(1/2)	(1/4)	(1/8)
		—	—	—
		1/8	1/16	1/32

Anti-IgM conjugate[b]

640	—	—	—
320	—	—	—
160	—	—	—
80	—	—	—
40	—	—	—

					(PEP)	
	320	—	—	—	—	—
(PT)	160	w+	w+	w+/±	w+	—
	80	+/++	+	+/w+	w+	—
	40	++	+/++	+	+/w+	—
	20	++/+++	++	+	+/++	—

IgA ANA	1/20	—	—	—	
NHS	1/10	—	—	—	
U/ml anti-IgG		—	—	—	
U/ml anti-IgM		(1)	(1/2)	(1/4)	
g/ml anti-IgM					
Dilution		1/8	1/16	1/32	

IgM						
ANA	1/10	++/+++	+++	+/++	+	±
NHS	1/10	—	—	—	—	—
		—	—	—	—	—
		1/4	1/8	1/16	1/32	1/64
		59	30	15	7	4
		1/32	1/64	1/128	1/256	1/512

Anti-Ig conjugate[b] (polyvalent C458)					(PEP)		
	640	—	w	—	—	—	—
(PT)	320	w	w	±/w	—	—	—
	160	w	w	w	w	—	—
	80	+/++	+	+/w	+/w	±/w	—
	40	++	++	+/++	+	w	—
IgG ANA	1/20	+++	+++	++	+	±/w	—
NHS	1/10	—	—				
U/ml anti-IgG		1/2	1/4	1/8	1/16	1/32	1/64
U/ml anti-IgM		(1/16)	(1/32)	(1/64)	(1/128)	(1/256)	(1/512)
Dilution		1/32	1/64	1/128	1/256	1/512	1/1024

	320	+/w	±/w	±/w	±	—
	160	+	+	w	+/w	—
	80	+/++	+	w	w	—
	40	++	++/+++	+	+/w	—
	20	+++	++	+/++	+/w	w/±
IgM ANA	1/10	+++	+++	+	+	w/±
NHS	1/10	±	—			
		NSS[a]				
		(8)	(4)	(1/4)	(1/8)	(1/16)
		1	1/2	1/32	1/64	1/128
		1/2	1/4	1/64	1/128	1/256

[a]Use dil., use dilution; NHS = normal human serum; U/ml = units/ml (see text page 19); NSS = nonspecific staining
[b]See Table 5 for listing of conjugate characteristics.

Table 5. Summary of Data on Conjugates and on Chessboard Titrations

	Conjugates used for titrations listed in Table 4		
	anti-IgG[a]	*anti-IgM*[a]	*anti-Ig*[a] *polyvalent*
1. Specificity (see Table 4)			
2. Assays for optical sensitivity (F/P) ratios			
a. Fluorescein	32.2	36.0	69.0
b. Protein	11.1	12.0	12.7
c. Weight F/P ratio	2.9	3.0	5.4
d. Molar F/P ratio	1.2	1.2	2.1
3. Antibody (Ab) concentration			
a. Anti-IgG U/ml	4–8[b]	<1 (neg)	16[b]
b. Anti-IgG μg/ml	0.9	neg	ND[c]
c. Anti-IgM U/ml	<1 (neg)	4–8[b]	2[b]
d. Anti-IgM μg/ml	neg	1.9	ND
4. Use dilution of conjugates for			
a. IgG-ANA	1/4 U/ml[d]	NR[c]	1/8 U/ml
b. IgG-ANA	or 56 μg/ml[d]	NR	ND
c. IgM-ANA	NR	1/8 U/ml	1/8 U/ml
d. IgM-ANA	NR	or 30 μg/ml	ND

[a]anti-IgG, Meloy Laboratories lot 77729; anti-IgM, Meloy Laboratories lot 77633; polyvalent anti-Ig, SUNY at Buffalo lot C-458.
[b]These unitage assays were performed with purified IgG or IgM preparations rather than with normal human sera, as suggested in the text.
[c]ND, not done; NR, no reaction observed.
[d]These values are maximal use dilutions based on the data in Table 4. Lower use dilutions can be used and are safer based on past experience. Concentrations should not be over 1/2 U/ml or 100 μg/ml, since they tend to give weaker reactions in some IF systems.
Note: Subsequent lots of anti-IgM conjugate from Meloy have failed to give comparable reactivity in unitage assays and in IF tests.

1. Regarding selection of antisera, they recommend a gel precipitation test assay with 1 mg/ml antigen (see the section below on "Unitage Assays"). Antisera with titers of 16 or more are deemed to be acceptable. This corresponds to the gel precipitation unitage assay with 1 mg/ml antigen that had been introduced in the 1960s by the principal author (6). While this is a useful primary screening method, the officially accepted criterion is that conjugates contain 10% specific antibody (23). Indirect IF tests with FITC-labeled monoclonal antibodies to human immunoglobulin give reactions comparable to those obtained with polyclonal antibodies of similar specificities (10).

2. Regarding specificity assessment, anti-Ig specific reagents and class-restricted ANA of the type described in Tables 4 and 5 are recommended (see the section on specificity tests below).

3. Regarding control of the degree of labeling, Chantler and Batty (10) suggest the use of absorbance ratios at 490/280 nm for primary screening (49). In our opinion, assays need to be performed with the approved methods of the National Committee for Clinical Laboratory Standards (NCCLS) (37), since these yield more reliable results.

4. Regarding assessments of potency, chessboard titrations are recommended (4,9,10). While these are of critical importance, it is clear that the data from antibody protein determinations and/or unitage assays (see point no. 1 above) must also be taken into consideration. Since the data on antibody protein concentrations should already be available for conjugates from reputable manufacturers, they should be used (see the section on "Basic Assays for Immunologic Sensitivity of Conjugates" Below).

Synopsis of Criteria for Selection of anti-Ig Conjugates by Immunopathology Laboratories

For reliably interpretable DIF and IIF tests with anti-Ig conjugates in diagnostic or research studies, the reagents selected should be provided with the data referred to in Table 2 (8,19). Such data are now provided with some commercial conjugates (see Appendix Section E for methods). This makes it possible to take three simple but highly effective steps to insure reliable reagents:

1. Check for the availability of the indicated data on specificity, total protein, F/P ratios, and antibody content. If these data are not provided or if the accepted assay methods (see below) are not used, that particular conjugate should not be purchased, and the desired reagent should be obtained from another manufacturer or from another source.

2. If the indicated data are supplied with the conjugates, they need to be examined to determine if the reagents have the desired characteristics. The four key factors to look for are as indicated in Table 2.

a) Specificity for Ig class(es) by methods described below.

b) Total conjugate protein: This should be about 10 mg/ml, except for affinity chromatography-purified reagents (see Appendix Section E2 for details).

c) Molar and weight F/P ratios: Molar ratios in the range of 1 to 4 are used for immunopathologic studies as indicated below (see Appendix Section E4 for methods). If weight F/P ratios are given, these can be converted to molar ratios by multiplying the weight F/P (in μg/mg) by 0.411.

d) The antibody content in milligrams of antibody per milliliter and U/ml or gel precipitation titers: The antibody-to-total protein ratio should be 0.1 or greater (i.e., >10%). However, reagents with a bit less antibody (i.e., down to 8%) are still functional. Gel precipitation alone is not adequate as indicated below.

3. If the data provided with a given lot of conjugate indicate that it has the desired characteristics and that it appears to merit examination in the laboratory, then at least one and, preferably, two types of evaluation tests need to be done.

a) Indirect IF titration (three doubling dilutions before and one after the endpoint is adequate) with a known positive serum in a reproducible test system, using at least the following three conjugate concentrations: 25, 50, and 100 g antibody/ml; or if appropriate unitage assays are available: 1/8, 1/4, and 1/2 U/ml. These three titrations should give either the same titer or fluctuations of not more than one doubling dilution in the endpoint.

b) If a properly standardized unitage assay is available (see below), this should be performed and compared, if possible, to the antibody protein assay and to the results of the above (step 1) three titrations. If this is performed and read as prescribed, then: 1) 1 U/ml is roughly equal to 0.2 mg/ml of antibody; 2) 1/2, 1/4, and 1/8 U/ml will give either the same titers or fluctuations of not more than one doubling dilution; and 3) unitage assays can be substituted for the the titrations and antibody protein assays in the selection of conjugates.

Specificity Assays

Tests for specificity of the anti-Ig and other conjugates used in immunofluorescence studies are of two types; those based on immunofluorescence serology and those based on precipitation or other serologic tests. Strictly speaking, those based on immunofluorescence are the only unequivocally valid ones. However, precipitation tests may be quite satisfactory or even the methods of choice for certain conjugates; for example, for assays of antifibrinogen conjugates (which cannot be used in immunofluorescence serology). On the other hand, immunofluorescence serology of the type shown in Tables 3 and 4 should be utilized more routinely.

Precipitation and Other Tests for Specificity Assays

For IgG-specific conjugates, immunoelectrophoresis with whole serum should give only the IgG line and no lines for IgM and IgA. This test could also be supplemented with gel diffusion tests. Specificity tests of anticomplement conjugates can be carried out with standard complement immunofluorescence serology.

Immunofluorescence Specificity Test of Anti-Ig Conjugates

Specificity tests of anti-Ig conjugates should be done with IIF tests using class-restricted antibodies. Table 4 summarizes the results of such specificity tests. The plateau titers of both the IgM and IgG class ANA were in the range of 160 to 320. The characteristics of the conjugates used in these specificity tests are listed in Table 5.

As seen in Table 6, all 16 ANA of sera from patients with systemic lupus erythematosus had predominantly IgG class ANA. These all had titers of 40 to 1280. For comparison, four normal sera were selected for the presence of ANA; titers ranged 10 to 40 using a polyvalent conjugate of the type shown in Tables 4 and 5. Of these four normal sera, one had predominantly IgG class ANA. The remaining three, were predominantly of the IgM class.

Assays for Optical and Immunologic Sensitivity of Conjugates

Since immunofluorescence tests are based on the optical properties of the F label, the optical sensitivity of conjugates depends on the number of F molecules per bound antibody molecule, and on the sensitivity of the optical system for detection of F.

Table 6. Immunoglobulin (Ig) Classes of ANA in Normal and Systemic Lupus Sera

Source of sera and ANA type	*Cases (no.)*	*Ig classes and titers of ANA*		
		IgG	*IgM*	*IgA*
Normal				
Mostly IgM	3	≤2.5	10–40	<2.5–5
Mostly IgG	1	10	2.5	<2.5
Systemic lupus				
Mostly IgM	0	—	—	—
Mostly IgG	6	40–160	2.5–40	2.5–40
(total 16)	10	320–1280	2.5–80	5–80

Basic Assays for Optical Sensitivity of Conjugates

The basic assays of a conjugate of a given specificity include protein (P) and fluorescein (F) content and their activity ratios; this ratio affords a measure of the optical sensitivity of a conjugate.

1. Total P assays by the biuret method give reliable values if done with appropriate controls (13,33). Since there are differences in the 280 nm extinction coefficients of various proteins, the biuret method should be used to determine for each type of protein preparation its particular extinction coefficient before the 280 nm readings can be used reliably for assays. Standard conjugates should be adjusted to 10 mg protein/ml (see Appendix Section E2 for details).

2. Total F assays according to the method of McKinney et al. (31) are based on 490 nm extinctions of conjugate dilutions made in N/10 NaOH and checked with a hydrolyzed F diacetate standard in N/10 NaOH. This method and the method for determining F/P ratios are the ones recommended by the NCCLS (37). Other methods based on extinction coefficients may not be accurate (see Appendix Section E1 for details.)

3. Fluorescein to protein (F/P) ratios calculated by standard methods (13,33; Appendix Section E4) must be restricted to a constant range for reproducible IIF tests for ANA or other antibodies. Low molar F/P ratios (e.g., 1.0:1.9) give "clean" ANA tests with low background staining, but somewhat lower intensities and titers of ANA. Somewhat higher molar F/P ratios (e.g., 2.0:3.9) give stronger intensities of IF staining and higher ANA titers (33), but give stronger background staining. Conjugates with a high molar F/P ratio (e.g. 4:7) give high NSS on tissue sections. Conjugates with even high molar F/P ratios (e.g., 10 or more) are used for bacterial fluorescent antibody studies and membrane immunofluorescence, but they give too much NSS to be of value in immunologic studies of tissues.

Basic Assays for Immunologic Sensitivity of Conjugates

Three types of assays of labeled specific antibodies may be used: 1) assays of mg of antibody using reference standards, 2) assays of milligram amounts of antibody without reference standards, and 3) rough approximation of labeled antibody concentrations.

The ratio of specific labeled antibody protein (Ab) to total labeled P or Ab/P ratios can be calculated quantitatively from assays that yield values on milligrams per milliliters of antibody. These are currently used in industry. As indicated below, recommendations of the World Health Organization (WHO) on commercial (and other) anti-Ig conjugates call for Ab/P ratios of 0.10; that is, 10% of labeled P should be antibody in acceptable conjugates. These Ab/P ratio determinations are needed to assess the acceptability of conjugates.

Laboratories that perform immunopathologic studies should use simple assays that give rough approximations of antibody concentrations. These serve as a check on both the validity of the information supplied by manufacturers and on the stability of the conjugates.

The major examples of the three above-mentioned types of sensitivity assays are as follows:

Assays of Milligrams of Antibody Using Reference Standards

Reverse radial immunodiffusion (RRID) affords the most commonly used method now for assays of mg Ab/ml (9). In essence, selected dilutions of reference standards with known concentrations of antibody, as well as selected dilutions of the conjugate to be assayed, are placed in wells in agar containing the antigen. The diameter plot of the rings of precipitation of the reference standard plotted versus its antibody concentration afford a basis for assaying unknown antiglobulins. This method (which is detailed in Appendix Section E3) requires the use of reference standards assayed by other methods.

Assays of Milligram Amounts of Antibody Without Reference Standards

Such assays, which constitute one of the most important contributions of the discipline of immunochemistry, are now well established (1,24). Interestingly, the first studies on labeled antigens and antibodies (20) were performed with a view toward quantitating antibody reactions. A procedure described recently by Huang et al. (24), which is based on photometric determination of the F content of labeled antibody molecules by affinity chromatography (FLAC), affords a highly reliable and functional method for assay of the concentration of IgG antibody in milligrams Ab per milliliter. Figure 2 illustrates the principles of the two types of affinity chromatography used in the FLAC assay method. As indicated in Figure 2, another type of IgG-coated bead serves as a means for determining both the total antibody bound (F) and the antibody F/P ratio. The above-mentioned NCCLS recommended methods for F assays, and F/P ratio determinations are used in this method. Since the F/P ratio of the affinity chromatography-purified, F-labeled antibodies is lower than the F/P ratio of the crude conjugate, this step is essential for valid assays of the milligrams Ab per milliliter concentration. This method of assay provides a means of obtaining or checking on the reference standards used in the above-mentioned RRID assay. Details of this FLAC method appear in Appendix Section F in this chapter.

Rough Approximations of Labeled Antibody Concentrations

Two simple and functional assays that give estimates of labeled antibody activity are chessboard titrations and unitage assays.

The above-mentioned plateau endpoint (PEP) of chessboard titrations (see Tables 4 and 5) gives a rough measure of antibody concentrations. Usually, the PEP falls in the range of about 10 to 26 μg antibody/ml. The PEP also affords a basis for selection of use dilutions. Because of the practical importance and potential pitfalls in unitage assays, details of the methods are given in the following subsection.

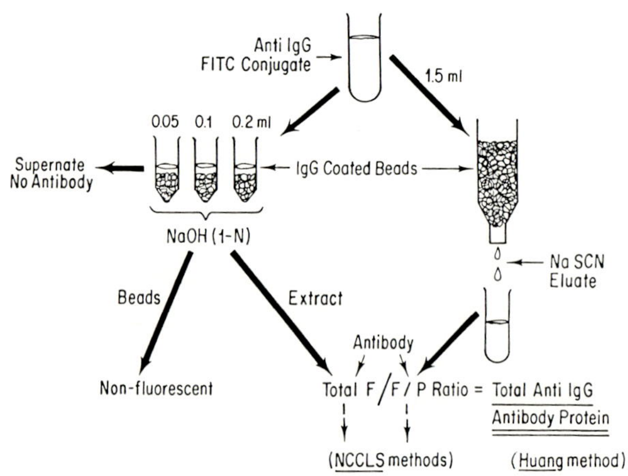

Figure 2. Principles of assay of fluorescein-labeled antibody concentration by affinity chromatography or FLAC assay. (Reprinted from Huang [24].)

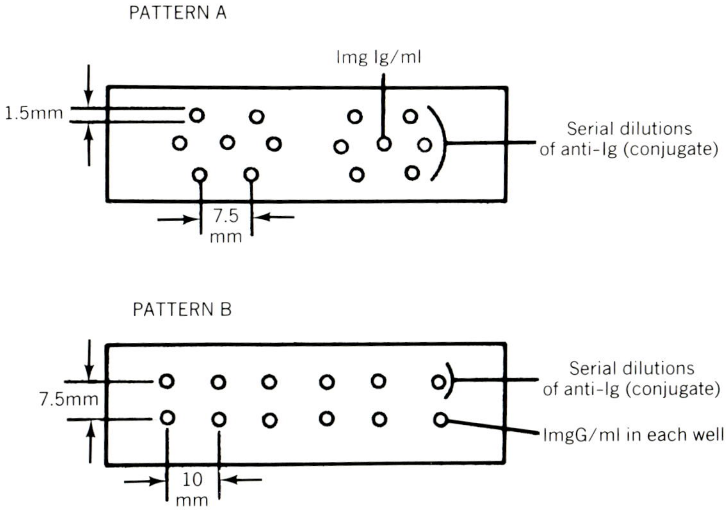

Figure 3. Templates for unitage assays. The templates are used to cut wells into agar for titrations of antiglobulin or antisera. The gel diffusion precipitation titers are expressed as U/ml or U/1% P. (Reprinted from Beutner EH, Chorzelski TP, Jordan RE: *Autosensitization in Pemphigus and Bullous Pemphigoid.* Charles C Thomas, Springfield, IL, 1970.)

Unitage Assays

These assays of conjugates are among the most useful laboratory methods in immunopathologic studies with labeled antibodies. Because of the problems entailed in the correct interpretation of the unitage assay, they merit a special discussion although the methods are very simple. In essence, a unitage assay is simply a gel precipitation titration of anti-Ig sera, globulin, or conjugates against 1 mg/ml of the homologous antigen using a standard template. While the RRID and/or the FLAC assays described above should be performed by manufacturers, unitage assays can and should be done in laboratories that perform immunopathologic studies. The key points that we need to stress for the effective use of unitage assays are:

1. The indicated procedure for the performance and, importantly, the reading and checking of procedures.
2. The use of the results of unitage assays together with a simple titration in selection of conjugates.

The indicated procedure is as follows: 1% Ion agar* is poured onto a microscope slide or some other suitable carrier to a depth of 1.5 nm. Wells are cut into the hardened agar by using one of the templates shown in Figure 3. For Pattern A, the central wells are filled with 1 mg/ml of human IgG, while for Pattern B, each well in one row is filled with IgG or whole human serum diluted to contain 1 mg IgG/ml. Serial twofold dilutions of conjugate or antiserum or immunoglobulin fraction of an antiserum are placed in the peripheral wells. *Pipettes must be changed for every dilution.* The plates are incubated at room temperature for 24 hours and read for the highest dilution that offers a visible line of precipitation. *This titer is the unitage* (e.g., a conjugate with a titer of 8 has 8 U/ml). Pattern B is now regarded as the template of choice for unitage

*Ion agar, Colab, Chicago Heights, IL 60411.

assays. Conjugates prepared from horse sera sometimes cannot be tested for unitage, because some fail to give precipitin lines under these conditions. The points that relate to the reading and checking of unitage assays are as follows. First, the endpoint of the precipitation lines must be read grossly by daylight (i.e., without staining or magnification or other methods of enhancement) to obtain a valid unitage. In effect, simply hold the plate up to a window and read it. Any enhancement of the sensitivity alters the titer, therefore changing the significance from that of a unitage to some unknown. Second, to check on the validity of the reading, unitage assay can be performed with commercial conjugates that are supplied with exact assay values on the antibody P concentration. The unitage should be such that:

$$\frac{\text{mg antibody protein/ml}}{\text{U/ml}} \approx \frac{\text{approximately 0.2 mg antibody}}{\text{unit}}$$

(i.e., 0.1 mg to 0.4 mg/unit)

For example, the data in Table 5 reveal the following:

a. for the anti-IgG conjugate

$$\frac{0.9 \text{ mg/ml}}{4\text{–}8 \text{ U/ml}} \approx 0.1 \text{ to } 0.2 \text{ mg/U}$$

b. for the anti-IgM conjugate

$$\frac{1.9 \text{ mg/ml}}{4\text{–}8 \text{ U/ml}} \approx 0.2 \text{ to } 0.4 \text{ mg/unit}$$

(The reason for the range of unitages is that repeat tests yielded somewhat variable results.)

Importantly, the values listed in Table 5 are in the expected range of 0.1 to 0.4 mg/U/ml of the conjugate. If the values fail to fall in this range, the unitage assays need to be repeated with a view toward finding possible sources of error; for example, the antibody protein given by the manufacturer of the commercial conjugate may be incorrect, the unitage assay was not performed and/or read correctly, or the antigen concentration was not adjusted correctly, etc. The antigen source and concentration for unitage assays is less critical than the method of reading the endpoint. To bring about a change of one doubling dilution in the titer of the antibody, it is necessary to change the concentration of the antigen by a factor of fourfold. In effect, a fluctuation of antigen concentration from, for example, 0.5 to 2 mg/ml would change the titer from 8 to 4, but a concentration range of 0.8 to 1.2 usually makes no difference or at the most, one doubling dilution. Thus, it is possible to get at least reasonable approximations of unitages by using a pool of normal human sera diluted according to the normal values of immunoglobulin concentration as a source of antigen. For example,

For IgG, dilute pooled normal human sera to 1/12.

For IgA and IgM, pooled normal sera can be used undiluted.

A somewhat more accurate method is to dilute human sera on the basis of their IgG, IgM, or IgA concentrations as determined by radial immunodiffusion assays. If purified preparations with known immunoglobulin concentrations are available (e.g., Table 5), these are useful but they are not necessary.

APPENDIX

A. CONJUGATE PREPARATION

Several methods for conjugate preparation have been described. The following brief outline is the method used by the authors. Conjugates prepared by this (or other) method(s) must be characterized as outlined previously in the section on "Criteria for Characterization, Selection, and Dilution of Anti-Ig Antibodies Conjugated with Fluorescein Isothiocyanate (FITC)." Globulins are prepared by ammonium sulfate fractionation as modified from Coons and Kaplan (11), and then conjugated by a modification of the method of Marshall et al. (30).

Fractionation of the serum to be conjugated is achieved by diluting the serum by 1:5 with PBS* and adding to it, drop by drop, an equal volume of 3.6 M ammonium sulfate, pH 7.0. The mixture is stirred for 1 hour. The precipitate formed is separated by centrifuging at 12,000 g for 10 minutes in a refrigerated (4°C) centrifuge. The supernatant is then decanted and discarded. The precipitate is resuspended and washed twice in 2 M ammonium sulfate. After each wash, the precipitate is separated by centrifuging (as above), and the supernatant is discarded. The gamma globulin precipitate is reconstituted to half the original serum volume with distilled water, and then dialyzed against 6 liters of 0.85% NaCl for 24 hours. To remove all ammonium sulfate, the 6 liter volume of saline is changed several times. Barium chloride (0.01 M) is used to check the dialysate for removal of all ammonium sulfate. Ammonium sulfate, if present, reacts with barium chloride to form a white precipitate. The final pH of the globulin is checked to assure neutrality.

Conjugation of serum globulins with fluorescein (F) is carried out as follows: The P concentration of the globulin solution is determined by the biuret method (17). The final volume of the conjugate is determined by the total P of the globulin; the conjugate should have a P concentration of 10 mg/ml. A globulin solution containing 300 mg of P, for example, can be used to prepare 30 ml of conjugate. Because optimal coupling of FITC to P occurs at pH 9.0 or greater, carbonate buffer (0.1 M Na_2CO_3, 0.4 M $NaHCO_3$, pH 9.5) equivalent to 15% of the total conjugate volume is added. The amount of FITC added is dictated by the desired F/P ratio. This has been determined empirically by Beutner et al. (9). Some of the values have been included in Table 7. The FITC is dissolved in a 10% carbonate buffer to a concentration of 1 mg FITC/ml of buffer. The total volume of globulin solution, carbonate buffer, and FITC solution is brought to the calculated total volume of conjugate by addition of 0.9% NaCl.

The globulin solution, carbonate buffer, and saline are first mixed together at 4°C, and the FITC solution is added by drops to the stirring mixture. This conjugate mixture is gently stirred for 24 hours at 4°C, and is finally dialyzed against large volumes of PBS with repeated buffer change until no free F is seen in the dialysate. Free F is revealed by examining the dialysate under ultraviolet (UV) light. When no fluorescence of the dialysate is seen, the conjugate is ready for characterization.

*PBS (phosphate buffered saline) ionic strength O.15N, pH 7.2 (unless otherwise indicated); 0.1165M NaCl + 0.0135M PO_4^{-3}. For PO_4^{-3}, use e.g. 1.47 g $Na_2H\ PO_4$ + 0.43 g $KH_2\ PO_4$ (anhydrous) per liter of glass distilled water.

Table 7. FITC Input Related to Molar F/P Ratio

Approximate molar F/P (±20%) desired	*Indicated input mg FITC/100 mg protein*
1.0	0.4
1.5	0.6
2.0	0.8
2.5	1.1
3.0	1.4
3.5	1.8
4.0	2.1
4.5	2.5
5.0	2.9

B. TRANSPORT MEDIUM FOR SHIPMENT OF SKIN BIOPSY SPECIMENS

The transport medium of Michel et al. (32) permits shipment of unfrozen skin biopsy specimens at ambient temperatures. Biopsy specimens that have been frozen cannot be handled with this medium.

1. Preparation of Buffer. Add 2.5 ml of 1 M potassium citrate buffer (pH 7.0), 5 ml of 0.1 M $MgSO_4$, and 5 ml of 0.1 M N-ethylmaleimide to 87.5 ml of distilled water. Adjust the final mixture to pH 7.0 with 1 M KOH.

2. Preparation of Fixative. Dissolve 55 g of $(NH_4)_2SO_4$ in 100 ml of buffer.

The final composition of the fixative is as follows:

$(NH_4)_2SO_4$	3.120 M
N-ethylmaleimide	0.005 M
$MgSO_4$	0.005 M
Citrate	0.025 M

3. Procedure for Use. a.) Place biopsy tissue into mixture solution. Do not freeze before putting in fixative. b.) On receipt by the laboratory of tissue in fixative solution, the biopsy specimen should be washed three times for 10 minutes in the buffer and frozen at −20°C. c.) The frozen tissue is processed the same as for standard immunofluorescence.

Notes: The final medium should be pH 7.0 to 7.2. Medium below about pH 6.4 or above pH 7.5 gives unsatisfactory results. The shelf life of the medium remains to be determined. It is clearly over 2 years.

The simplified fixative by Niedecken and Lange (38) is prepared by dissolving 55 g ammonium sulfate in 100 ml saline. Final solution was adjusted with 1 M sodium hydroxide (NaOH) to pH 7.4. The stability after preparation was at least 3 months at 4°C.

C. MOUNTING MEDIA, ANTIFADING AGENTS, AND STORAGE OF IMMUNOFLUORESCENT SLIDES

Mounting Media

There are basically two kinds of mounting media employed in immunofluorescent studies (12). One is buffered glycerine, which is prepared by mixing nine parts of glycerine with one part of PBS (pH 7.4).

The other kind of mounting medium is semipermanent and is useful in preserving the immunofluorescent-stained slide preparation for extended periods of time by preventing dehydration and other factors (42;) This medium can be prepared by mixing 20 g of polyvinyl alcohol (Gelvatol 20–30, Monsanto) with 80 ml of PBS (pH 7.2) for 16 hours at room temperature. At this time, add 40 ml of glycerol and stir for another 16 hours. Centrifuge the suspension at about 10,000 rpm for 15 minutes to remove undissolved materials. Test and adjust the pH to 7.2 and store at 4°C.

Antifading Agents

The intensity of fluorescence radiation is directly proportional to the excitation intensity, and the sensitivity can be increased by increasing the excitation intensity (discussed previously in the section on "Microscopy"). Associated with this increase in excitation intensity is the problem of rapid fading. This limits the analysis of fluorescent staining, especially when the staining is weak.

As shown in Figure 4, the rate of fading is a function of excitation intensity, and increases with an increase in magnification of the objective (43,44,46). The fading may be

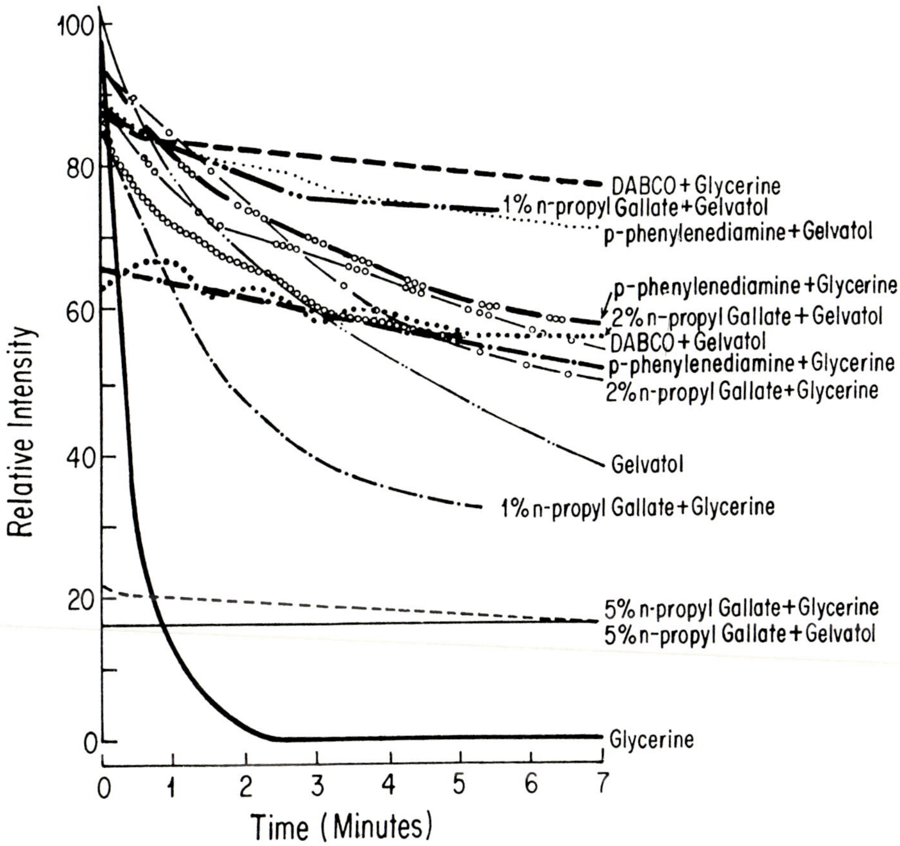

Figure 4. Fluorophotometric determination of the decay of fluorescent intensity of ANA reactivity on HEp-2 substrate slides mounted in buffered glycerine or Gelvatol (semipermanent) mounting medium with and without the presence of preservatives.

3. Gently swirl and warm on a hot plate until the FDA is completely solubilized.
4. Let cool to room temperature.
5. Quantitatively transfer the contents of the beaker to a 500 ml volumetric flask, using distilled water to rinse the beaker and bring the flask to volume. (This solution has been kept in a pyrex bottle protected from light for more than 2 years with no significant change in absorbance. Ordinary soft glass is not satisfactory for prolonged storage of this strong alkaline solution.)

A standard curve is constructed by:

1. Preparing appropriate dilutions of the above FDA reference standard solution (100 μg/ml) in 0.1 N sodium hydroxide to give a series of solutions of concentrations between 1 and 3 μg FDA/ml.
2. Obtaining absorbance (A) readings of these solutions at their λ_{max} near 495 nm, using the 0.1 N sodium hydroxide diluent as the blank.
3. Converting the FDA concentrations in micrograms per milliliter of each dilution to protein-bound concentrations in micrograms per milliliter by multiplying by the factor 1.066.*

$$\text{FDA } \mu\text{g/ml} \times 1.066 = \text{protein-bound FITC } \mu\text{g/ml}$$

4. And plotting the protein-bound FITC concentrations in micrograms per milliliter as the abscissa against the FDA absorbance readings as the ordinate.
5. Or (alternate to 3 and 4) calculating the extinction coefficient of FDA and dividing it by 1.066 to obtain the extinction coefficient of protein-bound FITC. The calculated value should be within 5% of the expected value of 0.195.

Example

$$\begin{aligned} E^{\mu g/ml}_{1\,cm} &= \lambda_{max} \text{ (near 490 nm)} \\ &= \frac{0.204}{1} \times \frac{1}{1.066} = 0.191 \text{ (for protein-bound FITC)} \end{aligned}$$

The FITC content of a conjugate is determined by:

1. Preparing an appropriate dilution of the conjugate in 0.1 N sodium hydroxide to give an A reading between 0.05 and 0.4 (in 10 mm cells) at maximum for the solution (near 495 nm). Use the diluent as the blank. If the A reading should be made on undiluted conjugates, the pH must be raised with 0.1 N NaOH to approximately pH 9.0.
2. Determining the concentration of protein-bound FITC in micrograms per milliliter from the standard curve, or calculating it from the extinction coefficient.
3. Multiplying this value by the dilution required for the A reading. The calculated value is the concentration of protein-bound FITC in the conjugate in micrograms per

*This relationship is based on the following: With a particular spectrophotometer, the extinction coefficient (E/μg 1 cm/ml) for protein-bound FITC was found to be 0.195, and for FDA was found to be 0.208. The extinction coefficient for FDA divided by the extinction coefficient for protein-bound FITC is the constant 1.066. Use of this factor and the standard curve, or extinction coefficient prepared with FDA, eliminates the effect of variation in spectrophotometers and relates all measurements of protein-bound FITC to the primary reference standard FDA.

milliliter. The concentration of FITC from the standard curve multiplied by the dilution of conjugate equals bound FITC in micrograms per milliliter.

2. Protein Concentration

The protein content of a conjugate is most readily calculated from biuret reactions with the serum proteins (30). A standard protein curve is prepared as follows:

1. Reagents
   a) Standard protein solution: Armour Laboratories or comparable standard solution of crystalline bovine albumin: 10 mg protein N/ml.
   b) Biuret reagent: Fisher Scientific Company (17).
2. Procedure
   a) Place the indicated amounts of 0.85% NaCl in each of 10 tubes.
   b) Prepare an initial dilution of 1:20 of the standard protein solution in 0.85% NaCl, and add the indicated volumes of the diluted standard to the tubes to make final dilution steps of 0:4, 1:4, 2:4, 3:4, and 4:4.
   c) Add 8 ml biuret reagent to each tube and mix well.
   d) Allow color development to proceed for 30 minutes at room temperature (25 to 30°C) before reading.
   e) Obtain A readings on a spectrophotometer at 560 nm.
   f) Plot A as the ordinate against milligrams per milliliter protein as the abscissa.

$$\text{mg/ml protein} = \frac{\text{Concentration standard} \times \text{N factor}}{\text{dilution of standard}}$$

(where N factor = 6.25) and determine protein N of unknown by graphic interpolations. Or (alternate to f) calculate extinction coefficient as:

$$E_{1\ \text{cm}}^{1\ \text{mg/ml}}\ 560\ \text{nm} = 0.28.$$

Example

1. Determine the protein concentration of the conjugate by making an initial dilution of 1:4 in 0.85% NaCl.
2. Add to this the biuret reagent, as previously described, to give a further dilution of 1:5 for a reaction mixture with a final dilution of 4 × 5 or 20-fold.
3. The optical density of the reaction mixture of 560 nm as measured in 1 cm cuvette = 0.20.
4. Calculate the total protein concentration of the conjugate from the above-mentioned extinction coefficient:

$$0.20 \times 20 \div 0.28 = 14.3\ \text{mg/ml}.$$

Determination of protein in FITC labeled conjugates (see the following notes)

Notes

1. This procedure was written for use with spectrophotometers requiring 10 mm cuvettes and a minimum volume for a reading of 6 ml. When smaller cuvettes are used,

smaller reaction mixture volumes may be prepared if the sample-to-biuret volume ratio of 1:5 remains constant (23). For example, a 2 ml diluted sample requires 8 ml of biuret; a 1 ml sample requires 4 ml biuret; a 0.5 sample requires 2 ml of biuret, etc.

2. The presence of high concentrations of FITC in the protein-biuret reaction mixture will alter readings at the wavelength setting of 540 nm used for the original biuret method. However, the reaction mixture gives approximately the same readings at 540 nm and 560 nm, and the slight shift in wavelength to 560 nm eliminates the interference of FITC absorption with the protein-biuret value.

3. Except under specially defined conditions, the ratio of A at 490 nm to A at 280 nm does not give a reliable measure of the degree of labeling. It does not measure actual F or P concentration. However, it can be used in certain research projects in which a constant form of labeled P is used under defined conditions. This ratio requires that the pH be specified to insure meaningful values. Certain preservatives used in conjugates absorb in the 280 nm region, and their presence further complicates the use of this method. Some examples of these are o-cresol, merthiolate, and phenol. Another drawback to the use of this method in some laboratories is the requirement of a spectrophotometer capable of measurements in the UV range.

4. Other methods of determining protein concentration may be used if they can be shown to be as reliable as the biuret method. It may also be calculated from independent determinations of N by the micro-Kjeldahl technique. However, the biuret method has been found to be simple, reliable, and free from interference by most substances commonly present in conjugates.

5. If serum proteins are fractionated with $(NH_4)_2SO_4$, they must be well dialyzed, since 0.08 M or greater concentration of the salt will interfere in the biuret test. If the ethanol fractionation procedure is used, the concentration of alcohol in the protein solution must be below 2.1% for protein determination by biuret. If turbidity-producing substances are present, they must be removed. The serum may be freed of lipids by treatment with ether (30).

6. It is suggested that: a) protein assays of conjugates be performed before addition of unlabeled protein, and b) the amounts of unlabeled proteins present in the final product be designated in milligrams per milliliter.

Extremely low concentrations of conjugated protein (below 2 mg/ml) are not diluted prior to the addition of the biuret reagent. Higher concentrations are appropriately diluted with 0.85% NaCl to obtain A readings of the reaction mixtures between 0.05 and 0.40 at 560 nm with 19 nm cells, or between 0.05 and 0.25 with 10 nm cells.

1. Prepare a blank tube containing 2 ml of 0.85% NaCl.
2. Dilute the conjugate to be tested with 0.85% NaCl, and place 2.0 ml in each of two separate tubes.
3. Add 8.0 ml of biuret reagent to each of the three tubes and mix well.
4. Allow color development to proceed for a minimum of 30 minutes to a maximum of 2 hours at 25 to 30°C.
5. Obtain A readings on a spectrophotometer at 560 nm, using the 0.85% NaCl blank to set the 0.0 A value.
6. Calculate the conjugated protein concentration as follows:

Conjugate dilution × mg/ml = mg/ml protein
(mg/ml from standard curve or calculated from extinction coefficient).

Preparation of Reagents

1. Biuret:
   a) Place 6 g sodium potassium tartrate ($NaKC_4H_4O_4 \cdot H_2O$; MW = 282.23) in a dry 1 liter volumetric flask and dissolve in about 300 ml of distilled water.
   b) Add 1.5 g $CuSo_4,5H_2O$ and dissolve by adding more distilled water up to a total volume of approximately 500 ml.
   c) With constant swirling, add 300 ml of 10% sodium hydroxide. (Prepare the NaOH from CO_2-free water that has been boiled and cooled in a stoppered flask with an attached $CaCl_2$ tube.)
   d) Dilute to the 1 liter mark with distilled water.
   e) Store in a paraffin-lined glass, polyethylene, or pyrex bottle.
   f) The reagent is stable for a considerable period of time, but must be discarded immediately if it shows signs of black or reddish precipitate.
2. Sodium chloride: 0.85% NaCl:
   a) Place 8.5 g NaCl in a dry 1 liter volumetric flask and dissolve in about 500 ml distilled water.
   b) Dilute to the 1 liter mark with distilled water and mix well.

3. Procedure for RRID Assays of Antibody Protein (5,9)

Diffusion Plates

1. a) Allow molten 2% Nobel agar and a 50 μg/ml solution of IgG (or other antigen to be tested) to equilibrate at 56°C.
   b) Mix equal volumes of the two.
   c) Pour to a depth of 1.5 mm onto a microscope slide.
   d) With a 1.5 mm punch, cut a row of 6 equidistant wells separated by at least 17 mm.
2. On each plate used, utilize three wells for serial two-fold dilutions of the reference standard (see below). Use the remaining three wells for serial dilutions of each test sample.

Reference Standard

1. Prepared as described in the literature (9) or as in section F below.
2. Reconstitute with 1 ml distilled water. Prepare dilutions of 1:2 and 1:4, etc., in isotonic saline. Freeze unused standard. Unused dilutions may be kept at 2°C for periods not exceeding 14 days.

Procedure of Test

1. In three wells, place the reference standard (undiluted, 1:2, 1:4, etc.). Care should be taken to uniformly fill each well level with the agar surface. Neither overfill nor underfill the wells. A slight overfill has less influence on the final results compared with the greater chance of error introduced by underfilling.
2. Similarly, place samples in the remaining three wells.
3. Place the plates in a moist chamber and allow them to diffuse at room temperature for 16 hours.

Reading of Test

1. If the precipitin ring is extremely light and difficult to read, the visibility can be improved by dipping the plate in 7.5% acetic acid for 1 to 2 minutes. Rinse the plate carefully and thoroughly in cold water, and then read immediately.
2. After incubation, remove the cover and measure the diameter of each precipitin ring by placing the plate beneath the eyepiece of a Behring Diagnostic Viewer or similar viewing device. Align one side of the ring with the zero mark on the grid, and measure the diameter of the precipitin ring to the nearest 0.1 mm. Alternatively, a dissecting microscope with a stage micrometer or eyepiece scale may be used.
3. Readings may be taken from both the horizontal and vertical axes if precipitin zones are not round. When this method is employed, the average diameter should be plotted.

Plotting of Data

1. On the log-log graph paper, the horizontal axis represents one diameter.
2. The vertical axis represents antibody expressed in milligrams per milliliter.
3. Plot the zone diameters of the reference standard and the concentration of each on the corresponding axis. Draw the straight line that best accommodates all three points.
4. Read antibody levels in the test samples and dilutions from the reference graph, and multiply values obtained by the dilution factor.

Interpretation of Results

1. For optimal results, the levels of the unknown samples must fall within the range of the reference curve. Dilution should be prepared accordingly, and some samples must be repeated for accurate assays.
2. Those samples facing above the highest reference will show decreasing values as the levels become greater. This phenomenon is accompanied by a reduction in accuracy. Similarly, as levels fall below the lowest standard, the results will become progressively less accurate, with a concomitant rise in results. These samples should be reassayed after an adjustment of the dilution.

4. Procedure for Calculating F/P, Ab/P, and Ab/F Ratios of Conjugates (3))

The following steps should be carried out:

1. The concentration of protein is expressed as milligrams of protein per milliliter of conjugate, with the protein determined by the biuret method.

2. The concentration of F is expressed as micrograms of bound FITC per milliliter of conjugate, with F determined by absorbance at λ_{max} (near 495 nm) and related to a pure FDA reference standard.

3. The F/P ratio expressed as micrograms FITC per milligram protein is measured by the above methods. To obtain this value, divide the protein-bound FITC concentration in micrograms per milliliter by the protein concentration in milligrams per milliliter, giving a w/w F/P ratio.

4. Since some workers are partial to the use of molar ratios, F/P ratios should be expressed in two ways. After the weight ratio is calculated, it may be converted to a molar ratio by multiplying the factor 0.411. The latter is derived from the expression

$$160{,}000/389 \times 10^{-3} = 0.411$$

where 160,000 is taken as the average molecular weight of gamma globulin, and 389 as the molecular weight of FITC.

5. Since this calculation of molar ratios entails some assumptions and since molar ratios are derived from weight ratios, the F/P ratios may be expressed as follows:

$$F/P = 5.1\ \mu g/mg = 5.1 \times 10^{-3}$$

$$\text{Estimated molar } F/P = 2.1 = (5.1 \times 0.411).$$

Neither the accuracy nor precision of the proposed FITC and protein analyses justifies the recording of more than two significant figures for F/P ratios.

6. Some workers prefer to check the FITC and protein assays reported by manufacturers. Thus, the results of these analyses should be listed individually, as well as in the form of F/P ratios in the product description. This information also aids in the prediction of conjugate characteristics.

7. Some manufacturers add unlabeled proteins to conjugates in order to increase specificity or stability. When this is done, it is necessary that: a) protein assays of conjugates should be performed before the addition of unlabeled protein; and b) the amount of unlabeled protein present in the final product should be designated in milligrams per milliliter.

8. The Ab concentration as determined by the RRID methods (see preceding Section 3) may be expressed either as micrograms per milliter or as milligram per milliliter, depending on the needs.

9. Ab/P ratios may be expressed as weight ratios (milligram/milligram). To obtain this value, divide the Ab concentration in milligrams per milliliter by the P concentration in milligrams per milliliter.

10. Following the same reasoning as for point 4 above, Ab/P ratios may be expressed as molar ratios. Ab/P (gram/gram) = Ab/P (molar), since 160,000 is taken as the molecular weight of both.

11. Ab/F ratios may be expressed as weight ratios (microgram/microgram). To obtain this value, divide the Ab concentration in micrograms per milliliter by the F concentration in micrograms per milliliter.

12. Following the same reasoning as for point 4 above, Ab/F ratios may be expressed as molar ratios. After the weight ratio is calculated, it may be converted to a molar ratio by multiplying it by the factor 0.411. This is derived as in point 4 above (without the 10^{-3}).

Example

$$Ab/F(\text{gram/gram}) = 82,$$

$$\text{estimated molar } Ab/F = 82/411 = 0.20.$$

F. Fluorescein-Labeled, Affinity Chromatography Assay*

This FLAC assay (24) for determining antibody content of conjugate has two components: the assay of the concentration of F bound to antibody as micrograms Ab F per milliliters and the determination of the F/P ratio of the labeled antibody.

$$\mu\text{g Ab F/ml/weight F/P}$$

$$(\text{in } \mu\text{g/mg}) \text{ of Ab} = \text{mg Ab/ml}.$$

The methods for antihuman IgG conjugates are given here. Comparable methods can be used for conjugates with other specificities if suitable antigen preparations are obtained.

Preparation of Absorbent Beads for Fluorescein-Labeled Antibody Concentration Assay

Preparation of Adsorbent. Forty-two milliliters packed CM-BioGel-A (Bio-Rad Laboratories, Richmond, CA) is covalently coupled with 737 mg of human fraction II according to the manufacturer's instructions. Briefly, after washing and equilibration in coupler buffer (PBS: 3.0 mM, pH 6.3), the gel is mixed for 30 minutes with 20 ml antigen solution (45 mg/ml in coupling buffer). Addition of 400 mg 1-ethyl-3-(3-diamethylaminopropyl) carbodiimide (EDAC) with constant adjustment of pH to 6.3 for 1 hour, followed by gentle overnight stirring, resulted in 98% coupling efficiency. The adsorbent is distributed into 1.5 ml polyethylene conical bottom microcentrifuge tubes at 0.3 ml packed gel per tube.

Determination of Antibody F/P Ratios

F/P Ratio Determination. Human Cohn fraction II (Miles Laboratories, Inc., Elkhart, IN) covalently coupled to agarose gel at 15 mg/ml packed gel and poured into Pasteur pipettes (2 ml packed gel each) serves as the ligand in a microscale affinity chromatography purification of conjugates. To each column 1.5 ml of conjugate is applied, followed by a wash with 5 ml of 1.4 M NaCl in PBS (0.01 M phosphate, 0.15 M NaCl; pH, 7.2). The bound antibody is eluted with 5 ml of 3 M NaSCN in PBS. The eluates are dialyzed for 24 hours in 4 liters of PBS (four changes), and are analyzed for F and P, using standard methods (31) for Ab F/P ratio determinations.

FLAC Assay of Fluorescein-Labeled Antibody Concentration

Conjugate Ab Assay. Figure 2 schematically outlines the method of Ab determination. The conjugate to be assayed is applied to adsorbent gel contained both in a Pasteur pipette column, as described above, and in microcentrifuge tubes (1.5 ml of conjugate in the former instance, and 0.2 ml of undiluted and 1:2 and 1:4 diluted samples in the latter). The pipette column-purified material, eluted from the beads as described above, affords a measure of the Ab F/P ratio. Adsorption of the specific Ab in the microcentrifuge tubes occurs over a period of 3 hours at room temperature with constant agitation. Examination of the supernatants by a capillary tube precipitation test for residual Ab indicates complete adsorption under these conditions. Washing the contents of each tube with 4 ml PBS removes unbound material. Overnight agitation at room temperature with 1 N NaOH (1.2 ml per tube) results in complete extraction of the bound F from the adsorbent, as revealed by nonfluorescence of the beads by UV microscopy. The supernatant extracts are assayed for F by the NCCLS-recommended method of McKinney et al. (31). The F content of each tube, when divided by the Ab F/P ratio, provides a measure of AbP per added volume of conjugate and, therefore, of AbP/ml.

*This section is adapted from the report of Huang, et al. (24) with permission of the N.Y. Acad. Sci.

G. Tests for Antiepithelial Antibodies

The antibodies to the intercellular (IC) areas of the skin and other stratified epithelia that cause pemphigus and the antibodies to the BMZ associated with various forms of pemphigoid are of critical importance in the diagnoses of these diseases.

Titers of IC antibodies are also of prognostic importance in proven cases of pemphigus. As indicated in Chapter 8, titers should be determined every 2 to 3 weeks until the disappearance of the pemphigus antibodies. Thereafter, serum studies may be repeated every 6 to 8 weeks until treatment is completed.

As indicated in the "Introduction" section of this chapter, such serum studies should be carried out by services that can perform these tests on a daily basis, not only because of the high costs of antigenic substrate, but because of the experience and resources needed to achieve and maintain reliable test procedures.

Monkey and Guinea Pig Esophagus Antigen

These are the recommended substrates. Sections should be prepared and used within 10 days to 2 weeks after sacrifice and quick freezing. Tissue and sections need to be stored at −70 to −80°C. Not all specimens are satisfactory. If the positive control sera fail to give the expected reactions, then another piece of fresh esophagus must be used. A suitable alternative to monkey esophagus is monkey tongue. Monkey lip can also be used, but it is generally less satisfactory because the amount of mucosa is often inadequate. In some studies, human esophagus has been used successfully, but many autopsy specimens must be tested to find a reactive one. Technically, this is not feasible for a routine service. Guinea pig alone can yield misleading results (47). It should be used together with monkey esophagus on the same slide. (See Chap. 9 Addendum.)

Sections of monkey esophagus should be cut at 4 μm for optimal sensitivity.

Positive Control Sera

Such sera, needed for each experiment, serve as a check on the titer and intensity of IC and BMZ staining. These control sera should be checked in other laboratories that perform such studies routinely to be sure that the expected sensitivity of reactions is obtained. Reference sera that have been checked in multiple laboratories are available through the ISIL.* To cut down on the number of control slides needed for each experiment, some laboratories that perform at least one experiment per day include only a standard IC antibody control serum, rather than both the IC and BMZ antibodies. Standard negative controls must be included with each experiment.

Other positive controls include the blood group antibodies needed for standard absorption studies and repeat test titrations of previous sera of pemphigus patients who are retested for a rise or fall in titers (see next page, "Standard protocol for screening").

Conjugate

This should be unabsorbed, antiwhole human IgG reagents with Ab/P ratios ≥ 0.1, molar F/P ratios ranging from 1.8 to 4.5, and dilutions containing about 25 to 50 μg Ab/ml. A preliminary chessboard titration based on antibody contents of the conjugate is advised before any conjugate is used for general screening of sera.

The actual dilutions of a conjugate with a selected specificity should be based on one or more of the following factors: 1) the antibody protein concentration, 2) the antibody unitage, and 3) the behavior of the conjugate in a chessboard titration. For conjugates

*International Service for Immunology Laboratories, 219 Sherman Hall, University of Buffalo, SUNY Medical School, Buffalo, NY 14214

recently purchased from a manufacturer, items 1 and 3 are recommended. If results are in doubt, items 2 and 3 may be recommended.

The following procedure may be used for calculating dilution steps required to obtain a desired Ab concentration from a conjugate with any given antibody concentration.

1. If μg Ab/ml is known:

$$\frac{\text{desired } \mu\text{g Ab/ml}}{\text{initial } \mu\text{g Ab/ml}}$$

$$= \frac{1}{x} = \text{dilution factor}$$

Proportion to use:

1 part conjugate + $(x - 1)$ parts diluent

Example:

$$\frac{\text{desired } 50\ \mu\text{g Ab/ml}}{\text{initial } 1200\ \mu\text{g Ab/ml}} = \frac{1}{24}$$

Proportions to use:

1 part conjugate + 23 parts diluent
Volume to use for 40 slide tests: about 4 ml
(Use about 0.1 conjugate dilution/slide)
0.2 ml conjugate + 4.6 ml diluent

2. If unitage is known:

$$\frac{\text{desired U/ml}}{\text{initial U/ml}}$$

$$= \frac{1}{x} = \text{dilution factor}$$

Example:

$$\frac{\text{desired } 1/4 \text{ U/ml}}{\text{initial } 4 \text{ U/ml}} = \frac{1}{16}$$

Proportions to use:

1 part conjugate + 15 parts diluent
Volume to use for 40 slide tests: about 4 ml
(Use about 0.1 ml conjugate dilution/slide)
0.3 ml conjugate + 4.2 ml diluent

Standard Protocols for Screening

These include the usual negative conjugate and serum controls and the positive control, which serves as a working standard for primary screening. Further controls are added as indicated in the following protocol.

PROTOCOL FOR PRIMARY SCREENING FOR EPITHELIAL ANTIBODIES

Slide no.	*Reagents tested* — *Sera*	*Dilutions*	IC *stain*	*BMZ stain*	*Interpretations and indications*
1	Buffered saline	–	–	–	Negative controls
2	Normal serum	1:10	–	–	acceptable.
3	IC control serum	1:10	+++	–	Expected titer is 80–160.
4		1:20	++	–	Thus, this
5		1:40	+	–	positive control
6		1:80	+	–	is acceptable.
7		1:160	±	–	
8	Patient 1 serum	1:10	weak	–	Pemphigus-like
9		1:20	±	–	antibodies are
10		1:40	Weak	–	suspected. Check
11		1:80	Weak	–	with biopsy (see
12		1:160	±	–	Chap. 8).
13	Patient 2 serum	1:10	–	+	Suggestive of
14		1:20	–	±	pemphigoid. Check
15		1:40	–	–	skin biopsy specimen if

Slide no.	Reagents tested: Sera	Reagents tested: Dilutions	IC stain	BMZ stain	Interpretations and indications
16		1:80	−	−	possible.
17		1:160	−	−	
18	Patient 3 serum	1:10	−	++	Consistent with a
19		1:20	−	++	diagnosis of
20		1:40	−	+	pemphigoid.
21		1:80	−	−	
22		1:160	−	−	
23	Patient 4 (first	1:10	+++	−	Suggestive of
24	serum of patient)	1:20	+++	−	pemphigus. Do
25		1:40	++	−	blood group antigen
26		1:80	++	−	absorption. Get
27		1:160	+	−	endpoint (see next section).

If the negative controls (slides 1 and 2) and positive controls (slides 3 to 7) yield the expected results, the test is acceptable. The normal serum (slide 2) then serves as a control for comparisons with 1:10 and 1:20 dilutions, while the buffered saline (slide 1) is compared with patient sera diluted to 1:40 or greater.

The weak to ± reactions of the serum of patient 1 are typical of pemphigus-like antibodies. To check on this, a biopsy specimen of the edge of a fresh lesion should be examined for IC deposits of IgG. The serum of patient 2 yielded a weak basement membrane reaction suggestive of pemphigoid and serum 3 yielded a stronger one, as indicated in the above protocol. Skin biopsy specimen confirmation is helpful, particularly for weak, doubtful reactions.

Patient 4, whose serum was tested here for the first time, gave an IC reaction highly suggestive of pemphigus. To minimize the chances of error, this serum should be absorbed with blood group antigen, as indicated in the following section.

Absorption with Blood Group Antigens

This absorption serves to differentiate between the IC staining of the epithelium caused by true pemphigus antibodies and by antibodies to the so-called blood group A and/or B antigens. These stain blood vessels as well as the IC areas.

Preparation of Horse Stomach Absorption

Absorption with red blood cells of groups A and B does not, however, remove these antibodies in all cases. On the other hand, absorption with horse stomach homogenates does remove both the reactivity with the blood vessels and some pemphigus-like antibodies. The procedure for preparing the horse stomach homogenate is as follows: 1) wash out contents of stomach by rinsing in PBS, 2) open stomach and strip the inner mucosal lining from the rest of the stomach, 3) mince the mucosa with scissors into small pieces and place in preweighed beaker, 4) weigh the mucosa and add to it two times that volume of PBS, 5) process in a blender until a homogeneous suspension is formed, 6) pass homogenate through cheesecloth in order to remove large pieces of tissue, and 7) Store aliquots of filtered suspension in freezer until needed, marking each aliquot with date of preparation.

To check on the test system, a serum with a high titer of blood group B antibodies that give a ++ to +++ staining reaction of the IC areas of the epithelium is selected as a positive control (see slides 3 to 6 in the following protocol). This serum, when absorbed with the above-mentioned blood group B antigen, should give essentially a negative reaction (slides 7 to 10 in the following protocol).

PROTOCOL FOR DIFFERENTIATION BETWEEN BLOOD GROUP ANTIBODIES AND PEMPHIGUS ANTIBODIES BY ABSORPTION

Slide no.	*Reagents tested*		*IC stain*	*BMZ stain*	*Interpretation and indications*
	Sera	*Dilutions*			
1	Buffered saline	–	–	–	Negative controls
2	Normal serum	1:10	–	–	acceptable.
3	Blood group B	1:10	+++	–	Expected reaction of
4	control serum	1:20	++	–	blood group B
5		1:40	+	–	antibodies (blood
6		1:80	–	–	vessels also stain
					on slides 3 & 4).
7	Absorbed[a] blood	1:10	±	–	Expected absorption
	group B control	1:20	±	–	of blood group B
8	serum	1:40	–	–	antibodies.
9		1:80	–	–	Absorbent is
10					acceptable.
11	Patient 4	1:10	+++	–	Endpoint of IC stain-
12		1:80	++	–	ing is 320.
13		1:160	+	–	
14		1:320	+	–	
15		1:640	–	–	
16	Absorbed patient	1:10	+++	–	Absorption fails to
17	4 serum	1:80	++	–	remove IC staining.
18		1:160	+	–	Consistent with
19		1:320	+	–	diagnosis of
20		1:640	–	–	pemphigus.

If the expected results are obtained as in the above protocol, then the absorption studies with the patient serum are acceptable. As indicated in the protocol, both the unabsorbed and the absorbed serum of patient 4 had a titer of IC antibodies of 320. This may be regarded as consistent with a diagnosis of pemphigus.

The blood group antibody and absorption controls must be carried out with each absorption test of a patient serum. Blood group antibodies also stain the capillaries in the musculature of the esophagus sections. However, this alone is not a reliable criterion, since weak blood group antibody reactions occur only in the IC areas of the epithelium.

Follow-up Studies on Sera of Pamphigus Patients

Such studies are needed to detect changes in titer of IC antibodies. Since titers on a single serum may vary by one (and occasionally by two) dilutions between two experiments, new sera should be tested, together with the preceding sera of the same patients that were tested before. Thus, sera of new cases that have been checked by absorption with blood group antigen (as indicated in the preceding section), as well as sera sent for follow-up studies, need to be stored at −70°C for at least 6 months.

The following protocol affords an example of a comparison of findings obtained with the first and second serum of a pemphigus patient. Since follow-up studies are usually carried out, together with primary screening for epithelial antibodies in a routine service, the standard negative and positive controls are listed as for the first protocol.

PROTOCOL FOR FOLLOW-UP STUDIES ON SERA OF A PEMPHIGUS PATIENT

Slide no.	*Reagents tested*		*IC stain*	*BMZ stain*	*Interpretations and indications*
	Sera	*Dilutions*			
1	Buffered saline	–	–	–	Negative controls
2	Normal serum	1:10	–	–	are acceptable.
3–7	IC control serum	1:10–	+++	–	(As for first proto
		1:160	±	–	col) acceptable.
8	Patient 4 (first	1:80	++	–	Titer of 320 repro-
9	serum	1:160	+	–	duced; acceptable test.
10		1:320	+	–	
11		1:640	–	–	
12	Patient 4 (second	1:40	++	–	Titer of 80. Signi-
13	serum)	1:80	+	–	ficant drop in titer.
14		1:160	–	–	
15		1:320	–	–	
16		1:640	–	–	

The dilutions of the first serum of the patient that were retested were selected to include not only the endpoint of 320, but also one dilution beyond (1:640) and two before (1:80 and 1:160). The second, or follow-up, serum is tested at the same dilutions, as well as one more below. Readings are best made by comparing comparable dilutions of the two sera to verify changes in pemphigus antibody activity. In the example given in the protocol, the tests revealed a drop in titer of 2 doubling dilutions.

A change of one doubling dilution in follow-up studies of a pemphigus patient is regarded as being of marginal or doubtful significance. A change of two or more doubling dilutions is significant if the above protocol, with repeat testing, is used. Since follow-up studies are done on patients under treatment, a significant rise in titer is rarely encountered. Thus, the protocol is designed to detect primarily a fall in titer.

Tests for the Herpes Gestationis (HG) Factor

These are indicated in suspected cases of herpes gestationis (HG), and entail an indirect complement immunofluorescence test of patients' sera. The reactants include:

1. The BMZ antigen of human skin, monkey esophagus, and monkey lip. Both human skin and monkey esophagus are used as antigenic substrate for the detection of the HG factor. Also Verrando, et al. (47a) report that human uterus is the substrate of choice.

2. Patients' sera with complement-fixing BMZ antibodies; that is, HG factor. This serves as a positive control serum.

3. Human complement in the form of a fresh normal serum diluted in a tris buffer with added Ca^{2+} and Mg^{2+} (each at 0.0025 M). Normal serum separated, aliquoted, frozen in less than 2 hours after collection, and diluted 1:10 immediately before use may

be employed for this purpose. Each batch of frozen aliquots must be checked with a known positive control serum before use in tests for the HG factor.

4. Conjugated anti-C3 or anti-C4 may be used, but anti-C3 reagents are more sensitive indicators. Either a high or medium F/P ratio conjugate can be used, although the latter affords a somewhat lower sensitivity than the above-described indirect test for BMZ antibodies; it gives somewhat less NSS of the stratum granulosum (and it can also be used for biopsy specimen studies). Anti-C3 conjugates can be assayed for their unitage with a 1:1 dilution of normal serum, and should be diluted to 1/4 U/ml for the HG factor assay. Standard PBS washings follow treatment with each of the reagents (2, 3, and 4).

PROTOCOL FOR HG FACTOR ASSAY ON MONKEY LIP BY INDIRECT COMPLEMENT IMMUNOFLUORESCENCE

Slide no.	*Reagents tested*[a] *Sera*	*Dilutions*	*Complement*[b]	*BMZ stain*	*Interpretations and indications*
1	Tris buffer	–	–	–	Negative controls
2		–	×	–	acceptable.
3	HG control serum	1:1	–	±[c]	
4		1:4	–	±	
5	HG control serum	1:4	×	+++	HG factor control,
6		1:8	×	++	expected titer 32.
7		1:16	×	++	Thus, this positive
8		1:32	×	+	control is
9		1:64	×	–	acceptable.
10	Patient 1 serum	1:1	×	–	Patient 1 serum is
11		1:4	×	–	negative.
12		1:8	×	–	
13		1:16	×	–	
14	Patient 2 serum	1:1	×	+++	Patient 2 serum has
15		1:4	×	++	an HG factor titer
16		1:8	×	+	of 8.
17		1:16	×	–	

[a]All sera including the HG control are heat activated at 56°C for 30 minutes and diluted in Tris buffer with Ca^{2+} and Mg^{2+} added.
[b]Complement is fresh normal serum diluted in the same diluent immediately before use in the same buffer (x, complement).
[c]This control may give a weak reaction.

REFERENCES

1. Bergquist NR, Norberg R: Determination of specific antibody content of fluorescein conjugates by radioimmunoabsorption. *J Immunol Methods* 5:275–282, 1974.
2. Beutner EH (Ed): Defined immunofluorescent staining. *Ann NY Acad Sci* 177, 1971, 529 pp.
3. Beutner EH: Defined immunofluorescence staining: Past progress, present status and future prospects for defined conjugates. In Beutner EH (Ed): Defined Immunofluorescent Staining. *Ann NY Acad Sci* 177:506–526, 1971.
4. Beutner EH, Binder WL, Kumar V: State of the art of immunofluorescence techniques in

tissues. In Keitges PW, Nakamura RM (Eds): *Diagnostic Immunology: Current and Future Trends.* College of the American Pathologists, Skokie, IL, 1980, pp. 89–99.

5. Beutner EH, Deng J-S, Shu S, et al: Studies on defined immunofluorescence in clinical immunopathology. 3. Past progress, some new methods and prospects for the future. *Ann NY Acad Sci* 254:573–591, 1975.
6. Beutner EH, Holborow EJ, Johnson GD: Quantitative studies of immunofluorescent staining. I. Analysis of mixed immunofluorescence. *Immunology* 12:327–337, 1967.
7. Beutner EH, Krasny S, Kumar V, et al: Prospects and problems in the definition and standardization of immunofluorescence. I. Present levels of reproducibility and disease specificity of antinuclear antibody tests. In Beutner EH, Nisengard RJ, Albini A (Eds): Defined Immunofluorescence and Related Chemical Methods. *Ann NY Acad Sci* 420:28–54, 1983.
8. Beutner EH, Nisengard RJ, Kumar V: Defined immunofluorescence: Basic concepts and their application to clinical immunodermatology. In Beutner EH, Chorzelski TP, Bean SF (Eds): *Immunopathology of the Skin,* ed. 2. Wiley, New York, 1979, pp. 29–75.
9. Beutner EH, Wick G, Sepulveda M, et al: A reverse immunodiffusion assay for antibody protein concentration in antisera or conjugates to human IgG. In Holborow EJ (Ed): *Standardization in Immunofluorescence.* Blackwell, Oxford, UK, 1970, pp. 165–169.
10. Chantler S, Batty I: Quality control of fluorescein isothiocyanate-labeled reagents. In Beutner EH, Nisengard J, Albini B (Eds): Defined Immunofluorescence and Related Cytochemical Methods. *Ann NY Acad Sci* 420:68–73, 1983.
11. Coons AH, Kaplan MH: Localization of antigen in tissue cells. II. Improvements in a method for detection of antigen by means of fluorescent antibody. *J Exp Med* 91:1, 1950.
12. Couser WG, Lewis EJ: Laboratory suggestion. A method for preservation of immunofluorescence in renal tissue. *Am J Clin Pathol* 6:873, 1974.
13. Cuatrecasas P: Protein purification by affinity chromatography. Derivitization of agarose and polyacrylamide beads. *J Biol Chem* 245:3059, 1970.
14. Deacon WE, Lucas JB, Price EV: Fluorescence treponemal antibody absorption (FTS-ABS) test for syphilis. *JAMA* 198:624, 1966.
15. Giloh H, Sedat JW: Fluorescence microscopy: Reduced photobleaching of rhodamine and fluorescein protein conjugates by n-propyl gallate. *Science* 217:1252–1255, 1982.
16. Goldman M: *Fluorescent Antibody Methods.* Academic Press, New York, 1968, 303 pp.
17. Gornall A, Bardawill C, David M: Determination of serum proteins by means of the biuret reactions. *J Biol Chem* 177:751, 1949.
18. Haiijman JJ: *Quantitative Immunofluorescence Microscopy: Methods and Application.* Publ. Inst Exp Gerontology Rijswijk Netherlands, 1977.
19. Hebert GA, Pittman B, McKinney RM, et al: The preparation and physicochemical characterization of fluorescent antibody reagents. US Dept of Health, Education and Welfare, Center for Disease Control, Atlanta. 1972.
20. Heidelberger M: Recognition of antibodies as labeled globulins. In Beutner EH, Nisengard RJ, Albini B (Eds): Defined Immunofluorescence and Related Cytochemical Methods. *Ann NY Acad Sci* 420:1–4, 1983.
21. Hijmans W, Schaeffer M (Eds): Fifth international conference on immunofluorescence and related staining techniques. *Ann NY Acad Sci* vol. 254, 1975, 627 pp.
22. Holborow EJ (Ed): *Standardization in Immunofluorescence.* Blackwell, Oxford, UK, 1970, 282 pp.
23. Holborow EJ (Ed): Report by a subcommittee on the discussion of requirements for specification of antiimmunoglobulin conjugates that took place during the conference. In Holborow EJ (Ed): *Standardization in Immunofluorescence.* Blackwell, Oxford, UK, 1970, p 275.
24. Huang JG, Beutner EH, Kumar V: Prospects and problems in the definition and standardization of immunofluorescence. II. A quantitative assay for antibody protein of FITC-labeled anti-IgG conjugates. In Beutner EH, Nisengard RJ, Albini B (Eds): Defined Immunofluorescence and Related Cytochemical Methods. *Ann NY Acad Sci* 420:55–61, 1983.
25. Johnson GD, Davidson RS, McNameeke G, et al: Fading of immunofluorescence during microscopy. A study of the phenomenon and its remedy. *J Immunol Methods* 55:231–242, 1982.

26. Kaplan DS, Picciolo GL: IF standardization by quantitative microfluorometry. II. Reduction in fading by reducing agents. *Immunol Commun* 12:107, 1983 (abstract).
27. Kawamura A: *Fluorescent Antibody Techniques and Their Application.* University Park Press, Baltimore, 1969, 203 pp.
28. Kawamura A: *Fluorescent Antibody Techniques and Their Application,* ed. 2. University of Tokyo Press, Tokyo, 1977, 292 pp.
29. Knapp W, Holubar K, Wick G (Eds): Immunofluorescence and Related Staining Techniques. Elsevier/North Holland, Amsterdam, 1978, 363 pp.
30. Marshall JD, Eveland WC, Smith CW: Superiority of fluorescein isothiocyanate (Riggs) for fluorescent antibody technic with a modification of its application. *Proc Soc Exp Biol Med* 98:898, 1958.
31. McKinney RM, Pearce GW, Spillane JT: Fluorescein diacetate as a reference color standard in fluorescent antibody studies. *Anal Biochem* 9:474–476, 1964.
32. Michel B, Milner Y, David K: Preservation of tissue fixed immunoglobulins in skin biopsies of patients with lupus erythematosus and bullous diseases. *J Invest Dermatol* 59:449–452, 1973.
33. Nairn RC: *Fluorescent Protein Tracing,* ed. 1. Williams and Wilkins Co., Baltimore, 1962, 280 pp.
34. Nairn RC: *Fluorescent Protein Tracing,* ed. 2. Williams & Wilkins, Baltimore, 1964, 335 pp.
35. Nairn RC: *Fluorescent Protein Tracing,* ed. 3 Williams & Wilkins, Baltimore, 1969, 503 pp.
36. Nairn RC: *Fluorescent Protein Tracing,* ed. 4. Churchill Livingstone, New York, 1976, 648 pp.
37. National Committee for Clinical Laboratory Standards: *Determinants of Fluorescein/Protein Ratios in Flourescein Isothiocyanate Labeled Protein.* August 1975. Villanova, Pa.
38. Niedecken HW, Lange CE: Simplified fixative medium for direct immunofluorescence in skin biopsies. *J Am Acad Dermatol* 12:828–831, 1985.
39. Nisengard R, Beutner EH. Quantitative studies of immunofluorescence staining. 4. Nonspecific staining by free fluorescein and labelled protein. *Int Arch Allergy Appl Immunol* 43:383–389, 1972.
40. Ploem J: A study of filters and light sources in immunofluorescence microscopy. *Ann NY Acad Sci* 177:414–429, 1971.
41. Ploem J: Immunofluorescence microscopy. In Beutner EH, Chorzelski TP, Bean SF, et al (Eds): *Immunopathology of the Skin,* ed. 1. Dowden, Hutchinson and Ross, Stroudsburg, PA, 1973, 248–270.
42. Rodriquez J, Deinhardt F: Preparation of a semi-permanent mounting medium for fluorescent antibody studies. *Virology* 12:316–317 1960.
43. Schauenstein K, Bock G, Wick G: Factors influencing fluorescence properties of free and protein-bound fluorochromes macro- and microfluorometric observations. In Knapp W, Holubar K, Wick G: *Immunofluorescence and Related Staining Techniques.* Elsevier/North Holland, Amsterdam, 1978, pp. 81–95.
44. Schauenstein K, Bock G, Wick G: The use of lasers to determine the fluorescence characteristics of fluorescein derivatives. In Wick G, Traukk KN, Schauenstein K (Eds): *Immunofluorescence Technology—Selected Theoretical and Clinical Aspects.* Elsevier, New York, 1982, p 27.
45. Skeete MVH, Black MM: The evaluation of a special liquid fixative for direct immunofluorescence. *Clin Exp Dermatol* 2:49–56, 1977.
46. Thomson LA, Hageage GJ: Evaluation of excitation light sources for incident immunofluorescence microscopy. *App Microbiol* 30:616–624, 1975.
47. Ullman S, Harberg P, Nielsen R: Anti-basement membrane antibodies in sera from patients without bullous pemphigoid. *Acta Dermatol* 55:305, 1975.
47a. Verrando P, Hsi B, Yeh GJ, et al. Herpes gestationis sera recognize the amniotic epithelial basement membrane. *J Invest Dermatol* 86:513, 1986 (abstract).
48. Weller TH, Coons AH: Fluorescent antibody studies with agents of varicella and herpes zoster propagated in vitro. *Proc Soc Exp Biol Med* 86:789, 1954.
49. Wells AF, Miller CE, Nadel MK: Rapid fluorescein and protein assay method for fluorescent antibody conjugates. *Appl Microbiol* 14:271–275, 1966.
50. Wick G, Baudner S, Herzog F: *Immunofluorescence.* Die Medizinische Verlagsgesellschaft, Marburg/Lahn, West Germany, 1978, 120 pp.

2 Standardization of Antinuclear Antibody and Other Immunofluorescent Tests Used in Immunopathologic Studies of the Skin

Ernst H. Beutner
Vijay Kumar
Susan A. Krasny
Tadeusz P. Chorzelski

INTRODUCTION

This chapter deals with the major factors in the standardization of immunologic tests used in the diagnosis of connective tissue and bullous diseases. We focus primarily on the antinuclear antibody (ANA) tests because other diagnostically relevant immunofluorescent (IF) and other immunologic tests have received less attention from the viewpoint of standardization. In effect, the data on the standardization of ANA tests provide a model for analyzing other relevant IF systems, such as the indirect IF (IIF) tests for the bullous diseases and the direct IF (DIF) studies of skin biopsy specimens. We need to consider the reason for this attention to the ANA and its nature before we can address the actual data on standardization. Since the methods of analysis reviewed in the sections on "Analysis of ANA Titer Reproducibility" and "Disease Specificity on ANA Tests on Different Substrates" are of interest to some but not all readers, this chapter provides an overview in the following sections: "Introduction," the subsection on "Conclusions Regarding Reproducibility of ANA Titrations," and the "Summary."

Use of trade names is for identification only and does not constitute endorsement by the Public Health Service, by the U.S. Department of Health and Human Services, or by the International Service for Immunology Laboratories.

Relevance of ANA in the Diagnosis of SLE

According to "The 1982 Revised Criteria for the Classification of Systemic Lupus Erythematosus" (19), one of the added criteria is the presence of "an abnormal titer of (ANA) . . . in the absence of . . . 'drug induced lupus' syndrome." According to this report by Tan et al., the fulfillment of 4 of the 11 revised American Rheumatism Association (ARA) criteria in a given patient is essentially diagnostic of systemic lupus erythematosus (SLE). As Manu pointed out (16), this means that all 11 criteria are equal; but after reanalyzing the data on the 11 criteria, he finds that "some are more equal than others." Specifically, according to their reanalysis (16) of the data of Tan et al. (19), the two highest levels of discrimination (i.e., relative sensitivity and specificity levels) in the diagnosis of SLE are achieved by tests; first for an "immunologic disorder," and second for ANA. Some of the tests for an immunologic disorder (which include the detection of either lupus erythematosus [LE] cells or antidouble [d] stranded DNA antibodies, or anti-Sm antibodies or biological false-positive tests for syphilis for 6 months or more) will be considered from the standpoint of standardization at the end of this chapter.

The relevant data (19) are as follows:

	Sensitivity	*Specificity*	*Discrimination*
Immunologic disorder	0.85	0.93	2.512
Antinuclear antibody	0.99	0.49	2.301
Other 9 criteria	from 0.18 to 0.86	from 0.37 to 0.99	from 0.748 to 1.927

where:

$$\text{sensitivity} = \frac{\text{true positive results}}{\text{total patients with the disease}}$$

$$\text{specificity} = \frac{\text{true negative results}}{\text{total patients without the disease.}}$$

The discrimination that is calculated from the sensitivity and specificity (17) is the highest for those criteria that are of the greatest value for differential diagnosis. In effect, the detection of an abnormal ANA titer is highly relevant in the diagnosis of SLE.

Clough et al. (12) reached a similar conclusion in a study comparing findings on 87 SLE cases to another "rheumatology control population" of 73 cases. According to their data on ANA, the sensitivity (0.99) and specificity (0.69) of this test is such that its absence constitutes a *negative* score. That is, a negative ANA is given a negative score of 1.8 if a positive score of 4 is needed to establish a diagnosis of SLE. Indeed, a negative ANA is commonly regarded as a basis for excluding a diagnosis of SLE, although it is obviously not always true; ANA-negative SLE cases do occur (see Chap. 33). As Levin et al. (15) indicate in their statistical comparison of the sensitivity of 1971 with 1982 ARA criteria for the classification of SLE, the increased sensitivity of the revised criteria is due to the immunologic tests that were added; that is, to the ANA, anti-dDNA and anti-Sm.

While the primary focus on the standardization of the ANA and other serologic tests used in the diagnosis of SLE seems to be well justified, the actual work that has been done in this area still leaves much to be desired, particularly from the viewpoint of dermatologists. (The reasons for this assessment are given below in the section on "Analysis of ANA Titer Reproducibility" and in Chap. 29.)

Role of ANA as a Trigger of the Autoimmune Repair Mechanism and as a Diagnostic Sign of SLE

ANA occur, at least in most and probably in all, normal adult sera (see Chap. 7 for some background on this point). For example, a single commercially available ANA test kit using KB cells (see section below on "Disease Specificity of ANA Tests on Different Substrates") in tests of normal human sera, starting at a 1:10 dilution, and an antihuman IgG conjugate revealed ANA in 62 of 91 (68%) of the sera tested in titers of 10 to 40. There is little doubt that at least some of the 29 "negatives" would yield ANA titers in the range of 1 to 5, particularly if the conjugate used is polyvalent and if multiple substrates are employed. Such tests, however, were not done because this is out of the diagnostically relevant range of studies.

Since ANA occurs at least in most and probably all, normal adult sera, we need to ask what their function is. While there are no systematic studies of this basic biological question, there is one set of general and one set of specific observations that afford useful clues.

In general, physiologic autoantibodies have the following properties: 1) they usually occur in all normal adult sera; 2) they fail to bind in vivo to their producers' homologous antigens in normal unaltered tissue; and 3) they do bind to their homologous antigens in altered, or injured, or dead tissue of the autoantibody producer in vivo. The function of physiologic autoantibodies with these properties appears, as indicated in Chap. 7, to be the triggering of autoimmune repair mechanisms or "ARM cascades." That is, such antibodies appear to aid in the removal of damage tissue components.

Specifically, most but not all ANA appear to fulfill each of the above-listed criteria for physiologic autoantibodies. That is: 1) They occur in normal sera as described above. 2) Most, but not all, ANA fail to bind to normal nuclei in vivo or in tissue culture. Among the exceptions are the ANA in mixed connective tissue disease (MCTD) that seem to bind in vivo and in tissue culture (see Chap. 7 for review). 3) In lesional skin, binding of immunoglobulin (usually IgG and/or IgM) to epidermal nuclei is seen at times. Considering the essentially universal occurrence of ANA, this can best be explained by the in vivo binding of ANA to its producers' epidermal nuclei in areas of cellular injury or death. These observations indicate that most ANA probably serve to trigger ARM cascades. Systematic studies of these observations and interpretations are clearly needed.

In a study using commercial mouse kidney sections, five selected normal sera were tested for ANA with specificities for IgG, IgA, and IgM class antibodies. Four of the five sera had predominantly IgM class ANA, and one was predominantly IgG class. Only one of the five ANA was exclusively of the IgM class. In the same study, 10 of 10 ANA in SLE sera were predominantly of the IgG class. In the test system used, the ANA of the selected normal sera ranged from 5 to 40, whereas the selected SLE sera had ANA titers of 160 or more.

Obviously, in the diagnostic use of ANA tests, the conditions employed in the test system must be adjusted to achieve maximum sensitivity and specificity. For example, as per the above-mentioned study of 5 normal and 10 SLE sera, conjugated antibodies that detect IgM need to be minimized or eliminated. The exact conditions needed to achieve optimal sensitivity and specificity vary from one test system to another. Precise definition of each component of the test system (i.e., substrate, conjugate, and controls [2,7]) is needed to attain both optimal conditions and reproducibility.

ANALYSIS OF ANA TITER REPRODUCIBILITY

Established statistical methods for the evaluation of the reproducibility of serologic and other clinical laboratory tests (22) were applied to the indirect IF titrations of ANA by Taylor and Fulford of the Centers for Disease Control (CDC) in 1980 (21). The methods entail the following calculations:

$$\overline{X}_G = \text{geometric mean} \qquad \log \overline{X}_G = \frac{\log x}{n}$$

$$S_G = \text{geometric standard deviation} \log S_G = \sqrt{\frac{(\log x - \log \overline{X}_G)^2}{n-1}}$$

$$\text{Variance} = (\log_2 S_G)^2 = \left(\frac{\log_{10} S_G}{\log_{10^2}}\right)^2$$

where: x = titer
n = number of titrations.

The $\overline{X}_G$ and S_G values afford objective modes for expressing the reproducibility of ANA titers. Twofold dilutions used in titrations constitute $\log_2$ increments. Thus, the above-listed "variance" affords a useful mode of expression for variability.

The traditional assumption of serologists—that titer differences of two doubling dilutions are significant—must be checked by such objective criteria as pointed out by Taylor (20).

In reality, in some laboratory studies, a single doubling dilution difference may be significant, while in others, differences of two doubling dilutions may be nonsignificant. To assess precision objectively, multiple replicate-coded samples need to be tested by a laboratory in a double-blind format. The calculated S_G values afford a measure of the intralaboratory precision. A simplified version of the probability table developed by Taylor for assessing probabilities from S_G values (20) and revised by him in this chapter is given in Table 1.

Intralaboratory Reproducibility of ANA Titers

Data on intralaboratory precision based on the average S_G values obtained by selected laboratories in three diagnostically important IIF tests (23) are as follows:

1. ANA: $S_G = 1.72$.
2. Herpes simplex virus: $S_G = 1.880$.
3. Cytomegalovirus: $S_G = 2.152$.

As may be seen from the data listed in Table 1, these mean intralaboratory precision values indicate the following:

1. ANA: a confidence level of about $p < 0.01$ may be ascribed to an eightfold titer difference on the average.
2. Herpes simplex virus antibodies: an eightfold titer difference is significant at a confidence level of $p < 0.05$ on the average.

Table 1. Ratio of Results Between Two Serologic Test Results Required for Statistical Significance with Selected S_G[a] Values for Intralaboratory Precision

Selected S_G values (precision)	*Ratios of results required for significant differences*			*Variances for S_G values*
	$p < 0.05$[b]	*$p < 0.01$*	*$p < 0.001$*	
1.160			twofold	0.046
1.210		twofold		0.076
1.284	twofold[c]			0.130
1.346			fourfold	0.184
1.464		fourfold		0.303
1.561			eightfold	0.413
1.649	fourfold			0.521
1.772		eightfold		0.681
2.117	eightfold			1.171

Modified from Taylor (20).

[a]S_G, Standard deviation of geometric mean titers.

[b]$p < 0.05$, Probability of random sampling errors is less than 0.05.

[c]Twofold differences between titers. For example, if replicate tests of a serum yield the S_G value of 1.40 (i.e., a value less than 1.464), then a fourfold titer difference (e.g., 40 vs. 160) is significant at a confidence level of $p < 0.01$, but not at a level of $p < 0.001$.

3. Cytomegalovirus antibodies: an eightfold titer difference is, on the average, almost but not quite significant at the $p \sim 0.05$ level.

The limitations on the ANA data are that these values are for:

1. Multiple reference laboratories (some have lower S_G values than others, as seen below),
2. Multiple manufacturers of ANA kits (some have lower S_G values than others),
3. Intralaboratory, not interlaboratory, precision (the interlaboratory precision level is much lower).

Point 1 above, regarding the intralaboratory precision, is illustrated by a double-blind study undertaken by the principal author's laboratory (5) in cooperation with the CDC under the following conditions. A total of 20 S_G values were determined with four replicate-coded samples of five reference sera tested on each of four antigenic substrates; that is, human cells, mouse fibroblasts, mouse kidney, and mouse liver. The 20 S_G values (determined at the CDC) were: 4 at 1.000, 7 at 1.414, 6 at 1.492, 2 at 1.761, and 1 at 1.942; the mean S_G value was 1.416. Consequently, a fourfold titer change between paired samples was deemed to be statistically significant at the 99% confidence level. Since this S_G value of 1.416 compares favorably with the mean S_G value of 1.72 for ANA tests reported by Taylor (23) (see beginning of this section), this indicates that some laboratories have higher S_G values than others.

The sources of ANA test systems appear to be a contributing factor to the high S_G values for intralaboratory precision observed in some test systems. The S_G values for eight identified major ANA kit manufacturers were 1.36, 1.47, 1.51, 1.54, 1.55, 1.57, 1.60, and 1.83. In contrast, the intralaboratory precision S_G values for noncommercial ANA test systems was 1.98; and for other minor commercial kits, the S_G was 2.14. In effect, the intralaboratory reproducibility achieved with the major commercial kits was consistently better than that attained with noncommercial kits, or with the less commonly used kits. Of the total of 313 laboratories that participated in this CDC study (21), 233 used one of the eight major ANA kits, 60 used noncommercial ANA tests, and 20 used less common ANA kits. Of the 313 laboratories that participated, 301 did replicate tests permitting evaluation of intralaboratory variances.

The reason for the above-listed range of S_G values from 1.36 to 1.83 for the intralaboratory variability of ANA titers is not clear (8). It seems clear, however, that manufacturers should attempt to determine what these values are for their ANA kits. And if the S_G is over 1.649 (as indicated in Table 1, this is the maximum S_G allowable to ascribe significance at a $p < 0.05$ level to two doubling dilutions difference in titers), the manufacturer should attempt to determine the reason for the high S_G value and attempt to remedy the problem. It is noteworthy in this connection that the manufacturer of the ANA test system that gave the above-listed value of $S_G = 1.83$ has withdrawn this ANA kit from the market, partly because of this problem of reproducibility.

Interlaboratory Reproducibility of ANA Titers

The comparisons of the interlaboratory with the intralaboratory precision in ANA titrations, depicted graphically in Figure 1, provides an overview of the relative reproducibility of ANA tests with kits from the eight manufacturers in the above-mentioned CDC study (2). For the kits that use cell culture preparations as antigens, a significant correlation appeared between the inter- and intralaboratory variances (5). This indicates that some factor(s) in the manufacture or use of the various kits employed played a role(s) in both the inter- and intralaboratory reproducibility attained. No correlation was found between the inter- and intralaboratory precision of ANA titers obtained with four kits that employ tissue sections (Fig. 1), apparently because there was little difference in the intralaboratory variances. However, marked (over threefold) differences in the interlaboratory variances were found. From this, it appears that manufacturers of ANA kits need to monitor not only the intralaboratory precision of their ANA kits as suggested above, but also the interlaboratory precision.

Figure 2 depicts graphically data (5) from the above-mentioned CDC study (21) on the frequency with which ANA titers were obtained with one "unknown" serum. This serum was examined as coded duplicates by the 233 laboratories that used one of four types of antigenic substrates from one of eight manufacturers, or by the laboratories that used noncommercial ANA test systems. This comparison of titer frequencies affords a graphic caricature of the effects of substrates on the detection of ANA. Obviously, this serum gave predominantly negative reactions on mouse fibroblasts, but significant ANA titers on the other three types of commercial ANA substrates; and, importantly, either negative findings or significant titers in noncommercial ANA test systems. Table 2 lists the key data on the five ANA test systems depicted in Figure 2. Note that while the S_G values of the four types of commercial ANA kits ranged from 2.39 to 3.63, the S_G value for noncommercial ANA test systems is 47.7. The corresponding range of variation in ANA titers—one S_G above or below the mean titer ($\overline{X}$)—is over 2000, as indicated in Table 2. Such a test system is obviously useless. Since most ANA do not give such a broad range of titer variation in different test systems, this may be regarded as a distortion or caricature. However, this is not uncommon, as indicated below in the section on "Disease Specificity of ANA Tests on Different Substrates." Thus, we must conclude that there is no such thing as an "ANA titer of a serum," but

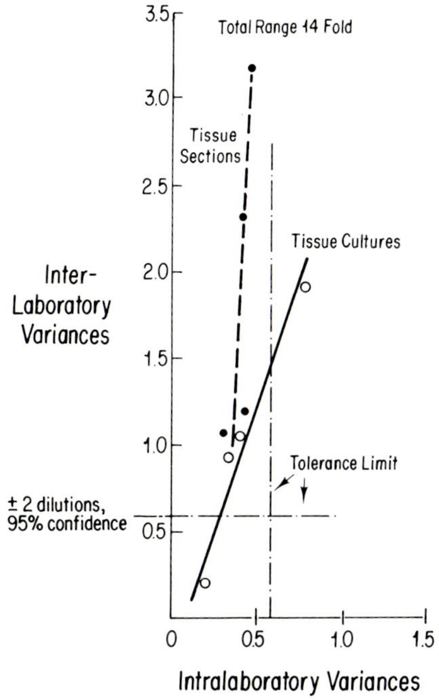

Figure 1. Comparisons of inter- and intralaboratory variances of ANA titers obtained with one reference serum in tests performed by 233 laboratories employing one of eight widely used commercial ANA kits: four with tissue sections and four with cell cultures. A significant correlation appeared between the inter- and intralaboratory variances with the four ANA kits that used cell culture preparations. The dotted lines signify the 95% ($p < 0.05$) confidence levels in the significance of fourfold (two doubling dilutions) differences in titers (see Table 1 for explanations). (This figure is a Modification [with permission from the New York Academy of Sciences] of Figure 1 in Beutner et al. [5].)

only an *ANA titer of a serum on a given substrate.* In effect, each test system must be evaluated separately.

The values for variances plotted in Figure 1 reveal that the intralaboratory precision of ANA tests with seven of eight commercial kits is within the tolerance limits of two doubling dilutions (fourfold) for a confidence level of $p < 0.05$ in the significance of titer differences. The kit that did not fall within these limits has been taken off the market. The precision of the interlaboratory variances did not allow for this level of confidence in this comparison. As may be seen by comparing Table 1 and Figure 1, most (five of eight) ANA kits yield interlaboratory variances that are close to or within a ± 3 doubling dilution (eightfold) range at a confidence level of 95% ($p < 0.05$).

The specific conclusions we may reach from the data in Figure 2 are as follows:

1. Commercial ANA kits yield greater precision in ANA titrations; that is, titers are more reproducible than noncommercial ANA test systems.
2. Each antigenic substrate differs in ANA sensitivity; thus, reports of ANA titers must designate the substrate used.
3. The current level of precision in ANA titrations of some commercial kits is in need of significant improvement to reach S_G levels at or below 2.117.

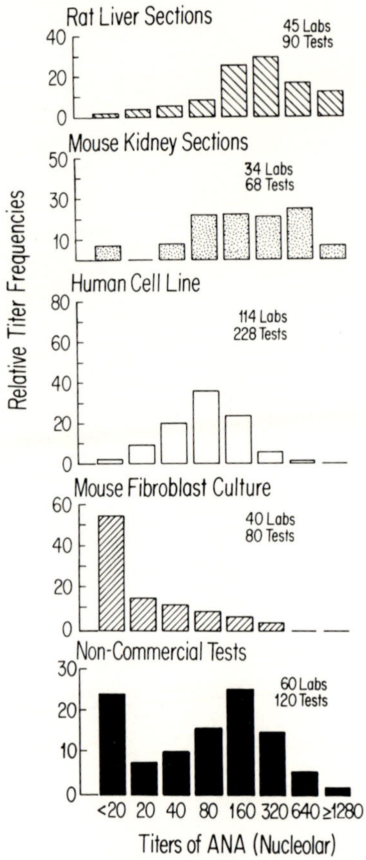

Figure 2. Frequency of ANA titers of one serum with nucleolar antibodies from a systemic sclerosis patient in tests on four types of antigenic substrates (commercial rat liver sections, mouse kidney sections, human cell cultures, and mouse fibroblast cultures) and noncommercial ANA test systems. Data on the significance of the differences observed are summarized in Table 2.

4. Two groups of factors need to be addressed to achieve improvement in the precision of titers achieved with ANA kits: The quality of kits and the reliability with which the test is performed. (The latter is dealt with in the next subsection.)

Programs for Improvement in the Precision of ANA Titrations

The "Performance Evaluation Program" of Behring Diagnostics* (9) serves as an example, in this chapter, of current efforts of the ANA kit industry to improve precision of ANA titrations (6). The findings in this program can be compared to the CDC study of 1980 (21), because the methods of analysis are the same (see preceding sections on "Analysis of ANA Titer Reproducibility" for formula for $\overline{X}$, S_G, and variance calculations, and also data in Table 1 for their use). This program entails quarterly mailings to participants of the following types of materials.

*Behring Diagnostics, 10933 N. Torrey Pines Rd, La Jolla, CA 92037.

Table 2. Analyses of Data on ANA Titer Frequencies Obtained with a Single Unknown Serum "N" by 305 Laboratories on Five Types of ANA Substrates[a]

Summary of data and their analyses	*Substrates for ANA tests*				
	Sections		*Cell cultures*		*Non-commercial ANA tests*
	Rat liver	*Mouse kidney*	*Human cells*	*Mouse fibroblasts*	
No. of manufacturers	3.0	1.0	3.0	1.0	60.0
No of labs using substrates	45.0	34.0	114.0	40.0	60.0
No. of titrations of serum N	90.0	68.0	228.0	80.0	120.0
Geometric mean ANA titers ($\bar{X}$)	254.0	180.8	76.4	14.5	86.7
Geometric standard deviation (S_G)	2.97	3.63	2.39	3.53	47.7
Titer range from $\bar{X} \times S_G$ to $\bar{X}/S_G$ expressed as *x*-fold	8.8×	13.2×	5.7×	12.5×	2275×

[a]See Figure 2 for graphs of titer frequencies.

1. Optical standard slides with microbeads of graded intensities of fluorescence, notably, 100%, 50%, 25%, 12.5%, 6.25%, 2%, and 0%. These slides provide a measure of the sensitivity of the fluorescence microscope; for example, in the studies of Molden et al. (17). This assumes importance because of the variations in light sources, filter systems, and optical systems employed.

2. Prestained multiple wells of slides using different sera or different serum dilutions for staining by IIF. This serves to evaluate the operators' capacity to distinguish positives from negatives, to identify the diverse ANA (and other antibody) patterns that may be encountered, and under some conditions to read endpoints of titrations correctly.

3. Unknown sera. These serve to evaluate the technician's ability to perform tests correctly.

Evaluation of participants' responses in these three parts of this performance evaluation program is based on a system that scores 50% for ANA patterns and 50% for ANA titers. The overall scores in five successive quarterly evaluation programs have shown some improvement (9). However, S_G values for ANA titers for all participants over this period were 2.19, 2.54, 2.05, 2.27, and 2.20. While the reproducibility for the whole group (71 to 124 of laboratories) has changed little and has stayed over the 2.028 level (see Table 1), some improvement is seen among "reference laboratories" that had performed well (≥90% scores) in previous performance evaluations. The S_G values for "reference laboratories" in four successive evaluations were 2.72, 1.58, 1.86, and 1.90. At least the latter three are within the tolerance range of 2.028 or less. Obviously, more improvement is needed in the future.

Conclusions Regarding the Reproducibility of ANA Titrations

The general conclusions that can be reached from the data reviewed in the preceding three subsections and that have been reached by others are as follows.

1. Reports on ANA titers without reference to the type of test system used or the manufacturer have limited significance, because the range of mean titers ($\overline{X}_G$) is great. Upon reviewing the data from the special study on ANA (21), Taylor et al. concluded that "It seems incredible that a physician could make much use of test data such as these when results depend on the test kit being used."

2. Commercial ANA kits afford some hope for attaining interlaboratory reproducibility in ANA titers; noncommercial ANA test systems do not. The range of interlaboratory reproducibility of most ANA kits is near ±3 doubling dilutions (eightfold) at a confidence level of $p < 0.05$, at least in the hands of well-qualified laboratories. Intralaboratory reproducibility should be within the two doubling dilutions (fourfold) range.

3. The precision that can be attained in titrations with the various available commercial ANA kits differs markedly. Regardless of whether this is a function of the quality of the manufactured ANA kit components or the methods used to perform the tests in clinical laboratories, the manufacturers of the kit need to assume responsibility for the reproducibility of the test. More specifically, this includes the following:

   a) Consistent reactivity of antigenic substrate.
   b) Fluorescein (F) labeled antihuman IgG conjugates with little or no IgM cross-reactivity, constant fluorescein-to-protein (F/P) ratio, and constant antibody protein concentration (see Chap. 1 for details).
   c) Realistic positive and negative control sera.
   d) Educational programs relevant to the significance, performance, and interpretation of ANA tests, including detailed data on the normal values and "cut-off titers" (see next section).
   e) Performance checks to assist users in identifying and overcoming problems in achieving reliable results. Considerably more needs to be done by manufacturers in these areas to improve ANA test precision.

4. Reference sera are needed for standardization studies with:

   a. Identified specificities of the ANA.
   b. Known titer ranges on given substrates as determined by multiple reference laboratories.

5. If ANA titers on a given substrate are determined by reliable laboratories in which reproducibility has been checked, then interpretable studies can be undertaken on the diagnostic specificity and sensitivity, as specified in the "Introduction" section of this chapter.

6. The findings summarized here serve to confirm and extend previous literature reports on substrate specificity on ANA. For example, Blaszczyk et al. (10) reported that although SLE sera yield comparable results on primate, a rodent tissue section, ANA of scleroderma patients react preferentially with primate tissues. The anticentromere antibodies that react with multiplying cells afford a classic example of tissue specificity (18). Burnham (see Chap. 36) stresses the importance of substrates for the detection of several ANA (e.g., those associated with drug-induced SLE).

Table 3. Examples of Cut-Off Titers[a] for ANA Based on Frequencies and Titers of ANA in Sera of Blood Donors[b]

Substrate source and short notation	*HEp-2 cells (Antibodies, Inc.)*	*HEp-2 cells (Behring Diagnostics)*	*Mouse liver (Meloy Laboratories)*	KB cells *(Electro-nucleonics)*
Mean titers ($\bar{X}$)	5.05	5.19	5.12	8.31
Standard deviation (S_G)	1.08	1.21	1.13	1.47
Cut-off titers: 99.9% conf. lim.				
Calculated[a]	6.87	11.12	8.35	38.81
Actual[a]	10.0	20.0	10.0	40.0
Lowest significant titer	20.0	40.0 (20.0)	20.0	80.0
SLE serum Q[c] ANA titer	10.0	10.0	10.0	20.0

[a]Calculated cut-off titers: $\bar{X} \times S_G^4$ for 99.9% confidence limits. For the calculations of $\bar{X}$ and S_G negative ANA, for example, 1:10 is considered as a titer of 5. Actual cut-off titer is the next highest actual doubling dilution in the dilutions series employed.
[b]See Figures 3A and 4A for actual data on ANA titers in sera of blood donors.
[c]A serum from what appears to be an ANA-negative SLE case.

DISEASE SPECIFICITY OF ANA TESTS ON DIFFERENT SUBSTRATES

As indicated in the "Introduction" section of this chapter, the 1982 revised ARA criteria for SLE (19) include as the 11th criterion "An abnormal titer of ANA. . ." Several reports (12,15,16) present data that point to the diagnostic value of this inclusion of ANA titers as a diagnostic criterion.

It is evident from the data presented in the preceding section that each antigenic substrate must be evaluated separately to determine exactly what constitutes "an abnormal titer of ANA. . ." (19, Chap. 29). The data presented in this section reveal that even for a given antigenic substrate, each commercial ANA kit should be evaluated separately to establish the "cut-off titer" for an abnormal ANA. The need for the latter is reinforced by some of the data reviewed in this section.

Methods of Analysis

The criterion we recommend for determining what constitutes an "abnormal ANA titer" in tests with a given commercial ANA kit is to perform tests with about 100 sera of blood donors (4). The ANA titer ranges observed provide the data base for calculating* ANA

*Calculating cut-off titers: The next highest dilution that is four standard deviations over the geometric mean titer of the normal sera is the cut-off titer; that is, the next doubling dilution over the value of $\overline{X} \times S_G^4$ is the cut-off titer. This is for a 99.9% confidence limit. For the calculations of $\overline{X}$ and S_G, "negatives" are calculated as the next lowest dilution; for example, <10 = 5 (see also the footnote of Table 3).

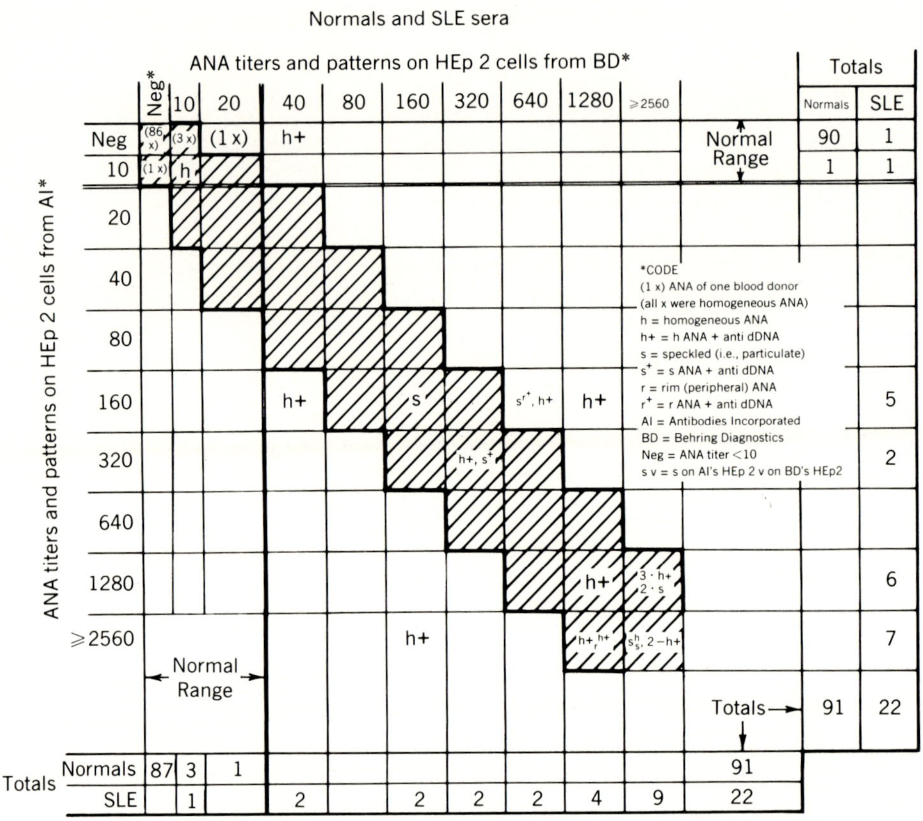

Fig. 3A

Figure 3. A. Comparisons of HEp-2 cell preparations from two sources (Behring Diagnostics, BD; Antibodies Inc., AI) as antigenic substrates for ANA titer and pattern determinations. Negative controls: blood donors (91 subjects) (See Table 3 for analyses of cut-off titers); and positive controls: systemic lupus (22 cases). B. Comparisons of HEp-2 cell preparations from the same two sources as Figure 3A for ANA titer and pattern determinations: Acrosclerosis (25 "A" cases) and cases with most or all "CREST" signs (27 "C" cases). (Reprinted from Beutner, et al. [4]. © copyright 1985, CV Mosby.)

"cut-off titers" for diagnostic studies of SLE (Fig. 3A and 4A; Table 3). These "cut-off titers" may also be compared to ANA titer ranges observed in other diseases, such as scleroderma (Figures 3B and 4B). Details of the methods used in the studies illustrated in Figures 3 and 4 (4,7) were as follows: Sera tested include: 1) 22 from SLE cases; 2) 91 blood donors, including approximately equal numbers of males and females and samplings from each decade from the 20s to the 60s; 3) 25 from acrosclerosis; and 4) 27 from "CREST" syndrome cases.

ANA tests were performed on five types of tissue culture cells and on three types of tissue sections using an antihuman IgG conjugate with a total protein (P) content of 10.6 mg/ml, a molar F/P ratio of 2.4, and an antibody content of 8 U/ml and 2.46 mg

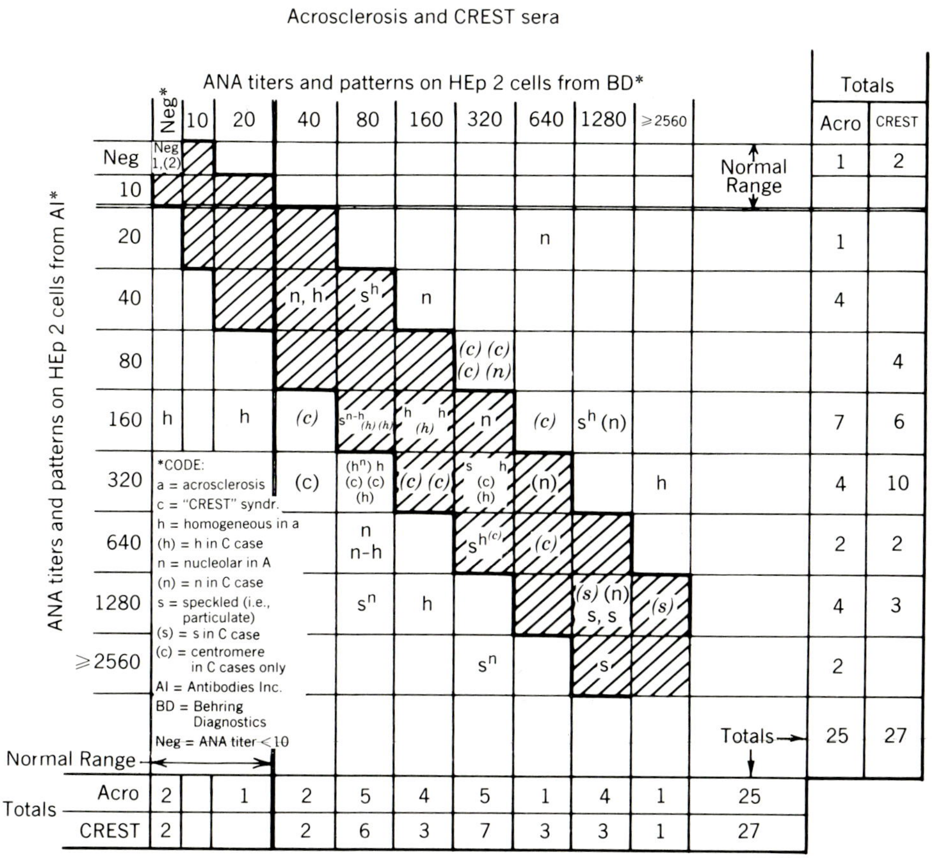

Fig. 3B

antibody/ml (7a). This conjugate was diluted 1:32 to contain 0.25 U/ml or 77 μg/ml for use. The five types of tissue culture cells included human HEp-2 from Behring Diagnostics (BD) and Antibodies, Inc. (AI), and human KB cells from Electronucleonics (EN) and Meloy Laboratories (ML).*

The tissue sections included mouse kidney from BD, mouse liver sections from ML, and monkey esophagus supplied by the IF Testing Service.†

All sera were tested on six of the substrates, and most were tested on KB cells of ML and the mouse fibroblast cells. The methods prescribed in the CDC proficiency tests (21) were employed as described above.

*BD, Behring Diagnostics, 10933 North Torrey Pines Rd., La Jolla, CA 92037; AI, Antibodies, Inc., P.O. Box 442, Davis, CA 95617; EN, Electronucleonics, 4809 Auburn Ave., Bethesda, MD 20814; and ML, Meloy Laboratories, 6715 Electronic Dr., Springfield, VA 22151.

†IF Testing Service, 963 Kenmore Ave., Buffalo, NY 14223.

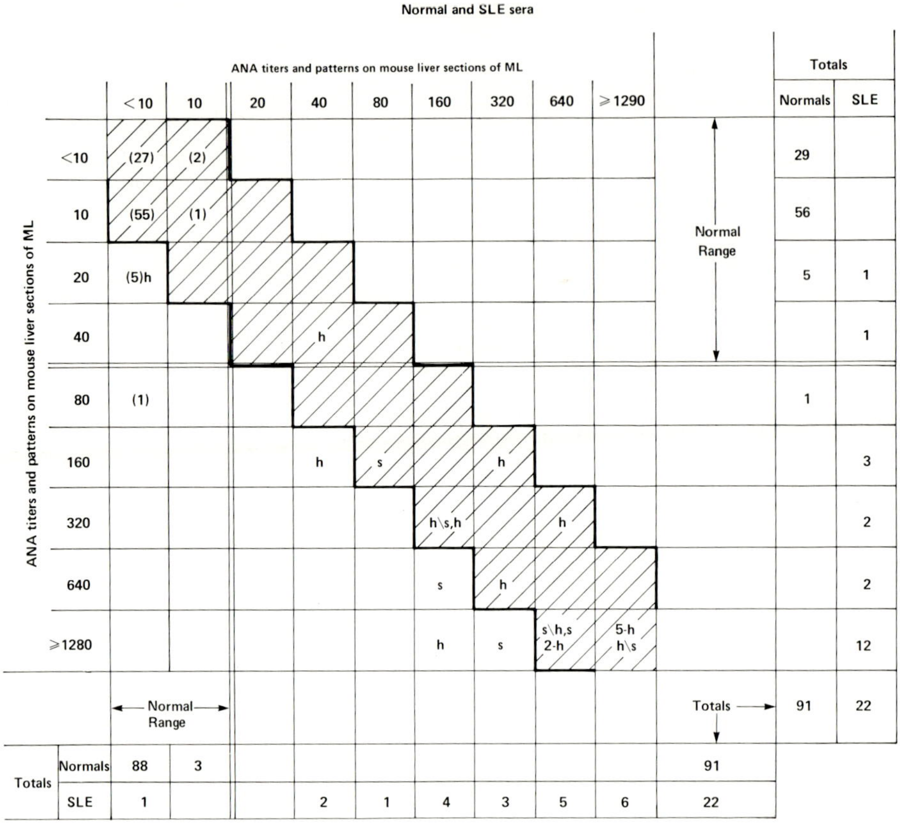

Fig. 4A

Figure 4. A. Comparisons of mouse liver sections from ML (Meloy Laboratories) with a KB cell preparation from EN (Electronucleonics) as antigenic substrates for ANA titer and pattern determinations. Negative controls: blood donors (91 subjects) (see Table 3 for analyses of cut-off titers); and positive controls: systemic lupus (22 cases). (*Note:* Use code in Fig. 3A; ML, Meloy Laboratories.) B. Comparisons of mouse liver sections with a KB cell preparation as antigenic substrates for ANA titer and pattern determinations. Acrosclerosis (25 "A" cases) and cases with most or all "CREST" signs (27 "C" cases). (*Note:* Use code in Figure 3B; use ML and EN as in Fig. 4A; (c), centromere pattern [i.e., ACA] in CREST sera.)

Divergence of Findings with Different ANA Test Systems

The frequency of ANA in sera of blood donors and the distribution of their titers varies for different antigenic substrates. Table 3, for example, lists the ANA cut-off titers on the four antigenic substrates shown in Figures 3A and 4A. (See footnote in Table 3 for description of method of calculating cut-off titers.) An inspection of these figures and the data in Table 3 reveals that although HEp-2 cells and mouse liver sections have calculated cut-off titers in the range of 11 to 15 and actual cut-off titers of 10 to 20, the actual cut-off titer for KB cells from EN was 40. An example of the value of these cut-off titers is seen in the ANA titers of serum Q from an SLE patient on these four substrates. The titers were 10, 10, <10 (negative), and 20. (This patient's serum is included in Figs. 3A and 4A.) The comparison of these titers with the "lowest signifi-

Acrosclerosis and CREST sera

ANA titers and patterns on mouse liver sections of ML (columns); ANA titers and patterns on KB cells of EN (rows)

KB cells of EN \ Mouse liver of ML	<10	10	20	40	80	160	320	640	≥1280		Totals Acro	Totals CREST
<10										Normal Range		
10	(h)	h									1	1
20	(h)			n\s							1	1
40	(c)				h						1	1
80	(3-c)n	(c\h) n\h		(n)							2	5
160	(c)	(c\h)n	2-h (c\h)	(c\s)	2-h		(n)				5	5
320	(2-c)		(c\h)	h,n	(n)	(2-h)	2-n	s			5	6
640	h				n\h,(h)	(h),h					3	2
≥1280	(c)				(c\h,n)	(h,)s	(s)s,h	s,h	(s)2-h		7	6
	Normal Range									Totals	25	27
Totals Arco	2	3	2	3	4	2	4	3	2	25		
Totals CREST	10	2	2	2	4	4	2	–	1	27		

Fig. 4B

cant titers" listed in Table 3 shows that this SLE patient is ANA negative. Without knowledge of the cut-off titers on these substrates, this serum could be misinterpreted as a weak positive ANA.

HEp-2 cells from two sources gave comparable titers and patterns of ANA with most SLE sera (Fig. 3A), and with most progressive systemic sclerosis (PSS) sera (Fig. 3B). Minor differences did occur. The BD HEp-2 cells gave a slightly higher frequency of ANA with normal sera (Fig. 3A). However, most sera with nucleolar antibodies (9 of 13 sera) reacted preferentially with the BD HEp-2 cells (Fig. 3B). The remaining sera with nuclear antibodies reacted equally well with the two HEp-2 cell preparations. None reacted preferentially with the "AI" HEp-2 preparations. This is another manifestation of the phenomenon illustrated in Figure 2.

As indicated in Figure 4B, mouse liver sections failed to react with anticentromere antibodies (ACA), as had been reported by Moroi et al. (18). While the human KB cells of EN reacted approximately as well as HEp-2 cells, the cut-off titers of EN's KB cells were significantly higher. Another type of preparation of KB cells that were produced by ML have a lower cut-off titer, but give weaker ACA reactions. Mouse fibroblast culture cells of ML fail to react with ACA, as do mouse kidney secretions from BD (18). Interestingly, monkey esophagus sections give minimal ACA reaction in the basal cell layer of the mucosa. Of the various substrates examined, the HEp-2 cell preparations were the antigens of choice for the detection of ACA.

The conclusions from these studies support and extend some of the conclusions from the CDC studies of Taylor et al. (20). Notably, the sensitivity of each antigenic substrate used for ANA tests needs to be evaluated separately. Even the same substrate from different sources needs to be evaluated separately. In effect, the correct expression of an ANA test result should include not only titers, patterns, and (as indicated above) the type of substrate, but also (as shown here) the source of the substrate.

STANDARDIZATION OF OTHER TESTS USED IN IMMUNOPATHOLOGIC STUDIES OF THE SKIN

It would be highly desirable to reexamine all tests used in immunologic studies of the skin from the viewpoints of: 1) their intra- and interlaboratory reproducibility, 2) the programs for improving their precision, and 3) the studies that evaluate objectively their diagnostic sensitivity and specificity by laboratories that have achieved acceptable levels of precision in intralaboratory comparisons (3). Obviously, the attainment of such objectives requires judicious selections of priorities and long-range planning of needs. The CDC studies on standardization of ANA (21) tests were undertaken because of the high priority these tests had been given. At this time in the development of the field, we need to consider further priorities. Among the various systems under consideration, the anti-dDNA antibody tests merit a high priority because of their general medical import in the diagnosis of SLE (12,15,16,19). From the viewpoint of immunopathology of the skin, it would obviously be highly desirable to promote the standardization of all IF studies of biopsy specimens and serum tests, particularly for the antibodies of pemphigus and pemphigoid as well as for the IgA class endomysial antibodies of dermatitis herpetiformis and celiac disease (see Chaps. 27 and 28). However, the volume of tests needed for diagnostic studies is too small to justify the types of analyses done on ANA tests. Thus, some special arrangements will have to be made to achieve better standardization.

The following subsections present preliminary observations relevant to the standardization of some of the above-mentioned tests used in immunopathology of the skin.

IF Tests for dDNA Antibodies: Preliminary Observations on Standardization

The diagnostic needs for anti-dDNA antibody tests are comparable to and dealt with in the same publications as the needs for ANA tests (15,16,19). Similarly, the best hope for standardization of anti-dDNA antibodies, at present, is for the diagnostic kit industry to undertake programs for improvements in precision of these antibody determinations that are comparable to those now in progress for ANA (see above). The IIF tests for anti-dDNA antibodies using smears of *Crithidia luciliae* (1), which are widely used now, lend themselves to inclusion in such programs for improvement in precision.

Two factors that cause false-positive dDNA antibody tests by IIF are interference due to binding of low-density lipoproteins (LDL) to the *C. luciliae* (14) and some unusual antihistone antibodies (13). In a preliminary study of a group of 31 randomly selected sera that gave positive IF reactions on *C. luciliae,* it was found that about half of the sera that were positive only at a dilution of 10 (3 of 6) became negative upon absorption with dextrane sulfate; whereas in sera with anti-DNA antibody titers of 20 or more, only 1 of 25 sera was negative upon absorption for LDL or histones. One of the 31 sera gave negative reactions on 0.1 N HCl-treated preparations of *C. luciliae* (according to the method of Deng [13] for removing histones), suggesting that the antibodies might be directed to histones rather than to DNA in this case.

The procedures used were as follows:

1. Removal of LDL (14): Mix 0.2 ml of patient serum with 0.05 ml of a 5% dextran sulfate solution, and add 0.15 ml of phosphate-buffered saline (PBS) and 0.1 ml of a 1 M $CaCl_2$ solution. Allow to stand at 4°C for 60 minutes. Centrifuge 1500 rpm for 15 minutes in a tabletop centrifuge to remove the precipitate of lipoproteins. Test the supernatant by standard IF methods for dDNA antibodies.
2. Removal of histones from *C. luciliae* smears (13). Place standard smears of *C. luciliae* in 0.1 N HCl solution for 30 minutes. Rinse with PBS; give slide a quick rinse in H_2O and allow to air dry for 2 minutes. Perform the standard dDNA antibody procedure by IF with one modification. A conjugate with an Evans blue counterstain is useful, because the HCl-treated *C. luciliae* are more autofluorescent.

In our opinion, any standardization work on IF tests for dDNA antibodies should include these or other comparable procedures for avoiding these types of false-positives.

IF Tests for Antiepithelial Antibodies of Pemphigus and Pemphigoid: Preliminary Observations on Standardization

The diagnostic importance of IF tests for the antiepithelial antibodies of pemphigus and pemphigoid (see Chaps. 8 and 10) plus the prognostic value of pemphigus antibody titer determinations (see Chaps. 8 and 9) mandate careful standardization of test procedures. The data of Krasny et al. in Chapter 9 on the relative precision of five antigenic substrates for the detection of pemphigus antibodies reconfirms the previous reports that monkey and guinea pig esophagus are the antigens of choice (13a; see also Chap. 9 and addendum). It must be stressed that quality assurance tests with positive control sera with known titers of pemphigus antibodies and negative control sera need to be performed not only on each new piece of tissue, but with each IF test performed with the section of it. Unless each of these quality assurance tests give the expected titers with a control serum, the tests with the other sera are not valid.

Monkey esophagus or oral mucosa is also the antigen of choice for the detection of the basement membrane zone (BMZ) antibodies of pemphigoid. Figures 5A and 5B summarize the results of a series of two-dimensional titrations of five sera with BMZ antibodies on mucosa and hair follicle and skin BMZ on monkey lip, guinea pig lip, and (for three of the five sera) rabbit lip (11). All five sera yielded maximal or near maximal titers on monkey lip sections. This was true of none of the other eight antigenic substrates examined. Two of the BMZ antibodies failed to react with any of the rabbit or guinea pig tissues. Two of the five sera (serum B in Fig. 5A and serum E in Fig. 5B) yielded doubtful reactions with monkey skin, but unequivocal positives with monkey lip mucosa. The finding that two sera (D and E in Fig. 5B) yielded higher titers on guinea pig lip mucosa than on monkey lip mucosa is offset by the above-mentioned negative reactions of sera B and C on all guinea pig tissues.

The conclusion—not only from these studies on BMZ antibodies of pemphigoid (Figs. 5A and 5B) and from studies on intercellular antibodies of pemphigus (Chap. 9), but also from studies on the IgA class antibodies to the endomysium associated with dermatitis herpetiformis and celiac disease (Chaps. 27 and 28)—is that the antigenic substrate of choice for serum studies on vesiculo-bullous diseases is monkey esophagus sections. This conclusion is confirmed by the findings in the initial performance evaluation of tests for antiepithelial antiantibodies described below.

For the standardization of IF tests of sera for vesiculo-bullous diseases, commercially standardized kits with monkey esophagus sections, conjugates, and control sera (all

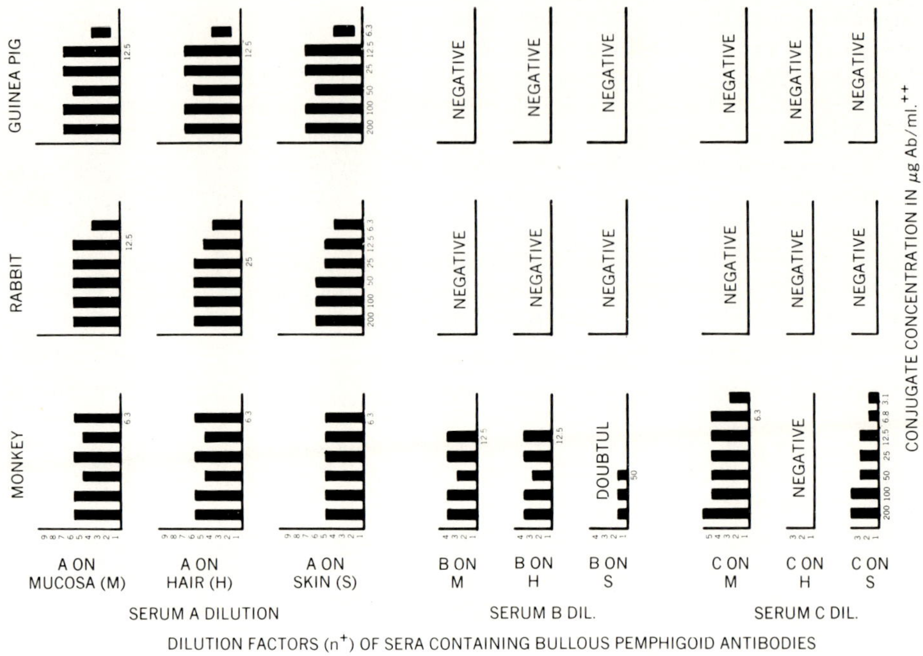
GUINEA PIG
RABBIT
MONKEY
NEGATIVE
DOUBTUL
A ON MUCOSA (M)
A ON HAIR (H)
A ON SKIN (S)
B ON M
B ON H
B ON S
C ON M
C ON H
C ON S
SERUM A DILUTION
SERUM B DIL.
SERUM C DIL.
DILUTION FACTORS (n+) OF SERA CONTAINING BULLOUS PEMPHIGOID ANTIBODIES
CONJUGATE CONCENTRATION IN μg Ab/ml.++

Fig. 5A

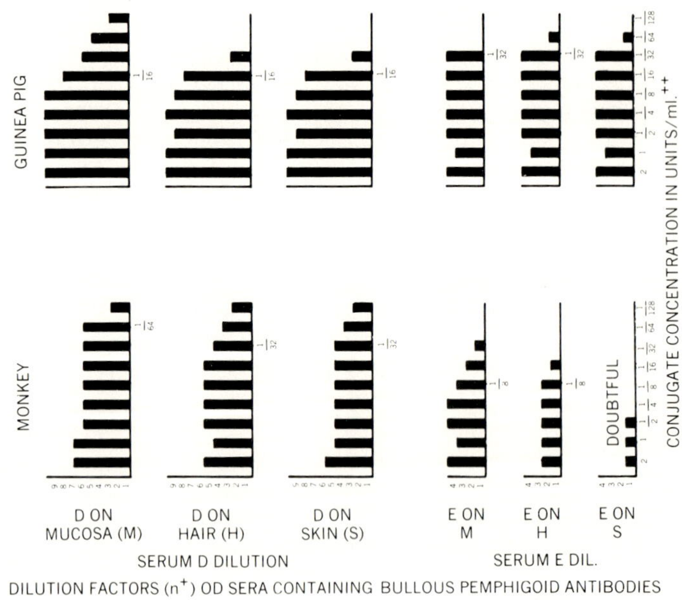
GUINEA PIG
MONKEY
DOUBTFUL
D ON MUCOSA (M)
D ON HAIR (H)
D ON SKIN (S)
E ON M
E ON H
E ON S
SERUM D DILUTION
SERUM E DIL.
DILUTION FACTORS (n+) OD SERA CONTAINING BULLOUS PEMPHIGOID ANTIBODIES
CONJUGATE CONCENTRATION IN UNITS/ml.++

Fig. 5B

Figure 5. Chessboard titrations (11) of five bullous pemphigoid sera with BMZ antibodies on sections of monkey, guinea pig lip, or (for three of the five sera) rabbit lip. A. Readings of reactions of serums A, B, and C were made for the IF staining of the BMZ of the mucosa (M), hair follicle (H), and skin (S) of monkey rabbit or guinea pig lip sections. Serum dilutions tested were as follows:

*n (Dilution factor)	1	2	3	4	5	6	7	8	9
real dilutions	1:10	1:20	1:40	1:80	1:160	1:320	1:640	1:1280	1:2560

The anti-IgG conjugate was assayed for antibody protein by reverse radial immunodiffusion [7], and the initial conjugate dilution was adjusted to contain 200 μg antibody protein/ml. Each serum dilution was tested with conjugate dilutions containing the following concentrations (in μg protein/ml) of antibody protein:

**200, 100, 50, 25, 12.5, 6.3, 3.1 μg/ml

The antibody protein concentration at the plateau endpoints (see note below) is noted in Figure 5A for each of the 14 chessboard titrations in which the BMZ antibodies of the bullous pemphigoid patients gave a plateau titer.
*(*Note:* The plateau titers [or titer ranges] of BMZ antibodies are the constant titer or titer ranges obtained with serial dilutions of conjugate. For example, in Fig. 5A, serum B on the hair follicle has a plateau titer range of 2 to 3 when expressed as dilution factors, or real titers of 10 to 20; or for serum C on mucosa, a plateau titer range of 160 to 320.) The plateau endpoint (7) is the lowest concentration of conjugated antibody that still gives a plateau titer. Plateau endpoints in all chessboard titrations are expected to fall in the range of 3.1 to 25 μg/ml of antibody protein. All but one of the values in Figure 5A fall into this range. The exception is in the chessboard titration with serum B on skin, which gave an apparent plateau endpoint of 50 μg/ml and a plateau titer of 10. The reason is probably that 1:10 was the highest dilution tested. Thus, if the plateau titer range had been 5 to 10, the conjugate plateau endpoint would be missed. B. Readings of sections of serums D and E were made for the IF staining of the BMZ of the M, S, and H, as in Fig. 5A, using monkey and guinea pig lip sections. Serial serum dilutions were tested with serial dilutions of conjugate adjusted in accordance with the unitage of the conjugate. One unit or the highest dilution of conjugate that gives a grossly visible line of precipitation in a standard gel diffusion (7) assay corresponds to about 200 μg/ml of antibody protein, as determined by reverse radial immunodiffusion (the assay used for Fig. 5A). The plateau endpoints of conjugate are expected to fall in the range of 1/8 to 1/64 U/ml of labeled antibody. (Figs. 5A and 5B are reprinted from Chorzelski and Beutner [11].)

monitored with well-controlled quality assurance procedures) would be highly desirable; unfortunately, such kits are not available.

Initial Performance Evaluations of Tests for the Antibodies of Pemphigus and Pemphigoid

Table 4 summarizes qualitative and quantitative analyses of the results obtained in the initial performance evaluations of tests for the antibodies of pemphigus and pemphigoid carried out in 1971 and 1973. Qualitatively, the frequency of false-negatives in the 1971 study was 3% for monkey esophagus sections (1 of 33 comparisons), 33% for guinea pig esophagus sections (4 of 12 comparisons), and 25% for human skin (2 of 8 comparisons). The frequency of false-positives in the 1973 study was one of five comparisons for blood group antibodies.

Table 4. Qualitative and Quantitative Analyses of Titer Variations Obtained in Tests for Antiepithelial Antibodies in 13 Laboratories Using Three Antigenic Substrates (19 Test Systems)

			Qualitative Frequencies of false-negatives					
			Case W pemphigus		*Case K pemphigus*		*Case B pemphigoid*	
Substrates used for IF tests	*No. of tests*	*No. of labs*	Neg/*Total*	*Percent neg*	*Neg/Total*	*Percent neg*	*Neg/Total*	*Percent Neg*
Monkey esophagus[a]	10–12	10	0/12	0%	1/11	9%	0/10	0%
Guinea pig esophagus[a]	4	3	0/4	0%	4/4	100%	0/4	0%
Human skin[a]	2–3	2–3	0/3	0%	2/3	66%	0/2	0%
			Case P pemphigus		*Case R pemphigoid*		*Blood group antibodies*	
Monkey esophagus[b]	5	4	0/5	0%	0/5	0%	4/5	80%

	No. of tests	No. of lbs	Quantitative Geometric mean titers ($\overline{X}$) and their standard deviations (S_G)					
			Case W		Case K		Case B	
			$\bar{X}^c$	$S_G{}^c$	$\bar{X}$	S_G	$\bar{X}$	S_G
Monkey esophagus[a]	12	1	538	1.82	37.6	2.72	845	1.79
Guinea pig esophagus[a]	4	3	121	1.86	<10.0	1.0	761	1.94
Human skin[a]	2–3	2–3	127	2.88	12.6	4.96	320	1.0
			Case P		Case R		Blood group	
			$\bar{X}$	S_G	$\bar{X}$	S_G	$\bar{X}$	S_G
Monkey esophagus[b]	5	4	28.3	3.32	158	5.68	7.58	2.53

[a] 1971 study.
[b] 1973 study.
[c] $\bar{X}$, Geometric mean titer.
S_G, Standard deviation of $\bar{X}$.

The quantitative analyses of these data show that the geometric mean titers ($\overline{X}$) of the pemphigus antibodies were higher on monkey esophagus sections than on the human skin or guinea pig esophagus (Table 4).

These findings indicate that at least some of the studies carried out in 1971 show a level of precision that is in an acceptable range; that is, S_G values below 2.028 (see Table 1). The problems with these findings are as follows:

1. The only tests for false-positives (1973 blood group antibodies) showed one of four participating laboratories failed to distinguish the control from the true positive pemphigus antibodies. Obviously, more studies of this type must be done and such problems must be overcome.
2. Little has been done since these studies were carried out over 1 decade ago.

Ideally, manufacturers of well-standardized kits with monkey esophagus sections should offer performance evaluation tests of the type shown in Table 4 at 3 to 6 month intervals. Without such regular precision checks, reliable diagnostic tests cannot be performed by laboratories associated with dermatology clinics.

SUMMARY

The presence of an abnormal titer of ANA is the 11th criterion for the diagnosis of SLE according to the 1982 revised ARA criteria. The diagnostic reliability of ANA tests is second only to that of the tests for an immunologic disorder (the 10th criterion). The ANA test aids in the exclusion of SLE because of its high diagnostic sensitivity (99%). The ANA test, however, has low specificity (49 to 65%). Most, if not all, normal sera contain low titers of ANA, mostly of the IgM class. Their in vivo reactions with nuclear debris probably serve as triggers for an ARM. Because of the diagnostic value of ANA and their presence in normal sera, standardization of test procedures is vital. The best standardization available is attained with manufactured ANA kits. Established methods of statistical analysis of the degree of standardization were first used by the CDC, and later by some ANA kit manufacturers. These reveal that most, but not all, ANA kits yield titers that are reliable within two doubling dilutions. But this is not true for noncommercial ANA test systems. That is, a twofold titer difference is within the limits of error of most commercial ANA kits. For noncommercial systems and some commercial kits, however, the range of error is even greater. In our opinion, it should be the responsibility of ANA kit manufacturers to bring the precision of their kits up to at least this minimal level of reliability and, if possible, to improve on this. The 1980 CDC study documents the fact that there is no such thing as an "ANA titer of a serum," but only an *ANA titer of a serum on a given substrate;* "from a given source" should be added.

Studies of disease specificity by a laboratory with a documented ability to attain expected levels of titer and pattern precision with ANA kits show the following. Each ANA kit must be evaluated separately for its normal serum "cut-off titer," and for its sensitivity for SLE. Even the same substrate from different manufacturers may give divergent "cut-off titers" with normal sera. These govern both the sensitivity and the specificity of ANA tests. Of the eight substrates compared, the most suitable were two ANA kits with HEp-2 cells (a human laryngeal carcinoma).

Standardization studies comparable to the ones that have been done on ANA kits need to be done on other test systems that are important for immunopathologic studies of the skin. Since such studies require much time and effort, it is necessary at this juncture to set priorities. Two possible candidates for such studies are the IF tests on *C. luciliae* smears for anti-dDNA antibodies and the test on monkey esophagus sections for the antiepithelial antibodies of pemphigus, pemphigoid, and epidermolysis bullosa, as well as for the IgA class antiendomysial antibodies of dermatitis herpetiformis and celiac disease. Preliminary studies demonstrate that methods for anti-dDNA antibody detection should include procedures for eliminating two identifiable types of false-positives, and that monkey esophagus is the substrate of choice for the detection of the above-mentioned antiepithelial antibodies. The best hope for full objective evaluations of the reproducibility of such tests is for manufacturers of kits to undertake standardization studies, preferably with the methods of analysis used by the CDC for evaluations of ANA kits.

REFERENCES

1. Aarden LA, de Groot ER, Feltkamp TE: Immunology of DNA. III. *Crithidia luciliae,* a simple substrate for the determination of anti-ds-DNA with the immunofluorescence technique. *Ann NY Acad Sci* 254:505–515, 1975.
2. Beutner EH: Defined immunofluorescence staining: Past progress, present status and future prospects for defined conjugates. In Beutner EH (Ed): Defined Immunofluorescent Staining. *Ann NY Acad Sci* 177:506–526, 1971.
3. Beutner EH, Chorzelski TP, Kumar V: Selection of laboratories for accurate diagnosis in immunodermatology. In *Clinics in Dermatology* (in press).
4. Beutner EH, Krasny SA, Chorzelski TP, et al: Evaluation of methods for detection of anti-centromere antibodies and other ANA. *J Am Acad Dermatol* 12:289–295, 1985.
5. Beutner EH, Krasny SA, Kumar V, et al: Prospects and problems in the definition and standardization of immunofluorescence. I. Present levels of reproducibility and disease specificity of antinuclear antibody tests. In Beutner EH, Nisengard RJ, Albini BA (Eds): Defined Immunofluorescence and Related Cytochemical Methods. *Ann NY Acad Sci* 420: 28–54, 1983.
6. Beutner EH, Kumar V, Greenlee P: Basics in standardization and practical applications of immunofluorescent microscopy. Standardization of antinuclear antibody tests. In Aloisi R, Hyun J (Eds): *Immunodiagnostics.* Alan R. Liss, New York, 1983, pp 49–70.
7. Beutner EH, Nisengard RJ, Kumar V: Defined immunofluorescence: Basic concepts and their application to clinical immunodermatology. In Beutner EH, Chorzelski TP, Bean SF (Eds): *Immunopathology of the Skin,* ed. 2. Wiley, New York, 1979 pp. 29–75.

7a. Beutner EH, Sepulveda MR, Barnett EV: Quantitative studies of immunofluorescent staining. II. Relationships of characteristics of unabsorbed antihuman IgG conjugates to their specific and non-specific staining properties in an indirect test for antinuclear factors. *WHO Bull* 39:587–606, 1968.

8. Beutner EH, Wolff HH: Summary of workshop on immunofluorescence and immunoelectron microscopy techniques. In Kukita A, Seiji M (Eds): *Proceedings of XVIth International Congress of Dermatology.* University of Tokyo Press, Tokyo, 1983, pp 593–597.
9. Binder WL, Cohan P, Rippe D, et al: Antinuclear antibody (ANA) standardization by performance evaluation (proficiency) program. In *ASM Abstracts, 84th Annual Meeting.* 1984, p 72.
10. Blaszczyk M, Jablonska S, Beutner EH, et al: Substrate specificity of antinuclear antibodies (ANA) in scleroderma. *J Invest Dermatol* 68:191–193, 1977.
11. Chorzelski TP, Beutner EH: Factors contributing to occasional failures in the laboratory diagnosis of bullous pemphigoid by indirect immunofluorescence. *Br J Dermatol* 86:111–117, 1972.
12. Clough JD, Elrazak M, Calabrese LH, et al: Weighted criteria for the diagnosis of systemic lupus erythematosus. *Arch Intern Med* 144:281–285, 1984.
13. Deng J-S, Sontheimer RD, Lipscomb MF, et al: Anti-histone antibodies (AHA) can bind to the *Crithidia luciliae* (CL) kinetoplast (KIN). *Clin Res P* 255A, 1984 (abstract).

13a. Feibleman C, Stolzner G, Provost TT: Pemphigus: Superiority of monkey esophagus in the determination of pemphigus antibody. *Arch Dermatol* 117:561–562, 1981.
14. Kumar V, Krasny SA, Beutner EH: Specificity of *Crithidia luciliae* method for detecting anti nDNA antibodies. Effect of absorption for lipoproteins. *Immunological Investigations* 14, 199–210, 1985.
15. Levin RE, Weinstein A, Peterson M, et al: A comparison of the sensitivity of the 1971 and 1982 American Rheumatism Association criteria for the classification of systemic lupus erythematosus. *Arthritis Rheum* 27:530–538, 1984.
16. Manu P: Receiver operating characteristic curves of the revised criteria for the classification of systemic lupus erythematosus. *Arthritis Rheum* 26: 1054–1055, 1983 (letter to the editor)
17. Molden DP, Nakamura RM, Tan EM: Standardization of immunofluorescence test for autoantibody to nuclear antigens ANA: Use of reference sera of defined antibody specificity. *Am J Clin Pathol* 82:57–66, 1984.
18. Moroi Y, Peebles C, Fritzler MJ, et al: Autoantibody to centromere (kinetochore) in scleroderma sera. *Proc Natl Acad Sci* 77, 1627–1631, 1980.
19. Tan EM, Cohen AS, Fries JF, et al: The 1982 revised criteria for the classification of systemic lupus erythematosus. *Arthritis Rheum* 25:1271–1277, 1982.
20. Taylor RN: Measurement of variation and significance in serologic tests. In Beutner EH, Nisengard RJ, Albini BA (Eds): Defined Immunofluorescence and Related Cytochemical Methods. *Ann NY Acad Sci* 420:13–21, 1983. (*Note:* Revisions in the mode of analyses have been suggested by Taylor and may be reported by him at a later date.)
21. Taylor RN, Fulford KM: *Proficiency Testing: Summary Analysis; Diagnostic Immunology; Special Study—Antinuclear Antibodies.* Centers for Disease Control, PHS, HMS, Atlanta, 1980, pp. 1–14.
22. Taylor RN, Fulford KM: *Theory and Application of the CDC Diagnostic Immunology Proficiency Testing Program.* Centers for Disease Control, Atlanta, 1981.
23. Taylor RN, Fulford KM: External quality control and standardization in labeled immunoassay. In Beutner EH, Nisengard RJ, Albini BA (Eds): Defined Immunofluorescence and Related Cytochemical Methods. *Ann NY Acad Sci* 420:22–27, 1983.

3
Monkey Esophagus: A Unique Antigenic Substrate in Immunodermatology

Vijay Kumar
Ernst H. Beutner

INTRODUCTION

Since the initial discovery of intercellular (IC) antibodies in the sera of pemphigus patients, it has been found that of all animal substrates tested, monkey esophagus is the most reliable and reproducible substrate for detecting IC antibodies in pemphigus vulgaris (11,13,29,34). Immediately following the above discovery, it was found that monkey lip (13) or esophagus is also an ideal substrate for detecting antibasement membrane zone antibodies in patients with pemphigoid (26,44). Now we know that monkey esophagus is not only the substrate of choice for detecting pemphigus and pemphigoid antibodies, but also that it has been employed for detecting other autoantibodies, as summarized in Table 1. The reason so many antibodies can be detected on monkey esophagus is that it contains not only stratified squamous epithelium, but also smooth and skeletal muscles, blood vessels, connective tissue, etc. (17). This makes monkey esophagus a uniquely useful substrate in the determination of autoantibodies in immunodermatology.

As mentioned in Chapter 2, it is of utmost importance that in order to obtain reproducible results, one must use the well-defined immunofluorescent (IF) system in performance of these test systems. Microscope optics and conjugate specificities are among the many factors that may influence the specificity and sensitivity of the IF test systems. This chapter will focus on the IF staining patterns observed on monkey esophagus, since descriptions of them are scattered throughout this volume.

BULLOUS DISEASE ANTIBODIES

The various bullous disorders with autoimmune etiology (Chap. 8) include pemphigus (Chaps. 9 to 13), pemphigoid (Chaps. 15 to 19), epidermolysis bullosa acquisita (EBA), (Chapter 20), linear IgA bullous dermatosis (LABD), and chronic bullous disease of childhood (CBDC) (see Chaps. 22 and 23). The most recent findings suggest that dermatitis herpetiformis (DH) may also have an autoimmune etiology (see Chaps. 27

Table 1. Type and Significance of Antibodies as Detected on Monkey Esophagus

Disease	*Type of antibody*	*Esophagus structures stained*	*Tissue of choice*	*Clinical significance*
A. Bullous diseases				
Pemphigus	Intercellular (IC)	Intercellular areas of epithelial cells	Monkey esophagus	Positive in virtually all active cases of pemphigus (≥90%). IgG class antibody
Pemphigoid (BP)	Basement membrane zone (BMZ)	BMZ of stratified epithelial cells	Monkey esophagus	Positive in ~ 70% of BP and in 10% of cicatricial pemphigoid patients, IgG class.
Epidermolysis bullosa acquisita (EBA)	BMZ	BMZ of stratified epithelial cells	Monkey esophagus	BMZ antibodies of IgG class positive in ~ 25% of EBA patients, but in low titers.
Herpes gestationis (HG)	BMZ, HG factor	BMZ of stratified epithelial cells	Monkey esophagus	BMZ antibodies of IgG class positive in -20%. Avidly complement fixing Ab. HG factor (BMZ antibodies) as detected by indirect complement IF).
Linear IgA bullous dermatosis (LABD)	BMZ	BMZ	Monkey esophagus	IgA class antibodies to the BMZ in 7–33% of LABD patients. More frequently positive in benign chronic bullous disease of childhood.

	Dermatitis herpetiformis (DH)	Antiendomysial (EmA)	Smooth muscle bundles	Monkey esophagus	IgA class antibodies in 70–80% of DH patients. Usually positive in all active cases. Titers parallel the degree of gut involvement.
		Antigliadin (AGA)	Intercellular areas of epithelial cells on gliadin-treated sections	Monkey esophagus	Virtually positive in all active cases of DH. Also positive in pemphigus, pemphigoid, other diseases, and even in normals.
B.	Connective tissue diseases				
	Systemic lupus erythematosus (SLE) Mixed connective tissue disease (MCTD) Progressive systemic sclerosis (PSS) Poly/dermatomyositis	Antinuclear	Nuclei of all epithelial and myoid cells	Mouse kidney and liver sections, HEp-2 cells	90–95% positivity in SLE, 100% in MCTD, 60–90% in PSS, and up to 60% in poly/dermatomyositis.
	CREST[a] syndrome	Centromere	Nuclei of basal cells of the epithelia	HEp-2 cells	Most patients with CREST.

(*Continued*)

Table 1. *(Continued)*

Disease	*Type of antibody*	*Esophagus structures stained*	*Tissue of choice*	*Clinical significance*
C. Others				
Chronic active hepatitis	Smooth muscle antibodies (SMA)	Muscularis mucosa of the lower 1/3 of the esophagus	Mouse kidney/stomach	Present in 60–70% of patients with chronic active hepatitis, and also positive in certain cases of primary biliary cirrhosis.
Myasthenia gravis (MG)	Skeletal muscle	Upper 1/3 of the muscularis mucosa	Any skeletal muscle	Titers of 80 or greater are present in 30% of MG patients and in 95% of MG patients with associated thymoma.
Allergic drug reaction Burn toxemia Bone marrow grafts	Basal cell	Basal cell layer of epithelium	Most stratified epithelia	10% of patients with drug reactions or bullous diseases.
Malignancy, autoallergic eczema	Cytoplasmic	Cytoplasm of epithelial cells (homogeneous)	Monkey esophagus or other epithelia	High titers in patients with certain malignancies.
Primary biliary cirrhosis	Mitochondrial	Cytoplasm of epithelial cells (granular)	Mouse or rat kidney	Positive in ≥90% of patients with primary biliary cirrhosis
D. Antibodies of no known diagnostic significance	Blood group	Intercellular areas of epithelial cells	Monkey esophagus	
	Pemphigus-like (PLA)	Intercellular areas of epithelial cells	Monkey esophagus	Post burn, drug reactions, skin transplants, etc.

[a]CREST, calcinosis, Raynaud's syndrome, esophageal immotility, sclerodactyly, and telangiectasis.

and 28). In all of the above disorders, immunohistologic studies on monkey esophagus have been very useful in detecting various autoantibodies in the sera of these patients.

Pemphigus

Pemphigus was the first skin disorder in which circulating autoantibodies to the IC substances of epithelial cells were demonstrated by indirect immunofluorescence (IIF) on monkey esophagus and other mucosal tissues (11,13); they are of the IgG class. Intercellular antibodies as detected by IIF on monkey esophagus as the antigenic substrate (Fig. 1) are found to be positive in almost all active cases of pemphigus. However, there can be some time intervals during which IIF studies are negative in active pemphigus cases (24,65). These IC antibodies can also be negative in pemphigus patients during remission. Most of the investigators found a positive correlation between the IC antibody titer and disease activity (29,30,35,62,67,77). However, some investigators did not find such correlation with the disease activity (8,46). As discussed in Chapter 9, this may be due to the time of sampling etc. While there have been some conflicting results (4, 22, 34), recent studies of Sabolinski, et al. (66a) have shown a dual substrate of monkey esophagus and guinea pig esophagus to be optimum in detecting IC antibodies (Chap. 9 addendum). Monkey esophagus is more sensitive for detecting IC antibodies of pemphigus vulgaris and guinea pig esophagus is best for detecting antibodies of pemphigus foliaceus.

Pemphigus-like and "Blood Group" Antibodies

In addition to the pemphigus antibodies, two other groups of antibodies may also mimic the type of IC staining observed in pemphigus patients; notably the so-called "blood

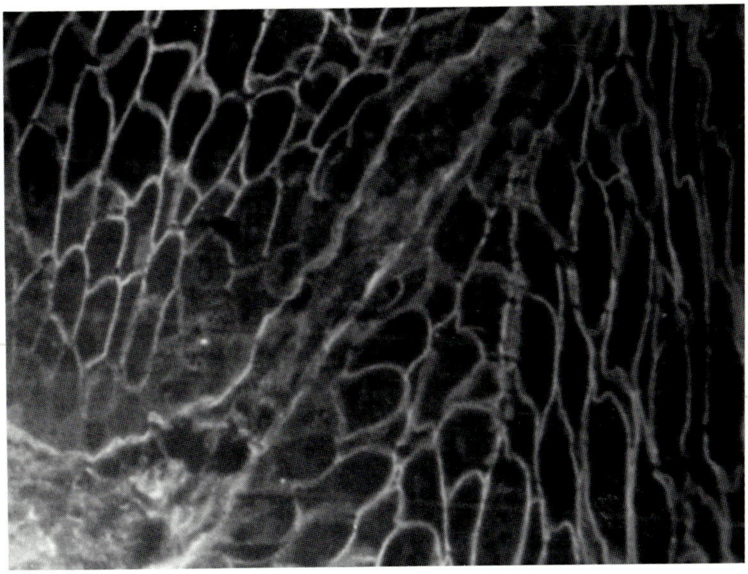

Figure 1. Indirect IF staining of monkey esophagus sections with a pemphigus serum. Note a continuous linear intercellular staining (112×).

group" antibodies and pemphigus-like antibodies (PLA). Antibodies to "blood group" antigens not only give an IC staining of the type associated with pemphigus, they also react with blood vessels (Fig. 2). The failure of red blood cells of type A or B to remove such antibodies raises questions on whether they are directed to blood group antigens. However, the staining associated with these so-called "blood group" antibodies can be removed by absorbing with horse stomach suspension (14). Sera should be routinely absorbed regardless of the presence of blood vessel staining.

The sera of certain patients with burns, drug reactions, and other diverse insults to the epidermis may have antibodies that give staining similar to pemphigus antibodies (9,48,52,56). They are not true pemphigus antibodies and are referred to as PLA. Some of the properties that differentiate pemphigus antibodies from PLA are listed in Table 2.

Pemphigoid

Antibodies to the basement membrane zone (BMZ) as detected by IIF are present in 60 to 80% of bullous pemphigoid patients (Fig. 3) (Chap. 8). This incidence may vary depending upon the tissue employed as the antigenic substrate. Chorzelski et al. have found that antibodies to BMZ may sometimes exhibit species and organ specificity

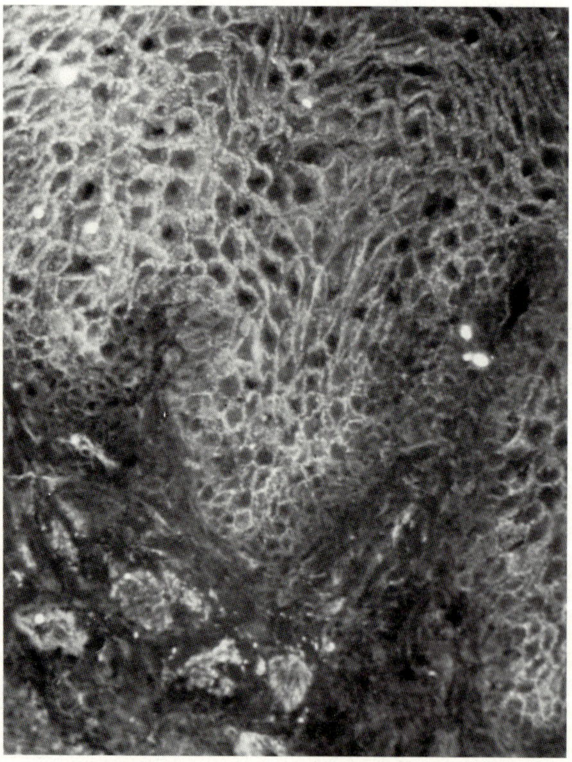

Figure 2. Intercellular (granular) and blood vessel staining of monkey esophagus due to blood group antibodies (56×).

Table 2. Differentiation of Pemphigus from Pemphigus-like Antibodies

Characteristics observed	*Pemphigus antibodies*	*Pemphigus-like antibodies*
in vivo DIF[a] skin biopsy studies of IgG in the epidermis associated with acantholysis	Mostly positive IC binding of antibodies	Negative
in vitro binding and induction of acantholysis of mucosal skin explants	Positive, especially when serum titers are 80 or greater	Negative even at high titers
complement-fixing ability as detected by indirect complement IF method (this is not a well-defined method)	Not present, in some cases, may be weakly positive, but in lower titers than indirect IF titers	Present in most, but may not be in all cases

[a]Direct immunofluorescence.

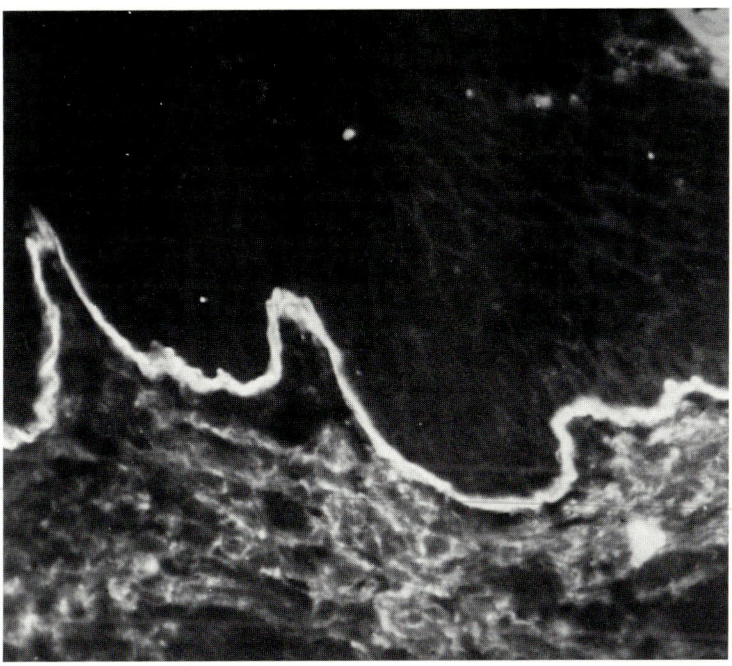

Figure 3. Basement membrane staining for IgG with a serum from pemphigoid patient, as revealed by IIF (112×).

(23,28). They also found monkey esophagus to be a reliable antigenic substrate for detecting anti-BMZ antibodies. Occasionally, sera of certain patients may give a prozone reaction, being negative at low dilutions and becoming positive when tested at higher dilutions (Fig. 4). As discussed in detail in Chapters 8 and 15, the incidence of anti-BMZ antibodies varies. For example, anti-BMZ antibodies are present in 50% and 30% in vesicular and erythematous pemphigoid patients, respectively, but the incidence is less than 10% in cicatricial pemphigoid. About 25% of patients with EBA have antibodies to another BMZ antigen. The antibodies are primarily of the IgG class; in one-half of pemphigoid patients, BMZ antibodies fix complement. Even though both direct immunofluorescent (DIF) and IIF findings are very similar both in pemphigoid and EBA, it is necessary to differentiate the two from each other, as corticosteroid treatment is contraindicated in EBA. To make such a differentiation, one may either study the localization of type IV collagen or laminin antigen by IF, as detailed in Chapter 21, or by binding characteristics of the BMZ antibodies on monkey esophagus split sections (Fig. 5; Table 3; Chap. 20). Preliminary observations in this laboratory suggest that *some,* but not all, sera that give "EBA"-type patterns are from EBA cases. In herpes gestationis (HG), serum studies for the presence of anti-BMZ antibodies are usually negative (Chaps. 8 and 19). However, in about one half of HG patients, there is a factor in the serum that fixes complement at the BMZ by the indirect complement IF tests (47,66; Chap. 19). This so-called "HG factor," as we now know, is an avidly complement-fixing IgG class antibody to the BMZ (45,47). Because of its low concentration in the serum, it could not be detected by IIF methods. As discussed above, antibodies to the BMZ are usually of the IgG class and, to a lesser extent, of the IgA class except in LABD, in which IgA predominates. These IgA class anti-BMZ antibodies have been reported in 7 to 33% of LABD patients (see Chaps. 22 and 23).

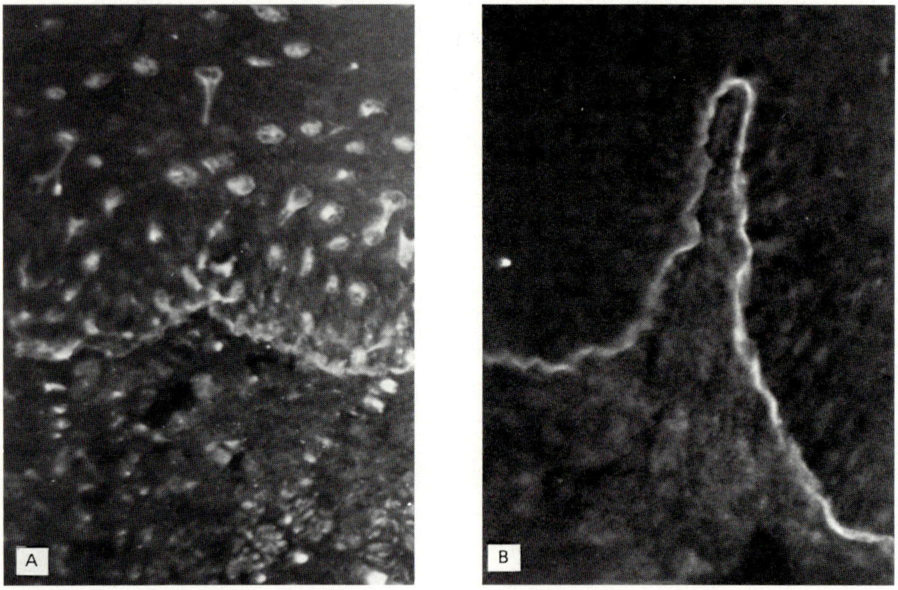

Figure 4. Indirect staining on monkey esophagus: Prozone effect. A. negative staining at the BMZ with a low 1:10 dilution of the serum. B. BMZ staining at a higher dilution (1:80) (112×).

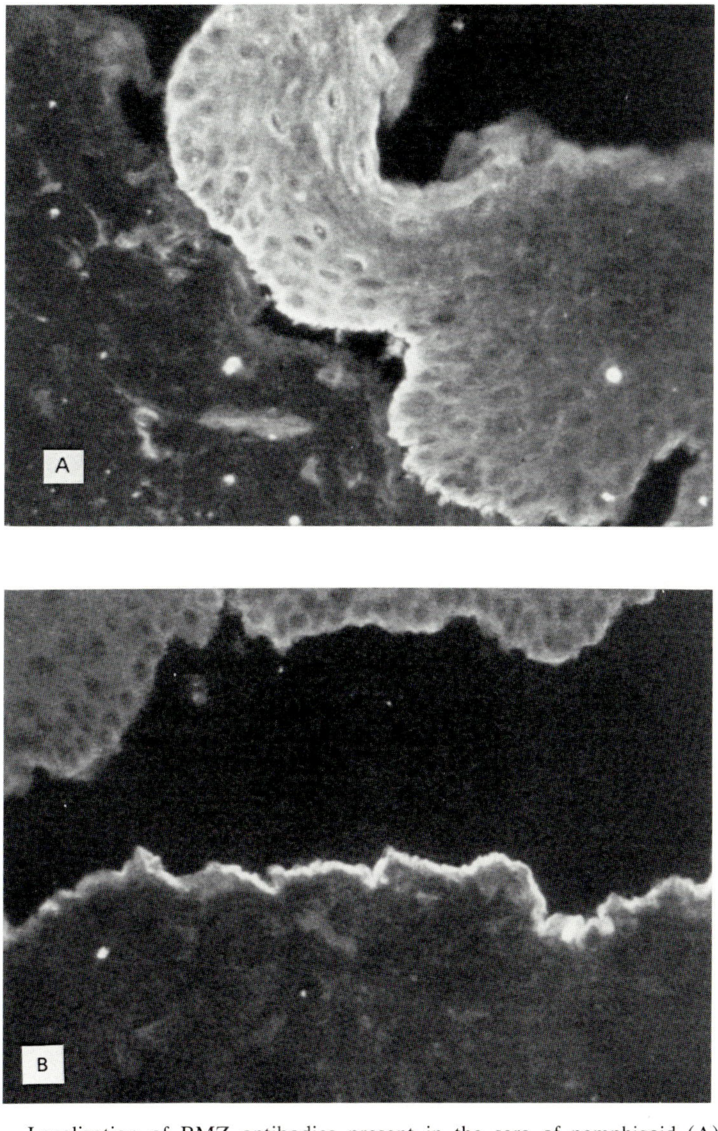

Figure 5. Localization of BMZ antibodies present in the sera of pemphigoid (A) or EBA patients (B) by IIF on split sections of monkey esophagus (112×).

According to Leonard et al. (Chap. 23), most patients with CBDC are positive for IgA class BMZ antibodies, as compared with LABD patients in whom they occur rarely. However, others have not confirmed this (see Chap. 22).

Dermatitis Herpetiformis

The presence of antigliadin and antireticulin antibodies has been associated with dermatitis herpetiformis (DH) (see Chaps. 25 and 26). Antigliadin antibodies could be detected

Table 3. Immunohistochemical Differentiation of Epidermolysis Bullosa Acquisita from Bullous Pemphigoid

Localization	*Localization of antigenic determinants on split skin sections upon staining with sera from patients with*	
	Bullous pemphigoid	*Epidermolysis bullosa acquisita*
Floor	−	+
Roof	+	−

on monkey esophagus sections by first treating these sections with an aqueous solution of gliadin followed by incubation of these sections with the patient's serum. The binding of antigliadin antibodies is then detected by IIF, as detailed in Chapter 28. Two types of staining could be seen: one staining both the IC areas of epithelial cells similar to the type associated with pemphigus (Fig. 6A), and the other staining both the IC areas of epithelial cells and the interfibrillar regions of the smooth muscle bundles (Fig. 6B). Only the latter is due to antigliadin antibodies. The first type of staining seems to be due to blood group antibodies, since it could be removed by absorption with horse stomach (14). Antigliadin antibodies are found in most active cases of DH, and the antibody titers seem to fluctuate with disease activity (57,60,70,75,76). However, these antibodies are not disease specific and have been found in celiacs, other bullous dermatoses such as pemphigus and pemphigoid, and even in controls (54). These antibodies are primarily of the IgG class.

An IgA class autoantibody found in the sera of DH and celiac patients is the antiendomysial antibody (anti-EmA). These antibodies react with the endomysial lining of smooth muscle bundles and are best detected by IIF on monkey esophagus. As shown in Figure 7, the best reactivity is seen with the muscularis mucosa adjacent to the mucosal epithelium. These antibodies are detectable in virtually all active cases of DH and celiac patients. In addition, the antibody titer parallels the degree of gut involvement (25,76; Chap. 27). The titers fluctuate with the disease activity and fall when the patient is on a gluten-free diet. These antibodies are of the IgA class, and thus may be synthesized in the gut mucosal lymphoid system.

CONNECTIVE TISSUE DISEASE ANTIBODIES

This group primarily constitutes patients with systemic lupus erythematosus (SLE), mixed connective tissue disease (MCTD), systemic sclerosis (SS), and polymyositis. The most common serologic studies include tests for antinuclear antibodies (ANA).

Antinuclear Antibodies

Antinuclear antibodies (ANA) are antibodies directed against multiple antigens located in the nuclei of many tissues studied. Even though mouse or rat kidney and liver sections or tissue culture cell substrates such as HEp-2 have been recognized as the substrates for detecting ANA, these antibodies could also be detected on monkey

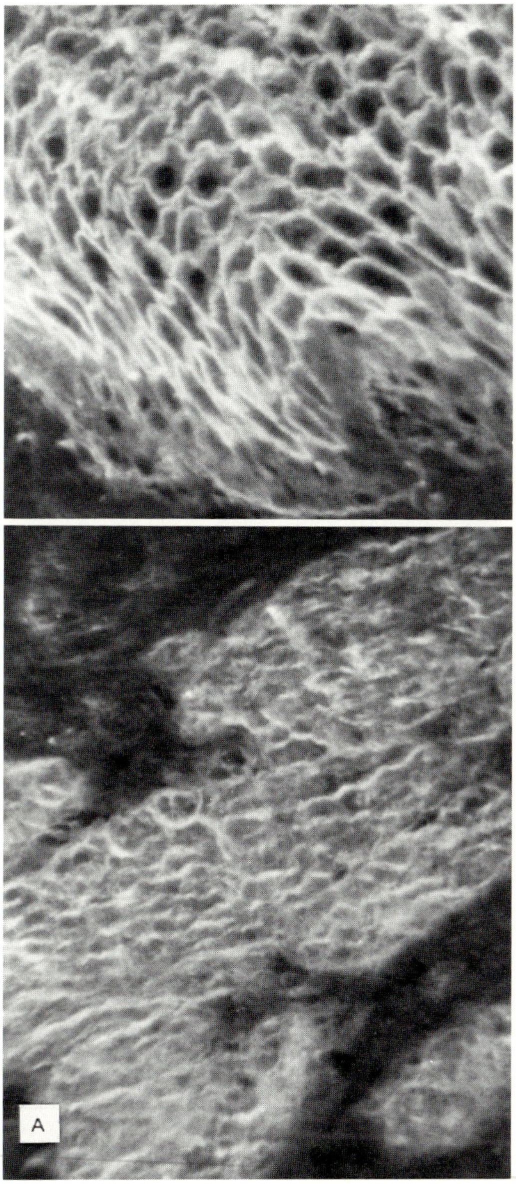

Figure 6. Intercellular staining on gliadin-treated monkey esophagus sections due to: A. Anti-gliadin (there is a staining of both the intercellular areas and also of the muscularis mucosa); B. Blood group antibodies (112×).

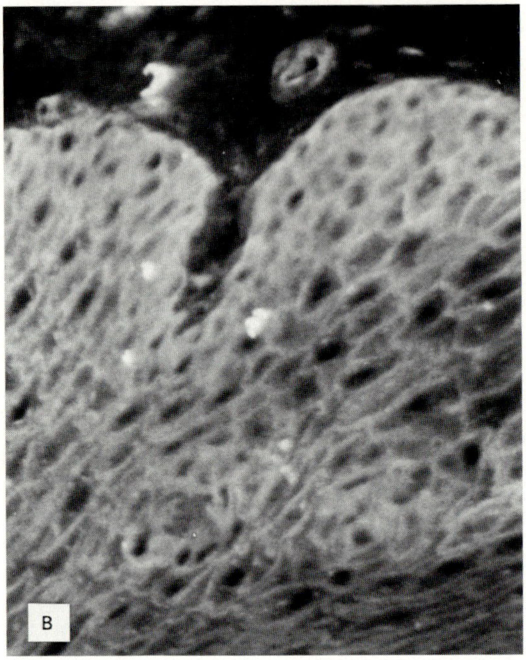

Figure 6 (continued)

esophagus sections. We have observed that ANA titers, when tested on monkey esophagus, are very similar to the one tested on the recommended substrates (12; Chap. 2). However, ANA patterns may vary on monkey esophagus compared to other substrates (16). In addition, these antibody patterns may not be easily readable on monkey esophagus.

The various ANA patterns that could be easily read are homogeneous, speckled, and nucleolar (Fig. 8). As discussed in detail elsewhere (Chap. 36), the homogeneous pattern has been associated with antibodies to deoxyribonucleoprotein and to DNA, especially when present in high titers. The peripheral pattern is produced primarily by antibodies to nDNA. The speckled pattern is produced by antibodies to saline-extractable acidic nucleoproteins. The nucleolar staining pattern is associated with 4-6S nucleolar RNA. In addition, another very fine speckled staining pattern associated with CREST syndrome, a benign subset of scleroderma, could also be detected on monkey esophagus (Fig. 9). Human tissue culture substrates such as HEp-2 cells are the ideal substrate for recognizing this staining pattern. These antibodies react with the centromeric proteins of the chromosomal material (27).

ANA especially in titers of 160 or higher, are found in patients either with SLE, MCTD, scleroderma, or in very few cases of rheumatoid arthritis (50). In addition to the nontissue specificity of most ANA, in systemic scleroderma, ANA can be substrate specific in certain cases. Jablonska and Blaszczyk and their associates reported ANA positivity in 97% of scleroderma patients on monkey esophagus, as compared to 62% on rat liver sections (16,39), thus suggesting ANA testing on two different substrates.

The presence of ANA in low titers has been observed in normal subjects and in patients with certain other noncollagen disorders. The presence of ANA in coexistence

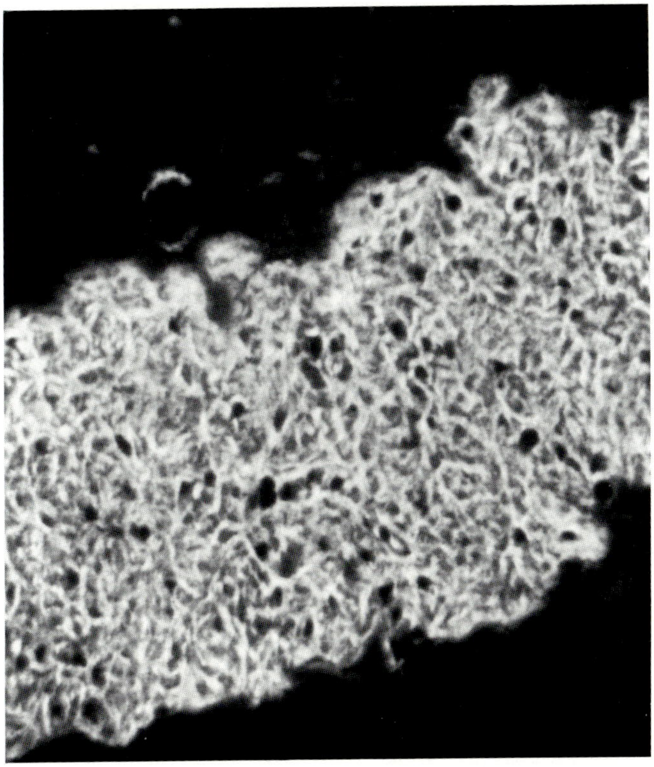

Figure 7. Staining of the endomysial lining of the smooth muscle on monkey esophagus for IgA class antiendomysial antibodies (112×).

with other autoantibodies, such as in pemphigus and pemphigoid, may give rise to an interference phenomenon in the detection of other antibodies (7,53,61).

OTHER ANTIBODIES

This group includes antibodies of patients with chronic active hepatitis (CAH), primary biliary cirrhosis (PBC), myasthenia gravis, and certain malignancies and autoallergic diseases. The antibodies found in the sera of these patients include the following groups.

Antismooth muscle antibodies

Antismooth muscle antibodies (ASMA) are both nonspecies- and nonorgan-specific antibodies. Even though the most common substrate for detecting ASMA is rat stomach, other tissues such as monkey esophagus can also be used. The distribution of muscle characteristic on monkey esophagus varies, being skeletal in the upper third and

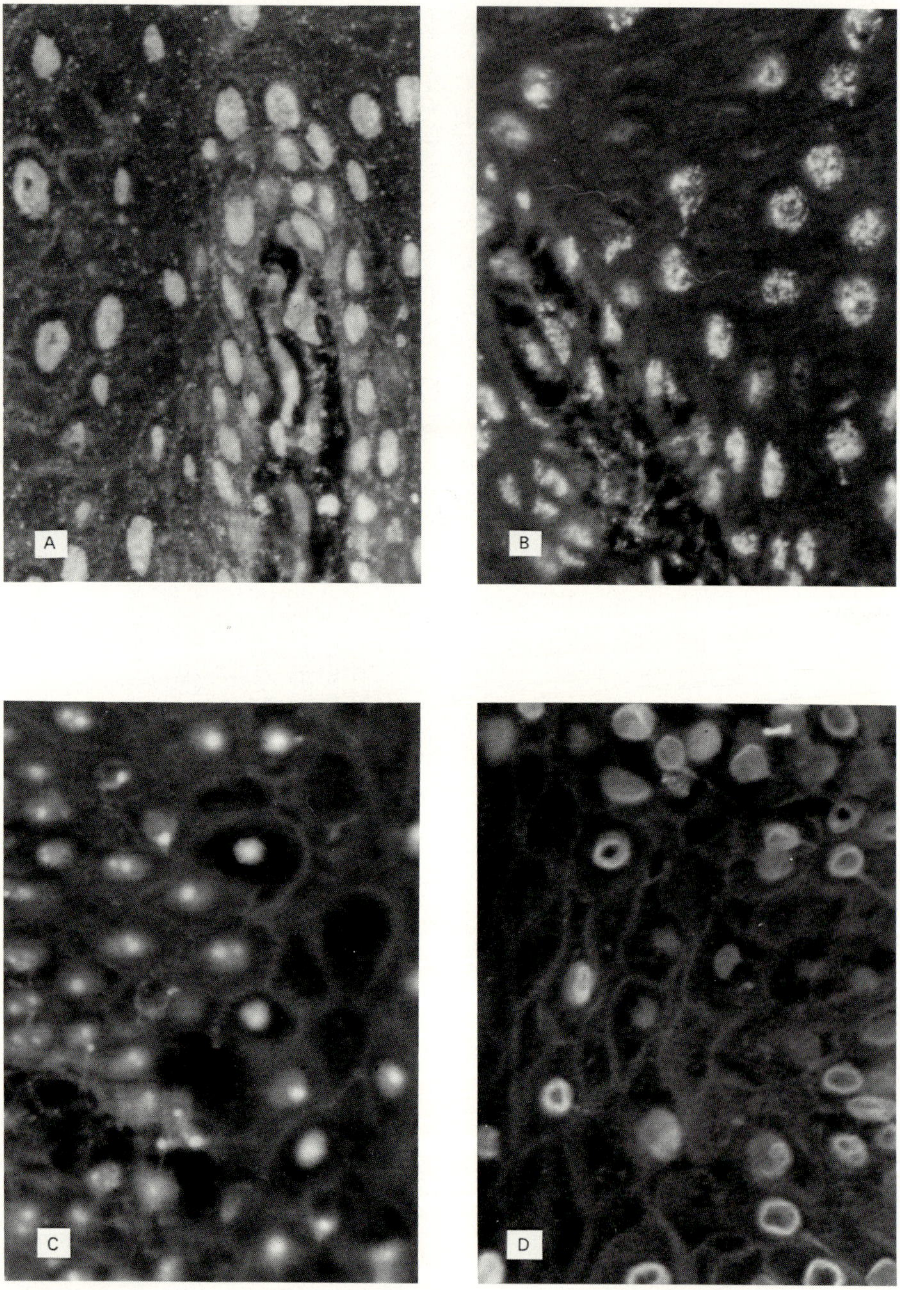

Figure 8. Antinuclear antibody staining on monkey esophagus. A. homogeneous; B. speckled; C. nucleolar; D. peripheral (224×).

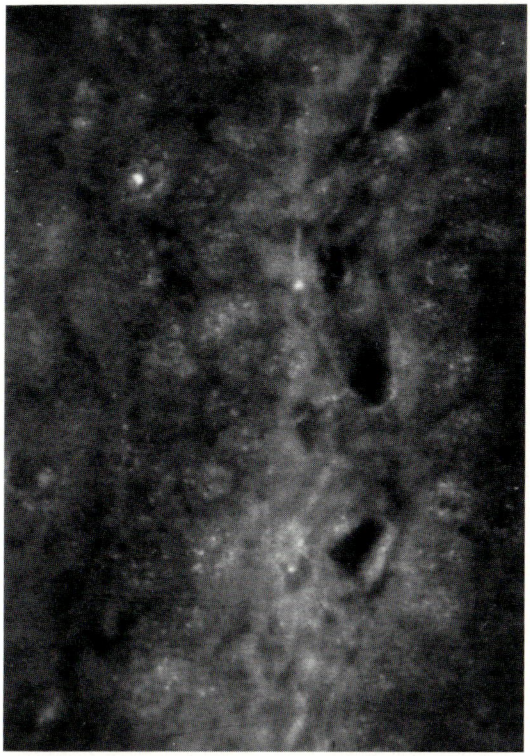

Figure 9. Anticentromere antibody staining on monkey esophagus. Note a very fine granular staining, especially of the basal cell layer (112×).

smooth in the lower third, and a mixture of the two in the middle portion (51). Thus, ASMA are best detected in the sections of the middle or lower third of the esophagus (Fig. 10).

ASMA occur in patients with CAH, PBC, acute viral hepatitis, infectious mononucleosis, many other diseases, and even in normal subjects (5–7,32,38,40,49,59,72).

The presence of ASMA in titers of 40 or more are found primarily in CAH. The incidence of ASMA varies; in normal subjects, it has been reported as 15 to 20%. This may, to a large extent, be due to antigenic substrate variations and to variations in the starting dilutions tested. The incidence of ASMA in CAH varies from 50 to 90%. ASMA occurs in 25% of patients with PBC, 87% with acute viral hepatitis, 81% with infectious mononucleosis, 73% with Burkitt's lymphoma, 23% with Hodgkin's disease, 5% with myeloproliferative disorders, and about 14% with warts.

ASMA can be of both IgG and IgM classes. The common occurrence of low titers of ASMA in normal sera suggests that they may be physiologic autoantibodies. The coexistence of elevated titers of ANA with ASMA are indicative of lupoid hepatitis. When positive, these antibodies should be titrated on mouse kidney-stomach or other appropriate tissue sections.

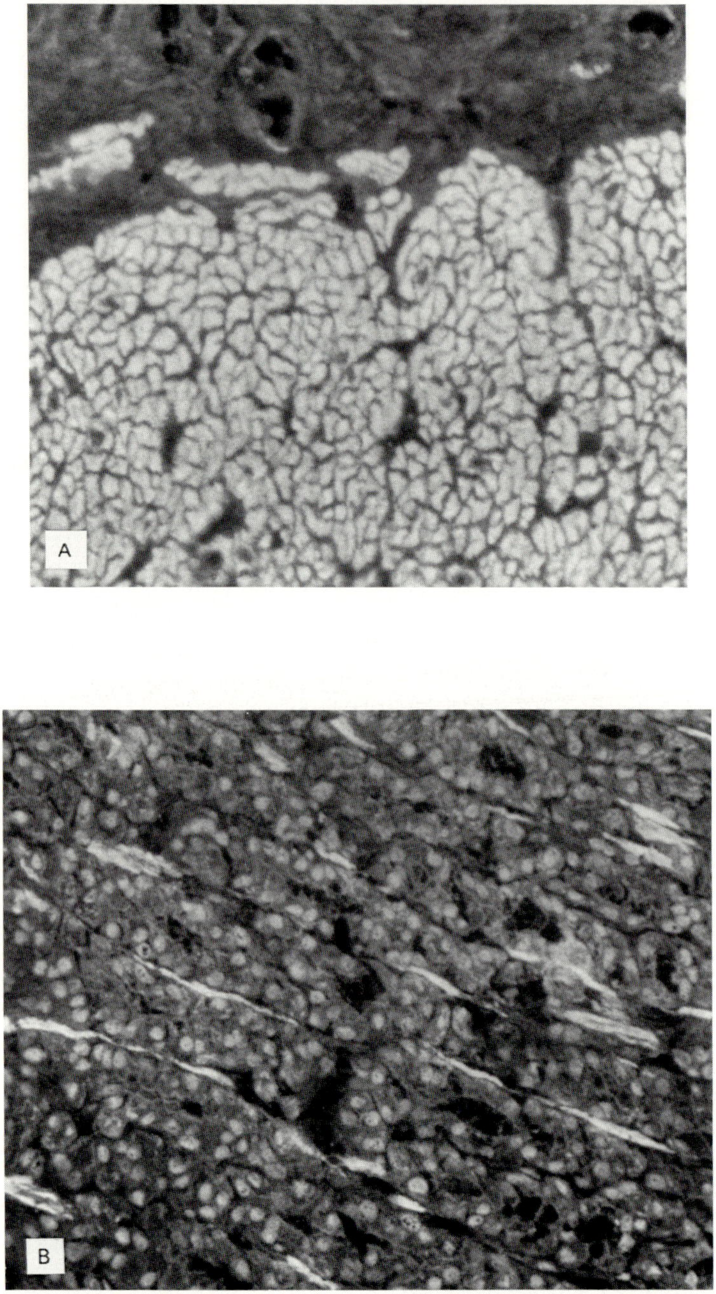

Figure 10. Indirect IF staining showing a homogeneous staining of: A. The sarcoplasm of the smooth muscle fibers; B. Muscle fibers of the mucosal epithelium (224×).

Antimitochondrial antibodies

Antimitochondrial antibodies (AMA) are a heterogeneous group of antibodies that are primarily non-tissue- and nonspecies specific, even though species-specific AMA have been reported (74). These antibodies are usually detected by IIF methods on mouse kidney-stomach sections. They can also be detected on monkey esophagus sections as coarse granular staining that could easily be mistaken for ANA (Fig. 11). If found to be positive, their reactivity and titer should be checked on mouse kidney sections.

AMA of five different specificities have been found in different clinical manifestations as tabulated below (Table 4). The presence of AMA, especially in high titers, are highly suggestive of a diagnosis of PBC. AMA are found in 90 to 95% of PBC patients and in very low numbers in other diseases, such as CAH and cryptogenic cirrhosis (10). PBC-specific mitochondrial antigen is present on the inner mitochondrial membrane and could be separated from the mitochondrial ATPase activity (55). Recently, it has been shown to be an adenine nucleotide translocator protein (71).

Anticytoplasmic antibodies

Antibodies to the cytoplasm, as detected by IIF on stratified epithelial cells (Fig. 12), are directed against a family of antigens (1,3,19–21,33,68,69). These antigens are tissue

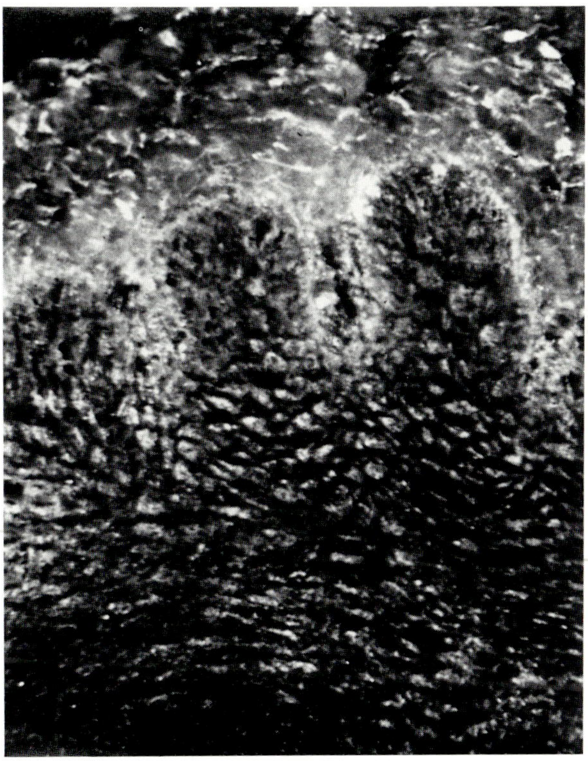

Figure 11. A granular cytoplasmic staining due to antimitochondrial antibodies (112×).

Table 4. Heterogeneity of Antimitochondrial (AMA) Antibodies as Revealed by Their Reactivity by Indirect Immunofluorescence

		Immunofluorescent staining							
		Kidney[a]			*Stomach*[a]				
Classification	*Diseases*	P_1	P_2	P_3	*D*	*PC*	*CC*	*Staining pattern*	*Nature of antigen*
M1	Syphilis (active secondary)	+	+	+	++	±	±	Diffuse[b]	Cardiolipin
M2	PBC (primary biliary cirrhosis)	+	+	+	+++	+++	w	Granular	Trypsin and mersalyl sensitive, inner mitochondrial membrane-associated antigen
M3	PLE (pseudolupus syndrome)	++	++	++	++	+++	w	Homogeneous(?)	Trypsin and mersalyl insensitive on outer membrane
M4	CAH (chronic active hepatitis)	+	+	+	+++	+++	w	Granular	Trypsin and mersalyl insensitive—may be more than one antigen, one on outer membrane
M5	Various collagen diseases and autoimmune hemolytic anemia	++	++	+	±	±	–	?	Trypsin and mersalyl insensitive outer membrane

[a]PC, parietal cells; CC, chief cells; P, proximal tubules; and D, distal tubules.
[b]Ethanol, 95% fixative, abolishes the reactivity.

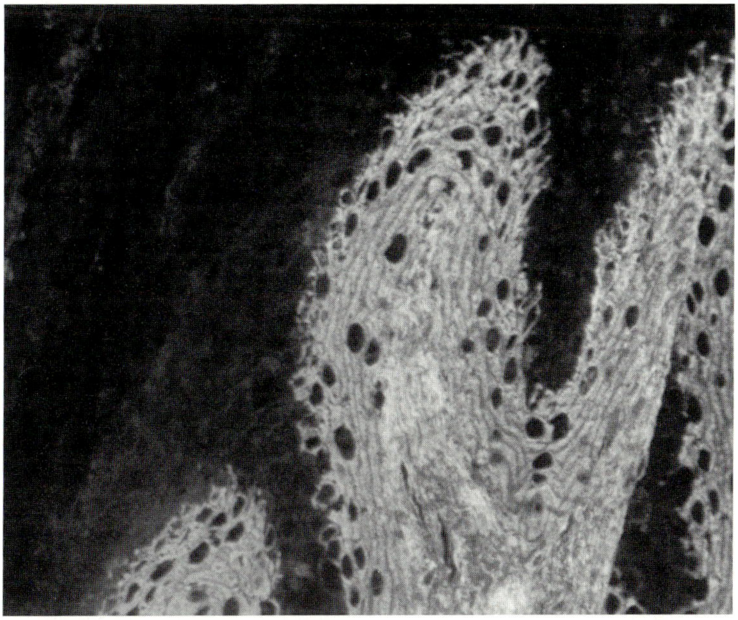

Figure 12. Indirect IF staining of monkey esophagus mucosa for cytoplasmic (homogeneous) staining (224×).

specific, but not species specific (Chaps. 41 and 42). An upper epidermal cytoplasmic (UEC) pattern is seen in equal frequencies (20%) both in normal human sera and in the sera of melanoma patients. Generalized epidermal cytoplasmic (GEC) staining, on the other hand, is found 2.5 times more often in melanoma patients than in normal control patients (18). Ackermann-Schopf found UEC staining in 86% of normal controls, whereas GEC staining was observed in sera of 9.5% of normal patients, in 29% of malignant melanoma patients, in 20% of patients with basal cell carcinoma, and in 16% of squamous cell carcinoma patients (2). We have observed four patients with cytoplasmic staining in titers of 40 or greater, and all four were found to have certain malignancies. These antibodies may be directed against keratin, as antikeratin antibodies raised in rabbits gave GEC staining (64; Chap. 42).

Didierjean and Saurat found that the sera obtained from bone marrow graft recipients who were positive for cytoplasmic antibodies also reacted with Hassall's corpuscles of the thymus (31, Chap. 40). The cross-reactivity of the cytoplasmic antibodies with the stratum corneum antibodies (reviewed in Chapters 39 and 41) has been confirmed in our laboratories.

Antibasal cell antibodies

Three types of anticytoplasmic antibodies directed against UEC, GEC, or the basal cell cytoplasm (BCC) have been observed. The first two, as already discussed above, are present in normal populations and in certain malignancies. The BCC antibodies are found in allergic skin reactions triggered by drugs, in burn toxemia, and in bone marrow graft recipients (42; Chap. 41).

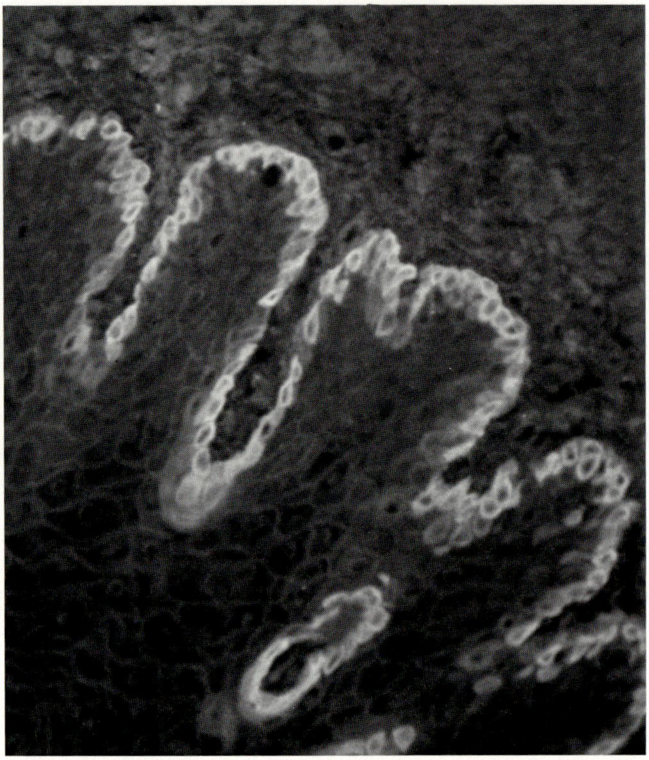

Figure 13. Basal cell cytoplasmic staining of the mucosal epithelial cells as revealed by IIF (224×).

The BCC antibodies exhibit organ specificity, but not species specificity, as they could be detected on stratified epithelia of different species (Fig. 13). However, there may be some differences in the quantity of these antigens expressed (41,43). Even though the precise nature of antigen reactive with BCC antibodies is not determined, it may be a calcium-binding protein of the type described by Saurat et al. (68). Skin calcium-binding protein is of cytoplasmic origin, and antibodies raised in rabbits against this antigen react with the BCC of stratified epithelia from guinea pig, rabbit, mouse, and humans.

Antiskeletal muscle antibodies

Myasthenia gravis is an autoimmune disease characterized by the presence of antibodies to acetylcholine receptors and to striations of the skeletal muscle (15,36,37). Strauss and coworkers (73) discussed the presence of skeletal muscle antibodies in the sera of patients with myasthenia gravis by IIF (Fig. 14). These antibodies are organ specific, but not species specific, as they react with cross-striations of skeletal muscles from many species. When tested on monkey esophagus, one must use the upper or middle third of the esophagus, in which adequate amounts of skeletal muscle fibers are present (51).

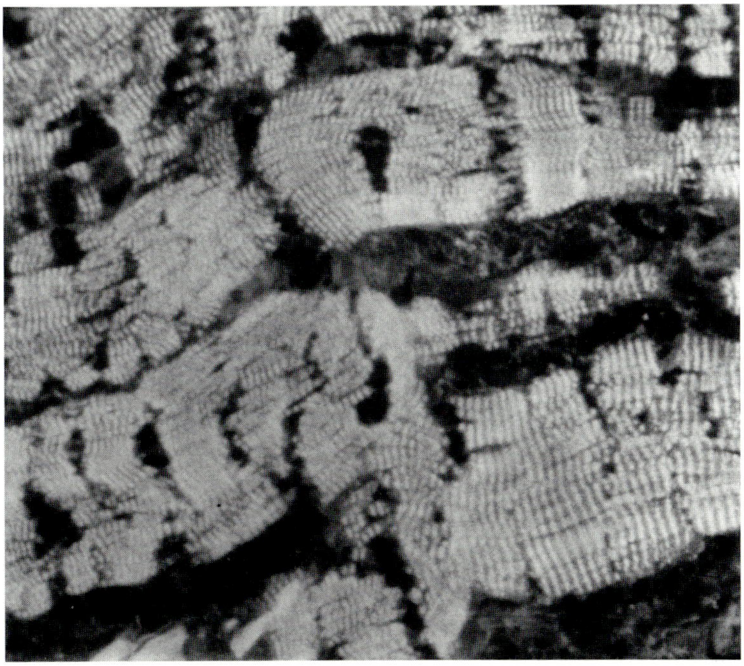

Figure 14. Indirect IF staining of cross-striations of the skeletal muscles localized primarily in the upper third of monkey esophagus (224×).

Antibodies against skeletal muscle are present in virtually all myasthenic patients with thymoma, and in 77% of thymoma patients without clinical symptoms of myasthenia gravis. Titers of 10 to 20 have been reported in 11% of myasthenic patients without thymoma and in 10% of normal control patients, whereas titers of 40 or greater are found primarily in patients with myasthenia gravis and thymoma. Those patients who are positive for antiskeletal muscle antibodies with thymoma are at a high risk for developing myasthenia gravis afterwards. Intervals of up to 22 years have been reported where myasthenia gravis developed in patients with a diagnosis of thymoma (58,63).

There seens to be an increased association of myasthenia gravis with other autoimmune diseases such as pemphigus (see Chaps. 8 and 10).

SUMMARY

Monkey esophagus is the antigenic substrate of choice for detecting antibodies of pemphigus, pemphigoid, and EBA, as well as the IgA class anti-EmA. In addition, it also detects other antibodies such as those to gliadin, ANA, ASMA, AMA, cytoplasmic, basal cell, and skeletal muscle antibodies. While monkey esophagus is the antigenic substrate of choice for serum studies on pemphigus, pemphigoid, HG, LABD, EBA, DH, and celiac disease, all studies must be done with proper controls to be acceptable and of diagnostic value.

REFERENCES

1. Abel EA, Bystryn J-C: Epidermal cytoplasmic antibodies: Incidence and type in normal persons and patients with melanoma. *J Invest Dermatol* 66:44–48, 1976.
2. Ackermann-Schopf C: Antibodies to basal epidermal cells in patients with basal or squamous cell carcinoma. *Arch Dermatol Res* 257:157–161, 1976.
3. Ackermann-Schopf C, Ackermann A, Terasaki PI, et al: Natural and acquired epidermal autoantibodies in man. *J Immunol* 112:2063–2067, 1974.
4. Acosta E, Ivanyi L: Comparison of the reactivity of various epithelial substrates for the titration of pemphigus antibodies by indirect immunofluorescence. *Br J Dermatol* 107:537–541, 1982.
5. Ajdukiewicz AB, Dudley FJ, Fox RA, et al: Immunological studies in an epidemic of infective short-incubation hepatitis. *Lancet* 1:803–805, 1972.
6. Andersen P, Small JV, Sobieszek A: Studies on the specificity of smooth muscle antibodies. *Clin Exp Immunol* 26:57–66, 1976.
7. Andersen P, Thestrup-Pedersen K, Ladefoged K: Studies of smooth muscle antibodies in acute hepatitis. *Acta Pathol Microbiol Scand C* 84:365–371, 1976.
8. Anderson HJ, Newcomer VD, Landau JW, et al: Pemphigus and other diseases. Results of indirect intercellular immunofluorescence. *Arch Dermatol* 101:538–546, 1970.
9. Ansel J, Petrozzi JW, Kumar V: Possible drug-induced pemphigus-like antibodies with the clinical manifestations of erythema multiforme. *Arch Dermatol* 119:1006–1009, 1983.
10. Berg PA, Baum H: Serology of primary biliary cirrhosis. *Springer Seminars Immunopathol* 3:355–373, 1980.
11. Beutner EH, Jordon RE: Demonstration of skin antibodies in sera of pemphigus vulgaris patients by indirect immunofluorescent staining. *Proc Soc Exp Biol Med* 117:505–510, 1964.
12. Beutner EH, Krasny SA, Chorzelski TP, et al: Evaluation of methods for detection of anti-centromere antibodies and other antinuclear antibodies. *J Am Acad Dermatol* 12:289–295, 1985.
13. Beutner EH, Lever WF, Witebsky E, et al: Autoantibodies in pemphigus vulgaris. Responses to an intercellular substance of epidermis. *JAMA* 192:682–688, 1965.
14. Beutner EH, Nisengard RJ, Kumar V: Defined immunofluorescence: Basic concepts and their application to clinical immunodermatology. In Beutner EH, Chorzelski TP, Bean SF (Eds): *Immunopathology of the Skin,* ed. 2. Wiley, New York, 1979, pp. 29–75.
15. Beutner EH, Witebsky E, Ricken D, et al. Studies of autoantibodies in myasthenia gravis. *JAMA* 182:46–58, 1962.
16. Blaszczyk M, Jablonska S, Beutner EH, et al: Substrate specificity of antinuclear antibodies (ANA) in scleroderma. *J Invest Dermatol* 68:191–193, 1977.
17. Bloom W, Fawcett DW: The esophagus and stomach. In Bloom W, Fawcett DW (Eds): *Textbook of Histology,* ed. 2. Saunders, Philadelphia, 1975, pp 639–657.
18. Burnham TK: The upper and general epidermal cytoplasmic immunofluorescent patterns. *J Invest Dermatol* 69:223–230, 1970.
19. Burnham TK: Two epidermal cytoplasmic immunofluorescent patterns detected by indirect immunofluorescence. *J Invest Dermatol* 62:100–106, 1974.
20. Bystryn J-C, Frances C: Cytoplasmic differentiation antigens of human epidermal cells. *Transplantation* 27:392–396, 1979.
21. Bystryn J-C, Nash M, Robins P: Epidermal cytoplasmic antigens: II. Concurrent presence of antigens of different specificities in normal human skin. *J Invest Dermatol* 71:110–113, 1978.
22. Chorzelski TP, Beutner EH: Factors contributing to occasional failures in demonstration of pemphigus antibodies by the immunofluorescence test. *J Invest Dermatol* 53:188–191, 1969.
23. Chorzelski TP, Beutner EH: Factors contributing to occasional failures in the laboratory diagnosis of bullous pemphigoid by indirect immunofluorescence. *Br J Dermatol* 86:111–117, 1972.
24. Chorzelski TP, Beutner EH, Jablonska S, et al: Report by Judd KP, Lever WF: Correlation of Antibodies in Skin and Serum with Disease Severity in Pemphigus. *Arch Dermatol* 116:1228–1229, 1980 (letter to the editor).

25. Chorzelski TP, Beutner EH, Sulej J, et al: IgA anti-endomysium antibody. A new immunological marker of dermatitis herpetiformis and coeliac disease. *Br J Dermatol* 111:395–402, 1984.
26. Chorzelski TP, Jablonska S, Beutner EH: Pemphigoid. In Beutner EH, Chorzelski TP, Bean SF (Eds): *Immunopathology of the Skin,* ed. 2. Wiley, New York, 1979, pp 243–255.
27. Chorzelski TP, Jablonska S, Beutner EH, et al: Anti-centromere antibody: An immunological marker of a subset of systemic sclerosis. *Br J Dermatol* 113:381–389, 1985.
28. Chorzelski TP, Beutner EH: Autoantibodies in some bullous diseases. *Ann NY Acad Sci* 177:224–226, 1971.
29. Chorzelski TP, von Weiss JF, Lever WF: Clinical significance of autoantibodies in pemphigus. *Arch Dermatol* 93:570–576, 1966.
30. Creswell SN, Black M, Bhogal B, et al: Correlation of circulating intercellular antibody titers in pemphigus with disease activity. *Clin Exp Dermatol* 6:477–483, 1981.
31. Didierjean L, Saurat JH: Epidermis and thymus. Similar antigenic properties in Hassall's corpuscle and subsets of keratinocytes. *Clin Exp Dermatol* 5:395–404, 1980.
32. Farrow LJ, Holborow EJ, Johnson GD, et al: Autoantibodies and the hepatitis associated antigen in acute infective hepatitis. *Br Med J* 2:693–695, 1970.
33. Faure M, Eisinger M, Bystryn J-C: Decreased expression of epidermal cytoplasmic antigens in cultured human keratinocytes. *J Invest Dermatol* 76:347–351, 1981.
34. Feibelman C, Stolzner G, Provost T: Pemphigus vulgaris. Superior sensitivity of monkey esophagus in the determination of pemphigus antibody. *Arch Dermatol* 117:561–562, 1981.
35. Fitzpatrick RE, Newcomer VD: The correlation of disease activity and antibody titers in pemphigus. *Arch Dermatol* 116:285–290, 1980.
36. Grob D (Ed): Myasthenia gravis. *Ann NY Acad Sci* vol. 274, 1976, 682 pp.
37. Grob D (Ed): Myasthenia gravis. Pathophysiology and management. *Ann NY Acad Sci* vol. 377, 1981, 902 pp.
38. Holborow EJ, Hemsted EH, Mead SV: Smooth muscle autoantibodies in infectious mononucleosis. *Br Med J* 3:323–325, 1973.
39. Jablonska S, Chorzelski TP, Blaszczyk M, et al: Immunologic phenomena in scleroderma. In Beutner EH, Chorzelski TP, Bean SF (Eds): *Immunopathology of the Skin,* ed. 2. Wiley, New York, 1979, pp 363–380.
40. Johnson GD, Holborow EJ, Glynn LE: Antibody to smooth muscle in patients with liver diseases. *Lancet* 2:878–879, 1965.
41. Joost T van: Incidence of circulating antibodies reactive with basal cells of skin in drug reactions. *Acta Dermatovener* 54:183–188, 1974.
42. Joost T van: Serum antibodies with affinity to the cytoplasm of epidermal basal cells. In Beutner EH, Chorzelski TP, Bean SF (Eds): *Immunopathology of the Skin,* ed. 2. Wiley, New York, 1979, pp 473–488.
43. Joost T van, Asghar SS, Cormane RH: Skin reactions caused by phenylbutazone. *Arch Dermatol* 110:939–933, 1974.
44. Jordon RE, Beutner EH, Witebsky E, et al: Basement zone antibodies in bullous pemphigoid. *JAMA* 200:751–756, 1967.
45. Jordon RE, Heine KG, Tappeiner G, et al: The immunopathology of herpes gestationis. Immunofluorescence studies and characterization of "HG factor." *J Clin Invest* 57:1426–1433, 1976.
46. Judd KP, Lever WF: Correlation of antibodies in skin and serum with disease severity in pemphigus. *Arch Dermatol* 115:428–432, 1979.
47. Katz S, Hertz KC, Yaoita H: Herpes gestationis. Immunopathology and characterization of the HG factor. *J Clin Invest* 57:1434–1441, 1976.
48. Krasny SA, Beutner EH: Experimental production of intercellular antibodies in monkeys. In Beutner EH, Nisengard RJ, Albini A (Eds): Defined Immunofluorescence and Related Cytochemical Methods. *Ann NY Acad Sci,* 420:343–352, 1983.
49. Kumar V, Beutner EH: Immunohistology of human autoantibodies on monkey esophagus. In Beutner EH, Chorzelski TP, Bean SF (Eds): *Immunopathology of the Skin,* ed. 2. Wiley, New York, 1979, pp 77–91.

50. Kumar V, Beutner EH: Autoimmunity and the skin. In Cruse JM (Ed): *Concepts in Immunopathology*. Karger, Basel, 1985, pp 318–353.
51. Kumar V, Beutner EH, Chorzelski TP: Distribution of monkey esophagus antigens reactive with IgA class antibodies in the sera of dermatitis herpetiformis patients. *Arch Dermatol Res* 276:293–296, 1984.
52. Kumar V, Beutner EH, Chorzelski TP, et al: Report by Nishikawa T, Kurihara S, Harada T, et al: Capability of Complement Fixation of Pemphigus Antibodies In Vitro. *Arch Dermatol Res* 263:239, 1978 (letter to the editor).
53. Kumar V, Binder WL, Schotland E, et al: Coexistence of bullous pemphigoid and systemic lupus erythematosus. *Arch Dermatol* 114:1187–1190, 1978.
54. Kumar V, Lerner A, Jain N, et al: Are antigliadin antibodies (AGA) specific for coeliac disease? *J Pediatr Gastroenterol Nutr* 3:815, 1984 (letter to editor).
55. Kumar V, Malviya AN, Beutner EH, et al: Mitochondrial antibodies—Heterogeneity and effects on mitochondrial respiration. *J Clin Lab Immunol* 2:325–328, 1979.
56. Kumar V, Yarbrough C, Beutner EH: Complement fixing intercellular antibodies in a case of cicatricial pemphigoid. *Arch Dermatol* 116:812–814, 1980.
57. Lane AT, Huff JC, Zone JJ, et al: Class-specific antibodies to gluten in dermatitis herpetiformis. *J Invest Dermatol* 80:402–405, 1983.
58. Lattes R: Thymoma and other tumors of the thymus. *Cancer* 15:1224–1260, 1962.
59. Lidman K: Clinical diagnosis in patients with smooth muscle antibodies. *Acta Med Scand* 200:403–407, 1976.
60. Ljunghall K, Lööf L, Grimelius L, et al: Dermatitis herpetiformis: Relation between circulating antibodies against reticulin and gluten, small intestinal mucosal status and absorptive capacity. *Acta Dermatovener* 63:27–34, 1983.
61. Maize JC, Dobson RL, Provost TT: Pemphigus and myasthenia gravis. *Arch Dermatol* 111:1334–1339, 1975.
62. O'Loughlin S, Goldman GG, Provost T: Fate of pemphigus antibody following a successful therapy. *Arch Dermatol* 114:1769–1772, 1978.
63. Oosterhuis HJGH, Feltkamp TEW, van Rossum AL, et al: HL-A antigens, autoantibody production and associated diseases in thymoma patients with and without myasthenia gravis. *Ann NY Acad Sci* 274:468–474, 1976.
64. Osborn M: Intermediate filaments as histologic markers: An overview. *J Invest Dermatol* 81:104s–109s, 1983.
65. Peck SM, Osserman KE, Weiner LB, et al: Studies in bullous diseases. Immunofluorescent serologic tests. *N Engl J Med* 279:951–958, 1968.
66. Provost TT, Tomasi TB Jr: Evidence for complement activation via the alternate pathway in skin diseases. I. Herpes gestationis, systemic lupus erythematosus and bullous pemphigoid. *J Clin Invest* 52:1779–1787, 1973.
66a. Sabolinski ML, Beutner EH, Krasny S, et al. Substrate specificity of anti-epithelial antibodies of pemphigus vulgaris and pemphigus foliaceus sera in immunofluorescence tests on monkey and guinea pig esophagus sections. J Invest Dermatol (in press)
67. Sams WM, Jordon RE: Correlation of pemphigoid and pemphigus antibody titers with activity of disease. *Br J Dermatol* 84:7–13, 1971.
68. Saurat JH, Diderjean L, Galoppin L, et al: Antibodies with affinity to the cytoplasm of keratinocytes produced after bone marrow transplantation in man. A review. In Thivolet J, Schmitt D (Eds): *Cutaneous Immunopathology,* vol. 80. INSERM, Paris, 1978, pp 77–92.
69. Saurat JH, Gluckman E, Didierjean L, et al: Anticorps anticytoplasme des cellules de l'epiderme humain. *Ann Dermatol Vener* 104:121, 1977.
70. Savilahti E, Perkko M, Kalimo K, et al: IgA anti-gliadin antibodies: A marker of mucosal damage in childhood coeliac disease. *Lancet* 1:320–321, 1983.
71. Schultheis HP, Berg P, Klingenberg M: The mitochondrial adenine nucleotide translocator is an antigen in primary biliary cirrhosis. *Clin Exp Immunol* 54:648–654, 1983.
72. Shu S, Nisengard RJ, Hale WL, et al: Incidence and titers of antinuclear, antismooth muscle and other autoantibodies in blood donors. *J Lab Clin Med* 86:259–265, 1975.
73. Strauss AJL, Segal BC, Hsu KC, et al: Immunofluorescence demonstration of muscle binding,

complement fixing serum globulin fraction in myasthenia gravis. *Proc Soc Exp Biol Med* 105:184–191, 1960.

74. Swana GT, Swana MR, Bottozzo GF, et al: A human specific mitochondrial antibody. Its importance in the identification of organ specific reactions. *Clin Exp Immunol* 28:517–525, 1977.
75. Unsworth DJ, Kieffer N, Holborow EJ, et al: IgA anti-gliadin antibodies in coeliac disease. *Clin Exp Immunol* 46:286–293, 1981.
76. Valnio E, Kalimo K, Reunala T, et al: Circulating IgA and IgG anti-gliadin antibodies to dermatitis herpetiformis detected by enzyme-linked immunosorbent assay. *Arch Dermatol Res* 275:15–18, 1983.
77. Weissmann V, Feuerman EJ, Joshua H, et al: The correlation between the antibody titers in sera of patients with pemphigus vulgaris and their clinical state. *J Invest Dermatol* 71:107–109, 1978.

4
Immunoelectron Microscopy and the Quantitation of Selected Immunohistochemical Methods

Immunoelectron microscopy (IEM) plays a significant role in selected aspects of immunopathologic studies of the skin (see Chaps. 8, 15, 20, and 23). It frequently employs horseradish peroxidase (HRP) labeling, as indicated in the first part of this chapter. HRP-labeled antibodies can be visualized in immunohistochemical studies by both light and electron microscopy. Two aspects of such studies are selected for inclusion in this chapter. The first part provides an overview of immunoelectron microscopic procedures, including both established methods such as HRP labeling and newer ones. The second part of this chapter delves into quantitative analyses of HRP labeling using selected multistep immunocytochemical techniques. Such quantitation is of central importance for generating a sound foundation for the use of HRP labeling in immunopathologic studies.

IMMUNOELECTRON MICROSCOPY TECHNIQUES: AN UPDATE

Boris Albini
Karl Holubar
Suyu Shu
Klaus Wolff

INTRODUCTION

Immunofluorescent (IF) staining procedures are well established in routine diagnostic and research immunodermatology (8,24; Chaps. 8 and 29). These techniques are now defined and standardized enough (see Chaps. 1 and 2) to provide for adequate specificity and sensitivity of reactions and for reproducibility and economy of tests. Nevertheless, IF techniques have some disadvantages: 1) fading of fluorescence (even though, recently, embedding media, e.g. a semipermanent mounting medium containing Elvanol [36], allow prolonged storage at the cost of some decrease in initial fluorescence intensity); 2) autofluorescence, which may interfere with specific staining; 3) nonspecific localization of the fluorochrome-antibody conjugates in tissues due to the negative charge of the dyes; 4) poor resolution at high magnification and restriction of IF staining procedures to light microscopy; and 5) the necessity of using special microscopes for reading the specimens. Because of these limitations, other methods of immunohistology have been explored. Thus, antibodies have been labeled with radioactive nuclides and used in autoradiography. This technique has the advantage of high sensitivity, and can be used in both light and electron microscopy (EM). However, the resolution is rather poor, especially at the ultrastructural level. Ferritin, a metalloprotein, has been used extensively for ultrastructural studies (40). It gives good resolution, but its large size substantially impairs tissue penetration and virtually prevents its use for localization of intracellular antigens. Heavy metals (e.g., mercury and uranium) have been used as markers in EM (41). These techniques were reported to be hampered by reduction of antibody reactivity upon adsorption of heavy metal to protein. However, the use of colloidal gold, proposed in 1971 by Faulk and Taylor (12), has recently been standardized, and it seems to be an excellent marker for immunoelectron microscopy (IEM) (see below). For scanning EM, preparations of antibodies adsorbed to latex particles have been used successfully (27). Currently, the most widely used markers for immunohistology besides fluorochromes are enzymes (1,11,41) and colloidal gold (17,23). The principles of both techniques have been reviewed widely in recent years (5,16,33,34). Basic considerations are discussed below. Potential application of these and other techniques to dermatologic problems are illustrated by a number of contributions in this volume (15,26) and by the corresponding chapter in the previous editions of this book (2).

In the enzyme-antibody methods, an antibody that is specific for the antigen to be detected is linked to an enzyme. An antigenic preparation (tissue sections or preparations of cells) is then allowed to react with the specific antibody. The antibody is localized at the site of antigens. The enzyme, which is linked to the antibody, subsequently catalyzes a specific reaction, transforming an inconspicuous substrate into a dye and/or an electron-opaque moiety. The end-product of this reaction is the histologic marker for the antigen-antibody reaction, as it precipitates at the site of the antigen. Enzymes may be linked covalently to antibodies, using a bivalent or multivalent coupling agent ("labeled enzyme-antibody method"). Alternatively, the antibodies that are specific for an antigen and for peroxidase may be linked by using immunologic mechanisms on the tissue section ("unlabeled enzyme-antibody method").

According to Sternberger (41), a reagent used in enzyme-antibody methods should be evaluated according to the following criteria:

1. The enzyme should be easily detectable by a cytochemical method, preferably one applicable to both light and electron microscopy. In order to provide high resolution, the enzyme reaction product should not diffuse away from the production site. The cytochemical substrate should have a high turnover number, with the enzyme in neutral buffers, which do not induce severe tissue damage.
2. The enzyme should be available in pure form.
3. Conjugation with immunoglobulin should not abolish enzyme activity, although it may impair it.
4. The enzyme should be fairly stable in a neutral solution.
5. The enzyme should have a relatively small molecular weight, since a small enzyme-conjugated antibody penetrates tissue better than a large enzyme-conjugated antibody.

6. Substrate-related enzymes should not be endogenous constituents of the tissues examined.

Monodispersed colloidal gold adsorbed to proteins is currently being used for a number of applications in IEM. Often, staphylococcal protein A is labeled in preference to antibodies. Using gold particles of two distinct sizes, double "staining" procedures can be performed with colloidal gold probes. In the following subsections, IEM employing enzymes, including horseradish peroxidase and colloidal gold probes, are discussed.

MARKERS AND ANTIBODIES

Enzyme Antibody Methods

Table 1 summarizes some characteristics of enzymes used in immunohistology. Alkaline phosphatase may be used for IEM. The wide distribution of endogenous enzyme, however, often poses annoying problems. Thus, alkaline phosphatase is very well suited for enzyme-linked immunosorbent assay (ELISA), but has not established itself firmly as a marker in immunohistology. Most widely used in IEM is horseradish peroxidase (HRP).

Horseradish Peroxidase

HRP is an oxidoreductase that catalyzes the transfer of hydrogen atoms from a donor (e.g, diamin) to an acceptor molecule (e.g., H_2O_2). It consists of an apoenzyme and protoporphyrin IX. HRP has an M_w of 40,000. It contains 1.27% iron. It is important to note that 70% ethanol or 10% buffered formalin do not impair the activity of HRP, but sodium azide does (11). Pure HRP has an RZ* value of 3. Only preparations of HRP with RZ higher than 2.5 should be used for enzyme immunohistology (11).

HRP is detected in histochemistry by a variety of reagents. For immunohistology, the method described by Graham and Karnovsky (18) is universally accepted. Under the influence of HRP, 3,3 diamino-benzidine (DAB) (a carcinogen) is oxidized in the presence of H_2O_2. The end-product is a polymer of DAB that has undergone cyclization. This end-product, which is rich in conjugated double bonds, appears with a brown color in normal light microscopy. After reaction with osmium tetroxide, it becomes electron-opaque. For optimal staining, DAB has to be well solubilized and used as a saturated solution in the presence of 0.001% H_2O_2. Optimal results are obtained if preparations are incubated with DAB for 15 to 60 minutes at room temperature or for 1 to 2 hours at 4°C.

Colloidal Gold

Monodispersed gold sols are obtained by reduction of an aqueous solution of chloroauric acid. The reducing agent can be varied and influences the size of the colloidal gold particles obtained. Use of phosphorus-saturated ether renders gold particles roughly 3 to 5 nm in diameter (12). Larger particles (10 to 15 nm) are obtained by reduction with sodium ascorbate, and particles with a diameter of 15 to 150 nm are harvested after reduction with sodium citrate (14,22). Whereas the largest particles are useful in light microscopy and scanning EM, gold particles measuring 3 to 20 nm seem optimal for

*RZ, Reaktionszahl (reaction number).

Table 1. Enzymes used in immunohistology

Trivial name	*Systemic name*	*Enzyme commission number*	*Source*	M_w	*pH Optimum*	*Class of protein*
Cytochrome C			Horse heart	12,000	5.0–8.0	Hemoprotein
Glucose oxidase	(beta-D-glucose:oxygen 1-oxireductase)	1,1,3,4	*Aspergillus niger*	160,000	4.0–7.0	Flavoprotein
Microperoxidase			Cytochrome C	1600	5.0–8.0	Hemepeptide
Peroxidase	(Donor:hydrogen-peroxide oxireductase)	1,11,1,7	Horseradish	40,000	7.0	Hemoprotein
Phosphatase, acid	(Orthophosphoric monoester phosphohydrolase II)	3,1,3,2	Wheat germ	55,000	4.0–5.5	
Phosphatase, alkaline	(Orthophosphoric) monoester phosphohydrolase I)	3,1,3,2	Chicken intestine	100,000	8.0–9.0	Zinc-metalloprotein
			Escherichia coli	85,000 (dimer:180,000)	8.0	Zinc-Mg-protein
Tyrosinase	(Monophenol, dihydroxy phenylalanin:O_2 oxidoreductase)	1,14,18,1	Mushrooms	128,000	6.0–7.0	Copper-metalloprotein

transmission EM. The methodology to obtain gold sols is described in laboratory protocols in the appendix of De Mey (10). Further reduction of gold particles by silver lactates increases their black color (21). As mentioned above, colloidal gold can be used in scanning EM, since it is an excellent emitter of secondary electrons.

Gold conjugates are becoming available commercially*; many of these preparations, however, may show large variations in size and tend to be rather large.

Antibody Preparations

For immunohistology, highly purified antisera should be used. The purification is best accomplished by the use of affinity chromatography (46). Crude antibody preparations increase significantly the amount of nonspecific staining and decrease the actual sensitivity of the method.

The availability of monoclonal antibodies (MCA) (30) has greatly improved IEM. The homogeneity of monoclonal preparations contributes to reduction of background staining. The monospecificity allows for reaction with one single epitope. However, the avidity of some MCA may be very low, and conjugation of MCA of the IgM class may be difficult. Most importantly, the monospecificity of MCA may paradoxically decrease the specificity for whole macromolecules. The epitope detected by the MCA used may not be present on all molecules of a defined species; for example, some of the MCA to IgD do not react with all the IgD molecules in a preparation; alternatively, an epitope may be shared by a number of molecular species; for example, a common epitope has been suggested to exist on DNA and cardiolipin. Since epitopes seem to be rather small (e.g., a few amino acids of a peptide), it does not seem surprising that cross-reactive epitopes may occur widely in nature. Monoclonals may be envisioned as "reading" letters of the immunologic alphabet, and polyclonal antibody preparations as syllables or words. Thus, in solving some problems of immunohistology, it may be advantageous to mix, prior to conjugation with markers, a number of MCA to obtain a well-defined polyclonal reagent.

TECHNIQUES FOR IMMUNOELECTRON MICROSCOPY

Tissue Fixation

In immunoenzyme methods for light microscopy, either unfixed frozen sections may be used or the same fixatives may be used as for IF staining procedures.

In specimens to be used for EM, the quest for a fixation becomes more problematic (1). A well-preserved ultrastructure is essential; but at the same time, the penetration of the tissue by the reagents should be as effective as possible. In addition, as with all immunohistology, the preservation of antigenicity is crucial for the outcome of the staining. Since alcohol and acetone destroy the ultrastructure (even though they provide good penetrability of tissue) and since glutaraldehyde preserves the ultrastructure, but inhibits penetration of tissues and destroys its antigenicity, only a compromise offers a workable solution. Thus, at present, 2 to 4% buffered paraformaldehyde, with or without 0.2% picric acid, is a commonly accepted fixative. Skin specimens are best cut in cubes (2 mm in diameter) and fixed for 1 hour at 4°C in 3% paraformaldehyde in 0.1 M phosphate-buffered saline (PBS) at pH 7.5. The fixative should contain 8.5% sucrose.

*For example, Geometric Data, Wayne, PA.

With the improved sensitivity of IEM, however, it is often possible to use tissues fixed in glutaraldehyde. For the detection of glycoprotein antigens, the periodate-lysine-paraformaldehyde fixative of MacLean and Nakane (29) seems, at present, to yield the best results. It is necessary to search for the optimal fixative for each single experiment. The interested reader is referred to monographs on fixation for EM for a better understanding of the basic mechanisms involved.

With epithelial antigens, both fixation and preservation of antigenicity are rather difficult to achieve. All the known fixation procedures inactivate the antigens relevant to pemphigus vulgaris and pemphigoid (45). Keratohyalin granule antigen and human-wart antigen, on the other hand, retain their antigenicity after fixation.

Endogenous HRP

Strong HRP reactivity is detectable in leukocytes, macrophages, and erythrocytes stained by the Graham and Karnovsky technique. Melanocytes, although known to possess HRP activity, do not exhibit staining after incubation with DAB (45). Therefore, the skin is very well suited for the use of HRP-antibody methods. In general, the background is much "cleaner" in HRP-antibody-reacted skin sections than in skin sections incubated with fluorochrome conjugates (Fig. 1). Even though some reports have been published showing nonspecific staining of nuclei, it seems that only very high concentrations of HRP-antibody preparations give such staining. Endogenous peroxidase can be blocked by simple procedures; for example, by periodate oxidation and by use of methanol and H_2O_2 or phenylhydrazine (20,43). It seems useful to also note that

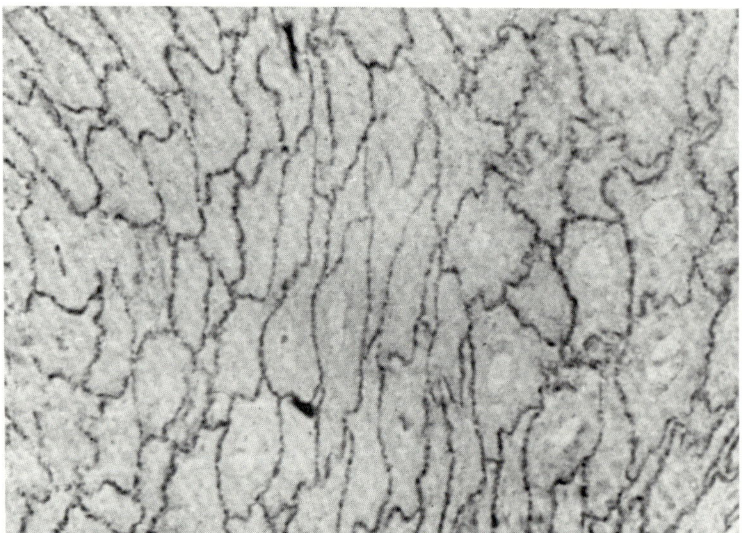

Figure 1. Indirect staining of monkey esophagus sections as antigenic substrate with pemphigus intercellular antibody and horseradish peroxidase antihuman IgG conjugate. (1000,× From Shu and Albini [38].)

alkaline phosphatase has been blocked successfully by incubation with levamisole or by periodate oxidation (6).

Controls

As in all immunohistologic methods, it is impossible to properly interpret the staining reactions with HRP and DAB, or IEM using colloidal gold probes, without controls. Controls must be performed with each test.

For the direct technique, these include: 1) the tissue incubated with an unrelated HRP- or colloid gold antibody conjugate, and 2) an unrelated tissue incubated with the same conjugate. For the indirect technique, the controls include: 1) the tissues incubated only with the conjugate, but without the serum to be tested, and 2) the tissues incubated with a normal serum from the same species from which the test serum or antibody are taken.

Added controls have to be performed when a new system is established. These controls are: 1) the inhibition of staining reaction by preincubation with unlabeled antiserum of the same specificity as that of the HRP- or colloidal gold antibody conjugate, although it should be kept in mind that inhibition may be accomplished by unrelated antibodies through steric hindrance; 2) the absorption of conjugate by the specific antigen; 3) when HRP is used, the incubation of the tissue section with DAB alone to control for endogenous peroxidase; and, if feasible, 4) the destruction of the antigen (e.g., of collagen by incubation with collagenase), repeating the test with this antigen-depleted preparation. In addition, parallel staining with a fluorochrome-conjugated antibody of the same specificity may be advantageous. Immunohistologic reactions should always first be performed and standardized using light microscopy. This is much more efficient and cost-effective than attempts to establish and define an IEM procedure by testing immediately at the ultrastructural level. Fortunately, both HRP and colloid gold techniques can be used with both light and electron microscopy.

Coupling of Markers to Proteins

Markers have to be linked to antibodies to achieve visualization of immunologic reactions. HRP can be linked covalently to antibody ("labeled enzyme-antibody staining") or antigen, and colloidal gold particles can be adsorbed to proteins. HRP may also be used in the "unlabeled enzyme-antibody method" without conjugation prior to staining; instead, in this procedure, the conjugation is established by immunologic reaction in the tissue.

A number of special procedures for indirect staining can be useful in EM. These methods usually increase sensitivity and allow for the use of more or less "universal" reagents; that is, reagents that can be applied to a number of "first-layer" antibodies. Cammisuli and Wofsy (7) have described a hapten sandwich technique. Antibodies are labeled with haptens, and antihapten antibodies are coupled to markers. All antibodies carrying a specific hapten can thus be visualized with one antihapten antibody marker conjugate. Since a large number of haptens interacts with one molecule of antibody, sensitivity of staining can be markedly enhanced. Finally, two antibodies with distinct specificities derived from the same animal species may be haptenized with two distinct haptens, and then used in double-staining procedures.

Another promising indirect staining method is the avidin-biotin method (19). The large egg white glycoprotein avidin binds the vitamin biotin with an extremely high binding constant (10^{15} per mol). Antibodies can be biotinilyzed with very good preservation of antigen-binding reactivity. Avidin can be coupled to fluorochromes, HRP, ferritin, or colloidal gold, and thus can visualize the site of the interaction of the biotinilyzed antibody with antigen. In addition, biotin may be interacted with the markers, rather than avidin; since avidin has four binding sites for biotin, large complexes can form composed of antigen-antibody coupled to biotin-avidin-biotin marker conjugate, enhancing the detectability of the reaction. Interactions of avidin with tissue biotin may be blocked (47).

Finally, staphylococcal protein A, a molecule reacting with the Fc portion of many immunoglobulin species (Table 2), may be coupled to a marker, thus yielding a homogeneous and stable "universal" reagent. Staphylococcal protein A is especially suited for use with colloidal gold (see below). Most recently, Fc-binding components have been characterized that are obtained from streptococci (35). These may soon be applied to immunohistology.

Labeled Enzyme-Antibody Staining

In the labeled enzyme-antibody methods, antigens are detected by antibodies coupled covalently to enzymes. In direct tests, antibodies coupled to HRP are allowed to react

Table 2. Reactivity of Staphylococcal Protein A and Streptococcal (Group C) Fc Receptors

Species	*Class of immunoglobulin*	*Protein A*	*Streptococcal Fc Receptor*
Man	IgG1	+	+
	IgG2	+	+
	IgG3	0	+
	IgG4	+	±
	IgM	±	
	IgA1	0	
	IgA2	±	
	IgD	0	
	IgE	0	
Mouse	IgG1	±	
	IgG2a	+	
	IgG2b	+	
	IgG3	0	
	IgM	0	
	IgA	0	
	IgE	0	
Rabbit	IgG	+	+
Rat	IgG	+	0
Guinea Pig	IgG	+	
Horse	IgG	+	
Sheep	IgG	±	+
Goat	IgG	±	+
Pig	IgG	+	+
Chicken	IgG	0	
Cow	IgG	0	+

with antigens present in tissues or cells. HRP-conjugated antibodies to immunoglobulins may also be used to detect antibody reactivity in sera, tissue eluates, or body fluids. In this "indirect test," tissue or cell preparations are first incubated with the serum to be tested for specific antibodies, and then the preparation is reacted with HRP-antiimmunoglobulin conjugates.

Conjugation of HRP with Antibodies

Originally, HRP and antibodies were incubated with a coupling agent, notably pp difluoro mm dinitrodiphenylsulfone (FNPS) (32) or glutaraldehyde (3). The conjugates obtained by this one-step method, however, were not very satisfactory. The linking agents establish not only links between HRP and the antibody, but also between molecules of antibodies or between molecules of HRP. To cope with these difficulties, two-step procedures have been developed for the conjugation of HRP with an antibody. Peroxidase is first reacted with glutaraldehyde and, in a second step, the peroxidase-aldehyde is reacted with the immunoglobulin (4). Similarly, carbohydrate moieties of HRP may be oxidized with sodium periodate to form aldehyde groups. In a second step, these aldehyde groups of the peroxidase react with α and η amino groups of the IgG (31). In this two-step procedure, it is claimed that 90 to 95% of the IgG used in the conjugation mixture is labeled with peroxidase (31).

HRP-antibody conjugates have M_w higher than 200,000. Using cytochrome c instead of HRP reduces somewhat the M_w. If microperoxidase (the active site of cytochrome c, with M_w 1600) is coupled to Fab fragments of the antibody, the M_w of conjugates may be decreased significantly, i.e. to 40,000 or 50,000. The preparation of microperoxidase, however, is somewhat laborious, and the end products are of variable quality.

To achieve defined staining with HRP conjugates, standardization of the components and procedures is necessary. It is crucial to characterize the HRP-antibody conjugate used.

The specificity of the antibody used may be tested in immunoprecipitation tests and in immunoelectrophoresis; methods developed to test specificity of a fluorescein isothiocyanate (FITC) conjugated antibody may also be used for HRP conjugates (see Chap. 1). The degree of labeling of antibodies, which reflects the staining efficiency per antigen-combining unit, may be estimated from the molar ratio of HRP to gamma globulin or antibody content (38). Total protein estimates, as used with FITC conjugates, are rather unsatisfactory, since HRP itself is a protein. Gamma globulin content may be estimated easily by means of radial immunodiffusion assays or rocket electrophoresis. Antibody content may be evaluated by the radial immunodiffusion assay (see Chap. 1) or by nephelometry. The HRP content is more difficult to evaluate. The HRP enzymatic activity is quantified by the "purpurogallin assay" (44). This test gives the most accurate data, but requires some experience and equipment for chemical work. Furthermore, it is time consuming. Radial immunodiffusion with anti-HRP serum incorporated into agar is a simple method, which gives less accurate but satisfactory results. The optimal working dilution of HRP conjugates may be found in direct tests by using a dilution series on the same antigenic substrate, and in indirect tests by testing the conjugate in chessboard titrations as described for FITC conjugates. The plateau titer and plateau endpoint behave in the same way in both FITC and HRP conjugate systems (38). When tested at the light microscopy level, HRP (in the one-step method) and FITC conjugates of the same antibody preparation showed comparable sensitivity in indirect tests (Fig. 2).

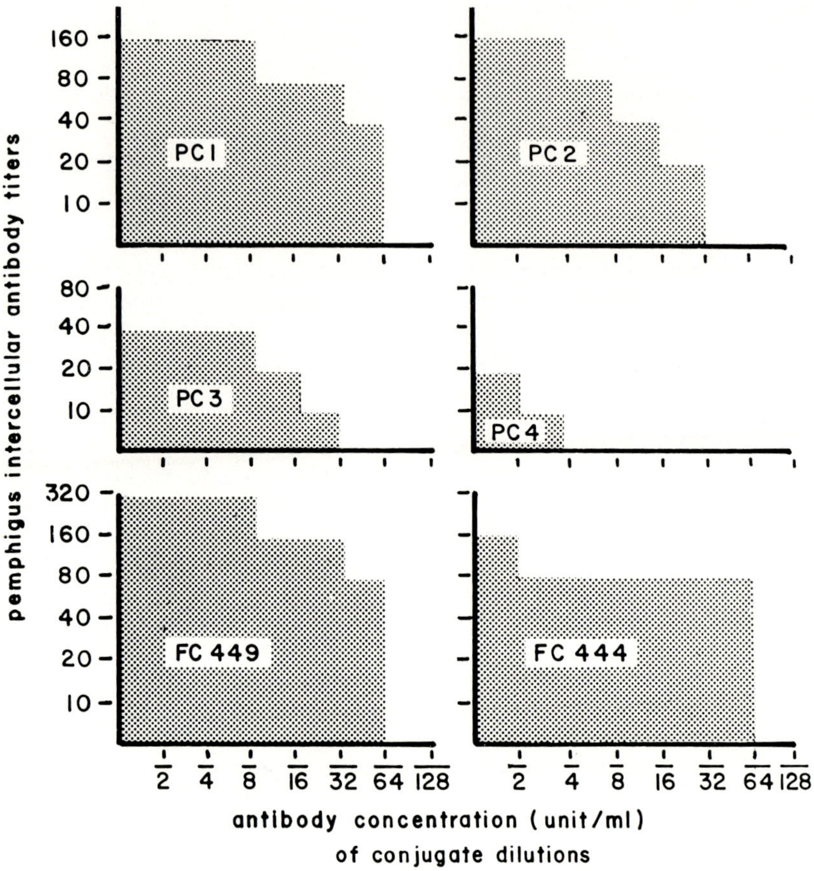

Figure 2. Chessboard titration of a serum containing pemphigus intercellular antibody with four horseradish peroxidase antihuman IgG conjugates and two FITC conjugates on monkey esophagus sections. (From Shu and Albini [38].)

Unlabeled Enzyme-Antibody Methods

Classic procedures of HRP conjugation to antibody produce molecules with a markedly decreased antibody activity. The penetration into tissue of HRP-antibody conjugates is more difficult than the penetration of immunoglobulins or HRP alone, because of the larger molecular size. Therefore, immunoenzyme techniques using unconjugated HRP antibodies have been developed (28). In these methods HRP is linked by a bridge consisting of two antibody molecules (Fig. 3). The final product of the HRP-mediated reaction is formed around the site of the specific antigen. This method is generally called the "triple-layer technique." It has yielded excellent results, as indicated in the second part of this chapter. Its main handicap is the difficulty in eluting antiperoxidase antibodies from the affinity chromatography column essential to purify the crude antiserum. Mostly low-affinity antibody is eluted; therefore the efficiency of the technique is greatly hampered (41).

A modification of this method, using peroxidase-antiperoxidase (PAP) complexes instead of antiperoxidase antibody and peroxidase in two steps, merits consideration in

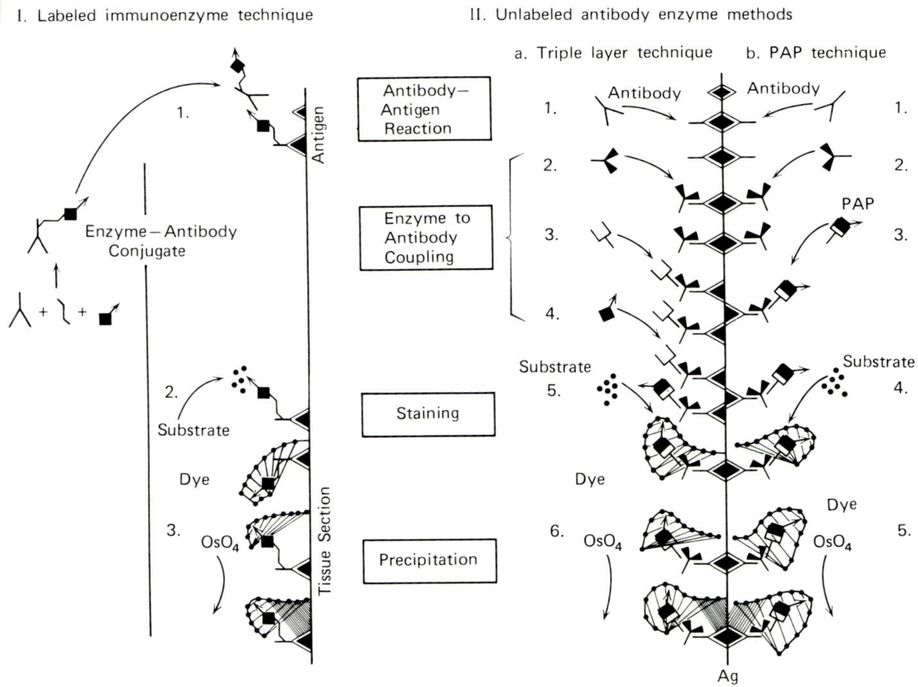

Figure 3. Labeled and unlabeled antibody enzyme methods.

Table 3. Immunohistologic Methods

	Use in			*Penetration*		*Resolution*		
Label	*LM*[a]	*EM*[b]	*Economy*	*EM*	*Sensitivity*	*LM*	*EM*	*Stand.*[c]
FITC	X		++++		++	++		+++
Rhodamine	X		++++		+	++		++
Autoradiography	X	X	+	+++	+++	+	+	±
Ferritin C[d]	(X)	X	++	+	++	(++)	+++	±
H[e]	(X)	X	+	++	++	(++)	+++	±
Enzymes L[f]	X	X	++	+	++	++	+	±
U[g]	X	X	+	+++	++++	+++	++++	±
Colloidal gold	X	X	++	++	+++	++	+++	±

[a]LM, Light microscopy.
[b]EM, Electron microscopy.
[c]Stand., Degree of standardization achieved.
[d]C, Conjugated ferritin to antibodies.
[e]H, "Hybrid" immunoferritin technique.
[f]L, Labeled antibody method.
[g]U, Unlabeled antibody method.

future studies on the immunopathology of the skin. If peroxidase is added to the elution fluid, antiperoxidase antibodies are eluted readily from the columns, and no selection of low-avidity antibodies is observed (41). Notwithstanding the fact that PAP is larger in size than the antibody or HRP alone, excellent results have been obtained with this technique in EM; antigens, including *Treponema pallidum,* ACTH, cartilage collagen in chickens, and type- and group-specific viral determinants have been detected (41).

The sensitivity of the PAP method seems to be 100 to 1000 times higher than IF staining or autoradiography, and therefore the reagents may be used in much higher dilutions than in many other methods of immunohistology.

Adsorption of Colloidal Gold to Proteins

The adsorption of colloidal gold to proteins is influenced by gold particle size, protein concentration, and pH. The ionic concentration of the buffer should be kept as low as possible during the reaction. Optimal adsorption is achieved with proteins that remain soluble at low salt concentration and a pH near their isoelectric point; these characteristics are best shown by staphylococcal protein A. Protein aggregates should be eliminated just prior to incubation with colloidal gold. Free protein, which may compete for binding sites with the labeled product, as well as unreacted gold particles are eliminated from the gold-protein conjugate by centrifugation. The conjugates are stored, after addition of 50% glycerol, at 4°C or at a temperature below the freezing point. A more detailed review and the necessary references are given by De Mey (10).

IMMUNOELECTRON MICROSCOPY FOR DETECTION OF CELL SURFACE MARKERS

Monoclonal antibodies (MCA) to cell surface markers are widely used in the analysis of inflammatory and lymphoid cell accumulations in tissue, as well as for the definition of Langerhans cells (LC) of the skin (13,25,37). The Langerhans cells, deriving from the bone marrow, have been shown to be able to replace monocytes in presenting antigens to T cells (42). Their role in contact allergy (39) and allograft rejection (32) has been well established. Since the routine fixatives affect cell surface markers detected by the OKT series of MCA (8), tissues should be used unfixed for incubation with the reagents. Obviously, cell surface markers can also be studied in cell suspension prepared from the epidermis (9).

Optimal results in immunohistology can be obtained only if in each specific case, the best technique is selected. Table 3 gives a rough outline of some preparations to be considered. It is based on the authors' own experience and does not make any claims for universal validity.

REFERENCES

1. Andres GA, Hsu KG, Seegal BC: Immunologic techniques for the identification of antigens or antibodies by electron microscopy. In Weir DM (Ed): *Handbook of Experimental Immunology.* Blackwell, Oxford, UK, 1978.
2. Albini B, Holubar K, Shu S, et al: Enzyme antibody methods in immunodermatopathology. In Beutner EH, Chorzelski TP, Bean SF (Eds): *Immunopathology of the Skin.* ed. 2. John Wiley, New York, 1979, pp. 93–134.
3. Avrameas S: Coupling of enzymes to protein with glutaraldehyde. Use of the conjugates for the detection of antigens and antibodies. *Immunochemistry* 6:43, 1969.

4. Avrameas S: Enzyme markers: Their linkage with proteins. *Histochem J* 4:321, 1972.
5. Beutner EH, Nisengard RJ, Albini B (Eds): Defined immunofluorescence and related cytochemical methods. *Ann NY Acad Sci* vol. 420, 1983.
6. Bulman AS, Heyderman E: Alkaline phosphatase for immunochemical labelling: Problems with endogenous enzyme activity. *J Clin Pathol* 34:1349, 1981.
7. Cammisuli S, Wofsy L: Hapten-sandwich labelling III. Bifunctional reagents for immunospecific labelling of cell surface antigens. *J Immunol* 117:1695, 1976.
8. Chu AC, Bhogal B, Black MM: Immunocytochemistry in Dermatology. In Polak JM, VanNoorden S (Eds): *Immunochemistry*. Wright PSG, Bristol, UK, 1983, p. 302.
9. Chu AC, Eisinger M, Lee JS, et al: Immune-electron microscopic identification of Langerhans cells using a new antigenic marker. *J Invest Dermatol* 78:177, 1982.
10. De Mey J: Colloidal gold probes in immunocytochemistry. In Polak J, VanNoorden S (Eds): *Immunocytochemistry*. Wright PSG, Bristol, UK, 1983, p. 82.
11. Essner E: Hemoproteins. In Hayat MA (Ed): *Electron Microscopy of Enzymes: Principles and Methods,* vol. 2. Van Nostrand Reinhold, New York, 1973, p 1.
12. Faulk WP, Taylor GM: An immunocolloid method for the electron microscopy. *Immunochemistry* 8:1081, 1971.
13. Fithian E, Kung P, Goldstein G, et al: Reactivity of Langerhans cells with hybridoma antibody. *Proc Natl Acad Sci USA* 78:2541, 1981.
14. Frens G: Controlled nucleation for the regulation of particle size in monodispersed gold suspensions. *Nature Phys Sci* 241:20, 1973.
15. Gammon WR, Wilson BD, Briggaman RA: Epidermolysis bullosa acquisita. This volume, chap. 20.
16. Gonda, MA: Immunoelectronmicroscopy. In Atassi MZ, van Oss CJ, Absolom DR (Eds): *Molecular Immunology*. Dekker, New York, 1984, p. 477.
17. Goodman SL, Hodges GM, Trejdosiewics L, et al: Colloidal gold markers and probes for routine application in microscopy. *J Microscopy* 123:201, 1981.
18. Graham RC, Karnovsky MJ: The early stages of absorption of injected horseradish peroxidase in the proximal tubules of mouse kidney: Ultrastructural cytochemistry by a new technique. *J Histochem Cytochem* 14:291, 1966.
19. Guesdon JL, Ternynck T, Avrameas S: The use of avidin-biotin interact in immunoenzymatic techniques. *J Histochem Cytochem* 27:1131, 1979.
20. Heyderman E: Immunoperoxidase techniques in histopathology: Applications, methods and controls. *J Clin Pathol* 32:971, 1979.
21. Holgate CS, Jackson P, Cowan PN, et al: Immunogold-silver staining—a new method of immunostaining with enhanced sensitivity. *J Histochem Cytochem* 31:938, 1983.
22. Horisberger M: Evaluation of colloidal gold as a cytochemical marker for transmission and scanning electron microscopy. *Biol Cellul* 36:253, 1979.
23. Horisberger M, Rosset J: Colloidal gold, a useful marker for transmission and scanning electron microscopy. *J Histochem Cytochem* 25:295, 1977.
24. Jablonska S, Beutner EH, Michel B, et al: Uses for immunofluorescence tests of skin and sera. *Arch Dermatol* 111:371, 1975.
25. Kung PC, Goldstein G, Reinherz EL, et al: Monoclonal antibodies defining distinctive human T cell surface antigens. *Science* 206:347, 1979.
26. Leonard JN, Haffenden GP, Ring NP, et al: Linear IgA bullous dermatosis in adults—the St. Mary's view. This volume, chap. 23.
27. Linthicum SD, Sell W, Wagner RM, et al: Scanning immunoelectronmicroscopy of mouse B and T lymphocytes. *Nature* 252:173, 1974.
28. Mason TE, Phifer RF, Spicer SS, et al: An immunoglobulin enzyme bridge method for localizing tissue antigens. *J Histochem Cytochem* 17:563, 1969.
29. McLean I, Nakane PK: Periodate-lysine-paraformaldehyde fixative—a new fixative for immunoelectronmicroscopy. *J Histochem Cytochem* 22:1077, 1974.
30. Milstein C, Galfre G, Secher DS, et al: Monoclonal antibodies and cell surface antigens. *Cell Biol Internatl Rep* 3:1, 1979.

31. Nakane PK, Kawaoi A: Peroxidase-labeled antibody. A new method of conjugation. *J Histochem Cytochem* 22:1084, 1974.
32. Nakane PK, Pierce GB: Enzyme-labeled antibodies: Preparation and application for the localization of antigens. *J Histochem Cytochem* 14:929, 1966.
33. Polak JM, VanNoorden S (Eds): *Immunocytochemistry.* Wright PSG, Bristol, UK, 1983.
34. Polak JM, VanNoorden S: *An Introduction to Immunocytochemistry: Current Techniques and Problems. Microscopy Handbooks 11.* Oxford University Press, Oxford, 1984.
35. Reis KJ, Ayoub EM, Boyle MDP: Streptococcal Fc Receptors I. Isolation and partial characterization of the receptor from a group C streptococcus. *J Immunol* 132:3091, 1984.
36. Rodriguez J, Deinhardt F: Preparation of a semi-permanent mounting medium for fluorescent antibody studies. *Virology* 12:316, 1960.
37. Rowden GR: Expression of Ia antigens on Langerhans cells in mice, guinea pigs and man. *J Invest Dermatol* 75:22, 1980.
38. Shu S, Albini B: Quantitative studies of peroxidase labeled antibody. I. Indirect staining system analyzed by chessboard titration. *J Immunol Meth* 13:341, 1976.
39. Silberberg I, Baer RL, Rosenthal SA: The role of Langerhans cells in contact allergy. 1. An ultrastructural study in actively induced contact dermatitis in guinea pigs. *Acta Derm Vener* 54:321, 1974.
40. Singer SJ: Preparation of an electron-dense antibody conjugate. *Nature* 185:1523, 1959.
41. Sternberger LA: *Immunocytochemistry.* Prentice-Hall, Englewood Cliffs, NJ, 1974.
42. Stingl G, Katz SI, Clement L, et al: Immunological functions of Ia-bearing epidermal Langerhans cells. *J Immunol* 121:2005, 1978.
43. Straus W: Inhibition of peroxidase by methanol and by methanol-nitroferricyanide for use in immunoperoxidase procedures. *J Histochem Cytochem* 19:682, 1971.
44. Sumner JB, Gjessing EC: A method for the determination of peroxidase activity. *Arch Biochem* 2:291, 1974.
45. Tappeiner G, Heine K, Jordon RE: Presence of immune complexes in pemphigus vulgaris sera as demonstrated by a Clq-binding assay. *Clin Res* 23:231A, 1975.
46. Triftshauser C, Hayden DW, Beutner EH: Procedures for the immunization of goats with human immunoglobulins and complement. *Int Arch Allergy Appl Immunol* 38:315, 1970.
47. Wood GS, Warnke R: Suppression of endogenous avidin-binding activity in tissues and its relevance to biotin-avidin detection systems. *J Histochem Cytochem* 29:1196, 1981.

QUANTITATIVE ANALYSES OF SELECTED UNLABELED ENZYME IMMUNOHISTOCHEMISTRY METHODS

Teresa Krainska

INTRODUCTION

The background and principles of the unlabeled enzyme-antibody methods are given in the first part of this chapter. This addendum summarizes both the results of quantitative analyses of the concentrations of the reagents used in two variants of these techniques (1–3) and their relationship to the results obtained. Based on these analyses, I make specific recommendations on optimal conditions.

Supported by a grant from the Warsaw Academy of Science.

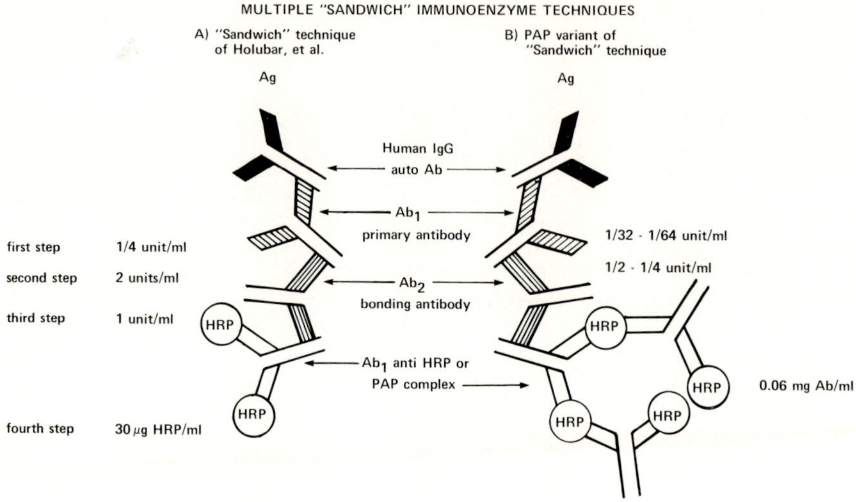

Figure 1. Concentrations of reagents recommended for unlabeled multistep immunoenzyme technique.

METHODS FOR UNLABELED ENZYME IMMUNOCHEMISTRY

One key factor for standardized methods is the activity of antibodies used in consecutive steps of the immunologic reaction. This may be expressed as units per milliliter of antibody activity. Units are defined in Chapter 1. Figures 1 specifies the optimal activity level for two variants of the multistep method.

Two examples of the "sandwich" method (1–4), which are listed as Type A and Type B in Table 4, are as follows:

	Type A	*Type B*
First step Ab_1	Rabbit antihuman	Goat antihuman
Second step Ab_2	Goat antirabbit	Rabbit antigoat
Third step	Rabbit anti-HRP or (PAP rabbit)	Goat anti-HRP or (PAP goat)

In this "sandwich" method of Holubar (1,2), it has been established that the optimal activity of antibodies (primary antibody: Ab_1) in the first step corresponds to about 0.25 U/ml; in the second step (for the bonding antibody; Ab_2), it is about 2 U/ml. The antibody activity in the third step (antibody directed against HRP) should be 1 U/ml. In the last step, 30 μg of HRP/ml is recommended.

A more suitable method for immunohistochemical reaction is the so-called peroxidase-antiperoxidase immune complexes or PAP method (3).

For optimal concentration of the antibodies reacting in consecutive steps, the following parameters should be taken into consideration:

1. Concentration and immunologic activity of Ab_1 and Ab_2.
2. Concentration of Ab_3 bound in PAP complex (the data provided by the company) and the concentration and enzymatic activity of peroxidase in PAP complex (enzymatic activity of HRP should be checked before use).

Table 4. Chessboard Titration of Immersions in First and Second Steps of PAP Method

Type A							Type B						
"Primary" Ab_1 rabbit IgG antihuman IgG		*"bonding" Ab_2 goat IgG antirabbit IgG*					*"Primary" Ab_1 goat IgG anti-human IgG (FITC)*		*"bonding" Ab_2 rabbit IgG antigoat IgG*				
Dilution	*Protein (Initial 10 mg/ml)*	*Ab activity (Initial 8 U/ml*	*Dilution: 1:16 IgG mg/ml: 0.17 U/ml: 1/4*	*1:32 0.08 1/8*	*1:64 0.04 1/16*	*PBS*	*Dilution*	*Protein (Initial 12.2 mg/ml)*	*Ab activity (Initial 16 U/ml)*	*Dilution: 1:16 IgG mg/ml: 0.1 U/ml: 1/2*	*1:32 0.05 1/4*	*1:64 0.02 1/8*	*PBS*
1:32	0.31	1/4	−	−	−	−	1:64	0.2	1/4	−	−	−	−
1:64	0.15	1/8	−	±	±	−	1:128	0.1	1/8	−	−	−	−
1:128	0.07	1/16	++	+	±		1:256	0.05	1/16	+	+	−	−
1:256	0.035	1/32	+++	++	+	−	1:512	0.025	1/32	+++	++	±	−
1:512	0.017	1/64	+++	++	+	−	1:1024	0.012	1/64	+++	+	±	−
1:1024	0.008	1/128	++/+	+	±		1:2048	0.006	1/128	+	−	−	−
	PBS		−	−	−	−		PBS		−	−	−	−
PAP complex Miles No. 862 (Rx), 0.046 mg Ab/ml							PAP complex Miles No. 667 (goat), 0.04 mg Ab/ml						

Table 5. Correlation Between Concentration of Antibodies and Enzymatic Activity in PAP Complexes and Results of Staining (Third Step) PAP Complex (Miles Lot No. 862)

	IgG mg/ml	0.09	0.046	0.023	0.01
	HRP mg/ml	0.12	0.06	0.03	0.015
	Purpurogallin U/ml	18.5	9.2	4.6	2.3
	ANA 1:320	+++	+++	++	±
	ANA 1:640	+++	+++	++/+	±
Serum	ANA 1:1280	+++	+++	+	−
dilution	ANA 1:2560	++	++/+	±	−
	ANA 1:5120	±	−	−	−
Controls	NHS 1:40	±	−	−	−
	PBS	−	−	−	−

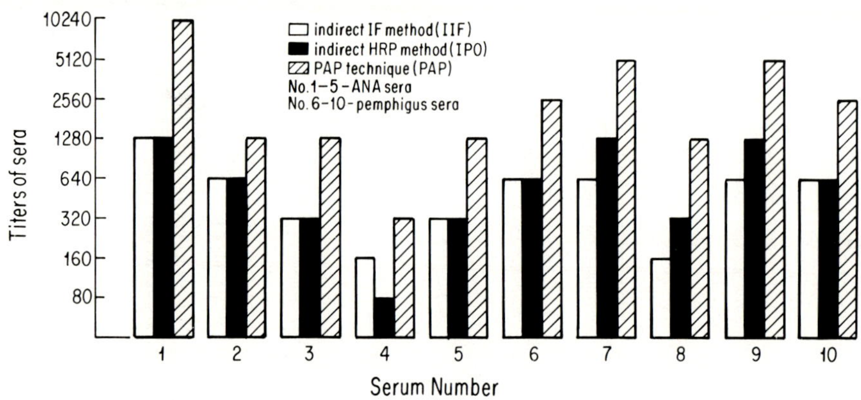

Figure 2. Titers of 10 sera as determined by three immunocytochemical methods.

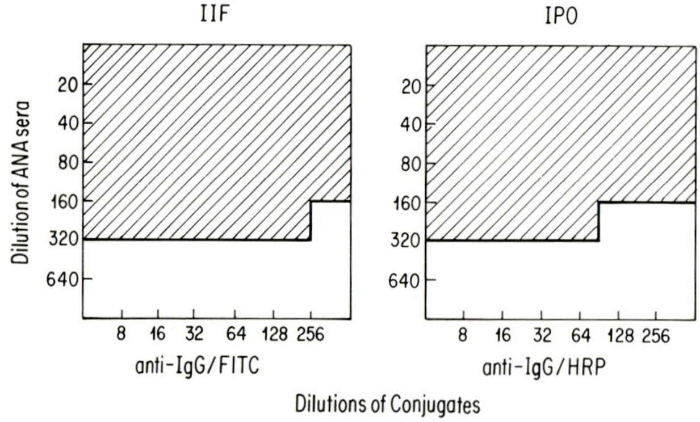

Figure 3. Chessboard titration with ANA containing serum with serial dilutions of FITC- and HRP-labeled antihuman IgG antibodies

The optimal immunologic activity of antibodies in the PAP method has been established for:

(see also Table 4).

Ab_1 1/32 to 1/64 U/ml (0.024 to 0.019 mg P/ml)

Ab_2 1/2 to 1/4 U/ml (0.1 to 0.17 mg Ab/ml)

The concentration of antiperoxidase antibody bound to peroxidase in commercial PAP complex (Miles) should be 0.090 to 0.046 mg Ab/ml, and the enzymatic activity of peroxidase should correspond to 9.2 to 18.5 purpurogallin U/ml (see Table 5).

It should be stressed that the excess or too low concentration of antibodies and too low enzymatic activity of peroxidase may result in false-negative findings. If Ab_1 is labeled with FITC, its antigenicity goes down and double concentrations of Ab_2 should be used.

SENSITIVITY OF METHODS

The sensitivity of the IIF and IPO* methods as compared to the PAP technique, using antinuclear antibodies (ANA) and pemphigus antibodies on monkey esophagus shows that the latter is four to eight times more sensitive (Fig. 2).

The chessboard titrations with a serum containing ANA depicted in Figure 3 show that the results obtained with IIF and IPO methods are comparable.

REFERENCES

1. Holubar K: Detection of immunoglobulins in skin of bullous dermatoses with a super sandwich technique. *Ann NY Acad Sci* 254:223, 1975.
2. Holubar K, Wolff K, Konrad K, et al: Ultrastructural localizations of immunoglobulins in bullous pemphigoid skin. *J Invest Dermatol* 64:220, 1975.
3. Sternberger LA: *Immunocytochemistry.* Prentice-Hall, Englewood Cliffs, NJ, 1974.
4. Sternberger LA, Hardy Ph Jr, Cuculis JJ, et al: The unlabeled antibody enzyme method of immunohistochemistry. Preparation and properties of soluble antigen-antibody complexes (horseradish peroxidase-anti-horseradish peroxidase) and its use in identification of spirochetes. *J Histochem Cytochem* 18,315:33, 1970.

*See abbreviations list at beginning of volume.

5
The Detection of Circulating Immune Complexes

Thomas J. Lawley
Kim B. Yancey

INTRODUCTION

The role of immune complexes in the pathophysiology of cutaneous diseases has received notable attention in the past few years (16,32). This is partly due to the development of a variety of relatively sensitive assays that will detect circulating immune complexes (CIC) in biological fluids (15). Immune complexes, for the purpose of discussion, can be divided into two broad categories. First, there are immune complexes formed in situ. In this situation, circulating antibody binds to a tissue-fixed antigen to form an immune complex, which remains at the site of antigen-antibody interaction. Examples of this type of immune complex formation would include the binding of circulating antibody to the respective relevant antigens in pemphigus vulgaris, bullous pemphigoid, and herpes gestationis (HG). The other broad category of immune complexes are those formed in the fluid phase and circulating freely before being cleared from the circulation or depositing in tissues and causing tissue damage. Examples of diseases associated with this type of immune complex include various forms of leukocytoclastic angitis and serum sickness. In this chapter, we will concentrate on a review of the methods of detection of CIC. Several of the most widely used immune complex assays will be discussed in detail as well as the interpretation of results generated by these assays.

An issue that should be dealt with at the outset is that none of the assays widely used for the detection of CIC are antigen specific. This means that both false-positive and false-negative results can occur in all assay systems. Additionally, it must be noted that even if CIC are detected in a given situation, it does not necessarily mean that the CIC are important in the pathogenesis of the disease process. The CIC may be formed secondary to ongoing tissue destruction, or they may be totally unrelated to the disease. Therefore, interpretation of results should be made with these caveats in mind. Despite these potential drawbacks, the development of reliable assays for CIC and their subsequent implementation in a variety of disease states have demonstrated that CIC are much more common than initially suspected. They have been detected not only in diseases where one might reasonably expect them, such as systemic lupus erythematosus (SLE), serum sickness, and necrotizing vasculitis, but also in a wide variety of infectious, neoplastic, and miscellaneous nonrheumatologic conditions where CIC were not thought to be important. Evidence that CIC play a role in the pathogenesis of a given disease depends upon several factors: 1) demonstration of CIC in most patients with the disease; 2) demonstration of substantial levels of CIC by several different assays that depend upon different immunochemical characteristics of the immune complexes; 3) correlation between immune complex levels and disease activity; and 4) evidence of deposits of immune complexes in target organs. There is little question that any disease fulfilling all these criteria is mediated at least in part by CIC. In most situations, only one or two of these criteria are met and, subsequently, the role of immune complexes is much less clear.

The reason that the detection of CIC is of scientific and clinical interest is that CIC can cause tissue damage and may also influence the immune response. The evidence that CIC can induce clinical disease first evolved from the observations of von Pirquet and Schick (30). In the early 1900s, they noted that almost all individuals who were injected with substantial amounts of horse antiserum to diphtheria toxin developed a syndrome characterized by fever, leukopenia, arthralgias, and urticaria that they termed serum sickness. Since this syndrome developed 8 to 12 days after the patients were first exposed to the horse serum, von Pirquet and Schick felt that the reaction was not due to a direct toxic effect of the antiserum, but rather to an immune response in the host. They suspected that host factors were combining with horse proteins and that the products of this interaction were in some way responsible for the clinical syndrome in their patients. It was not until the 1950s that significant scientific insights were achieved in this area, when Germuth and Dixon developed animal models of serum sickness in rabbits (6,9). In Dixon's model of "one-shot" serum sickness, a radiolabeled foreign protein was injected intravenously into nonimmune rabbits and its removal from the circulation was monitored. In addition, the interaction of the foreign protein with inflammatory mediators and the clinical condition of the rabbits were also studied. It was found that on about day 8, as the concentration of foreign antigen slowly decreased due to normal degradative processes, several events occurred more or less simultaneously. First, the concentration of the foreign antigen in the serum of the rabbits began to fall precipitously. Likewise, CIC began to form that contained the foreign protein as antigen, and serum complement levels began to fall. Shortly thereafter, the animals became ill, developing carditis, arteritis, and glomerulonephritis. Examination of the affected tissues by immunofluorescence (IF) techniques revealed the deposition of antigen, antibody, and complement in areas of tissue damage. These experiments provided direct evidence for the role of CIC in the pathogenesis of serum sickness.

These in vivo observations stimulated interest in immune complexes and raised questions about the properties of these immunoreactants that influence their biological function. For example, both antigen valence and antibody valence can greatly affect how an immune complex will behave in vivo. A large multivalent antigen has more antibody binding sites, is better able to form cross-links within the immune complex matrix, and thus will tend to form larger immune complexes than small univalent antigens. Although these large immune complexes are usually efficiently removed from the circulation by the reticuloendothelial system, they are also more likely to cause tissue damage.

Antibody class is also an important determinant of the biological behavior of immune complexes. Immune complexes that contain IgM or IgG (subclasses 1, 2, or 3) can activate the classic complement pathway, whereas IgA immune complexes are able to activate complement only through the alternative pathway. In contrast, IgD and IgE are not thought to activate the complement system efficiently. A recent series of in vitro observations suggest that immune complexes may also be modified by the complement system to form complexes with different immunochemical and biological properties. Miller and Nussenzweig, and subsequently other investigators, have noted that precipitated or insoluble immune complexes may be solubilized by complement (25,31). Specifically, it appears that bound immune complexes may interact with alternative pathway complement components, which results in the incorporation of large amounts of the C3b fragment of C3 into the lattice of the immune complex. This causes disruption of the existing precipitated immune complexes and results in the formation of smaller, soluble immune complexes with altered antigen-antibody ratios that have decreased affinity for Fc IgG and C3 receptors on cell membranes. The exact relevance of these observations to the in vivo situation is not clear, but these findings underscore the complexity of the types of interactions involving these mediators.

Not only are the characteristics of antigen and antibody important in determining the fate of immune complexes, but their molar ratio at the time of formation is also critical (Fig. 1). Immune complexes formed at antigen-antibody equivalence, slight antibody excess, or slight antigen excess are larger than those formed at large antigen or large antibody excess. These larger complexes are usually removed from the circulation rapidly. Immune complexes formed at moderate antigen excess are intermediate in size and

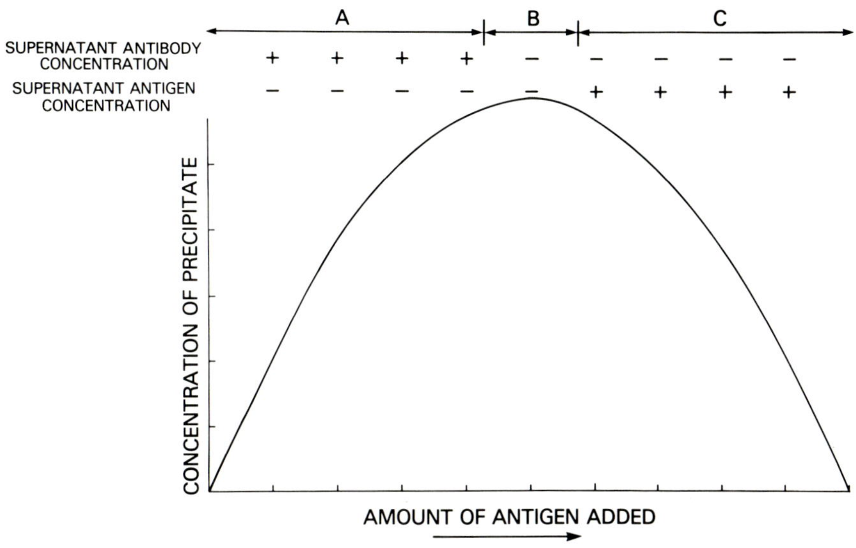

Figure 1. Schematic representation of a precipitin reaction. Increasing amounts of antigen are incubated with a constant volume of antibody, and the resultant immune complexes form immunoprecipitates that can be removed by centrifugation. The supernatants and the precipitates can then be analyzed for their content of antigen and antibody. A. Immune complexes formed in antibody excess consist of Ab_nAg_1 where n equals the number of antibody molecules bound to each molecule of antigen. At large antibody excess, n is an estimate of antigen valence. Immune complexes decrease in size as the ratio of antibody to antigen increases due to decreased lattice formation. B. At equivalence, large, heavily cross-linked immune complexes form and precipitate. Theoretically, no free antigen or antibody remain in the supernatant. C. In antigen excess, antibody-binding sites are saturated, the complex Ag_2Ab tends to predominate, and the size of immune complexes decreases as lattice formation is limited by antibody availability. (With permission from Yancey KB, Lawley TJ: Circulating immune complexes: Their immunochemistry, biology, and detection in selected dermatologic and systemic diseases. *J Am Acad Dermatol* 10:711, 1984.)

are thought to have maximal pathogenic potential, since they are able to activate complement efficiently yet are not as rapidly cleared from the circulation as complexes formed at equivalence.

The reticuloendothelial system (RES), also known as the mononuclear phagocyte system, is responsible for the removal of CIC from the circulation. The RES consists of tissue-fixed macrophages in the liver, spleen, lung, lymph nodes, kidney, and other organs, as well as in circulating phagocytic cells. Immune complexes bind to cell surface receptors for the Fc portion of IgG or to receptors for complement, especially C3. In most instances, phagocytosis seems to occur via the Fc IgG receptor, although under certain circumstances, phagocytosis mediated by C3 receptors can also occur. Mannik and coworkers have demonstrated that large immune complexes are removed from the circulation more efficiently than small complexes, that most are removed by the liver, and that saturation of the RES by injection of large amounts of immune complexes can prevent the efficient clearance of even large immune complexes (21,22). This can result in prolonged circulation of the large-size and intermediate-size immune complexes, tissue deposition of the immune complexes, and tissue damage.

The precise events that result in tissue damage following immune complex deposition are not known. However, available evidence suggests that immune complexes leave blood vessels following separation of the tight junctions between endothelial cells lining the vessel walls. This separation, in certain animal models of vasculitis, appears to be caused by vasoactive amines such as histamine or serotonin, which can be generated by triggering the release of mast cell contents, or by factors released from platelets or neutrophils. Once the immune complexes have lodged in the vessel walls, they may activate the complement system, resulting in the generation of a number of biologically active cleavage fragments. Of special interest is C5a, which is the 11,000 dalton cleavage fragment of C5. C5a is a potent chemoattractant for polymorphonuclear neutrophils, and is a potent anaphylatoxin that causes mast cell degranulation with release of a variety of soluble mediators including histamine. The accumulation of neutrophils in the area of immune complex deposition is followed by their phagocytosis of immune complexes, as well as by the release of their lysosomal enzymes. These enzymes, including elastase, kinin-activating enzymes, and others, are all potentially damaging to tissue and may lead to destruction of the blood vessel wall.

IMMUNE COMPLEX ASSAYS

The purpose of this section is to provide an overview of a selected number of immune complex assays currently available. Several of the more commonly used assays are described in some detail. The reader should keep in mind the fact that none of these assays is antigen specific, and that all of them may generate both false-positive and false-negative results. The specific substances or conditions that can commonly generate spurious results often vary from assay to assay and are discussed for those assays presented in detail.

Physical Methods

Cryoprecipitation

An early technique for detecting antigen-antibody complexes was that of examining serum for the presence of a cryoprecipitate. This visible, insoluble protein precipitate may form when serum remains at 4°C for 12 to 96 hours. Cryoprecipitates often represent relatively insoluble macromolecular immune complexes present in serum. However, they may also represent monoclonal proteins such as IgG or IgM cryoglobulins, cryo-Bence-Jones proteins, or even cryoprecipitable IgA. Mixed cryoglobulins—cryoprecipitable proteins which on analysis are found to be composed of two different immunoglobulin classes—are often associated with connective tissue disease and may themselves represent CIC that are cold insoluble (2,10). They are usually present in relatively small amounts, and often have anticomplementary (i.e., complement-fixing ability) or rheumatoid factor-like activity. The cryoprecipitation technique has the important advantage of simplicity, although care must be exercised in drawing and processing the blood to ensure that its temperature does not fall below 37°C prior to testing. Its major defects are that it lacks sensitivity and specificity, since not all CIC are cryoprecipitable. For these reasons, other more sensitive and specific tests have been developed.

Polyethylene Glycol Precipitation

Polyethylene glycol (PEG), at appropriate concentrations, will preferentially precipitate macromolecular immunoglobulin leaving uncomplexed immunoglobulin in solution. Antigen-antibody complexes have decreased solubility at 4°C, particularly when they are composed of relatively large protein aggregates. This relative insolubility can be greatly increased by the addition of PEG. Although this PEG precipitation method is a more sensitive assay than simple cryoprecipitation, the conditions of precipitation are critical. Several immune complex assays that use PEG precipitation have been described. In one method, 0.1 ml of serum is mixed with 0.1 ml of a 4% solution of PEG in phosphate-buffered saline (PBS) and is incubated for 1 hour at 4°C (4). The pellet is washed with 2% PEG and resuspended in 0.1 ml of PBS. The IgG, IgA, and IgM concentrations in the resuspended precipitate are measured and compared to the concentrations present in serum. The percentage of immunoglobulins precipitated by 4% PEG in excess of two standard deviations from the normal mean is considered to be in the form of immune complexes. While quite easily performed, lack of sensitivity and specificity are drawbacks of this technique.

Other physical methods of immune complex detection that are rarely used because they are either cumbersome or technically difficult include analytic and preparative ultracentrifugation and gel filtration techniques (15).

BIOLOGICAL METHODS

Complement-Dependent Assays

Since one of the best known features of IgG- and IgM-containing CIC is their ability to fix complement, this property has been used to devise various assays to detect their presence. Three basic complement-immune complex interactions have been used to detect CIC. The first group uses the ability of IgG- and IgM-containing immune complexes to bind Clq (a subcomponent of Cl) into the lattice of the complex. The second group uses the ability of a bovine protein known as conglutinin to bind to the C3bi fragment of C3 present in immune complexes. The third type of assay system uses the ability of solid-phase antibody to bind to complement already fixed in the immune complex lattice.

^{125}I-Clq Binding Assay

The ^{125}I-Clq binding test is based on the ability of purified human Clq (M.W. 400,000) to bind noncovalently to immune complexes whose antibody is either IgG_1, IgG_2, IgG_3,

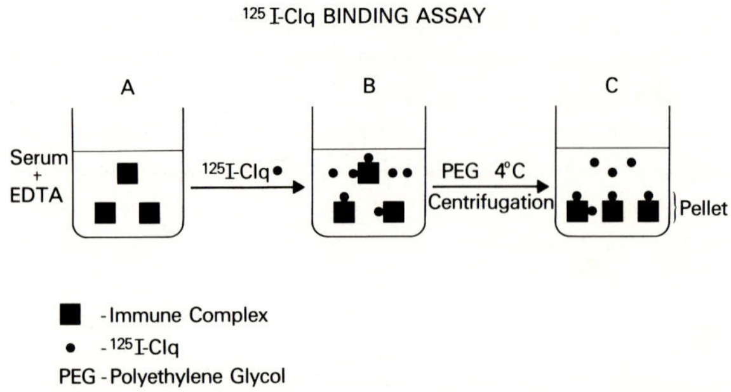

Figure 2. ^{125}I-Clq binding assay. This assay is performed by mixing human serum samples with ethylenediaminetetraacetic acid (EDTA) to dissociate native Cl into subcomponents Clq, Clr, and Cls. This dissociation presumably allows incorporation of ^{125}I-Clq into native Cl bound to immune complexes in the test sample. Free Clq is separated from Clq bound to immune complexes by precipitation with PEG at 4°C. Sample tubes are then centrifuged, and the amount of radioactivity precipitated is used as an index of IgG- or IgM-containing circulating immune complexes present in the test sample.

or IgM (Fig. 2) (27). The assay is performed by mixing human serum with ethylenediaminetetraacetic acid (EDTA), in order to dissociate native Cl into the subcomponents Clq, Clr, and Cls. Presumably, this dissociation facilitates exchange between the exogenous ^{125}I-Clq added and the native Clq,r,s complex, which may be bound to the complexes in the serum sample. The EDTA-serum mixture is then allowed to react with ^{125}I-Clq. Free Clq is then separated from Clq bound to immune complexes by precipitation with PEG, and the amount of radioactivity precipitated is quantitated. Results can be expressed as percentage of ^{125}I-Clq precipitated, or it can be referred to a standard curve generated by reacting ^{125}I-Clq with normal human serum containing various amounts of aggregated human gamma globulin (AHG) and expressed as microgram equivalents of AHG. The test is sensitive, highly reproducible, and does not give false-positive results in sera containing bacterial endotoxin or DNA, since these substances are quite soluble in the low-strength PEG solution used in this assay. However, heparin and other anticoagulants will cause falsely elevated values in this assay.

Clq Solid-Phase Assays

The solid-phase Clq radioassays use purified C1q that has been attached to the sides of plastic test tubes in which test sera are subsequently incubated (13,18). A radiolabeled or enzyme-linked antihuman immunoglobulin is added, and the antiserum binds immunoglobulin in the immune complexes that have attached to the solid-phase C1q. The amount of label bound is a measure of the immune complex level in the serum. These assays are immunoglobulin specific, because the indicator substance is a heavy chain-specific anti-immunoglobulin. Substances such as DNA, endotoxin, and polyanions will not cause false-positive results, but the presence of rheumatoid factors in the test serum will interfere with the assay.

Conglutinin-Binding Assays

Conglutinin is a high molecular weight (M.W. 750,000), nonimmunoglobulin protein found in certain bovine sera. Conglutinin will bind to a particular cleavage product of C3 known as C3bi. Since the conversion of immune complex-bound C3b to C3bi takes place within a matter of minutes and the conglutinin has a strong affinity for immune complex-bound C3bi, several immune complex assays have been developed using solid-phase conglutinin (3,7). Plastic tubes are coated with purified conglutinin, and test sera are incubated in them. Immune complexes with bound C3bi will adhere to the test tube-bound conglutinin. A radiolabeled, purified anti-IgG antibody is added, and the amount of radioactivity remaining after thoroughly washing the reaction tubes is a measure of immune complexes in the test sera. These assays are sensitive and easy to perform, but because of the relatively short half-life of C3bi (1 to 8 hours) before it is converted to C3d, they will detect only part of the immune complexes that have bound C3.

Solid-Phase Anti-C3 Assay

In this assay, the $F(ab')_2$ fragment of an antihuman C3 antibody is bound to a solid-phase matrix (29). The test serum is incubated with the solid-phase anti-C3, and then radiolabeled antihuman IgG is added. The amount of radioactivity bound is an indicator of the amount of C3-containing IgG CIC present in the test serum. This assay is sensitive and not affected by nonimmune complex substances such as polyanions, endotoxin, or rheumatoid factor.

Anti-C3 ELISA Assay

A variation of the anti-C3 assay devised by Hall uses enzyme-linked immunosorbent assay (ELISA) technology (Fig. 3) (12). In this system, antiserum to human C3 and its various fragments is bound to the bottom of plastic wells. After incubation with an appropriate dilution of the test serum, peroxidase-conjugated antibody, which is specific for the heavy chain of an immunoglobulin class (IgG, IgM, or IgA), is added. Bound antibody then undergoes color development by adding a diaminobenzidene-containing medium, and the amount of absorbance at 492 nm is a measure of the amount of immune complexes contained in the serum sample.

IMMUNOGLOBULIN-DEPENDENT ASSAYS

Reactions with Rheumatoid Factors

Rheumatoid factors (RF) are IgM or IgG immunoglobulins that bind to antigenic sites on IgG molecules. RFs bind more avidly to aggregated IgG or IgG complexed with antigen than to monomeric IgG, and can thus be used to detect CIC. The RF protein molecules may be polyclonal or monoclonal in type. Polyclonal RFs (pRFs) are found in the sera of patients with rheumatoid arthritis (RA) and also in some patients with other CTDs. Monoclonal rheumatoid factors (mRFs) are found in the sera of some patients with lymphoproliferative diseases. Radioimmunoassays employing mRF and pRF that are quite sensitive and reproducible have been developed. A double-antibody radioimmunoassay, with pRF acting as the primary antibody and rabbit antihuman IgM as the secondary antibody, has been described (5). Immune complexes of the IgG type will bind to pRF, and thus inhibit the precipitation of aggregated ^{125}I-IgG by the antihuman IgM. A solid-phase radioimmunoassay using mRF has also been developed (20). In this test, purified mRF is conjugated to microcrystalline cellulose, and is then mixed with the test serum and aggregated ^{125}I-IgG. The degree of inhibition of binding of the aggregated ^{125}I-IgG to the solid-phase mRF is used as a measure of the amount of immune complexes in the test serum. Another assay employing mRF is that described by Lurhuma et al. (19). This is based on the ability of immune complexes to inhibit the agglutination of IgG-coated latex particles. Gabriel and Agnello have used a sensitive

DETECTION OF CIRCULATING IMMUNE COMPLEXES BY ELISA

1. Goat anti-human C3 adsorbed to plate
2. Human Serum added
3. Goat anti-human IgA, IgG, or IgM (peroxidase conjugated) added
4. Enzyme substrate added and $O.D._{492}$ determined

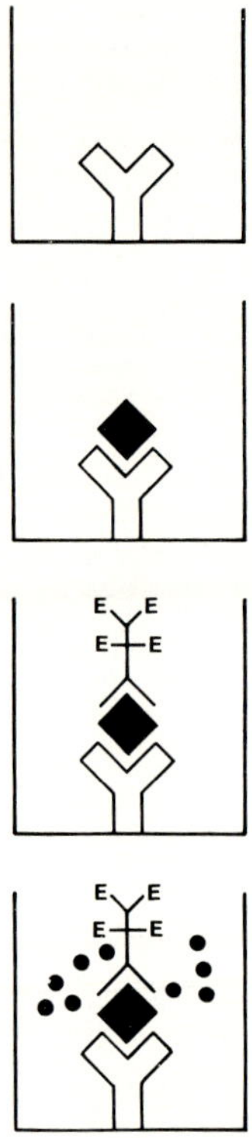

Figure 3. Anti-C3 ELISA assay. In this assay, antiserum to human C3 is bound to the bottom of plastic wells. After incubation with diluted test serum, the wells are washed and then reacted with enzyme-linked (E) antibody directed against the heavy chain of a specific human immunoglobulin class (e.g., peroxidase-conjugated goat antihuman IgG, IgA, or IgM). After the wells are washed once again, the enzyme-bound indicator antibody undergoes color development by adding diaminobenzidene-containing medium. The absorbance (optical density, O.D.) at 492 nm is a measure of the amount of C3-containing immune complexes present in the test sample.

radioimmunoassay in which immune complexes are detected by measuring the amount of inhibition of binding of radiolabeled monoclonal RF to IgG-coated Sepharose particles (8). All of these assays will detect CIC of the IgG type, regardless of their complement-fixing ability. However, the presence of high concentrations of IgG in the test serum, as well as the presence of RF, may adversely affect the test results.

Reactions with Other Antiglobulins

Another assay uses a substance called anti-antibody (AA). AAs are IgM antibodies of either rabbit or human origin capable of combining with structurally altered IgG. They are quite rare, may occur in seemingly normal individuals, and appear to be different from rheumatoid factors, in that they will not combine with aggregated human IgG and that they have specificity for the $F(ab')_2$ fragment of IgG. A test for CIC using AA and the principle of inhibition of agglutination has been described (24).

ASSAYS USING Fc OR C RECEPTORS ON CELLS

Raji Cell Assays

One of the most widely used, sensitive immune complex assays is the Raji cell radioimmunoassay (33,34) (Fig. 4). Raji cells are lymphoblastoid cells that have surface receptors for complement and the Fc portion of IgG, but do not express membrane-bound immunoglobulin. The Fc receptors are thought to be either of low avidity or few in number, while the complement receptors are large in number or of high avidity. Recent studies have determined that the complement receptors on Raji cells include receptors for Clq, C3b, C3bi, and C3d. Thus, immune complexes that have activated complement (either the classic or alternative pathways) and have components in their matrices will bind to the surface of Raji cells.

Briefly, the Raji cell radioimmunoassay is performed by incubating an appropriately diluted test serum with a fixed number of viable Raji cells. After thoroughly washing the Raji cells, they are reacted with radiolabeled antibody to human IgG. The Raji cells are again washed, and the amount of radioactivity associated with the Raji cells is determined. The amount of immune complexes present in the test serum is calculated using a standard curve that is generated by incubating Raji cells with aliquots of normal human serum to which various known amounts of heat-aggregated gamma globulin have been added. Another method of quantitating the results of the Raji cell radioimmunoassay is one in which a large panel of normal sera is used to define an upper 95% confidence limit for the normal range of values. Each time the assay is performed, representative normal sera are processed along with test sera, and the upper limit of normal is redefined. The assay has proved to be highly sensitive and reproducible. One of the drawbacks of the Raji cell assay is that in certain connective tissue diseases, such as SLE, IgG antilymphocyte antibodies are present in the circulation and may bind to the surface of Raji cells. The binding of these warm reactive IgG antibodies, which apparently have auto- or allospecificity to cell surface antigens, will cause false-positive results in the Raji cell assay (1).

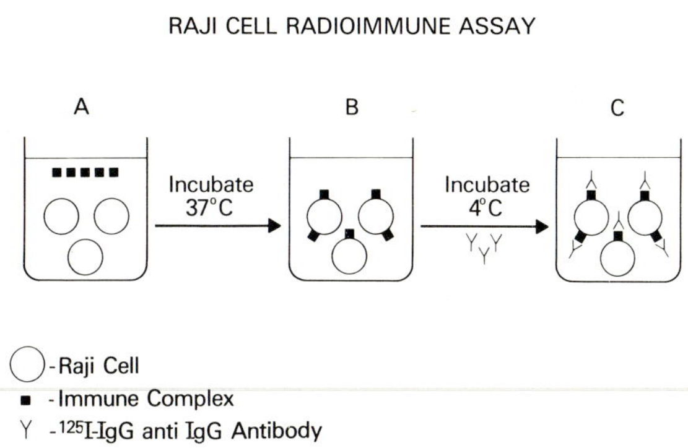

Figure 4. IgG Raji cell radioimmune assay. In this assay, a fixed number of Raji cells are mixed with each test serum sample at 37°C. During this incubation, C3-containing immune complexes bind to the surface of the Raji cells via their C3 receptors. The Raji cells are then washed thoroughly and incubated with a radiolabeled antibody directed against human IgG. Unbound radiolabeled antibody is removed by washing, and the amount of radioactivity associated with the Raji cells is used as an index of IgG-containing circulating immune complexes present in the test sample.

Macrophage Uptake Inhibition

An immune complex assay using guinea pig peritoneal exudate cells has been developed (28). In this assay, test sera are incubated with both guinea pig peritoneal exudate cells and radiolabeled aggregated human gamma globulin. The amount of inhibition of phagocytosis of the radioactive gamma globulin by the test serum is a measure of the amount of immune complexes in the serum sample.

Platelet Aggregation Method

Circulating immune complexes (CIC) are complexes capable of interacting with the surface of human platelets and causing their aggregation. The exact mechanism of the aggregation is not clear, but the interaction between soluble complexes and the platelet surfaces seems to be mediated by the Fc portion of IgG, since damage to the Fc region or the presence of RF will inhibit the reaction. The platelet aggregation test consists of incubating fresh, washed human platelets suspended in buffer with serial dilutions of test sera in microtiter plates at 4 to 8°C for 18 to 24 hours, and then examining them for aggregation (26). The assay is sensitive in detecting large (19S or greater) immune complexes, but false-positive results can occur since anti-platelet antibodies, viruses, aggregated gamma globulin, heparin, thrombin, and certain proteolytic enzymes can produce platelet aggregation under these test conditions.

Inhibition of Antibody-Dependent Cell-Mediated Cytotoxicity

Antibody-dependent cell-mediated cytotoxicity occurs when antibody-coated, radiolabeled target cells are lysed by nonsensitized lymphocytes. The lysis depends upon the interaction of the immunoglobulin on the surface of the target cell with the Fc receptor of the lymphocytes. The reaction can be inhibited by substances that will preferentially bind to the Fc receptor of the lymphocytes (for example, immune complexes). Thus, immune complex assays have been developed that measure competitive inhibition of antibody-dependent cell-mediated cytotoxicity (14). These assays tend to be sensitive, but can be adversely affected by RF. Also, the complement system of the test serum must be inactivated by heating or incubation with EDTA. Some evidence suggests that this assay preferentially detects noncomplement-fixing immune complexes.

ASSAYS USING STAPHYLOCOCCAL PROTEIN A

Protein A is a staphylococcal cell wall component that binds to the Fc portion of IgG_1, IgG_2, and IgG_4, as well as to some IgA and IgM. This property has been used to develop several different immune complex assays. One assay uses heat-killed, formalin-fixed Cowan I strain *Staphylococcus aureus* to detect immune complexes (23). The test serum is reacted with 5% PEG (6000). The precipitate is resolubilized and incubated with a known concentration of protein A. After washing, rabbit IgG is added to saturate the IgG binding sites. A radiolabeled rabbit antihuman IgG is then added, and the amount of radioactivity bound is measured. This assay is sensitive and unaffected by heparin and immunoglobulin concentrations, but is influenced by the presence of rheumatoid factor.

ASSAYS FOR DETECTING IgA-CONTAINING IMMUNE COMPLEXES

Most of the above-mentioned assays are designed to detect IgG-containing immune complexes. Some assays, especially those depending on physical properties or on complement-protein interactions, are capable of detecting both IgG- and IgM-containing immune complexes. Until recently, there have been no sensitive radioimmunoassays to detect IgA-containing immune complexes. Since IgA-containing immune complexes may be involved in the pathogenesis of diseases such as Henoch-Schönlein purpura, Berger's disease, gluten-sensitive enteropathy, and dermatitis herpetiformis, there has been significant interest in developing IgA immune complex assays. Recently, several radioassays have been developed that detect circulating IgA immune complexes. One type, termed the IgA Raji cell radioassay, uses Raji cells and purified radiolabeled antihuman IgA antisera (11). It will detect IgA-containing immune complexes that have activated the complement system. The other type is an assay that uses rabbit IgM antihuman IgA antiserum, and that measures immune complexes by inhibition of agglutination (17). The anti-C3 ELISA assay previously described has also been adapted to detect IgA-containing CIC (12).

SUMMARY

In the past few years, a large number of assays for the detection of CIC have been developed. These assays have proved useful in expanding our understanding of immune complex disease and the interactions of immune complexes with the afferent and efferent limbs of the immune response. However, these assays have not proved to be useful in the diagnosis of specific diseases. This is partly due to the unexpectedly large number of diseases in which immune complexes have been detected. Additionally, the use of these assays to define the antigen present in immune complexes has been extremely difficult. Studies to precisely define the components of immune complexes as well as the interactions of CIC with elements of the RES and specific soluble mediators of inflammation are currently underway.

REFERENCES

1. Anderson CL, Stillman WS: Raji cell assay for immune complexes. Evidence for detection of Raji-directed immunoglobulin G antibody in sera from patients with systemic lupus erythematosus. *J Clin Invest* 66:353, 1980.
2. Brouet JC, Clauvel JP, Danon F, et al: Biologic and clinical significance of cryoglobulins. *Am J Med* 57:775, 1974.
3. Casali P, Bossus A, Carpentier NA, et al: Solid-phase enzyme immunoassay or radioimmunoassay for the detection of immune complexes based on their recognition by conglutinin: Conglutinin-binding test. *Clin Exp Immunol* 29:342, 1977.
4. Chia D, Barnett EV, Yamagata, J et al: Quantitation and characterization of soluble immune complexes precipitated from sera by polyethylene glycol (PEG). *Clin Exp Immunol* 37:399, 1979.
5. Cowdery JS, Treadwell PE, Fritz RB: A radioimmunoassay for human antigen-antibody complexes in clinical material. *J Immunol* 114:5, 1975.
6. Dixon FJ, Feldman JD, Vazquez JJ: Experimental glomerulonephritis. The pathogenesis of a

laboratory model resembling the spectrum of human glomerulonephritis. *J Exp Med* 113:899, 1961.

7. Eisenberg RA, Theofilopoulos AN, Dixon FJ: Use of bovine conglutinin for the assay of immune complexes. *J Immunol* 118:1428, 1977.
8. Gabriel A, Agnello V: Detection of immune complexes. *J Clin Invest* 59:990, 1977.
9. Germuth FG Jr: A comparative histologic and immunologic study in rabbits of induced hypersensitivity of the serum sickness type. *J Exp Med* 97:257, 1953.
10. Grey HM, Kohler PF: Cryoimmunoglobulins. *Semin Hematol* 10:87, 1973.
11. Hall RP, Lawley TJ, Heck JA, et al: IgA-containing immune complexes in dermatitis herpetiformis, Henoch-Schönlein purpura, systemic lupus erythematosus and other diseases. *Clin Exp Immunol* 40:431, 1980.
12. Hall RP, Lawley TJ: Characterization of circulating and cutaneous IgA immune complexes in patients with dermatitis herpetiformis. *J. Immunol.* 135: 1760–1765, 1985. .
13. Hay FC, Nineham LJ, Roitt IM: Routine assay for detection of immune complexes of known immunoglobulin class using solid phase Clq. *Clin Exp Immunol* 24:396, 1976.
14. Jewell DP, MacLennan ICM: Circulating immune complexes in inflammatory bowel disease. *Clin Exp Immunol* 14:219, 1973.
15. Lawley TJ: Methods of detection of circulating immune complexes. In Fauci AS (Ed): *Clinics in Immunology and Allergy,* vol. 1. Saunders, Philadelphia, 1981, p 383.
16. Lawley TJ, Hall RP: Circulating immune complexes in dermatologic disease. *Springer Semin Immunopathol* 4:221, 1981.
17. Levinsky RJ, Barratt TM: IgA immune complexes in Henoch-Schönlein purpura. *Lancet* 2:100, 1979.
18. Lunde MN: A Clq enzyme-linked immunosorbent assay (ELISA) for immune complexes using polyethylene glycol. *Am J Trop Med Hyg* 32:392, 1983.
19. Lurhuma AZ, Cambiaso CL, Masson Pl, et al: Detection of circulating antigen-antibody complexes by their inhibitory effect on the agglutination of IgG coated particles by rheumatoid factor or Clq. *Clin Exp Immunol* 25:212, 1976.
20. Luthra HS, McDuffie FC, Hunder GC, et al: Immune complexes in sera and synovial fluids of patients with rheumatoid arthritis: Radioimmunoassay with monoclonal rheumatoid factor. *J Clin Invest* 56:458, 1975.
21. Mannik, M: Physicochemical and functional relationships of immune complexes. *J Invest Dermatol* 74:333, 1980.
22. Mannik M, Arend WP: Fate of preformed immune complexes in rabbits and rhesus monkeys. *J Exp Med* 134:195, 1971.
23. McDougal JS, Redecha PB, Inman RD, et al: Binding of immunoglobulin G aggregates and immune complexes in human sera to Staphylococci containing protein A. *J Clin Invest* 63:627, 1979.
24. Milgrom F, Kano K: Comparison of various procedures for detection of antigen-antibody complexes. *Intern Arch Allergy Appl Immunol* 56:224, 1978.
25. Miller GW, Nussenzweig V: A new complement function: Solubilization of antigen-antibody aggregates. *Proc Natl Acad Sci USA* 72:418, 1975.
26. Myllyla G: Aggregation of human blood platelets by immune complexes in the sedimentation pattern test. *Scand J Haematol* 19(Suppl):1, 1973.
27. Nydegger UE, Lambert PH, Gerber H, et al: Circulating immune complexes in the serum of systemic lupus erythematosus and in carriers of hepatitis B antigen. Quantitation by binding to radiolabeled Clq. *J Clin Invest* 54:297, 1974.
28. Onyewotu II, Holborow EJ, Johnson GD: Detection and radioassay of soluble circulating immune complexes using guinea pig peritoneal exudate cells. Nature 248:156, 1974.
29. Pereira AB, Theofilopoulos AN, Dixon FJ: Detection and partial characterization of circulating immune complexes with solid-phase anti-C3. *J Immunol* 125:763, 1980.
30. Pirquet CF von, Schick B: *Die Serumkrankheit.* Deuticke, Leipzig, 1905.
31. Takahashi M, Takahashi S, Brade V, et al: Requirements for the solubilization of immune aggregates by complement. The role of the classical pathway. *J Clin Invest* 62:349, 1978.

32. Theofilopoulos AN, Dixon FJ: The biology and detection of immune complexes. *Adv Immunol* 28:89, 1980.
33. Theofilopoulos AN, Wilson CB, Bokisch VA, et al: Binding of soluble immune complexes to human lymphoblastoid cells. II.Use of Raji cells to detect circulating immune complexes in animal and human sera. *J Exp Med* 140:1230, 1974.
34. Theofilopoulos AN, Wilson CB, Dixon FJ: The Raji cell radioimmune assay for detecting immune complexes in human sera. *J Clin Invest* 57:169, 1976.

6
Langerhans Cell and T-Cell Subset Identification Using Monoclonal Antibodies: Immunocytochemical Methods in Light and Electron Microscopy Applied on Human Skin

Jean Thivolet
Daniel Schmitt

This chapter reports the various methods used to identify, in tissue sections or cell suspensions, T-cell subsets and Langerhans cells (LC). In light microscopy, the immunofluorescence (IF) and different immunoperoxidase [IP] techniques (indirect immunoperoxidase, avidin biotin [A-B] amplification) are reported. In immunoelectron microscopy (IEM), the IP labeling and immunogold technique are supplemented by various methods of cell biology (obtaining cell suspension from normal epidermis, cell subset enrichment). In addition, the possibility of quantitative studies using these techniques is discussed. Finally, recent results obtained in cutaneous pathology using these methods are reported (T-cell subsets and LC in inflammations and tumors of the skin).

INTRODUCTION

In normal skin as well as in cutaneous lesions, the exact nature of infiltrating mononuclear cells is difficult to establish using conventional light- or electron-microscopy (EM).

The immunocytochemical identification of immunoglobulin-producing cells (B-cell lineage) has been carried out using conventional anti-immunoglobulin (anti-Ig) antisera in immunofluorescence (IF) and/or peroxidase (Po) procedures. Similarly, direct evidence has been obtained on the nature of T cells by using rosetting techniques (8), enzyme histochemistry with α-naphthyl-acetate esterase (48), and immunohistochemical techniques using specific conventional antisera against human T-lymphocyte surface antigens (HTLA) (1, 81).

More recently, hybridoma technology has permitted the production of murine monoclonal antibodies (MCA) that are specific for different T-cell surface antigens and are characteristic of different subsets of T lymphocytes. Such antibodies are more specific and sensitive and offer a means to establish the exact phenotype of the cells in mononuclear infiltrates including Langerhans cells (LC).

Efficiency of MCA has first been proven in normal lymphoid tissues and human intestinal mucosa. Since then, MCA have been applied to the study of skin biopsy specimens, and have become a useful tool in cutaneous immunohistochemistry. Moreover, some recent immunoelectron microscopic (IEM) investigations have been carried out with the aid of MCA, giving new data on the mapping of cell-surface antigens. In this chapter, we will briefly review the recommended methods and give some examples of typical findings in cutaneous diseases of T-cell subsets and LC at the light and electron microscopic levels.

METHODOLOGY

On frozen sections, IF has some disadvantages. Lability of IF preparations and poor morphologic detail, even if a fluorescent counterstaining is used, may give rise to some difficulty in correlating histologic features with the fluorescent labeling. This is one of the reasons why IF was not initially accepted by pathologists.

The peroxidase-antiperoxidase (PAP) technique adapted for paraffin sections has been proposed to overcome some of the disadvantages of IF. Initial optimism for this approach was tempered by the evidence of frequent false-negative and/or erroneous results. Some studies compared the use of frozen and paraffin sections for typing lymphomas. Results confirmed the necessity of using frozen sections as substrates for accurate detection of surface immunoglobulins and differentiation lymphocyte cell surface antigens.

The immunoperoxidase (IP) test on frozen sections, using either PAP or avidin biotin peroxidase complex (ABC) procedures, has been subsequently developed as an alternative for IF. Finally, IP and IF techniques applied to frozen sections gave comparable results.

Handling Skin Biopsy Specimens and Tissue Processing

Results of immunohistochemistry (IHC) in cutaneous pathology as well as in other applications depend on good conservation of antigens under study. Lymphocytes and LC bear very fragile glycoprotein differentiation antigens that are destroyed after even a light fixation. Immunoglobulins present on B lymphocytes and related cells are more resistant. However, various fixatives undoubtedly alter or destroy immunoglobulins. Many studies have confirmed the necessity of using frozen sections as substrates for accurate study of both lymphocytes and LC. Enzyme digestion with trypsin or pronase improves results in cases of immunoglobulin staining on previously fixed tissues, but optimum detection of lymphocytes requires frozen rather than paraffin sections. Thus, the requirements for fresh and quick-frozen biopsy specimens cannot be overcome.

The following technique may be proposed*: Human skin biopsy specimens must be processed immediately after surgical removal. Representative 2 mm square blocks are divided with a sharp knife, and are placed in and completely surrounded by embedding medium (OCT compound, Miles Laboratories) in avilight plastic capsules prior to freezing in liquid nitrogen. The capsules are stored below −20°C until sectioned. Similar blocks are fixed for IEM and for standard light microscopy. Cryostat sections for IF or IP are cut at 4 to 6 μm and fixed in cold acetone before storage and staining.

IF and IP Procedures

Light Microscopy

Antibodies Against Immunocompetent Cells (currently used; see Table 1)

Indirect Immunofluorescence (IIF). Frozen sections of 4 to 5 μm are fixed in acetone (10 minutes at −20°C), incubated with the appropriate MCA diluted in phosphate-buffered saline (PBS) at 37°C for 45 minutes, and rinsed in PBS twice for ten minutes. Sections are then incubated in fluorescein isothiocyanate (FITC) conjugated goat antimouse Ig (MELOY, 1:20) at 37°C for 45 minutes, rinsed twice in PBS, and mounted in buffered glycerin (36).

Indirect Immunoperoxidase (Fig. 1). The same procedure can be used with Po conjugate correctly diluted in PBS (45 minutes at 37°C) instead of the FITC conjugate. After washing, the Po activity of the conjugate is revealed by 3,3′ diaminobenzidine with H_2O_2, which gives a brown deposit at the site of fixation of MCA. (See below for details on amino ethyl carbozol [AEC] [91].)

Immunoperoxidase with the Avidin Biotin System (ABS). The commercially available Vectasin ABS kit can be used. Frozen sections are incubated with two blocking reagents: hydrogen peroxide (0.3% in PBS) and normal serum (for 40 minutes) to reduce nonspecific background staining. Sections are then sequentially incubated for 1 hour at 37°C with: 1) the MCA produced in mice, 2) a biotinylated antimouse IgG, and 3) the Vectasin avidin biotin complexes conjugated with Po. After each incubation, slides are washed for 20 minutes, and the peroxidase activity of the AB complexes is revealed by addition of AEC for 10 minutes. Sections can be counterstained with Mayer's hematoxylin solution and mounted with Aqua mount medium (35,91,99).

Cell Quantification in Epidermis. The slides could be viewed under an IF microscope or light microscope (IP), and positive cells could be counted by means of an ocular square grid covering (under 40× objective magnification) 0.0576 mm^2 of skin section surface. Each grid slide was divided into 10 parts so that the grid field contained 100 smaller squares. A total of 40 adjacent grid fields of epidermal sections can be examined on two slides, each bearing three skin sections for each skin specimen and MCA used. This represents about 9.6 mm of continuous section. The exact proportion between IF^- and IF^+ epidermal cells depends on epidermal thickness. In addition, only cellular bodies exhibiting bright fluorescence and a dark nucleus should be counted as positive (36).

*See also Addendum of this chapter for a "protocol" of an alternative group of techniques used for studies of lymph nodes; these entail the use of the transplant medium described in Chapter 1.

Table 1. Antibodies Directed against Immunocompetent Cells

	Origin	*Specificity*	*Produced by*
T101	Mouse	All circulating	Hybritech (U.S.)
OKT3		T lymphocytes	Ortho (U.S.)
Leu1			Becton Dickinson (U.S.)
OKT4	Mouse	Helper T cells	Ortho (U.S.)
Leu3a			Becton Dickinson (U.S.)
OKT8	Mouse	Suppressor	Ortho (U.S.)
Leu2a		cytotoxic T cells	Becton Dickinson (U.S.)
OKT6	Mouse	Common thymocytes	Ortho (U.S.)
BL6		LC	Immunotech (France) (103)
BL2	Mouse	HLA-DR Ag	Immunotech (France)
OKIa			Ortho (U.S.)
Anti-HLA-DR			Becton Dickinson (U.S.)
HTLA†	Rabbit	T lymphocytes	Mérieux (France)

†Polyclonal antibodies

Ultrastructural Immunocytochemistry

Materials

Lymphocyte suspensions. Mononuclear cells are separated from peripheral blood by "Ficoll-Paque" (Pharmacia) density centrifugation (6).

Langerhans cell suspensions. Single-cell suspensions can be prepared from freshly removed normal human skin (plastic surgery; breast or abdominal). Briefly, trimmed skin is split-cut with a keratotome set at 0.1 mm. The resulting slices are treated for 30 minutes at 37°C with 0.3% trypsin (Difco, Detroit MI) in buffer (0.68% NaCl; 0.04% KCl; 0.1% glucose; 0.22% $NaHCO_3$; pH, 7.3.). The epidermis is detached from the dermis with fine forceps. Isolated epidermal samples are pooled in minimum essential medium (MEM, Gibco, Glasgow, U.K.) supplemented with 20% fetal calf serum (FCS), and repeatedly blown in and out of a 5 ml pipette. After filtration through sterile gauze, the suspended cells are centrifuged for 20 minutes at 400 g. The collected cells were resuspended in RPMI 1640 (Gibco, Glasgow, U.K.) supplemented with 15% heat-inactivated A-B human serum, 20 mmol/l hepes buffer, 2 mmol/l L-glutamine, and antibiotics. Following a triple wash in the RPMI medium, the cells are counted and the viability is estimated by trypan blue exclusion. Viability, after trypsinization, is 85% or higher; after 18 hours, maintenance exceeded 75% (24,79).

Enrichment of epidermal cell (EC) suspensions (LC-enriched suspensions)

1. The panning method (with anti-HLA-DR or OKT6 MCA) (80,102). For IEM studies, DR-positive or $OKT6^+$ EC are enriched using a modification of the plate technique described by Wysocki and Sato (102). Briefly, plastic plates (Corning, NY) are coated with affinity-purified goat antimouse Ig (Tago, Inc., Burlingame, U.S.). Concurrently, isolated EC are incubated with the correctly diluted MCA for 1 hour at room temperature, and then washed twice in PBS. Then, 3 ml of the cell suspensions at a concentration of 5 to 6 × 10^6/ml are applied to a single goat antimouse Ig-coated plate. After 60 minutes the supernatant is removed. The adherent cells are then re-

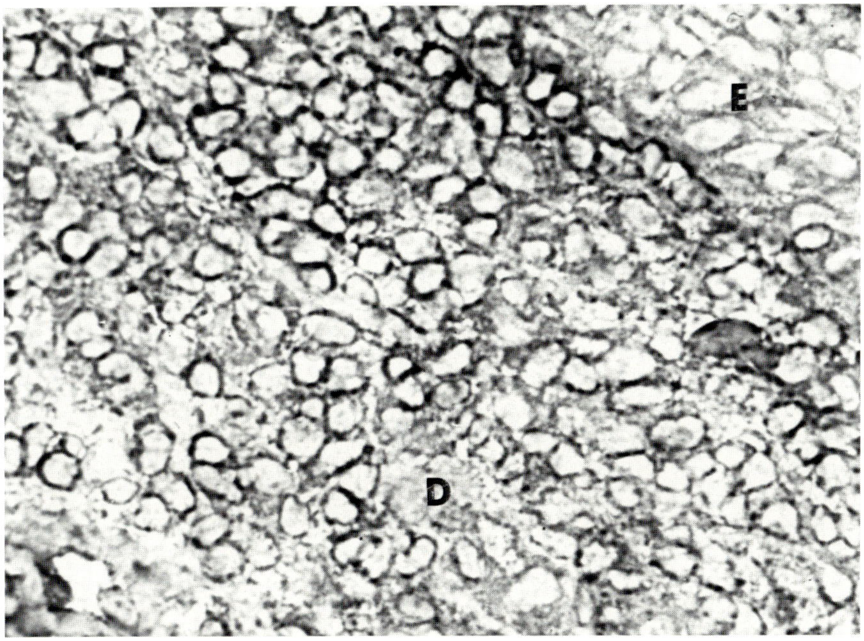

Figure 1. Indirect IP method in light microscopy, showing identification of T lymphocytes infiltrating the upper dermis (D), using specific antibodies and a peroxidase conjugate in a case of discoid lupus erythematosus (E, epidermis) (800×).

moved by repeated scraping with a rubber policeman and are processed for imunogold labeling (15,24).

2. Ficol-Hypaque gradient (17). LC enrichment is obtained by Ficoll-Hypaque (Pharmacia France SA, Le Chesnay, France) sedimentation. Dispersed skin cells (4×10^6 cells/ml) in TC 199 (Gibco, Glasgow, U.K.) supplemented with 20% FCS are layered on the gradient and centrifuged for 30 minutes at 400 g at 4°C. The lymphoïd-like cells at the interface are washed and resuspended in PBS, pH 7.2.

Immunocytochemistry

Immunoperoxidase

1. On skin sections (61). Both 15 and 4 μm cryostat sections of unfixed and prefixed (3% paraformaldehyde) tissue are mounted on glass slides. The former are then fixed in 3% paraformaldehyde; subsequently, all sections are washed in PBS for 20 minutes at room temperature. Incubation with the antibodies for 30 minutes is carried out, followed by gentle washing in PBS. The specimens are then incubated with the Fab-Po conjugate directed against the first Ig for 30 minutes. Washing is then carried out in PBS for 30 minutes before fixation with 2% glutaraldehyde in sodium cacodylate buffer for 15 minutes at room temperature. The tissue is then washed in sodium cadodylate buffer twice for 10 minutes and in Tris-HCl buffer for a further 10 minutes.

Po activity is revealed by Graham-Karnovsky medium (34) (10 mg of 3,3 diaminobenzidine [DAB] in 10 ml of Tris-HCl buffer with 0.1% hydrogen peroxide). The specimens are once more washed in PBS for 30 minutes. The stained 4 μm sections are mounted in buffered glycerin and examined by light microscopy.

The 15 μm sections are postfixed in 1% osmium tetroxide in sodium cacodylate buffer for 10 minutes, washed in distilled water, and hydrated in successive 5 minute baths of 25%, 50%, 70%, 95%, and 100% alcohol. The sections are then covered by a mixture of 100% alcohol and epoxy resin for 1 hour, and with pure resin overnight followed by the final inclusion compound for 1 hour. A gelatin capsule containing the final inclusion compound is inverted over the sections on the slide, so that the section is included in continuous resin from slide to capsule. The specimens are then polymerized in a 60° oven for 2 to 3 days. The gelatin blocks including the embedded sections are separated from the glass slides by gentle heating.

Ultrathin sections are observed by EM with or without counterstaining.

2. On cell suspensions (13, 82). Polyclonal-monoclonal antibodies are used at working dilution for 30 minutes at 37°C on cells fixed by 3% paraformaldehyde. The murine antibodies, fixed on the cell surface, are revealed by a Po conjugate at a 1:20 dilution for 30 minutes at 37°C. The Po activity is revealed with the Graham-Karnovsky medium (34) (see above). The cells are postfixed for 20 minutes with osmium tetroxide, and embedded in epoxy medium. Ultrathin sections are examined without staining with a Hitachi HU12A electron microscope. Some sections are poststained with lead citrate and uranyl acetate for standard examination.

3. Avidin Biotin method Fig. 2) (60). Immunocytochemical staining is carried out after fixation in 3% paraformaldehyde on 20μm cryostat section and on chopped tissue specimens. OKT8 antibody (produced by Ortho, Raritan, NY) is directly conjugated with biotin; 50 μg biotinyl-N-hydroxysuccinimide ester reacted with 1 mg/ml antibody in 0.1 M $NaHCO_3$ buffer at 25°C for 4 hours. The tissue specimens are incubated with the biotinylated antibody (diluted at 1:5) at 37°C for 1 hour. Subsequently, an avidin-Po complex is used (1:20 dilution, incubation for 1 hour at 37°C; Medac, Hamburg, FRG). After reaction with 3′, 3′ diamino-benzidine (Sigma, St. Louis, MO), cryostat sections and chopped tissue specimens are included in epoxy medium. Ultrathin sections are examined before and after poststaining with uranyl acetate and lead cytrate.

Immunogold procedure (Figs. 3 and 6). In the past few years, colloidal gold-labeled immunoreagents have been used in EM to label cell surface antigens on cell suspensions (19,21,22,38), cell monolayers (88), and ultrathin plastic-embedded (74) or frozen sections (see also Chap. 4). Various advantages of this method could be noted: 1) the absence of nonspecific absorption of gold markers on cell surfaces; 2) the possibility of poststaining ultrathin sections without changes in the immunolabeling contrast and of a double labeling using gold particles of different sizes (32,45–47). Furthermore, colloidal gold allows a quantitative evaluation of surface markers based on the direct counts of particles located in close apposition to the plasma membrane (46,47,55).

1. Immunogold-labeling procedure on cell suspensions (84–86). The EC suspensions are fixed in 3% paraformaldehyde in PBS buffer. After washing, antibodies are applied to specimen cells for 30 minutes at 37°C. The antibodies, fixed on the cell surface, are identified by the use of immunoglobulin labeled with gold granules (Janssen Pharm., Beerse Belgium) applied at a 1:2 dilution for 1 hour at 37°C. After washing in PBS, the cells are postfixed for 20 minutes with 2% glutaraldehyde in cacodylate buffer, and then for 20 minutes with 1% osmium tetroxide and embedded in epoxy medium. Ultrathin sections are examined after or without poststaining with lead citrate and uranyl acetate.

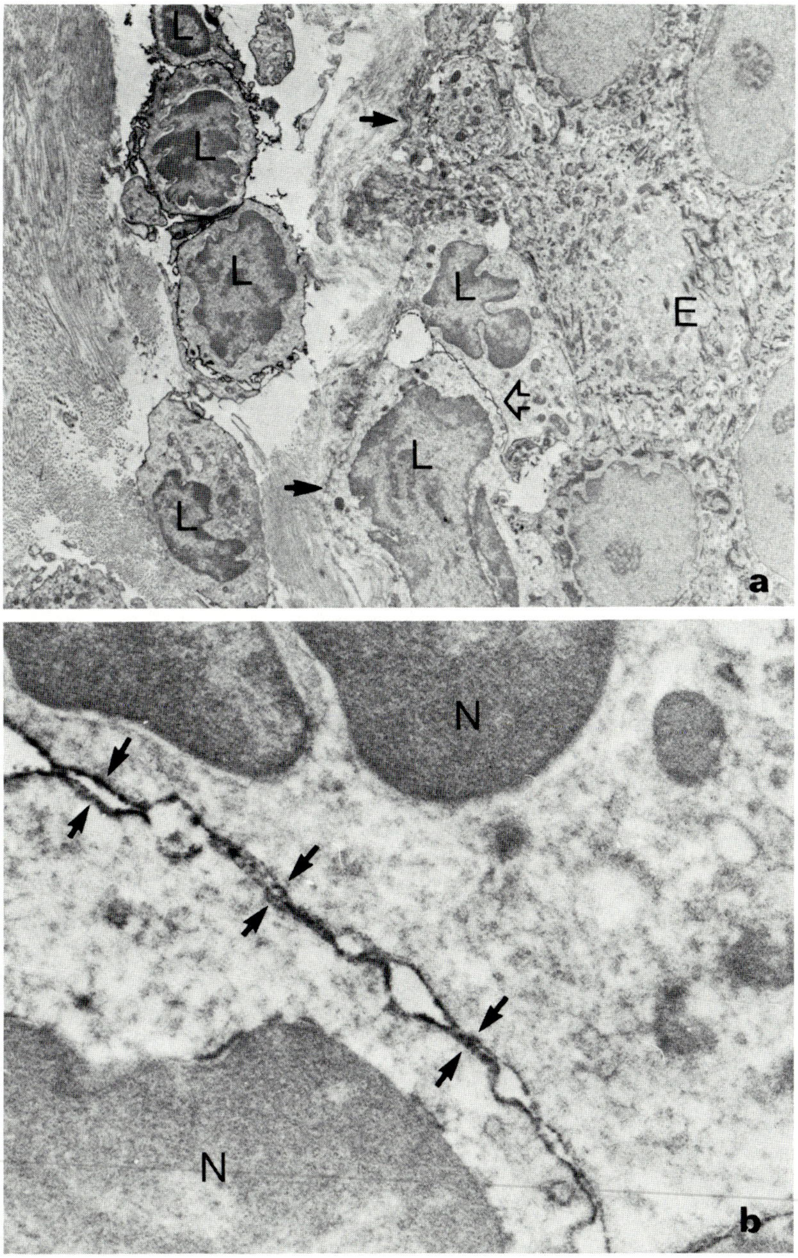

Figure 2. A. Avidin-biotin-peroxidase system showing low magnification of the epithelial mesenchymal interface in oral lichen planus. There are several OKT8-positive lymphocytes (L) in the stroma and the epithelium (E). Arrows point to the basal membrane zone. There is discontinuous staining of the cell membrane, with focal concentration between adjacent lymphocytes (open arrow) and poststaining with lead utrate and uranyl acetate (5200×). B. Detail of the pronounced staining (arrows) between two lymphocytes within the epithelium (N, nucleus) (21,000×). (Courtesy of Dr. Thomas Loening, Hamburg.)

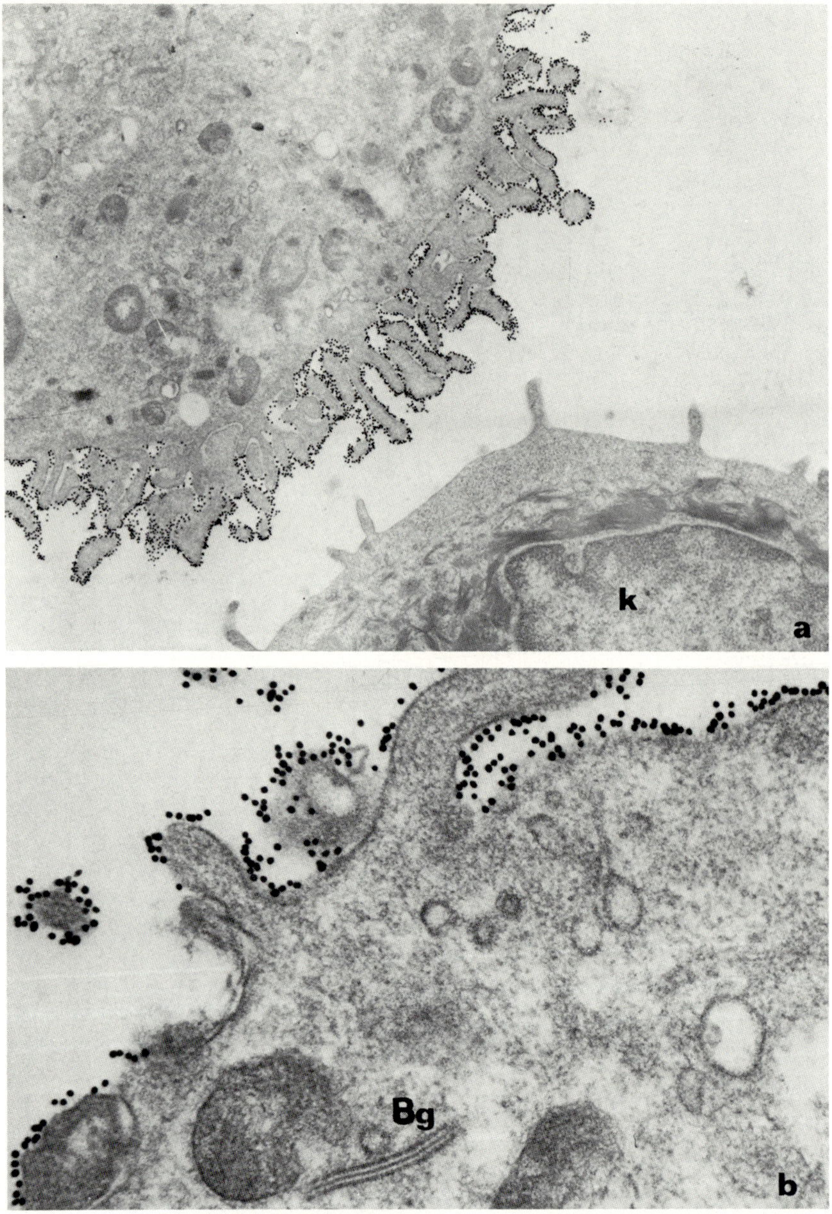

Figure 3. A. Immunogold technique with indirect ultrastructural identification of T6 antigen-expressing cell in an epidermal cell suspension by the use of OKT6 monoclonal antibody and a gold conjugate with particles 20 nm in diameter. Note the absence of gold granules on the keratinocyte surface (K) (20,000×). B. Detail of the electron-dense gold particles fixed along the cell surface of a Langerhans cell (with typical Birbeck granule, Bg) (62,000×).

2. Quantitative analysis of surface labeling. As demonstrated by Horisberger (45) and Lafferty et al. (55), the number of antigenic sites may be estimated from the densities of gold particles bound to the surface, keeping in mind that steric hindrance resulting from the size of the label allows exclusion of amplification phenomenon.

The number of gold particles along the circumference of the cell membrane is counted to determine the extent of surface labeling. Mean and standard errors for each morphologic group are determined. The cells analyzed are those sectioned near their midplane to minimize tangential membrane sections and to provide a uniform morphologic comparison between cells. Labeling data are reported as the mean number of gold particles per micrometer of membrane (gp/μm). Particle counts are obtained from at least 10 cells in each population.

The approximate number of cell surface antigenic sites can be estimated from the number of gold particles per micrometer according to the method of Trucco and de Petris (94,95). This method was applied to the quantitative analysis of HLA-DR antigen expression by human LC (17).

APPLICATIONS

Normal Skin

When samples of normal skin are examined with MCA-to-leukocyte subpopulations, a small number of lymphocytes appears in the dermis. All these cells are labeled with pan-T cell antibodies. If we connsider the T-helper or T-suppressor cytotoxic origin, both populations appear to be scattered throughout the dermis with some tendency to a perivascular localization.

OKT6, BL6, and anti-HLA-DR MCA give an intense staining of epidermal dendritic cells (LC) (28,43,59,68,104).

T-Lymphocyte Subpopulations and Skin Lesions

Nontumoral Lesions

Human Skin Tuberculin Reaction (79). After 48 and 96 hours of intradermal purified protein derivative (PPD) injections in human skin, the majority of the T lymphocytes infiltrating the skin reacted with MCA specific for the helper-induced phenotype, and a few with MCA reacting with the suppressive-cytotoxic cells. In addition, a large percentage of cells express the HLA-DR antigens.

Erythema Multiformis (66). In lesions, the number of OKT8+ cells is greater than the number of OKT4+ cells. In addition, the number of $OKT6^+$ cells increases in the upper and lower dermis.

Cutaneous Sarcoidosis (9). Skin lesions of patients with systemic and cutaneous sarcoidosis show a large number of infiltrating cells that react with anti-T-MCA. In addition, the majority of T cells show a reactivity with anti-helper inducer MCA ($OKT4^+$). Rare suppressor-cytotoxic T cells can be observed ($OKT8^+$). These results suggest the importance of helper T cells in the formation of the sarcoid granuloma.

Graft Versus Host Reaction (GVH) and Skin (33,57). In skin lesions of chronic GVH reaction infiltrates, the large majority of lymphoid cells express the phenotype T8 of the suppressor cytotoxic T cells.

In addition, the expression of HLA-DR antigens by keratinocytes in skin lesions of GVH is actually accepted by the majority of authors (53,56,67).

T-Cell Subsets in Allograft Rejection (5). Both major T-cell subsets, $T4^+$ and T8, infiltrate human skin allografts. $T4^+$ cells are predominant in the graft dermis and graft bed. In contrast, $T8^+$ cells are relatively more numerous in the epidermis and hair follicles. Rejection probably proceeds by two apparently independent pathways: 1) direct contact killing of graft epithelial cells, presumably by immunologically specific T8-positive cytotoxic cells; and 2) injury of microvascular endothelium of both the graft and graft bed with secondary graft infraction.

Lichen Planus (4,20,33,54,63). Skin lesions of lichen planus are characterized by the presence of lymphocytes infiltrating the dermis, which are stained by the MCA reacting with the T-cell lineage. In addition, the majority of the infiltrating cells also stained with anti-T4-MCA. The majority of the lymphoid cells express the HLA-DR antigens. In addition, the DR specificity also seems to be expressed by the keratinocytes above the dermal infiltrate.

Tumoral Lesions

Wart Lesions (11). In wart lesions showing a dermal infiltrate, OKT4- and OKT8-positive T-cell populations are present, suggesting the existence of a local cellular immune reaction.

Epidermal Tumors (Basal and Squamous Cell Carcinoma, Malignant Melanoma) (25). In these types of epidermal tumors, the use of MCA for T-cell subsets demonstrates that the infiltrating lymphoid cells around the tumors are mainly of the cytotoxic-suppressor type ($T8^+$).

Sézary Syndrome and Mycosis Fungoides (Cutaneous T-cell Lymphoma) (Fig. 4). In this field, correlations of established criteria of cellular morphology with the newer immunologic markers, particularly the increasing range of MCA, have been of considerable value (14,54,83,96–98).

Mycosis fungoides and Sézary syndrome are considered by many to be closely related processes, possibly two parts of a continuous spectrum of cutaneous T-cell lymphomas. There is abundant evidence that the neoplastic cells in mycosis fungoides and Sézary syndrome have a helper cell function, based on observations that these cells are able to facilitate Ig production by B cells in vitro. More recently, evidence derived from the use of MCA with specificity against the helper cell phenotype has substantiated the belief that these conditions represent neoplasms of helper T cells (41,44,54,58,82).

The panel of MCA applied to sections of skin from patients with mycosis fungoides revealed several other departures from the norm. For example, in cases of mycosis fungoides, more than 80% of the infiltrating lymphocytes appeared to be positive with HLA-DR antibody, possibly reflecting a state of "activation" of the infiltrating neoplastic lymphocytes (2,42,43,65).

Proof that the neoplastic cells infiltrating the skin in mycosis fungoides are, in fact, helper cells has been difficult to obtain, since extraction of these cells from skin—at least in sufficient numbers for assays of helper function or for studies of surface pheno-

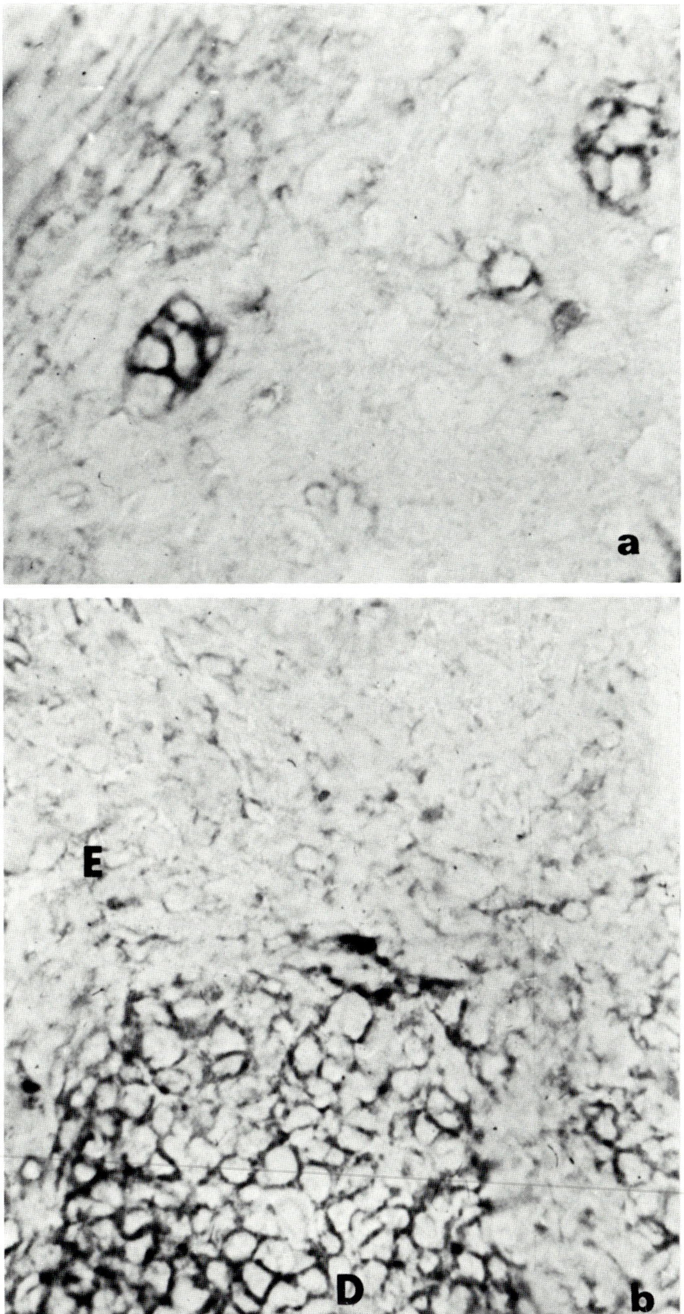

Figure 4. Mycosis fungoides, skin lesion. Identification of tumoral T cell by indirect immunoperoxidase technique in the epidermis (A) and in the dermis (B) (E, epidermis; D, dermis) (800×).

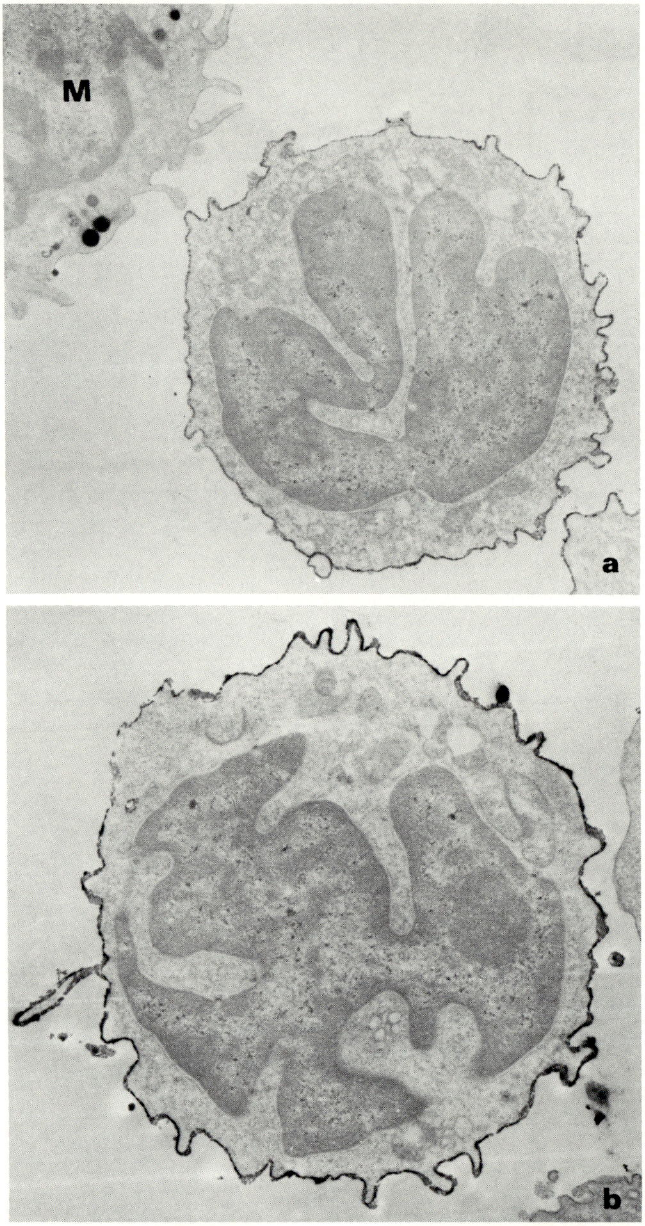

Figure 5. A. Circulating Sézary cells, indirect immunoperoxidase technique, with identification of T3 antigen by OKT3 MCA on the surface of the Sézary cell. Note the absence of T3 activity on the membrane of the adjacent monocyte (M) (with peroxidase-positive cytoplasmic granules) (12 000×). B. Reactivity of a Sézary cell with OKT4 MCA. (12 000×).

type using cell suspensions—has proved to be a problem. However, direct labeling of the neoplastic cells within tissue sections, using IP techniques, circumvents this problem and provides a means of examining the phenotypic marking of the neoplastic cells in situ. Both IF and IP techniques have been applied to frozen sections for this purpose; both techniques give similar results, demonstrating quite clearly that the majority of the lymphoid cells within the skin in mycosis fungoides and Sézary syndrome express the helper-inducer phenotype (OKT4 or Leu 3) (12,82,92,100).

LC and MCA

Surface Markers

HLA-DR Antigens and HLA-ABC Antigens. Numerous studies have shown that some epidermal cells express HLA-DR (or Ia-like) antigens (37,51,76). Two types of HLA-DR-positive cells have been defined in normal human epidermis: 1) LC with Birbeck granules, and 2) the indeterminate cells without Birbeck granules (77,78). HLA-DR (Ia-like) antigens are considered to be highly specific markers for LC and their putative precursors in normal human epidermis.

Recently, HLA-ABC antigens were demonstrated on the surface of normal epidermal dendritic mononuclear cells (7).

T6 Antigens (Revealed by OKT6 or BL6 MCA) (Fig. 6) (103). More recently, OKT6 MCA which react with a surface antigen of cortical thymocytes, have been shown to bind specifically to human LC in the epidermis (29,69). This OKT6 MCA has been largely used to identify LC in skin sections (23,43,59,68,70) and in epidermal cell suspensions (13). Immunogold recently was used in the identification of LC in EM (84,85,104).

T4 Antigens (Revealed by OKT4 MCA) (Fig. 7). Moreover, the reactivity of normal and pathologic human LC with MCA specific for T4 antigens usually shared by circulating helper T lymphocytes has been reported recently (71,102). In a recent paper, we discussed use of an indirect immunogold technique in EM to compare the respective density of cell membrane determinants revealed by OKT6 and OKT4 on normal human LC in suspensions through a direct quantification of gold particles fixed on the cell membrane. Under EM examination, 12.9 ± 3.5 gold granules were noted per cell section on OKT4-positive LC, whereas 236.8 ± 23.5 granules were counted per cell section on OKT6-reactive cells (86).

These results confirm the reactivity of human LC with OKT4 MCA, and demonstrate a marked quantitative difference on LC surface between their antigenic determinants recognized by either OKT6 or OKT4 MCA.

Existence of Circulating T6⁺ Cells (Table 2). The specificity of OKT6 for peripheral blood mononuclear cells was examined by IIF and ultrastructural immunogold labeling using normal peripheral blood (PB) cells.

Some rare PB mononuclear cells (approximately 1%) express T6 antigen on their membrane surface, as determined by light microscopy and cytofluorometry. Electron microscopic examination of immunogold-labeled cells reveals that OKT6-positive cells are dendritic, lacking the Birbeck granules, and express variable densities of the membrane T6 antigen (18).

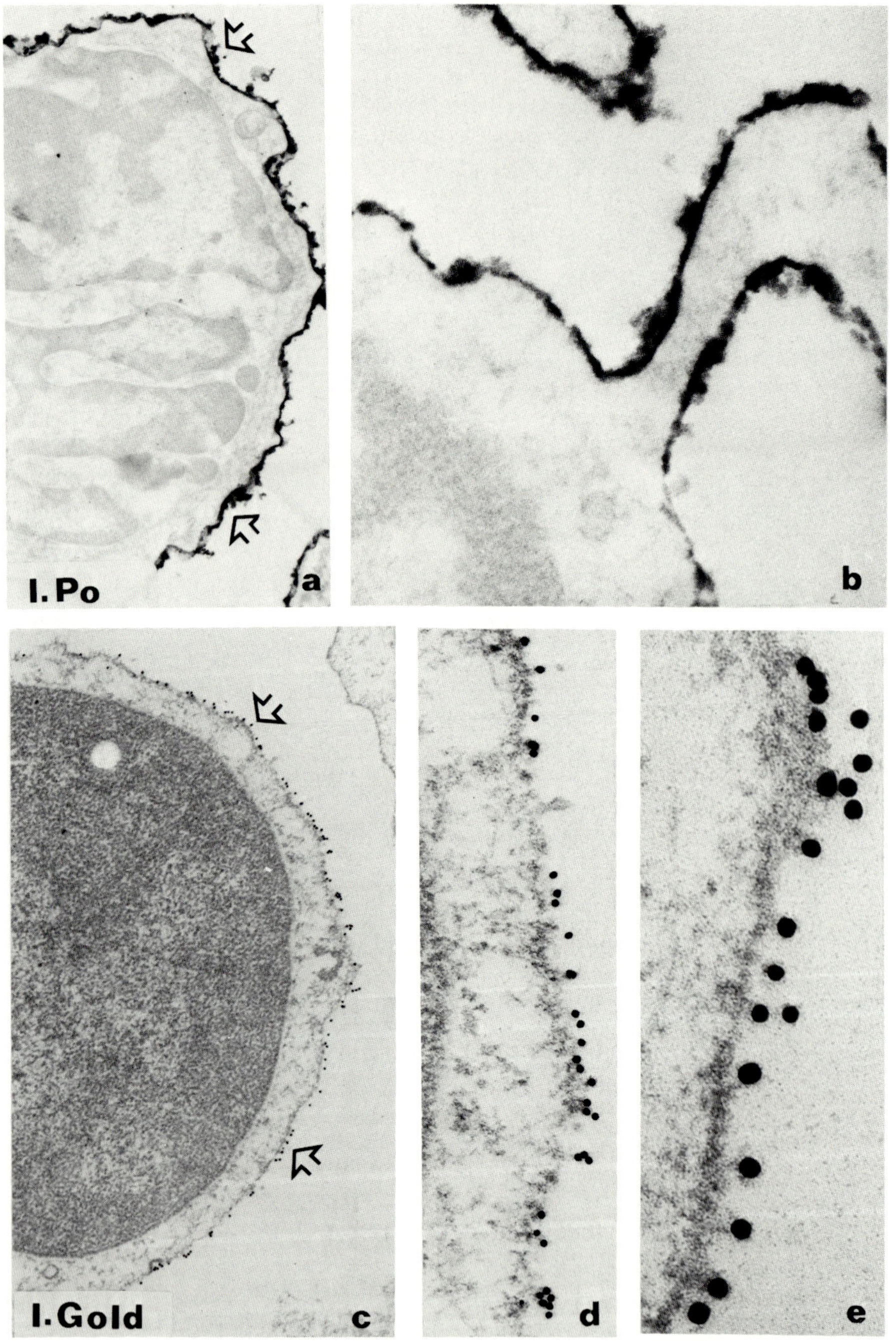

Figure 6. Immunoultrastructural labeling of a surface Ag expressed by a lymphocyte using the indirect immunoperoxidase technique (arrow) (I.Po) (A, B) and using the immunogold technique (I. Gold) (arrow) (C, D, E) with increasing magnifications.

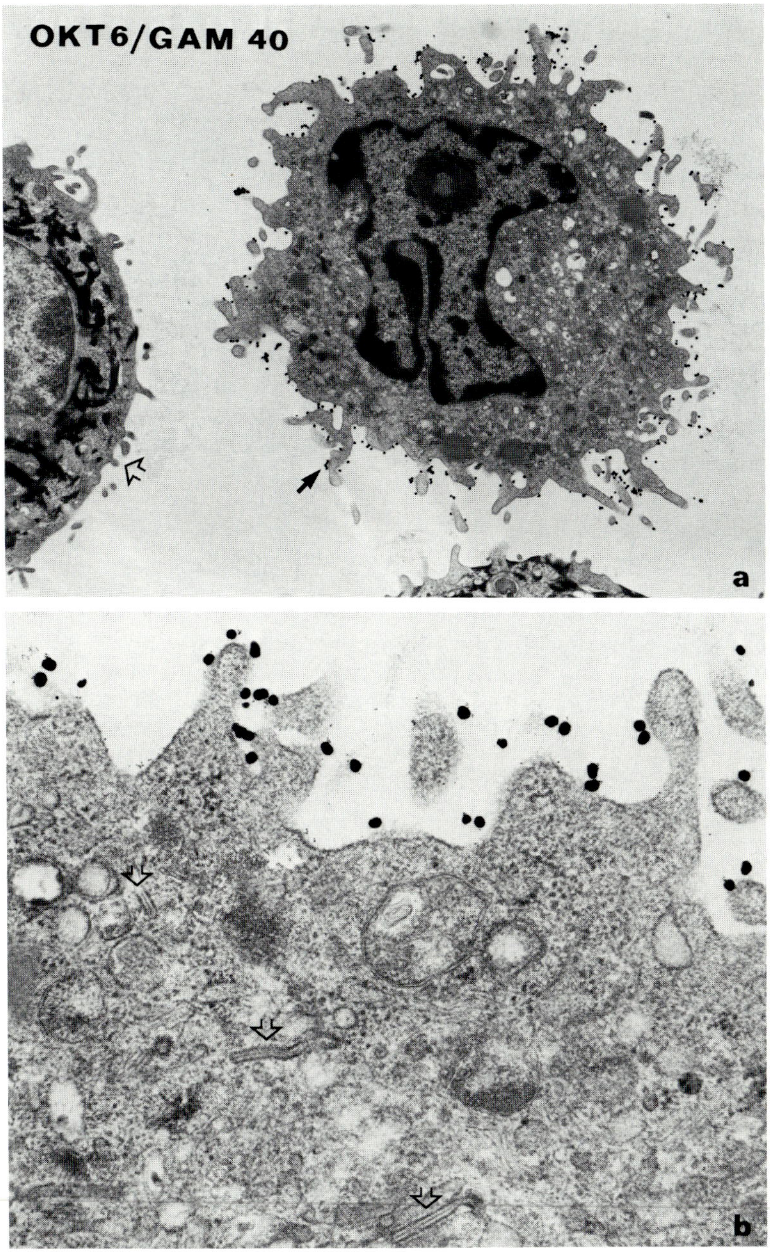

Figure 7. a) Immunogold labeling of a Langerhans cell for OKT4 MCA positivity using a gold conjugate with 40 nm ϕ gold particles. The arrow points to the punctate pattern of the colloidal gold particles along the cell membrane. Note the absence of gold along the keratinocyte (open arrow) (9600×). b) High magnification of the membrane labeling of a Birbeck granule-containing cell (open arrows) (48,000×).

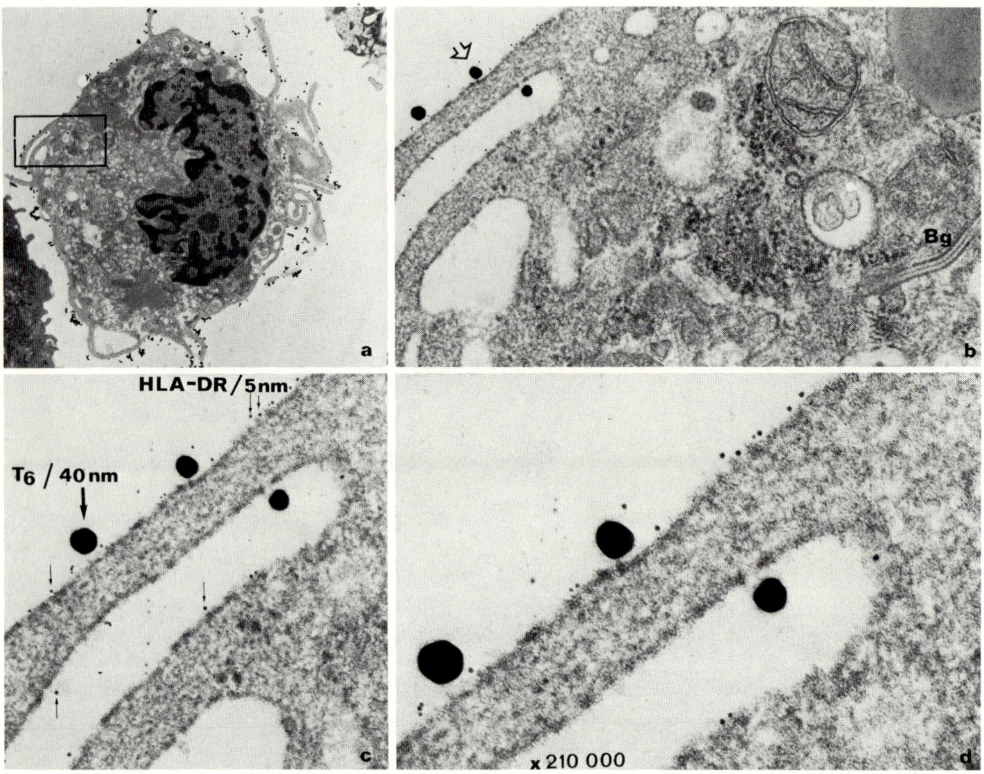

Figure 8. a) Double immunogold labeling of human Langerhans cells. Isolated dendritic epidermal cells were labeled successively with 40 nm gold granules, indicating the presence of T6 antigen, and with 5 nm gold granules labelled with anti-HLA-DR MCA (BL2). Note the absence of gold particles on an adjacent keratinocyte (9800×). b. OKT6$^+$ and BL2$^+$ reactive EC showing ultrastructural characteristics of LC (Birbeck granules unstained, Bg) (48,000×). c, d) 40 nm and 5 nm gold particles do not interact with each other and are exclusively located in close apposition with the cytoplasmic membrane (100,000× and 210,000×, respectively).

Table 2. Characterization of Peripheral Blood Mononuclear Leukocytes with Monoclonal Antibodies. Values are Means ± SD (n = 6). Fluorescent-labeled Cells Were Examined with Either a Fluorescence Microscope or a Cytofluorograph

	Fluorescence microscopic analysis			*Cytofluorometric analysis*		
Subject's age (yr)	*OKT3$^+$ (%)*	*OKM1$^+$ (%)*	*OKT6$^+$ (%)*	*OKT3$^+$ (%)*	*OKM1$^+$ (%)*	*OKT6$^+$ (%)*
1–13	53.5 ± 13.4	16.3 ± 4.3	1.8 ± 1.2	64.5 ± 7.4	16.4 ± 1.7	1.0 ± 1.2
20–26	55.7 ± 6.4	17.1 ± 3.6	0.6 ± 0.7	63.8 ± 6.5	19.7 ± 7.5	1.3 ± 0.9

From Dezutter-Dambuyant, et al. (18).

LC Subpopulations

Existence of Two DR-expressing Cell Populations in Normal Human Epidermis. HLA-DR antigens are only expressed by LC and indeterminate cells in normal human epidermis. IIF and ultrastructural immunogold labeling were used to study the HLA-DR expression by means of two anti-DR MCA.

Freshly dispersed DR-positive epidermal cells express different densities of DR antigens on their membrane surface. Approximately 25% of DR-positive cells are strongly labeled by anti-DR MCA, and 75% are weakly stained. After 18 hours in complete culture medium before labeling, no significant difference in these percentages are observed. The lymphoid-like LC-enriched cells obtained by Ficoll-Hypaque centrifugation were processed for cell sorting, which revealed two populations of DR-positive EC: strongly labeled cells (30.8 %) and weakly labeled cells (69.2 %).

Using indirect ultrastructural immunogold labeling, DR-positive cells may be divided into two types according to the density of DR sites on cell membrane: 1) type DR^+ which is a weak surface labeling by electron-dense gold particles (8.8±3.0/μm) and cytoplasmic Birbeck granules identifying such cells as typical LH; and 2) type Dr^{3+}, which is a strong membrane immunogold labeling (38.9 ± 4.6gp/μm) of either Birbeck granule-containing cells or Birbeck granule-lacking cells. The gold particles bound to the cell membrane were used to quantify the number of HLA-DR sites expressed on each cell type: 1×10^5 sites on Dr^+ and 5×10^5 on Dr^{3+} cells (17).

Subpopulations Defined by the Simultaneous Detection of T6 and HLA-DR Antigens. In dispersed EC suspensions, these membrane antigens may distinguish three antigen-positive EC subsets by means of double IF labeling: 97.3 ± 1.2% of the labeled cells are DR(+)/T6(+), while 2.2 ± 0.9% are DR(+)/T6(−) and 0.5 ± 0.6% are DR(−)/T6(+). IEM with gold particles confirms the coexistence of T6-positive and T6-negative epidermal cells (Table 3) Fig. 8 (16).

Advantages of Immunogold Labeling (Fig. 6)

An ultrastructural immunogold labeling was recently developed for better identification of LC surface antigens (84). Since the first report by Page-Faulk and Taylor (72), this immunogold method has been extensively used (45). Various advantages of this method were noted: the absence of nonspecific absorption of gold granules on the cell surface, the possibility of poststained ultrathin sections without changes in the immunolabeling

Table 3. Simultaneous Detection of T6 and DR Antigen-bearing Epidermal Cells in Normal Human Skin

Antigen-positive cells (phenotype)	*Crude EC suspensions %(a)*	*Enriched EC suspensions %(a)*
DR(+)	99.5 ± 0.6	99.7 ± 0.4
T6(+)	97.8 ± 0.9	97.2 ± 1.1
DR(+)/T6(+)	97.3 ± 1.2	96.9 ± 0.9
DR(+)/T6(−)	2.2 ± 0.9	2.8 ± 1.1
DR(−)/T6(+)	0.5 ± 0.6	0.3 ± 0.4

(a) %, $\frac{\text{Antigen-positive cells}}{\text{Total labeled cells}} \times 100$ expressed as mean ± SD.

contrast, and the ability of a double labeling using gold particles of different sizes. Furthermore, colloidal gold allows a quantitative approach to surface antigens based on the direct count of particles located in close apposition to the plasma membrane (46,47,55).

The binding of gold particle-conjugated antibody to membrane antigens is primarily determined by the size of the granule. In addition, no direct relationship can be established between the number of bound particles and the number of antibody-binding sites, except if the binding occurs when the granules have a size below 12 to 20 nm. In fact, because of steric hindrance, the accessibility of the gold granule-conjugated antibody to receptors depends upon the size of the gold particles. With particles of a large diameter (40 nm), the number of granules fixed on the cell surface largely minimizes the real number of antigenic sites revealed by the immunogold conjugate (46).

For example, Figure 8 shows the simultaneous detection of T6 and HLA-DR antigens on the surface of normal LC obtained in suspension. In addition, this double labeling can be performed on EA rosette-forming LC, in which the Fc receptors for IgG are visualized by erythrocytes coated with IgG (Fig. 9) (part I) (part II).

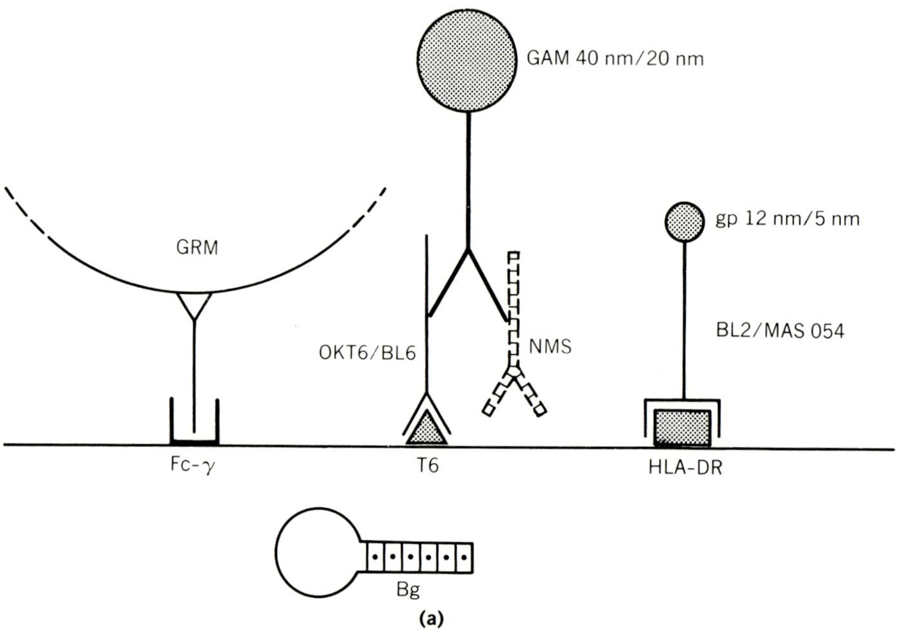

(a)

Figure 9. Human Langerhans cell. a) Simultaneous identification of Fc receptors, T6 and HLA-DR antigens, and Birbeck granules in the same cell. b) Visualization of Fc receptors for IgG using IgG-coated erythrocytes 16,000×. (Inset, rosette-forming cell with IgG-coated red blood cells 2800×.) c,d) Double immunogold labeling of T6 (large gold granules 20 nm in diameter) and HLA-DR (small gold granules 12 nm in diameter) (Bg, Birbeck granule) (48000× and 100,000×, respectively).
OKT6/BL6, anti-T6 MCA; BL2/MAS 054, anti-HLA-DR MCA; GRM, sheep erythrocytes; Fcφ receptors for Fc fragment of IgG; Bg, Birbeck granules; NMS, normal mice serum; GAM 40 nm/20 nm, goat Ig antimice Ig labeled with gold granules of 40 nm or 20 nm in diameter; gp 12 nm/5 nm, gold particles of 12 nm; or 5 nm in diameter

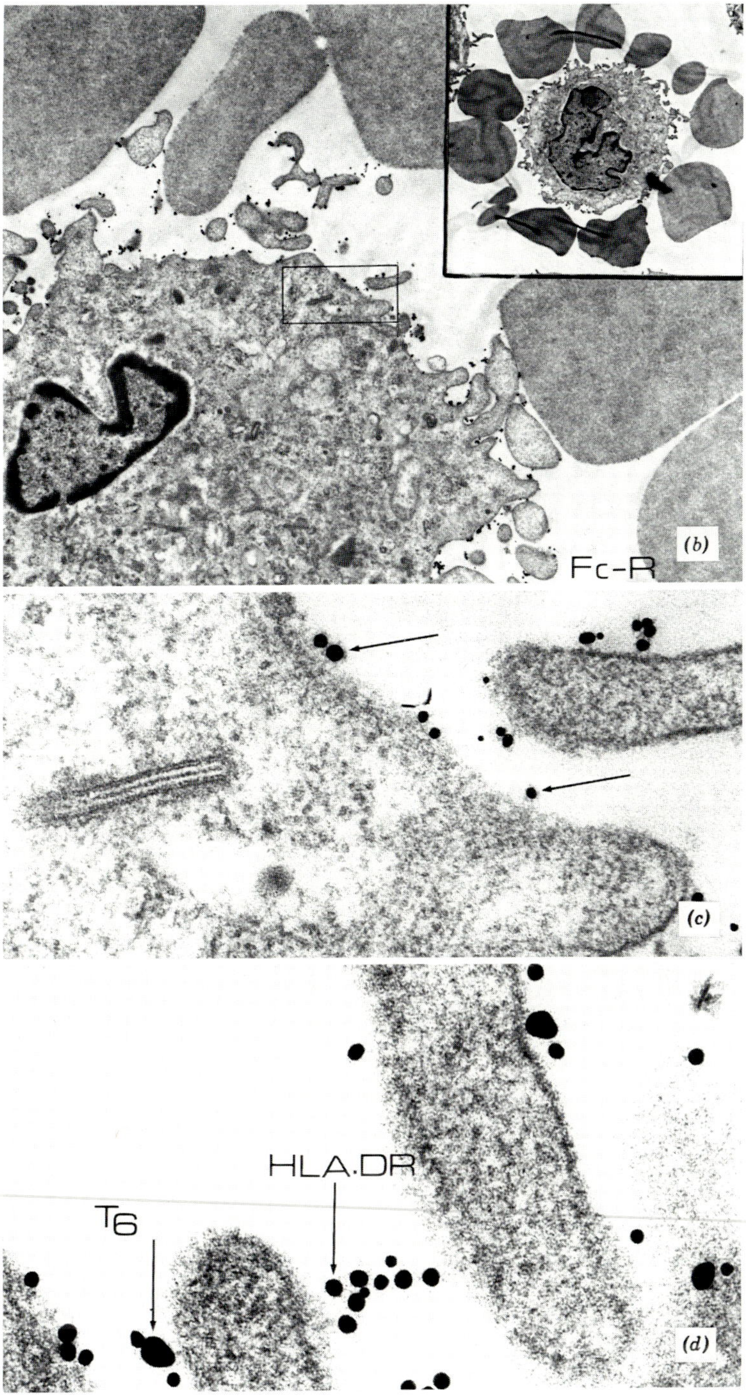
(b)
Fc-R
(c)
HLA.DR
T6
(d)

LC and Nontumoral Lesions

LC and Aging and Chronic Sun Exposure (3,90). In the skin of old adults with chronic actinic damage, the number of LC is significantly decreased. In addition, significantly fewer LC are observed in exposed versus covered skin. The decreased number of LC on the sun-damaged skin of elderly individuals may play a critical permissive role in the development of cutaneous carcinoma.

LC and Psoralen Ultraviolet A (PUVA) Therapy. PUVA therapy decreases the number of LC in the epidermis (from 704 ± 58 cells/mm^2 to 195 ± 173 cell/mm^2 after a single PUVA dose of 5 J/cm^2) (52,73). Ninety percent of LC had disappeared after 2 weeks of treatment with PUVA (8-MOP). The number of LC return to normal within 3 weeks after cessation of therapy; LC disappeared only with the combination of PUVA and 8-MOP (31).

LC and Aromatic Retinoids. In lichen planus (27), recent results show an increase in the number of LC after treatment with oral retinoids. In psoriasis (36), changes in the number and distribution of OKT6- and HLA-DR-positive cells in the involved epidermis are corrected by oral retinoid treatment.

LC and Sarcoidosis (30). LC play a role in cell-mediated immune reactions that are often depressed in sarcoidosis. In comparison to normal skin, the epidermis overlaying noninvolved sarcoidal- and Kveim-reactive skin contains significantly fewer detectable HLA-DR and T6 antigen-bearing LC. The reductions within noninvolved skin are most pronounced in patients with multisystem disease.

LC and Cutaneous Lupus Erythematosus (LE) (89). In cutaneous LE lesions, LC are less dendritic, more irregularly distributed, and present in fewer numbers when compared with those in adjacent normal skin.

LC and Lichen Planus (LP) (26). The in situ immunologic typing of LC in LP lesions demonstrates that the number of dendritic cells in epidermis is greater in involved skin than in noninvolved skin. In recent lesions, LC are more abundant than in older lesions.

LC and Allergy Patch Tests (50). In minimum positive allergic and toxic patch tests, no differences are observed in the appearance of LC or in the number of LC mononuclear cells contact after 24, 48, and 78 hours.

LC and Cutaneous Lymphoid Infiltrates (64). OKT6-positive cells are identified in the dermis in various cases of atrophic parapsoriasis and lymphomatoid populations.

LC and Skin Tumors

LC and Wart Lesions (11). In most cases, the density of LC is markedly reduced in wart epidermis, as compared to normal epidermis. In some lesions showing an inflammatory infiltrate around the tumor, the number of LC is high in both the dermis and epidermis.

LC and Epidermal Carcinoma (25). In basal and squamous cell carcinomas, the LC identified by OKT6 or BL6 MCA can be observed in the epidermis overlapping the tumor masses, and also within the proliferative tissue.

LC and Cutaneous T-Cell Lymphomas. In skin lesions of mycosis fungoides (MF) and Sezary syndrome, the MCA reacting with LC allows identification of dendritic cells in the dermis of skin lesions (12,92,93). These results are confirmed by standard EM (49).

In skin lesions of MF, quantitative studies using MCA have shown an increase in the number of LC in the dermis and epidermis (44,62).

Histiocytosis X and LC

HX Cell Phenotype. HX cells are abnormal proliferations of LC. The existence of T6 antigens on the membrane of HX cells is now clearly established (10,39,75,87). The expression of T4 antigens by these tumoral cells has been recently reported (40,71).

Using the IP technique, Murphy et al. (71) studied the reactivity of normal human LC and tumoral cells of histiocytosis X with various MCA directed against T3, T4, T6, and T8 antigens. In their study, LC reacted only with anti-T6 MCA (OKT6), whereas HX cells showed a reactivity with both anti-T6 and anti-T4 MCA (respectively, OKT6 and OKT4 MCA). On HX cells, OKT4 produced a focal membrane staining strikingly less intense by IEM than that of OKT6. Lastly, normal LC and HX cells did not react with OKT3 and OKT8 MCA.

On the other hand, Wood et al. (101) studied the reactivity of various MCA (anti-leu 3a/3b, OKT4, and anti-T4) with LC, HX cells, and other cells of the mononuclear phagocyte lineage using IIF on tissue sections or cell suspensions. The microscopic observation and the fluorescent-activated cell sorter analysis showed that the reactivity of LC and HX cells with OKT4 and anti-T4 MCA was less intense than that noted with OKT6.

Recently, Harrist suggested that the presence of T4-T6-positive cells in cutaneous disease may be a marker for abnormal LC. The demonstration of T4 Ag on the surface of normal LC shows the absence of relationship between this phenotype ($T4^{+}T6^{+}$) and abnormalities of LC (39).

CONCLUSIONS

Immunohistologic techniques used with the express purpose of combining immunologic parameters with morphologic criteria for recognition of normal and abnormal cells are in their infancy. The cases reported in this chapter illustrate the remarkable potential of these methods at the light or elecron microscopic level when combined with the exquisite specificity of MCA. Clearly, a field of study has been opened for exploration by dermatopathologists.

Immunocytologic stains depend not only upon the quality of the antibodies, but also on the integrity of the antigens studied. Labile antigens, which do not survive fixation or processing, may be successfully demonstrated on cryostat sections. However, the number of antigens successfully demonstrated in paraffin sections continues to grow. The diagnostic role of some antigens is yet to be established, while for others, antibodies of possible diagnostic value are yet to be discovered. The availability of kits containing essential matched reagents with specificity against many of these antigens greatly enhances the potential of these immunolabeling procedures for diagnostic as well as research studies.

REFERENCES

1. Alario A, Ortonne JP, Schmitt D, et al: Lichen planus: Study with anti-human T lymphocyte antigen (HTLA) serum on frozen tissue sections. *Br J Dermatol* 98, 601–604, 1978.

2. Alero-Thomas J, Janossy G, Graham-Brown RA, et al: The relationship between T lymphocyte subsets and Ia-like antigen positive non-lymphoid cells in early stages of cutaneous T cell lymphoma. *J Invest Dermatol* 78:169–176, 1982.
3. Berman B, Chen VL, France DS, et al: Anatomical mapping of epidermal Langerhans cell densities in adults. *Br J Dermatol* 109:553--558, 1983.
4. Bhan AK, Harrist TJ, Murphy GF, et al: T cell subsets and Langerhans cells in lichen planus: In situ characterization using monoclonal antibodies. *Br J Dermatol* 105:617–622, 1981.
5. Bhan AK, Mihm MC, Dvorak HF: T cell subsets in allograft rejection. In situ characterization of T cell subsets in human skin allografts by the use of monoclonal antibodies. *J Immunol* 129:1578–1583, 1982.
6. Boyum A: Separation of leukocytes from blood and bone marrow. *Scand J Clin Lab Invest* 21(Suppl 97):77–89, 1968.
7. Bronstein BR, Murphy GF, Harrist TJ, et al: Location of HLA-A, B, C, antigens in dendritic cells of normal human skin: An immunoelectron microscopic study. *J Invest Dermatol* 80:481–484, 1983.
8. Brubaker D, Whiteside TL: Localization of human T lymphocytes in tissue sections by a rosetting technique. *Am J Pathol* 88:323–332, 1977.
9. Buecher SA, Winkelmann RK, Banks PM: T-cell subsets in cutaneous sarcoidosis. *Arch Dermatol* 119:728–732, 1983.
10. Cambazard F, Fernandez-Bussy R, Schmitt D, et al: Identification immunohistologique des cellules de l'histiocytosis X. Intérêt diagnostic. *Ann Dermatol Venereol* 110:33–40, 1983.
11. Chardonnet Y, Beauve P, Viac J, et al: T-cell subsets and Langerhans cells in wart lesions. *Immunol Lett* 6:191–196, 1983.
12. Chu A, Kung I, Edelson R: Dermal Langerhans cells in cutaneous lymphoma: An in situ study using monoclonal antibodies. *J Invest Dermatol* 76:324(A), 1981.
13. Chu A, Eisinger M, Soolee JI, et al: Immunoelectron microscopic identification of Langerhans cells using a new antigenic marker. *J Invest Dermatol* 78:177–180, 1982.
14. Chu AC, Robinson D, Smith NP, et al: The Sézary cell. A morphologically distinct by non-specific cell type. *J Invest Dermatol* 80:332–333, 1983.
15. Czernielewski J, Faure M, Schmitt D, et al: In vitro mixed skin cell lymphocyte culture reaction (MSLR) in man: Analysis of the epidermal cell and T cell subpopulations. *Clin Exp Immunol* 50:426–433, 1982.
16. Dezutter-Dambuyant C, Faure M, Schmitt D, et al: Simultaneous detection of T6 and HLA-DR antigens distinguishes three cell subpopulations in dispersed normal human epidermal cells. *Immunol Lett* 7:203–207, 1984.
17. Dezutter-Dambuyant C, Cordier G, Faure M, et al: Quantitative evaluation of two distinct cell populations in normal human epidermis which express HLA-DR antigens. *Br J Dermatol* 1984 (in press).
18. Dezutter-Dambuyant C, Schmitt D, Faure M, et al: Detection of OKT6-positive cells in normal peripheral blood (without visible Birbeck granules). *Immunol Lett 8*:121–126, 1984.
19. De Mey J, Moermans M, De Waele M, et al: The IGS (Immuno Gold Staining) method used with monoclonal antibodies. In Peters H (Ed): *Prot Biol Fluids*. Pergamon Press, Oxford, 1982, pp 943–947.
20. De Panfilis G, Manara G, Sansoni P, et al: T-cell infiltrate in lichen planus. Demonstration of activated lymphocytes using monoclonal antibodies. *J Cut Path* 10:52–58, 1983.
21. De Waele M, De Mey J, Moeremans M, et al: Colloidal gold as a marker for the light microscope detection of leukocyte cell surface antigens with monoclonal antibodies. *J Clin Immunol* 2:24S–31S, 1982.
22. De Waele M, De Mey J, Moeremans M, et al: Immunogold staining method for the light microscopic detection of leukocyte cell surface antigens with monoclonal antibodies: Its application to the enumeration of lymphocytes subpopulations. *J Histochem Cytochem* 31:376–381, 1983.
23. Dubertret L, Picard O, Bagot M, et al: Specificity of monoclonal antibody anti-T6 for Langerhans cells in normal human skin. *Br J Dermatol* 106:287–289, 1982.
24. Faure M, Frappaz A, Schmitt D, et al: Role of HLA-DR bearing Langerhans and epidermal

indeterminate cells in the in vitro generation of alloreactive cytotoxic T cells in man. *Cell Immunol* 83–271–279, 1984.

25. Fernandez-Bussy R, Cambazard F, Mauduit G, et al: T-cell subsets and Langerhans cells in skin tumours. *Eur J Cancer Oncol* 19:907–913, 1983.
26. Fernandez-Bussy R, Schmitt D, Gaucherand M, et al: Lichen planus: Evaluation of cells in skin lesions and of T-lymphocyte subsets in blood. *J Dermatol* 10:17–24, 1983.
27. Fernandez-Bussy R, Schmitt D, Mauduit G, et al: Effects of aromatic retinoid (Ro 10–9359) on Langerhans cells in lichen planus. Arch Dermatol Res 275:105–108, 1983.
28. Fithian E, Kung P, Goldstein G, et al: Reactivity of Langerhans cells with hybridoma antibody. *Proc Natl Acad Sci USA* 78:2541–2544, 1981.
29. Fithian E, Kung P, Goldstein G, et al: Reactivity of Langerhans cells with hybridoma antibody. *Proc Nat Acad Sci USA* 4:2541–2544, 1981.
30. Fox JL, Berman B, Teirstein AS, et al: Quantitative of cutaneous Langerhans cells of sarcoïdosis patients. *J Invest Dermatol* 80:472–475, 1983.
31. Friedmann PS, Ford G, Ross J, et al: Reappearance of epidermal Langerhans cells after PUVA therapy. *Br J Dermatol* 109:301–307, 1983.
32. Geuze H, Slot J, Van Der Ley P, et al: Use of colloidal gold particles in double labelling immunoelectromicroscopy of ultrathin frozen tissue sections. *J Cell Biol* 89:653–665, 1981.
33. Gomes MA, Schmitt D, Souteyrand P, et al: Lichen planus and chronic graft versus host reaction. In situ identification of immunocompetent cell phonotypes. *J Cut Pathol* 9:249–257, 1982.
34. Graham RC, Karnovsky MJ: The early stages of adsorption of injected horseradish peroxidase in the proximal tubules of mouse kidney. Ultrastructural cytochemistry by a new technique. *J Histochem Cytochem* 14:291–302, 1966.
35. Guesdon JL, Ternynck T, Avrameas S: The use of avidin-biotin interacton in immunoenzymatic techniques. *J Histochem Cytochem* 27:1131–1134, 1979.
36. Haftek M, Faure M, Schmitt D, et al: Langerhans cells in skin from patients with psoriasis: Quantitative and qualitative study of T6 and HLA-DR antigen expressing cells and changes with aromatic retinoid administration. *J Invest Dermatol* 81:10–14, 1983.
37. Hammerling GJ, Mawve G, Goldberg E, et al: Ia on spermatozoa, macrophages, and epidermal cells. *Immunogenetics* 1:428–437, 1975.
38. Hannah J, Langley M, Naeim F: Immunogold staining method for identification and subclassification of lymphoid cells and their malignant counterparts. *Lab Invest* 48:32(A), 1983.
39. Harrist TJ, Bhan AK, Murphy GF, et al: Histiocytosis X: In situ characterization of cutaneous lesions. *J Invest Dermatol* 78:354–355, 1982.
40. Harrist TJ, Bhan AK, Murphy GF, et al: In situ characterization of cutaneous infiltrates with monoclonal antibodies. *Am J Clin Pathol* 79:294–300, 1983.
41. Haynes BF, Metzgar RS, Minna JD, et al: Phenotypic characterization of cutaneous T cell lymphoma. Use of monoclonal antibodies to compare with other malignant T cells. *N Engl J Med* 304:1319–1323, 1981.
42. Haynes BF, Hensley LL, Jegasothy BV: Differentiation of human T lymphocytes: II. Phenotypic difference in skin and blood malignant T cell in cutaneous T cell lymphoma. *J Invest Dermatol* 78:323–326, 1982.
43. Holden CA, Morgan EW, MacDonald DM: A technique for immunoultrastructural identification of T6-positive Langerhans cells and indeterminate cells in mycosis fungoides. *J Invest Dermatol* 79:382–384, 1982.
44. Holden CA, Morgan EW, MacDonald DM: The cell population in the cutaneous infiltrate of mycosis fungoides: In situ studies using monoclonal antisera. *Br J Dermatol* 106:385–392, 1982.
45. Horisberger, M: Evaluation of colloidal gold as a cytochemical marker for transmission and scanning electron microscopy. *Biol Cellulaire* 36:253–258, 1979.
46. Horisberger M, Tacchini-Von Lanthen M: Stability and steric hindrance of lectin labeled gold markers in transmission and scanning electron microscopy. In Boghansen TC, Spengler GA (Eds): *Lectins: Biology, Biochemistry, Clinical Biochemistry,* vol. 3. W. de Gruyter (Hawthorne) 1983, pp 189–198.

47. Horisberger M, Vauthey M: Labelling of colloidal gold with protein. A quantitative study using -lactoglobulin. *Histochemistry* 80:13–18, 1984.
48. Howmark A: Acid alpha naphtyl acetate esterase staining of T lymphocytes in human skin. *Acta Dermatol Venereo (Stockholm)* 57:497–502, 1977.
49. Jimbow K, Chiba M, Horikoshi T: Electron microscope identification of Langerhans cells in the dermal infiltrates of mycosis fungoides. *J Invest Dermatol* 78:102–107, 1982.
50. Kanerva L, Rankt A, Mustakallio K: Langerhans cell-mononuclear cell contacts are not specific for allergy in patch tests. *Br J Dermatol* 109(Suppl 25):64–67, 1983.
51. Klareskog L, Tjernlund U, Forsum U, et al: Epidermal Langerhans cells express Ia antigens. *Nature* 268:248–250, 1977.
52. Koulu L, Jansen CT: Effect of oral methoxsalen photochemotherapy on human Langerhans cell number. *Arch Dermatol Res* 274:79–83, 1982.
53. Krueger GG, Daynes RA, Robert CK, et al: Migration of Langerhans cells and the expression of Ia on epidermal cells following the grafting of normal skin to nude mice. Immune Deficient Animals. 4th Int. Workshop Exp. Res. Chexbers, 1982. *Expt Cell Biol* 52:97–102, 1984.
54. Kung PC, Berger CL, Goldstein G, et al: Cutaneous T cell lymphoma: Characterization by monoclonal antibodies. *Blood* 52:261–268, 1981.
55. Lafferty MD, Ackerman GA, Dunn CDR, et al: Ultrastructural immunocytochemical localization of presumptive erythropoietin binding sites on developing erythrocytic cells of normal human bone marrow. *J Histochem Cytochem* 29:49–56, 1981.
56. Lampert IA, Suitters AJ, Chisholm PM: Expression of Ia antigen on epidermal keratinocytes in GVH disease. *Nature* 293:149, 1981.
57. Lampert IA, Janossy G, Suitters AJ, et al: Immunological analysis of the skin in GVH disease. *Clin Exp Immunol* 50:123–131, 1982.
58. Laroche L, Bach JF: T-cell imbalance in nonleukemic and leukemic cutaneous lymphoma defined by monoclonal antibodies. *Clin Immunol Immunopathol* 20:278–285, 1981.
59. Loening Th, Caselitz J, Seifert G, et al: Identification of Langerhans cells: Simultaneous use of sera to intermediate filaments, T6 and HLA-DR antigens or oral mucosa, human epidermis and their tumours. *Virchows Arch A* 398:119–128, 1982.
60. Loening Th, Schmitt D, Becker WM, et al: Application of the biotin-avidin system for ultrastructural identification of suppressor/cytotoxic lymphocytes in oral lichen planus. *Arch Dermatol Res* 272:177–180, 1982.
61. MacDonald DM, Schmitt D, Germain D, et al: Ultrastructural demonstration of T cells in cutaneous tissue using specific anti-human T-cell antiserum. *Br J Dermatol* 99:641–646, 1978.
62. MacKie RM, Turbitt ML: Quantification of dendritic cells in normal and abnormal human epidermis using monoclonal antibodies directed against Ia and HTA antigens. *J Invest Dermatol* 81:216–220, 1983.
63. McMillan EM, Martin D, Wasik R, et al: Demonstration in situ of T cells and T cell subsets in lichen planus using monoclonal antibodies. *J Cut Pathol* 8:228–234, 1981.
64. McMillan EM, Wasik R, Everett MA: In situ demonstration of OKT6-positive cells in cutaneous lymphoid infiltrates. *Am Acad Dermatol* 5:274–279, 1981.
65. McMillan EM, Wasik R, Peters S, et al: OKT9 reactivity in mycosis fungoides and large plaque (atrophic) parapsoriasis. *Cancer* 51:1403–1407, 1983.
66. Margolis RJ, Tonnesen MG, Harrist TJ, et al: Lymphocyte subsets and Langerhans cells/Indeterminate cells in erythema multiforme. *J Invest Dermatol* 81:403–406, 1983.
67. Mason DW, Dallman M, Barclay AN: GVH disease induces expression of Ia antigen in rat epidermal cells and gut epithelium. *Nature* 1981.
68. Murphy GF, Bhan AK, Sato S, et al: A new immunologic marker for human Langerhans cells. *N Engl J Med* 303:370–371, 1981.
69. Murphy GF, Bhan AK, Sato S, et al: Characterization of Langerhans cells by the use of monoclonal antibodies. *Lab Invest* 45:465–468, 1981.
70. Murphy GF, Bhan AK, Harrist TJ, et al: In situ identification of T6-positive cells in normal human dermis by immunoelectron microscopy. *Br J Dermatol* 108:423–431, 1983.
71. Murphy GF, Harrist TJ, Bhan AK, et al: Distribution of cell surface antigens in histiocytosis

X: Quantitative immunoelectron microscopy using monoclonal antibodies. *Lab Invest* 48:90–97, 1983.

72. Page-Faulk W, Taylor GM: An immunocolloid method for the electron microscope. Immunochemistry 8:1081–1083, 1971.
73. Ree K: Reduction of Langerhans cells in human epidermis during PUVA therapy. A morphometric study. *J Invest Dermatol* 78:488–492, 1982.
74. Roth J, Bendayan M, Orci L: Ultrastructural localization of intracellular antigens by the use of protein-A-gold complex. *J Histochem Cytochem* 26:1074–1081, 1978.
75. Rousseau-Merck MF, Barbey S, Jaubert F, et al: Reactivity of histiocytosis X cells with monoclonal antibodies. *Pathol Res Prac* 177:8–12, 1983.
76. Rowden G, Lewis MG, Sullivan AK: Ia antigen expression on human epidermal Langerhans cells. *Nature* 268:247–248, 1977.
77. Rowden G: Immunoelectron microscopic studies of surface receptors and antigens of human Langerhans cells.*Br J Dermatol* 1977. 97:593–608.
78. Rowden G, Phillips TM, Lewis MG: Ia antigen in indeterminate cells of the epidermis: Immunoelectron microscopic studies of surface antigens. *Br J Dermatol* 100:531–542, 1979.
79. Scheynius A, Klareskog L, Forsum U: In situ identification of T lymphocyte subsets and HLA-DR expressing cells in the human skin tuberculin reaction. *Clin Exp Immunol* 49:325–330, 1982.
80. Scheynius A, Klareskog L, Forsum U, et al: Enrichment of epidermal Langerhans cells: Studies with a monolayer technique and flow cytometry sorting. *J Invest Dermatol* 82:452–455, 1982.
81. Schmitt D, Alario A, Thivolet J: In situ characterization of tissue lymphoid cells of cutaneous infiltrates using specific membrane antigens. *Clin Exp Dermatol* 4:161–173, 1979.
82. Schmitt D, Souteyrand P, Brochier J, et al: Phenotype of cells involved in mycosis fungoides and Sézary syndrome (blood and skin lesions): Immunomorphological study with monoclonal antibodies. *Acta Dermatol Venereol (Stockholm)* 62:193–199, 1982.
83. Schmitt D, Thivolet J: Use of monoclonal antibodies specific for T cell subsets in cutaneous disorders: II. Immunomorphological studies in blood and skin lesions. *J Clin Immunol* 2:1115–1195, 1982.
84. Schmitt D, Faure M, Dezutter-Dambuyant C, et al: Ultrastructural immunogold staining of Langerhans cells. *J Invest Dermatol* 80:344–345, 1983.
85. Schmitt D, Faure M, Dezutter-Dambuyant C, et al: Ultrastructural immunogold labelling of human Langerhans cells enriched epidermal cell suspensions. *Arch Dermatol Res* 276:27–32, 1984.
86. Schmitt D, Faure M, Dezutter-Dambuyant C, et al: Distribution of T4 and T6 surface antigens on human Langerhans cells: Quantitative immunoelectronmicroscopic comparison using monoclonal antibodies and colloidal gold method. *Br J Dermatol 111,* 655, 1986.
87. Schuler G, Stingl G, Aberer W, et al: Histiocytosis X cells in eosinophilic granuloma express Ia and T6 antigens. *J Invest Dermatol* 80:405–409, 1983.
88. Sieber-Blum M, Sieber F, Yamada K: Cellular fibronectin promotes adrenergic differentiation of quail neural crest cells in vitro. *Exp Cell Res* 133:285–295, 1981.
89. Sontheimer RD, Bergstresser PR: Epidermal Langerhans cell involvement in cutaneous lupus erythematosus. *J Invest Dermatol* 79:237–243, 1982.
90. Thiers BH, Maize JC, Spicer SS, et al: The effects of aging and chronic sun exposure on human Langerhans cell populations. *J Invest Dermatol* 82:223–226, 1984.
91. Thivolet J, Faure M: Immunohistochemistry in cutaneous pathology. *J Cut Pathol* 10:1–32, 1983.
92. Thivolet J, Schmitt D, Souteyrand P, et al: Les cellules des lymphomes épidermotropes (mycosis fongoïde et syndrome de Sézary). Etude grâce aux anticorps monoclonaux. *Nouv Presse Méd* 11:3033–3038, 1982.
93. Tjernlund U: Immunological markers of Langerhans cells in mycosis fungoides skin lesions. *Acta Dermatol Venereol (Stockholm)* 62:241–243, 1982.
94. Trucco M, De Petris S: Determination of equilibrium binding parameters of monoclonal

antibodies specific for cells surface antigens. In Lefkovits I, Pernis B (Eds): *Immunological Methods.* Academic Press, New York, 1981, pp 1–26.

95. Trucco M, De Petris S, Garotta G, et al: Quantitative analysis of cell surface HLA structures by means of monoclonal antibodies. *Human Immunol* 3:233–242, 1980.
96. Van Der Loo EM, Cnossen J, Meijer CJLM: Morphological aspects of T cell subpopulations in human blood: Characterization of the cerebriform mononuclear cells in healthy individuals. *Clin Exp Immunol* 43:506–516, 1981.
97. Van Der Loo EM, Meijer CJLM, Scheffer E, et al: The prognostic value of membrane markers and morphometric characteristics of lymphoid cells in blood and lymph nodes from patients with mycosis fungoides. *Cancer* 48:738–744, 1981.
98. Van Vloten WA: Dutch Mycosis fungoides study group, in Goos M, and Christophers E (Eds): *Lymphoproliferative Diseases of the Skin.* Springer-Verlag, Berlin, 1982, pp 260–265.
99. Warnke R, Levy R: Detection of T and B cell antigens with hybridoma monoclonal antibodies. *J Histochem Cytochem* 28:771–776, 1980.
100. Willemze R, Graaf-Reitsma B de, Cnossen J: Characterization of T-cell subpopulations in skin and peripheral blood of patients with cutaneous T-cell lymphomas and benign inflammatory dermatoses. *J Invest Dermatol* 80:60–66, 1983.
101. Wood GS, Warner NL, Warnke RA: Anti-Leu 3/T4 antibodies react with cells of monocyte/macrophage and Langerhans lineage. *J Immunol* 131:212–216, 1983.
102. Wysocki LJ, Sato VL: Panning for lymphocytes: A method for well selection. *Proc Natl Acad Sci USA* 75:2844–2850, 1978.
103. Yonish-Rouach E, Viac J, Schmitt D, et al: Preparation of monoclonal anti-human thymocyte antibodies: Unexpected markers of epidermal cells. In Serrou B, Rosenfeld C, and Daniels J (Eds): *Current Concepts in Human Immunology and Cancer Immunomodulation.* Elsevier/North Holland, Amsterdam, 1982, pp. 55–62.
104. Yonish-Rouach E, Schmitt D, Viac J, et al: Monoclonal anti-thymic cell antibodies detecting epidermal cells. *Thymus* 6:67–78, 1984.

ADDENDUM: PROTOCOL RECOMMENDED FOR IMMUNOCYTOCHEMICAL STUDIES OF LYMPH NODE SECTIONS*

A. SPECIMEN COLLECTION

Lymph nodes must be processed not more than 20 minutes after removal. More rapid processing is preferable.

B. INITIAL PROCESSING

Small pieces with one dimension of 5 mm or less should be used. Three alternative methods may be employed for initial processing.

1. Immediate quick freezing. See below for details. This is the method of choice.
2. Hold moistened (not wet) gauze on ice for not more than 2 hours enroute to laboratory for quick freezing.

*These recommendations (2) were generated by participants in the Summary Session at the end of the Immunohistochemical Expo organized by John Kateley on October 14–15, 1984. This session was chaired by Julius Elias, the consensus compiled by Ernst H. Beutner, and the edited version (2) reproduced here with permission of the publisher.

3. Place in Michel's transport medium (3) with pH properly adjusted (1) for not more than about 1 week (3). When washing out the ammonium sulfate, gentle washing for not more than 10 minutes should be used. Before quick freezing, the excess fluid should be removed by blotting.

C. QUICK FREEZING

Before freezing tissue, cover it with OTC† to prevent drying. Regardless of the method of initial processing, the methods for quick freezing include the following (listed in the order of preference).

1. Liquid nitrogen. The tissue should be in a tube or some other appropriate container to prevent direct contact with liquid nitrogen. Such contact causes problems with cracking.
2. A mixture of solid CO_2 (dry ice) and an appropriate organic solvent (acetone, petroleum ether, or ethanol). It is critically important that tissue be in a tube or other container to prevent contact with solvents. Such contact destroys antigens completely.
3. CO_2 jets that quick freeze at outlet from CO_2 tanks.
4. Cold bars in cryostats. This is the least desirable quick freezing method because of the slow freeze they induce and the resultant problems.

D. CUTTING

Mount the tissue in OTC for preparing cryostat sections. Cut at 4 to 6 μm thickness. (If storage is desired, see point F.) If problems arise with sections floating off of slides, use coated slides. Coating can be done by, for example, dipping slides into 1% Elmer's glue in distilled water or other appropriate adhesive agent and allowing to dry.

E. DRYING SLIDES

Before fixation or other processing, dry slides. In a dry climate, 10 minutes at room temperature is adequate. In more humid climates, 10 minutes in a dessicator may be used. Some workers recommend 2 hours or overnight at room temperature. Importantly, if slides in sealed containers are stored in a freezer or refrigerator, the container needs to be brought to room temperature before opening it to prevent the deposition of condensation moisture on the previously dried section.

F. STORAGE OF TISSUE BLOCK

If storage is desired after cutting, coat cut edge of block with OTC, cover with foil, put into zip-lock bag with chips of ice and store in freezer at temperatures of −30°C or less, not at −20°C. Do not store in frost-free freezer. Tissues can be pulled from storage and recut up to three times. They can be kept for at least 6 months if handled properly.

†OTC, Lab Tek Products, Naperville, IL 60540.

G. ACETONE FIXATION

Fix in dry acetone for 10 to 20 minutes. Fix not more than 40 slides in a Coplin jar of acetone to prevent accumulation of water. Screwcap Coplin jars may be used for the same reason. Some workers recommend use of cold acetone. If cold acetone is used, accumulation of condensation moisture must be prevented. If slides are stored under refrigeration before use in immunohistochemical studies, they must be placed in an airtight container to prevent condensation of moisture on removal.

H. IMMUNOCYTOCHEMICAL TESTS

Frozen sections prepared by the above-mentioned methods may be used for any of the diverse types of immunocytochemical methods, including the indirect, PAP, ABC, and other methods. Details of methods are described elsewhere (2). The following specifics were discussed.

1. If a peroxidase label is used, it is necessary that the DAB should be clear. It is soluble up to about 5 mg/ml of tris buffer. The concentrations used may range, from example, from 2 to 10 mg of DAB/10 ml, depending on the sensitivity desired.
2. For immunoenzyme labels or for colloidal gold (which are read with light microscopy), a hematoxylin counterstain may be used for 3 minutes.
3. Mounting of stained slides may be done in a polyvinyl alcohol (gelvatol) glycerol mixture (4), which hardens in a few days to give semipermanent slides. (See Chap. 1, page 22.) These can be stored for several months at 4°C.
4. Controls should include a section that is not treated with a primary specific antibody. Other controls depend on the test system used, circumstances, and the user's discretion.

REFERENCES

1. Beutner EH, Nisengard RJ, Kumar V: Defined immunofluorescence: Basic concepts and their application to clinical immunodermatology. In Beutner EH, Chorzelski TP, Bean SF (Eds.): *Immunopathology of the Skin,* ed. 2. Ed., Wiley, New York, 1979, pp 29–75.
2. Elias JM, LeNeve D, Beutner EH, et al. Optimal conditions for demonstrating human lymphocyte differentiation antigens. A working protocol for the immunohistochemical analysis of a lymph node biopsy. *J Histotechnology* 8: 201–203, 1985.
3. Michel B, Milner Y, David K: Preservation of tissue fixed immunoglobulins in skin biopsies of patients with lupus erythematosus and bullous diseases. Preliminary report. *J Invest Dermatol* 59:449–452, 1973.
4. Rodriquez J, Deinhardt F: Preparation of a semi-permanent mounting medium for fluorescent antibody studies. *Virology* 12: 316–317, 1960.

7
Pathologic and Physiologic Autoimmunity and the Autoimmune Repair Mechanism

Ernst H. Beutner
Roger K. Cunningham
Tadeusz P. Chorzelski

INTRODUCTION

Basic Postulates of Studies on Autoimmunity

The basic postulates for studies on autoimmunity, from the viewpoint of the strict immunopathologist, are as follows:

1. All forms of autoimmunity are immunologically specific responses to identifiable antigens, as demonstrated by in vitro tests for antibodies or delayed-type hypersensitivities. They differ from all other forms of immunity in that they are reactive with their tissue component producers, that is, with *identifiable self-antigens in the in vitro tests.*
2. The principal feature of all forms of autoimmunity, from the viewpoint of the producers and from the standpoint of their unique biological significance, is their *potential to undergo in vivo reactions* and to produce physiologic and/or pathologic changes. The de facto ability of each type of autoimmunity to fulfill this potential with physiologic and/or pathologic effects needs to be documented.
3. The corollary needs for studies based on the first two postulates relating to autoimmunity are as follows:
   a) To determine whether a given type of in vitro reaction is *immunologically specific* for an identifiable antigen;
   b) If so, to determine whether it is *autoimmune;*
   c) If so, to determine whether any *in vivo reactions* can be detected in their producers' normal tissue or altered self;
   d) If so, to determine the physiologic/pathologic/biochemical *effects* of *in vivo reactions* on their producer;

e) If effects can be determine, assess *the biological role* (*s*) of the autoimmune response;
f) If points a and b are established, to determined *the cause* (*s*) of the autoimmunity; and
g) If points a to f are established adequately, to determine what types of theories on autoimmunity are applicable.

Primary Classification of Responses to Autosensitization

From the viewpoint of an individual who develops an autoimmune response and from the standpoint of the immunopathologist, the above points 3c and 3d are the most important; that is: 1) What in vivo reactions occur between their self-antigens and their autoantibodies (or autoreactive delayed-type hypersensitivity)? 2) What effects do such in vivo reactions have on the individual? Studies of these two questions permit us to classify autoimmune responses into two types: physiologic and pathologic. Table 1 affords a primary classification of host response to autosensitization into the three major categories: no response, physiologic, and pathologic autoimmunity. This section affords descriptions of these three types of responses. The criteria for distinguishing between physiologic and pathologic autoimmunity appear in the below section on "Differentiation of Pathologic from Physiologic Forms of Autoimmunity" on page 159.

"Horror Autotoxicus"

Most commonly, no immune response develops to immunization with self-antigens. This is what Ehrlich (30) referred to as horror autotoxicus, or what Burnet (21, 23) referred to as self-tolerance. Burnet ascribed this self-tolerance to clonal deletion induced by antigen excess. However, as indicated below (see section on "Tolerance and Autoimmunity"), present-day findings clearly demonstrate that tolerance to delayed type hypersensitivities is, at least under some circumstances, an active process mediated by three types of T suppressor (Ts) cells and soluble Ts factors, including anti-idiotype antibodies. The latter, which are themselves a type of physiologic autoantibodies, are currently receiving much attention (66, 68). Clearly a third possible explanation for failures in developing autoimmunity that has been advanced also merits attention: notably, the lack of antigenic stimulation due to rapid degradation of antigens by endogenous hydrolytic enzymes of antigen-processing macrophages (37, 38).

Physiologic Autoimmunity

The second most common response to self-antigens is that autoantibodies or autoreactive delayed-type hypersensitivity develop readily in essentially all normal subjects. These physiologic autoantibodies are directed to hidden self-antigens, and are implicated as triggering agents of the "autoimmune repair mechanism" (see below). We may classify these into two groups: 1) those found in some, but not all, normal adult sera, but readily elicited in all normal subjects; and 2) those found in all normal adult sera. Examples of the first are Wassermann antibodies and rheumatoid factor (RF). We cannot preclude the possibility that these and other physiologic autoantibodies occur in most or all normal adult sera in titers too low to detect by present methods.

Examples of the universal type of physiologic autoantibodies are the antibodies to stratum corneum (SC), which have been studied in this and other laboratories (11, 12, 41, 44; Chap. 41), and the antibodies to the T antigens of red blood cells. Burnet (22) advances the view that the latter are not true autoantibodies (he calls them "nonself"), because neuraminic acid sequesters these antigens in fresh red blood cells and because no neur-

Table 1. Types of Autoimmunity and Their Characteristics

Types of responses to autoimmunization	*Characteristics of responses and examples*
A. No autoimmunity develops. ("Self-tolerance")	This is the most common response. It may be due to self-recognition, immune paralysis, and/or degradation of antigens by hydrolytic enzymes.
B. Autoimmunity is readily developed in normal subjects to some antigens. These tend to be hidden or altered or novel. These autoimmune responses may be	These are the next most common responses. Most have no pathologic effects; a few do under abnormal conditions.
1. Found in some but not all normal subjects prior to immunization.	e.g., rheumatoid factor, IgM antibodies to altered IgG; Wassermann antibodies to cardiolipins.
2. Universal; i.e., found in essentially all normal subjects.	e.g., antibodies to T antigens of red cells; stratum corneum (SC) antibodies to SC proteins and carbohydrates
C. Pathologic autoimmune responses are usually to antigens that occur in reactive forms in *normal* tissue. They may be caused by	These are the most rare. Most can cause pathologic changes.
1. Abnormal antigenic stimuli.	e.g., thyroglobulin autoimmunity in experimental thyroiditis; pemphigus antibodies associated with Brazilian pemphigus.
2. Abnormal immune responsiveness.	SLE and related connective tissue disease and animal models of them; e.g., NZB/NZW F1 hybrids.

aminidase is known to occur in the body. This is not a tenable interpretation because the antigen is present in all red blood cells. Also, as stressed below, aging red blood cells constantly shed neuraminic acid, thus exposing such "senescence" antigens. The role of this mechanism in the removal of senescent erythrocytes is illustrated in Figure 1. Since neuraminidase serves to reveal senescence antigens, excesses of this enzyme may cause fatal hemolytic episodes, as shown in Figure 2. In reality, most forms of autoimmunity may be classified with these anti-T antibodies as physiologic types. The basic relationships between such immune responses and their hidden self-antigens are illustrated in Figure 3.

Pathologic Autoimmunity

Pathologic autoimmune responses, which are the most rare, fall into two categories as we have stressed before (8): 1) those induced by abnormal antigenic stimuli; 2) and those caused by abnormal immune responsiveness. The latter includes systemic lupus

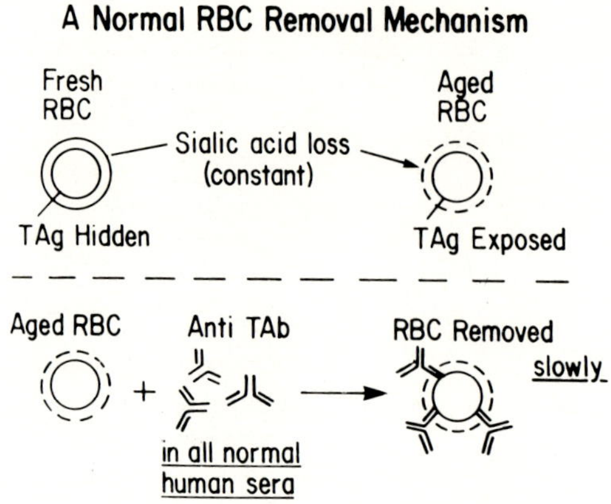

Figure 1. A classic example of an autoimmune repair mechanism or ARM. A normal mechanism for the removal of senescent red blood cells (RBC). Freshly formed RBC, when released from the bone marrow, have a sialic (neuraminic) acid coating that "hides" the antigens. We refer to these as TAg. The TAg are hidden or *H-self*. Throughout their life, the erythrocytes shed sialic acid. Thus, as these RBC age, their TAg become exposed. Therefore, the senescent RBC can react with the anti-T antibodies (Anti-TAb), which are present in all adult normal human sera. Once the aged erythrocytes have reacted with the anti-TAb, they are quickly phagocytosed by the macrophages. This is an ARM cascade. More extensive binding of anti-TAb to RBC can lead to their lysis in the presence of complement.

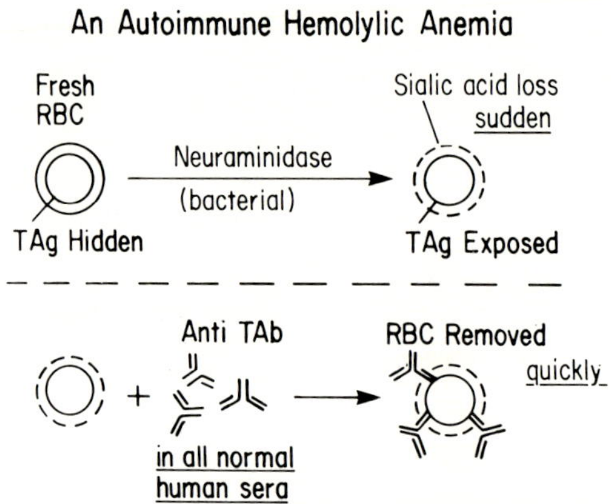

Figure 2. A classic example of a dysfunction of an ARM cascade. A form of autoimmune hemolytic anemia caused by a combination of an abnormally rapid exposure of TAg (an *H-self* component of RBC) and their reaction with the normal universal anti-TAb. Certain factors, such as neuraminidase formed by pneumococci, can cause a sudden loss of sialic acid from the surface of erythrocytes and a resultant rapid exposure of their TAg. This, in turn, causes the rapid binding of the universal TAb that normally aid in the removal of senescent RBC. The resultant rapid removal of the RBC causes a hemolytic anemia that may be fatal.

erythematosus (SLE) and its variants, systemic sclerosis (SS), mixed connective tissue disease (MCTD), and Sjogren's syndrome, plus SLE-like diseases in experimental animals such as the NZB/NZW F1 hybrid mice (16). In these conditions, many diverse and unusual physiologic as well as pathologic autoimmune responses appear (49). Figure 4

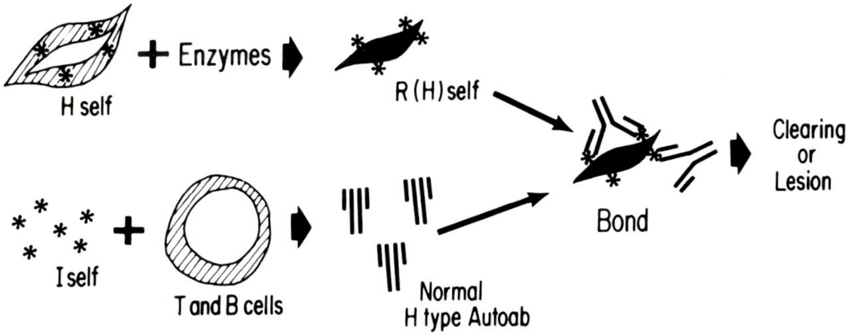

Figure 3. The relationships are shown that are obtained in physiologic forms of autoimmunity that normally trigger the autoimmune repair mechanism or ARM, and that may at times also give rise to pathologic changes (e.g., see Fig. 1 and 2). Hidden or *H-self* antigens can convert to reactive *R(H)-self* forms as a result of trauma, autolytic enzymes, senescence, or other unknown factors. Normal *H-type autoab* are shown that can be present in all normal sera (e.g., antibodies to T antigens of red cells; see the section in this chapter on "Senescence Antigens and Polyagglutinability") or stratum corneum antibodies (see Chap. 42), or antibodies that may be stimulated by the action of normal autologous immunogenic or *I-self* antigens on normal immunocompetent T and B cells (e.g., rheumatoid factor). These normal *H-type autoab* bind to the R (H)-self to promote the clearing of the latter. Such in vivo reactions may, at times, give rise to pathologic changes (e.g., in hemolytic anemia) produced by autoantibodies to the T antigens of red blood cells (see Fig. 2), and possibly also in psoriasis. Most, but not all, autoantibodies are of the *H type*. Thus, the prime function of autoimmunity appears to be the triggering of ARM cascade. (Modified from Beutner EH, Chorzelski TP, Binder WL [8].)

illustrates the basic relationships that are obtained in such autoimmune abnormalities. Most current theories on autoimmunity focus on such abnormalities.

Most truly pathologic autoantibodies occur either by themselves or with a narrowly circumscribed group of other autoimmune responses, as in pemphigus, phemphigoid, and myasthenia gravis. Importantly, these are directed to self-antigens, which are accessible in the fresh normal state of the tissue as illustrated in Figure 5.

Aims of this Chapter

The authors' objectives in writing this chapter are threefold: 1) to review briefly the historic background on immunohistochemical and other serologic findings that aid in the differentiation of pathologic from physiologic forms of autoimmunity; 2) to review briefly the criteria for documenting the role of the physiologic forms in the "autoimmune repair machanisms" (9), as illustrated by some immunohematologic studies; and 3) to relate these findings to some of the present-day concepts on tolerance to self and nonself. The methods of study govern the insights gained. Defined immunofluorescence (IF) (13) and other immunohistochemical studies of the antibody producer's tissue afford both uniquely suitable methods for studies of in vivo reactions and sound bases for generating realistic criteria for evaluation of host response to autoantibodies to tissue-fixed antigens. The ultimate goal of this chapter is to stress these criteria.

QUESTIONS ON THE PATHOLOGIC SIGNIFICANCE OF AUTOIMMUNITY

Even a cursory review of some of the divergent assumptions made in discussions of autoimmunity clearly point to the need for objective criteria for classifying autoimmune responses into at least two major categories.

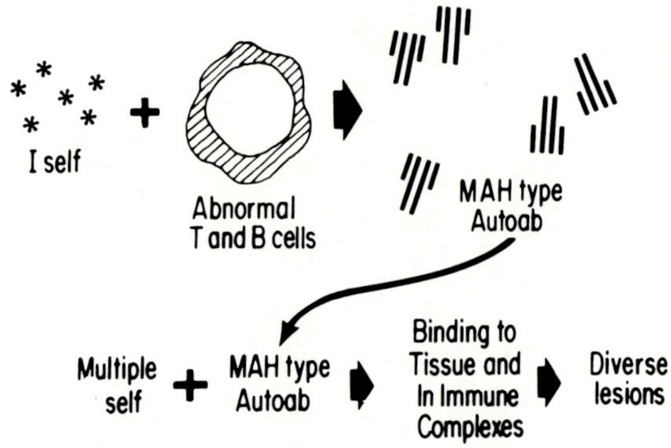

Figure 4. An overview of immunologic disturbances that appear to be caused by *abnormal T and B cell* functions of the type implicated in SLE. Diverse antigenic stimuli (I-self) that fail to elicit abnormal autoimmune responses in immunologically normal individuals appear to give rise to *m*ultiple *A*-type and *H*-type autoimmune responses (i.e., *MAH-type autoantibodies*). These, in turn, react in vivo with their *multiple R-self* antigen, which may present either in the form of normal, reactive, *A-self* antigens or reactive forms of hidden self or a *R(H)-self* form. Diverse pathologic changes arise from these in vivo reactions, either as a result of tissue-specific reactions with *A-self* (e.g., red cell autoantibodies) or immune complexes (e.g., lupus nephritis resulting from immune complexes, most notably DNA-anti-DNA complement deposition in the glomeruli). (Modified from Beutner EH, Chorzelski TP, Binder WL [8].)

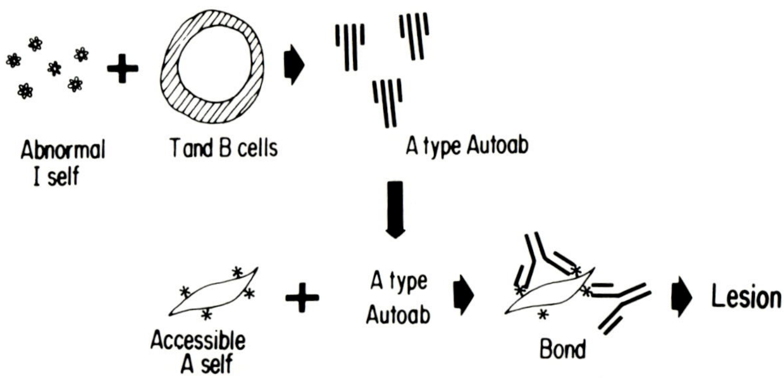

Figure 5. Shown are the basic etiology and pathogenesis of changes caused by autoantibodies or autoreactive cell-mediated immune responses that are induced by abnormal antigenic stimulus. This *abnormal I-self* may, for example, be an infectious agent with cross-reactive antigenic determinants. This is postulated for Brazilian pemphigus foliaceus. Also, abnormal processing of altered skin antigens might produce the *I-self* in some forms of nonendemic pemphigus foliaceus that are triggered by burns. Changes in red blood cells triggered by α-methyl-dopa might cause the formation of anti-e (Rh) autoab. In either type of situation, the normal immunocompetent T and B cells produce anti-A-self responses (to accessible tissue antigens), commonly in the form of antibodies (i.e., *A-type autoantibodies*). Their in vivo reaction with normal *accessible* or *A-self* antigens frequently results in pathologic changes. (Modified from Beutner, EH, Chorzelski TP, Binder WL [8].)

Historic Perspectives on the Pathologic Significance of Autoimmunity

The diversity of autoimmune responses has led to the development of divergent theories. Most theories assume that all forms of autoimmunity play pathogenic roles (22, 23, 30, 70). These include the "horror autotoxicus" concepts of Ehrlich and Morgenroth (30) and the interpretation of this concept by Witebsky et al. (70), as well as the forbidden clone theories of Burnet (22, 23). Many modern theories still make such assumptions; for example, Nossal (54) and most contributors to a recent conference on "Immunologic Tolerance to Self and Non-Self" (6). At the other extreme are the views and concepts of Boyden (20), Grabar (37, 38), Kay and Makinodan (43), and Talal (68), which stress the physiologic role of autoimmune responses. As Kay and Makinodan (43) indicate, "it is now necessary to distinguish between 'physiologic' autoimmunity which performs regulatory functions and 'pathologic' autoantibody which contributes to a destructive disease process." Talal (68), on the basis of studies on autoanti-idiotype and other forms of autoimmunity, concluded that "Self-recognition, far from being a forbidden event, now appears to be a major principle upon which the immune system is founded." Talal recognizes that while most autoantibodies play physiologic roles, some have pathologic effects, but he addresses himself only to theories on etiologic mechanisms (61, 68). None of these concepts or theories set forth the bases for differentiating between physiologic and pathologic forms of autoimmunity; none addresses the dual role that physiologic autoimmunity may play; that is, physiologic and pathologic (see Figs. 1 to 3). To cope with these problems, we have focused attention previously (8–10), and now primarily, on the effect that in vivo reaction of autoantibodies or autoreactive T cells have on their producers. An understanding of the nature of the effects of these in vivo reactions is not only the most important question from the viewpoint of the individual who has produced the immune response, but is a prerequisite for a realistic and functional understanding of the unique feature of all forms of autoimmunity; that is, their specificity for fixed or fluid antigens of the tissues of their producers.

Differentiation of Pathologic from Physiologic Forms of Autoimmunity

The basic difference between pathologic and physiologic forms of autoimmunity lies in their capacity to undergo in vivo reactions with their producers' self-antigens. Pathologic autoantibodies, such as the ones that cause pemphigus, are directed to *accessible* or *A-self* antigens; these exist in a reactive form in normal intact tissue (see Fig. 5). Such autoantibodies can be identified by their capacity to undergo in vivo reactions with normal tissue. It must be kept in mind, however, that not all in vivo reactions of autoantibodies with normal tissue components trigger pathologic changes; for example, the antiribonucleoprotein (anti-RNP) antibodies found in MCTD, SS, and SLE (see Chap. 31 to 33) bind in vivo, but produce only subtle (2, 3) or not (35) detectable changes. Physiologic forms of autoimmunity, on the other hand, are directed to *hidden* or *H-self* antigens, which occur in nonreactive forms under normal conditions, but which can be converted to reactive, R(H)-self forms when they become altered; for example, due to senescence, injury, infection, other insults, or selective alterations (see Fig. 3). Autoantibodies to H-self antigens may occur either on fluid or fixed tissue components. Examples of autoantibodies to H-self-type antigens of fluid tissue components are RF, which binds to IgG altered by immunologic reactions (50), and conglutinin, which fixes to complement components altered by binding to immune complexes (40).

Examples of tissue-fixed H-self-type antigens to which physiologic autoimmunity exists include components of membranes of red blood cells (33, 55, 69; see also section below on "Senescence Antigens and Polyagglutinability: Examples of Autoimmunity to the Erythrocyte") and the horny layer of the skin (10–12, 41, 44; Chap. 41), and the cytoplasm of the prickle cell layer of the epidermis (1, 14, 58; Chaps. 40 and 41) and nuclei of all cells for most but not all antinuclear antibodies (9, 15). While most concepts and theories of autoimmunity focus on its pathologic roles, most autoantibodies, as indicated above and in Table 1, are directed to H-self types of antigens and should more realistically be considered as mediators of physiologic functions.

One of the most useful means of differentiating autoimmune responses to tissue-fixed antigens of the A-self-type from those of the H-self type is by organ culture studies. Those directed to A-self antigens bind into cultures of normal unaltered tissue components as they do in vivo, while antigens of the H-self type in such cultures of intact unaltered tissues fail to react with their homologous autoantibodies as illustrated in Table 2.

Autoimmunity to both A-self and H-self components share some key features. Importantly, all forms of true autoimmunity can and must be demonstrable by in vitro tests with the tissue antigens of their producers. Autoimmunity to both A- and H-self can be detected by the same types of serologic procedures or in vitro tests for delayed type hypersensitivity; that is, they entail comparable humoral or cellular types of immune responses. In all forms of autoimmunity, the specific tissue antigens can and should be identified, and the immunologic specificity for said antigens needs to be documented.

While it is not possible to determine by serologic tests or other in vitro tests alone whether an autoimmune response is directed to A-self or H-self, these two forms of

Table 2. Similarities and Differences Between Physiologic and Pathologic Autoantibodies

Characteristics	*Pathologic autoantibodies*	*Physiologic autoantibodies*
Identification of autoimmunity (similarities)		
Serologic reaction mediators	IgG or other Ig[a] class antibodies	IgG or other Ig class antibodies
Complement (C) fixation	Some but not all fix C	Most fix, C
In vivo and tissue culture reactivity of autoantibodies (differences)		
Types of autoimmunity based on producers' reactions	Reactive with A self-type antigens in normal tissue	Nonreactive with H self-type antigens in unaltered tissue
Reactivity with unaltered tissue in culture	Reactive	Nonreactive
Frequency of occurrence and induction (differences)		
Occurrence in population	Highly disease specific; not usually found in normal subjects	May occur either in all or many normal subjects
Induction of immune responses	Usually difficult to induce	Readily inducible

[a]Ig, immunoglobulin.

autoimmunity differ in a number of fundamental respects. Table 2 lists the most basic similarities and differences between autoantibodies to A-self-type and H-self-type antigens (compare also Figs. 3 and 5).

ROLE OF PHYSIOLOGIC AUTOANTIBODIES IN THE AUTOIMMUNE REPAIR MECHANISM (ARM)

One of the first physiologic autoimmune responses to be subjected to detailed analytic studies are those directed to the T antigens of red blood cells (RBC) (see Fig. 1 and 2). Since RBC can serve as an excellent model for analyses of autoimmunity, the following sections on polyagglutinability afford a review of the subject. The understanding derived from these studies can be applied to noncirculating, tissue-fixed antigens by use of defined immunohistochemical methods, such as combinations of direct (DIF) and indirect (IIF) IF methods, together with tissue culture studies and other appropriate serologic procedures. Stated briefly, studies of polyagglutinability and "senescence antigens" of RBC indicate that anti-T autoantibodies and/or other antibodies to RBC surface antigens normally sequestered by neuraminic acid serve to aid the removal of senescent RBC (see section below on "Senescent Antigens and Polyagglutinability: Examples of Autoimmunity to the Erythrocyte"). We may think of this as a removal or a repair mechanism triggered by the autoantibodies; that is, an autoimmune repair mechanism (ARM).

Studies with defined IF (and other labeled antibody techniques) of autoimmune responses, particularly to tissue-fixed H-self-type antigens, afford an independent group of methods that can provide soundly based criteria for evaluating the physiologic or pathologic roles of autoantibodies. These indicate that ARM may be operative in other tissues such as the skin. For fluid antigens, other methods are needed, but comparable ARM's are operative.

Two types of physiologic autoantibodies reactive with skin components serve to illustrate the need for criteria for evaluating their function; notably, the stratum corneum (SC) antibodies and the antibodies to cytoplasmic components of the epidermis. These are now recognized as being the same antibodies (Chap. 41). A set of criteria to aid in characterization of such autoantibodies and their triggering effects on ARM cascades in both the normal state and in dysfunctions of ARMs had been reported previously (10). These *ARM criteria* are set forth in greater detail here:

1. Demonstrate and characterize an autoimmune response to H-self. That is, demonstrate by in vitro serologic test methods the immunologic specificity of the tissue antibodies, characterize their antigen by these methods, show that the antigen occurs in the tissue of the antibody producer, test for frequency of occurrence in normal sera, and demonstrate that they fail to react in vivo with the normal, newly formed H-self-type antigens in tissue culture. Such immune responses are either present or readily elicited in all normal subjects.

2. Identify the biochemical and/or anatomic nature of the sequestering factors; that is, the factors causing the antigens to be of the H-self type.

3. Demonstrate in vivo reactions of the autoantibodies with altered or degraded forms of the H-self antigens; this may provide some indirect evidence for the triggering effect of the autoantibodies on an ARM cascade.

4. Demonstrate the biological significance of and mechanism of the implicated ARM in terms of:

(a) Its effect on normal repair. (This remains to be done for most anti-H-self responses. For those in which there is acceptable evidence, the ARM should be regarded as a phenomenon rather than a thesis.)

(b) If an ARM does affect repair, what mechanisms are involved?

(c) The cause of the development of the autoimmunity. (This merits separate consideration.)

5. If dysfunction of an ARM cascade is implicated in the pathogenesis or etiology of a disease or in healing defects, demonstrate what the nature of this dysfunction is.

SENESCENCE ANTIGENS AND POLYAGGLUTINABILITY: EXAMPLES OF AUTOIMMUNITY TO THE ERYTHROCYTE

Autoantibodies to erythrocytes were the first form of autoimmunity to be recognized (45). Autoantibodies to RBC still provide a uniquely suitable model for studies on autoimmunity, because cell suspensions of unaltered erythrocytes are readily accessible in essentially pure form in volumes adequate to permit detailed studies by diverse methods. Such studies provide valuable clues and insights into the general nature of autoimmunity. For example, since the antibodies of autoimmune disorders involving the erythrocyte are bound in vivo, it is a relatively easy task to obtain the tissue involved and to elute the antibodies from the unaltered cells. Frequently, antibodies are also present in excess free in the individual's serum. Thus, the picture that can be obtained from these specimens, in many respects, is "cleaner" than the more complex situation present in other tissues. Just as for other tissue, autoimmunity to the erythrocyte can be divided into two types: frankly pathologic (as appears in cases of autoimmune hemolytic anemias) and "natural" or physiologic antibodies. This last group will be discussed below. There are distinct differences in these varieties. The autoimmune hemolytic anemias are acquired, cause obvious symptoms, and are now thought to arise from a breakdown in normal tolerance (see section below on "Tolerance and Autoimmunity"). The antibodies involved are usually IgG and cause the rapid, premature removal of the erythrocytes to which they are bound. In the present context, however, these are of less interest than the natural physiologic type of autoreactivity, and they will not be considered further.

Nonpathogenic Autoantibodies

Of primary concern in this discussion are the normally nonpathologic antibodies that are involved in the normal process of removing senescent RBC from the circulation. Such antibodies appear during the first year of life in the circulation of all persons, and are a part of the homeostatic mechanisms of the normal human body. Their formation may be due either to endogenous antigenic stimulation such as senescent erythrocytes or to some exogenous stimulation such as bacteria that have cross-reactive antigens. It is entirely possible that both mechanisms may be operative.

Autoagglutination of RBC by serum of the same individual was described from the beginning of studies on blood groups. Landsteiner (46) showed that such autoagglutinins are present in the serum of all normal adults, but could be demonstrated only when the cell-serum mixture was incubated at temperatures less than 37°C. Thus, although antibodies that can react are present in each individual's circulation, they fail to do so in vivo because the body temperature is too high for the reaction to occur and consequently do no harm. In rare instances, individuals, for unknown reasons, fail to maintain the thermal restriction and produce antibodies (or antigens) that react close to normal body temperature with consequent hemolysis and anemia. This condition is termed cold hemagglutinin disease. The role of the cold agglutinin in normal individuals is not known, but it is tempting to suggest that since the structure with which the antibodies react is masked in the erythrocyte by neuraminic acid (48), which is lost as the RBC ages, the cold agglutinin can react with older cells and provide a signal for their removal in senescence.

Polyagglutinability

A more studied case of the role of autoantibodies in maintaining homeostasis can be found by examination of cases of polyagglutination. The term refers to a situation in which the erythrocytes of an individual are agglutinated by the serum of all, or nearly all, persons, including his own. The condition arises due to an abnormality of the erythrocyte and should be distinguished from panagglutination, in which the serum of an individual agglutinates the cells of all other humans.

Erythrocytes can become polyagglutinable both in vivo and in vitro. In either case, receptors that are normally hidden on the surface of the cell are exposed, and thus can react with physiologic antibodies that are present "naturally" in all normal human sera. Such an event can be brought about in one of two ways: 1) in some cases, the erythrocytes are modified by microbial products; 2) in others, the condition arises spontaneously, and often without discernible cause. There is a suggestion that some types of polyagglutinability are due to a failure in the marrow to produce RBC with normal amounts of neuraminic acid (see below).

T Activation

Polyagglutination was first systematically investigated by Thomsen in 1926, although the phenomenon had previously been reported by Huebener, who did not recognize the significance of his finding. Thomsen eventually turned the work over to an assistant, Friedenreich, who in 1930 published a monograph on the subject (34). The phenomenon thus acquired the rather unwieldy caption of the "Huebener-Thomsen-Friedenreich" phenomenon; this has largely been replaced by the term "T activation," which we will use here.

The work of Thomsen and Friedenreich showed that T activation occurs when erythrocytes are exposed to certain bacteria, or to culture filtrates in which these had been growing; they acquired the property of becoming agglutinable by all normal adult human sera. The action of enzymes produced by the bacteria in cleaving material from the RBC exposes an antigen T, which then can react with naturally occurring anti-T antibodies in serum. Although absent in the newborn, IgM antibodies arise in the first year or so of life and persist throughout life.

T activation can occur in vivo in patients with infections or by other mechanisms as indicated above. Exposed T receptors can lead to severe hemolytic anemias and, as well, make blood grouping and transfusion difficult. The cells of the patient are found to agglutinate with all reagent sera. T activation that occurs in vitro (e.g., in a bag of blood that has become contaminated with bacteria) can lead to severe transfusion reaction; its severity is related to the capacity of anti-T antibodies to avidly fix complement. In both cases, a bacterial (or it can be viral) neuraminidase cleaves neuraminic acid from glycoprotein of the erythrocyte surface and exposes an otherwise hidden T receptor.

The T receptor is not restricted to erythrocytes, but can be demonstrated on the surface of neuraminidase-treated lymphocytes, tumor cells, and other normal tissue (63). Furthermore, the T antigen is widely distributed in mammals, and is phylogenetically probably very old.

Newly "born" erythrocytes are richly endowed with neuraminic acid residues on the cell surface glycoproteins and glycolipids. However, as the cells age, neuraminic acid is constantly shed from the termini of the oligosaccharide side chains of the outer surface. Thus, as RBC age, they lose their normal negative charge, electrophoretic mobility, and increasingly acquire T reactivity. They also become much smaller than new cells. It has been postulated that the life of the erythrocyte, some 100 to 120 days, is actually determined by the eventual exposure of a critical number of T receptors (47). These receptors then react with the animal's own anti-T antibodies and complement. The terminal components of complement (C5–C9) are then inserted into the membrane, which disturbs the normal osmotic equilibrium of the cell. It has been shown that T, anti-T reactions in the presence of complement, when the numbers of T receptors are low, result in an extremely slow lysis of the affected cells (some 15 minutes). Thus, rather than lysing in the circulation, the prelytic swollen cell may be trapped in the sinusoids of the spleen and removed. Alternatively, the cell could be expected to be removed simply by the normal phagocytic events that occur when opsonized particles pass through the spleen. Anti-T complement-mediated lesions may also be involved in controlling the proliferation of nucleated cells that have altered surface sialic acid and exposed T receptors due to metabolic defect or malignancy.

In recent years, there has been a reawakening of interest in the T, anti-T blood group system. The interest has been stimulated by the finding that the T antigen of humans is related to another alloantigenic system in the RBC; namely, the MN system. This antigen system consists essentially of two alloantigens, M and N, coded by genes that are inherited in a normal Medelian fashion. The genes are codominant. Thus, with anti-M and anti-N sera, three genotypes can be identified: MM, MN, and NN. Alloantibodies can be found to the antigens (although relatively rare) in the sera of patients who have been immunized by transfusion. Since human antisera are difficult to find, the usual practice has been to prepare anti-M and anti-N reagents by injecting the appropriate cells into rabbits and then absorbing the resultant serum to a monospecific reagent. For example, to prepare an anti-M serum, one would immunize with MM cells and later absorb the resulting antiserum with NN cells to remove the antihuman RBC antibodies that the rabbits also produce. The first step in the story of the M, N, and T relationship arose from just such procedures. It was commonly thought initially that while anti-M sera were quite easy to prepare, anti-N sera were difficult because when absorbing anti-N sera with MM cells, the anti-N activity was slowly removed as well as the other agglutinins. This property led many investigators, but principally Springer and associates (62, 63), to begin an investigation that has ramified far from the original intentions. The original studies (62) demonstrated that treatment of isolated M substance with neuraminidase converted the antigenicity of the isolated sialoglycoprotein from M to N, with a concomitant release of free neuraminic acid. Thus, N activity was part and parcel both M and N substance; but in M cells, it was buried behind an additional terminal neuraminic acid residue. Removal of this moiety revealed the otherwise occult N activity. The reason that M cells could remove both anti-M and anti-N activity from rabbit anti-N sera was that not all sialoglycoproteins of the human M erythrocyte bear a terminal neuraminic acid residue, although most do. The minor fraction of unsubstituted N substance could then react with anti-N antibodies. This was not the case; however, in the reverse situation, absorption of rabbit anti-M sera with N cells was straightforward because the N-absorbing cells had only N structures on their surface.

This contention was shown experimentally when it was demonstrated that mild neuraminidase treatment could convert M substance to N. A similar effect could also be produced by simple mild acid hydrolysis as well. The terminal residue present on the N-specific sialoglycoprotein was B-galactose, either as terminal nonreducing groups of one branched chain, or as separate termini on different chains. Further work revealed an unexpected result. If the treatment of M substance with neuraminidase was more vigorous, or N substance itself was further treated with this enzyme under appropriate conditions, N activity was lost and T activity appeared. The disappearance of N, of course, was accompanied by a release of free neuraminic acid. These experiments then showed the remarkable fact that M and N antigens were the structures that covered an underlying T activity present on the same macromolecule. A precursor molecule, in this case, is converted in the individual human to blood group antigen M, N, or MN, depending upon inherited sialotransferase enzymes.

Tn Polyagglutinability

In the discussion above of T activation, only the classic form of activation was mentioned. It now becomes important to introduce another type of polyagglutinability first described by Moreau et al. (53). This form of polyagglutination (Tn) has never been duplicated in vitro. The RBC react with almost all human adult sera, and even with those completely absorbed with T-activated cells. The condition usually is found by accident in apparently normal health individuals, but can also be associated with disorders such as leukemia or myeloproliferative disease. The polyagglutination can last for years, but has been known to disappear spontaneously or after the administration of cytotoxic drugs. Often, only a proportion of the cells of a given individual are agglutinable. Examination of the anti-Tn agglutinable subpopulation of erythrocytes reveals that they are very deficient in neuraminic acid. The neuraminic acid content of the nonagglutinable cells (by anti-Tn) is also reduced, but not nearly to the extent of the agglutinable cells. The thought is that since Tn activation has no apparent relationship to infection of any kind, the neuraminic acid deficiency is not due to its enzymatic removal, but to a failure or deficiency in the bone marrow synthesis of the erythrocytes. It is of some note, however, in the present context, that in the sera of most normal adults, antibodies with anti-Tn specificity can be easily demonstrated to exist in addition to the anti-T antibodies already mentioned. Tn activation can take two courses: one pathologic and the other benign. Clear-cut anemia is present in some cases, although it is not known whether the foreshortened life span of the erythrocytes in those patients is a result of destruction by anti-Tn antibodies of the patient's own circulation, or simply a shortened intrinsic life span of the cells. Reversion of Tn-activated erythrocytes to normal is accompanied by clinical improvement in the patient (42). The condition is not inherited.

Tn activation, although rare, fits neatly into the chemical scheme that begins with the removal of neuraminic acids to reveal the occult T antigen that owes its activity to a terminal β-galactose residue. When T antigen is treated with β-galactosidase, Tn antigen is expressed as free β-galactose is released. Thus, hidden under the T antigen is a second layer of occult antigen, Tn. Tn antigen possesses a terminal α-N-acetyl-galactosamine residue upon which its serologic specificity resides. Removal of this residue with appropriate enzymes renders the molecule serologically inert to any known agglutinins. The stepwise degradation pathway of M substance is shown in Figure 1. It should be mentioned that, in addition to degradation, experiments beginning with Tn substance have shown that when the appropriate glycosyl or neuraminyl transferases and activated monosaccharides are provided, the reverse synthesis of M through T and N can be accomplished.

Tk Polyagglutinability

A further type of polyagglutinability was described by Bird and Wingham in 1972 (19) that differs from T and Tn, since normal human adult sera that had been absorbed with T- and Tn-activated cells still reacted with the cells of these donors. The condition was termed Tk polyagglutination and was shown to be a mild, transient, and reversible state that was thought to accompany bacterial infection. The neuraminic acid content of Tk-activated cells is within normal limits. The work on Tk, however, led to the introduction of lectins into the research on polyagglutination. This was an important step forward, since on the practical level, these reagents allow a more ready identification of the various polyagglutinable states. Even more importantly, however, the idea emerged that the reactions of T-related structures with lectins indicated that the anti-T of normal human serum contained mixed specificities. It should be kept in mind that the reactions with lectins have their counterpart in all normal human sera, where analogous antibodies of similar specificity can be found. Thus, the use of plant agglutinins has enabled the identification of previously undetected subspecificities of autoantibodies that react with aging cells.

Reactions with Lectins

The first lectin to be used was that of *Arachis hypogea,* more popularly known as the peanut. Saline protein extracts of the peanut were found to react with T- and Tk-activated erythrocytes, but not with cells that were Tn activated. Tn-activated cells, however, could be identified by their reaction with a lectin obtained from seeds of *Dolichos biflorus,* horse gram. This lectin is normally used to identify the ABO subgroup A1, but was also found to specifically react with group O and B cells, when they were from individuals with Tn polyagglutinability.

The *Dolichos* lectin also reacts with the cells found in still another rare form of polyagglutinability known as Cad polyagglutinability. First described in Japan, Cad was named by Cazal et al. (25), who demonstrated that Cad is a dominant inherited character. Others later showed that Cad was, in fact, an abnormally powerful case of the blood group antigen Sd(a) known previously by the name of "super sid" and symbolized as Sd(a^{++}). The Sd(a) antigen is very common and is present in about 90% of random individuals. Furthermore, minute amounts of anti-Sd(a) are present in the serum of the vast majority of individuals, and the agglutinating power of a given donor's serum is inversely related to the strength of the person's own Sd (a) antigen (57). In the case of Cad polyagglutinability, the individual has received a gene that codes for a highly active enzyme that produces larger than normal amounts of the Sd(a) antigen so that these cells will now react with the anti-Sd(a) in the serum of most individuals, but that normally cannot be demonstrated easily because the antigenic distribution on most erythrocytes is too sparse to support agglutination. The terminal sugar, N-acetylgalactosamine, is required for Sd(a) activity; hence, also for Cad polyagglutinability. The molecule that bears the antigen varies widely in molecular weight, is glycoprotein, and is widely distributed in the body. The antigen is shed in the urine and is difficult to separate from accompanying ABO and Lewis blood group activity. Furthermore, the antigen is found in at least 12 species of mammals, although it is apparently absent in birds.

The problem with polyagglutinability has always been to sort out which variety is present in a given instance. Since there is a range of naturally occurring antibodies encountered in normal human serum, the tendency has been to look more toward the use of lectins in an attempt to isolate the specificities involved. Unlike antibodies, lectins have very narrow spectra of reaction specificity. Lectins can often be inhibited by monosaccharides, which is seldom possible with antibodies. Thus, wholesale screenings of lectins have been undertaken, and a battery of these have been found that can be used to sort out the serologic reactions of polyagglutinable cells (18). In addition to the peanut and *Dolichos,* lectins extracted from species of the genus *Salvia* are used. A summary of the reactions is shown in Table 3.

Senescence Antigens

Although the role of Sd(a) and Tn in the aging and subsequent removal of erythrocytes is, thus far, only suggested by the data, the role of T seems beyond doubt. An additional dimension, however, has been added by the study of the so-called senescence antigen (43). This antigen is a surface glycoprotein present on the surface of human and animal erythrocytes, platelets, embryonic kidney cells, and adult liver cells. The antigen is not normally expressed on the erythrocyte, but appears on the surface of senescent or damaged cells. An antibody that reacts with this antigen can be isolated from the surface of the oldest fraction of circulating RBC, but not from freshly formed cells. The antibody in this case was identified as an IgG (unlike the antibodies of the previously described polyagglutinability), and causes the rapid phagocytosis of old cells. The oldest RBC have approximately 100 molecules of such IgG on their surface per cell. The IgG antibody is an autoantibody that cannot react with younger cells, because the senescence antigen is not exposed and is presumably cryptic until the cell ages. There is evidence to suggest that the senescence antigen, in this case, is a breakdown product derived from the major sialoglycoprotein fraction of the cell. Mature erythrocytes cannot synthesize protein; hence, the idea that the senescence antigen is derived from the

Table 3. Reactions Between Selected Reagents and Polyagglutinable Erythroctyes

Reagent used	*Normal cells*	*Polyagglutinable cells*		
		T	*Tn*	*Cad*
AB serum	−	+	+	+
Arachis lectin	−	+	−	+
Dolichos lectin[a]	−	−	+	+
Bauhinia lectin	−	?	+	−

[a]Group A_1 and A_1B excepted.

modification or breakdown of an existing structure seems most probable. Unfortunately, the relationship of the senescence antigen to the antigens responsible for polyagglutinability is not known. However, it is tempting to speculate that these represent an IgG form of one of the already known specificities described above. To put a name on the antibody, of course, does not detract from the important role that such an antigen would play in maintaining homeostasis of the mammalian body through an immunologic surveillence (Fig. 1).

T Antigen in Malignancy

One cannot leave the topic under discussion without at least a passing reference to the possible importance of polyagglutinability and senescent antigenic changes in tumor immunity. This work, largely due to Springer and colleagues (63), has given important insights and possible leads in understanding the role of such antigens in tumor immunology. Using anti-M and anti-N sera, these workers were able to demonstrate the appropriate MN phenotypes in mammary tissue taken from patients. More surprising, however, was the presence of T activation in malignant tissue, but not in benign tumors. The T and Tn antigens were found to be present on the surface of all invasive tumors tested. Furthermore, in patients with malignancy, the anti-T antibodies were severely depressed. The titers of anti-T were seen to rise in patients after surgical removal of the tumor. When extracts containing T antigen were used to skin test the patients, most responded vigorously with a strong T-cell-mediated, delayed hypersensitivity reaction. This presumably showed that the anti-T titers had dropped because the tumor was taking up the antibody, since they clearly had mounted an immune response to their tumors when assessed in the T-cell limb of the immune response. Other patients with benign lesions of the mammary gland showed no such depression of anti-T titers nor did they show response to intradermal challenge with isolated T antigen. Thus, the evidence strongly suggests that the antigens involved in polyagglutinability and senescence may well play an important role in protection against tumor development in mammals.

TOLERANCE AND AUTOIMMUNITY

Tolerance or the failure to develop immune responses following exposure to antigens or haptens is, on the one hand, a prime focus of attention in studies of regulatory mechanisms of the immune system; on the other hand, it also needs to be considered from the viewpoint of the behavior of the antigens.

Tolerance as an Active Process

Burnet and Fenner in 1949 (24) anticipated the existence of immunologic tolerance as a result of contact with foreign antigens during embryonic life. Billingham et al. (17) are generally credited with the discovery of self-tolerance in newborn mice in 1949, and Felton and Ottinger (31) with the description of immune paralysis in adult mice in 1942. Chase (27), on the other hand, traces the original observations on tolerance to Frei (32), who reported in 1928 that persons injected intravenously with neosalversan could not be sensitized by intradermal injections, although such injections induced hypersensitivity in normal volunteers. Comparable induction of tolerance to neosalversan and salversan in guinea pigs was intimated by Sultzberger (64, 65) in 1929, but could not be confirmed until Chase (26) used a modified protocol in 1946. Thus, tolerance is referred to (28) as the "Frei, Sultzberger, Chase phenomenon" by some workers. Independent observations on allogeneic tolerance in chick embryos were also made by Hasek (39).

Burnet (22), in 1959, proposed that immune tolerance is due to clonal deletion. On the one hand, a growing body of evidence indicates that at least in some experimental models, it is an active process (4, 27, 29, 59, 60). On the other hand, some experimental models such as Möller et al. (52), which uses antigenic and nonantigenic forms of dextran, yield results pointing to antigen excess as the tolerance-inducing factor. It is not surprising, therefore, that some workers such as Polak (56) now find responses suggestive of clonal deletion by intravenous injections with haptenized macrophages; but following comparable injections of hapten alone, the tolerance induced appears to be an active process.

Since tolerance to cell-mediated immunity (CMI) is more readily induced, it is referred to as low-zone tolerance; and humoral immunity, which does not respond as readily to tolerizing treatments, is referred to as high-zone tolerance. Indeed, it remains to be determined whether complete tolerance to humoral immunity, which cannot be broken, is in fact inducible.

The adoptive transfer of tolerance to CMI into virgin mice with viable syngeneic cells from tolerized animals affords a model system that lends itself well to analytic studies. These reveal that Ts cells are responsible for the active induction of tolerance (5,36,71), that these cells elaborate T-suppressor factors or TsF (66,67), and that multiple cell types are involved in the suppression of the afferent and efferent arms of the CMI responses. Based on an analysis of the literature, Benaceraff et al. (7) recently classified these into: 1) Ts_1 and TsF_1, which suppress the afferent arm or inducive phase of the immune responses; and 2) Ts_2, TsF_2, Ts_3, and TsF_3, which suppress the efferent arm or response phase, with the TsF_2 acting via anti-idiotype effectors.

Tolerance and the Autoimmune Repair Mechanism

On the one hand, the sophisticated studies on the mechanism of tolerance—which appear to have been activated by the Nobel prizes awarded to Medaward and Burnet in 1960 for their work on acquired immunologic tolerance and to Jerne in 1974 for his theory on immune regulation—shed increasing light on the mechanisms of active induction of tolerance, in particular, and immune responses, in general. On the other hand, some of the underlying assumptions related to autoimmunity need to be modified. For example, the leading report in the conference on "Immunologic Tolerance to Self and Non-Self" of the New York Academy of Science (59) is predicated on the assumptions that "the immune system does not overtly respond to its own antigens" and "that this process of 'self tolerance' is an active one." While such statements are partly true, they fail to take cognizance of three factors, the first of which relates to tolerance itself, the second to physiologic autoimmunity, and the third to the difference between self and nonself. The first two merit discussion here.

1. First, more than one mechanism may be involved in the induction of tolerance. In addition to the two above-mentioned mechanisms of clonal deletion (22) (or other mechanisms related to antigen excess [52]) and the active processes involved in some forms of tolerance involving Ts cells (4,27), the biochemical degradation considered by Grabar's "transporteur" theory (37) merits consideration. He advances the view that since hydrolytic enzymes of the body degrade self-antigens more rapidly than nonself or foreign antigens, this can account for the greater antigenicity of nonself antigens.

Stated simply, self tolerance can conceptually be attributed to: 1) active processes mediated by Ts cells and TsF of different types; 2) a chronic state of antigen excess causing clonal deletion or immune paralysis; or 3) a chronic state of antigen paucity due either to lack of access or to rapid degradation by hydrolytic enzymes of antigen-processing cells. Each of these alternative explanations merits consideration. Documentation of an active process rests primarily on experimental studies of delayed-type hypersensitivity or contact allergies to foreign haptens (36,66). The induction of tolerance of humoral immune responses to true self-antigens that cannot be broken by altered antigens has not been demonstrated. Thus, in the absence of further evidence, it is not tenable to ascribe all of the tolerance to the many self-antigens to which no autoimmunity has been detected to the activity of Ts cells. The second alternative, notably that excess quantities of self-antigens can tolerize, requires that the amounts of normal self-antigen and each of their antigenically distinct, normal degradation products be available to the immunocompetent cells in concentrations adequate to induce tolerance. Some observations on naturally occurring autoantibodies to the Rh antigens of erythrocytes in blister fluids, but not in serum (51), suggest that such a mechanism may be operative for some accessible self-antigens. However, these are antigens readily detectable in the bloodstream. Even an antigen present in the bloodstream in low concentration (e.g., thyroglobulin) fails to induce tolerance, as evidenced by the ready induction of thyroglobulin autoantibodies (70). Thus, it appears that antigens which tolerize by their high concentration need to be present not merely in detectable amounts in the bloodstream, but in amounts adequate to induce tolerance. It seems doubtful if this holds true for most of the self-antigen to which no autoimmunity develops, since there are too many for all to be present in tolerizing concentrations in the bloodstream. The third explanation, notably the lack of access of immunocompetent cells to immunizing dosages of most self-antigens, requires that the hydrolytic enzymes of the parenchymal, stromal, and inflammatory cells (including the macrophages that process antigens) degrade most self-antigens with a speed that prevents them from becoming immunogens. While this thesis (like the other two) remains to be proven, it is clearly at least as tenable as the others.

2. Second, all normal adults do, in fact, have numerous physiologic autoantibodies to hidden self-antigens. We need to retain a flexible frame of mind to seek and find the reasons for the formation of such "physiologic" autoantibodies. We implicate them as triggering agents of the ARM, as indicated above. A tenable working hypothesis for their genesis is as follows. Since the formation of physiologic autoantibodies appears to play a significant role in the removal of damaged tissue, it follows that it would be detrimental to the organism if it develops hydrolytic enzymes that can degrade these hidden self-antigens to nonantigenic forms before an immune response can be raised to them. If this is true, then the quantity of the nondegraded immunogenic forms of hidden self-antigens that can interact with macrophages and T-helper cells also assumes importance in the normal development of physiologic autoantibodies. The amounts obviously cannot be so high that they induce high-zone tolerance (regardless of the mechanism involved) or so low that no immune response is raised. As indicated above, studies are needed to determine whether self-tolerance is due to an active process of Ts cells, to antigen excess (or clonal deletion), or to an absence of adequate concentrations of immunogenic self-antigens. An important corollary to the latter interpretation is that the evolutionary development of appropriate types and concentrations of hydrolytic enzymes degrade most self-antigens, but a deficiency in a few may account for the fact that autoimmunity normally develops to only a few hidden self-antigens. It is obvious that we need to gain a better understanding of the autoimmunity that exists or develops readily in the normal state before we can gain a meaningful understanding of pathologic dysfunctions of ARMs.

REFERENCES

1. Ackermann-Schopf C, Ackermann R, Terasaki PI, et al: Natural and acquired epidermal autoantibodies in man. *J Immunol* 112:2063–2067, 1974.
2. Alarcon-Segovia D, Ruiz-Arguelles A, Fishbein E: Antibody to nuclear ribonucleoprotein penetrates live human mononuclear cells from Fc receptors. *Nature* 271:67–69, 1978.
3. Alarcon-Segovia D, Ruiz-Arguelles A, Llorente L: Antibody penetration into living cells. II. Antiribonucleoprotein IgG penetrates into T lymphocytes causing their deletion and the abrogation of suppressor functions. *J Immunol* 122:1855–1862, 1979.
4. Asherson GL, Zembala M: The role of the T acceptor cell in suppressor systems. Antigen-specific T suppressor factor acts via a T acceptor cell; this releases a nonspecific inhibitor of the transfer of contact sensitivity when exposed to antigen in the context of I-J. *Ann NY Acad Sci* 392:71–88, 1982.
5. Asherson GL, Zembala M, Barnes MR: The mechanism of immunological unresponsiveness to picryl chloride and the possible role of antibody mediated depression. *Clin Exp Immunol* 9:111–121, 1971.
6. Battisto JR, Claman HN, Scott DW (Eds): Immunologic tolerance to self and non-self. *Ann NY Acad Sci* 392:1–433, 1982.
7. Benacerraf B, Greene MI, Sy MS, et al: Suppressor T cell circuits. *Ann NY Acad Sci* 392:300–308, 1982.
8. Beutner EH, Chorzelski TP, Binder WL: Nature of autoimmunity: Pathologic versus physiologic responses and a unifying concept. In Beutner EH, Chorzelski TP, Bean SF, (Eds): *Immunopathology of the Skin,* ed. 2. Wiley, New York, 1979, pp 147–180.
9. Beutner EH, Cunningham RK: Autoimmunity. In Stone J (Ed): *Dermatologic Immunology and Allergy,* CV Mosby, St. Louis, 1985, pp 125–142.
10. Beutner EH, Dabski K, Jablonska S, et al: Stratum corneum antigens: Their role in psoriasis and in the autoimmune repair mechanism. In Marks R, Plewig G (Eds): *Stratum Corneum,* Springer-Verlag, Heidelberg, 1983, pp 92–111.
11. Beutner EH, Jablonska S, Hebborn P, et al: Autoimmunity in psoriasis. This volume, chap. 42.
12. Beutner EH, Jablonska S, Jarzabek-Chorzelska M, et al: Studies in immunodermatology. VI. IF studies of autoantibodies to the stratum corneum and of in vivo fixed IgG in stratum corneum of psoriatic scales. *Int Arch Allergy* 48:301–323, 1975.
13. Beutner EH, Kumar V, Krasny SA, et al: Defined IF in immunodermatology. This volume, chap. 1.
14. Beutner EH, Rhodes EL, Holborow EJ: Autoimmunity in chronic bullous skin diseases. Immunofluorescence staining of three types of antibodies to skin in sera of patients with pemphigus, bullous pemphigoid and in other human sera. *Clin Exp Immunol* 2:141–151, 1967.
15. Beutner EH, Sullivan M, Barnes G, et al: Studies of *in vivo* reactions of nuclear antibodies. In Grabar P, Miescher P, (Eds): *Mechanisms of Cell and Tissue Damage Produced by Immune Reactions, IInd International Symposium on Immunopathology,* Benno Schwabe, Basel, 1961, pp 331–336.
16. Bielschowsky M, Goodall CM: Origin of inbred NZ mouse strain. *Cancer Res* 30:834–836, 1970.
17. Billingham RE, Brent L, Medawar PB: Actively acquired tolerance of foreign cells. *Nature (London)* 172:603–605, 1953.
18. Bird GWG: Complexity of erythrocyte polyagglutinability. In Mohn JF, Plunkett RW, Cunningham RK, et al (Eds): *Human Blood Groups,* Karger, Basel, 1977, pp 335–343.
19. Bird GWG, Wingham J: Tk. A new form of red cell polyagglutination. *Br J Haematol* 23:759–763, 1972.
20. Boyden S: Pathology: Autoimmunity and inflammation. *Nature* 201:200–201, 1964.
21. Burnet FM: Autoimmune disease. 2. Pathology of the immune response. *Br Med J* 2: 720–725, 1959.
22. Burnet FM: *The Clonal Selection Theory of Acquired Immunity.* Cambridge Univ Press, Cambridge, 1959, 209.
23. Burnet FM: Autoimmune disease as a breakdown in immunological homeostasis. In *Cellular Immunology,* Cambridge University Press, Cambridge, 1970, 255.

24. Burnet FM, Fenner R: *The Production of Antibodies.* Macmillan, Melbourne, 1949, pp 1–142.
25. Cazal P, Morris J, Canbel J, et al: Polyagglutinabilité héréditaire dominante antigèn privé (Cad) correspondant à un anticorps public et à une lectine de *Dolichos biflorus. Revue fr Transf* 11:209–221, 1968.
26. Chase MW: Inhibition of experimental drug allergy by prior feeding of the sensitizing agent. *Proc Soc Exp Biol Med* 61:257–259, 1946.
27. Chase MW: The induction of tolerance to allergenic chemicals. *Ann NY Acad Sci* 392:228–247, 1982.
28. Chase MW, Battisto JR, Ritts RE: Acquisition of immunologic tolerance via simple allergenic chemicals. In *Conceptual Advances in Immunology and Oncology, 16th Annual Symposium on Fundamental Cancer Research,* Harper & Row, New York, 1963, pp 395–416.
29. Diener E, Diner UE, von Borstel RC, et al: Can experimental B cell tolerance serve as a model for self tolerance? *Ann NY Acad Sci* 392:35–44, 1982.
30. Ehrlich P, Morgenroth J: Ueber haemolysine Dritte mitteilung. *Berliner Klin Wochenschr* 37:453–458, 1900.
31. Felton LP, Ottinger BS: Pneumococcal polysaccharide as a paralysing agent on the mechanism of immunity in white mice. *J Bacteriol* 43:94–95, 1942 (abstract).
32. Frei W: Ueber willkürliche Sensibilisierung gegen chemisch definierte Substanzen. I. Mitteilung: Untersuchungen mit Neosalvarsan am Menschen. *Klin Wochenschr* 7:539–542, 1928. (Reference from [26] above.)
33. Friedenreich V: Fortgesetzte untersuchungen über bakterielle Umformung der isoagglutinatorischen Verhaltnisse der Blutkorperchen in vitro. *Acta med Scand* 26:308, 1927.
34. Friedenreich V: *The Thomsen Hemagglutination Phenomenon.* Levin & Munksgaard, Copenhagen, 1930, pp 1–128.
35. Galoppin L, Saurat JH: In vitro study of the binding of antiribonucleoprotein antibodies to the nucleus of isolated living keratinocytes. *J Invest Dermatol* 76:264–267, 1981.
36. Gershon RK, Kondo H: Infectious immunological tolerance. *Immunology* 21:903–914, 1971.
37. Grabar P: Hypothesis. Auto-antibodies and immunological theories: An analytical review. *Clin Immunol Immunopathol* 4:453–466, 1975.
38. Grabar P: Is autoimmunity an aberration of physiological mechanisms? In Milgrom F, Albini B (Eds). *Immunopathology. Proceedings of the 6th International Convocation on Immunology,* Karger, Basel, 1979, pp 1–6.
39. Hasek M: Vegetative hybridization of animals by joining their blood circulations during embryonic development. *Cs Biol 2:* 265–277, 1953 (in Czech.). (Reference from Hraba, T, et al: *Ann NY Acad Sci* 392:47–54, 1982.)
40. Hole NH, Coombs RRA: The conglutinating phenomenon. III. *J Hygiene* 45:497–503, 1947.
41. Jablonska S, Chorzelski TP, Jarzabek-Chorzelska M, et al: Studies in immunodermatology. VII. Four compartment system studies of IgG in stratum corneum and of stratum corneum antigen in biopsies of psoriasis and control dermatoses. *Int Arch Allergy* 48:324–340, 1975.
42. Jiji RM, Jahn EFW, Bilenki LA: Tn activation with acquired A-like antigen associated with pancytopoenia and "ringed" sidero-blasts. *Proceedings 26th Annual Meeting, American Association of Blood Banks.* Bal Harbour, FL 1973, p 112.
43. Kay MMB, Makinodan T: Immunobiology of aging: Evaluation of current status. *Clin Immunol Immunopathol* 6:394–413, 1976.
44. Krogh HK, Tönder O: Stratum corneum antigens and antibodies. In Beutner EH, Chorzelski TP, Bean SF (Eds): *Immunopathology of the Skin,* ed., 2. Wiley, New York, 1979, pp 413–425.
45. Landsteiner K: Ueber Agglutinationser-scheinungen normalen menschichen Blutes. *Wien Klin Woch* 14:1132–1134, 1901.
46. Landsteiner K, Sturli A: Ueber die Hämagglutinine normalen sera. *Wien Klin Woch* 15:38–40, 1902.
47. Lauf PK: Blood group antigens and membrane permeability in erythrocytes of man and ruminants. In Mohn JF, Plunkett RW, Cunningham RK, et al (Eds): *Human Blood Groups.* Karger, Basel, 1977, pp 383–393.
48. Lisowska E, Duk M: Effect of modification of amino groups of human erythrocytes on M, N and Nvg blood group specificities. *Vox Sang* 28:392–397, 1975.

49. Miescher PA, Paronetto F, Lambert PH: Systemic lupus erythematosus. In Miescher PA, Muller-Eberhard HJ (Eds): *Textbook of Immunopathology,* ed. 2. Grune & Stratton, New York, 1976, pp 963–1001.
50. Milgrom F, Witebsky E: Studies on the rheumatoid and related serum factors. I. Autoimmunization of rabbits with gamma globulin. *JAMA* 174:56–63, 1960.
51. Milgrom F, Wozniczko G, Dudziak Z: Physiological production of auto-antibodies. *Allgemeine Pathol u Bakteriol* 20:373–381, 1957.
52. Möller G, Bergstedt S, Dai S, et al: The degree of clonal elimination in various types of specific immunological unresponsiveness. *Ann NY Acad Sci* 392:23–33, 1982.
53. Moreau R, Dausset J, Bernard J, et al: Anémie hémolytique acquise avec polyagglutinabilitié des hématies par us nouveau facteur présent dans le serum humain normal (anti-Tn). *Bull Soc Med Hop, Paris, Seance,* May 17, 569–587, 1957.
54. Nossal GJV: Unifying concepts of tolerance and immune regulation. In Ogra PL, Jacobs D (Eds): *Regulation of the Immune Response—Proceedings of the 8th International Convocation on Immunol.* Karger, Basel, 1982, pp 1–11.
55. Pirofsky B: *Autoimmunization and the Autoimmune Hemolytic Anemias.* Williams & Wilkins, Baltimore, 1969.
56. Polak L: Self molecules in induction of hypersensitivity and tolerance in DNCB contact sensitivity in the guinea pig. *Ann NY Acad Sci* 392:90–106, 1982.
57. Sanger R, Race RR: Discussion: Journée d'etudes sur la membrane du globule Rouge. *Nouv Revue fr Hémat* (*Paris*) 11:878–884, 1971.
58. Saurat JH, Didierjean L: The immunotracing of keratinocyte subsets. In Marks R, Plewig G (Eds): *Stratum Corneum.* Springer-Verlag, Heidelberg, 1983, pp 135–143.
59. Scott DW, Darrow TL, Grouix B: Recognition and regulation by modified self. *Ann NY Acad Sci* 392:1–7, 1982.
60. Sehon AH: Suppression of IgE antibodies with conjugates of haptens or allergens and synthetic hydrophilic polymers. *Ann NY Acad Sci* 392:55–69, 1982.
61. Smith JB, Talal N: Significance of self recognition and interleukin-2 for immunoregulation, autoimmunity and cancer. *Scand J Immunol* 16:269–278, 1982.
62. Springer GF, Desai PR: Human blood group MN and precursor specificities: Structural and biological aspects. *Carbohydr Res* 40:183–192, 1975.
63. Springer GF, Desai PR, Yang HJ, et al: Interrelations of blood group M and precursor specificities and their significance in human carcinoma. In Mohn JF, Plunkett RW, Cunningham RK, et al (Eds): *Human Blood Groups.* Karger, Basel, 1977, pp 179–187.
64. Sultzberger MB: Zur Frage der experimentellen Salvarsan Ueberempfindlichkeit. *Klin Wochenschr* 8:253–254, 1929. (Reference from [26] above.)
65. Sultzberger MB: Hypersensitiveness to neoarsphenamine in guinea pigs: Experiments in prevention and desensitization. *Arch Dermatol Syphilis* 20:669–697, 1929. (Reference from [26] above.)
66. Sy MS, Dietz MH, Germain, RN, et al: Antigen and receptor driven regulatory mechanisms. IV. Idiotype bearing I-J suppressor T cell factor (TsF) induced second order suppressor T cells (Ts-2) which express anti-idiotypic receptors. *J Exp Med* 151:1183–1195, 1980.
67. Tada TK, Okumura K, Taniguchi M: Regulation of homocytotropic antibody formation in the rat. VIII. An antigen specific T cell factor that regulates anti-haptene homocytotropic antibody response. *J Immunol* 111:952–961, 1973.
68. Talal N: Autoimmunity and the immunologic network. *Arthritis Rheum* 21:853–861, 1978.
69. Thomsen O: Ein vermehrungsfähiges Agens als Veranderer des isoagglutinatorischen Verhalten der roten Blutkörperchen, eine bisher unbekannte Quelle der Fehlbestimmungen. *Z Immunol Forsch* 52:85, 1927.
70. Witebsky E, Rose NR, Terplan K, et al: Chronic thyroiditis and autoimmunization. *JAMA 164*: 1439–1447, 1957.
71. Zembala M, Asherson GL: T cell suppression of the T cell phenomenon of contact sensitivity. *Nature* (*London*) 244:227–228, 1974.

Section IIA

VESICULO-BULLOUS DISEASES

8
Clinical Significance of Immunofluorescence Tests of Sera and Skin in Bullous Diseases: A Cooperative Study*

Editors

Ernst H. Beutner

Tadeusz P. Chorzelski

Stefania Jablonska

Contributors

Samuel F. Bean
Maria Blaszczyk
Thomas K. Burnham
Mark V. Dahl
Lionel Fry
Nancy L. Furey
James Gilliam
Karl Holubar
Susan Krasny
Vijay Kumar
Rona M. Mackie
Beno Michel
Thomas T. Provost
W. Mitchell Sams
Denny L. Tuffanelli
Hiroaki Ueki
Hideo Yaoita

INTRODUCTION

Immunofluorescence (IF) studies afford valuable adjuncts to clinical and histologic examinations, particularly in vesiculo-bullous and connective tissue diseases, and to some extent also in immune complex disturbances and certain other skin diseases. Both serum studies by indirect IF (IIF) tests and skin biopsy specimen examinations by direct IF (DIF) staining can provide diagnostic information, as indicated in Table 1.

*Adapted from Beutner, EH, Chorzelski, TP, Jablonska, S, Eds. Immunofluorescence tests. Clinical significance of sera and skin in bullous diseases. *Int. J. Dermatol.* 24: 405, 1985 with permission of the Int. J. Dermatol.

Table 1. Bullous Diseases: Summary of the Diagnostic Significance of Serum and Biopsy Findings

Bullous diseases	*Serum findings IIF*[a]	*Biopsy findings DIF*[a]	*Relevance of IF*[a] *Findings*
Pemphigus, all forms	IC antibodies (over 90%)	IC deposits of IgG[b]	IIF and/or DIF diagnostic
BP[a] (and some other forms of pemphigoid)	BMZ antibodies, IgG about 70% of BP	IgG and/or C[a] *in BMZ*[a] linear; sometimes other Ig[a] and F[a]	DIF and/or IIF diagnostic
Cicatricial pemphigoid and Brunsting-Perry variety of CP[a]	BMZ antibodies, IgG about 10%	IgG and/or C in BMZ linear	DIF or IIF diagnostic
Herpes gestationis	BMZ antibodies, IgG about 20%; HG[a] factor about 50%	most C, some Ig in BMZ linear	DIF or IIF diagnostic
"Linear IgA bullous dermatosis"	BMZ antibodies, IgA about 10%	IgA linear at BMZ; also F, rarely C	DIF diagnostic
Dermatitis herpetiformis, typical	IgA-EmA[a] in about 70%; AGA[a] in about 60%	IgA; also F and C granular or fibrillar in dermal papillae; over 90%	DIF diagnostic IIF characteristic
Epidermolysis bullosa acquisita	BMZ antibodies, IgG about 30%	BMZ linear Ig and/or C	DIF and/or IIF diagnostic
Desquamative gingivitis	(see Table 3)		

[a]IF, Immunofluorescence; DIF, direct IF; IIF, indirect IF; IC, intercellular areas of stratum spinosum; BMZ, basement membrane zone; Ig, immunoglobulin; F, fibrin or fibrinogen; C, complement; HG factor, Herpes gestationis factor; CP, cicatricial pemphigoid; BP, bullous pemphigoid; IgA-EmA, IgA antiendomysial antibodies; AGA, antigliadin antibodies.
[b]If negative findings are obtained, it is due to the site biopsied; that is, old lesions are negative. Also, inactive cases usually give negative results.

SPECIMENS, METHODS OF HANDLING, AND NATURE OF FINDINGS

Serum Samples

Blood samples of about 10 ml should be taken without an anticoagulant; for example, into a red top Vacutainer* tube or into a dry test tube. Separated serum should be sent for laboratory studies. Some laboratories request sterile serum. If facilities for separating serum are not available, clotted blood can be sent to laboratories at ambient temperature.

Indirect IF studies and other serologic procedures entail in vitro tests with normal tissue components for specific antibodies (19), as indicated in Table 1. Serum studies of complement involve assays of total hemolytic activity or quantitative tests for specific complement components (89).

Biopsy Sites

Direct IF studies entail examination of frozen sections of biopsy specimens for deposits of immunoglobulins, complement components, and fibrinogen with fluorescein-labeled antibodies to these serum components. Findings may be "diagnostic" or "suggestive but not diagnostic," or just "nondiagnostic," depending on the diseases under consideration, as indicated in Table 1. Optimal results of DIF studies can only be obtained by appropriate selection of biopsy sites. Since immunoreactants may be present in one area, but not another, in such diseases as pemphigus, pemphigoid, and dermatitis herpetiformis (DH), it is sometimes necessary to perform a second biopsy procedure to establish a diagnosis.

Studies of vesiculo-bullous diseases call for biopsy procedures primarily of clinical normal or nonbullous skin adjacent to lesions. Some experts prefer to obtain biopsy specimens of both normal skin and of the edge of a fresh vesiculo-bullous eruption. IF studies of most bullous diseases call for biopsy specimens of normal perilesional skin. If these give negative reactions, then any lesions that may be present can be examined by DIF staining. IF studies of lichen planus, porphyria, and erythema multiforme call for biopsy specimens of lesions; often, older lesions need to be examined. In contrast, IF studies of vasculities require examination of very fresh lesions or lesions recently induced by histamine injection (20). In psoriasis, early lesions with intact scales should be examined (see Chap. 42).

METHODS OF HANDLING BIOPSY SPECIMENS FOR IF STUDIES

The two methods now in general use are quick freezing, usually in liquid nitrogen, and Michel's transport medium (125, 137). Quick freezing is used more commonly in clinics that perform DIF studies, in their own laboratories. Several methods can be used (19). Since shipment of frozen biopsy specimens is costly and time consuming, physicians who do not have access to in-house IF testing services generally prefer to use the transport medium for handling specimens. Only ambient temperatures should be used for it, since frozen biopsy specimens cannot be used for IF studies if they are transferred to transport medium. Specimens can be sent to laboratories by first-class mail in transport medium.

*Becton, Dickinson, & Co., Rutherford, NJ.

Most findings on quick-frozen specimens versus those handled in the transport medium are comparable (125,137). One report by Skeete and Black (171) indicated that the IF-staining reactions diminish significantly in a few days in the transport medium. However, a cooperative study with these authors (Nisengard et al., unpublished results) suggests that initial failures may have been due to changes in the pH or in the transport medium. Some workers stress the fact that the architecture of the vascular bed becomes changed in specimens handled in transport medium. However, these pose no problems in interpreting immunopathologic findings. Importantly, immunopathologic changes of the epidermis and dermal epidermal junction appear to be affected little, if at all, by use of the transport medium.

NATURE OF FINDINGS IN PEMPHIGUS, PEMPHIGOID, AND HERPES GESTATIONIS

Pemphigus (113) can be distinguished from other dermatoses with acantholytic lesions by IF studies of serum and biopsy specimens (17,18,35,39,90) (Fig. 1 and 2). Similarly, true pemphigoid differs from erythema multiforme in that the latter may or may not have vascular deposits of IgM and/or C3 (see section below on "Other Bullous Diseases with immunocytochemical and/or immunopathologic findings in the skin"), while biopsy specimens of pemphigoid have basement membrane zone (BMZ) deposits of immunoreactants and sera contain circulating antibodies to a BMZ component. The antigens reactive with anti-BMZ antibodies of true pemphigoid are in the lamina lucida (166), while those of epidermolysis bullosa acquisita (EBA) are below the basal lamina (37,135,187). While most autoantibodies are physiologic (11,13), appearing in low titers

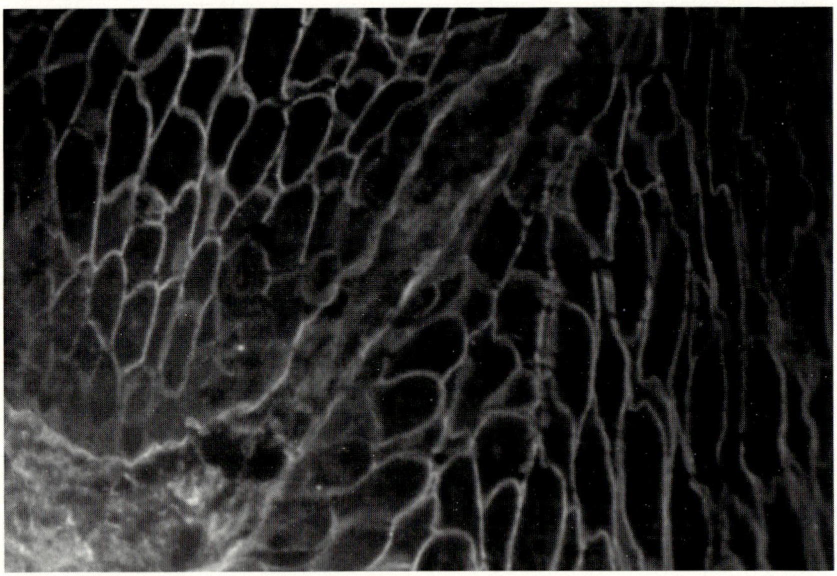

Figure 1. Indirect IF test on monkey esophagus section. Note the strongly positive IC staining. The BMZ reaction seen here is not significant. Such IC reactions are essentially diagnostic of pemphigus since PLA do not give both such strongly positive reactions and high titers in this case, 640 (800×).

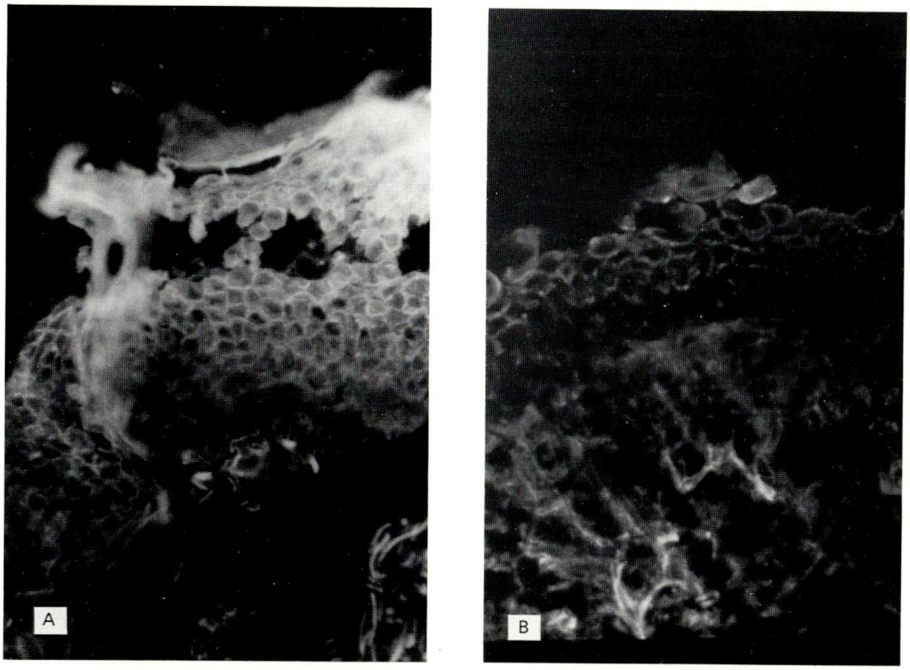

Figure 2. A. Direct IF of a lesion from a patient with pemphigus. The IF tests were carried out using an anti-IgG conjugate containing 16 U/ml (titer of 16 in a standard gel precipitation test), diluted 1:64, and using a molar F/P ratio of 2.5. Note that IgG binding to surface of keratinocytes at the floor of this intraepidermal bulla was exfoliated. No other immunoreactants were found (400×). B. Direct IF of a lesion from a patient with pemphigus. Note the strongly positive IC binding of IgG above and below the intraepidermal separation. This patient's skin biopsy specimen gave no reaction with IgM, IgA, or complement component (C3). Direct IF findings such as those found in this case are diagnostic of pemphigus (300×).

in many or all sera, the antibodies of pemphigus and pemphigoid are pathologic and disease specific.

Clinically, some cases of pemphigus, pemphigoid, DH, and linear IgA bullous dermatosis (also called chronic bullous disease of childhood [CBDC] when it occurs in children) resemble each other so closely that they cannot be distinguished unequivocally without both histologic and immunopathologic laboratory studies of biopsy and serum specimens. Judd et al. (93,94) and Lever (114) express the view that only DIF studies of biopsy specimens are indicated in pemphigus. However, other studies (29; Chap. 9) indicate that the results obtained by the IIF studies by these authors are due to technical problems, including times at which blood specimens are taken and use of inappropriate antigenic substrate. Examination of IF findings in 106 confirmed cases of pemphigus (Chap. 9) yielded the following distribution of findings: Direct IF positive, indirect IF negative: 9 cases (8.5%). Direct IF negative, indirect IF positive: 28 cases (26.4%). Direct IF positive, indirect IF positive: 69 cases (65.1%).

Thus, in this sampling of 106 cases of pemphigus from diverse clinics, serum studies gave positive findings more frequently than did biopsy studies. In effect, two schools of thought now prevail. One holds that IF studies only of biopsy specimens are indicated

(93,94,114). The other stance is that both serum and biopsy studies are indicated in various combinations (28,88,117). The difference in philosophy appears to lie largely in the methods used for performing serum studies. A major factor in the methods is the availability of monkey esophagus sections. As has been shown repeatedly, a good quality of sections of monkey esophagus or other monkey-stratified squamous cell mucosa is the antigenic substrate of choice for the IIF detection of the antibodies of pemphigus and pemphigoid (18,26,88,117,143). Studies in press when this chapter went into print (Sabolinski ML, Beutner EH, Krasny SA, et al. Substrate specificity of anti-epithelial antibodies of pemphigus vulgaris and pemphigus foliaceus sera in IF tests on monkey and guinea pig esophagus sections. J Invest. Dermatol) indicate that two substrates, monkey and guinea pig esophagus, are superior for the detection of antibodies in pemphigus foliaceus. Also, the IgA class antiendomystial antibodies (anti-EMA) associated with DH that have been described (30,38) can be best detected on monkey esophagus sections. In effect, if serum studies on sections of monkey and guinea pig esophagus are available, these should be done. The technical problem of how to obtain fresh monkey and guinea pig esophagus sections of a good quality remains to be resolved. In cases of severe bullous eruptions in which the diagnosis is not certain (e.g., Stevens Johnson or Lyell syndrome versus pemphigus or pemphigoid), simultaneous IF studies of both biopsy specimens and serum are indicated since time factors are important in such cases and either or both types of studies can yield decisive findings. Regardless of the times at which serum studies are started, the indication for follow-up IIF tests depend on the outcome of the initial studies. If the diagnosis is pemphigoid, herpes gestationis (HG) or linear IgA bullous dermatosis, no further serum studies are needed. On the other hand, if the diagnosis is pemphigus, follow-up serum studies are indicated (28), as indicated below.

Pemphigus

Serum studies for pemphigus antibodies are indicated in all forms of pemphigus according to many experts (18,26,82,88,117,143); that is, pemphigus vulgaris, pemphigus vegetans, pemphigus foliaceus (including the Brazilian form), and pemphigus erythematosus, as well as in atypical cases such as those referred to by some experts as pemphigus herpetiformis (28,72,81,145,185) and cases of eosinophilic spongiosis (68,104,172).

Serum Studies

Pemphigus antibodies that are pathogenic autoantibodies are demonstrable in virtually all active cases, if repeat tests are made with sera taken at different times (12,18,39,148). These are IgG class antibodies directed to the intercellular (IC) areas of stratified epithelia of mucous membranes and skin. The use of monkey esophagus sectins in a defined IF test system (19) gives the highest frequency of positive reactions (19,28,94). Titers as low as 10 or 20 in the presence of typical clinical and histologic findings may be regarded as consistent with pemphigus. With atypical findings, pemphigus antibody titers of more than 40 may be regarded as consistent with a diagnosis of pemphigus. Even then, confirmation by DIF tests is recommended. Circulating pemphigus antibodies cannot be detected in cases in full remission. They may be difficult to detect in early cases when there are only a few lesions, and also in pemphigus herpetiformis. In cases of suspected early pemphigus with negative, weak, or questionable reactions for pemphigus antibodies, further sera should be examined. Figure 1 shows the reaction of pemphigus antibodies.

Pemphigus-like antibodies (PLA) may appear in low or moderate titers; for example, after extensive burns (2,177). They may coexist with true pemphigus antibodies

(102). They also occur in other conditions (94,147,177), and are found in normal persons (47), particularly with the more sensitive optical systems now in use. They usually disappear spontaneously. The persistence of PLA for several months should alert physicians to the possible development of true pemphigus. The differentiation of PLA from pemphigus antibodies depends on the examination of skin biopsy specimens; only true pemphigus lesions have IC IgG deposits, as seen by DIF (41). The IF complement fixation tests can also be helpful (102). Nishikawa and associates report that some (65,67,139) or all pemphigus sera (66) can fix complement to IC areas in vitro by complement IF tests, that in vivo binding of complement occurs in some but not all pemphigus lesions (140,141). However, complement is not needed to induce acantholysis in skin explants (124). All of these observations are consistent with those reported by others (28,48,88,124,167). Nishikawa and associates suggest, on the basis of their observations, that true pemphigus antibodies fix complement. This interpretation is open to question, because sera from nonpemphigus patients with PLA do fix complement in vitro (102), but do not bind or produce acantholysis in vivo or in tissue culture explants with stratified epithelium (4,100), as indicated in Table 2. On the one hand, Fab fragments of IgG from sera of patients with high titers of pemphigus antibodies can induce acantholysis (126). This leaves no doubt that complement is not needed for inducing acantholysis. On the other hand, an augmenting effect of complement in mediating the effect of pemphigus antibodies has not been ruled out completely, since hemolytic complement levels are low in blister fluids of pemphigus (89).

From a practical standpoint, the methodologies for complement IF tests have not been worked out as thoroughly as for IIF techniques. Nevertheless, complement IF tests using antihuman C3 conjugates and patients' sera serve to differentiate true pemphigus antibodies from PLA, although this is not an absolute criterion.

There is a general correlation between titers of pemphigus antibodies and the clinical condition. However, a single titer cannot be used as a basis for adjusting the dosage of drugs such as corticosteroids or immunosuppressants (83,143,146). For adjusting drug

Table 2. Examples of Typical Findings in Two Patients: One with Pemphigus and One with Erythema and Pemphigus-like Antibodies

	Findings in patients with	
	Pemphigus with pemphigus antibodies	*Erythema multiforme with pemphigus-like antibodies*
DIF	Positive IC[a] binding of IgG	Negative
IIF	160	160
Complement IF	Negative	40
Skin explant of normal mucosa in patients' sera:		
DIF	Positive IC binding of IgG	Negative (no reaction)
Histology	Acantholysis	No changes

From Fry (56) and Fry and Seah (57).
[a]Same as for Table 1.

dosage, both the clinical condition and changes in titers should be taken into account. Importantly, patients in apparent remission, but with persistent pemphigus antibodies, are more likely than seronegative patients to develop a relapse if therapy is withdrawn or dosages are lowered too rapidly, as illustrated in Figure 3 and demonstrated in Chapter 9. However, a rise in titer of two or more doubling dilutions of IC antibodies is frequently a sign of an impending relapse. Similarly, a fall in titer is an indication of effective control of the disease process. Repeated tests on sequential sera of patients to detect changes in titers may therefore be very helpful both in evaluating the clinical course and in the management of a patient with pemphigus. These tests may be performed preferably every 2 to 4 weeks until the disease is in remission. During remission, the tests may be repeated every 1 to 6 months. Figure 3 illustrates the relation of titers of IC antibodies to the extent of lesions in a representative patient with pemphigus vulgaris. A change in titer of either one or two or more doubling dilutions is within the limits of error, depending on the intralaboratory variance of a given laboratory (176). The latter should be established by double-blind evaluations of laboratories performed by an independent agency (see Chap. 2). Properly controlled laboratory procedures can reliably detect a change of one doubling dilution in a patient's antibody titer of old and new sera tested at the same time. In some studies (e.g., the initial serum studies of the case shown in Fig. 3), pemphigus antibodies appear in the absence of skin lesions. While findings of this type have, at times, been interpreted as discrepancies (94,114), the course of the disease process, as seen in Figure 3, indicates that changes in titers of pemphigus antibodies in tests that are performed properly are a prognostic sign (16,102,117). Thus, sequential serum studies of individual patients by appropriate IF methods can afford a useful aid in their management.

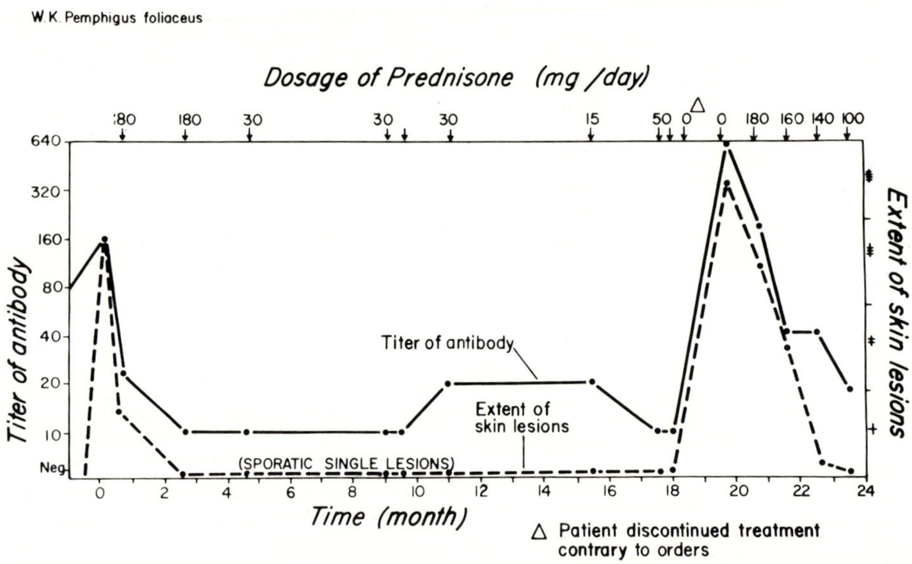

Figure 3. Relationship between the titer of antibody, extent of pemphigus lesions, and time and dosage of prednisone in a case of pemphigus foliaceus. In this case, the appearance and rise in titer of pemphigus antibodies either preceded or ran parallel to the extent of the skin lesions (see Chap. 9 for further details). (Reprinted from Beutner, Chorzelski, and Jordon [14].)

Skin Biopsy Studies

Intercellular deposits of IgG (Figs. 2A and 2B) can be demonstrated by IF in the epithelium of virtualy all patients with active pemphigus, although not all areas of the skin are positive. Especially in untreated cases of pemphigus, complement is bound to the IC areas together with the IgG in lesional ares (43,87). The finding of IC complement deposits in normal skin should not be mistaken as a sign of pemphigus, since such findings have been associated with other conditions, thus constituting false-positives (101). For IF examination, biopsy specimens should be obtained from the apparently normal skin adjacent ot a bulla. Biopsy specimens of bullae often yield misleading results because of secondary changes. If biopsy specimens of fresh bullae are obtained, they should be accompanied by a separate specimen from the adjacent uninvolved skin, or the specimens should be from an area that includes both the edge of a fresh lesion and the adjacent normal skin.

For immunopathologic studies of lesions on the mucous membranes, biopsy specimens should be obtained from the periphery of a fresh lesion, since the epithelium is usually extensively eroded in lesional areas, and therefore the IF reactions with epithelium usually are not detectable.

In pemphigus erythematosus, not only IC deposits of IgG, but also dermoepidermal junction deposits of a band of complement and sometimes of IgG may be demonstrable (6,36,59,144). IF at the dermal-epidermal junction can be demonstrated mainly in lesions localized on the face and other exposed areas. These findings occur less frequently on the trunk and other unexposed areas.

Biopsy procedures for IF studies are also indicated when there is difficulty in differentiating clinically and histologically between pemphigus vegetans and pyoderma vegetans, since acantholytic cells may occur in both disorders.

Immunopathologic studies of pemphigus patients with clinical features of DH show characteristic IF findings of pemphigus (28,72,81,145,185). While there had been some controversy on the classification of such cases (68), most experts who have seen such cases now accept the designation of pemphigus herpetiformis (37,38,185), if the clinical signs resemble those of DH and the IF findings confirm the diagnosis of pemphigus.

Atypical pemphigus may clinically resemble lupus erythematosus (LE), erythema annulare centrifugum, erythema multiforme, intertrigo, aphthous ulcers, or other disorders. In such cases, IF studies of sera and skin biopsy specimens establish the correct diagnosis. Skin specimens are also helpful in differentiating cases of subcorneal pustular dermatosis from early pemphigus erythematosus or foliaceus, since intercellular IF is positive only in true pemphigus.

Immunoflorescence is invariably negative in the normal skin of patients with familial benign chronic pemphigus of Hailey and Hailey and transient acantholytic dermatosis (24,62), and in other skin diseases with acantholysis (28). However, in lesional areas, some secondary changes detectable by DIF have been reported in transient acantholytic dermatosis (129,170). Such secondary changes occur in many types of skin lesions.

Pemphigoid

Both biopsy and serum studies are of critical value in the diagnosis of bullous pemphigoid (BP) (14,33). Biopsy studies and, to a lesser extent, serum studies are of vital importance in the diagnosis of other clinical forms of this disease. These include vesicular forms of pemphigoid; that is, cases that develop only small vesicles (8), erythematous form of pemphigoid with few bullae (28), nodular or acantholytic pemphigoid

(155,192), as well as pemphigoid coexistent with lichen planus or "lichen planus pemphigoides" (133)—with systemic lupus (103) and with other diseases (14). These are all characterized by IgG and/or C3 binding to the BMZ. Positive serum findings of anti-BMZ antibodies tend to appear less frequently than in the common BP form of the disease (33). Herpes gestationis (HG) also has many features in common with BP (see the section below on "Herpes gestationis").

Serum Studies

Antibodies to BMZ antigens of stratified epithelium are associated with pemphigoid. (Fig. 4.) Anti-BMZ antibodies occur both in the various forms of pemphigoid (18,33,35,90) and in EBA (37,184). As indicated in the section below on "Epidermolysis bullosa acquisita," the anti-BMZ antibodies are quite distinct from those of pemphigoid (33). The percentage of seropositive cases varies with the form of the disease (see Chaps. 15 and 16). In the bullous forms of the disease, about 60 to 80% are seropositive (8,184). In other forms of pemphigoid, the percentage of seropositive findings is lower. In the vesicular type, about 40% are seropositive, and about 50% in the erythematous variety (21). Some correlation occasionally appears between the titers of BMZ antibodies and the severity of pemphigoid in individual cases, but this is not a constant finding. Thus, fluctuations in titers cannot be used for prognostic or therapeutic purposes, as with pemphigus (3,14). Often antibodies cannot be detected early in the course of the disease. Also, the antibodies may persist in cases in remission. The percentage of patients with cicatricial pemphigoid who have circulating basement membrane antibodies is low (7,9,10,154; Chap. 17). The same holds true for the Brunsting-Perry variant called localized pemphigoid (7,122,123).

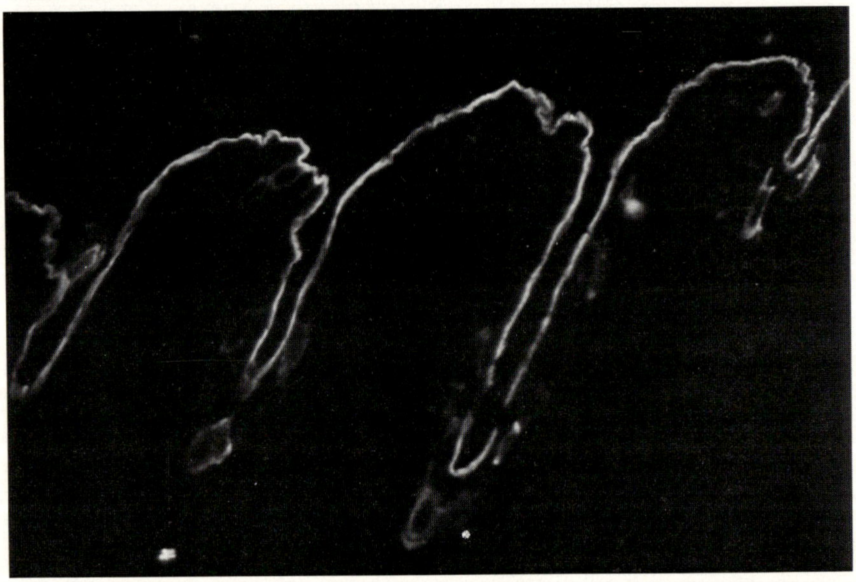

Figure 4. Indirect IF (same conjugate as in Fig. 1) reaction of anti-BMZ antibodies of a patient with BP on a section of monkey esophagus. The test was performed using a 1:20 dilution of the patient's sera. Such reactions have only been reported thus far with sera of patients with various forms of pemphigoid and in cases of EBA (see text for differentiation of the latter) (300×).

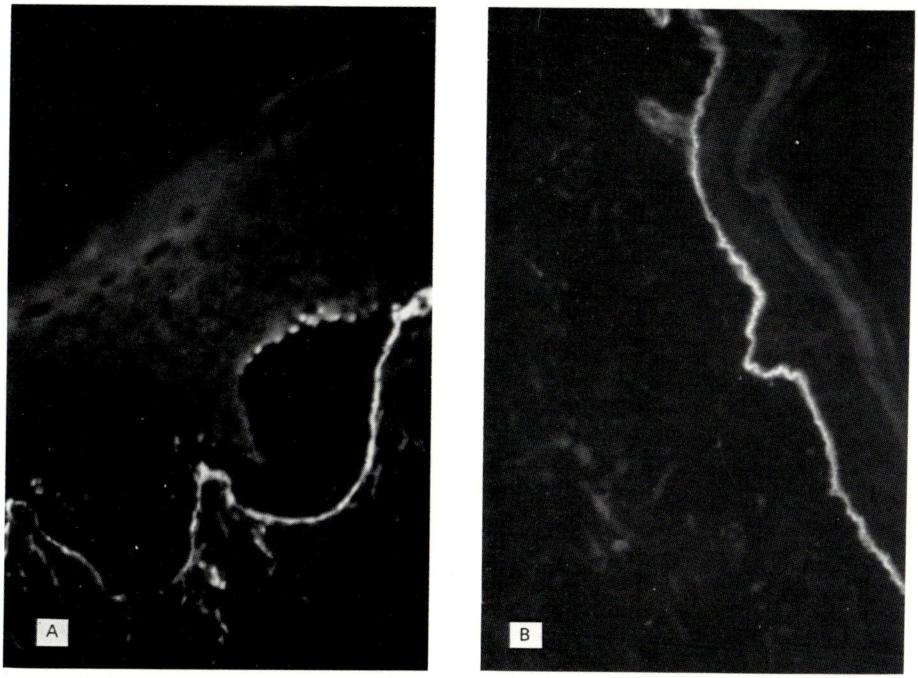

Figure 5. A. Direct IF test of a bullous lesion in a case of BP with the same type of conjugate as in Fig. 1. Note binding of IgG to the BMZ primarily at the floor of the bulla. This reaction pattern extended into the adjacent, less-involved area of the biopsy specimen, giving a pattern of the type shown in Figure 5B. Immunofluorescence tests with anticomplement (C3) conjugate gave a similar reaction pattern. Tests using anti-IgA and anti-IgM conjugates gave negative reactions. Such findings are essentially diagnostic of either a form of pemphigoid or of EBA (see Figs. 8A and 8B for differentiation of the latter) (300×). B. Direct IF test of normal skin near a subepidermal bulla stained by using an anti-IgA conjugate. IF tests for IgA reactions were performed with a conjugate (Kallestad) with the following characteristics: 4 units of specific antibody/ml, 1.85 ml of antibody, molar F/P ratio of 2.7 used at a dilution of 1:16. Note the strongly positive, sharply linear IgA binding to the BMZ. This biopsy specimen gave no reaction with anti-IgG, anti-IgM, or anticomplement conjugates. Such findings are diagnostic of linear IgA bullous dermatosis (300×).

Skin Biopsy Studies

Direct IF studies of skin or mucosal biopsy specimens reveal C3, IgG, and sometimes other Ig and/or fibrin deposits in the BMZ in cases of BP or its variants. (Fig. 5A). Biopsy specimens should be taken from apparently normal skin adjacent to a bulla. Older lesional specimens often yield negative findings, because the basement membrane is destroyed. If fresh bullae are available for a biopsy specimen, these may also be examined, but such specimens should be accompanied by a separate biopsy specimen of perilesional tissue. Sometimes it is necessary to examine serial sections of tissue near the bulla or to repeat the biopsy procedure.

Biopsy specimens from cicatricial pemphigoid patients with oral mucous membrane lesions should be obtained from the area adjacent to an erosion of bulla (9,122,123,138,162). Biopsy specimens from ocular lesions frequently give negative IF findings, but oral biopsies yield many positive diagnostic findings according to these authors. In the Brunsting-Perry type, if no fresh lesions are available, a biopsy specimen should be obtained partly from a scarred area for histopathologic studies, and partly from the adjacent normal skin for examination by DIF.

Herpes Gestationis

Immunofluorescence studies have shown that this vesiculo-bullous disease, which occurs during pregnancy or shortly thereafter, reacts like a variant of pemphigoid (22,75,80,157,188; Chap. 19). Thus, some physicians refer to it quite rightly as "gestational pemphigoid," which is a term that avoids unnecessary confusion with herpes.

Serum Studies

Circulating IgG class BMZ antibodies are usually not detectable in this disease, but some sera do bind complement to the BMZ as shown by complement IIF (150). This was originally thought to be due to a non-Ig serum factor, for which the term "HG factor" was proposed (156). The in vitro binding of complement at the BMZ is now recognized to be the result of IgG class BMZ antibodies that avidly fix complement and are usually not detectable by routine IF methods (91,96). One study suggests that HG factor and anti-BMZ antibodies are important for the prognosis of the fetus (108). However, more recent findings indicate that newborn infants are only affected transiently (32,169).

Skin Biopsy Studies

The DIF biopsy test is usually the most reliable method of diagnosis (157). That is, DIF tests are more reliable than IIF and histologic studies. As in BP biopsy specimens should be taken from the apparently uninvolved skin adjacent to lesions. In addition, specimens may be taken from the edge of lesions. Some workers prefer to take biopsy specimens from erythematous, preferably nonedematous lesions. Most commonly, DIF studies reveal C3 and other complement components in the BMZ (157). These may also be found in the newborn infant (32,108,169). Immune deposits may also be present in the walls of cutaneous vessels (84).

Epidermolysis Bullosa Acquisita

EBA, which has been recognized as a nosologic entity since 1904 (95), is a rare disease of adults that is not inherited (159). It differs from the other chronic bullous diseases considered here in several respects, most notably trauma induces bulla formation; the disease is usually accompanied by other diseases (e.g., diabetes, multiple myeloma, chronic lymphatic leukemia, and others), and importantly there is little or no response to treatment with corticosteroids. Positive DIF reactions occur in essentially all cases of EBA (37,135,184,187). Ultrastructurally, these are below the lamina densa (37,135,187), unlike the Ig deposits of pemphigoid which occur in the lamina lucida (37,60,166; Chap. 20).

Serum Studies

Serum studies are of interest in EBA, since they reveal the presence of circulating antibodies (primarily of the IgG class) to the BMZ (37,184) in some (25 to 36%) of the reported cases. While the IF reactions of these antibodies look like those of pemphigoid patients, the antigens with which they react are clearly distinct from those reactive with anti-BMZ antibodies of pemphigoid, not only in their ultrastructural localization, but also biochemically (21). Recent studies suggest that this clinically important difference can also be demonstrated by performing IF serum studies on sections of skin that have been separated or sheared at the lamina lucida (21). To do such studies, skin is submerged in 1 M NaCl for about 2 days or until the epidermis can be separated by gentle traction. The separated epidermis is rinsed in physiologic buffered saline, quick frozen, sectioned, and used for standard IF tests of the sera containing anti-BMZ antibodies (Chap. 20). Such tests with EBA sera yield reactions in or below the lamina densa, which adheres to the floor of the separation, while the anti-BMZ antibodies of true pemphigoid cases react either with the roof or partly with the roof, and partly with the floor of the 1 M NaCl-induced separation. This method reveals that some of the patients diagnosed as having typical "pemphigoid," have antibodies to component(s) of the lamina densa. This method of differentiation (which has been confirmed, in part, by some of the contributors) will probably be of considerable value in future development of the immunopathology of bullous diseases. In view of the recent findings on the regional variations in the expression of BP antigen in human skin (61), it seems probable that such studies will, in the future, be done routinely with skin from the flexor surfaces of the arm, leg, or thigh for the differentiation of anti-BMZ antibodies of the EBA type.

Skin Biopsy Studies

Direct IF tests of both lesional and adjacent, less involved skin reveal IgG and usually also other immunoglobulin (Ig), complement (C), and fibrin deposits in the BMZ in a linear pattern resembling that of pemphigoid. Survey of the limited literature suggests that multiple Ig and C components tend to occur more commonly in EBA than in pemphigoid (184). As mentioned above, immunoelectron microscopic (IEM) findings indicate that the immune deposits in EBA occur below the basal lamina (37,135,187), in contrast to pemphigoid. These findings, together with the electron microscopic (EM) and periodic acid Schiff (PAS) staining patterns that reveal bulla formation below the basal lamina, indicate clearly that EBA is distinct from pemphigoid (60,136). This distinction can also be demonstrated in diagnostic studies by performing "IF mapping" on sections of bullae with anti-type IV collagen or antilaminin antibodies (69,181; Chap. 21). These antigens appear in the roof of EBA bullae, but predominantly in the floor of pemphigoid bullae (compare Figs. 6A and 6B).

CLASSIFICATION OF SUBEPIDERMAL BULLOUS ERUPTIONS WITH IgA DEPOSITS

The classification of subepidermal bullous eruptions with IgA deposits has given rise to much confusion (8,25,27,34,42,52–54,56,57,73,74,97,158). The IF findings of Ig by Cormane (42), of IgA in a granular pattern by van der Meer (119), Chorzelski et al. (27), Fry and Seah (57), and others, and of C3 by Holubar et al. (73) and others have served to clarify the nosologic position of DH and have aided in clarifying the position of atypical forms with linear deposits of IgA in the BMZ. Some authors interpret the latter finding as a variant of BP (8,74,86), and others as a variant of DH (97). The suggestion that the finding of linear IgA deposits in the BMZ of adults is characteristic of linear IgA bullous dermatosis (LABD) (25) appears to be gaining general acceptance. Comparable findings in children are considered to be typical of chronic bullous disease of childhood (CBDC) (31). Some experts point to the self-clearing nature of the childhood form of the disease and to the more chronic nature of the adult form of LABD (111). However, since the adult and childhood forms of the disease appear to have comparable immunopathologic mechanisms (25), they are considered together

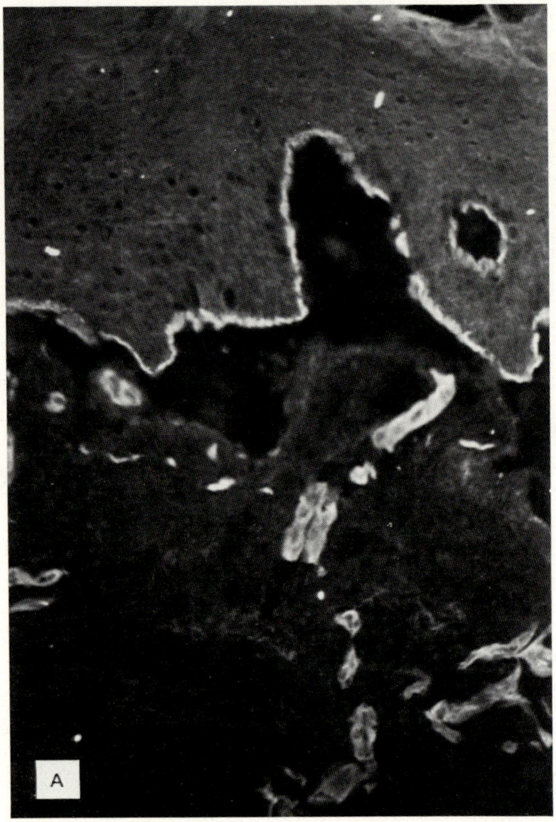

Figure 6. A. Skin biopsy specimen of a lesion of EBA tested by IIF for the localization of laminin. (Tests for laminin were performed with a rabbit antiserum to mouse laminin containing 0.25 mg/ml of specific Ig (obtained from Bethesda Research Laboratories) and diluted 1:100; this treatment was followed by a goat antirabbit conjugate with a molar F/P ratio of 2.4, containing 4 U/ml and diluted 1:16; i.e., to contain 0.25 U/ml.) Note that the laminin occurred in the roof of the bulla in this disease. This finidng serves to differentiate EBA from pemphigoid (300×). B. Indirect IF test of a lesion of a patient with BP for localization of laminin. Note the localization of the laminin in the floor of the bulla. This finding is characteristic of pemphigoid bulla (300×).

under the heading of LABD in this chapter, and the findings on DH are considered in a separate section. (For details, see Chapters 22 to 28.)

Linear IgA Bullous Dermatosis

This form of bullous eruption, which is now clearly distinguished from both DH and BP (25,111,118,131, Chaps. 22 and 23), is further divided into two types of the basis of the ultrastructural localization of the immune deposits according to some authors (63,190). According to these reports, IgA may occur either in the lamina lucida (as in BP) or below the basal lamina. However, reports from other laboratories (46,130,186) show

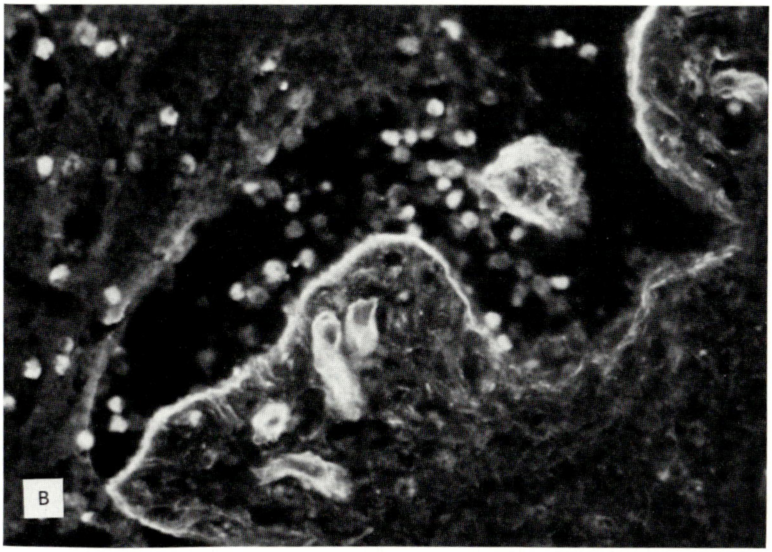

that the IgA deposits in single cases appear in both localizations. LABD is considered as a single entity in this chapter. Patients with this dermatosis respond to sulfones either alone or with corticosteroids (25). Interestingly, the same holds true to LABD in dogs (168).

Serum Studies

Routine tests for IgG class BMZ antibodies are indicated, since most LABD cases resemble BP and since these serum studies aid in differentiating BP from LABD. Circulating antibodies of the IgA class to the BMZ of monkey esophagus and/or skin occur in some of the LABD cases (120,151,191). These IgA class antibodies have been reported in variable but low frequencies (from 7 [191] to 33% [151]). Thus, serum studies for IgA class anti-BMZ antibodies prior to the detection of linear IgA deposits in biopsy specimens are not indicated for diagnostic studies.

Skin Biopsy Studies

Direct IF testing for IgA deposits in the BMZ (Fig. 5B) is the only method for establishing the diagnosis of LABD. This diagnosis assumes clinical importance for two reasons. One is that LABD patients do not have gluten-sensitive enteropathy (109), as do DH patients (56). Second, while such patients do initially respond to sulfones or sulfapyridine, as do DH patients (56), some of them require progressively higher doses; however, the combination of low doses of both sulfones (or sulfapyridine) and prednisone give excellent responses in such cases (25,34).

Direct IF studies of biopsy specimens of some patients with vesiculo-bullous eruptions yield a positive BMZ reaction for both IgA and IgG. In such cases, serum studies for IgG class antibodies are important. Also, the finding of C3 and of more strongly positive IgG deposits suggest a diagnosis of BP, while the detection of more strongly positive IgA deposits and an absence of C3 point to a probable diagnosis of LABD.

Dermatitis Herpetiformis

One of the most significant differences between LABD and DH is that DH is associated with gluten-sensitive enteropathy or celiac disease (31,56,109,112,182; Chaps. 24 to 28).

Serum Studies

The only disease-specific autoantibodies detected to date are the IgA class antiendomysial antibodies (IgA-EmA), which are directed to connective tissue components of smooth muscle of the gastrointestinal tract (Fig. 7) (30,38). These antibodies occur in about 70 to 80% of patients with DH and celiac disease (Chap. 27 and 28). The titers of IgA-EmA are proportional to the severity of enteropathy. Patients with DH or celiac disease also have antigliadin antibodies (AGA), but these are not disease specific (30,38,106,115,164,179,180; Chap. 28). The IgA class AGA are disease specific and more closely related to the severity of enteropathy than those of the IgG class (106,179). In view of the available data, not only biopsy studies but also studies for both IgA-EmA and AGA are indicated for a diagnosis of DH (38).

While some authors (56,57) report the finding of reticulin antibodies in DH, IF studies for them are not performed routinely, because these IgG class antibodies occur in only about 20 to 30% of DH cases and in some control sera. IgA class antireticulin antibodies have also been reported with a slightly elevated frequency in DH patients; that is, about 19% (116).

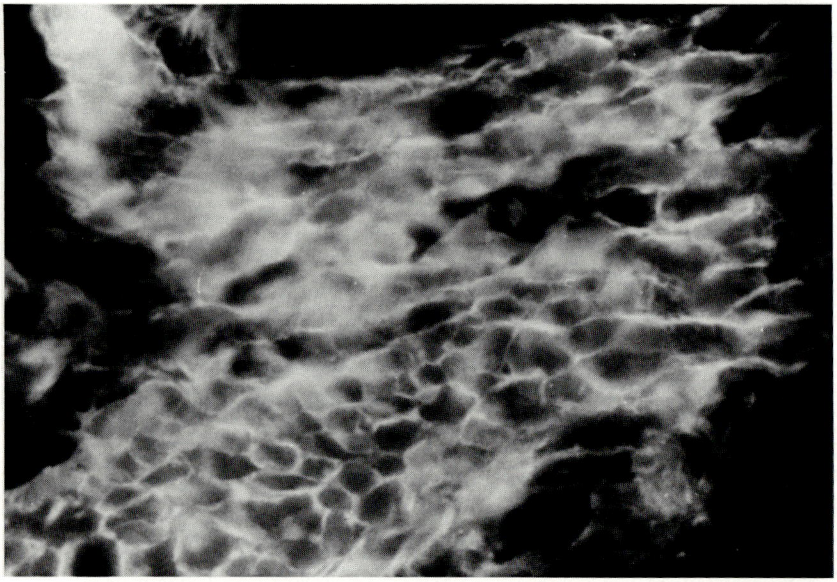

Figure 7. Indirect IF test with an anti-IgA conjugate (same anti-IgA conjugate as in Fig. 5B) and a 1:10 dilution of serum from a patient with DH on the smooth muscle layer of a section of monkey esophagus. Note the strong positive reactions of these IgA-EmA between and around the smooth muscle fibrils. These IgA-EmA are found only in DH, celiac disease (see Chaps. 27 and 28 for details). Their titer appears to be associated with the severity of enteropathy—not with the severity of the skin lesions (800×).

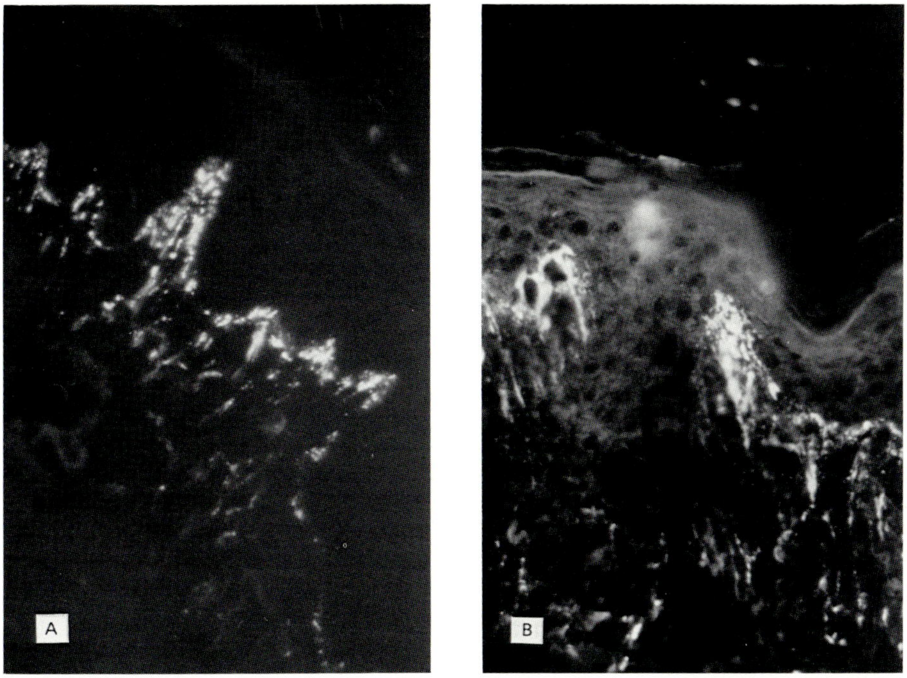

Figure 8. A. Direct IF test of a normal skin specimen from the buttock of a patient with DH with an anti-IgA conjugate (same anti-IgA conjugate as in Fig. 5B). Note the strongly positive, predominantly granular deposits of IgA in the dermal papillae. Tests using anti-IgG, anti-IgM, and anti-complement conjugates yielded negative reactions. These findings are essentially diagnostic of DH. They afford the most reliable means of documenting the diagnosis (300×). B. Same as in Figure 7A using a skin biopsy specimen from another DH patient with IgA deposits predominantly in a fibrillar pattern (300×).

Skin Biopsy Studies

Direct IF tests for granular or fibrillar IgA deposits (Fig. 8A and 8B) afford the most reliable method available of diagnosing DH (27,56,97,98,116). Selection of the biopsy site in patients with DH is of the utmost importance. Normal buttock skin is recommended (56,57); this may contain IgA deposits even in patients in remission. Perilesional skin may also be used (27). Since vesicular lesions themselves frequently yield negative IF results, biopsy specimens should be obtained from normal skin. While the immune deposits consist mainly or exclusively of IgA, papillary deposits of fibrin are also found frequently in cases in DH (184). Additional components may be IgG, IgM and/or IgD, fibrin, and C (27,42,73,98,116,119,134). Deposits of IgA and other Ig and C components in normal skin biopsy specimens of DH patients in the dermal papillae may have a granular, speckled, or fibrillar pattern (compare Figs. 8A versus 8B). IEM studies reveal comparable patterns (174,189). Fibrin deposits tend to be denser, often filling the entire papillae. The finding of granulr deposits of IgA alone or with other Ig and C in various patterns (which are commonly referred to as papillary) is diagnostic of DH (34,56,97).

OTHER BULLOUS DISEASES WITH IMMUNOCYTOCHEMICAL AND/OR IMMUNOPATHOLOGIC FINDINGS IN THE SKIN

Other bullous diseases are actually symptoms of multiple disturbances that can in many, but not all, cases be distinguished by IF studies of biopsy specimens without serum studies. This holds true of desquamative gingivitis and lichen planus pemphigoides. Certain other bullous dermatoses—notably hereditary forms of epidermolysis bullosa, lichen planus (Chap. 29), bullous eruptions in LE, porphyria, and erythema multiforme—have features that are recognizable by immunopathologic studies. While such immunologic features of these bullous diseases are of some diagnostic value, they do not have the high degree of disease specificity as the findings in pemphigus, pemphigoid and its variants, and DH. This also holds true of the DIF findings in psoriasis (Chap. 42).

Desquamative Gingivitis

This is a clinical condition in which diverse pathogenic mechanisms may be operative (55,138,153,160–162). Clinical, histologic, and IF studies of 100 randomly selected patients revealed that 35 were cases of cicatricial pemphigoid, 3 were pemphigus, 28 were lichen planus, 1 was a psoriasiform lesion (138), and 33 had no immunopathologically recognizable changes in terms of the diagnoses associated with clinical findings of desquamative gingivitis. More recent studies at the Mayo Clinic have yielded comparable findings (162). Chapter 18 summarizes both groups of findings. These findings point to the need for DIF studies of biopsy specimens in cases of desquamative gingivitis (see Table 3).

Epidermolysis Bullosa, Hereditary Forms ("IF mapping")

Selected immunocytochemical studies (which have nothing to do with the immune responses of the patients) can aid in the differentiation of hereditary forms of epidermolysis bullosa (EB) in clinical laboratory studies. That is, while none of the hereditary

Table 3. Etiologies of Desquamative Gingivitis and DIF Findings on Gingival Biopsy Specimens

Etiologies of desquamative gingivitis	*Percent of total*		*Serum findings*	*DIF findings*
	a	*b*		
Cicatricial pemphigoid	25	78	Anti-BMZ[c] 10%	BMZ deposits of IgG and/or C3
Lichen planus	28	2	None	Cytoid Ig[c], F[c], C3[c], Fibrin at DEJ[d]
Pemphigus	3	2	anti-IC[c] AB, −50%	IC deposits of IgG also on lesions
Psoriasis	1	—		
Idiopathic	33	17	None	No specific findings

[a]Data from Nisengard and Neiders (138).
[b]Data from Rogers, Sheridan, Nightingale (162).
[c]Same as for Table 1.
[d]DEJ, dermal epidermal junction.

forms of EB have been found to have specific autoantibodies or immunopathologic features (159), IF studies of biopsy specimens with reagents for the detection of anti-type IV collagen and antilaminin, however, are of differential value. Both of these components of the basal lamina give positive reactions in the roof of the bullae of dermolytic dystrophic forms of EB; in junctional and epidermal (EB simplex) forms of these mechano-bullous diseases, however, the reactions appear in the floor of the bullae (70). The anti-BMZ antibodies of BP, when used as immunocytochemical markers, have yielded divergent results (70,165). This may be due to differing specificities for the BMZ found in pemphigoid antibodies of different patients. (See Chapter 21.)

Lichen Planus Pemphigoides (or Bullosus) Versus Lichen Planus and Bullous Pemphigoid

There is some confusion concerning the terminology of bullous lesions in lichen planus. There are cases that have clinical, histologic, and IF findings suggesting both lichen planus (LP) and BP. In such cases, biopsy specimens in areas near subepidermal bullae reveal linear IgG and/or C3 deposits at the BMZ. Also, circulating IgG class antibodies occur in some cases (40,133,163,173). These findings together with IEM localization of immune deposits in the lamina lucida (71) correspond to BP. However, a recent report suggests that the circulating antibody is not directed towards BP antigens, since it is not reactive with it in the immunodiffusion test (107). The characteristic IF features of LP may be superimposed on the findings of the pemphigoid type or other type with distinctive antigens in this disease.

Direct IF studies of skin biopsy specimens of LP lesions characteristically reveal cytoid (or colloid) bodies stained for IgM, and frequently also for IgG, IgA, and/or fibrin; in some lesions, fibrin deposits also occur at the dermal-epidermal junction (1,5,127). Most reports question the antibody nature of the Ig deposits. However, this has not been ruled out by elution studies (127); it is possible that these deposits are in vivo-bound physiologic autoantibodies to keratinocyte cytoplasms, which aid in the removal of damaged epidermal cells (15: Chaps. 7, 39, and 42).

The finding of Ig and fibrin deposits, particularly in clusters of large cytoid bodies, are characteristic of LP, but they are not disease specific (1,5,127). They also appear in other dermatoses with hydropic degeneration of the basal layer, such as LE. Cytoid bodies also occur commonly in lesions of BP. Not all bullous eruptions in cases of LP can be classified as coexistent LP and pemphigoid. Some have only the immunopathologic features of LP with no evidence of coexistent BP, as defined clinically and histologically (bullous lesions exclusively within the involved skin), as well as by DIF and IIF. These cases should be classified as LP pemphigoides or bullosus (78).

Bullous Eruptions in Systemic Lupus Erythematosus (SLE): Bullous Pemphigoid Coexistent with SLE Versus Bullous LE

Cases of coexistence of SLE with BP with IF features of each have been reported (92,103,121,128), although not all cases have been adequately documented clinically and immunologically. In one well-documented case with clinical features of both diseases, the demonstration of antibodies to the BMZ required tissue cultures of skin explants in the patient's serum (103) because of the interference of the strongly positive IF band in the biopsy studies and of the interference of high titers of antinuclear antibodies (ANA) with the serum studies. In another documented case of SLE with bullous lesions (See chapter 20.), in vivo nucleolar IgG deposits and sharp linear BMZ binding of IgG and C3, as well as serum findings of nucleolar antibodies and anti-Sm antibodies, point again to a possible coexistence of these two diseases. However, such coexistence should not be confused with the occasional occurrence of ANA in typical cases of BP.

Cases of bullous LE of the type described by Pedro and Dahl (149) and Jacoby and Abraham (85), which are referred to also as Rowell syndrome (79), have no immunologic signs of pemphigoid, but only IF findings of LE. According to Gammon et al. (58), tests of of both normal and lesional skin biopsy specimens of such patients with bullous SLE in organ culture show more complement-dependent leukocyte migration than normal lesional skin of patients with nonbullous SLE (58). This points to a role for immune complexes in blister formation. The higher frequency of linear Ig deposits in the noninvolved skin of patients with bullous LE, than in matched SLE patients without bullae (58), raises a question about the possible role of in vivo-bound antibodies to the BMZ. Earlier studies revealed that acid eluates of skin from two of three (105) and two of four (183) fatal cases of SLE contained anti-BMZ antibodies. However, the IEM demonstration of the linear IgG deposits below the basal lamina (64,142) resemble the findings in EBA (37,135,187), rather than pemphigoid (37,166). This led Gammon and associates (58) to conclude that cases reported as LE coexistent with pemphigoid (92,103,121,128) may be LE coexistent with a variant of EBA (see Chap. 20 for details). This view is now widely accepted.

Vesiculo-bullous eruptions clinically simulating DH were also reported (64,85,152). Such eruptions were not localized to places typical of DH; but the histologic picture with neutrophil microabscesses was consistent with DH. However, IF findings did not reveal granular papillary IgA deposits characteristic of DH. The immunopathologic picture had some features of both BP and LE, since there were not only granular Ig and C3, but also linear immune deposits (64,85,152).

Some cases were responsive to corticosteroids. However, cases reported by Hall (64), Szabo et al. (175), and four patients of Chorzelski responded to sulfones. In contrast to typical DH, a proportion of cases required sulfones intermittently, and withdrawal did not always result in relapse.

In one of our patients, linear deposits consisted mainly of IgA, but not in all biopsy specimens and not in all relapses. This is in accordance with findings of Hall et al. (64). Importantly, some patients of Hall et al. (64) also had leukocytoclastic vasculitis in skin biopsy specimens. In one vesiculo-bullous eruption coexisting with SLE, circulating anti-BMZ antibodies were detectable. Regardless of the nosologic position of this vesiculo-bullous eruption in SLE, it is important to note that sulfones may be the treatment of choice. It is stressed that besides these vesiculo-bullous forms simulating DH or vesicular BP, the true coexistence of DH and LE has been repeatedly reported (132,178).

Porphyria

Porphyria cutanea tarda (PCT) and other forms of porphyria may present with subepidermal bullae. Immunofluorescent tests of skin biopsy specimens in porphyria reveal immune deposits in the walls of enlarged blood vessels in the papillary dermis and at the dermal-epidermal junction (44,45,49). Such findings appear in PCT, erythropoietic protoporphyria, variegate porphyria, coproporphyria (44,45,49,50), and in tetracycline-induced photosensitization (51). The immune deposits in the vessel walls and in the junctional region consist primarily of IgG, and not infrequently IgM, C, fibrin, and occasionally IgA. Reports in the literature on these immune deposits justifiably raise questions about their antibody nature. However, elution and other immunologic studies to prove this point have not been done as yet.

The frequency of typical DIF findings in active lesions is close to 100%. In uninvolved areas of the skin of patients with active disease, the frequencies of such findings drop to about 50%. DIF findings of porphyria should be confirmed by urine or serum porphyrin assays.

Erythema Multiforme

Bullous erythema multiforme and its variants, Stevens-Johnson disease and Lyell's toxic epidermal necrolysis are bullous disorders largely of unknown etiology. At least in some cases, immune complex disturbances are implicated. Immune deposits, mostly IgM and C3 in the walls of superficial dermal vessels, have been reported to occur in lesional skin areas (23,77,99). However, these are not disease-specific findings. The immune deposits are reported to occur most commonly in early lesions (99). However, in sequential examinations before, during, and after the appearance of lesions in 26 cases, none were found to have specific intravascular deposits (110). Other surveys of immune deposits in vessels in the upper dermis yield positive findings in 4 of 12 (33%) (77) to 20 of 23 (87%) (99) of the cases examined. Serum studies by Clq-binding assays (77) or by monoclonal rheumatoid factor assay (23) revealed circulating immune complexes in up to half of the cases of erythema multiforme (23,77,110). A critical review of the literature on this disease (76) indicates that DIF studies serve primarily to rule out pemphigoid, DH, and pemphigus in the differential diagnosis.

REFERENCES

1. Abell E, Presbury DG, Marks R, et al: The diagnostic significance of immunoglobulin and fibrin deposition in lichen planus. *Br J Dermatol* 93:17–24, 1975.
2. Ablin R, Milgrom F, Kano K, et al: Pemphigus-like antibodies in patients with skin burns. *Vox Sang.* 16:73–75, 1969.
3. Ahmed AR, Maize JC, Provost TT: Bullous pemphigoid. Clinical and immunologic follow-up after successful therapy. *Arch Dermatol* 113:1043–1046, 1977.
4. Ansel J, Petrozzi JW, Kumar V: Possible drug induced pemphigus-like antibodies with the clinical manifestation of erythema multiforme. *Arch Dermatol* 119:1006–1009, 1983.
5. Baart de la Faille-Kuyper EH, Baart de la Faille H: An immunofluorescence study of lichen planus. *Br J Dermatol* 90:365–371, 1974.
6. Bean SF, Lynch FW: Senear-Usher syndrome (pemphigus erythematosus). Immunofluorescent studies in a patient. *Arch Dermatol* 101:642–645, 1970.
7. Bean SF, Michel B: Cicatricial pemphigoid. In Beutner EH, Chorzelski TP, Bean SF, et al (Eds): *Immunopathology of the Skin: Labeled Antibody Studies.* Dowden, Hutchinson, Ross, Stroudsburg, PA, 1973, pp. 55–63.
8. Bean SF, Michel B, Furey N, et al: Vesicular pemphigoid. *Arch Dermatol* 112:1402–1404, 1976.
9. Bean SF, Rogers RS III, Jordon RE, et al: Cicatricial pemphigoid. In Beutner EH, Chorzelski TP, Bean SF (Eds): *Immunopathology of the Skin.* ed. 2. Wiley, New York, 1979, pp 257–263.
10. Bean SF, Waisman M, Michel B: Cicatricial pemphigoid. Immunofluorescent studies. *Arch Dermatol* 106:195–199, 1972.
11. Beutner EH, Binder WL, Jablonska S, et al: Nature of stratum corneum autoantibodies, antigens and antigen conversion and their role in healing and in psoriasis. In Marks R, Christophers E (Eds): *The Epidermis in Disease.* MTP Press, Lancaster, UK, 1981, pp 577–583.

12. Beutner EH, Chorzelski TP, Bean SF, et al. (Eds): *Immunopathology of the Skin: Labeled Antibody Studies.* Dowden, Hutchinson, Ross, Stroudsburg, PA, 1973, pp 1–461.
13. Beutner EH, Chorzelski TP, Binder WL: Nature of autoimmunity: Pathologic versus physiologic responses and a unifying concept. In Beutner EH, Chorzelski TP, Bean SF (Eds): *Immunopathology of the Skin,* ed. 2. Wiley, New York, 1979, pp 147–180.
14. Beutner EH, Chorzelski TP, Jordon RE: *Autosensitization in Pemphigus and Bullous Pemphigoid.* Charles C Thomas, Springfield, IL, 1970, pp 1–194.
15. Beutner EH, Cunningham RK: Autoimmunity. In Stone J (Ed): *Dermatologic Immunology and Allergy.* CV Mosby, St Louis, 1984, pp 125–142.
16. Beutner EH, Jablonska S, Jarzabek-Chorzelska M, et al: Studies in immunodermatology. VI. IF studies of autoantibodies to the stratum corneum and of in vivo fixed IgG in stratum corneum of psoriatic lesions. *Int Arch Allergy Appl Immunol* 48:301–323, 1975.
17. Beutner EH, Jordon RE: Demonstration of skin antibodies in sera of pemphigus vulgaris patients by indirect immunofluorescent staining. *Proc Soc Exp Biol Med* 117:505–510, 1964.
18. Beutner EH, Lever WF, Witebsky E, et al: Autoantibodies in pemphigus vulgaris. Responses to an intercellular substance of epidermis. *JAMA* 192:682–688, 1965.
19. Beutner EH, Nisengard RJ, Kumar V: Defined immunofluorescence: Basic concepts and their application to clinical immunodermatology. In Beutner EH, Chorzelski TP, Bean SF (Eds): *Immunopathology of the Skin,* ed. 2. Wiley, New York, 1979, pp 29–75.
20. Braverman IM, Yen A: Demonstration of immune complexes in spontaneous and histamine-induced lesions and in normal skin of patients with leukocytoclastic angitis. *J Invest Dermatol* 64:105–112, 1975.
21. Briggaman RA, Gammon WR, Inman AO, et al: Heterogeneous nature of bullous pemphigoid-like IgG associated basement membrane zone disorders. *J Invest Dermatol* 80:364, 1983 (abstract).
22. Bushkell LL, Jordon RE, Goltz RW: Herpes gestationis: New immunological findings. *Arch Dermatol* 110:65–69, 1974.
23. Bushkell LL, Mackel SE, Jordon RE: Erythema multiforme: Direct immunofluorescence studies and detection of circulating immune complexes. *J Invest Dermatol* 74:372–374, 1980.
24. Chalet M, Grover RW, Ackerman AB: Transient acantholytic dermatosis. *Arch Dermatol* 113:431–435, 1977.
25. Chorzelski TP, Bean SF, et al: Linear IgA bullous dermatosis: Adult and childhood forms. In Beutner EH, Chorzelski TP, Bean SF (Eds): *Immunopathology of the Skin,* ed. 2. Wiley, New York, 1979, pp 316–323.
26. Chorzelski TP, Beutner EH: Factors contributing to occasional failures in demonstration of pemphigus antibodies by the IF test. *J Invest Dermatol* 53:188–191, 1969.
27. Chorzelski TP, Beutner EH, Jablonska S, et al: Immunofluorescence studies in the diagnosis of dermatitis herpetiformis and its differentiation from bullous pemphigoid. *J Invest Dermatol* 56:373–380, 1971.
28. Chorzelski TP, Beutner EH, Jablonska S: The role and nature of autoimmunity in pemphigus: Clinical significance of pemphigus antibodies. In Beutner EH, Chorzelski TP, Bean SF (Eds): *Immunopathology of the Skin,* ed. 2. Wiley, New York, 1979, pp 183–229.
29. Chorzelski TP, Beutner EH, Jablonska S, et al: Letter to the Editor on Judd and Liver: Correlation of antibodies in skin and serum with disease severity in pemphigus. *Arch Dermatol* 116:1228–1229, 1980.
30. Chorzelski TP, Beutner EH, Sulej J, et al: IgA-endomysium antibody. A new immunological marker of dermatitis herpetiformis and coeliac disease. *Br J Dermatol* 111:395–402, 1984.
31. Chorzelski TP, Jablonska S: IgA linear dermatosis of childhood (chronic bullous disease of childhood). *Br J Dermatol* 101:535–542, 1979.
32. Chorzelski TP, Jablonska S, Beutner EH, et al: Herpes gestationis with identical lesions in the newborn. *Arch Dermatol* 112:1129–1131, 1976.
33. Chorzelski TP, Jablonska S, Beutner EH: Pemphigoid. In Beutner EH, Chorzelski TP, Bean SF (Eds): *Immunopathology of the Skin,* ed. 2. Wiley, New York, 1979, pp 243–255.
24. Chorzelski TP, Jablonska S, Beutner EH, et al: Linear IgA bullous dermatosis. In Marks R,

Christophers E (Eds): *The Epidermis in Disease.* MTP Press, Lancaster, UK, 1981, pp 557–583.

35. Chorzelski TP, Jablonska S, Blaszczyk M: Immunopathologisch Untersuchungen bei der subcornealen pustulosen Dermatose Sneddon-Wilkinson. *G Ital Dermatol* 107:809–820, 1966.
36. Chorzelski TP, Jablonska S, Blaszczyk M: Immunopathological investigation in the Senear-Usher syndrome. (Co-existence of pemphigus and lupus erythematosus.) *Br J Dermatol* 80:211–217, 1968.
37. Chorzelski TP, Petkow L, Dabrowski J, et al: Epidermolysis bullosa acquisita (EBA). *Der Hautarzt* 36:487–490, 1981.
38. Chorzelski TP, Sulej J, Tchorzewska H, et al: IgA class endomysium antibodies in dermatitis herpetiformis and coeliac disease. In Beutner EH, Nisengard RJ, Albini B (Eds): *Defined Immunofluorescence and Related Cytochemical Methods.* Ann NY Acad. Sci, New York, 1983, pp 325–334.
39. Chorzelski TP, von Weiss JF, Lever WF: Clinical significance of autoantibodies in pemphigus. *Arch Dermatol* 93:570–576, 1966.
40. Collins NJ, Dowling JP: Lichen planus and bullous pemphigoid. *Austr J Dermatol* 23:9–13, 1982.
41. Cooperative Study: Uses for immunofluorescence tests of skin and sera. *Arch Dermatol* 111:371–381, 1975.
42. Cormane RH: Immunofluorescent studies of the skin in lupus erythematosus and other diseases. *Pathol Eur* 2:170–180, 1967.
43. Cormane RH, Chorzelski TP: "Bound" complement in the epidermis of patients with pemphigus vulgaris. *Dermatologica* 134:463–466, 1967.
44. Cormane RH, Szabo E, Hauge LS: Immunofluorescence of the skin: The interpretation of the staining of blood vessels and connective tissue aided by new techniques. *Br J Dermatol* 82(Suppl 5):26–53, 1970.
45. Cormane RH, Szabo E, Hoo TT: Histopathology of the skin in acquired and hereditary porphyria cutanea tarda. *Br J Dermatol* 85:531–539, 1971.
46. Dabrowski J, Chorzelski TP, Jablonska S, et al: The ultrastructural localization of IgA deposits in chronic bullous disease of childhood (CBDC). *J Invest Dermatol* 72:291–295, 1979.
47. Dahl MV, Katz SI, Scott RM, et al: Viral studies in pemphigus. *J Invest Dermatol* 62:96–99, 1974.
48. Deng JS, Beutner EH, Shu S, et al: Pemphigus antibody action of skin explants. Kinetics of acantholytic changes and stability of antigens in tissue cultures of normal monkey skin explants. *Arch Dermatol* 113:923–926, 1977.
49. Epstein JH, Tuffanelli DL, Epstein WL: Cutaneous changes in porphyrias. A microscopic study. *Arch Dermatol* 107:689–698, 1973.
50. Epstein JH, Tuffanelli DL, Epstein WL: Cutaneous porphyrias and porphyria-like cutaneous changes induced by drug photosensitization. In Beutner EH, Chorzelski TP, Bean SF (Eds): *Immunopathology of the Skin,* ed. 2. Wiley, New York, 1979, pp 445–471.
51. Epstein JH, Tuffanelli DL, Seibert JS, et al: Porphyria-like cutaneous changes induced by tetracycline hydrochloride photosensitization. *Arch Dermatol* 112:661–666, 1976.
52. Esterly NB, Furey NL, Kirschner RS, et al: Chronic bullous dermatosis of childhood. *Arch Dermatol* 113:42–46, 1977.
53. Faber WR, Joost TH van: Juvenile pemphigoid. *Br J Dermatol* 89:519–522, 1973.
54. Feuerman EJ, Metzker A, Varsano I: Dermatitis herpetiformis in childhood. *J Israel Med Assoc* 88:114–118, 1975.
55. Forman L, Nally FF: Oral non-dystrophic bullous eruptions mainly limited to the gingivae: a mechano-bullous response. *Br J Dermatol* 96:111–117, 1977.
56. Fry L: Dermatitis herpetiformis: Basic findings. in Beutner EH, Chorzelski TP, Bean SF (Eds): *Immunopathology of the Skin,* ed. 2. Wiley, New York, 1979, pp 283–301.
57. Fry L, Seah PP: Dermatitis herpetiformis. In Fry L, Seah PP (Eds): *Immunological Aspects of Skin Diseases.* Wiley, New York, 1974, pp 22–65.
58. Gammon WR, Briggaman RA, Inman AO III, et al: Evidence supporting a role for immune

complex-mediated inflammation in the pathogenesis of bullous lesions of systemic lupus erythematosus. *J Invest Dermatol* 81:320–325, 1983.

59. Gianetti A: Studies in Senear-Usher syndrome. *Arch Dermatol Forsch* 248:287–292, 1974.
60. Gibbs RB, Minus HR: Epidermolysis bullosa acquisita with electron microscopic studies. *Arch Dermatol* 111:215–220, 1975.
61. Goldberg DJ, Bystryn JC: Regional variations in the expression of bullous pemphigoid antigen in human skin. *J Invest Dermatol* 80:365, 1983 (abstract).
62. Grover RW: Transient acantholytic dermatosis. Electron microscopic study. *Arch Dermatol* 104:26–37, 1971.
63. Haffenden GP, Ring NP, Leonard J, et al: Immuno electron microscopical studies in patients with linear IgA deposits. *J Invest Dermatol* 80:363, 1983 (abstract).
64. Hall RP, Lawley TJ, Smith HR, et al: Bullous eruption of systemic lupus erythematosus: Dramatic response to dapsone therapy. *Ann Intern Med* 97:165–170, 1982.
65. Hashimoto T, Nishikawa T, Kurihara S, et al: Complement fixing pemphigus antibodies. *Arch Dermatol* 114:1191–1192, 1978.
66. Hashimoto T, Sugiura M, Kurihara S, et al: In vitro complement activation by intercellular antibodies. *J Invest Dermatol* 78:316–318, 1982.
67. Hashimoto T, Sugiura M, Kurihara S, et al: Experimental acantholysis by complement-fixing intercellular antibodies. *Arch Dermatol Res* 273:129–135, 1982.
68. Hashimoto T, Sugiura M, Kurihara S, et al: Atypical pemphigus showing eosinophilic spongiosis. *Clin Exp Dermatol* 8:37–40, 1983.
69. Hintner H, Fritsch PO, Foidart JM, et al: Expression of basement membrane zone antigens at the dermo-epibolic junction in organ cultures of human skin. *J Invest Dermatol* 74:200–204, 1980.
70. Hintner H, Stingl G, Schuler G, et al: Immunofluorescence mapping of antigenic determinants within the dermal-epidermal junction in mechanobullous diseases. *J Invest Dermatol* 76:113–118, 1981.
71. Hintner H, Tappeiner G, Hönigsmann H, et al: Lichen planus and bullous pemphigoid. *Acta Dermatovener* 59(Suppl 85):71–76, 1979.
72. Holubar K, Beutner EH: Pemphigus vs. acantholytic herpetiformis dermatitis. *Arch Dermatol* 109:408, 1974 (abstract).
73. Holubar K, Doralt M, Eggerth G: Immunofluorescence patterns in dermatitis herpetiformis. Investigations on skin and intestinal mucosa. *Br J Dermatol* 85:505–510, 1971.
74. Honeyman JF, Honeyman AR, De la Parra MA, et al: Polymorphic pemphigoid. *Arch Dermatol* 115:423–427, 1979.
75. Hönigsmann H, Stingl G, Holubar K, et al: Herpes gestationis. Fine structural pattern of immunoglobulin deposits in the skin in vivo. *J Invest Dermatol* 66:382–392, 1976.
76. Huff JC, Weston WL, Tonnesen MG: Erythema multiforme: A critical review of characteristics, diagnostic criteria and causes. *J Am Acad Dermatol* 8:763–775, 1983.
77. Imamura S, Yanase K, Taniguchi S, et al: Erythema multiforme: Demonstration of immune complexes in sera and skin lesions. *Br J Dermatol* 102:161–166, 1980.
78. Ingber A, Feureman EJ: Letter to the Editor on Mora et al. Lichen ruber pemphigoides: Clinical and immunofluorescent findings in four cases. *J Am Acad Dermatol* 9:606, 1983.
79. Jablonska S, Blaszczyk M, Chorzelski TP: Syndrome de Rowell-Lupus erythematosus avec des lesions coexistantes de type crytheme. *Med Hygiene* 30:1390–1393, 1972.
80. Jablonska S, Chorzelski TP, Beutner EH, et al: Immunologic phenomenon in herpes gestationis. *Arch Dermatol Forsch* 252:267–274, 1975.
81. Jablonska S, Chorzelski TP, Beutner EH, et al: Herpetiform pemphigus. A variable pattern of pemphigus. *Int J Dermatol* 14:353–359, 1975.
82. Jablonska S, Chorzelski TP, Beutner EH, et al: Indications, methods and concepts for immunopathologic studies. In Beutner EH, Chorzelski TP, Bean SF (Eds): *Immunopathology of the Skin,* ed. 2. Wiley, New York, 1979, pp 3–28.
83. Jablonska S, Chorzelski TP, Blaszczyk M: Immunosuppressants in the treatment of pemphigus. *Br J Dermatol* 83:315–323, 1970.

84. Jablonska S, Chorzelski TP, Maciejowska E, et al: Immunologic phenomenon in herpes gestationis. Their pathologic and diagnostic significance. *J Dermatol* 2:149–158, 1975.
85. Jacoby RA, Abraham AA: Bullous dermatosis and systemic lupus erythematosus in a 15 year old boy. *Arch Dermatol* 115:1094–1097, 1979.
86. Jones RR, Goolamali SK: IgA bullous pemphigoid. A distinct blistering disorder. *Br J Dermatol* 102:719–725, 1980.
87. Joost Th van, Cormane RH, Pondman KW: Direct immunofluorescent study of the skin and occurrence of complement in pemphigus. *Br J Dermatol* 87:466–474, 1972.
88. Jordon RE: Immunohistopathology of the skin. In Rose NR, Friedman H (Eds): *Manual of Clinical Immunology*. American Society for Microbiology, Washington, DC, 1976, pp 701–709.
89. Jordon RE: The complement system in pemphigus and bullous pemphigoid. In Beutner EH, Chorzelski TP, Bean SF (Eds): *Immunopathology of the Skin,* ed. 2. Wiley, New York, 1979, pp 135–145.
90. Jordon RE, Beutner EH, Witebsky E, et al: Basement zone antibodies in bullous pemphigoid. *JAMA* 200:751–756, 1967.
91. Jordon RE, Heine KG, Tappeiner G, et al: The immunopathology of herpes gestationis. Immunofluorescence studies and characterization of "HG factor." *J Clin Invest* 57:1426–1433, 1976.
92. Jordon RE, Muller SA, Hale WL, et al: Bullous pemphigoid associated with systemic lupus erythematosus. *Arch Dermatol* 99:17–25, 1969.
93. Judd KP, Lever WF: Correlation of antibodies in skin and serum with disease severity in pemphigus. *Arch Dermatol* 115:428–432, 1979.
94. Judd KP, Mescon H: Comparison of different epithelial substrates useful for indirect immunofluorescence testing of sera from patients with active pemphigus. *J Invest Dermatol* 72:314–319, 1979.
95. Kablitz E: Ein Beitrag zur Frage der Epidermolysis bullosa traumatica. (Hereditary et Acquisita.) Thesis, University of Rostock, Rostock, GDR, 1904.
96. Katz SI, Hertz KC, Yaoita H: Herpes gestationis: Immunopathology and characterization of the HG factor. *J Clin Invest* 57:1434–1441, 1976.
97. Katz SI, Lawley TJ: Dermatitis herpetiformis: Recent advances. In Beutner EH, Chorzelski TP, Bean SF (Eds): *Immunopathology of the Skin,* ed. 2. Wiley, New York, 1979, pp 303–313.
98. Katz SI, Strober W: The pathogenesis of dermatitis herpetiformis. *J Invest Dermatol* 70:63–75, 1978.
99. Kazmierowski JA, Wuepper KD: Erythema multiforme: Immune complex vasculitis of the superficial cutaneous microvasculature. *J Invest Dermatol* 71:366–369, 1978.
100. Krasny SA, Beutner EH: Experimental production of intercellular antibodies in monkeys. In Beutner EH, Nisengard RJ, Albini B (Eds): *Defined Immunofluorescence and Related Cytochemical Methods.* Ann NY Acad Sci, New York, 420: 1983, pp 343–352.
101. Krasny SA, Kumar V, Tarfare N, et al: Intercellular complement C3 binding in normal skin of patients without pemphigus. *J. Am. Acad. Dermatol.* 14: 52–58, 1986.
102. Kumar V, Beutner EH: Complement-fixing intercellular antibodies. *Arch Dermatol* 117:528, 1981.
103. Kumar V, Binder WL, Schotland E, et al: Coexistence of bullous pemphigoid and systemic lupus erythematosus. *Arch Dermatol* 114:1187–1190, 1978.
104. Lagerholm B, Frithz A, Borglund E: Light and electron microscopic aspects of pemphigus herpetiformis (eosinophilic spongiosis) in comparison with other acantholytic disorders. *Acta Dermatovener* 59:305–314, 1979.
105. Landry M, Sams WM Jr: Systemic lupus erythematosus. Studies of the antibodies bound to skin. *J Clin Invest* 52:1871–1880, 1973.
106. Lane AT, Huff JC, Zone JJ, et al: Class-specific antibodies to gluten in dermatitis herpetiformis. *J Invest Dermatol* 80:402–405, 1983.
107. Lang PG, Maize JC: Coexisting lichen planus and bullous pemphigoid or lichen planus pemphigoides. *J Am Acad Dermatol* 9:133–140, 1983.

108. Lawley TJ, Stingl G, Katz SI: Fetal and maternal risk. Factors in herpes gestationis. *Arch Dermatol* 114:552–555, 1978.
109. Lawley TJ, Strober W, Yaoita H, et al: Small intestinal biopsies and HLA types in dermatitis herpetiformis patients with granular and linear IgA skin deposits. *J Invest Dermatol* 74:9–12, 1980.
110. Leigh IM, Mowbray JE, Levene GM: Recurrent erythema multiforme. An immune complex-mediated vasculitis? *Br J Dermatol* 109(Suppl 24):22, 1983 (abstract).
111. Leonard J, Haffenden GP, Ring NP, et al: Linear IgA disease in adults. *Br J Dermatol* 107:301–316, 1982.
112. Leonard J, Haffenden GP, Tucker W, et al: Gluten challenge in dermatitis herpetiformis. *N Engl J Med* 308:816–819, 1983.
113. Lever WF: Pemphigus. *Medicine* 32:1–123, 1953.
114. Lever WF: Pemphigus and pemphigoid. *J Am Acad Dermatol* 1:2–31, 1979.
115. Ljunghall K, Lööf L, Grimelius L, et al: Dermatitis herpetiformis: Relation between circulating antibodies against reticulin and gluten, small intestinal mucosal status and absorptive capacity. *Acta Dermatovener* 63:27–34, 1983.
116. Ljunghall KI, Scheynius A, Forsum U: Circulating reticulin autoantibodies of IgA class in dermatitis herpetiformis. *Br J Dermatol* 100:173–176, 1979.
117. Maize JC, Provost TT: Value of immunofluorescent techniques in studies of bullous disease. *Am J Dermatopathol* 5:67–72, 1983.
118. Marsden RA: The treatment of benign chronic bullous dermatosis of childhood and dermatitis herpetiformis and bullous pemphigoid beginning in childhood. *Clin Exp Dermatol* 7:653–663, 1982.
119. Meer JB van der: Granular deposits of immunoglobulins in the skin of patients with dermatitis herpetiformis. An immunofluorescent study. *Br J Dermatol* 813:493–503, 1969.
120. Meer JB van der, Remme JJ, Nefkens MJJ, et al: IgA antibasement membrane antibodies in a boy with pemphigoid. *Arch Dermatol* 113:1462, 1977.
121. Meyer A, Jenni Ch, Krebs A: Diagnostic problems associated with the coexistence of bullae diseases and systemic lupus erythematosus. *Dermatologica* 153:57–64, 1976.
122. Michel B: Localized chronic pemphigoid of Brunsting-Perry: Its relationship to bullous pemphigoid. In Beutner EH, Chorzelski TP, Bean SF (Eds): *Immunopathology of the Skin,* ed. 2. Wiley, New York, 1979, pp 265–271.
123. Michel B, Bean SF, Chorzelski TP, et al: Cicatricial pemphigoid of Brunsting Perry. *Arch Dermatol* 113:1403–1405, 1977.
124. Michel B, Ko CS: Effect of pemphigus and bullous pemphigoid sera and leukocytes on normal skin in organ culture: An in vitro model for the study of bullous diseases. *J Invest Dermatol* 62:541, 1974 (abstract).
125. Michel B, Milner Y, David K: Preservation of tissue fixed immunoglobulins in skin biopsies of patients with lupus erythematosus and bullous diseases. Preliminary report. *J Invest Dermatol* 59:449–452, 1973.
126. Michel B, Schiltz JR: In vitro studies on the mechanism of acantholysis in pemphigus. Organ culture and cell suspension studies. In Beutner EH, Chorzelski TP, Bean SF (Eds): *Immunopathology of the Skin,* ed. 2. Wiley, New York, 1979, pp 231–242.
127. Michel B, Sy EK: Tissue-fixed immunoglobulins in lichen planus. In Beutner EH, Chorzelski TP, Bean, SF, et al (Eds): *Immunopathology of the Skin. Labelled antibody Studies.* Dowden, Hutchinson, Ross, Stroudsburg, PA, 1973, pp 182–193.
128. Miller JF, Downham TF, Chapel TA: Coexistent bullous pemphigoid and systemic lupus erythematosus. *Cutis* 21:368–373, 1978.
129. Millus JL, Doyle JA, Muller SA: Positive cutaneous IF if Grover's disease. *Arch Dermatol* 116:515, 1980 (abstract).
130. Miyagawa S, Kiriyama Y, Shirai T, et al: Chronic bullous disease with coexistent circulating IgG and IgA anti-basement membrane zone antibodies. *Arch Dermatol* 117:349–353, 1981.
131. Mobacken H, Kastrup W, Ljunghall K, et al: Linear IgA dermatosis: A study of ten adult patients. *Acta Dermatovener* 63:123–128, 1983.

132. Moncada B: Dermatitis herpetiformis: In association with system lupus erythematosus. *Arch Dermatol* 109:723–725, 1974.
133. Mora RG, Nesbitt LT, Brantley JB: Lichen planus pemphigoides: Clinical and immunofluorescent findings in four cases. *J Am Acad Dermatol* 8:331–336, 1983.
134. Mustakallio KK, Blomqvist K, Laioho K: Papillary deposition of fibrin, a characteristic of initial lesions of dermatitis herpetiformis. *Ann Clin Res* 2:13–18, 1970.
135. Nieboer C, Boorsma DM, Woerdeman MJ, et al: Epidermolysis bullosa acquisita. *Br J Dermatol* 102:383–392, 1980.
136. Nieboer C, Boorsma DW, Woerdeman MJ: Immunoelectron microscopic findings in cicatricial pemphigoid: Their significance in relation to epidermolysis bullosa acquisita. *Br J Dermatol* 106:419–422, 1982.
137. Nisengard RJ, Blaszczyk M, Chorzelski TP, et al: Immunofluorescence of biopsy specimens. Comparison of methods of transportation. *Arch Dermatol* 114:1329–1332, 1978.
138. Nisengard RJ, Neiders M: Desquamative lesions of the gingiva. *J Periodontol* 52:500–510, 1981.
139. Nishikawa T, Kurihara S, Harada T, et al: Capability of complement fixation of pemphigus antibodies in vitro. *Arch Dermatol Res* 260:1–6, 1977.
140. Nishikawa T, Kurihara S, Harada T, et al: Capability of complement fixation by in vivo bound antibodies in pemphigus skin lesions. *Clin Exp Dermatol* 3:57–60, 1978.
141. Nishikawa T, Sugiura M, Hashimoto T, et al: Demonstration of β1H globulin in pemphigus. *Acta Dermatovener* 63:39–41, 1983.
142. Olansky AJ, Briggaman RA, Gammon WR, et al: Bullous systemic lupus erythematosus. *J Am Acad Dermatol* 7:511–520, 1982.
143. O'Loughlin S, Goldman GC, Provost TT: Fate of pemphigus antibody following successful therapy. *Arch Dermatol* 114:1769–1778, 1978.
144. Orfanos CE, Gartmann H, Mahrle G: Zur Pathgenes des pemphigus erythematosus. Übergang eines chronischen Discoiden erythematodes in einem Pemphigus erythematosus (Senear-Usher). *Arch Dermatol Forsch* 240:317, 1971.
145. Parodi A, Nunzi F, Rebora A: Urticaria as presenting manifestations of pemphigus herpetiformis. *Dermatologica* 164:278–283, 1982.
146. Peck SM, Osserman KE: Studies in bullous disease: Treatment of pemphigus vulgaris with methotrexate, two patients (one with concurrent myasthenia gravis). *J Mt Sinai Hosp* 36:71–76, 1969.
147. Peck SM, Osserman KE, Rule AH: Intercellular antibodies. Presence in *Trichophyton rubrum* infection. *J Invest Dermatol* 58:133–138, 1972.
148. Peck SM, Osserman KE, Weimer LB, et al: Studies in bullous diseases. Immunofluorescence serologic tests. *N Engl J Med* 279:951–958, 1968.
149. Pedro SD, Dahl MV: Direct immunofluorescence of bullous systemic lupus erythematosus. *Arch Dermatol* 107:118–120, 1972.
150. Pehamberger H, Gschnait F, Konrad K, et al: Bullous pemphitgoid, herpes gestationis and linear dermatitis herpetiformis: Circulating anti-basement membrane zone antibodies; in vitro studies. *J Invest Dermatol* 74:105–108, 1980.
151. Pemhamberger H, Konrad K, Holubar K: Circulating IgA antibasement membrane antibodies in linear dermatitis herpetiformis (Duhring): Immunofluorescence and immunoelectron microscopic studies. *J Invest Dermatol* 69:490–493, 1977.
152. Pennys NS, Wiley HE III: Herpetiform blisters in systemic lupus erythematosus. *Arch Dermatol* 115:1417–1428, 1979.
153. Person JR, Rogers RS III: Bullous and cicatricial pemphigoid. Clinical histopathologic and immunologic correlations. *Mayo Clin Proc* 52:54–66, 1977.
154. Person JR, Rogers RS III, Jordan RE: Cicatricial pemphigoid with circulating anti-basement membrane antibodies. *Dermatologica* 154:90–97, 1977.
155. Provost TT, Maize JC, Ahmed AR, et al: Unusual subepidermal bullous diseases with immunologic features of bullous pemphigoid. *Arch Dermatol* 115:156–160, 1979.
156. Provost TT, Tomasi TB: Evidence for complement activation via the alternate pathway in

skin diseases. I. Herpes gestationis, systemic lupus erythematosus and bullous pemphigoid. *J Clin Invest* 52:1779–1787, 1973.

157. Provost TT, Yaoita H, Katz SI: Herpes gestationis. In Beutner EH, Chorzelski TP, Bean SF (Eds): *Immunopathology of the Skin,* ed. 2. Wiley, New York, 1979, pp 273–282.
158. Prystowsky S, Gilliam JN: Benign chronic bullous dermatosis of childhood. *Arch Dermatol* 112:837–838, 1976.
159. Roenigk HH, Ryan JG, Bergfeld WF: Epidermolysis bullosa acquisita. *Arch Dermatol* 103:1–10, 1971.
160. Rogers RS III, Perry HO, Bean SF, et al: Immunopathology of cicatricial pemphigoid: Studies of complement deposition. *J Invest Dermatol* 68:39–43, 1977.
161. Rogers RS III, Sheridan PJ, Jordan RE: Desquamative gingivitis. Clinical, histopathologic and immunopathologic investigations. *Oral Surg* 42:316–327, 1976.
162. Rogers RS III, Sheridan PJ, Nightingale SH: Desquamative gingivitis. Clinical, histopathologic, immunopathologic and therapeutic observations. *J Am Acad Dermatol* 7:729–735, 1982.
163. Saurat JH, Guinepain MT, Didierjean L, et al: Coexistence d'un lichen planus et d'une pemphigoide bulleuse. *Ann Dermatol Venerol* 104:368–374, 1977.
164. Savilahti E, Perkko M, Kalimo K, et al: IgA anti-gliadin antibodies: A marker of mucosal damage in childhood coeliac disease. *Lancet* i:320–322, 1983.
165. Schachner I, Lazarus GS, Dembitzer H: Epidermolysis bullosa hereditaria letalis. *Br J Dermatol* 96:51–58, 1977.
166. Schaumburg-Lever G, Rule A, Schmidt-Ulrich B, et al: Ultrastructural localization of in vivo bound immunoglobulins in bullous pemphigoid—A preliminary report. *J Invest Dermatol* 64:47–49, 1975.
167. Schlitz JR, Michel B: Effect of pemphigus autoantibodies on human epidermal cells in organ or suspension culture. *J Invest Dermatol* 66:279, 1976 (abstract).
168. Scott DW, Manning TO, Lewis RM: Linear IgA dermatoses in the dog: Bullous pemphigoid, discoid lupus erythematosus and a subcorneal pustular dermatitis. *Cornell Vet* 72:394–402, 1982.
169. Shornick JK, Bangert JL, Freeman RG, et al: Herpes gestationis: Clinical and histologic features of twenty-eight cases. *J Am Acad Dermatol* 8:214–224, 1983.
170. Simon RS, Bloom D, Ackerman AB: Persistent acantholytic dermatosis. A variant of transient acantholytic dermatosis (Grover's disease). *Arch Dermatol* 112:1429–1431, 1976.
171. Skeete MVH, Black MM: Evaluation of a special liquid fixative for direct immunofluorescence. *Clin Exp Dermatol* 2:49–56, 1977.
172. Sneddon IB: Bullous eruptions. In Rook A, Wilkinson DS, Ebling FJG (Eds): *Textbook in Dermatology,* ed. 3, vol. 2. Blackwell, Oxford, UK, 1972, pp 1441–1481.
173. Sobel S, Miller R, Shatin H: Lichen planus pemphigoides. *Arch Dermatol* 112:1280–1283, 1976.
174. Stingl G, Hönigsmann H, Holubar K, et al: Ultrastructural localization of immunoglobulins in skin of patients with dermatitis herpetiformis. *J Invest Dermatol* 67:507–512, 1976.
175. Szabo E, Sandor H, Kovacs L: Coexistent atypical bullous pemphigoid and systemic lupus erythematosus. *Br J Dermatol* 104:71–75, 1981.
176. Taylor R: Measurement of variation and significance in serologic tests. In Beutner EH, Nisengard RJ, Albini B (Eds): *Defined Immunofluorescence and Related Cytochemical Methods.* Ann NY Acad Sci, New York, 1983, pp 13–21.
177. Thivolet J, Beyvin AJ: Recherches par immunofluorescence d'autoanticorps sériques vis-à-vis des constituants de l'épiderme chez les brules. *Experientia* 24:945–946, 1968.
178. Thomas JR III, Su DWP: Concurrence of lupus erythematosus and dermatitis herpetiformis. A report of nine cases. *Arch Dermatol* 119:740–745, 1983.
179. Unsworth DJ, Kieffer N, Holborow EJ, et al: IgA anti-gliadin antibodies in coeliac disease. *Clin Exp Immunol* 46:286–293, 1981.
180. Valnio E, Kalimo K, Reunala T, et al: Circulating IgA and IgG anti-gliadin antibodies to dermatitis herpetiformis detected by enzyme-linked immunosorbent assay. *Arch Dermatol Res* 275:15–18, 1983.

181. Weber L, Krieg T, Müller PK, et al: Immunofluorescent localization of type IV collagen and laminin in human skin and its application in junctional zone pathology. *Br J Dermatol* 106:267–273, 1982.
182. Weinstein WM: Latent celiac sprue. *Gastroenterology* 66:489–493, 1974.
183. Wierzchowiecki MO, Quismorio FP, Friou GJ: Immunoglobulin deposits in skin in systemic lupus erythematosus. *Arthr Rheum* 18:77–82, 1975.
184. Wilson BD, Birnkrant AP, Beutner EH, et al: Epidermolysis bullosa acquisita: A clinical disorder of varied etiologies. *J Am Acad Dermatol* 3:280–291, 1980.
185. Winkelmann RK, Roth HL: Dermatitis herpetiformis with acantholysis or pemphigus with response to sulfonamides. *Arch Dermatol* 82:385–390, 1960.
186. Yamasaki Y, Hashimoto T, Nishikawa T: Dermatitis herpetiformis with linear IgA deposition. Ultrastructure localization of in vivo bound IgA. *Acta Dermatovener* 62:401–405, 1982.
187. Yaoita H, Briggaman RA, Lawley TJ, et al: Immunoelectronmicroscopic localization of in vivo bound IgG in skin of patients with epidermolysis bullosa acquisita. *J Invest Dermatol* 72:269, 1979 (abstract).
188. Yaoita H, Gullino M, Katz SI: Herpes gestationis. Ultrastructure and ultrastructural localization of in vivo bound complement. *J Invest Dermatol* 66:383–388, 1976.
189. Yaoita H, Hertz KC, Katz SI: Dermatitis herpetiformis: Immunoelectron microscopic and ultrastructural studies of a patient with linear deposition of IgA. *J Invest Dermatol* 67:691–695, 1976.
190. Yaoita H, Katz SI: Immunoelectronmicroscopic localization of IgA in skin of patients with dermatitis herpetiformis. *J Invest Dermatol* 67:502–506, 1976.
191. Yaoita H, Katz SI: Circulating IgA anti-basement membrane antibodies in dermatitis herpetiformis. *J Invest Dermatol* 69:558–560.
192. Yung CW, Soltani K, Lorincz AL: Pemphigoid nodularis. *J Am Acad Dermatol* 5:54–60, 1981.

9
Specificity and Sensitivity of Indirect and Direct Immunofluorescent Findings in the Diagnosis of Pemphigus

Susan A. Krasny

Ernst H. Beutner

Tadeusz P. Chorzelski

INTRODUCTION

Since the demonstration by immunofluorescence (IF) of circulating intercellular (IC) antibodies in the serum of pemphigus patients by Beutner and Jordon (6), and of the binding of these antibodies in vivo in pemphigus patients and passively sensitized monkeys by Beutner, Lever, Witebsky et al. (7), there has been both indirect and direct evidence for the correlation of antibody titers with disease severity. In early passive transfer studies, Wood and coworkers (51) demonstrated a correlation between the ability of sera injected into monkeys to cause experimental lesions and the titers of pemphigus antibodies (see Chap. 11). Similarly, the injection into neonatal mice of IgG fractions from sera of patients with pemphigus demonstrated that high titers of pemphigus antibodies were most effective in producing acantholysis, and the titers of circulating IC antibodies in mouse serum correlated with the severity of the disease induced (4) (see Chap. 11 and 12).

In the organ culture model for the study of the pathogenicity of pemphigus antibodies, both the binding of these antibodies and the development of histologic changes depended upon the concentration of antibody (24,48) (see Chap. 13).

The work on this report was supported by the IF Testing Service, Buffalo, NY, and in part by a grant from the Summerhill Foundation.

Editors' note: Dr. Walter Lever was invited to present his views on this topic in the form of an accompanying chapter. Unfortunately, he could not prepare such a chapter for reasons of health. The readers are referred to his reports cited in the references for this chapter for statements on his viewpoints.

An early study on single serum samples from pemphigus patients indicated that there was an association of IC antibody titers and disease activity (7). Subsequent follow-up studies with serial serum samples confirmed these earlier findings. Titers of pemphigus antibodies of individual patients fluctuated directly with changes in clinical condition (8–10). Chorzelski et al. (10) provided the first evidence of a rise in IC antibody titer preceding a flare in disease, and thus raised the possibility of the prognostic significance of titer determinations. Importantly, the above studies used monkey esophagus as a substrate for the indirect immunofluorescence (IIF) test. Since these early reports, other investigators have repeatedly demonstrated the correlation of IC antibody titers with the clinical severity of the disease (27,30,35,36,40–42,44,46,47,50).

However, some authors have questioned the use of serial titrations as a guide to therapy or an indicator of prognosis, although they agree that high antibody titers indicate severe disease activity and that low titers reflect less severe disease or remission (13,19).

Some investigators have taken exception to the finding of even general correlation between IC antibody titers and disease activity (3,28,29). They describe both a high percentage of pemphigus patients with low antibody titers in the presence of extensive disease and others in whom antibody titers were high with only minimal or no disease activity. Because of these latter findings, Judd and Lever (28) claim the IIF test is not reliable for evaluating the status of pemphigus patients; thus, it is inferior to direct immunofluorescence (DIF) as a diagnostic test (see addendum to this chapter). However, the antigenic substrate used for IIF studies was guinea pig esophagus—not the monkey esophagus recommended in previous studies. Nevertheless, this judgment of the superiority of DIF over IIF for the diagnosis of pemphigus has been refuted by several studies (7,10,36,40). However, these reports included only small numbers of patients.

This chapter summarizes results of double-blind studies using five antigenic substrates to examine larger numbers of pemphigus cases. The results: 1) strongly support the correlation of pemphigus antibody titer with disease severity, especially when monkey esophagus is used as a substrate; 2) affirm the usefulness of serial titrations of pemphigus antibodies in the prognosis and treatment of this disease; and 3) emphasize the importance of both IIF as well as DIF studies for the diagnosis of pemphigus. We stress the need for proper technique for IIF studies of patients' sera and for methods of analysis as these may account for the problems encountered in demonstrating comparable correlations in other laboratories.

CORRELATION OF PEMPHIGUS ANTIBODY TITERS AND SEVERITY OF DISEASE

Experimental Design

We have examined 111 serum samples from 11 pemphigus cases including 4 males and 7 females. The number of blood specimens per patient ranged from 6 to 25 with an average of 10 per patient. The interval between the collection of serum specimens averaged 3.6 weeks. All cases were confirmed pemphigus by clinical, immunopathologic and histologic studies. All patients were in an active stage of their disease when first included, with the time of onset ranging from 3 weeks to 5 years prior to this study. Seven patients were on therapy when the study began whereas 4 initially were not receiving treatment. Seven patients had pemphigus vulgaris, 2 had pemphigus foliaceus and one was diagnosed as having pemphigus vegetans. Interestingly, one patient (LES) converted from pemphigus vulgaris to pemphigus foliaceus during the period of observation. (See also Addendum B on Page 246).

At the time each serum sample was obtained, the patient was graded for extent and activity of disease according to the following criteria:

Oral Mucosa

	Extent	*Activity*
±	Isolated abortive erosion(s)	Isolated new erosion(s)
+	Few persistent erosions and/or bullae	Few new erosions and/or bullae
++	Numerous erosions and/or bullae	Numerous new erosions and/or bullae
+++	Most of the mucosa involved	New lesions constantly appearing with some tendency towards healing
++++	Whole oral mucosa involved including lips, in some cases also the larynx	No tendency towards healing

Skin

	Extent	*Activity*
±	Isolated lesions	Isolated new lesions
+	Few lesions	Few new lesions
++	Numerous lesions	Numerous new lesions
+++	Widespread lesions over half the body surface	New lesions constantly appearing with some tendency towards healing
++++	Generalized lesions (erythroderma)	No tendency towards healing

IC antibody titers for all serum samples were determined by standard methods as previously described (see Chap. 1). Importantly, every test included a titer control; that is, a positive control serum with a known titer of IC antibodies. Without such titer controls, IIF tests are not valid. In our studies, a selected serum of patient LES served as this control. This reference serum is available through ISIL.* Five different substrates were used in an IIF test with a goat antihuman IgG conjugate: both heavy and light chain specific (molar fluorescein-to-protein ratio [F/P] = 2.5; antibody [Ab] protein [P] = 2.46 mg/ml; Ab/P = 0.23). All serum samples from one patient were tested simultaneously on each substrate in order to eliminate variations in technique and reading as a source of error in accounting for differences in titer. Monkey esophagus, rabbit esophagus, guinea pig esophagus, and human skin were chosen as substrates because they are commonly used as sources of pemphigus antigen for IIF testing. Dog esophagus was included because of a special interest in pemphigus antigen from this animal. All esophagus specimens were obtained from newly sacrificed animals. Each substrate used represents tissue from a single animal. The human skin was a fresh surgical biopsy specimen from normal breast tissue. All tissues were immediately frozen

*ISIL, International Service for Immunology Laboratories, 219 Sherman Hall, SUNY at Buffalo, Buffalo, NY 14214.

in liquid nitrogen, stored at −70°C, and used within 1 month. Each tissue sample was checked with the reference pemphigus serum having a known titer of IC antibodies.

Because blood group antibodies, in addition to reacting with blood vessels, can stain the IC areas of epithelial tissue resulting in a false test for pemphigus antibodies, all sera giving blood vessel staining were absorbed with a homogenate of horse stomach mucosa containing blood group antigens. Additional sera not reacting with the blood vessels were also chosen at random for absorption so that for each patient, at least two serum samples were absorbed.

The complement immunofluorescence (CIF) studies described in the section on "Studies Eliminating Pemphigus-like Antibodies (PLA) as a Possible Explanation for Discrepancies Between High Antibody Titers and Low Disease Activity" were performed as follows. Briefly, all sera were inactivated for 30 minutes at 56°C, and twofold serial dilutions were made in Tris buffer containing Ca^{2+} and Mg^{2+} ions (each at 0.0025 M). After monkey esophagus sections had been incubated for 30 minutes with diluted sera and then washed in phosphate-buffered saline (PBS), fresh normal human serum was added as a source of complement. This serum was diluted at 1:20 in Tris buffer and incubated on the sections for 30 minutes. After a second PBS wash, a goat antihuman complement C3 conjugate (Kallestad; molar F/P = 2.47; Ab protein = 1.71 mg/ml; Ab/P = 0.14) at a 1:32 dilution was added, and the sections were again incubated for 30 minutes. This was followed by a final wash in PBS for 30 minutes.

Negative controls consisted of sections incubated in Tris buffer, normal human serum, and the reference pemphigus serum both with and without complement added. The positive control serum was from a patient with erythema multiforme and contained pemphigus-like antibodies (PLA) (see the section referred to in the paragraph above and its accompaning table). This serum gave a negative reaction with an anti-C3 conjugate when no complement was added, but it had an IC antibody titer of 80 to 160 when incubated with fresh human serum as a source of complement.

Staining Patterns, Staining Intensities, and Antibody Titers on Different Epithelial Substrates

Figure 1 illustrates the type of IC staining reaction seen on each of the five substrates. Note that with the exception of human skin, there is little difference in the linear staining seen on all substrates. The staining reaction on human skin is more diffuse, and with some sera (not shown here), it is more granular. Great variability occurred from patient to patient and from substrate to substrate in the intensity of IC staining reactions. In general, the strongest were always observed on monkey esophagus. In Table 1, the serum from patient LES reacted with comparable staining intensity on all substrates tested. In contrast, although serum from JAG reacted on both monkey and dog esophagus with comparable titers, the intensity of the staining was much weaker on dog esophagus. The intensity of staining reactions on the remaining substrates was also weak. The greatest contrast in staining reactivity, illustrated in Table 1 by serum from CEJ, occurred with the sera of two patients (see also Table 2). These sera were positive on monkey esophagus, but were negative on all other substrates tested. Weakly positive or negative staining reactions were not due to the poor quality of substrate, as demonstrated by the positive control sera. Precautions, as described in the previous section, were taken to ensure tissue suitability. Specifically, since many serum samples from patient LES, including the one used in Table 1, reacted with comparable staining intensities and titers on all substrates, one of these served as a titer control.

Table 1. Comparison of Intensity of Staining of IC Antibodies on Various Epithelial Substrates Used in an IIF Test

	Intensity of IC Staining on				
Pemphigus serum dilutions	*Monkey esophagus*	*Rabbit esophagus*	*Guinea pig esophagus*	*Human skin*	*Dog esophagus*
LES 1/10[a]	++	+	++	+	+
20	++	+	++	+	+
40	++	+	+	+	+
80	+	+	+	+	+
160	+	+	+/w	+	w
320	+	+	+/w	w	w
640	+	w	w	−	−
1280	w/±	−	−		
2560	−				
Titers	640	640	640	320	320
JAG 1/10[b]	++	w	w	w	+
20	++	w	w	w	+
40	++	w	w	w	+
80	+	w	w	w	w
160	+	−	−	±	w
320	+			−	w
640	+/w				w
1280	−				w
2560					−
Titers	640	80	80	80	1280
CEJ 1/10[c]	++	−	−	−	−
20	++				
40	++				
80	++				
160	+				
320	+				
640	w				
1280	−				
2560	−				
Titers	640	<10	<10	<10	<10

[a]LES, 11-21-78.
[b]JAG, 6-29-79.
[c]CEJ, 6-27-79.

An additional check on the suitability of the human skin specimen was performed. Representative sera that were found to be positive or negative on human skin were sent to Thomas Burnham, M.D., Henry Ford Hospital, Detroit, MI. This laboratory routinely uses human skin for the determination of pemphigus antibody titers. Their results were in complete agreement with those obtained for this study in terms of positive and negative findings. Minor differences occurred between the titers observed in the two laboratories. As a further check, multiple sites of monkey skin, including flexor and extensor surfaces of arms and legs, were compared for relative reactivity with IC antibodies of pemphigus patients. No differences were observed.

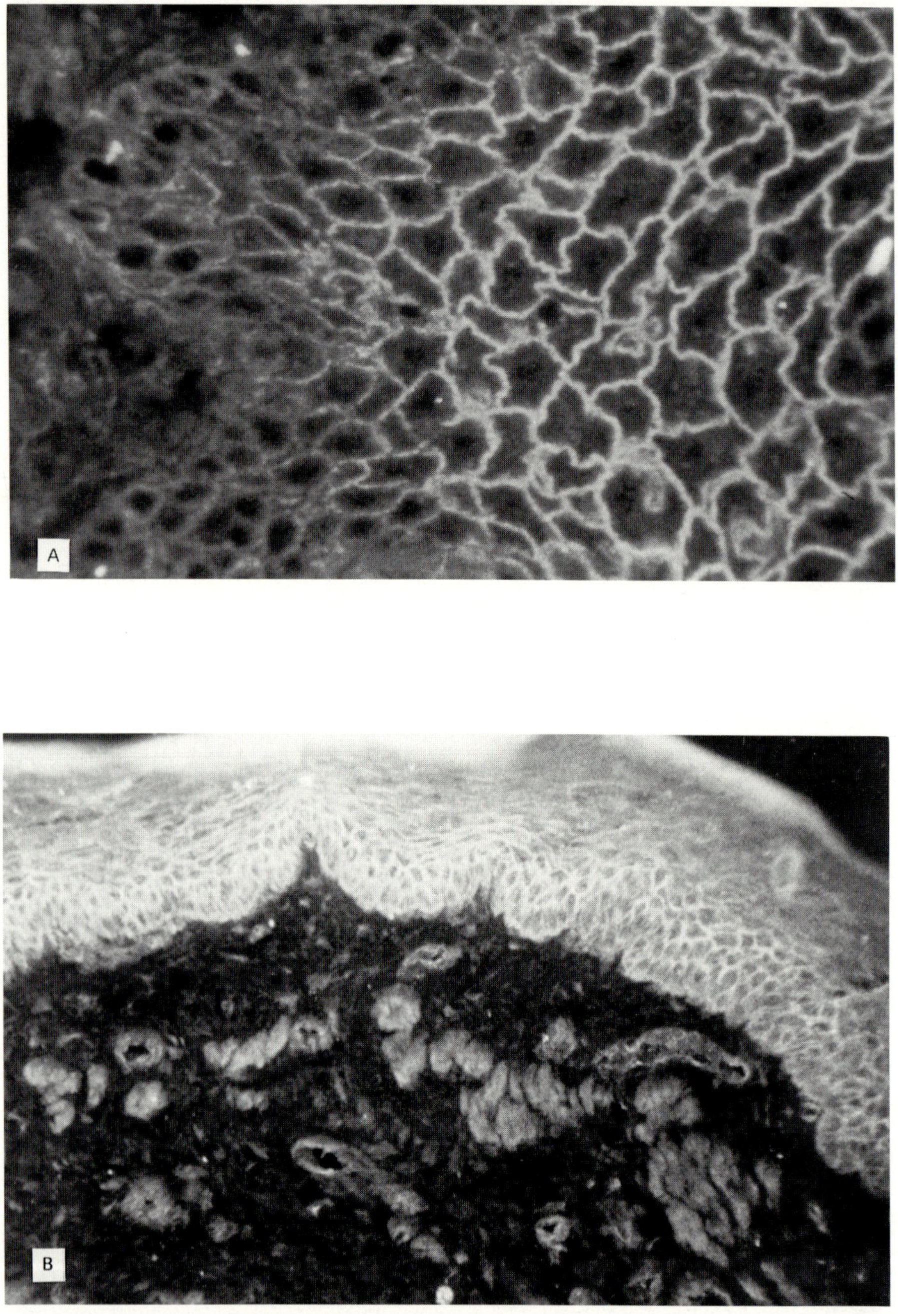

Figure 1. Intercellular staining by pemphigus antibodies on various epithelial substrates, with an anti-IgG conjugate in an IIF test with serum LES (11-21-78) 1/20 on (A) monkey esophagus (400×), (B) rabbit esophagus (200×), (C) guinea pig esophagus (400×), (D) human skin (400×), and (E) dog esophagus (200×).

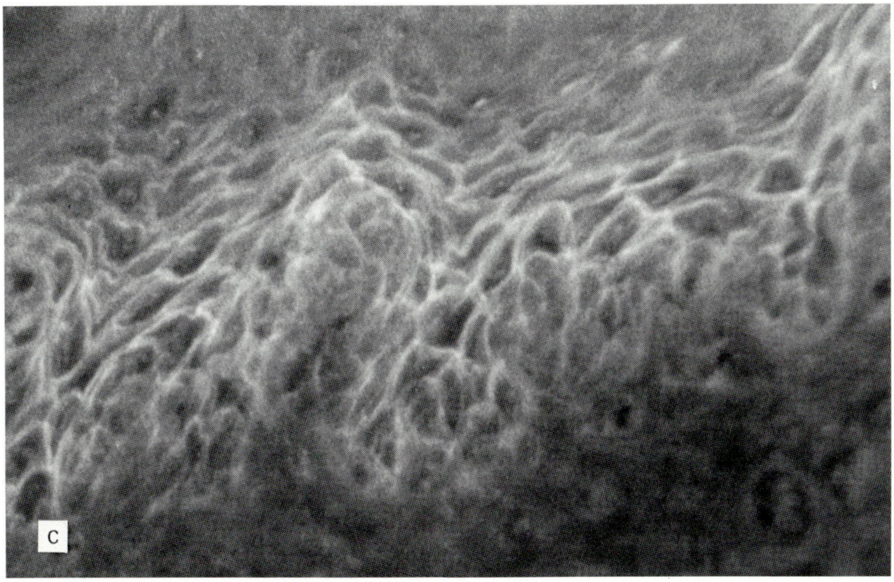
C

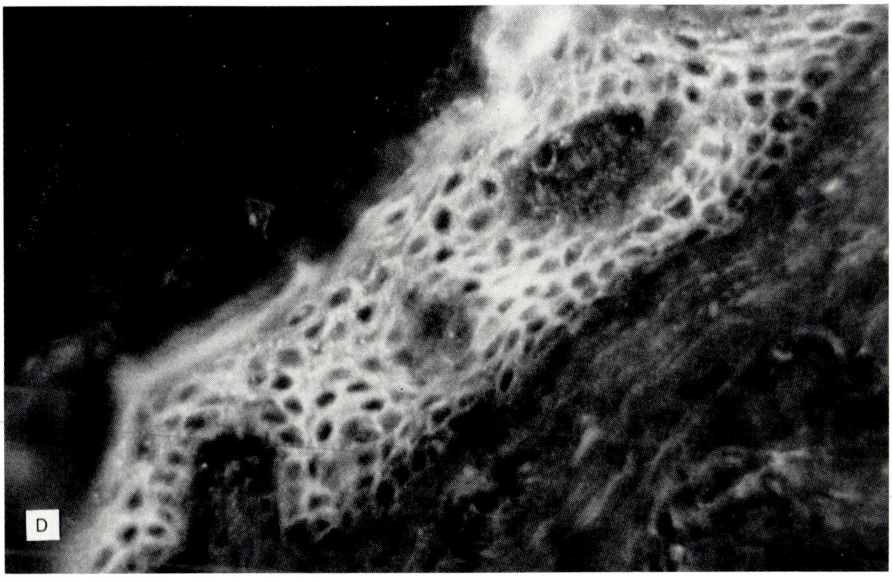
D

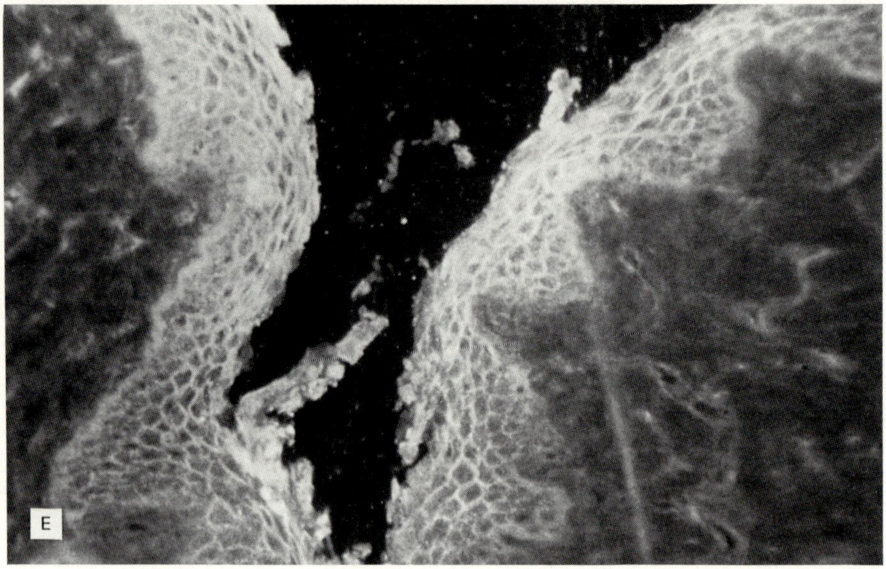

Finally, no significant change in IC-staining intensity or antibody titer was observed after absorption of sera with horse stomach homogenate. However, as expected, any blood vessel staining was abolished.

Table 2 lists the IC antibody titers on the five substrates tested for each of the serum samples from all 11 pemphigus patients. Also included is the clinical condition and the treatment of each patient at the time the serum was collected. The sera of three patients (CEJ, ORN, and SWI) were consistently negative on guinea pig esophagus, human skin, and dog esophagus. The sera of an additional three patients (NAU, ZAL, and CZA) were also negative on human skin. Importantly, while all patients observed to be negative for serum IC antibodies on monkey esophagus were also negative on all other substrates examined, the converse did not hold true.

Table 3 shows the number of sera from 11 pemphigus patients that were positive for IC antibodies on each of the epithelial substrates examined, as compared to the results obtained by Judd and Mescon in a similar study (29). It is readily evident that the highest frequency of positive sera was obtained using monkey esophagus. This percentage is significantly higher than for any other substrate tested in our study: $p < 0.005$ by chi square analysis. Importantly, the frequency of sera positive on monkey esophagus was higher in this study than in that of Judd and Mescon ($p < 0.005$). There was no significant difference in the frequency of findings on rabbit or guinea pig esophagus. In contrast, the frequency of sera that were positive on human skin was much less in this study compared to the frequency determined by Judd and Mescon ($p < 0.005$). We feel that precautions need to be taken to ensure the suitability of substrates. Specifically, each substrate must, as indicated above, be checked with positive control sera with known titers. There is no indication whether the Judd and Mescon study (29) included such titer controls. Also the type of pemphigus plays a role. (See page 246).

Determination of Correlation of Disease Severity with Pemphigus Antibody Titers on Different Epithelial Substrates

To evaluate the relation of IC antibody titers to disease activity, two approaches were used. One was based on analyses of correlations of the data listed in Table 2; these are described in this section. The other was based on comparisons of the last of the serum studies listed in Table 2 with absorptions in clinical follow-up studies, as described in the following section on "Prognostic Value of Determining IC Antibody Titers."

Three different methods were used to determine the correlations of disease severity with the IC antibody titer on each substrate tested; notably, the Spearman rank correlation coefficient (r_s), the coefficient of correlation (r), and an inspection method. The r_s and r values were calculated as described in standard statistic textbooks. The inspection method was performed as follows. With the data in Table 2, graphs were constructed for each patient showing the changes over time in disease severity versus IC antibody titer on each of the five substrates tested. Figure 2 shows these changes for four representative patients. The number of disease flares and remissions for each patient were identified from inspection of the graphs. Then for each patient and substrate tested, the following was determined with only a two doubling dilution or greater change in titer considered as being significant.

1. The number of times there was a concurrent disease flare-up or remission and pemphigus antibody titer change; that is, remission and negative antibody titer, low disease severity ($\leq$+) and low antibody titer ($\leq$40), and high disease activity ($\geq$++), and high antibody titer ($\geq$80).
2. The number of times there was a rise in:
   a) Antibody titer preceding a flare-up in disease by 1 month or less; or
   b) Following a flare-up within 1 month or less.
3. The number of times there was a drop in:
   a) Antibody titer preceding a remission; or
   b) Following remission.

Also included were the number of times there was:

4. No change in antibody titer, but a change in disease activity;
5. No change in antibody titer and no change in disease activity;
6. Change in antibody titer and no change in disease activity; and
7. Change in antibody titer and change in disease activity.
8. Discrepancies in antibody titers and disease activity were also noted; that is, high antibody titer and low disease activity or remission, and vice versa.

A positive score of 1 was assigned to each of the following steps above: 1, 2a, 3, 5, and 7, whereas a negative value was given to 2b, 4, 6, and 8. The scores for each patient and each substrate were then tabulated. A positive score indicated correlation, whereas a zero or negative value meant a lack of correlation.

Almost all patients showed agreement in correlation determined by all three methods with a few exceptions. Patient CEJ demonstrated correlation by the Spearman rank correlation test, with titers determined on guinea pig esophagus, human skin, and dog esophagus. However, the titers of all these sera were negative (i.e., <10) despite the patient having an active disease. This same test also yielded a correlation of disease severity and antibody titer on monkey esophagus for patient CZA despite her being in remission and her sera demonstrating high IC antibody titers.

Table 2. Changes in IC Antibody Titers and Disease Severity in 11 Pemphigus Patients

Patient	Date	Drug dose (mg)			Extent of lesions	Activity of lesions	IC antibody titers on				
		*Pred**	*Cycl**	*Imu**			*ME**	*RE**	*GPE**	*HS**	*DE**
KOW[a] (PV)*	11-03-79	–	–	–	+++	+++	1280	640	640	80	320
	11-13-79	100	100		+	+	640	640	640	80	320
	11-29-79	80	100		+	+	640	<10	ND*	ND	160
	12-05-79	80	100		–	–	160	ND	ND	ND	ND
	1-04-80	80/0**	100/0**		–	–	10	<10	<10	<10	<10
	3-14-80	35	100/0		–	–****	<10	<10	<10	<10	<10
LES[a] (PV)	11-21-78	100		150***	++++	++++	640	640	1280	320	320
	11-30-78	100		150***	++++	++++	320	320	320	80	160
	12-07-78	100	100		++++	++++	640	1280	320	640	320
	12-15-78	80	200	***	++	+	160	320	40	160	160
	12-22-78	80	200	***	+	±	80	40	<10	160	10
	12-29-78	80	100		±	–	160	320	10	160	80
	4-25-79	50	100/0	***	+	+	80	320	40	320	40
	5-11-79	50	100/0		+	++	80	80	20	80	40
	5-22-79	50	100/0	***	+	+	160	320	640	320	<10
	6-01-79	50	100/0		+++	±	160	320	160	40	<10
	6-07-79	50	100/0		++	–	160	640	10	20	<10
	6-22-79	50	50		++	–	160	320	80	10	<10
	6-29-79	50/0	50		++	±	40	80	40	40	<10
	7-17-79	40/0	50/0		+	+	40	320	80	80	10
	8-01-79	30/0	100/0		++	+	160	160	160	160	10
	8-08-79	30/0	100/0		++	+	640	320	320	160	<10
	8-15-79	25/0	100/0		++/+	+	160	320	320	160	20
	8-22-79	20/0	100/0		++	±	160	640	320	160	20
	8-29-79	20/0	100/0		++	±	80	320	320	80	40
	9-05-79	20/0	100/0		++	±	160	320	80	40	80
	9-21-79	20/0	100/0		±	±	160	320	160	160	160
(PF)*	10-10-79	20/0	100/0		±	±	40	320	40	40	20
	10-19-79	20/0	50/0		+	±	40	80	40	40	40
	11-14-79	20/0	50/0		+	+	80	1280	1280	160	1280
	1-04-80	50/0	50/0		++	+****	160	320	320	160	320

ZAL[b] (PF)	8-08-79	–	–	–	++++	+++	160	640	160	<10	320
	8-15-79	100	100		++++	++	160	1280	1280	<10	2560
	8-22-79	100	100		+++	+++	160	640	160	<10	640
	10-10-79	80/30	100		±	–	10	40	20	<10	<10
	10-16-79	80/20	100/0		±	–	10	10	10	<10	<10
	10-24-79	80/15	100		±	–	10	10	10	<10	<10
	10-31-79	60/0	100/0		±	–	<10	<10	<10	<10	<10
	11-13-79	30	40/0		+	±	<10	<10	<10	<10	<10
	11-23-79	40	50/0		–	–	<10	<10	<10	<10	<10
	1-04-80	30	50/0		–	–****	<10	<10	<10	<10	<10
NAU[c] (PVeg)*	10-31-79	–	–	–	++	++	320	320	<10	<10	640
	11-07-79	100	100		++	++	640	640	80	<10	640
	11-13-79	100	100		++	++/+	640	640	80	<10	1280
	1-04-80	60	100/0		±	+	320	40	<10	<10	640
	2-22-80	40/0	50/0		±	±	160	160	40	<10	640
	4-25-80	40/0	50/0		+	+	320	160	80	<10	1280
	5-30-80	30	100/0		+	+	320	160	160	<10	1280
	6-02-80	30	50/0		+	+****	320	160	<10	<10	640
CZA[d] (PV)	8-03-79	15		50	+	+	320	<10	<10	<10	<10
	8-31-79	15/0		50/0	–	–	160	20	<10	<10	<10
	9-28-79	15/0		50/0	–	–	160	<10	<10	<10	<10
	10-19-79	10/0		50/0	–	–	160	<10	<10	<10	<10
	11-23-79	10/0		50/0	–	–	40	40	<10	<10	10
	12-28-79	10/0		50/0	–	–	160	10	<10	<10	40
	4-18-79	10/0		50/0	–	–	320	20	<10	<10	20
	5-30-80	70/0		50/0	–	–****	320	40	<10	<10	40
SWI[e] (PV)	6-29-79	5/wk*		25/wk	–	–	10	20	<10	<10	<10
	7-27-79	5/wk		25/wk	+	+	20	10	<10	<10	<10
	8-24-79	5/wk		25/wk	+	±	20	10	<10	<10	<10
	9-21-79	5/wk		25/wk	–	–	<10	10	<10	<10	<10
	2-22-80	5/wk		25/wk	–	–	<10	10	<10	<10	<10
	3-21-80	5/wk		50/wk	–	–	20	20	ND	ND	<10
	4-18-80	5/wk		25/wk	–	–****	<10	10	<10	<10	<10

(Continued)

Table 2. *(Continued)*

Patient	Date	Drug dose (mg)			Extent of lesions	Activity of lesions	IC antibody titers on				
		Pred*	Cycl*	Imu*			ME*	RE*	GPE*	HS*	DE*
KOZ[f] (PV)	10-09-79	100			+++	++	10,240	10,240	640	80	1280
	10-16-79	100			±	−	5120	320	320	80	1280
	10-24-79	100			±	−	10,240	20	320	40	1280
	10-31-79	100			+	+	5120	640	160	<10	640
	11-07-79	100			+	+	10,240	640	160	160	640
	11-21-79	100	100		±	±	1280	320	320	80	160
	11-29-79	80	100		±	±	20,480	2560	160	320	320
	12-05-79	80	100		±	±	1280	640	ND	ND	ND
	12-12-79	60	100/0		−	−	640	160	40	<10	160
	1-04-80	50	100/0		±	−****	320	80	40	<10	40
CEJ[g] (PV)	6-27-79	−	−	−	++	++	640	<10	<10	<10	<10
	7-04-79	100	100		+	+	320	<10	<10	<10	<10
	7-11-79	100	100		+	+	320	<10	<10	<10	<10
	7-17-79	100/65	100		+	+	160	<10	<10	<10	<10
	7-25-79	100/50	100		−	−	80	<10	<10	<10	<10
	7-31-79	100/45	100		+	+	160	<10	<10	<10	<10
	8-08-79	100/15	100		+	+	160	<10	<10	<10	<10
	9-08-79	60/10	100		+	±	20	<10	<10	<10	<10
	10-10-79	50/0	100/0		±	±****	640	20	<10	<10	<10
ORN[g] (PV)	6-29-79	40/0		50/0	±	+	80	<10	<10	<10	<10
	7-30-79	100		100	+	+	80	<10	<10	<10	<10
	8-24-79	35		50/0	++	+	40	<10	<10	<10	<10
	10-01-79	40/0		100/0	+	±	160	<10	<10	<10	<10
	11-16-79	30/0	50/0		++	++	80	<10	<10	<10	<10
	3-14-80	30/0	50/0		++	++	320	<10	<10	<10	<10
	4-14-80	40/0	50/0		±	±	160	<10	<10	<10	<10
	5-16-80	30/0	50/0		+	±****	160	<10	<10	<10	<10

SIL[g] (PF)	7-17-79	50	–	100/0	+	+	80	<10	640	20	160
	9-21-79	30/0		50/0	±	±	80	80	640	<10	320
	10-19-79	30/0		50/0	+	±	80	320	320	40	640
	10-26-79	30/0		50/0	±	±	80	160	80	<10	320
	2-22-80	20/0		50/0	±	++	80	320	160	80	160
	3-21-80	60/0		50/0	+	+	2560	2560	2560	<10	5120
	5-30-80	60/0		50/0	±	–****	80	320	320	40	640
JAG[g] (PV)	6-29-79	5/0		25/0	±	+	640	80	80	80	1280
	7-30-79	5/0		25/0	–	–	1280	160	40	10	320
	9-21-79	5/0		25/0	–	–	2560	320	80	<10	1280
	10-26-79	5/0		25/0	–	–	640	80	80	<10	320
	11-30-79	5/0		25/0	–	–	320	<10	80	<10	80
	1-04-80	5/0		25/0	±	–	1280	320	80	40	640
	3-07-80	5/0		25/0	–	–	1280	320	ND	ND	2560
	4-04-80	5/0		25/0	–	–	10,240	ND	ND	ND	ND
	5-13-80	5/0		25/0	±	±	640	160	160	40	640
	5-16-80	5/0		25/0	–	–****	640	160	160	160	640

*Pred, prednisone; Cycl, cyclophosphamide; Imu, Imuran (azothioprene); ME, monkey esophagus; RE, rabbit esophagus; GPE, guinea pig esophagus; HS, human skin; DE, dog esophagus; PV, pemphigus vulgaris; PF, pemphigus foliaceus; PVeg, pemphigus vegetans; and ND, no data.

**80/0 or 80/15, etc. = alternate-day therapy using (e.g.) 80 mg and 0 mg or 80 mg and 15 mg on alternate days; 5/wk or 25/wk = mg/wk.

***Plasmapheresis.

****While Tables 3 to 5 focus primarily on comparisons and analyses of the data up to this point in time, Table 6 lists clinical follow-up data on each of these patients over a 4 yr period; Tables 7 to 9 focus on analyses of the data in both Table 2 and Table 6.

[a]Correlation of disease activity with IC antibody titers on all five substrates.

[b]Correlation of disease activity with IC antibody titer on four substrates: ME, RE, GPE, and DE.

[c]Correlation on ME and RE.

[d]Correlation on GPE and HS.

[e]Correlation only on ME.

[f]Correlation only on RE.

[g]No correlation on any substrate.

Table 3. Frequency of Pemphigus Sera Positive for IC Antibodies in an IIF Test on Various Epithelial Substrates

	No. patients with positive sera		*No. sera tested*		*No. sera positive*		*% Sera positive*	
Substrate	*Authors*[a]	*Judd*[b]	*Authors*	*Judd*	*Authors*	*Judd*	*Authors*	*Judd*
Monkey esophagus	11	9	111	50	104	26	94[c]	52
Rabbit esophagus	10	10	104	50	79	33	76	66
Guinea pig esophagus	7	10	105	50	63	38	60	76
Human skin	5	10	102	50	43	37	42	74
Dog esophagus	7	ND[d]	104	ND	60	ND	57	ND

[a]Study included a total of 11 pemphigus patients.
[b]Results of study by Judd and Mescon (29) of 10 pemphigus patients.
[c]The frequency of sera positive on monkey esophagus by IIF is significantly higher than on other substrates tested by the authors at $p < 0.005$ by chi square analysis. The frequency of sera positive on monkey esophagus is also higher in the authors' study than in the study of Judd and Mescon ($p < 0.005$). The frequency of positive results on human skin in the authors' study is significantly less ($p < 0.005$) than the frequency obtained by Judd and Mescon.
[d]No data.

The graphs in Figure 3 are the lines of best fit that can be constructed for disease severity versus IC antibody titers determined on monkey esophagus, knowing the value of r. Patients demonstrating a correlation of disease severity with IC antibody titer are shown in Figure 3A, whereas those for whom no correlation was obtained up to the initial cut-off date are shown in Figure 3B. Note in Figure 3A that even though the serum IC antibody titers correlated with disease activity for all patients, the antibody titers varied greatly from patient to patient with the same clinical activity. For this reason, the analyses for correlation had to be done on an individual basis, rather than on the entire population of pemphigus patients being examined. The latter has been done in previous studies (13,17,28,29,50). Most importantly, the inspection of the graphs of antibody titer versus disease severity over time is a better method for determining correlation, as it is the only one taking into account the dynamics of the disease. This latter method, similar to that used by Barada and coworkers (5), affords insights into the predictability of disease flare-up or remission by IC antibody titer. This cannot be done using the Spearman rank test or the coefficient of correlation. With the inspection method, it becomes evident that apparent discrepancies between disease severity and antibody titer serve as indicators of disease flare-up or remission, rather than as instances of lack of correlation.

Table 4 lists pemphigus patients according to the substrate on which their serum antibody titer correlated with disease severity. Correlation was assigned if positive correlation was demonstrated by two of the three methods used. More than one-half of the patients examined demonstrated correlation with antibody titers determined on one or more substrates. There seems to be individual variation as to which substrate used to detect pemphigus antibodies best demonstrates correlation of antibody titer and disease severity. The serum antibody titers of patient KOW show a correlation regardless of which substrate is used. In other patients, demonstration of correlation of antibody titers is limited to fewer substrates. Patients SWI and NAU show correlation of anti-

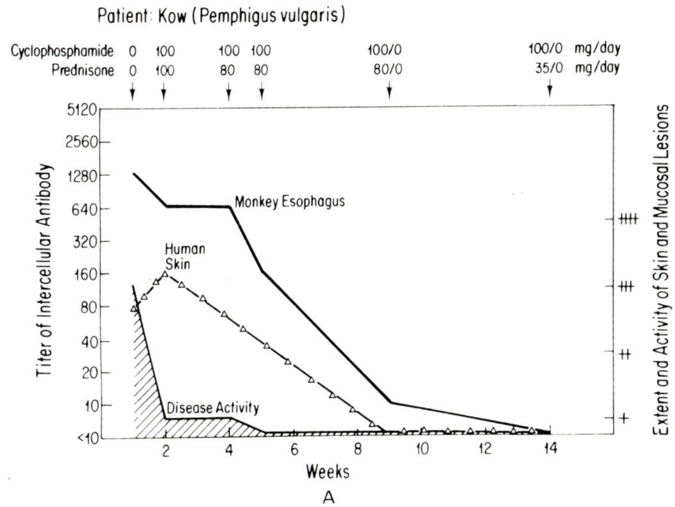

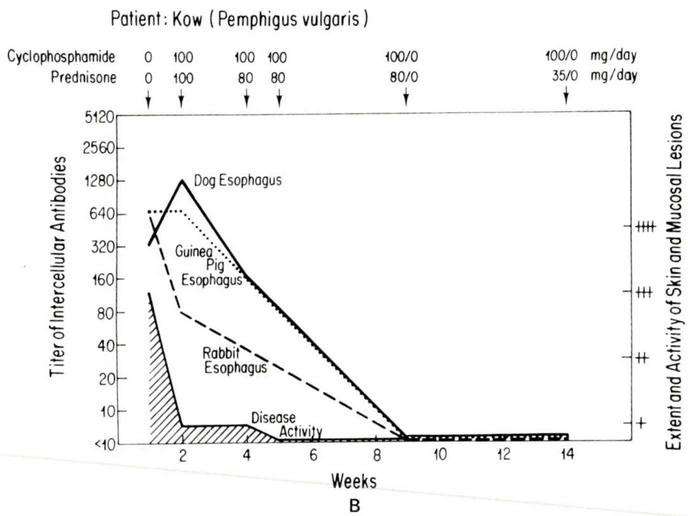

Figure 2. Graphs of IC titers versus extent and activity of clinical disease in four pemphigus patients. A, B. KOW: Correlation of disease severity and antibody titer on all epithelial substrates tested. C. LES: Correlation on monkey esophagus. In addition, this patient's antibody titer demonstrated correlation with disease severity on rabbit esophagus and guinea pig esophagus (not shown). D. NAU: Correlation on monkey and rabbit esophagus only; note that pemphigus antibodies from this patient were nonreactive with human skin. E, F. SIL: No correlation on any substrate at the time of the serum studies. However, clinical follow-up studies showed that this patient did relapse.

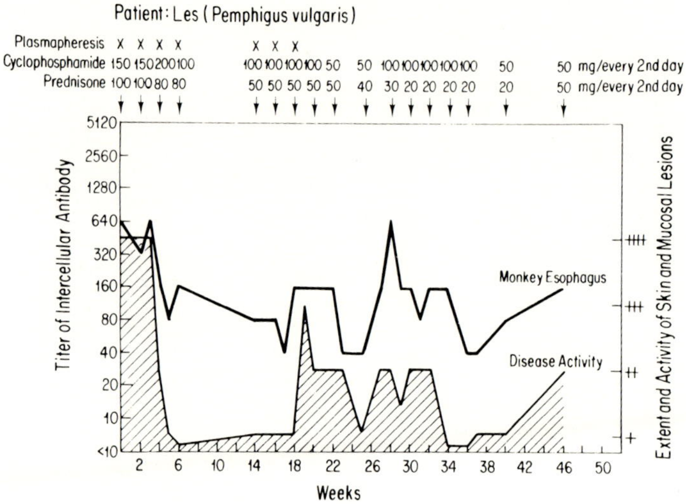

C

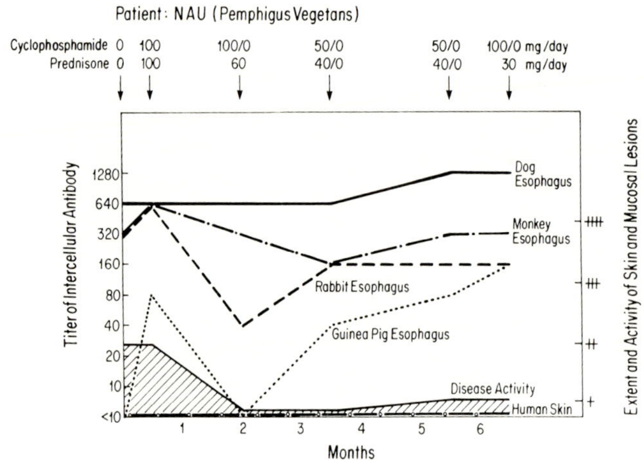

D

body titer and disease activity only when titers are determined on monkey esophagus or rabbit esophagus. Moreover, correlation up to the original cut-off date of this study can be demonstrated for the greatest number of patients when either of these two substrates is used. However, when the follow-up clinical data are factored in, the use of monkey esophagus sections alone gives the best correlation (see the following section for details).

Table 5 summarizes the results of the three methods used to determine correlation. In all three, the greatest number of patients demonstrated correlation when monkey esophagus was used to determine pemphigus antibody titers, although there was no statistical difference between the frequency of correlation on monkey esophagus and guinea pig or rabbit esophagus. The use of guinea pig esophagus to determine pemphigus antibody

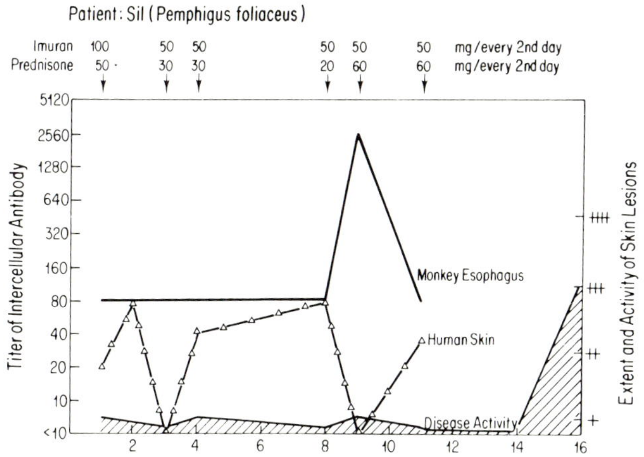

E

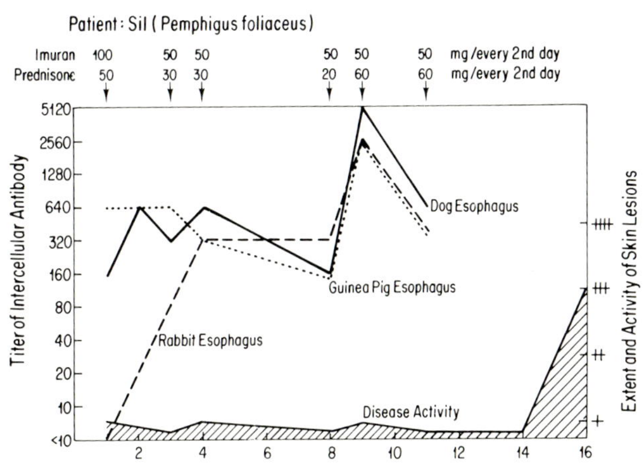

F

titers in Judd and Lever's study (28) may very well explain their failure to demonstrate correlation of disease severity and antibody titer. In another publication, Judd and Mescon (29) reported that monkey esophagus was better than guinea pig esophagus, rabbit esophagus, or human skin because of its higher rank correlation coefficient. With the methods employed in this study, we have also seen the superiority of monkey esophagus. Many previous reports in the literature have advocated the use of monkey esophagus over other substrates (11,17,40). Most recently, a study by Feibleman et al. (17) compared the IC antibody titers on both monkey esophagus and guinea pig esophagus in 16 pemphigus patients. The sera from five patients with active disease failed to demonstrate IC antibody titers on guinea pig esophagus despite positive titers on monkey esophagus. Four patients who we examined yielded similar results. In no case did the opposite occur; that is, there

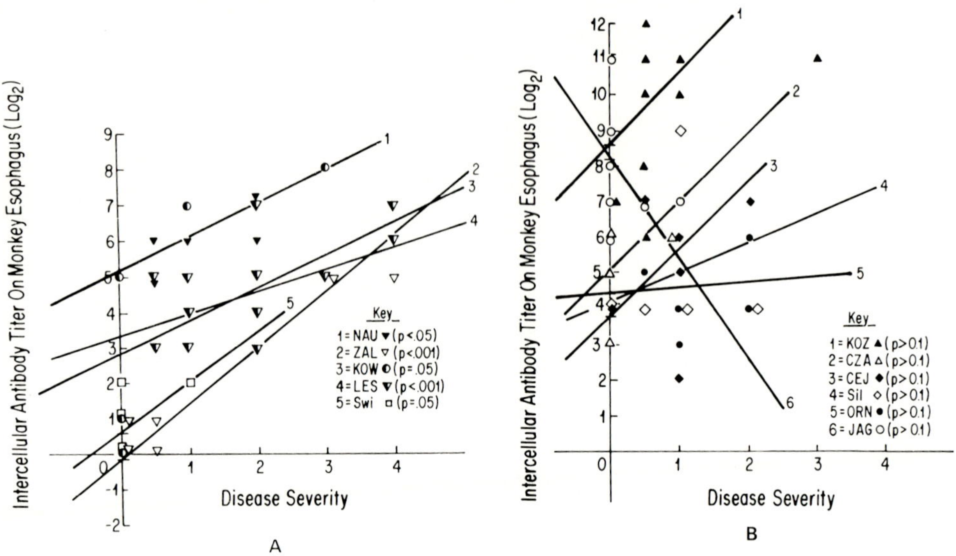

Figure 3. Diagram of IC antibody titer on monkey esophagus versus disease severity showing line of best fit generated from calculation of coefficient of correlation. A. Patients demonstrating correlation of disease severity and IC antibody titer. B. Patients demonstrating no correlation of disease severity with IC antibody titer.

Table 4. Listing of Individual Pemphigus Patients According to the Substrate on Which Their Serum Antibody Titer Correlated with Disease Severity

Patient	*No. Substrates correlated on/ total no. substrates*	*Money esophagus*	*Rabbit esophagus*	*Guinea pig esophagus*	*Human skin*	*Dog esophagus*
KOW	5/5	X[a]	X	X	X	X
LES	4/5	X	X	X	—[a]	X
ZAL	4/5	X	X	X	—[c]	X
NAU	2/5	X	X	—	—[c]	—[b]
CZA	2/5	—[b]	—[b]	—	—	—[b]
SWI	1/5	X	—	—[c]	—[c]	—[c]
KOZ	1/5	—[b]	X	—[b]	—[b]	—[b]
CEJ	0/5	—[b]	—[b,c]	—[c]	—[c]	—[c]
ORN	0/5	—[b]	—[c]	—[c]	—[c]	—[c]
SIL	0/5	—[b]	—[b]	—[b]	—[b]	—[b]
JAG	0/5	—[b]	—	—[b]	—	—[b]
Totals		5 (+6[b])	5 (+3[b])	3 (+3[b])	1 (+1[b])	3 (+5[b])

[a]X, Correlation of pemphigus antibody titer and disease severity; −, no correlation.
[b]Patients' sera positive for high titers of pemphigus antibody at the end of the study with remission or low disease activity. Each of these patients suffered relapses 3 days to 4 mo after the last serum (and the initial cut-off date) for these analyses. (See section on "Prognostic Value of Determining Intercellular Antibody Titers" and Table 6 for further details).
[c]Patients' sera negative for pemphigus antibodies throughout most of the study, but clinical activity present most of the time.

Table 5. Summary of Results From Three Methods Used to Determine Correlation of Antibody Titer with Clinical Severity for 11 Pemphigus Patients

	Number (and percentage) of cases with positive correlations			
Substrate	r_s[a] (%)	r[a] (%)	*Inspection*[b] (%)	*Average (%)*
Monkey esophagus	6[a] (55)	5 (45)	5 (45)	5.3 (48)
Rabbit esophagus	5 (45)	4 (36)	4 (36)	4.3 (39)
Guinea pig esophagus	5 (45)	4 (36)	3 (27)	4.0 (36)
Human skin	5 (45)	2 (18)	1 (9)	2.7 (24)
Dog esophagus	4 (36)	3 (27)	1 (9)	2.7 (24)

[a]r_s, Spearman rank correlation coefficient; r, coefficient of correlation.
[b]Inspection of graph for each patient of pemphigus antibody titer versus disease severity for relationships of antibody titer to disease flares and remissions; that is, concurrent, precede, follow. See text for complete explanation.

were no patients with active disease whose serum pemphigus antibody titers were negative on monkey esophagus but positive on other substrates. Judd and Mescon had 7 of 10 patients in this category, which accounts for their low frequency of sera positive on monkey esophagus (52%) compared to the 94% found in this study. These discrepancies in the frequency of positive findings emphasize the necessity of titer controls to ensure the suitability of monkey tissue employed in the IIF test.

Other investigators have favored substrates other than monkey esophagus. Acosta and Ivanyi (2) recommend the use of human tonsil for detecting pemphigus antibodies. However, only a small number of serum samples were tested. Even so, IIF tests on guinea pig esophagus consistently gave the lowest titers when compared to human tissue or monkey esophagus. In another study of five pemphigus patients, Gligora (20) demonstrated no significant difference between human tonsil and monkey esophagus for determining the titers in sera from four pemphigus patients. All sera were negative on guinea pig tissue. Other authors have used rabbit esophagus (9) and human skin (13,30) for routine IIF testing for pemphigus antibodies. In earlier studies, Katz et al. (30) found human skin to be superior to rabbit esophagus. In contrast, we have observed that the frequency of correlation of disease severity and IC antibody titer determined on rabbit esophagus was second only to monkey esophagus. In addition, the second highest frequency of positive sera (Table 3) was detected using rabbit esophagus.

Factors other than choice of substrate may have contributed to the failure of Judd and Mescon (29) and Judd and Lever (28) to establish correlation of disease activity and pemphigus antibody titer. Serum samples taken at 2 to 3 month intervals may result in a failure to detect a rise in antibody titer preceding a flare-up in disease. Intervals of 1 to 3 weeks are recommended until remission occurs. Then intervals of 1 to 2 months are recommended for a period of about 6 months. Practically speaking, serum studies should be done at every visit to the clinic or office. This is verified by the relapses observed in the clinical follow-up examinations of patients who had IC antibodies but little or no clinical activity up to the initial cut-off date, as indicated in the following section.

Prognostic Value of Determining IC Antibody Titers

We have been able to obtain 4 year follow-up data on the clinical condition of all 11 patients included in this study. These findings are reported in Table 6. All five patients

Table 6. Long-Term Clinical Follow-up on 11 Pemphigus Patients

Patient	*Date of last serum sample in study*	*Last titer in study*[a]	*Last recorded level of disease activity in study*	*Relationship of antibody titer to disease activity*[b]	*Dates of clinical follow-up*	*Clinical follow-up*	*Time of relapse*[c]	*Total no. of patients*
KOW	3-14-80	<10	Remission	C	4/80 to 6/84	Stable & complete remission		
ZAL	1-04-80	<10	Remission	C	2/80 to 6/84	Stable & complete remission		3
SWI	4-18-80	<10	Remission	C	5/80 to 6/84	Stable & complete remission		
NAU	6-02-80	320	Moderate	C	7/80	Relapse		
					9/80	Relapse		
					1981 to 6/84	Severe relapse	1 mo	2
LES	1-04-80	160	Moderate	C	1/80 to 6/84	Never complete remission		
KOZ	1-04-80	320	Low	NC	1/18/80 to 6/84	Severe relapse; occasional erosions on mucous membranes	14 days	

JAG	5-16-80	640	Low	NC	8/80 to 6/84	Moderate relapse; occasional erosions on oral mucosa	2 mo	
CZA	5-30-80	320	Remission	NC	8/80	Severe relapse	2 mo	6
					2/82	Severe relapse		
					to 6/84	Occasional exacerbations		
CEJ	10-10-79	640	Low	NC	11/79	Moderate relapse	1 mo	
					12/79	Remission		
					1/80 to 6/84	Complete remission		
					10/82	Off treatment		
ORN	5-13-80	160	Low	NC	5/16/80	Moderate relapse		
					7/13/80	Severe relapse	3 days	
					Early 1984	Severe relapse		
SIL	5-30-80	80	Low	NC	9/26/80	Severe relapse		
					11/07/80	Very severe relapse		
					Early 1983 to 6/84	Moderate relapse; occasional exacerbations	4 mo	

[a]Monkey esophagus as substrate.
[b]C, correlation; NC, no correlation.
[c]Time after cut-off of initial study; that is, time after last serum study and exam.

who had demonstrated a correlation of antibody titer on monkey esophagus with disease severity continued to show this correlation. Of these five, three who had negative (<10) titers and had been in remission when the study ended continued in remission over the next 4 years. O'Loughlin et al. (40) have reported similar results. During a 6 year period, 6 of 17 (35%) patients had prolonged remission with negative antibody titers while off therapy. An additional seven patients (for a total of 76%) displayed complete suppression of their clinical disease, as well as minimal pemphigus antibody titers of 10 or less. The results of O'Loughlin et al. and our study do not support the findings of Fitzpatrick and Newcomer (19). The latter investigators reported that the occurrence of a negative titer during complete remission was of no particular prognostic importance, because 70% of these patients had a disease flare-up after an average of 8.9 months. In our studies, two of the five patients who continued to demonstrate correlation of antibody titer and disease activity occasionally experienced relapses of their disease over the 4 year follow-up period. Importantly, all six of the patients who had not demonstrated correlation of disease severity and antibody titer when monkey esophagus was used as a substrate developed clinical relapses of their disease within 3 days to 4 months after completion of the last serum study. Moreover, these six patients had all consistently demonstrated high antibody titers but low disease activity or remission. These follow-up studies emphasize that patients in remission or with low disease activity and with significant titers of IC antibodies may be expected to have a relapse. Therefore, any evaluation of the correlation of antibody titer and disease activity must include a study of the dynamics of the disease. Because of the variable lag periods in relapses, it is frequently difficult to make such evaluations purely with statistical analyses. Persistence of high IC antibody titers despite low clinical activity should alert the physician to an impending relapse in disease. Similar observations have been noted by O'Loughlin et al. (40). Penneys (44) reported that all attempts to stop therapy in pemphigus patients clinically free of disease, but with detectable antibody titers, resulted in recurrence of disease. Moy and Jordan (37) are also of the opinion that a persistently high pemphigus antibody titer identifies patients who are more likely to relapse and require closer clinical observation.

Table 7 summarizes the frequency with which the IC antibody titer on various substrates correlated with disease severity or was predictive of disease severity both throughout the study and within the period of clinical follow-up. The frequency of concurrent correlation of antibody titer with disease flare-up was the same for monkey, rabbit, and guinea pig esophagus (60%). The use of human skin and dog esophagus resulted in a lower frequency of correlation. There was little difference among substrates in the concurrent correlation of antibody titer with disease remission except for human skin. The use of this substrate for IIF testing resulted in a lower frequency. The frequencies of concurrent correlation of antibody titer with disease flare-up did not differ significantly from the frequency with disease remission for any of the substrates except dog esophagus. For this substrate, there was better correlation of low antibody titers and low disease activity.

Significant differences occurred among substrates in the predictive value of a rise in antibody titers. Titers determined on monkey esophagus yielded the highest frequency (75%), followed by rabbit esophagus (50%). The IC antibody titers determined on guinea pig esophagus predicted disease flare-up at a much lower frequency. Our frequency for episodes of a rise in antibody titer (determined on monkey esophagus), which predicted a disease flare-up (75%), was much greater than the 25% reported by Fitzpatrick and Newcomer (19) and the 14% reported by Creswell et al. (13). We agree with Fitzpatrick and Newcomer that a twofold or greater decrease in titer only rarely

Table 7. Prediction of Disease Severity by Concurrent Change in Pemphigus Antibody Titer for 11 Patients

Substrate	*Episodes of disease flare*	*Episodes of disease remission*	*Episodes of concurrent correlation of disease flare with antibody titer (%)*	*Episodes of concurrent correlation of disease remission with antibody titer (%)*	*Episodes of rise in antibody titer preceding disease flare[a] (%)*	*Episodes of antibody titer drop preceding remission[b] (%)*	*Episodes of antibody titer drop following remission[c] (%)*
Monkey esophagus	12	11	3 (60)	7 (64)	9[d] (75)	0	4 (36)
Rabbit esophagus	12	11	3 (60)	6 (55)	6 (50)	0	5 (45)
Guinea pig esophagus	12	11	3 (60)	5 (45)	2 (17)	1 (20)	4 (36)
Human skin	12	11	1 (20)	2 (18)	2 (17)	2 (40)	2 (18)
Dog esophagus	12	11	1 (20)	5 (45)	3 (25)	1 (20)	4 (36)

[a]Rise in pemphigus antibody titer preceded disease flare by 3 days to 4 mo.
[b]Drop in pemphigus antibody titer preceded disease remission by 2–4 wk.
[c]Drop in pemphigus antibody titer followed disease remission by 1–3 wk.
[d]One patient (ORN) had a flare in disease followed 1 wk later by rise in antibody titer (data not included in this table).

precedes a remission. The frequency of decreases in antibody titer following remission was similar for all substrates, again with the exception of human skin, which was lower.

Table 8 indicates that for the substrates tested, almost all episodes of high antibody titer in the presence of low disease activity were predictive of a flare-up. Importantly, episodes of low antibody titer with high disease severity were not as predictive of remission when guinea pig or dog esophagus was used as a substrate.

Finally, Table 9 reflects the greater sensitivity of monkey esophagus as a substrate

Table 8. Frequency of Episodes of Discordant Pemphigus Antibody Titer and Disease Activity That Predicted Disease Flare or Remission

Substrate	*Total no. of episodes of high antibody titer and low disease activity or remission*	*Proportion of episodes that predicted flare*[a]	*Total no. of episodes of low antibody titer and high disease activity*	*Proportion of episodes that predicted remission*[b]
Monkey esophagus	10	9 of 10	0	0 of 0
Rabbit esophagus	6	6 of 6	0	0 of 0
Guinea pig esophagus	3	2 of 3	2	1 of 2
Human skin	2	2 of 2	2	2 of 2
Dog esophagus	4	3 of 4	3	1 of 3

[a]High pemphigus antibody titer preceded disease flare by 3 days to 4 mo.
[b]Low pemphigus antibody titer preceded disease remission by 1–2 wk.

Table 9. Changes in Disease Activity with or without Change in Antibody Titer

	Change in disease activity concurrent with		*No change in disease activity concurrent with*	
Substrate	*Correlative change in antibody titer (%)*	*No change in antibody titer (%)*	*Correlative change in antibody titer (%)*	*No change in antibody titer (%)*
Monkey esophagus	15 (94)	1 (6)[b]	17 (37)[a]	29 (63)
Rabbit esophagus	15 (65)	8 (35)[c]	17 (46)[a]	20 (54)
Guinea pig esophagus	10 (50)	10 (50)[c]	13 (33)[a]	26 (67)
Human skin	14 (64)	12 (46)[c]	17 (41)[a]	24 (59)
Dog esophagus	14 (64)	12 (46)[c]	14 (37)[a]	24 (63)

[a]Almost all accounted for by three patients (KOZ, SIL, JAG) who are in remission or have low disease activity with fluctuating pemphigus antibody titers.
[b]One patient (KOZ) with high pemphigus antibody titers and in remission.
[c]Almost all accounted for by one patient (ORN) whose serum is negative for pemphigus antibodies on all substrates except monkey esophagus.

for determining pemphigus antibody titers. Ninety-four percent of episodes of changes in disease activity were accompanied by significant correlative changes in antibody titer when monkey esophagus was used. Conversely, when there was no change in disease activity, the frequency of changes in antibody titer was low and approximately the same for all substrates. The high frequency of changes in disease activity accompanied by changes in antibody titer on monkey esophagus obtained in our study is in sharp contrast with the findings of Newcomer and Fitzpatrick (19). They found a correlative change in antibody titer with a change in disease activity in only 53% of cases. Creswell's (13) finding of a 28% change in clinical activity without a change in antibody titer on human skin is similar to our results for human skin.

Studies Eliminating Pemphigus-like Antibodies (PLA) as a Possible Explanation for Discrepancies Betwen High Antibody Titers and Low Disease Activity

Before the results of the long-term clinical follow-up studies were known, the patients' sera, which showed high antibody titers on monkey esophagus along with low disease activity or remission, were considered to possibly contain pemphigus-like antibodies (PLA). These are circulating IC antibodies found in the sera of many patients with a variety of diseases, including infections (43,45), burns (1), drug reactions (18), skin grafts (14), neoplasia (16), and occasionally in normal sera (15). They have also been demonstrated in various dermatoses such as erythema multiforme, bullous pemphigoid (BP) (23), cicatricial pemphigoid (12,34), and apparently even pemphigus itself (38). However, unlike true pemphigus antibodies, they do not bind in vivo. Previous studies by Kumar et al. (34) suggested that these PLA bind complement in a CIF test, but that true pemphigus antibodies do not. Nishikawa et al. have reported divergent results (21,22,38,39). In principle, in studies of sera with IC antibody titers of 80 or more on primate mucosa, organ culture studies with explants of comparable primate mucosa afford the most unequivocal distinction between PLA and true pemphigus antibodies, since only the latter bind to the viable explants of stratified epithelia (31,32).

The data in Table 10 show results of the sera study with true pemphigus antibodies and PLA by IIF and CIF tests and the reactions of these sera in an organ culture system (31,32). As expected, the sera from pemphigus patients were positive by standard

Table 10. Comparison of Serologic and Organ Culture Reactions of Pemphigus and PLA

	IC Antibody titer on monkey mucosa		*Biopsy DIF*	*Organ culture reactions*	
Sera	*IIF*	*CIF*	*(IC areas)*	*DIF-IC IgG binding (No. pos/No. tests)*	*Acantholysis (No. pos/No. tests)*
Pemphigus					
Les	160	<10	IgG	26/29 (90%)	16/25 (64%)
Pemphigus-like					
SKI[a]	640	40	Neg	0/4	0/4
BAG[b]	320	80–160	Neg	0/3	0/3
POL[c]	160	40	Neg	0/1	0/1
Total				0/8 (0%)	0/8 (0%)

[a]Patient with malignant lymphatic lymphoma in remission.
[b]Patient with erythema multiforme (drug induced).
[c]Patient with suspected LE not confirmed.

defined IIF tests. All sera in this group were negative for complement-fixing IC antibodies in the test system used. As previously documented, the IgG not only bound to the IC areas of an explant of monkey mucosa (Fig. 4A), but also caused acantholysis (Fig. 4C). In contrast to true pemphigus antibodies, PLA did fix complement in a CIF test (Fig. 5). Importantly, when sera with PLA served as a culture medium for explants of oral mucosa of monkeys, the PLA failed to bind to the mucosa (Fig. 4B) or to produce acantholytic changes (Fig. 4D).

The CIF and organ culture methods described above were used to determine the nature of IC antibodies in the sera of four of six patients with high IC antibody titers and low disease activity. As can be seen in Table 11, all four sera in question failed to fix complement in a CIF test, thus behaving as true pemphigus antibodies. In fact, all 111 serum samples from the 11 pemphigus cases were examined using this method and none were positive. All controls (as noted in Table 11 and the section on "Experimental Design") performed as expected. These data differ from those of Nishikawa et al.; they report that most pemphigus antibodies are capable of fixing complement in vitro (21,22,38,39). The difference in findings may be due to the fact that CIF test methods have not been defined, as have IIF methods.

Moreover, the four sera that we examined in an organ culture system were bound to the IC areas of mucosal explants (Fig. 6). Acantholysis was not observed at 48 hours with any of the sera, including the pemphigus control. These results are consistent with reactions of true pemphigus antibodies and not PLA. This conclusion was further strengthened with the finding, in subsequent clinical follow-ups, that each of these patients experienced a relapse in their disease within 3 days to 4 months (Table 6).

Summary

This study has provided evidence that monkey esophagus is the substrate of choice for detection of IC antibodies in cases of pemphigus, and that a correlation exists between the titer of these IC antibodies and the clinical severity of the disease. The bases for these conclusions are summarized in the following points: 1) Many pemphigus sera showing strong staining intensity on monkey esophagus in an IIF test were only weakly

Table 11. Serologic and Organ Culture Reactions of IC Antibodies From Selected Pemphigus Patients with Little or No Disease Activity

	IC Antibody titer on monkey mucosa		*Organ culture reactions DIF-IC IgG binding (No. pos/No. tests)*
Sera	*IIF*	*CIF*	
Controls			
Normal	<10	<10	0/4
Pemphigus	320	<10	4/4
PLA (BAG)	160	80	0/3[a]
Low disease activity			
CZA	320	<10	4/4
SIL	320	<10	4/4
JAG	320	<10	4/4
KOZ	320	<10	4/4

positive on the other epithelial substrates tested. 2) Thirty-six percent of patients with active disease were both positive for circulating IC antibodies on monkey esophagus and negative on other substrates. 3) Patients' sera that were negative for IC antibodies on monkey esophagus were not positive on other substrates tested. 4) The highest frequency of positive sera (94%) was found when monkey esophagus was used as a substrate in the IIF test. 5) With the three methods used to determine correlation of disease severity with IC antibody titer, more than half of the patients examined exhibited correlation using one or more substrate. 6) All discrepancies with monkey esophagus IC antibody titers were in patients with elevated titers and little or no disease activity; each of these patients had relapses within 4 months, and the greatest number of patients showed correlation of disease activity and antibody titer when monkey esophagus was used. 7) In patients who were followed long enough, a rise in IC antibody titer on monkey esophagus preceded a flare-up in disease 75% of the time. 8) Monkey esophagus exhibited a greater sensitivity than other substrates, as 94% of the changes in disease activity were accompanied by significant correlative changes in antibody titer when this substrate was used. And finally, 9) continued negative antibody titers over a period of 1 month or more were shown to be good prognostic indicators of prolonged remission of disease. (See Addendum B for role of pemphigus types.)

DIAGNOSTIC VALUE OF INDIRECT VERSUS DIRECT IMMUNOFLUORESCENCE IN PEMPHIGUS

Experimental Design

Judd and Lever have repeatedly questioned the value of IIF studies for the diagnosis of pemphigus (28,29). They found that less than 50% of pemphigus patients had circulating IC antibody titers,* whereas DIF was positive in 92% of cases (28). Since their IIF results were obtained on guinea pig esophagus and the results of the studies discussed at length in this chapter indicated that monkey esophagus is a superior substrate for detection of pemphigus antibodies, a retrospective study was done to determine what the incidence of DIF versus IIF would be with monkey esophagus as the substrate for IIF.

Biopsy specimens in Michel's transport medium and serum samples from 106 patients with active pemphigus were examined, respectively, by DIF for deposition of IgG, IgA, IgM, fibrin, and complement component C3 and by IIF tests with a goat antihuman IgG conjugate according to standard methods described previously in Chapter 1. The ranges of F/P ratios and antibody concentration for conjugates used over a 5 year period were as follows:

Conjugate	*Molar F/P*	*Antibody protein content (mg/ml)*
IgG	1.9–4.0	1.60–5.50
IgA	1.9–3.5	0.79–1.02
IgM	2.2–3.3	0.85–1.11
Fibrin	1.9–2.6	1.50–1.67
C3	2.4–4.6	0.70–1.16

*See footnote in Table 14 and Lever's point 1 in the "Addendum" to this chapter.

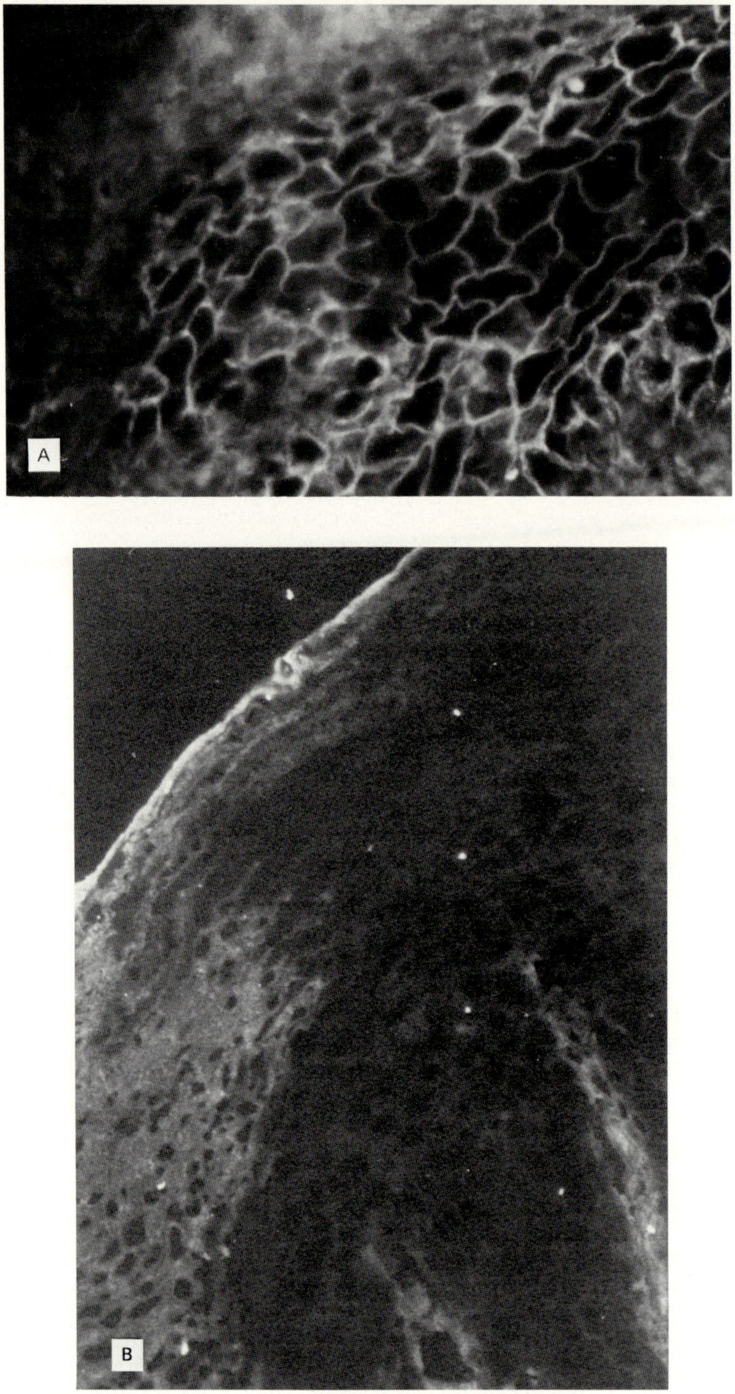

Figure 4. Organ culture reactions of pemphigus and PLA. A. Intercellular staining with an anti-IgG conjugate in a DIF test on a monkey mucosal explant incubated for 24 hours in serum (LES) containing pemphigus antibodies (400×). B. Absence of IC staining with an anti-IgG conjugate in a DIF test on a similar mucosal explant incubated for 24 hours in a serum (BAG) containing PLA (160×).

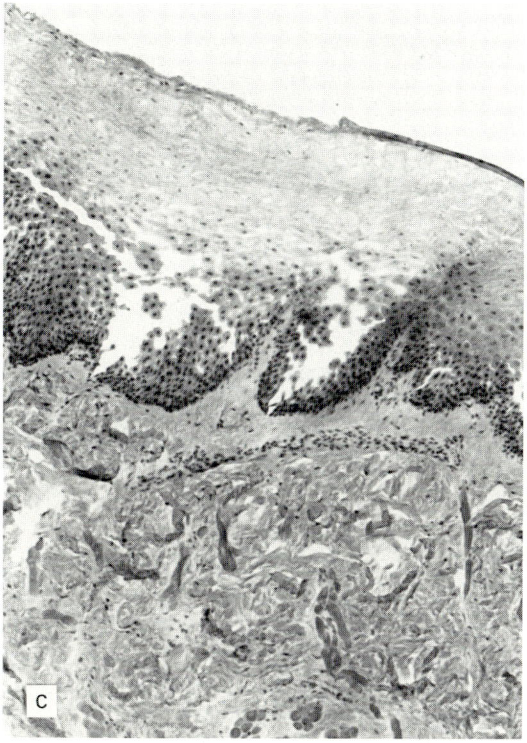

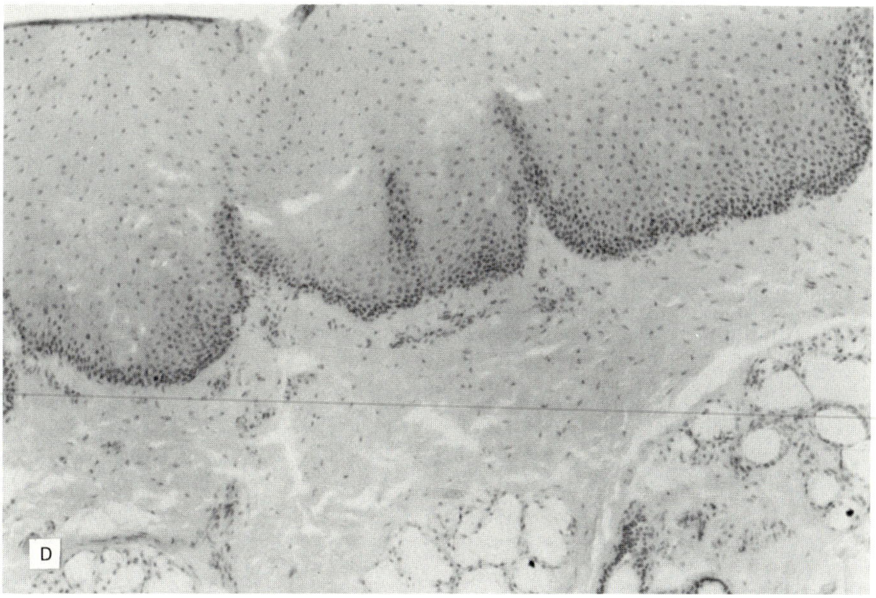

C. H & E stained section of an explant incubated for 72 hours in a serum (LES) containing pemphigus antibodies. Note the free acantholytic cells (160×). D. H & E stained section of an explant incubated for 72 hours in a serum (BAG) containing PLA. Note absence of acantholysis (100×).

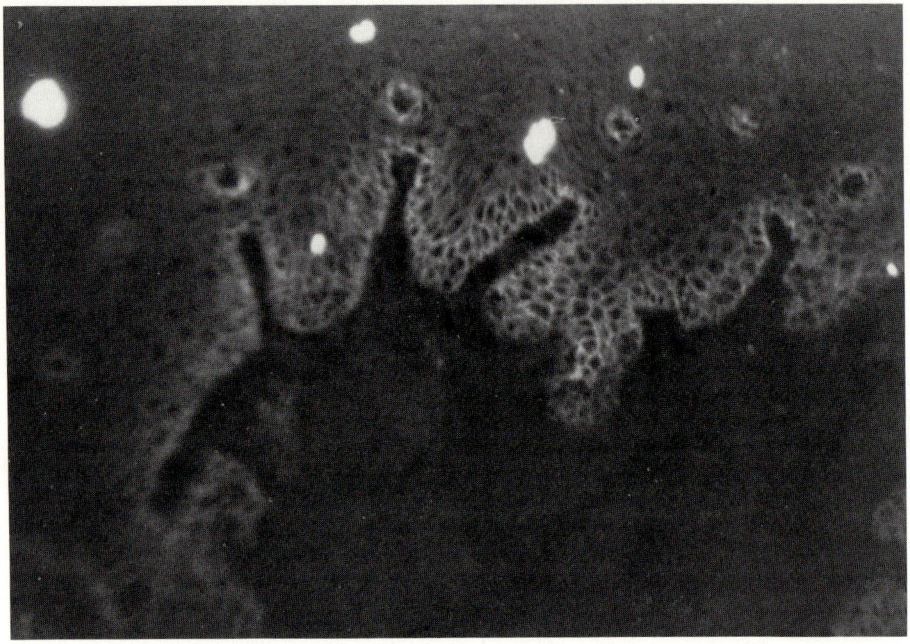

Figure 5. Intercellular staining on monkey esophagus mucosa using an anti complement component C3 conjugate with serum BAG 1/10 containing PLA. Source of complement was fresh human serum 1/20 (200×).

Approximately 63% of the biopsy specimens were examined with a substage illuminated fluorescence microscope with a mercury vapor lamp. Twenty-three percent were examined with this same microscope and an epi-illuminated microscope with a tungsten halogen lamp. Finally, 14% of the specimens were examined only with the latter fluorescent microscope.

The diagnosis of pemphigus was confirmed both clinically and histologically in all cases.

IIF Versus DIF Findings in Pemphigus Patients

Retrospective analysis (Table 12) over a 5 year period identified 69 cases (65.1%) that were positive by both DIF and IIF. Importantly, another 28 patients (26.4%) had circulating IC antibodies, but had negative biopsy results. Of the total 42 biopsy specimens from this group of patients, 17 (40.5%) were from mucosal sites and 25 (59.5%) were skin specimens. Lesional specimens made up 66.7% of the total 42 specimens, and the remaining 33.3% were from normal sites. Therefore, the high percentage of negative DIF findings could not be explained entirely by the fact that the majority of biopsy specimens came from mucosal or normal sites, which are often negative (see Table 13).

Significantly, only nine patients (8.5%) failed to reveal circulating IC antibodies, but were positive by DIF for in vivo-bound immune deposits. Therefore, a total of 97 patients (91.5%) had an initial serum sample positive for circulating IC antibodies. Only

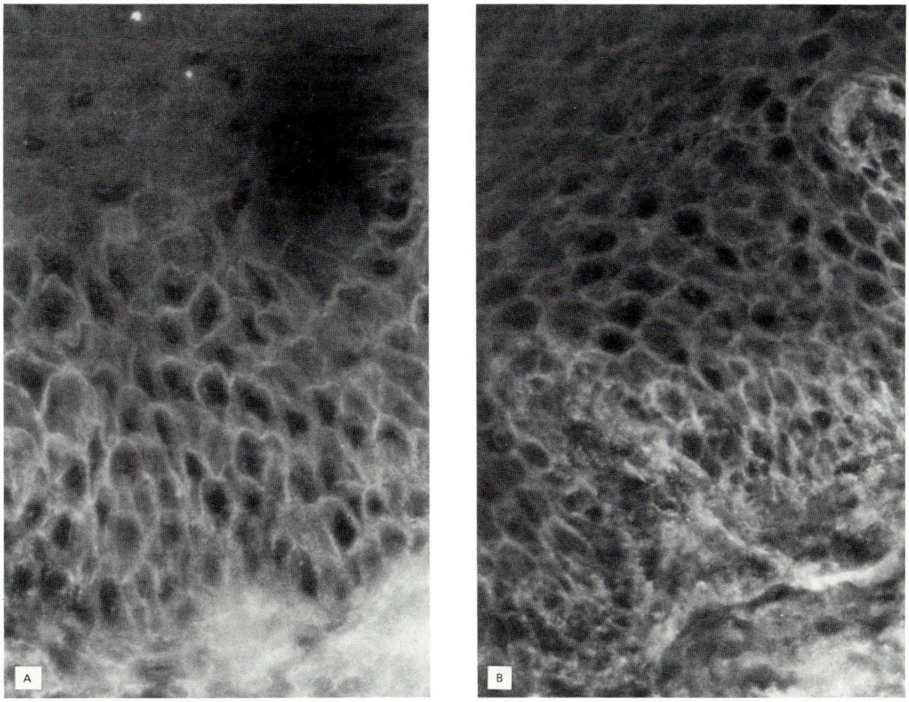

Figure 6. Intercellular binding using an anti-IgG conjugate in a DIF test on a monkey mucosal explant incubated for 24 hours in serum from (A) pemphigus patient (LES). This patient's IC antibody titers on monkey esophagus correlated with disease severity (400×). B. Intercellular binding under the same conditions as Figure 6A; only serum was from a patient (SIL). This patient's IC antibody titers did not correlate with disease severity on any substrate tested (400×).

Table 12. IIF and DIF Findings in Patients with Pemphigus

Findings by			
IIF[a]	*DIF*[b]	*No.*	*%*
Pos	Pos	69	65.1
Neg	Pos	9	8.5
Pos	Neg	28	26.4
Total Pos		97	92.5
	Total Pos	78	73.6
Total		106	

[a]Presence of circulating antibodies to the IC substance of epithelial tissue of monkey esophagus.
[b]Presence of bound IgG and, in some cases, also IgM/IgA and complement C3 in the IC areas of epithelial tissue. The presence of complement alone or of comparable deposits of IgM and/or IgA were not deemed positive findings.

Table 13. Comparison of Positivity of Biopsy Specimens From Skin and Mucosal Sites

		DIF+	
Biopsy Site	*No. of Biopsy Specimens*[a]	*No. pos*	*% pos*
Mucosa			
Total	29	12	41.4
Lesion	21[b]	9	42.9
Normal	8	3	37.5
Skin			
Total	115	89	77.4[c]
Lesion	85[b]	68	80.0
Normal	30	21	70.0
Lesion (mucosa & skin)	106	77	72.6[d]
Normal (mucosa & skin)	38	24	63.2

[a]Total of 144 biopsy specimens from 106 patients.
[b]Both mucosal and skin biopsy specimens were primarily from lesional sites (72.4% versus 73.9%).
[c]The number of skin specimens positive by DIF is significantly higher than mucosal specimens at $p < 0.005$ by chi square analysis.
[d]The number of lesional specimens positive by DIF is not significantly higher than normal specimens at $p > 0.250$ by chi square analysis.

78 (73.6%) of the patients were positive by DIF. Deposition of IgG in an IC pattern was demonstrated in all positive biopsy specimens. In no case was complement component C3 present as the sole immunoreactant.

When titers of IC antibodies in pemphigus patients with DIF positive results were compared to those in patients with DIF negative biopsy specimens, there was no difference in the geometric mean titer ($x_G = 90.7$ versus $x_G = 110.4$, respectively). We found no significant differences relating to age or sex. The data did reveal the known tendency for pemphigus to occur more frequently in older age groups (>40).

We observed a significantly greater number ($p < 0.005$ by chi square analysis) of skin biopsy specimens than mucosal specimens that were positive by DIF as shown in Table 13. Of the skin specimens, 77.4% were positive. This compares to only 41.4% of the mucosal specimens. The site of the mucosal biopsy specimens, whether lesional or normal adjacent tissue, did not influence the outcome of the specimen's being positive or negative. Almost the same percentage of lesional (as well as normal) mucosal specimens were found to be DIF positive; also, there was no difference seen in the percentage of DIF-positive lesional versus normal skin biopsy specimens.

Overall, the percentage of total DIF-positive lesional (skin and mucosa) biopsy specimens (72.6%) did not differ from that of the normal specimens (63.2%) ($p > 0.25$). Hence, there was no significant difference ($p > 0.25$) in the percentage of DIF-positive specimens if both lesional and normal biopsy specimens (65.5%) were submitted, or if only a lesional (78%) or a normal (62.5%) specimen was submitted alone.

Table 14 is a comparison of the number of pemphigus cases that were positive by IIF and DIF as reported by different investigators. For all studies in which monkey epithelium was used to determine the pemphigus antibody titer, the frequency of IIF positive findings was significantly higher ($p < 0.005$) than when guinea pig esophagus was used. In Judd and Lever's study (28), which employed guinea pig esophagus, the frequency of

Table 14. Number of Pemphigus Cases Positive by IIF and DIF as Reported by Different Investigators

Investigator	No. Cases	DIF+[a] No.	DIF+[a] %	IIF+[b] No.	IIF+[b] %	Substrates for IIF
Beutner et al. (7)	20	5[c]	100	14	70	Monkey lip
Chorzelski et al. (10)	35	ND		26	74	Monkey lip
Meurer et al. (36)	9	9	100	7	77	Monkey esophagus
O'Loughlin et al. (40)	17	17	100	16	94	Monkey esophagus
Judd and Lever (28)	63	58[d]	92[e]	31	49.2[f]	Guinea pig esophagus
Krasny et al.	106	78	73.6	97	91.5[g]	Monkey esophagus

[a]Presence of bound IgG and, in some cases, also IgM-IgA and complement C3 in the IC areas of epithelial tissue. The presence of complement alone, of comparable deposits of IgM and/or IgA, or of basement membrane deposits alone should not be deemed positive findings.
[b]Presence of circulating antibodies to the IC substance of epithelial tissue.
[c]Only 5 of the 20 cases were examined by DIF.
[d]Two patients showed IgG deposits along the BMZ rather than intercellularly. One patient had IgM and IgA deposits without IgG deposits.
[e]The number of cases positive by DIF studied by Judd and Lever is significantly greater than the number of cases studied by Krasny et al. at $p < 0.010$ by chi square analysis.
[f]As indicated in the addendum to this chapter, Dr. Lever stated that of the 35 cases with active pemphigus, 19 (54%) had circulating pemphigus antibodies. The remaining cases were inactive; according to Dr. Lever, the latter "included cases that had been free of lesions for many years."
[g]The number of cases positive by IIF on monkey esophagus is significantly greater than the number of cases positive on guinea pig esophagus at $p < 0.005$ by chi square analysis.

positive indirect findings was only 49.2% (see Lever's comments in the "Addendum"). This agrees with the less favorable results we observed with guinea pig esophagus and reported on earlier in this chapter.

The clinical condition of the patients may also explain the disparities in the IIF findings between these studies. Judd and Lever's patients were at various stages of disease activity; that is, from severe disease to remission. Most of the patients in our study were in an active phase of their disease. Thus, one would expect a higher frequency of positive IIF findings in these cases as the pemphigus antibody titer correlates with disease activity.

The percentage of cases that were positive (73.6%) by DIF in this study were significantly lower ($p < 0.01$ by chi square analysis) than the frequency observed by Judd and Lever (91.5%) and other investigators (see the "Addendum" for comments). In Judd and Lever's study, two patients showed IgG deposits along the basement membrane zone (BMZ) rather than intercellularly. One patient had IgM and IgA IC deposits without IgG deposition. In this study, the presence in the IC areas of complement alone or of comparable deposits of IgM and/or IgA, or BMZ deposits alone, were not deemed specific positive findings for pemphigus since such findings do occur in other diseases.

Our study differed also in that both lesional and normal skin and mucosal biopsy specimens were submitted by physicians throughout the U.S., while in the other studies, specimens were taken in single centers according to standard protocols. For example, Judd and Lever examined only normal skin specimens. Since the biopsy specimens in this study were unselected, the results more realistically reflect the incidence of DIF-positive findings seen in a clinical reference laboratory. The lower frequency of DIF-positive findings in this study are probably the result of submitting biopsy specimens such as those from older lesions and mucosal lesions, which are frequently negative. Therefore, the routine use of IIF tests is indicated together with DIF studies for the diagnosis of pemphigus.

Frequency of Immunoreactants in Pemphigus Biopsy Specimens

We have also examined the incidence of immunoreactants in biopsy specimens that were positive by DIF and, whenever possible, compared them to the frequencies reported by other investigators (Table 15). Our results for lesional specimens are in close agreement with those reported by O'Loughlin et al. (40). Compared to our results, theirs was the next next largest study in terms of numbers of specimens examined. IgG alone and IgG with C3 were seen most frequently. Of the four studies shown that examined lesional specimens, only Meurer et al. (36) reported on the finding of C3 alone in three of nine specimens. Fibrin was also positive in these specimens, indicating that the lesions may have been very advanced.

We have reported on the finding of C3 alone in the IC areas of specimens from patients who did not have pemphigus (33). Specifically, 10 had IC deposits of C3 in normal skin. Half of these patients were diagnosed as having drug-related reactions. Three had connective tissue diseases and the remaining two had a neurodermatitis.

In Meurer's study, the high percentage of specimens that were positive for IgA (56%) was explained by the presence of high concentrations of locally synthesized IgA in oral mucosa. Similarly, in Jordan's study (26), the four specimens that stained for IgA were also from oral lesions. In contrast, in the present study, none of the specimens that revealed IgA staining were from oral mucosa. It is generally agreed that C3 deposition is present primarily in lesional specimens, and is more frequently found prior to the initiation of steroid treatment (25,26,49). This is reflected in our study by the lower incidence of C3 staining (16.7%) observed in the normal specimens. However, Judd and Lever (28) have reported a frequency of 53% of normal specimens that were positive for C3 staining. We have also observed a significantly lower incidence of IgM and/or IgA staining in normal specimens: 4.2% versus 41 to 46% found by Judd and Lever. In ours and other studies, 100% of the specimens have been positive for IgG in the IC areas. In Judd and Lever's study, the frequency for IgG was 94.8%. They identified one patient with pemphigus foliaceus whose specimen revealed IC deposition of IgM and IgA, but no IgG. Also included in their report were two patients with pemphigus vulgaris whose skin specimens showed IgG deposits along the BMZ. This is not a specific diagnostic finding for pemphigus.

Summary

We have found IIF tests to be of equal or greater value than DIF studies in the diagnosis of pemphigus, provided they are performed using monkey esophagus as a substrate. Importantly, 26.4% of the pemphigus cases we examined had circulating IC antibodies, but had negative biopsy specimen results; whereas only 8.5% failed to reveal circulating IC antibodies, but were positive by DIF. Moreover, specimens from mucosal sites tended to be more frequently negative by DIF, but the IIF results were positive in all cases examined. The IIF studies are also helpful where the proper biopsy site is in question or when the biopsy specimen is submitted from an advanced lesion.

Table 15. Immunoreactants in Biopsy Specimens From Pemphigus Patients Examined by DIF

	Lesion				*Normal*
Immunoreactants[a]	*Present study*[b] *No. (%)*	*Jordon (26) No. (%)*	*Meurer (36) No. (%)*	*O'Loughlin (40) No. (%)*	*Present study*[b] *No. (%)*
IgG only	50 (65)	0	0	11 (65)	20 (83.3)
IgG & C3	17 (22)	2 (33)	1 (11)	4 (23)	3 (12.5)
IgG & IgM/A	2 (2.6)	0	0	0	0
IgG, IgM/A & C3	8 (10.4)	4 (67)	5 (56)	2 (12)	1 (4.2)
C3 alone	0	0	3 (33)	0	0
IgG & C3 (Total)	25 (32.5)	6 (100)	6 (67)	6 (35)	4 (16.7)
Total biopsy specimens	77	6	9	17	24

[a]An IC staining pattern was observed in all specimens.
[b]Total of 101 of 144 specimens from 106 pemphigus patients were positive by DIF.

RECOMMENDATIONS

On the basis of the published data reviewed in this chapter and the new data presented here, the following recommendations regarding the performance and use of IF studies in the diagnosis and management of pemphigus cases are indicated.

1. Regarding the performance of IF studies for pemphigus:
   a) Indirect IF studies of patients' sera using monkey esophagus sections that give the expected titers of IC antibodies with titer controls need to be used with defined anti-IgG conjugates (see Addendum B for use of guinea pig esophagus.)
   b) Direct IF studies should be performed with standard defined conjugates.
2. Regarding specimens in IF studies for the diagnosis of pemphigus:
   a) The combination of IF studies of both serum and biopsy specimens for the reactions of pemphigus affords the highest level of diagnostic reliability.
   b) For biopsy studies, specimens should be taken from the edge of fresh lesions if they are present. Skin biopsy specimens are recommended, because they yield significantly more positives than mucosal specimens.
3. Regarding the prognostic use of serum studies for IC antibodies:
   a) Titers of pemphigus antibodies do correlate with disease severity, in most cases, and this correlation is best shown when monkey esophagus is used as a substrate.
   b) Continued negative titers of 1 month or more are good prognostic indicators of prolonged remission of disease.
   c) Persistence of high antibody titers despite low clinical activity should alert the physician to an impending relapse in disease. Lag periods before relapse vary from patient to patient.
   d) Serum samples should be taken at 1 to 3 week intervals until remission occurs. Then intervals of 1 to 2 months are recommended for about 6 months. In practice, serum studies should be done at every visit to the clinic or physician's office.

REFERENCES

1. Ablin RJ, Milgrom F, Kano K, et al: Pemphigus-like antibodies in patients with skin burns. *Vox Sang* 16:73–75, 1969.
2. Acosta E, Ivanyi L: Comparison of the reactivity of various epithelial substrates for the titration of pemphigus antibodies by indirect immunofluorescence. *Br J Dermatol* 107:537–541, 1982.
3. Anderson HJ, Newcomer VD, Landau JW, et al: Pemphigus and other diseases. Results of indirect intercellular immunofluorescence. *Arch Dermatol* 101:538–546, 1970.
4. Anhalt GJ, Labib RS, Voorhees JJ, et al: Induction of pemphigus in neonatal mice by passive transfer of IgG from patients with the disease. *N Engl J Med* 306:1189–1196, 1982.
5. Barada FA, Andrews BS, Davis JS, et al: Antibodies to Sm in patients with systemic lupus erythematosus. Correlation of Sm antibody titers with disease activity and other laboratory parameters. *Arthritis Rheum* 24:1236–1244, 1981.
6. Beutner EH, Jordan RE: Demonstration of skin antibodies in sera of pemphigus vulgaris patients by indirect immunofluorescent staining. *Proc Soc Exp Biol Med* 117:505–510, 1964.
7. Beutner EH, Lever WF, Witebsky E, et al: Autoantibodies in pemphigus vulgaris. Responses to an intercellular substance of epidermis. *JAMA* 192:682–688, 1965.
8. Beutner EH, Jordon RE, Chorzelski TP: The immunopathology of pemphigus and bullous pemphigoid. *J Invest Dermatol* 51:63–80, 1968.

9. Chorzelski TP, Jablonska S, Blaszczyk M: Autoantibodies in pemphigus. *Acta Dermatovenereol* 47:26–33, 1966.
10. Chorzelski TP, von Weiss JF, Lever WF: Clinical significance of autoantibodies in pemphigus. *Arch Dermatol* 93:570–576, 1966.
11. Chorzelski TP, Beutner EH: Factors contributing to occasional failures in demonstration of pemphigus antibodies by the immunofluorescence test. *J Invest Dermatol* 53:188–191, 1969.
12. Cram DL, Griffith MR, Fukuyama K: Pemphigus-like antibodies in cicatricial pemphigoid. *Arch Dermatol* 109:235–238, 1974.
13. Creswell SN, Black MM, Bhogal B, et al: Correlation of circulating intercellular antibody titers in pemphigus with disease activity. *Clin Exp Dermatol* 6:477–483, 1981.
14. Dahl MV, Katz SI, McGowen JH, et al: Pemphigus-like antibodies in sera of patients with thermal burns, gunshot wounds and skin grafts. *Milit Med* 139:196–198, 1974.
15. Dahl MV, Katz SI, Scott RM, et al: Viral studies in pemphigus. *J Invest Dermatol* 62:96–99, 1974.
16. Ead RD: Pemphigus-like antibodies: A report of two cases. *Br J Dermatol* 100:723–725, 1979.
17. Feibleman C, Stolzner G, Provost TT: Pemphigus: Superiority of monkey esophagus in the determination of pemphigus antibody. *Arch Dematol* 117:561–562, 1981.
18. Fellner MJ, Prutkin L: Morbilliform eruptions caused by penicillin. *J Invest Dermatol* 55:390–395, 1970.
19. Fitzpatrick RE, Newcomer VD: The correlation of disease activity and antibody titers in pemphigus. *Arch Dermatol* 116:285–290, 1980.
20. Gligora M: Epithelium of the human palatal tonsil used for new test antigen in IIF examination (for pemphigus, pemphigoid antibodies and ANA). *Dermatologica* 155:108–114, 1977.
21. Hashimoto T, Nishikawa T, Kurihara S, et al: Complement-fixing pemphigus antibodies. *Arch Dermatol* 114:1191–1192, 1978.
22. Hashimoto T, Sugiura M, Kurihara S, et al: *In vitro* complement activation by intercellular antibodies. *J Invest Dermatol* 78:316–318, 1982.
23. Heine KG, Kumar A, Jordan RE: Pemphigus-like antibodies in bullous pemphigoid. *Arch Dermatol* 113:1693–1695, 1977.
24. Hu CH, Michel B, Schlitz JR: Epidermal acantholysis induced *in vitro* by pemphigus autoantibody. *Am J Pathol* 90:345–351, 1978.
25. Jordon RE, Sams WM, Diaz G, et al: Negative complement immunofluorescence in pemphigus. *J Invest Dermatol* 57:407–410, 1971.
26. Jordan RE, Schroeter AL, Rogers RS, et al: Classical and alternate pathway activation of complement in pemphigus vulgaris lesions. *J Invest Dermatol* 63:256–259, 1974.
27. Jordon RE: Immunopathology. In Ahmed AR (moderator): Pemphigus: Current Concepts. *Ann Intern Med* 92:396–405, 1980.
28. Judd KP, Lever WF: Correlation of antibodies in skin and serum with disease severity in pemphigus. *Arch Dermatol* 115:428–432, 1979.
29. Judd KP, Mescon H: Comparison of different epithelial substrates useful for indirect immunofluorescence testing of sera from patients with active pemphigus. *J Invest Dermatol* 72:314–316, 1979.
30. Katz SI, Halprin KM, Inderbitzin TM: The use of human skin for the detection of antiepithelial autoantibodies. A diagnostic and prognostic test. *J Invest Dermatol* 53:390–399, 1969.
31. Krasny SA: Production and characterization of monkey antibodies to epithelial intercellular antigens: A comparison to human pemphigus antibodies and pemphigus-like antibodies. Doctoral Thesis, State University of New York at Buffalo, 1981, 205 pp.
32. Krasny SA, Beutner EH: Experimental production of intercellular antibodies in monkeys. *Ann NY Acad Sci* 420:343–352, 1983.
33. Krasny SA, Kumar V, Tarfare N, et al: Intercellular complement C3 binding in normal skin of patients without pemphigus. *J Am Acad Dermatol* 14:52–58, 1986.
34. Kumar V, Yarbrough C, Beutner EH: Complement-fixing intercellular antibodies in a case of cicatricial pemphigoid. *Arch Dermatol* 116:812–814, 1980.
35. Lever WF: Methotrexate and prednisone in pemphigus vulgaris. Therapeutic results obtained in 36 patients between 1961 and 1970. *Arch Dermatol* 106:491–497, 1972.

36. Meurer M, Millns JL, Rogers RS, et al: Oral pemphigus vulgaris. A report of ten cases. *Arch Dermatol* 113:1520–1524, 1977.
37. Moy R, Jordon RE: Immunopathology in pemphigus. In Ahmed JR (Ed). *Clinics in Dermatology,* vol. 1. Lippincott, Philadelphia, 1983, pp 72–81.
38. Nishikawa T, Kurihara S, Harada T, et al: Capability of complement fixation of pemphigus antibodies *in vitro. Arch Dermatol Res* 260:1–6, 1977.
39. Nishikawa T, Kurihara S, Hatano H: Comparison of *in vivo* and *in vitro* capability of complement fixation by pemphigus antibodies. *Dermatologica* 159:290–294, 1979.
40. O'Loughlin S, Goldman GC, Provost TT: Fate of pemphigus antibody following successful therapy. Preliminary evaluation of pemphigus antibody determinations to regulate therapy. *Arch Dermatol* 114:1769–1772, 1978.
41. Peck SM, Osserman KE, Weiner LB, et al: Studies in bullous diseases. Immunofluorescent serologic tests. *N Engl J Med* 279:951–958, 1968.
42. Peck SM, Osserman KE, Samuels AJ, et al: Studies in bullous diseases. Treatment of pemphigus vulgaris with immunosuppressives and leucovorin calcium. *Arch Dermatol* 103:141–147, 1971.
43. Peck SM, Osserman KE, Rule AH: Intercellular antibodies: Presence in a *Trichophyton rubrum* infection. *J Invest Dermatol* 58:133–138, 1972.
44. Penneys NS, Eaglstein WH, Indgin S, et al: Gold sodium thiomalate treatment of pemphigus. *Arch Dermatol* 108:56–60, 1973.
45. Quismorio FP, Rea TH, Levan NE, et al: Immunoglobulin deposits in lepromatous leprosy skin. *Arch Dermatol* 111:331–334, 1975.
46. Roenigk HH, Deodhar S: Pemphigus treatment with azathioprine. Clinical and immunologic correlation. *Arch Dermatol* 107:353–357, 1973.
47. Sams WM, Jordan RE: Correlation of pemphigoid and pemphigus antibody titers with activity of disease. *Br J Dermatol* 84:7–13, 1971.
48. Schlitz JR, Michel B: Production of epidermal acantholysis in normal human skin *in vitro* by the IgG fraction from pemphigus serum. *J Invest Dermatol* 67:254–260, 1976.
49. Van Joost T, Cormane RH, Pondman KW: Direct immunofluorescent study of the skin on occurrence of complement in pemphigus. *Br J Dermatol* 87:466–474, 1972.
50. Weissman V, Feuerman EJ, Joshua H, et al: The correlation between the antibody titers in sera of patients with pemphigus vulgaris and their clinical state. *J Invest Dermatol* 71:107–109, 1978.
51. Wood GW, Beutner EH, Chorzelski TP: Studies in immunodermatology. II Production of pemphigus-like lesions by intradermal injection of monkeys with Brazilian pemphigus sera. *Int Arch Allergy Appl Immunol* 42:556–564, 1972.

ADDENDUM A

EVALUATION BY WALTER F. LEVER

Originally, Dr. Walter Lever was invited to contribute Part I to a two-part chapter on pemphigus, with this chapter of Dr. Krasny's being Part II. While it was not possible for Lever to prepare Part I, he did kindly review this chapter in its final form. His comments are as follows*:

"(1) You state on page 233 [second sentence in section on "Diagnostic Value of Indirect Versus Direct Immunofluorescence in Pemphigus"] that less than 50% of my

*Editorial revisions are in brackets.

pemphigus patients had circulating antibodies. It is true that only 47% had circulating antibodies, but this included patients who had been free of lesions for many years. Of those with lesions, 19 patients were positive for circulating antibodies and 16 patients were negative, so that the percentage of positive IIF was 54% (Table 1 in the Judd and Lever paper; [28]).

"(2) I am surprised at the low percentage of DIF in your series, namely 73.6%, as compared with 90% in the Judd and Lever series carried out on *normal skin* of the patients. I suspect that some of your referring physicians allowed some of the specimens to stand around for some time, or perhaps the transport solution was not always perfect. To use these poor results as an argument for preference of IIF over DIF appears questionable to me.

"(3) I suspect after reading the paper of Feibelman et al. that monkey esophagus is preferable to guinea pig esophagus, if available; but these authors also state that the clinical status of patients is the most important determinant of treatment dosage.

COMMENTS OF BEUTNER AND KRASNY ON EVALUATIONS BY WALTER F. LEVER

Regarding point 1, we thank Dr. Lever for the added information. It is entered as a footnote in Table 14 and in the text.

Regarding point 2 (the evaluations of the data of Krasny et al. as "poor results"), obviously the data are accurate. The nature of the problem is well illustrated by a recent case that we studied. Biopsy specimens were sent to our laboratory from two physicians in short succession. The one was completely negative, and the other was strongly positive for intercellular IgG. Both were in transport medium. Clearly, some areas of the patient's skin are positive and others are negative. It takes a bit of experience to find the positive areas reliably. The high percentages of positives reported by others (7,36,40) are based on the use of multiple specimens in at least some examined cases. The data reported in this chapter are on *single* specimens. The frequency of 74% positives in our studies is a reliable datum for the conditions used by the average dermatologist who takes a single specimen using standard methods. Specimens that include the edge of lesions plus the adjacent clinically normal (or less involved) skin give the highest percentages of positives.

Regarding point 3, the statement made regarding the report of Feibelman et al. is taken out of context. These authors not only state that the clinical status of the patients is the most important determinant, but add: "However, our previous studies have indicated that monitoring antibody titers also gives valuable information regarding *potential* disease activity." We should also consider the information presented in this chapter regarding this latter point, since the data presented here are the most extensive and detailed that have been reported to date. They document the superiority of monkey esophagus sections to other tissues examined. Monkey esophagus sections are commercially available. (Some trivial savings affected by use of "homemade" sections from, e.g., guinea pig esophagus, obviously do not justify their use.) Most importantly, the data summarized in Tables 6 and 8 of this chapter indicate clearly that not only the clinical status of the pemphigus patients but also their titers of pemphigus antibodies need to be considered. As noted in Table 6, *all six patients with low or no disease activity, but with significant titers had relapses.* The time of the relapse varied from 3 days to 4 months. In contrast, *none of the cases of remission who had no detectable pemphigus antibody titers relapsed over the 4 year period of observation.* It is evident from these findings that *the indications for the optimal care of pemphigus patients is to monitor not only their clinical condition, but also their pemphigus antibody titer.*

E.H. Beutner
S. Krasny
T.P. Chorzelski

ADDENDUM B

Since this chapter and Addendum A were completed, studies by Michael Sabolinski in the laboratory of Ernst H. Beutner revealed that most sera from pemphigus vulgaris can be distinguished from most pemphigus foliaceus sera by their relative reactivity on monkey esophagus and guinea pig esophagus sections. Specifically, two studies (one open, one coded, but both still in preparation) reveal that pemphigus vulgaris sera react preferentially with monkey esophagus, while the sera of pemphigus foliaceus patients react more strongly with guinea pig esophagus. Accordingly, the data listed in Table 2 in this chapter have been analyzed for the relative titers of IC antibodies of these two substrates. The cases were classified into three groups: pemphigus vulgaris, pemphigus foliaceus, and the one case (LES) that changed from foliaceus to vulgaris. All sera listed in Table 2 were analyzed in accordance with the differential characteristics reported by Sabolinski. Titer differences (shown in Table 2) of one doubling dilution were considered to be nonsignificant, but differences of two or more dilutions were regarded as significant. The results of this analysis are summarized in Table 16.

The findings summarized in Table 16 substantiate the findings reported by Sabolinski. As indicated, most of the 60 sera from the eight pemphigus vulgaris patients listed in Table 2 yielded significantly higher titers on monkey esophagus, but none yielded higher titers on guinea pig esophagus. Conversely, none of the eight sera from the

Table 16. Differentiation of Pemphigus Vulgaris From Pemphigus Foliaceus by Their Relative Reactivity on Monkey and Guinea Pig Esophagus

	Sera (no. of cases)		
Relative reactivity on monkey and guinea pig esophagus sections	*Pemphigus vulgaris*	*Pemphigus foliaceus*	*Pemphigus foliaceus & vulgaris*
Higher titer on monkey esophagus	51	0	5
Higher titer on guinea pig esophagus	0	5	3
No significant difference	9	3	17
Total sera	60	8	25
(Total cases)	(8)	(2)	(1)

pemphigus foliaceus patients yielded higher titers on monkey esophagus, but most yielded higher titers on guinea pig esophagus. Analysis of the original data in terms of the intensity of staining of these sera on these two substrates (data not shown in Table 2 in this chapter) yielded comparable relationships. Importantly, the sera of the one patient who changed from foliaceus to vulgaris revealed variable results, as shown in Table 16. On reexamining the records of the individual titrations of a serum of this patient that had been studied by Michael Sabolinski, they were also found to be variable. In essence, it appears that the antibodies of pemphigus vulgaris differ from those of pemphigus foliaceus, and that the one patient (LES) who had both diseases has both types of antibodies.

Ernst H. Beutner

10
Relationship of Autoimmunity to Clinical Findings in Pemphigus

Tadeusz P. Chorzelski
Stefania Jablonska
Ernst H. Beutner

INTRODUCTION

Immunofluorescence (IF), including direct and indirect IF (DIF and IIF) (9,11), is generally accepted as a most reliable diagnostic criterion of pemphigus. With the use of IF, it was confirmed that previously recognized forms of pemphigus have a common underlying autoimmune mechanism. In addition, application of the IF method made it possible to detect new clinical types that had not been recognized previously. Thus, pemphigus can be presently classified into the following clinical types:

Main varieties (originally described):

Pemphigus vulgaris;
Pemphigus vegetans (a variant of pemphigus vulgaris);
Pemphigus erythematosus, or seborrhoicus; and
Pemphigus foliaceus, including fogo selvagem.

Recently described:

Pemphigus herpetiformis; and
Unclassified (atypical) forms.

In all of these types of pemphigus, circulating antibodies are directed against the surface antigens of keratinocytes (9,11). The frequency of their detectability depends, in part, on the substrate used for the IF reaction (see Chap. 9). However, in some atypical pemphigus cases, in drug- or burn-induced cases, and in early oral pemphigus

Supported in part by the Polish Academy of Sciences and in part by the Summerhill Foundation

Table 1. Relative Frequency of Various Types of Pemphigus

Pemphigus type	*No. of cases*	*Total (%)*
Vulgaris	95	46
Erythematosus	76	37
Foliaceus	9	4
Vegetans	10	5
Herpetiformis	13	6
Unclassified	2	1
Total	205	

vulgaris, intercellular (IC) antibodies may not be detectable on any substrate (18,54,66,72,96,108). The relative frequency of the above-listed clinical forms of pemphigus in our series is presented in Table 1.

The prevalence of pemphigus vulgaris, reported in the literature is almost 80% (57,90,92). This is more than the 46% observed in our studies. It is conceivable that some differences may be attributed to the ethnic and/or environmental factors (8,86,99).

Pemphigus erythematosus occurred in more than one-third of our patients. The other forms were rare. It should be stressed that differentiation between pemphigus erythematosus and foliaceus may be arbitrary, since both have superficial acantholysis. We have classified our cases as pemphigus erythematosus if lesions were present on the face and on light-exposed and/or seborrhoic areas. The clinical diagnosis of typical pemphigus is not difficult. There are, however, cases that may resemble other skin diseases, and the final diagnosis can only be established by IF. As seen in Table 2, the discrepancies between tentative clinical diagnosis of patients referred to us and IF findings was 13% for the whole group of 205 cases of pemphigus. Three percent of pemphigus vulgaris cases were misdiagnosed as pemphigoid. However, 10 cases referred to us as pemphigus were proven by IF to be bullous pemphigoid (BP) with positive circulating anti-BMZ antibodies in most of them (see Chap. 15). For pemphigus erythematosus, the clinical misdiagnosis was 13%, that is, the same frequency as for the entire pemphigus group. The pemphigus herpetiformis patients were diagnosed by referring doctors as dermatitis herpetiformis (DH), pemphigoid, lupus erythematosus (LE), etc. Clinical recognition of pemphigus herpetiformis was most difficult; this variety was misdiagnosed in all of the 13 cases included in this survey of 205 cases.

PEMPHIGUS VULGARIS

The site of initial involvement is most often the oral mucosa, which is involved at one time or another in almost all patients. Single or abortive painless lesions are not infrequently overlooked by patients and physicians. The patients are quite often referred to dermatologists from dentists or ear, nose, and throat specialists, sometimes only after the bullous lesions had appeared on the skin. Pemphigus vulgaris may be confined to the oral mucous membranes for several weeks or months, up to 1 year or more. Involvement of other mucous membranes has also been reported, such as the larynx and pharynx (13), esophagus (87), rectal mucosa (31), conjuctiva (6), and uterine cervix (73). The esophagus, larynx, and pharynx seem not to be infrequent sites of pemphigus

Table 2. Discrepancies Between Tentative Clinical Diagnosis and Confirmed Clinical and Laboratory Findings in 205 Pemphigus Cases

Tentative clinical diagnosis	*Total no. of misdiagnoses*	*Final diagnosis (based on clinical findings) among misdiagnosed cases*			
		Vulgaris	*Erythematosus*	*Herpetiformis*	*Unclassified*
Dermatitis herpetiformis	9		3	6	
Pemphigoid	10	3	3	3	1
Linear IgA bullous dermatosis	4			4	
Lupus erythematosus	2		2		
Dermatitis seborrhoica	1		1		
Intertrigo	1		1		
Total no. of misdiagoses / Total pemphigus cases	27/205 (13%)	3/95 (3%)	10/76 (13%)	13/13 (100%)	1/2

lesions (13,55,87). These patients may be undiagnosed if the disease starts in this location or is recognized as asymptomatic in the follow-up period. This may be the reason for the apparent discrepancies between persistence of IC antibodies and disease activity in some cases.

Oral pemphigus may also be misdiagnosed due to either abortive or aphthous-like changes. A mucosal biopsy specimen examined by direct IF is necessary for the final diagnosis. The specimens should be taken from normal mucosa, since lesional areas are usually devoid of epithelium or the epithelium is lost in processing.

In some rather exceptional cases confirmed by immunopathology and histology, erosions or aphthous-like lesions may regress spontaneously. For example, in three patients in our clinic, symptom-free intervals with no treatment were extended up to 3 years. We have not applied any therapy in these patients because they manifested long-lasting spontaneous remissions. In one of these cases, there was a single cutaneous blister on the forehead in the third year of observation, and this healed under local corticosteroid therapy. However, in general, oral pemphigus should be treated as soon as the diagnosis is confirmed by IF and histology, since prompt initiation of therapy may prevent cutaneous involvement (72), particularly in cases with circulating antibodies (Chap. 9).

Pemphigus lesions on the skin, as a rule, are positive for immune deposits in the IC substance of the epidermis (9,11). The biopsy specimen should be obtained preferably from the surrounding healthy skin, including part of the bulla (46). In this way, the section may be evaluated not only for immune deposits, but also for the architecture of the bulla. IgG is always detectable; other immunoglobulins may also be present occasionally. In early untreated cases, complement is often concomitantly bound, usually to the lower parts of the epidermis, and focally in areas where the acantholytic process begins (Table 3; 24,51–53). Complement disappears from the skin after therapy with corticosteroids is begun (25).

PEMPHIGUS VEGETANS

Two varieties of pemphigus vegetans have been recognized in old literature: 1) the Neumann type, with characteristic clinical and histologic features of pemphigus vulgaris and vegetations (Fig. 1); and 2) the Hallopeau type, with rare or no blisters, and with pustules evolving into vegetations and erosions (Fig. 2). In both types, the cutaneous

Table 3. Findings in 13 Cases of Pemphigus Herpetiformis

Findings	*Cases (No.)*	*Cases (%)*	*Comments*
DIF, IC IgG	13	100	All cases tested were also positive for C3
IIF, IC antibodies	5	38	
Histology, acantholysis	9	69	Acantholysis was sparse or absent
Treatment response			
Sulfones alone	1	8	
Corticosteroids + sulfones	7	54	
Corticosteroids alone or with immunosuppressants	5	38	Both given in low or high doses

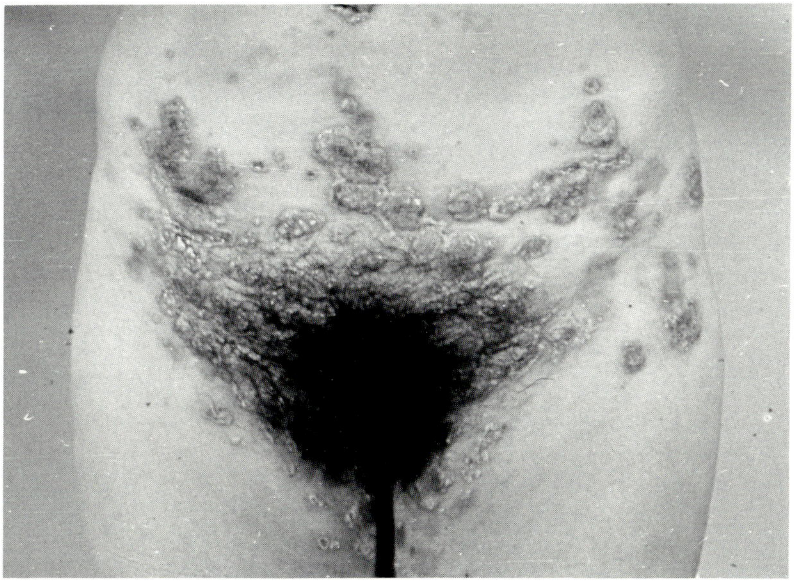

Figure 1. A case of Neumann-type pemphigus vegetans. Blisters and pustules with vegetations.

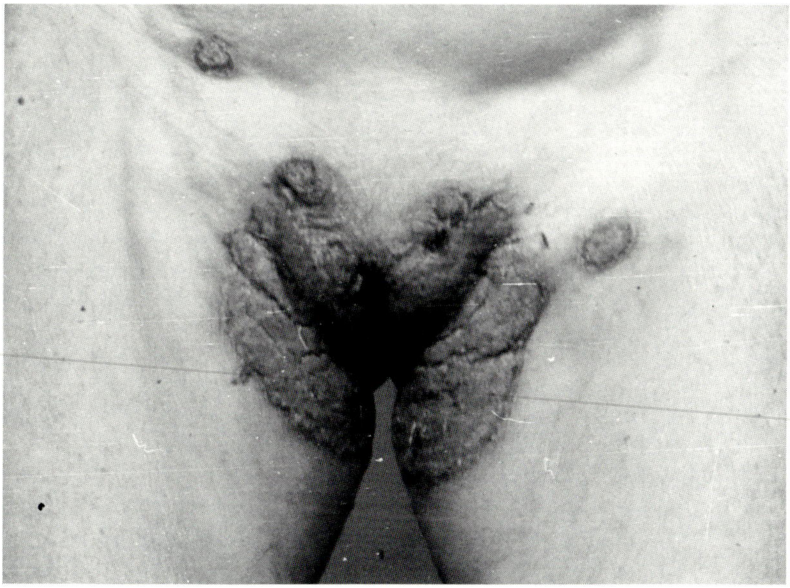

Figure 2. A case of Hallopeau-type pemphigus vegetans. Vegetations without evident pustules and blisters.

lesions are localized mainly in the axillary and inguinal folds and in traumatized areas. The Neumann type is usually more benign than pemphigus vulgaris, although it is, in reality, its variant. Still controversial is the nosologic position of the Hallopeau type, which has been originally described as vegatating pyoderma (pyodermite vegetante) and later regarded as a variant of the Neumann type by the same author; that is, as a true, although more benign, pemphigus (40). In both of these variants, oral lesions may be present; and in both, the histologic pattern is quite characteristic, with eosinophilic microabscesses and scant acantholysis in the lower parts of the proliferating epidermis. A most important finding is the presence of IC IgG deposits in a characteristic pattern and, in some cases, also circulating pemphigus antibodies (32,76,77).

Neumann-type cases regress under the regimen used in pemphigus therapy (corticosteroids and immunosuppressants), whereas in the Hallopeau type, dapsone seems to be a drug of choice that promptly controls cutaneous and oral lesions (83). While the Neumann and Hallopeau types, as shown by IF studies, should be regarded as a variant of pemphigus, there are reported anecdotal cases with vegetating lesions that are indistinguishable clinically from the Hallopeau type with eosinophilic microabscesses in histology. Those cases could not be classified as pemphigus, because DIF and IIF studies were negative and the patients responded dramatically to antibiotics. We believe that the name pyoderma vegetans should be confined exclusively to the cases with negative IF findings. The terms Neumann and Hallopeau types of vegetating pemphigus should be retained because of the differences in the course and responses to treatment.

PEMPHIGUS ERYTHEMATOSUS

This form of pemphigus was originally described by Senear and Usher (98) as an unusual type of pemphigus combining features of LE. The authors suggested two possibilities, either that manifestations resembling LE can occur as an atypical feature of pemphigus or that this syndrome combines two diseases—pemphigus and lupus. Early histologic studies have shown the presence of acantholysis that is characteristic of pemphigus (84); the classification as a form of pemphigus was finally established by IF studies (5,19,49). Detection of immunoglobulins and complement at the basement membrane zone (BMZ) of the light-exposed lesional skin (5,19,69,108) provided support for some relationship with LE. However, the IF pattern of LE, in addition to immune deposits characteristic of pemphigus, does not necessarily imply coexistence of the two diseases, but merely points to the concomitant presence of immunologic abnormalities of the LE type. The true association of pemphigus with LE is very rare, but some well-documented cases have been reported (12,19,101).

We have demonstrated immunoglobulins and complement at the dermal-epidermal junction in 80% of cases of skin specimens from exposed areas, and in about 20% of cases in biopsy specimens obtained from covered skin (49). The antinuclear antibodies (ANA) in our series occurred in about 30% of patients (49). The coexistent DIF findings of pemphigus and LE types in the skin were confirmed by other investigators (5,108). Some investigators did not detect ANA in serum (37). It should be stressed that pemphigus antibodies in cases with coexistent ANA may be undetectable due to the interference phenomenon (10,17). Interestingly, we have found this variety of pemphigus to be associated more frequently than pemphigus vulgaris with myasthenia gravis, thymoma, and other autoimmune disorders (19,47).

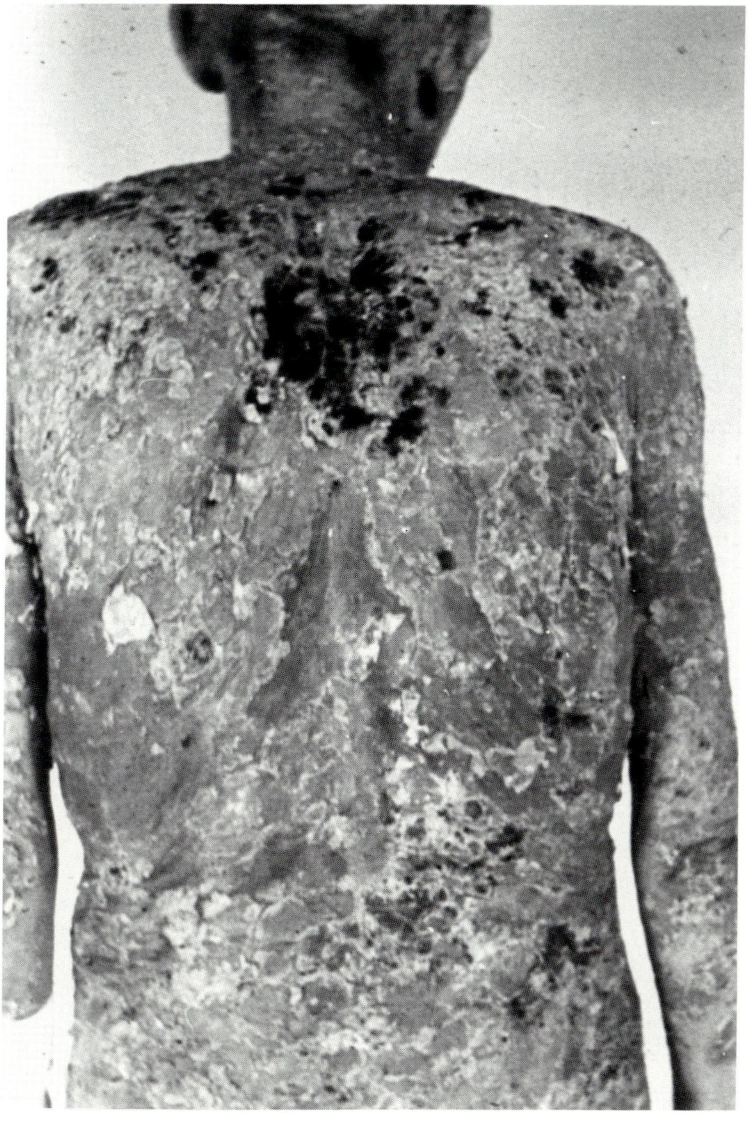

Figure 3. A case of pemphigus foliaceus. Erythematous and scaling lesions with erosions.

PEMPHIGUS FOLIACEUS

This variety, which is widespread and not infrequently generalized (Fig. 3) with superficial bullae and usually with subcorneal acantholysis, is related to pemphigus erythematosus. In the course of the disease, the clinical picture shows variations; and in some relapses, may resemble pemphigus erythematosus or pemphigus herpetiformis (Fig. 4). A possible similarity to DH may be the reason why, in the old literature, pemphigus

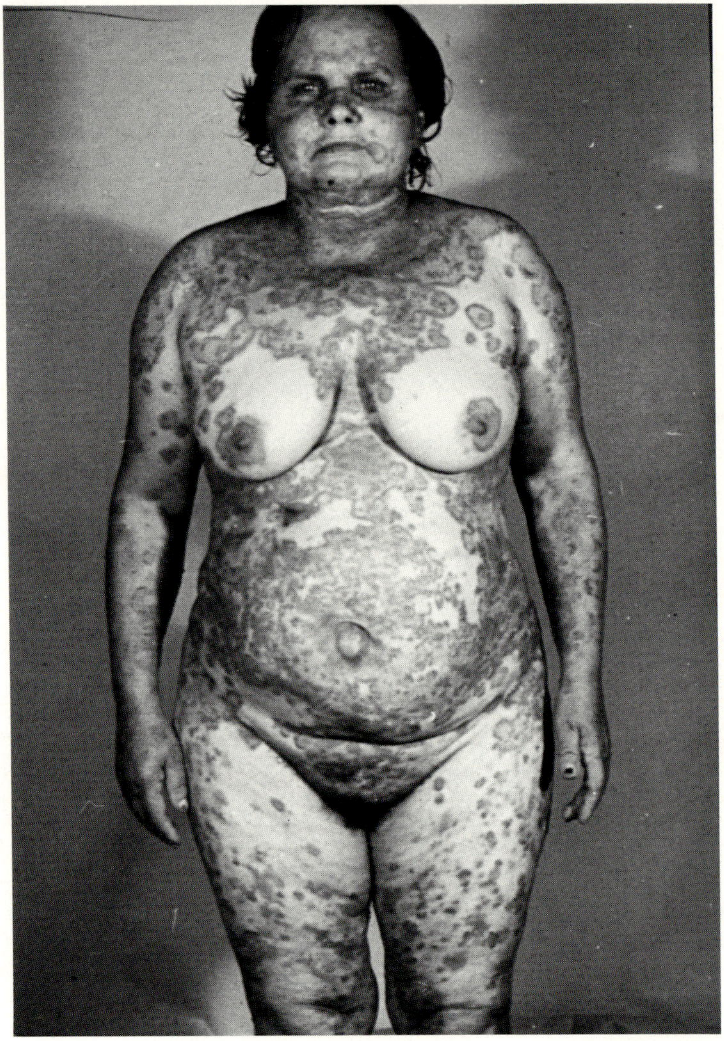

Figure 4. A case of pemphigus foliaceus. Erythematous and vesicular lesions with central clearing and peripheral spread.

and DH were regarded as two variants of the same disease (107,114). The immunopathology differs somewhat from that of pemphigus vulgaris. Frequently, the IC deposits of IgG are predominant in the superficial layers of the epidermis. This has been interpreted as a loss of the antigen from the lower layers of the epidermis since, in those cases, pemphigus vulgaris sera were also not reactive with those areas (14,89). On the other hand, recent immunoblot studies revealed differences between the antigens reactive with IC antibodies of pemphigus foliaceus and pemphigus vulgaris (103a). Interestingly, although oral mucosa is usually not involved, the DIF staining is positive for IC

IgG deposits (15). We have recently demonstrated differences in the specificity of pemphigus antibodies (see Addendum to Chap. 9).

The titers of pemphigus antibodies are usually high, probably due to the large extent of skin lesions. Periodically, in some relapses, circulating antibodies may be undetectable, especially if skin lesions are of the pemphigus herpetiformis type (see below).

SOUTH AMERICAN PEMPHIGUS FOLIACEUS (FOGO SELVAGEM)

This variety has all clinical, histologic, and immunologic features of pemphigus foliaceus. That is, there are no clinically and histologically detectable oral lesions, but immunopathology was found to be positive in all patients studied (15,102). In contrast to nonendemic pemphigus erythematosus, IF deposits at the dermal-epidermal junction are not found in cases of fogo selvagem with the features of pemphigus erythematosus (15). The difference between fogo selvagem and other forms of pemphigus is its endemic occurrence, which is suggestive of the role of environmental factors (see Chap. 11). An interesting observation, in this respect, was the presence of circulating pemphigus antibodies in some family members of the patients and in nonrelated individuals living in the same neighborhood (16).

PEMPHIGUS HERPETIFORMIS

Pemphigus herpetiformis, in large part, is a clinical diagnosis based on the appearance of the lesions (see Fig. 4). It is a form of true pemphigus in the sense that all cases give characteristic positive DIF findings. Most cases of pemphigus herpetiformis behave like variants of pemphigus foliaceus, with superficial acantholysis and without oral lesions. In the old literature, cases of pemphigus foliaceus with clinical features of DH were regarded as transitional forms between the two diseases (for historic review, see [107]). Similar cases were reported under different names: clinically typical "DH presenting acantholysis" (34,100), "dermatitis herpetiformis with acantholysis" or "pemphigus with response to sulfonamides" (116), and "pemphigus controlled by sulfapyridine" (97). Since the IF studies have finally solved the controversy, this unusual bullous disease should be regarded as a form of pemphigus. Because of the similarity to DH, the name "pemphigus herpetiformis" (48) is now widely accepted (4,39,62,82). The clinical features are variable, ranging from urticarial and erythematous (Fig. 5) to papular and vesicular lesions in herpetiform arrangement (Fig. 6). Both erythematous and urticarial lesions manifest central clearing and peripheral spreading (Fig. 4 and 6). In some cases, they may resemble fungal infections. A common histologic sign is eosinophilic spongiosis (4,30,39,82), with or without acantholysis. If acantholysis is present (see Table 3), it is usually superficial and scanty.

While a typical DIF pattern appears in all cases, circulating IC antibodies were detected in less than half of our cases (38%). The course of the disease is usually more benign than in pemphigus vulgaris. Since some cases respond to sulfones (4,39,82), it is reasonable to start treatment with this medication. A combined therapy with sulfones and corticosteroids may be beneficial in others, and some require high doses of corticosteroids and immunosuppressants, as in other forms of pemphigus (Table 3).

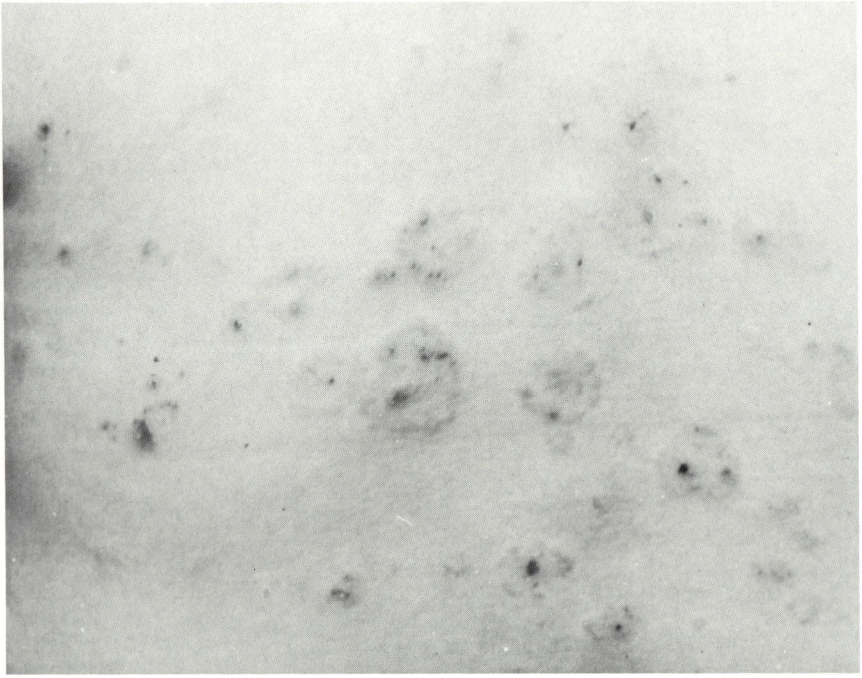

Figure 5. A case of pemphigus herpetiformis. Mostly urticarial lesions with small vesicles in periphery.

UNCLASSIFIED VARIETIES

These may present manifestations of urticaria (82), erythema multiforme (2), erythema centrifugum annulare (Fig. 7) (18,28,42), intertrigo (18), etc. These cases are clinically unrecognizable, and histology may not be diagnostic, since eosinophilic spongiosis (a common feature of these atypical forms) may not necessarily be accompanied by acantholysis. The diagnosis can be established only by IF studies. DIF may be decisive, because circulating antibodies are not infrequently undetectable.

INDUCED PEMPHIGUS

Changes similar to or identical with pemphigus were reported to be induced by external factors, mainly burns (8,18,20), and by drugs. Penicillamine or chemically related compounds (27,44) are the most common causative drugs. As seen in Table 4, the most frequent provoking factors in our series were burns and (secondly) penicillamine. The most common clinical form was pemphigus foliaceus or erythematosus, or transitional variety between the two (about 80% in our series). Bullae were occasional, rather flaccid, and with scaling and crusted lesions localized mainly on the trunk and proximal parts of extremities, not infrequently on the face and scalp. The less common clinical form was pemphigus vulgaris (2 of 11 cases in our series). Histology usually showed

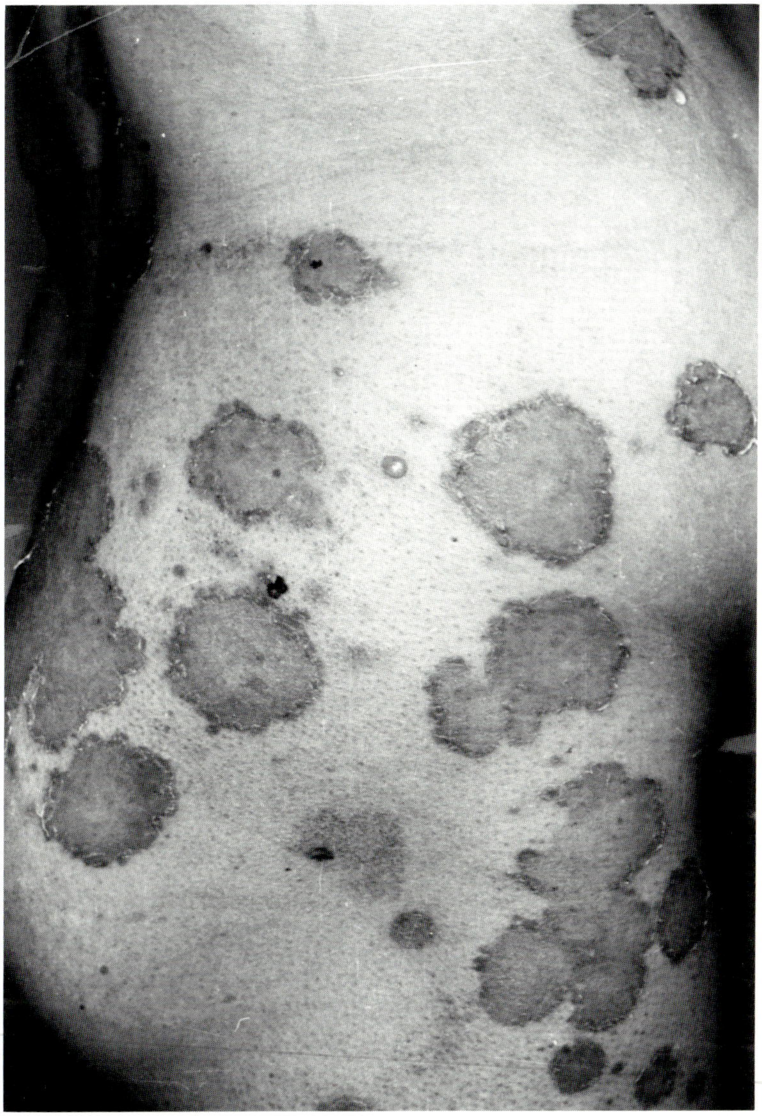

Figure 6. A case of pemphigus herpetiformis. Erythematous lesions with central healing and small vesicles in periphery.

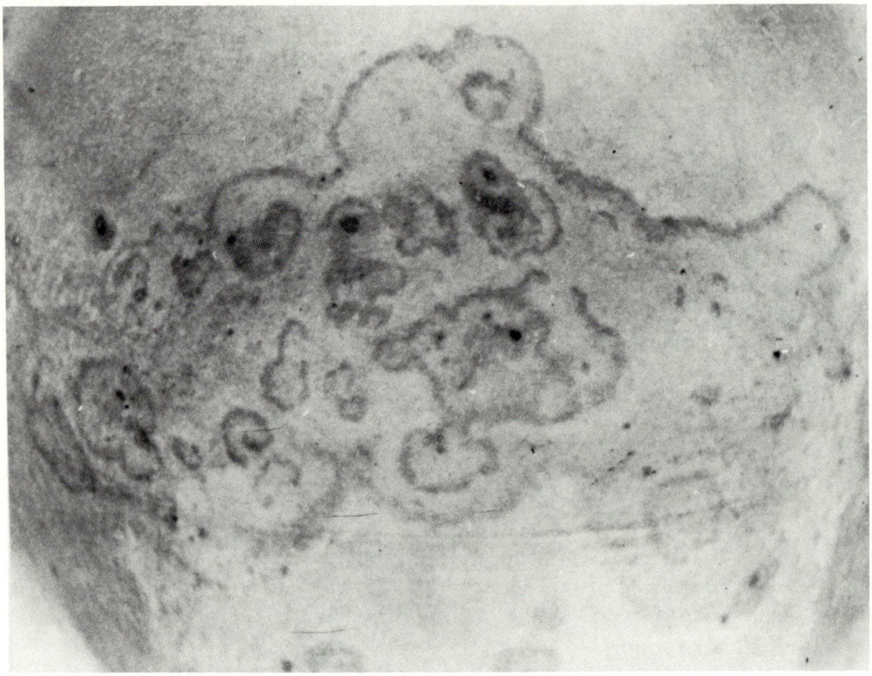

Figure 7. A case of unclassified pemphigus with erythema centrifugum annulare-type lesions.

Table 4. Findings in 11 Cases of Provoked Pemphigus

	Forms of pemphigus				*IF findings*	
	Cases (No.)	*Vulgaris*	*Erythematosus*	*Foliaceus*	*DIF pos.*	*IIF pos. (titers)*
Burn	7	2	4	1	7	5 (40–1280)
Butazolidine	1			1	1	1 (1280)
Drugs						
d-Penicillamine	3		1	2	3	1 (160)
Totals	11	2	5	4	11	7
Percentages		18	45	36	100	64

evident acantholysis, most pronounced in the upper parts of the epidermis, with the exception of two pemphigus vulgaris cases. In all patients, immune deposits were present in IC substance of the epidermis. In the majority of our cases (7 of 11), circulating IC antibodies were present in titers ranging from 40 to 1280. All lesions provoked by burns regressed after therapy with small doses of corticosteroids (40 to 60 mg). In one patient, local treatment with steroids was sufficient to control the disease. Pemphigus foliaceus provoked by butazolidine in a patient with rheumatoid arthritis was very severe and long-lasting, and it had to be treated with large doses of steroids. Pemphigus was induced by penicillamine in three patients with rheumatoid arthritis, and it had a rather mild course in two patients; one was resistant to treatment with low doses of corticosteroids.

Of 82 cases of penicillamine-induced pemphigus described in the literature up to 1983, 69% were pemphigus foliaceus, 15% were pemphigus vulgaris, 12% were pemphigus erythematosus, and a single case of pemphigus herpetiformis was described (54). Direct IF was reported to be negative in 7 of 25 patients (28%) in a survey by Santa Cruz et al. (96) and in 15% of 82 cases in a survey by Kaplan and Callen (54). The IC immune deposits were usually IgG and complement and rarely IgM; exceptionally, IgM was the only component (118). In most cases of pemphigus erythematosus, immune deposits were also present at the dermal-epidermal junction of light-exposed skin (50). Cases with negative DIF findings have also been reported (7,70), usually with IC antibodies in circulation, and sometimes in a high titer. It is conceivable that these were pemphigus-like antibodies (PLA), as suggested by Ansel (2) who reported a case with very high titers of complement-fixing IC antibodies and negative DIF findings. However, in general, IC antibodies were either absent in 50 to 65% (54) of cases or present in low titers. In some cases, both DIF and IIF findings were negative, although the clinical and histologic features were quite characteristic of pemphigus (36,110); these cases, of course, are open to question.

Penicillamine may have a nonimmunologic effect on the skin (91). As shown by Ruocco (91), skin tissue cultures grown in the presence of penicillamine develop acantholytic changes. Penicillamine is known to bind easily to sulfhydryl groups of the keratinocyte cell membranes, thereby impairing cell cohesion. This may induce the observed acantholysis. Alternatively, by modifying surface antigens of keratinocytes, it may evoke production of PLA or pemphigus antibodies.

It should be stressed that other drugs reported to induce pemphigus foliaceus or erythematosus have similar chemical structure. They include mercaptopropionylglycine used in cystinuria (66), thiopronine (1) or pyritinol used in rheumatoid arthritis (22), and captopril—a new, potent antihypertensive agent (81).

Pemphigus induced by penicillamine regressed in a majority of cases after discontinuation of therapy (26,74,106). Alternatively, it may take a milder course and may be easily controlled by low doses of corticosteroids within several weeks or months. However, in about 25 to 30% of cases (54), the disease persisted (35,60,70,108). In some cases, relapses may occur after a long symptom-free period (21). These cases require the same type of therapy as other forms of pemphigus (35,60). In brief, penicillamine clearly induces true pemphigus with typical clinical, immunologic, and histologic features. The available data suggest that it may induce clinical and histologic features of pemphigus without immunologic markers, with or without PLA, which are not bound in vivo.

PEMPHIGUS COEXISTENT WITH THYMOMA AND OTHER AUTOIMMUNE DISEASES

Coexistence of pemphigus with thymoma and myasthenia gravis has been repeatedly reported (10,23,43,45,47,56,67,68,79,88,93,103–105,109,112,115,117).

In our series of six cases, pemphigus foliaceus or erythematosus were the only forms associated with this syndrome. In the statistics given by Kaplan and Callen (54), pemphigus vulgaris was the most common variety (47%) among the reported cases; 37% were pemphigus erythematosus and 13% were pemphigus foliaceus. This discrepancy may be due to the criteria of recognition of pemphigus vulgaris.

In pemphigus of the erythematous or foliaceus type, immune deposits were not infrequently present at the dermal-epidermal junction, and ANA occurred in the circulation, as in SLE. And, indeed, overt SLE cases have been reported (12,19,49,54,61,101), as have other autoimmune disorders, mainly rheumatoid arthritis (29,33,62,78) and single cases of pernicious anemia (69).

Myasthenia gravis itself is an autoimmune disease in which antibodies against acetylcholine receptors seem to have a pathogenic potential proven by passive transfer experiments (64).

It has been suggested that spindle cell thymic tumors may be related to the concurrent development of pemphigus and myasthenia gravis (61). Antigenic similarities between thymic Hassall's bodies and keratinocyte constituents have been implicated in the induction of IC autoantibody formation. IC antibodies have also been reported to occur in cases of thymoma without clinical features of pemphigus (113). Whether these are true pemphigus antibodies or PLA remains to be determined.

Myasthenia gravis, as a rule, preceded the onset of pemphigus, and thymoma has been recognized in these patients before or after the appearance of skin lesions (12,19,45,49,117). Thymectomy is usually beneficial for myasthenia gravis, but pemphigus has been reported to either improve (32,50) or exacerbate after thymechtomy (112). However, neither the exact time of development of thymoma nor the beginning of pemphigus can be established precisely. Thymoma may not be detectable, and abortive superficial bullous lesions may be overlooked.

Thymectomy does not necessarily mean a complete removal of the tumor, since the scattered thymic satellites may exert their adverse immunologic activity regardless of whether the tumor is malignant.

Characteristic IF findings in pemphigus associated with myasthenia and/or thymoma are circulating IC, antistriated muscle, antinuclear antibodies and specific acetylcholine receptor antibodies (23,64,79).

Direct IF in skin, in and around the lesions, as a rule shows IgG bound to IC substances of the epidermis. In pemphigus foliaceus or erythematosus in light-exposed areas, immune deposits not infrequently are also present at the dermal-epidermal junction. In such cases, sun exposure may provoke an acute exacerbation (19,23,105,111). In one of our cases with myasthenia gravis and thymoma, a typical butterfly-like rash developed after sun exposure concurrently with other signs of systemic lupus erythematosus (SLE), including lupus nephritis. The coexistence of pemphigus with myasthenia gravis and thymoma seems not to be fortuitous, and the cases of this type provide further evidence for autoimmune pathomechanism of pemphigus.

PEMPHIGUS ASSOCIATED WITH NEOPLASIA

Malignancy associated with pemphigus includes carcinomas and lymphomas (38,58,63,75,85,94); for a review, see Kaplan and Callen (54). Although a long-lasting immunosuppressive therapy is known to enhance the incidence of neoplasia (41,59,65), there does not seem to be a causal relationship between such therapy and pemphigus. Neoplasias associated with pemphigus are of different types and are reported to occur in various organs (3,71,80,95). Most importantly, the frequency did not exceed the incidence for the age group of the patients (54). There is no evidence for antigenic components of any internal tumors that react with pemphigus antibodies. We had a case with pemphigus foliaceus-like clinical and histologic features, as well as a malignant and rapidly growing, convoluted lymphoblastic lymphoma of the mediastinum with no thymus involvement. Repeated IF studies of biopsy specimens and serum were negative for IgG IC deposits and circulating IC antibodies. Neither skin lesions nor the tumor were responsive to high dosages of corticosteroids and immunosuppressants, and the patient eventually died. The lack of response of bullous rash to such an aggressive therapy suggests a nonimmunologic mechanism of acantholytic disease having clinical and histologic signs of typical pemphigus.

In conclusion, there is, at present, no convincing evidence for a causal relationship between malignant tumors (other than thymoma) and true pemphigus.

COMMENTS ON PLASMAPHERESIS IN TREATMENT OF PEMPHIGUS

Plasmapheresis, as an adjunct to the treatment of pemphigus, was introduced by Ruocco et al. (91a) with a view toward decreasing levels of antibodies to the IC areas. It has been effective in a limited number of problem cases when used with conventional modes of treatment. Originally it was thought that plasmapheresis would remove IC antibodies, and that this would provide additional evidence for their pathogenic potential. It should be stressed, however, that the patients have to be concurrently treated with corticosteroids and/or immunosuppressive drugs. In reality, the level of the antibodies is even enhanced apparently by the rebound phenomenon after initial removal of the plasma (14a). This is a result of a feedback mechanism in the regulation of the antibody synthesis.

Since plasma exchange is an expensive procedure, only severe cases resistant to corticosteroids and immunosuppressants have been studied. There is no firm consensus as to how much, and in what time intervals, plasma should be removed. In most reports, large volumes of plasmapheresis (2 to 5 liters) were used with very good results (91a). In our own experience, small volumes of plasmapheresis (550 to 800 ml), performed once a week, were equally effective (12a), and this has been confirmed by Ruocco et al. (91a). One explanation for the observed similarity in responses to large and small volumes of plasmapheresis is that the feedback mechanism that stimulates cells to greater antibody synthesis also makes the cells more susceptible to the corticosteroids and immunosuppressants.

REFERENCES

1. Alinovi A, Benoldi D, Manganelli P: Pemphigus erythematosus induced by thiopronine. *Acta Dermat Venereol* 62:452, 1982.
2. Ansel J, Petrozzi JW, Kumar V: Possible drug-induced pemphigus-like antibodies with the clinical manifestation of erythema multiforme. *Arch Dermatol* 119:1006, 1983.
3. Basler RSW: Senear-Usher syndrome with parathyroid adenoma. *Br J Dermatol* 91:465, 1974.
4. Bauer R, Orfanos CE: Pemphigus herpetiformis: eine klinische Variante des Pemphigus vulgaris. *Hautarzt* 31:540, 1980.
5. Bean SF, Lynch FW: Senear-Usher syndrome/pemphigus erythematosus. Immunofluorescent studies in a patient. *Arch Dermatol* 101:642, 1970.
6. Bean SF, Holubar K, Gillett BB: Pemphigus involving the eye. *Arch Dermatol* 111:1484, 1975.

7. Benveniste M, Crouzet J, Homberg JC, et al: Pemphigus induits par la d-penicillamine dans la polyarthrite rhumatoïde. *Nouv Presse Med,* 4:3125, 1975.
8. Beutner EH, Chorzelski TP: Studies on etiologic factors in pemphigus. *J Cut Pathol* 3:67, 1976.
9. Beutner EH, Jordon RE: Demonstration of skin antibodies in sera of pemphigus vulgaris patients by indirect immunofluorescent staining. *Proc Soc Exp Biol Med* 117:505, 1964.
10. Beutner EH, Chorzelski TP, Hale WL, et al: Autoimmunity in concurrent myasthenia gravis and pemphigus erythematosus. *JAMA* 203:845, 1968.
11. Beutner EH, Lever WF, Witebsky E, et al: Autoantibodies in pemphigus vulgaris. *JAMA* 192:682, 1965.
12. Blanchet PH, Auffret N, Fauchard J, et al: Association of thymoma with pemphigus foliaceus, nephrotic syndrome and lupus biology. *Ann Dermatol Venereol* 108:471, 1981.
12a. Blaszczyk M, Chorzelski T, Daszynski J, et al: Plasmapheresis as a supplementary treatment in pemphigus. *Arch Dermatol Immunol Therap Exp* 29:763, 1981.
13. Block LJ, Caldarelli DD, Holinger PH, et al: Pemphigus of the air and food passages. *Ann Otol Rhinol Laryngol* 86:584, 1977.
14. Bystryn JC, Abel FL, De Feo D: Pemphigus foliaceus: Subcorneal intercellular antibodies of unique specificity. *Arch Dermatol* 110:857, 1972.
14a. Bystryn J-C: Adjuvant therapy of pemphigus. *Arch Dermatol* 120:941, 1984.
15. Castro RM, Roscoe JT, Prado Sampaio SA: Brazilian pemphigus foliaceus. In Ahmed AR (Ed): *Clinics in Dermatology,* Vol. 1. Lippincott, Philadelphia, 1983, pp 22–41.
16. Castro RM, Chorzelski TP, Jablonska S, et al: Antiepithelial antibodies in healthy people living in an endemic area of South American pemphigus foliaceus (fogo selvagem). Preliminary report. *Castellania* 4:111, 1976.
17. Chorzelski TP, Beutner EH: Factors contributing to the occasional failures of detection of pemphigus antibodies by indirect immunofluorescent test. *J Invest Dermatol* 53:188, 1969.
18. Chorzelski TP, Beutner EH, Jabłonska S: The role and nature of autoimmunity in pemphigus. In Beutner EH, Chorzelski TP, Bean SF (Eds): *Immunopathology of the Skin* ed. 2. Wiley, New York, 1979, pp 183–229.
19. Chorzelski TP, Jablonska S, Błaszczyk M: Immunopathological investigations in the Senear-Usher syndrome (coexistence of pemphigus and lupus erythematosus). *Br J Dermatol* 80:211, 1968.
20. Chorzelski TP, Jabłońska S, Beutner EH, et al: Can pemphigus be provoked by a burn? *Br J Dermatol* 85:320, 1971.
21. Chouvet B, Thivolet J, Bathias J, et al: Pemphigus induit par la d-pénicillamine. *Dermatololgica* 160:297, 1980.
22. Civatte J, Duterque M, Blanchet P, et al: Deux cas de pemphigus superficial induit par le pyritinol. *Ann Dermatol Venereol* 105:573, 1978.
23. Cooper A, Wells JV: Pemphigus foliaceus, myasthenia gravis, and thymoma in a patient with serological evidence of SLE. *Aust NZJ Med* 11:277, 1981.
24. Cormane RH, Chorzelski TP: "Bound" complement in the epidermis of patients with pemphigus vulgaris. *Dermatologica* 134:463, 1967.
25. Cram DL, Fukuyama K: Immunohistochemistry of ultraviolet induced pemphigus and pemphigoid lesions. *Arch Dermatol* 106:819, 1972.
26. Davies MG, Holt P: Pemphigus in a patient treated with penicillamine for generalized morphea. *Arch Dermatol* 112:1308, 1976.
27. Degos R, Touraine R, Belaich S, et al: Pemphigus chez un malaide traité par penicillamine pour malaide de Wilson. *Bull Soc Fr Dermatol Syph* 76:751, 1969.
28. Degos R, Civatte J, Belaich S, et al: Pemphigus avec aspect clinique d'erythème annulaire centrifuge de Darier et immage histologique de spongiose à éosinophiles. *Ann Dermatol Venerol* 105:861, 1978.
29. Diaz LA, Glamb RW, Silva J Jr: A syndrome of multiple immune autoreactivity. *Arch Dermatol* 116:77, 1980.
30. Emmerson RW, Wilson Jones E: Eosinophilic spongiosis in pemphigus. A report of unusual histological change in pemphigus. *Arch Dermatol* 97:252, 1968.

31. Epstein JH, Feigen GM, Epstein NN: Pemphigus vulgaris with lesions of the rectal mucosa. *Arch Dermatol* 78:36, 1958.
32. Faber WR, Neumann HAM, Flinterman J: Persistent vegetating and keratotic lesions in patients with pemphigus vulgaris during immunosuppressive therapy. *Br J Dermatol* 109:459, 1983.
33. Falk ES: Pemphigus foliaceus in a patient with rheumatoid arthritis and Sjögrens syndrome. *Dermatologica* 158:348, 1979.
34. Floden CH, Gentele H: A case of clinically typical dermatitis herpetiformis (M. Duhring) presenting acantholysis. *Acta Derma Venereol* 35:128, 1955.
35. From E, Frederikson P: Pemphigus vulgaris following d-penicillamine. *Dermatologica* 152:358, 1976.
36. Fulton RA, Thomson J: Penicillamine-induced bullous dermatosis. *Br J Dermatol* 107(Suppl 22):95, 1982.
37. Gianetti A: Immunofluorescence studies in the Senear-Usher syndrome. *Arch Dermatol Forsch* 248:287, 1974.
38. Good VD, Pasricha JS: Pemphigus and Hodgkins disease. *Br J Dermatol* 99:575, 1974.
39. Haensch R: Pemphigus herpetiformis. *Hautarzt* 30:418, 1979.
40. Hallopeau H: "Pyodermite végétante," ihre Beziehungen zur Dermatitis herpetiformis und dem Pemphigus vegetans. *Arch Dermatol u Syph* 43:289, 1898.
41. Harris CC: Malignancy during methotrexate and steroid therapy for psoriasis. *Arch Dermatol* 103:501, 1971.
42. Hashimoto T, Sugiura M, Kurihara S, et al: Atypical pemphigus showing eosinophilic spongiosis. *Clin Exp Dermatatol* 8:37, 1983.
43. Hatano H: Pemphigus erythematosus, myasthenia gravis and thymoma. *Jpn J Clin Dermatol* 25:1094, 1971.
44. Hewitt J, Leasana-Leibowitch M, Benveniste M, et al: Un cas de pemphigus induit par la D-penicillamine. Le pemphigus iatrogéne existe-til?. *Ann Med Interne* 122:1003, 1971.
45. Imamura S, Takigawa M, Ikai K, et al: Pemphigus foliaceus, myasthenia gravis, thymoma and red cell aplasia. *Clin Exp Dermatol* 3:285, 1978.
46. Jabłońska S, Chorzelski TP, Beutner EH: Indications for skin and serum immunofluorescence in dermatology. In Beutner EH, Chorzelski TP, Bean SF (Eds): *Immunopathology of the Skin,* Wiley, New York, 1979, pp 3–28.
47. Jabłońska S, Chorzelski TP, Lebioda J: Koexistenz von Pemphigus erythematosus und Myasthenia gravis. *Hautarzt* 21:156, 1970.
48. Jabłońska S, Chorzelski TP, Beutner EH, et al: Herpetiform pemphigus, a variable pattern of pemphigus. *Int J Dermatol* 14:353, 1975.
49. Jabłońska S, Chorzelski TP, Błaszczyk M, et al: Pathogenesis of pemphigus erythematosus. *Arch Dermatol Res* 258:135, 1977.
50. de Jong MCJM, Doeglas HMG, Dijkstra JWE: Immunohistochemical findings in a patient with penicillamine induced pemphigus. *Br J Dermatol* 102:333, 1980.
51. Joost van Th, Cormane RH, Pondman KW: Direct immunofluorescent study of the skin on occurrence of complement in pemphigus. *Br J Dermatol* 87:466, 1972.
52. Jordon RE: The complement system in pemphigus and bullous pemphigoid. In Beutner EH, Chorzelski TP, Bean SF (Eds): *Immunopathology of the Skin,* ed. 2. Wiley, New York, 1979, pp 135–145.
53. Jordon RE, Schroeter AL, Rogers RS III, et al: Classical and alternate pathway activation of complement in pemphigus vulgaris lesions. *J Invest Dermatol* 63:256, 1974.
54. Kaplan RP, Callen JP: Pemphigus associated diseases and induced pemphigus. In Ahmed AR (Ed): *Clinics in Dermatology,* vol. 1. Lippincott, Philadelphia, 1983, pp 42–71.
55. Kaplan RP, Touloukian J, Ahmed R, et al: Esophagitis dissecans superficialis associated with pemphigus vulgaris. *J. Am. Acad. Dermatol.* 4:682, 1981.
56. Kavli G: Pemphigus vulgaris and thymoma. A T-lymphocyte defect? *Br J Dermatol* 99:97, 1978.
57. Krain LS: Pemphigus—epidemiologic and survival characteristics of 59 patients, 1959–1973. *Arch Dermatol* 110:862, 1974.

58. Krain LS, Bierman SM: Pemphigus vulgaris and internal malignancy. *Cancer* 33:1091, 1974.
59. Krain LS, London J, Newcomer VD: Cyclophosphamide in the treatment of pemphigus vulgaris and bullous pemphigoid. *Arch Dermatol* 106:657, 1972.
60. Kristensen JK, Wadskov S: Penicillamine-induced pemphigus foliaceus. *Acta Dermatol Venereol* 57:69, 1977.
61. Kough EH, Barnes WT: Thymoma associated with erythroid aplasia, bullous skin eruption and the LE cell phenomenon. *Ann Intern Med* 61:308, 1964.
62. Lagerholm B, Frithz A, Borglund E: Light and electron microscopic aspects of pemphigus herpetiformis (eosinophilic spongiosis) in comparison with other acantholytic disorders. *Acta Dermatol Venereol* 59:305, 1979.
63. Lakaris GC, Papavasilion SS, Bovopoulac OD: Association of oral pemphigus with chronic lymphocytic leukemia. *Oral Surg* 50:244, 1980.
64. Lindstrom J: Autoimmune response to acetylocholine receptors in myasthenia gravis and its animal model. *Adv Immunol* 27:1, 1979.
65. Lowney ED: Antimitotic drugs and aggressive squamous cell tumors. *Arch Dermatol* 105:924, 1972.
66. Lucky PA, Skovby F, Thier SO: Pemphigus foliaceus and proteinuria induced by A-mercaptopropionylglycine. *J Am Acad Dermatol* 8:667, 1983.
67. Lynfield VL, Pertschuk LP, Zimmerman A: Pemphigus erythematosus provoked by allergic contact dermatitis. *Arch Dermatol* 108:690, 1973.
68. Maize JC, Dobson RL, Provost TT: Pemphigus and myasthenia gravis. *Arch Dermatol* 111:1334, 1975.
69. Maize JC, Green D, Provost TT: Pemphigus foliaceus, a case with serologic features of Senear-Usher syndrome and other autoimmune abnormalities. *J Am Acad Dermatol* 7:737, 1982.
70. Marsden RA, Hill H, Morvat AG, et al: Penicillamine-induced pemphigus. *Proc Roy Soc Med* 70:103, 1977.
71. McKee PH, McClelland M, Sondford JC: Co-existence of pemphigus, anti-skeletal muscle antibody and a retroperitoneal paraganglioma. *Br J Dermatol* 99:441, 1978.
72. Meurer M, Millns JL, Rogers RS, et al: Oral pemphigus vulgaris. A report of ten cases. *Arch Dermatol* 113:1520, 1977.
73. Mikhail GR, Drukker BH: Pemphigus vulgaris involving the cervix uteri. *Arch Dermatol* 95:496, 1967.
74. Morioka S, Ogawa H: Herpetiform pemphigus-like skin lesions induced by d-penicillamine. *J Dermatol* 7:425, 1980.
75. Muller SA, Herrmann ED, Winkelmann RK: Herpes simplex infections in hematologic malignancies. *Am J Med* 52:102, 1972.
76. Nelson CG, Apisarnthanarax P, Bean SF, et al: Pemphigus vegetans of Hallopeau. Immunofluorescent studies. *Arch Dermatol* 113:942, 1977.
77. Neumann HAM, Farber WR: Pyodermite vegetante of Hallopeau. Immunofluorescence studies performed in an early disease stage. *Arch Dermatol* 116:1169, 1980.
78. Neumann-Jensen B, Worsaae N, Dabelsteen E, et al: Pemphigus vulgaris and pemphigus foliaceus coexisting with oral lichen planus. *Br J Dermatol* 102:585, 1980.
79. Noguchi S, Nishitani H: Immunologic studies of a case of myasthenia gravis associated with pemphigus vulgaris after thymectomy. *Neurology* 26:1075, 1976.
80. Ortonne JP, Elbare P, Faure M, et al: Pemphigus vulgaire et pseudolymphome de Castleman. *Ann Dermatol Venereol* 110:662, 1983.
81. Parfrey P, Clement M, Vandenburg M, et al: Captopril-induced pemphigus. *Br Med J* 3:194, 1980.
82. Parodi A, Nunzi E, Rebora A: Urticaria presenting as manifestation of pemphigus herpetiformis. *Dermatologica* 164:278, 1982.
83. Pearson RW, O'Donoghue M, Kaplan SJ: Pemphigus vegetans. Its relationship to eosinophilic spongiosus and favorable response to dapsone. *Arch Dermatol* 116:65, 1980.
84. Percival GH: Diagnostic du pemphigus foliacée et du syndrome de Senear-Usher. *Arch Belges Dermatol Syph* 5:278, 1949.
85. Pisanti S, Garfunkel A: Kaposi's sarcoma. *J Oral Med* 25:89, 1970.

86. Pisanti S, Sharav Y, Kaufman E, et al: Pemphigus vulgaris: Incidence in Jews of different ethnic groups according to age, sex and initial lesions. *Oral Med* 38:382, 1974.
87. Rague CJ, Stein KM, Samitz MH: Pemphigus involving the esophagus. *Arch Dermatol* 102:371, 1970.
88. Ridley CM: Pemphigus vulagris, myasthenia gravis and membranous colitis. *Postgrad Med J* 46:168, 1970.
89. Rodriguez J, Bystryn JC: Pemphigus foliaceus associated with absence of intercellular antigens in lower layers of epidermis. *Arch Dermatol* 113:1696, 1977.
90. Rosenberg FR, Sanders S, Nelson CT: Pemphigus: A 20-year review of 107 patients treated with corticosteroids. *Arch Dermatol* 112:962, 1976.
91. Ruocco V, de Luca M, Pisani M, et al: Pemphigus provoked by d-penicillamine. An experimental approach using in vitro tissue cultures. *Dermatologica* 164:236, 1982.
91a. Ruocco V, Astarita C, Pisani M: Plasmapheresis as an alternative or adjunctive therapy in problem cases of pemphigus. *Dermatologica* 168:219, 1984.
92. Ryan JG: Pemphigus: A 24-year survey of experience with 70 cases. *Arch Dermatol* 104:14, 1971.
93. Safai B, Gupta S, Good RA: Pemphigus vulgaris associated with a syndrome of immunodeficiency and thymoma, a case report. *Clin Exp Dermatol* 3:129, 1978.
94. Saikia NK: Extraction of pemphigus antibodies from a lymphoid neoplasm and its possible relationship to pemphigus vulgaris. *Br J Dermatol* 86:411, 1972.
95. Saikia NK, MacConnell LFS: Senear-Usher syndrome and internal malignancy. *Br J Dermatol* 87:1, 1972.
96. Santa-Cruz DJ, Marcus MD, Prioleau PG, et al: Pemphigus-like lesions induced by d-penicillamine. Analysis of clinical, histopathological and immunofluorescence features in 34 cases. *Am J Dermatol* 3:85, 1981.
97. Seah PP, Fry L, Cairns RJ, et al: Pemphigus controlled by sulphapyridine. *Br J Dermatol* 89:77, 1973.
98. Senear FE, Usher B: An unusual type of pemphigus combining features of lupus erythematosus. *Arch Dermatol* 13:761, 1926.
99. Simon DG, Krutchkoff D, Kaslow RA, et al: Pemphigus in Hartford County, Connecticut from 1972 to 1977. *Arch Dermatol* 116:1035, 1980.
100. Sneddon I, Churg R: Pemphigus foliaceus presenting as dermatitis herpetiformis. *Acta Dermatol Venereol* 47:440, 1967.
101. Somorin AO, Agbakwu SN, Nwaefuna A: Systemic lupus erythematosus and pemphigus vulgaris preceded by depressive psychosis. *Central African J Med* 27:12, 1981.
102. Sotto MN, Shimizu H, Costa JM, et al: South American pemphigus foliaceus: Electron microscopy and immunoelectron localization of bound immunoglobulin in the skin and mucosa. *Br J Dermatol* 102:521, 1980.
103. Souteyrand P, Berthier-Boachon M, Thivolet J: Association pemphigus et thymome: Revue de la littérature et étiopathogénie. *Ann Dermatol Venereol* 108:457, 1981.
103a. Stanley JR, Koulu K, Thivolet Ch: Distinction between epidermal antigens binding pemphigus vulgaris and pemphigus foliaceus autoantibodies. *J Clin Invest* 74:313, 1984.
104. Stillman MA, Baer RL: Pemphigus and thymoma. *Acta Dermatol Venereol* 52:393, 1972.
105. Tagami H, Imamura S, Noguchi S, et al: Co-existence of peculiar pemphigus, myasthenia gravis and malignant thymoma. *Dermatologica* 152:181, 1976.
106. Tan SG, Rowell NR: Pemphigus like syndrome induced by d-penicillamine. *Br J Dermatol* 95:99, 1976.
107. Tappeiner J, Pfleger L: Pemphigus vulgaris-Dermatitis herpetiformis. Eine historische Streitfrage der Wiener dermatologischen Schule. *Arch klin exp Derm* 214:415, 1962.
108. Thorvaldsen J: Two cases of penicillamine-induced pemphigus erythematosus. *Dermatologica* 159:167, 1979.
109. Touraine R, Revuz J, Prost Y, et al: Pemphigus, myasthenia and thymoma. *Ann Med* 127:923, 1976.
110. Troy JL, Silvers DN, Grossman ME, et al: Penicillamine-associated pemphigus: Is it really pemphigus?. *J Am Acad Dermatol* 4:547, 1981.

111. Uhlin SR, Maiocco KJ, Bhatia SG: Pemphigus erythematosus and thymoma. *Cutis* 25:177, 1980.
112. Vetters JM, Saikia NK, Wood J, et al: Pemphigus vulgaris and myasthenia gravis. *Br J Dermatol* 88:437, 1973.
113. Whittingham S, MacKay IR: The pemphigus antibody and immunopathies affecting the thymus. *Br J Dermatol* 84:1, 1971.
114. Wiedmann A: Dermatitis herpetiformis-Pemphigus vulgaris. *Wien Med Wschr* 106:434, 1956.
115. Wilhelm T, Metz J, Deuchert K: Pemphigus erythematosus and malignant thymoma. *Hautarzt* 33:156, 1982.
116. Winkelmann RK, Roth HL: Dermatitis herpetiformis with acantholysis or pemphigus with response to sulfonamides. *Arch Dermatol* 82:385, 1960.
117. Yoshinaga H, Yamada JM, Imamura S: A case of pemphigus foliaceus associated with thymoma, myasthenia gravis, nephrosis, and red cell aplasia. *Jpn J Dermatol* 87:251, 1977.
118. Zone J, Ward J, Boyce E, et al: Penicillamine induced pemphigus. *JAMA* 247:2705, 1982.

11
Passive Transfer for Studies of Bullous Diseases: Review of Original Studies and Unpublished Comments on Brazilian Pemphigus

Philip S. Spencer
Ernst H. Beutner
Frederick Helm

INTRODUCTION

The original report on passive transfers of both intercellular (IC) antibodies of pemphigus and basement membrane zone (BMZ) antibodies of pemphigoid by Beutner et al. (4) in 1965 and by Chertok (8) revealed in vivo binding in normal monkey skin, but no acantholysis. While there were no formalized concepts on the nature of pathogenic versus physiologic autoimmunity at that time, as there are now (see Chapter 7), it was realized that these findings together with the observations on comparable reaction patterns in the normal skin of patients are highly suggestive phenomena. Those realizations stimulated several studies (1,2,10,11,17,18), which are reviewed here.

Some later reviews on the transfer of pemphigus (e.g., Chap. 12) refer to the work of Lindenberg in 1937 (13). This is not a tenable association of these observations,* which

The work on this report was supported in part by a grant from the Summerhill Foundation.

*Specifically, Lindenberg (13) reported that 1 to 6 weeks after the intratesticular injections of rabbits with about 1 to 2 ml of blood of Brazilian pemphigus patients, erosive lesions in the skin developed. (The skin had been pretreated with a depilatory agent.) However, these "infections" of pemphigus and psoriasis could not be transferred. The cause of the reported "psoriatic lesions" in guinea pigs is a matter of conjecture. One possible interpretation of the observed lesions of rabbits is that they were due to the passive transfer of pemphigus antibodies. This, however, is not tenable

deal with the "infectious" nature of both psoriasis and Brazilian pemphigus. While the findings of Lindenberg do not provide reproducible observations (i.e., evidence for neither the passive transfer nor infectious nature of Brazilian pemphigus), a previously unreported observation relevant to the infectious nature of the disease is discussed in the following section.

BRAZILIAN PEMPHIGUS: POSSIBLE TRANSMISSION BY RATS

At the time of the original immunofluorescent (IF) studies of Brazilian pemphigus foliaceus (BPF) by Beutner et al. (5), virtually all of the patients in the Sao Paulo hospital for pemphigus foliaceus, as well as the even larger number of BPF patients being treated on an outpatient basis, were from the Santo Amora district of the city (2). This suburb of Sao Paulo, in the vicinity of the city water reservoir at Guarapiranga, consisted largely of a middle-class residential area.

According to Castro et al. (6), BPF cases involved all ethnic groups in endemic areas. These authors refer to "the disappearance of the disease from areas of prior endemicity as the areas become developed," citing a report by Proenca in 1977 (14). Importantly, on visiting the endemic focus of BPF in Guarapiranga, Beutner learned from the father of a teenage girl who had recently contracted pemphigus that some sick rats were seen around the house at the time his daughter developed blisters. It was not possible to undertake a study of the rats at that time. In 1978, however, Beutner contacted the World Health Organization (WHO) in an effort to begin studies of rats from this endemic area of Brazil. An agreement was reached to collect rat tissue and blood for the study through the Pan American Health Organization (PAHO), but the project was cancelled. About 1 year later, Beutner was advised through a nonmedical personal contact living near the endemic area in Sao Paulo that "there were no rats and that there was no pemphigus." These observations raise the question as to whether the WHO-PAHO project to begin studies of pemphigus in rats in endemic areas may have stimulated a rat extermination program, and that this program led to the reported decline in BPF (14) in the endemic areas of the city. If so, the project achieved its WHO-PAHO goal.

This conjecture on the role of rats is consistent with a number of other published and unpublished observations, including the finding that pemphigus antibodies occur not only in BPF patients, but also in other members of households in which they live (7). This, and other observations, led us to the following working hypothesis regarding the epidemiology of BPF:

1. A viral agent "*X*," which can infect rats cross-reacts with or alters pemphigus antigen to stimulate the autoimmune response.
2. This viral agent *X* can be carried by some arthropod from rats to humans, but is not transmitted directly from person to person.

for several reasons. One is that the lesions appeared in 1 to 6 weeks. This differs from the microscopic lesions that were induced subsequently by intradermal injections of rabbits with sera of Brazilian pemphigus patients (1,10). These appeared in 24 to 48 hours and disappeared thereafter. Also, 1 to 6 weeks after the injection of human serum, the rabbit would develop antibodies to the human IgG. These would neutralize and prevent reactions of any human antibodies, including the pemphigus antibodies. Thus, if the findings of Lindenberg could be reproduced, it is doubtful if they would be attributable to the transfer of an autoantibody.

3. If this is true, then:
   a) Extermination of rats should lead to the disappearance of the endemic form of pemphigus referred to as BPF.
   b) Rats with clinical, immunologic, and histologic hallmarks of pemphigus should be demonstrable in endemic regions.

This working hypothesis assumes importance in light of the fact that other endemic foci may appear unexpectedly in the future. Since no explanation has been given in the current review (6) for the disappearance of BPF from the urban endemic foci in the south-central parts of Brazil, this working hypothesis may prove to be of value.

ORIGINAL PASSIVE TRANSFER STUDIES INTO MONKEYS

The original observations on pemphigus and pemphigoid antibodies (2,3) led Beutner et al. to undertake passive transfer studies of both (3). Specifically, they observed that the sera of most patients with pemphigus vulgaris contain antibodies to an IC substance of stratified squamous epithelium as demonstrated by indirect immunofluorescence (IIF) staining, and that similar IC localization of IgG occurred in the skin as demonstrated by direct immunofluorescence (DIF). Eight of 13 sera from patients with pemphigus vulgaris were found to contain antibodies to a substance at the surface of the epithelial cells, particularly in the stratum spinosum, as demonstrated by IIF staining. The reactions of four of these eight sera were deemed to be weakly positive or doubtful, while the remaining four sera yielded titers of 1:30 to 1:120 by IIF staining. The reactive antigen was found only in stratified squamous epithelium. A skin biopsy specimen of one of the antibody-producing patients with pemphigus vulgaris revealed the presence of bound gamma globulin on the surface of the epithelial cells in an apparently normal portion of the skin adjacent to a vesicle. This localization was identical to that obtained by IIF staining with the patient's serum. These observations led the investigators to study the passive transfer of pemphigus antibodies by intradermal injection of antibody-containing sera into monkeys (4,8). This injection resulted in binding of the antibodies in vivo on the surface of basal cells in a pattern comparable to that of the gamma globulin binding in the patients' own normal skin (see Fig. 1). There appeared to be a correlation between the sites of gamma globulin fixation and the characteristic histopathology of the skin diseases under consideration. However, the fixation of antibody to the antigen-containing site did not necessarily lead to the development of lesions. This was evident from the failure of the injected monkeys to develop blisters, and from the demonstration of fixed gamma globulin in IC epidermal areas of apparently normal skin of patients with pemphigus. Subsequently, Sams et al. (16) reported similar changes following intravenous injections of pemphigus antibodies. However, the conclusions they drew were different, as indicated below.

Evidence favoring an autoimmune etiology of the bullous pemphigoid (BP) (referred to in the original IF study simply as a subepidermal bullous disease) included the finding that: 1) the patients' sera contained anti-BMZ antibodies; 2) when these antibodies were passively injected intradermally into monkeys, they bound in vivo to their homologous antigen; and 3) comparable in vivo binding occurred in the patients' skin (3). In a subsequent report on the same patients with subepidermal bullae, as well as some additional cases of this type by Jordon et al. (12), they were identified as cases of BP. While the in vivo binding in the BMZ of passively sensitized monkeys had been demon-

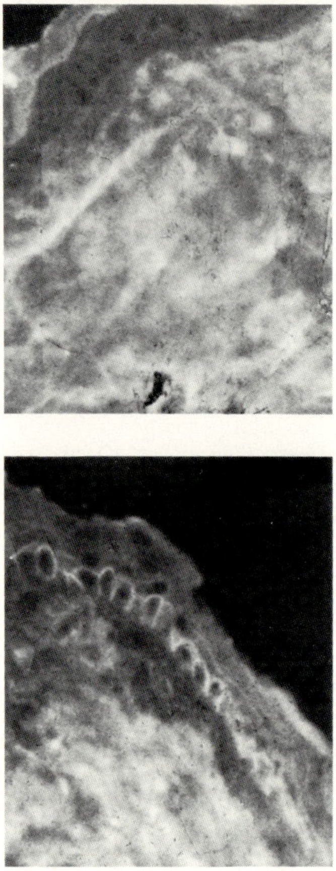

Figure 1. Intradermal (ID) injection of monkey sera with pemphigus serum. The photograph on the bottom shows an area of monkey skin that was injected with serum from a patient with pemphigus. The cells of the stratum spinosum did not demonstrate as much staining. The dermis was negative. The picture at the top is of a skin site injected with normal human serum; no evidence of IgG localization was found. (100×). (Reprinted from Chertok [8].)

strated, the question remained unanswered as to whether the disease process could be passively transferred with the circulating antibodies. However, by present criteria for the identification of pathologic and physiologic autoantibodies (see Chap. 7), the observations on passive transfer into monkeys described in this original report (3) do serve to identify the anti-BMZ antibodies as pathologic.

PASSIVE TRANSFER INTO RABBITS

Studies on the transfer of pemphigus antibodies into rabbits (1,10) yielded variable findings, while studies of transfer into monkeys gave unequivocal results. Specifically, studies by Chorzelski and Beutner (10) on rabbits noted that two factors appear to be required for the elicitation of acantholytic lesions: 1) A substance that increases permeability through the dermal-epidermal barrier to permit increased passage of the pemphigus antibodies into IC spaces of the epidermis (e.g., 2,4,dinitrochlorobenzene [DNCB]). 2) An enhancing factor(s) found in certain pathologic sera (e.g., sera from patients with pneumonia or tuberculosis). With the aid of these two factors, pemphigus-like lesions (intraepidermal acantholytic microbullae) were elicited between hair follicles in rabbit skin by intradermal injection of sera-containing pemphigus antibodies, but not by injection of other human sera. Observations made in further studies on the same system (1) revealed that the formation of intraepidermal acantholytic microbullae, which were histologically comparable to human pemphigus bullae, only occurred in the first of three groups of passive transfer experiments with rabbits. The formation of intraepidermal clefts with few or no free acantholytic cells demonstrable by IF, but not by histologic methods, did appear to be a reproducible phenomenon, provided the experiments were performed with fresh BPF sera with high titers (1:280 or greater). In numerous "blind readings" of sections stained for histologic studies or by the DIF staining methods, such cleft formation was never encountered in control biopsy specimens. Thus, they appeared to be immunologically specific. While these studies did not yield a reproducible histologic demonstration of the passive induction of pemphigus-like lesions in rabbits, they did afford the first direct indication that at least some fresh sera that contain high titers of pemphigus antibodies can incite the development of early changes detectable in immunopathologic examinations.

PASSIVE TRANSFER AND INDUCTION OF LESIONS IN MONKEYS

Further studies undertaken on monkeys (18) revealed that lesions could be produced in the epidermis with sera of BPF patients without the use of DNCB or other forms of secondary treatment. Specifically, intraepidermal acantholytic microbullae, which are completely comparable histologically to the characteristic lesions of human pemphigus, were produced in rhesus monkeys by multiple intradermal injections of sera from BPF patients (see Fig. 2). In addition, a correlation between the ability of sera to cause experimental lesions and titers of pemphigus antibodies became apparent in these studies (Fig. 3; Table 1).

Experimental transfer of pemphigus antibodies of patients suffering from pemphigus vulgaris into monkey oral mucosa elicited intraepithelial acantholytic lesions, if the sera had high titers, and three injections into the experimental respective sites were made. Multiple injections of control sera failed to elicit such reactions (see Fig. 3). These results were in contrast to those of a study by Sams and Jordon (16), in which rhesus monkeys received an intravenous transfusion with plasma from patients with pemphigus, and the binding of antibody to the monkey skin was followed by the IF technique. Transfusion of human pemphigus plasma into four monkeys failed to produce disease or lesions despite binding of antibody to the epidermal IC space. Wood (17) noted that when sera from pemphigus patients were transferred to monkeys by intradermal injection, IC antibody binding generally occurred, but lesions rarely formed following single injections. When the same sera were injected two or three times into the same skin site, intraepidermal acantholytic lesions characteristic of pemphigus formed. A direct correlation was established between the concentration of pemphigus antibodies in a serum and its ability to produce pemphigus-like lesions (Table 2).

Sams and Gleich (15) reported on three rhesus monkeys transfused with plasma from three different patients with pemphigoid. The antibody bound firmly to the BMZ, as determined by DIF, but again no clinical or histologic lesions developed. Traumatizing

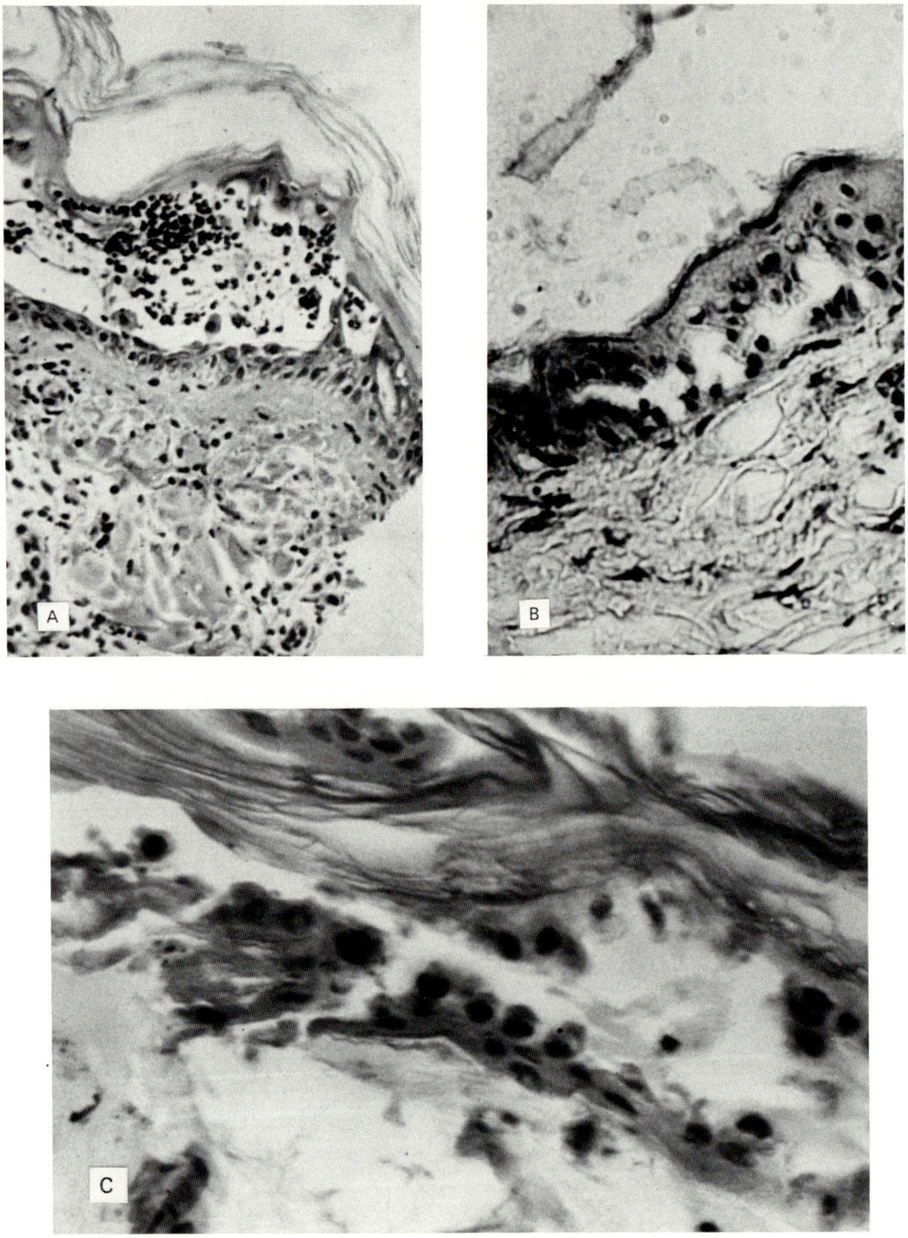

Figure 2. Depicts histologic findings in skin biopsy specimens obtained at various times following ID injections with BPF sera to control sera. A. Histologic section of monkey skin site injected three times (0, 3, and 7 hours) with 0.2 ml of a BPF serum; a biopsy specimen was obtained at 24 hours. Suprabasal microbulla containing single, free epidermal cells as well as numerous PMN can be seen (250×). B. Same as for Figure 2A. Note suprabasal cleft with partially isolated epidermal cells in some areas. Adherence of the roof to the floor can also be seen in several spots (500×). C. Comparable to Figure 2A with only two injections at 0 and 3 hours, and biopsy procedure at 7 hours. Intraepidermal microbulla with partially or completely separate epidermal cells in the upper layer of the epidermis is depicted (500×). (From Beutner EH, Chorzelski TP, Jablonska S: The nature of pemphigus antibodies and antigens. In *Immunopathology of the Skin,* ed. 2 Wiley, New York, 1979, pp 196–229.)

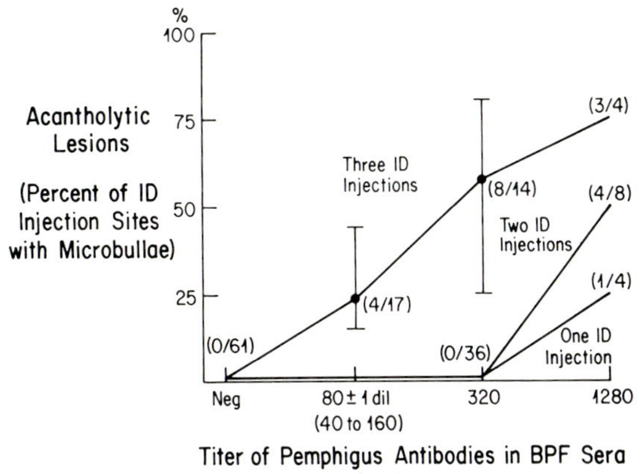

Figure 3. Graphic synopsis of data listed in Table 1. The development of acantholytic lesions is dose-dependent in two respects: 1) the frequency of lesion formation increases with increasing numbers (1, 2, or 3) of ID injections; and 2) the frequency of lesions following three ID injections increases with the titer of the antibodies. None of the control sera yielded acantholytic lesions (61 controls injected three times, plus 19 controls injected 1 or 2 times).

Table 1. In Vivo Binding of Pemphigus Antibodies and Suprabasal Acantholytic Formation Following Intradermal Injections of Monkeys with BPF

		Appearance of acantholytic microbullae 3 h or more after last ID injection of serum					
		One injection		*Two injections*		*Three injections*	
Sera injected intraepidermally	*IIF[a] titers of pemphigus antibodies*	*No. of sites*	*No. with bullae*	*No. of sites*	*No. with bullae*	*No. of sites*	*No. with bullae*
BPF[a] 1	1280	4	1	8	4	4	3
BPF 2	320	22	0			5	4
BPF 3	320	11	0			5	3
BPF 4	320	3	0	4	0	4	1
BPF 5	160	1	0	4	0	7	1
BPF 6	160	1	0	4	0	5	2
5 other BPF sera	40–160	3	0	11	0	5	1
45 control sera		8	0	11	0	61	0

[a]IIF titers-IIF staining of BPF sera in tests performed on sections of monkey skin under standard defined conditions

From Beutner EH, Chorzelski TP: Experimental studies on autosensitization in bullous diseases and on transfer of pemphigus. In *Immunopathology of the Skin,* ed. 1. 1973.

the skin when antibody binding was maximal also failed to produce lesions. However, these investigators considered (15) that prolonged exposure of basement membrane to continued high levels of antibody may be required for bullae to develop. This corresponds to the above-mentioned finding reported earlier by Beutner et al. (3) (Fig. 1).

Holubar et al. (11) found that the passive transfer of IgG fractions, as well as sera from patients with pemphigus vulgaris, can elicit intraepithelial lesions at the sites of multiple intramucosal injections of monkey lips (see Fig. 4). Thus, the role of serum

Table 2. Suprabasal Acantholytic Lesion Formation and In Vivo Fixation of Pemphigus Antibody (PAb) Following Intramucosal Injections of Monkey Lip Sites Under Various Conditions

Condition of Testing	No. of monkeys tested	*Histologic studies* — *Biopsy specimens with suprabasal lesions*		*IF studies* — *Biopsy specimens with IC-bound PAb*	
		PAb inj[a]. *(pos/total[a])*	*Control inj[a].* *(pos/total)*	*PAb inj.* *(pos/total)*	*Control inj.* *(pos/total)*
Number of injections[b]					
1 or 2 injections	4	0/6	0/6	9/9	0/6
3 injections	7	6/15	0/8	16/17	0/13
Time after 1st injections[c]					
9–12 h	2	0/3	0/1	4/4	0/6
14–17 h	3	1/7	0/5	5/6	0/5
21–24 h	2	5/5	0/2	7/7	0/2
Totals		6/21	0/14	25/26	0/19

[a]PAb inj.-sites injected with PAb containing sera or their IgG fractions; pos/total-positive sites/total sites; Control inj.-sites injected with control sera.

[b]Injections were made at 0, 3, and 6 or 7 h.

[c]Pemphigus sera and IgG fractions prepared from them had PAb titers of 160 to 2560. Controls in experiments in which suprabasal cleft formation occurred included sera from SLE and BP cases and IgG from normal sera. The times given are from the first injection to the time of sacrifice and biopsy procedure.

From Beutner EH, Chorzelski TP: Experimental studies on autosensitization in bullous diseases and on transfer of pemphigus. In *Immunopathology of the Skin*, ed. 1. 1973.

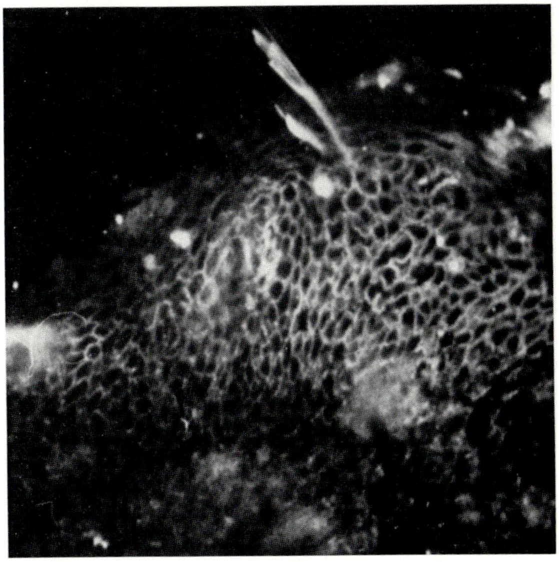

Figure 4. Direct IF staining of monkey lip mucosa for IgG at a site injected according to the schedule described for Table 2. The conjugate characteristics were molar F/P 1.7; Ab/P 2.6. The concentration of labeled anti-IgG antibody used for IF staining was 50 μg/ml. Note strong IC fluorescence throughout the prickle cell layer (200×). (From Beutner EH, Chorzelski TP, Jablonska S: The nature of pemphigus antibodies and antigens. In *Immunopathology of the Skin,* ed. 2. Wiley, New York, 1979, pp 196–229.)

proteins other than Ig in the triggering of lesion formation could be ruled out. However, IC IgG, but not participation of complement, could be detected in the lip mucosa at the injection sites. The only detectable fixation of complement occurred at the basement membrane (see Fig. 5). Throughout these studies on passive transfer into monkey skin (18), rabbit skin (1,10), and monkey lip (11) with BPF or pemphigus vulgaris sera, the development of acantholytic lesions was preceded by the in vivo binding of the pemphigus antibodies. One can refer here to the binding of the antibodies, rather than to the IC deposits of IgG because of the negative results in controls used in all of these studies. In some lesional areas in the human disease, IC complement deposits appeared at the sites of acantholytic bullae. This finding may be compared to the relationship that occurs in tissue culture (see Chap. 13) and in humans: 1) Complement does not play a role in the induction of acantholytic changes in skin explants maintained in the presence of pemphigus antibodies; and 2) while IC complement deposits do occur in some (but not all) lesional areas of skin in active cases, they do not occur in the nonlesional skin of pemphigus patients. Thus, the complement binding appears to be a secondary event.

SUMMARY OF ORIGINAL STUDIES ON PASSIVE TRANSFER OF PEMPHIGUS AND PEMPHIGOID (9)

A dose-response relationship exists in the expression of the pathogenic potential of pemphigus antibodies, as seen in passive transfer studies in monkey skin and lip mucosa

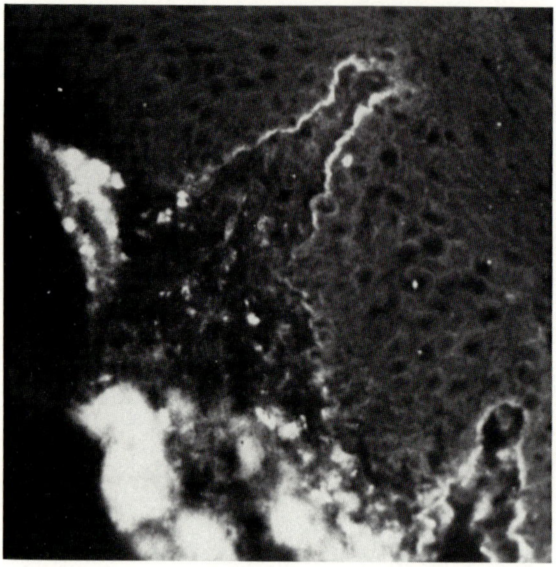

Figure 5. Direct IF staining of monkey lip mucosa for complement component C3 at a site comparable to the one shown in Figure 4. The characteristics of the reagents were as follows: The rabbit antihuman C3 (Netherlands Red Cross), which contained 1 U/ml was diluted to 1/4 U/ml. A goat antirabbit conjugate with the molar F/P ratio of 3.5, 8 U/ml, diluted 1/32 to a final concentration of 1/4 U/ml. Note staining at the BMZ and negative reaction of the IC areas. (From Beutner EH, Chorzelski TP, Jablonska S: The nature of pemphigus antibodies and antigens. In *Immunopathology of the Skin,* ed. 2. Wiley, New York, 1979, pp 196–229.)

(Fig. 3). Low doses yield only in vivo binding of pemphigus antibodies. High titers of pemphigus antibodies from patients with the Brazilian form of the disease occasionally yield acantholytic lesions following intradermal injections of rabbits. These same sera yield comparable lesions more regularly in monkey skin following multiple intradermal injections. Sera of patients with active pemphigus vulgaris and high titers of pemphigus antibodies also give rise to acantholytic lesions following multiple intramucosal injections. These observations provide unequivocable evidence for the pathogenicity of pemphigus antibodies.

The dose-dependent relationships in the induction of acantholysis in transfer studies in monkeys are comparable to the relationships of titers of pemphigus antibodies to responses: 1) In the human disease, fluctuations in the severity or extent of lesions in patients suffering from pemphigus parallel titer fluctuations (see Chap. 9); and 2) the titers of pemphigus antibodies parallel their capacity to induce the formation of acantholytic lesions in explants of skin in a tissue culture system (see Chap. 13).

A serum from an active case of pemphigus vulgaris that gave rise to unequivocal acantholytic lesions following intramucosal injections of monkey lip also yielded comparable changes in cultures of monkey skin explants. This observation, together with those noted above, points to a close relationship between the role of pemphigus antibodies in the induction of acantholysis in humans, in passive transfer, and in culture.

These findings have been confirmed and extended by more recent studies on the passive transfer of IC antibodies of pemphigus. Also, the basic observations on the in vivo reactivity of passively transferred BMZ antibodies of pemphigoid (4) have been confirmed, and they are being extended to studies pointing to their pathogenic potential, as indicated in Chapter 12.

These various observations on the passive transfer and organ culture studies of antibodies of pemphigus and pemphigoid have contributed to the development of new insights into the nature of autoimmunity.

REFERENCES

1. Beutner EH, Chorzelski TP, Jarzabek M, et al: Studies in immunodermatology. I. Passive induction of intraepidermal clefts in rabbits by transfer of sera from Brazilian pemphigus foliaceus patients. *Int Arch Allergy Appl Immunol* 42:545–555, 1972.
2. Beutner EH, Chorzelski TP, Jordon RE: *Autosensitization in Pemphigus and Bullous Pemphigoid.* Charles C Thomas, Springfield, IL, 1970, 194 pp.
3. Beutner EH, Jordan RE: Demonstration of skin antibodies in sera of pemphigus vulgaris patients by indirect immunofluorescent staining. *Proc Soc Exp Biol Med* 117:505–510, 1964.
4. Beutner EH, Lever WF, Witebsky E, et al: Autoantibodies in pemphigus vulgaris. Responses to an intercellular substance of epidermis. *JAMA* 192:682–688, 1965.
5. Beutner EH, Prigenzi LS, Hale WL, et al: Immunofluorescent studies of autoantibodies to intercellular areas of epithelia in Brazilian pemphigus foliaceus. *Proc Soc Exp Biol Med* 127:81–86, 1968.
6. Castro RM, Roscoe JT, Sampaio SAP: Brazilian pemphigus foliaceus. In Ahmed AR (Ed): *Clinics in Dermatology.* Lippincott, Philadelphia, 1983, pp 22–41.
7. Castro RM, Chorzelski TP, Jablonska S, et al: Antiepithelial antibodies in healthy people living in endemic areas of South American pemphigus foliaceus. *Castellania* 4:111–112, 1976.
8. Chertok BL: Skin testing of animals with sera from patients with pemphigus vulgaris using immunofluorescent techniques. Honors Thesis, School of Medicine, State University of New York at Buffalo, 1967.
9. Chorzelski TP, Beutner EH, Jablonska S: The role and nature of autoimmunity in pemphigus. In Beutner EH, Chorzelski TP, Bean SF (Eds): *Immunopathology of the Skin,* ed. 2. Wiley, New York, 1979, pp 183–229.
10. Chorzelski TP, Beutner EH, Jarzabek M: Passive transfer of pemphigus in experimental animals. *Int Arch Allergy* 39:106, 1970.
11. Holubar K, Chorzelski TP, Gauto M, et al: Studies in immunodermatology. III. Induction of intraepithelial lesions in monkeys by intramucosal injections of pemphigus antibodies. *Int Arch Allergy Appl Immunol* 44:631–643, 1973.
12. Jordan RE, Beutner EH, Witebsky E, et al: Basement zone antibodies in bullous pemphigoid. *JAMA* 200:751–756, 1967.
13. Lindenberg A: Quelques recherches tendant a etablir l'etiologie du pemphigus et du psoriasis. *Soc de Dermatologie et de Syphiligraphie 44:* 1956–1961, 1937.
14. Proenca NG: Declinio do penfigo foliaceo em Sao Paulo. *Rev Paul Med* 89:97–100, 1977.
15. Sams WM Jr, Gleich GH: Failure to transfer bullous pemphigoid with serum from patients. *Proc Soc Exp Biol Med* 136:1027–1031, 1971.
16. Sams WM Jr, Jordan RE: Pemphigus antibodies: Their role in disease. *J Invest Dermatol* 56:474–479, 1971.
17. Wood GW: Studies of the role of autoantibodies in the pathogenesis of pemphigus. Doctoral Thesis, State University of New York at Buffalo, 1971, 89 pp.
18. Wood GW, Beutner EH, Chorzelski TP: Studies in immunodermatology. II. Production of pemphigus-like lesions by intradermal injection of monkeys with Brazilian pemphigus sera. *Int Arch Allergy Appl Immunol* 42:556–564, 1972.

12
Recent Advances in Passive Transfer Studies of Bullous Diseases

Justin T. Roscoe
Grant J. Anhalt
Harish Patel
Luis A. Diaz

INTRODUCTION

The pemphigus group of diseases comprises all bullous dermatoses characterized by an intraepidermal acantholytic cleft (5,27) and by the presence of autoantibodies directed against antigens found in the intracellular substance (ICS) of the epidermis. Both criteria must be fulfilled. Certain genodermatoses, such as Darier's disease and Hailey-Hailey's disease, have acantholysis, but no autoantibodies (7). Conversely, autoantibodies against ICS components have been described after burns (1), certain drug eruptions (16), and when antiblood group antibodies are found (19). Yet only a few drugs, such as rifampin (18) and penicillamine (13), have been implicated in the formation of lesions. Passive transfer studies in pemphigus examine the relationship between the presence of autoantibodies that bind up to the ICS and the formation of such intraepidermal acantholytic clefts.

The previous chapter described the passive transfer studies (6,10,22,34,38) that were undertaken in response to the discovery by Beutner and Jordan (7) and Jordan et al. (23) of the pemphigus and pemphigoid antibodies, as well as the relationship of these studies to a report by Lindenberg (28) in the 1930s on the injection of rabbits and guinea pigs with sera or blood of Brazilian pemphigus or psoriasis patients.

The Athymic Nude Mouse Model

Buschard et al. (8) transplanted normal human oral mucosa onto adult athymic nude mice. Then 0.5 ml of high-titer pemphigus vulgaris (PV) serum or control serum was

This investigation was supported by U.S. Public Health Services Grant (R01-AM 32081, R01-AM 32599, R23-AM 32079, R23-AM 32490, and T32 AM07324 from the National Institutes of Health and by a gift from the Estee Lauder Corporation.

injected intraperitoneally. None of the control mice showed any alteration in their transplants. However, all 23 experimental animals showed positive staining of the ICS by direct immunofluorescence (DIF). Intracellular (IC) edema of varying degrees was observed in 15 mice, and three of these transplants showed suprabasilar splitting. This splitting was associated with the higher titer serum.

Since only 3 of the 23 mice developed lesions that could be detected histologically, and dealing with athymic nude mice is inherently difficult and artificial, a better mouse model would be useful. Perhaps manipulation of the titer, concentration, and duration of the autoantibodies could provide more definitive proof. The quantity of pemphigus antibodies (Pabs) given intravenously (IV) had probably been inadequate. Intradermal (ID) injections had been successful (see Chap. 11) because they had provided a locally greater quantity per mass of epithelial tissue. However, increasing the quantity of Pabs reaching the ICS posed a series of technical problems: 1) Plasma volume given IV had already been maximized, and heart failure would result if increased further; and 2) increasing the time of infusion would produce neutralizing antibodies in an immunocompetent animal.

The Neonatal Mouse Model

In the studies of Anhalt et al. (4), the neonatal mouse was chosen because it is: 1) Immunologically tolerant to foreign proteins such as IgG, but otherwise does not require special care with regard to infections; 2) small enough to require very little IgG per experiment, thus eliminating the need to remove large amounts of plasma from pemphigus patients; and 3) easier and cheaper to breed and handle than either monkeys or adult athymic nude mice. Next, an experimental protocol was established. IgG fractions are purified from higher titer pemphigus and normal human sera either by staphylococcal protein A (SPA) affinity chromatography or by 50% ammonium sulfate precipitation followed by ion exchange chromatography. After dialyzing against phosphate-buffered saline (PBS), the solution is pressure ultrafiltered to a final concentration of 50 to 100 mg IgG/ml, sterilized by passing through a Millipore filter, and then stored at −20°C or −70°C until use. This allows a very large amount of high-titer Pabs to be delivered in a small volume. Doses of 5 to 10 mg IgG/g body weight are injected intraperitoneally (IP) with a 30 gauge needle b.i.d. into 24 hour old Balb/c mice weighing approximately 1.5 grams (Fig. 1). When bullae erupt, the mice are heparinized and then sacrificed to obtain serum for IIF and IgG concentration, as well as tissue for DIF, hematoxylin and eosin (H&E) histopathology, and electron microscopy (EM). If no bullae appear, the mice are sacrificed 48 hours after the first injection.

PEMPHIGUS VULGARIS

Using the model outlined above, IgG from pemphigus vulgaris (PV) patients reproduced the clinical, histopathologic, ultrastructural, and immunologic characteristics of the disease. Both localized (Fig. 2A) and extensive (Fig. 2B) disease were seen, and the acantholytic nature of these was confirmed histopathologically. Three distinct histopathologic pictures were recognized: 1) Suprabasilar acantholytic clefting (Fig. 3A) (26); 2) intraepidermal polymorphonuclear vesiculation corresponding to the eosinophilic spongiosis of Emmerson and Wilson-Jones (Fig. 3B) (15); and 3) subgranular cell layer acantholysis, often with necrosis of affected keratinocytes (Fig. 3C). This latter effect was seen only with doses above 12 mg/g body weight/day. Electron microscopy

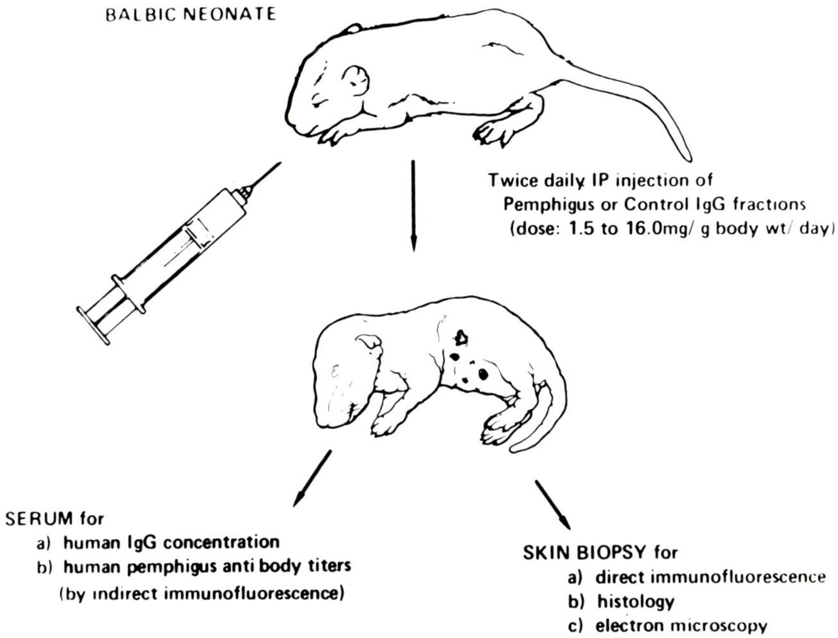

Figure 1. The neonatal mouse model applied to PV. The type of antibody, as well as titer and concentration, may be varied according to experimental design.

showed the characteristic widening of epidermal IC spaces and other ultrastructural changes of acantholysis, as previously reported by Hashimoto and Lever (20) (Fig. 4). Direct IF revealed the presence of human IgG bound to the mouse epidermal ICS (Fig. 5). The extent of disease correlated with both the dose of IgG (Fig. 6) and the Pabs titer (Fig. 7) injected; that is, a dose-response relationship can be demonstrated. Since the quantity of Pabs is a function of both IgG concentration and Pabs titer, this very strongly suggests that they are not merely an epiphenomenon, but the actual pathogenetic agent.

Two other studies have already proven the usefulness and broad applicability of this model. Peterson and Weupper (30) developed a procedure to purify pemphigus antigens (Pags) from normal human skin and then used it to immunize a rabbit. When indirect IF (IIF) of the rabbit serum was carried out, the pattern of binding was identical to that seen in human pemphigus. They then purified and concentrated the serum and injected it into neonatal mice, using the same method outlined above. Mice injected with this IgG concentrate developed clinically, histologically, and immunologically typical pemphigus. This fulfills the criteria outlined by Witebsky et al. (37) to conclusively establish the role of an autoantibody in the pathogenesis of any putative autoimmune disease.

BRAZILIAN PEMPHIGUS FOLIACEUS

Brazilian pemphigus foliaceus (BPF) (9) is found endemically in Brazil, where cases are clustered among individuals living in areas that have recently been converted from native vegetation to cultivated fields or along rivers, suggesting that a vector-mediated

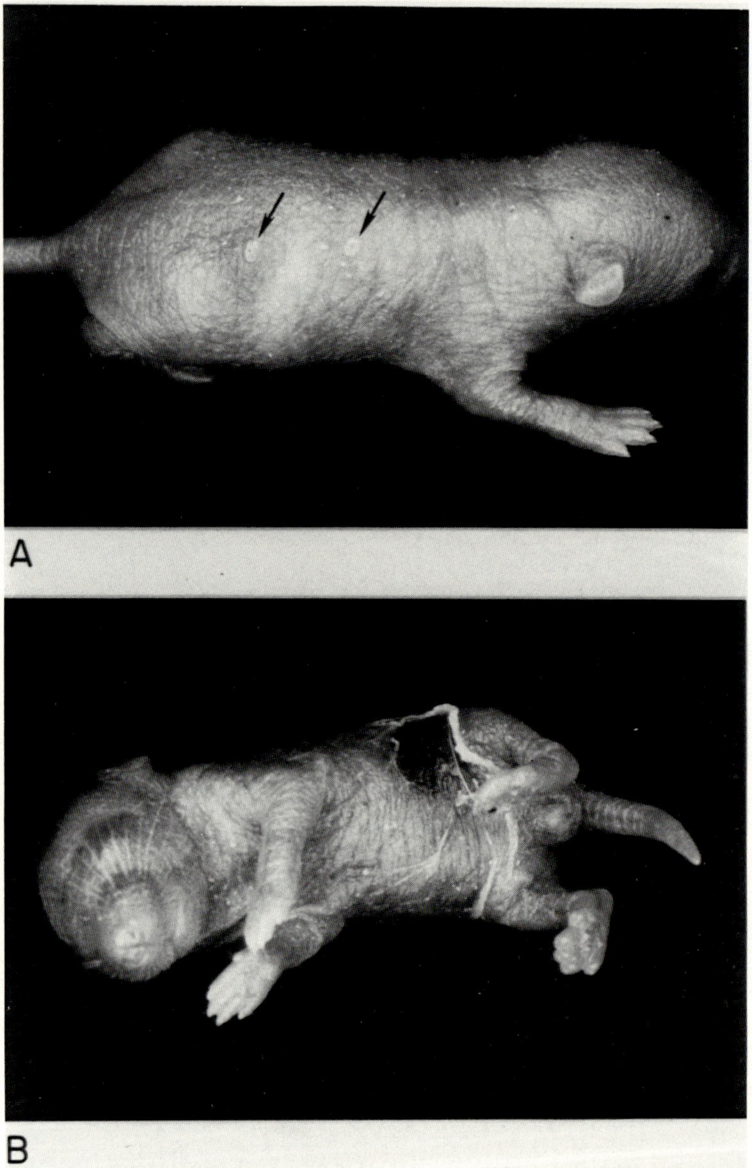

Figure 2. Clinical aspects of PV induced by passive transfer of autoantibodies to the neonatal mouse. A. Limited disease, with small blisters shown by the arrows. B. Extensive disease, with large erosion and extensive sloughing of the epidermis.

viral infection may be involved. BPF is distinguished clinically from PV not only by its peculiar epidemiology, but also by the extreme rarity of mucosal lesions, the greater tendency to generalize to exfoliative erythroderma, and the more favorable prognosis if left untreated. Histopathologically, the intraepidermal acantholytic cleft is usually at the

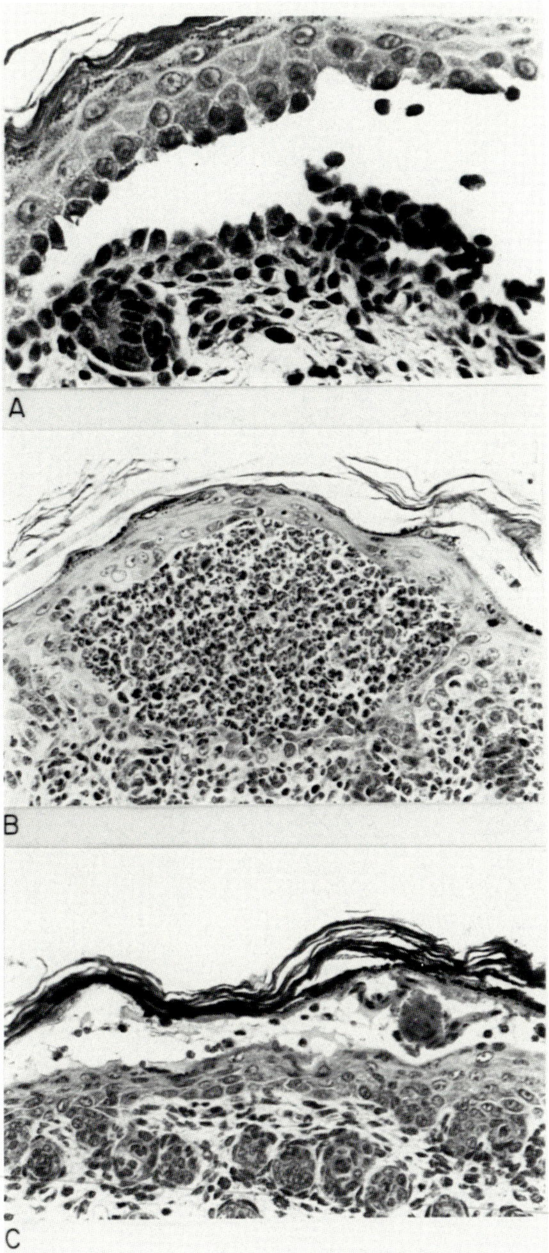

Figure 3. Histopathology of PV induced by passive transfer of autoantibodies to the neonatal mouse. A. Suprabasilar cleft. The row of "tombstones" is attached to the dermis, and acantholytic cells are free in the blister cavity (400×). B. Intraepidermal polymorphonuclear pustule. Because eosinophils and neutrophils vary in function among different species, this probably corresponds to the eosinophilic spongiosis of Emmerson and Wilson-Jones (100×). C. Subgranular acantholytic cleft. Since this occurred only at high doses, it may be due to a direct cytopathic effect of Pabs (100×).

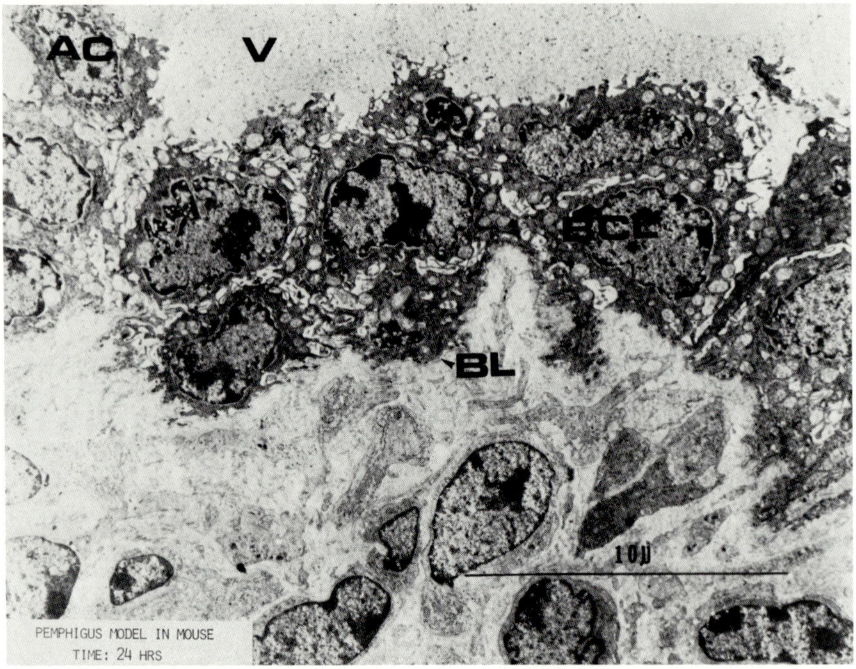

Figure 4. Electron micrograph of PV induced by passive transfer to the neonatal mouse. Note the acantholytic cells (AC) and the basal cells (BCL) that continue well attached to the basal lamina (BL) despite widening of the ICS between cells forming the vesicle (V) (47, 500×).

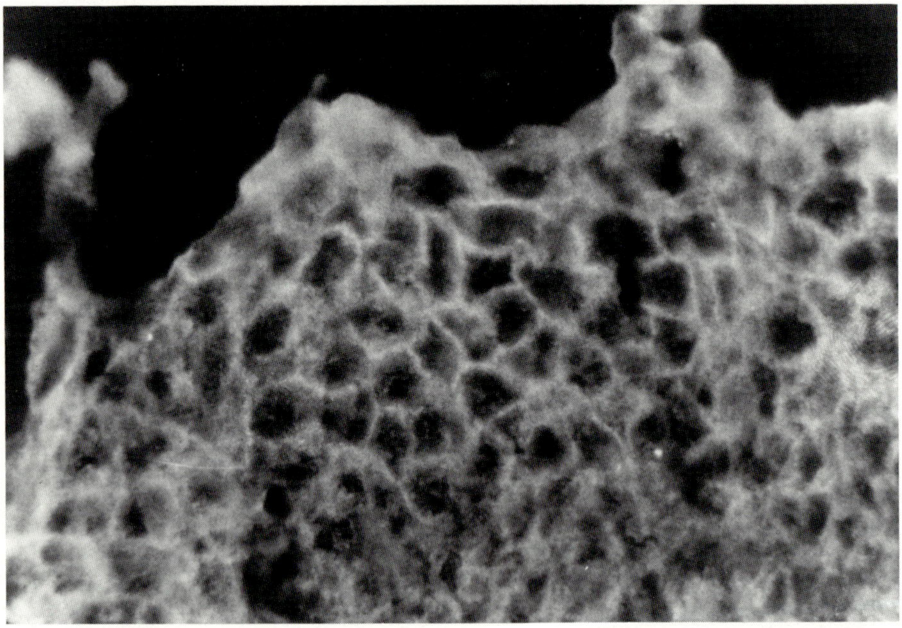

Figure 5. Direct IF revealing human IgG bound to mouse epidermal ICS in the typical reticulated pattern seen in the human disease (400×).

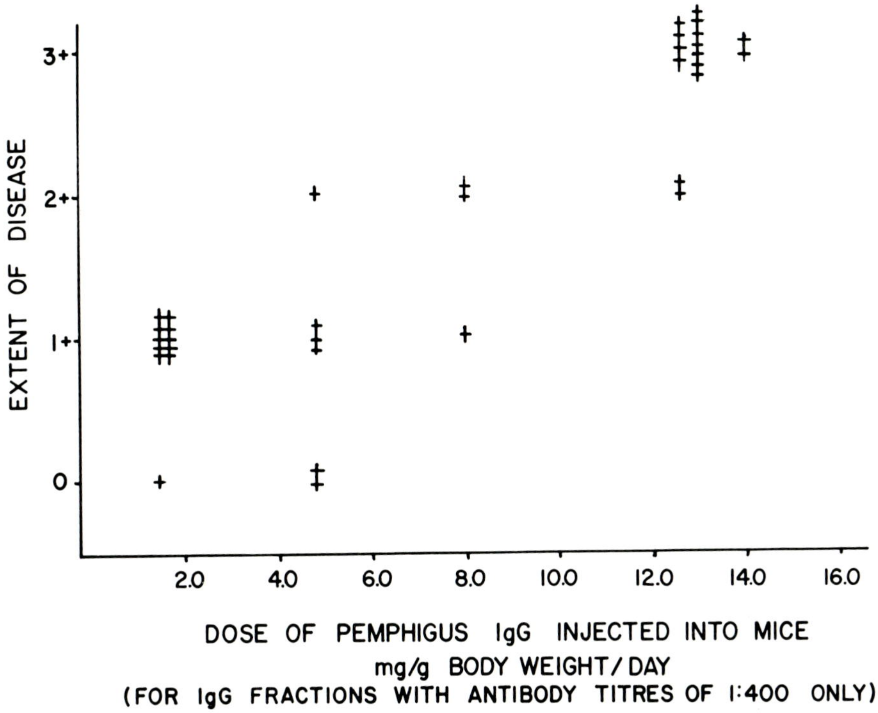

Figure 6. Relationship between dose of PV IgG injected into the neonatal mouse and disease extent. Each cross represents a neonatal mouse. Animals were graded as having no disease (0), minimal disease (1+), moderate disease (2+), or extensive disease (3+). The relationship is significant ($p < 0.002$ by chi square analysis).

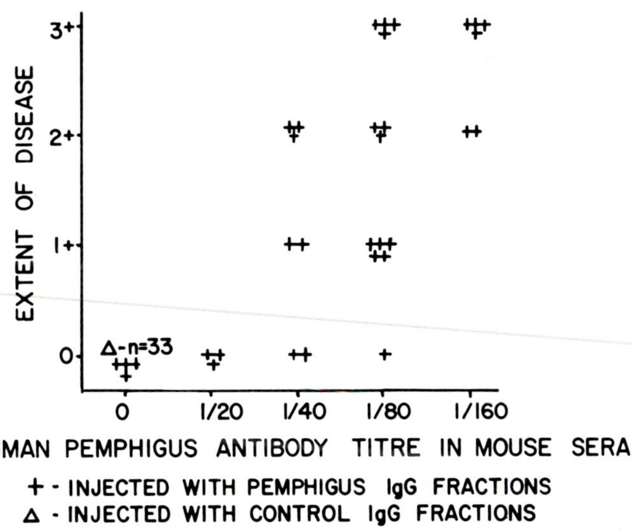

Figure 7. Relationship between PV antibody titer and extent of disease in the neonatal mouse. Each cross represents one animal. The grades for extent of disease are the same as in Figure 6. The relationship is highly significant ($p < 0.0001$ by chi square analysis).

granular layer, rather than at the suprabasilar region as in PV. Nonetheless, the acantholysis itself has proven to be indistinguishable even at the ultrastructural level (35). Despite the intraepidermal clefting and the generally higher Pabs titer, no differences have been found consistently on IF or immunoelectron microscopy (IEM).

Using the neonatal mouse model, our laboratory (32) has successfully reproduced BPF clinically (Fig. 8), histologically, ultrastructurally, and immunologically. Neonatal Balb/c mice were injected IP twice daily with IgG purified from serum of patients with BPF. The IgG was concentrated to 50 to 100 mg/ml and given twice daily in doses of 5

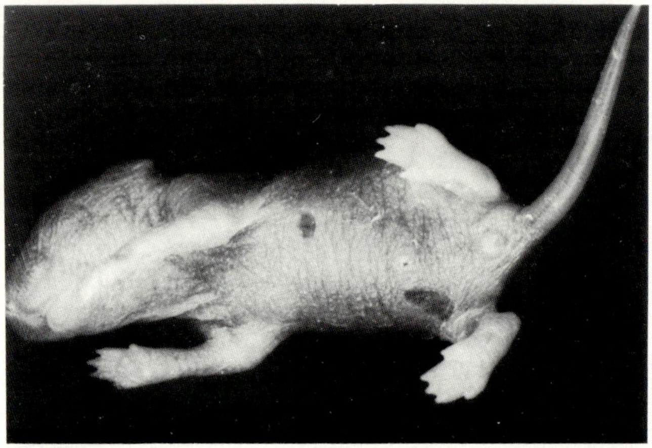

A

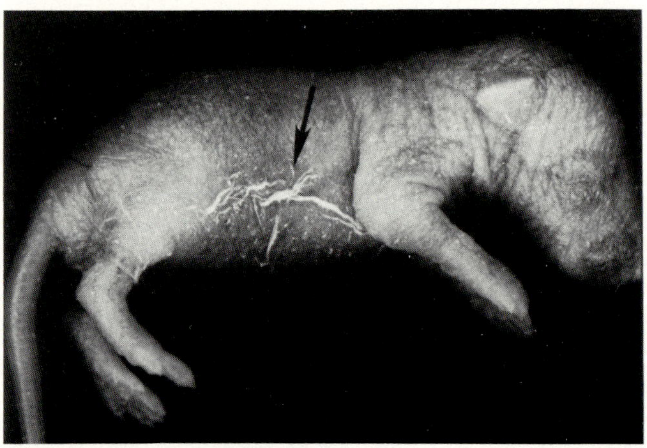

B

Figure 8. Clinical aspects of BPF induced by passive transfer to the neonatal mouse. A. Disease limited to small erosions that appear as dark spots on the underbelly of the neonatal mouse. B. Arrow points to sloughing of epidermis that is characteristic of extensive disease.

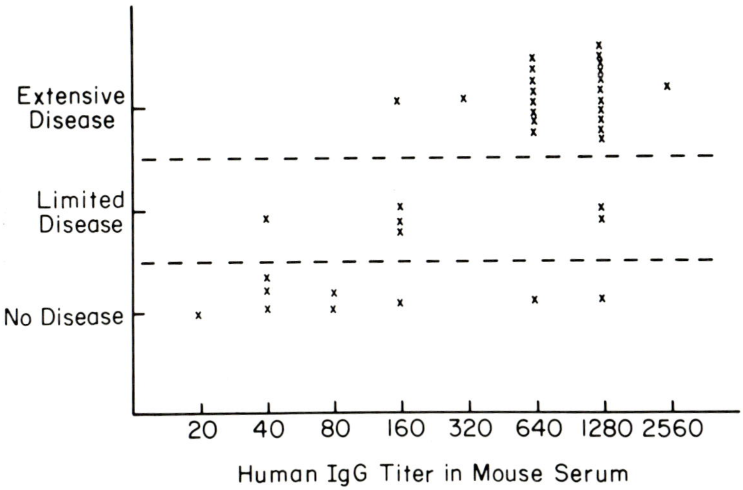

Figure 9. Relationship between titer and disease extent of BPF induced by passive transfer to the neonatal mouse. Each X represents one animal. Note that extensive disease is induced only by very high titers.

to 10 mg IgG/g body weight. A relationship between titer and disease extent similar to that demonstrated for PV was also seen (Fig. 9). Interestingly, as in the human disease, the most common clinical presentation was exfoliative erythroderma, although localized disease was ocasionally seen. Lower titers did not result in a lower level of cleavage, as had occurred with PV. Localized disease was as restricted to the granular cell layer as was the extensive sloughing seen in most mice, indicating a distinctive effect of these antibodies on granular cell adhesion.

BULLOUS PEMPHIGOID

Another blistering disease that has attracted a great deal of interest is bullous pemphigoid (BP). This chronic, yet frequently self-limited, bullous dermatosis commonly seen on the flexor surfaces of the elderly is characterized by subepidermal vesiculation in association with a predominately polymorphonuclear eosinophil infiltrate (36). There seems to be a defined sequence of pathologic events that begins with mast cell changes and the deposition of immunoreactants in the skin. IgG and C3 are usually seen as a linear band at the basement membrane zone (BMZ) of perilesional skin when examined by DIF (24). Deposition of IgE, alternate pathway components, and fibrin has been demonstrated by Provost and Tomasi (31). Transplacental transfer has not been reported, although some controversy about whether herpes gestationis (HG) is merely BP during pregnancy still exists (21); and HG has been reported to be transferred transplacentally (25). In addition, antibody titer does not correlate well with disease activity (11). Nonetheless, Gammon et al. (17) have shown in vitro that BP antibodies (BPabs) fix to sections of human skin and produce attachment of peripheral blood leukocytes along the BMZ after a source of complement is added. This rather substantial circumstantial and experimental evidence indicates that autoantibodies may play an important role. Passive transfer experiments can more directly examine the relationship between circulating autoantibodies that bind to the BMZ and the formation of subepidermal blisters.

As in pemphigus, an early in vivo experiment failed to induce blistering, but provided much useful data. Sams and Gleich (33) obtained plasma by plasmapheresis from three patients that had high titers of IgG directed against the BMZ. Two of the three sera fixed complement. Rhesus monkeys were intravenously injected with an amount of this BP serum equal to 25 to 30% of their own plasma volume. Despite attempts to faciliate the appearance of blisters by rubbing, ultraviolet (UV) light, or liquid nitrogen, no blisters formed that did not also occur in control animals subjected to the same trauma. The DIF examination did, however, reveal intense linear staining of the BMZ.

THE RABBIT CORNEA MODEL

Intradermal injections had been successful in pemphigus, apparently because they delivered high concentrations locally. Anhalt et al. (3) decided to use corneal epithelium as the target tissue, because it has no vascular supply or lymphatics and injected immunoglobulins would diffuse very slowly out of the stroma (2). Corneal epithelium is similar to epidermis, except that it does not keratinize. Furthermore, Cowen et al. (12) showed that BP antigen is found at the BMZ of dog cornea. Accordingly, sera from patients with well-characterized BP were obtained and IgG fractions were purified, concentrated, and sterilized, as described earlier for the neonatal mouse model. A variety of vertebrate squamous epithelia have been shown to have BP antigen at the BMZ (14). The New Zealand white rabbit was thus chosen and injected after being given 0.5% proparacaine topical anesthesia. A 30-gauge needle was used to introduce 0.05 ml of the prepared IgG concentrate into the anterior corneal stroma, producing an approximately 3 mm diameter central bleb. Normal human serum concentrate was used in one eye as a control, and the experimental BP serum concentrate was injected in the other eye. Slit lamp examinations by a single experienced observer were performed daily on the animals. None of the 32 control corneas had any lesions or inflammation other than slight scarring along the needle tract (Fig. 10A). At 48 hours after injection, 28 of 32 corneas injected with BPabs showed an inflammatory reaction (Table 1). This ranged from mild haziness of the anterior cornea to a circular opaque ring, with visible bulla formation and iritis with ciliary flush and aqueous cell and flare (Fig. 10B).

Table 1. Relationship Between IgG Concentration Injected, DIF Titer for BP Antibody and Complement Fixation, and the Ability to Induce Corneal Inflammation

Patients	*IgG concentration*	*BP antibody titer*	*Complement fixation titer*	*Corneas inflamed/injected*
A	38	1:400	1:100	17/17
B	20	1:3200	1:200	4/4
C	28	1:1600	1:200	2/2
D	34	1:3200	?	1/2
E	41	1:400	?	0/3
F	21	1:40	1:100	1/1
G	19	—	—	3/3
Total				28/32
Normal	36			0/32

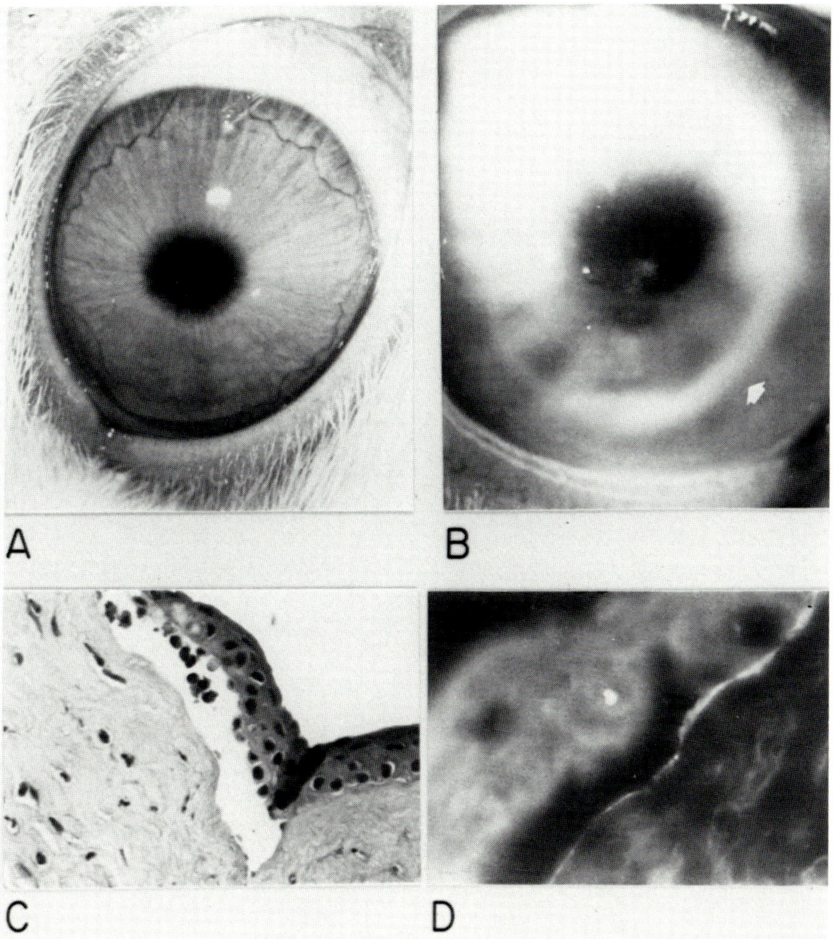

Figure 10. Bullous pemphigoid induced by passive transfer of autoantibodies into rabbit cornea. A. Eye injected with normal human IgG. B. Eye injected with IgG purified from serum of BP patients. C. Photomicrograph of H&E-stained section showing the subepithelial cleft (100×). D. Direct IF showing linear fluorescence at the BMZ (400×).

Animals were sacrificed at 72 hours, and their eyes were enucleated for histologic and immunofluorescence (IF) studies. H&E sections of the BPabs-injected corneas (Fig. 10C) showed engorgement of the limbal vessels with polymorphonuclear leukocytes, which also infiltrated the stroma and clustered at the epithelial-stromal interface. Subepithelial separation was seen, with inflammatory cells attached to the roof of the blister cavity. The DIF study showed linear deposition of IgG and C3 and the BMZ (Fig. 10D). None of these changes were seen in the control animals. The intracorneal injection of BPabs thus passively transferred BP in the rabbit cornea model.

Additional studies demonstrated that the intensity of the inflammatory response is dose related, but the IIF titer for IgG is not a reliable measure. The ability of that IgG fraction to fix complement did correlate with pathogenicity, with one exception, as seen in Table 1. Intradermal BPab injections into the rabbits' ears were not successful in producing clinical, histopathologic, or immunologic changes. This was interpreted as being due to the faster elimination of antibodies from that site.

THE GUINEA PIG MODEL

Naito et al. (29) used guines pigs as the in vivo counterpart to his in vitro experiments using human skin explants to study BP. Sera and blister fluid (BF) were obtained from two untreated patients with BP. An IgG fraction was obtained by SPA affinity chromatography using some BP serum. Hartley guinea pigs were injected intradermally with approximately 0.5 ml of BF, serum, or IgG from BP patients. BP serum that had been preincubated with human IgG antisera and a control solution of 0.9% NaCl were injected similarly. This dose was divided into 6 to 12 separate injections spread over the shaved skin of the animals' backs. Biopsy specimens were obtained from injection sites at 1, 3, 6, 12, 24, and 48 hours and then examined both histologically and by DIF. Although the DIF results were not reported, the histologic findings were clear.

Six hours after the injection of either BP sera or BF, a dermal-epidermal separation could be observed histologically, along with a mixed perivascular infiltrate consisting of neutrophils, eosinophils, and some lymphocytes. Pretreatment with antiserum to human IgG prevented the induction of lesions and resulted in skin as normal as those obtained after the control injections. However, normal human serum would have been a better control than 0.9% NaCl. Additional studies addressing this point and reporting the IF studies seem appropriate. Nonetheless, these observations suggest that BP IgG is the necessary initiating factor.

In our laboratory, concentrated IgG fractions from sera of patients with proven BP have been injected IP into neonatal Balb/c mice, as described earlier. Unlike pemphigus, repeated attempts to consistently induce cutaneous blistering have not been successful. It seems likely that BP IgG requires adequate interaction with other factors, such as complement, peripheral blood leukocytes, IgE, and mast cells. Since interactions among these components of the immune system vary somewhat among species, an attempt with other animals is warranted. Despite some progress with local models, further studies are still needed to develop an adequate parenteral passive transfer model for BP.

SUMMARY

The following will summarize recent advances that have been made using passive transfer of autoantibodies to study their role in the bullous diseases.

1. Pemphigus
   a) Intraperitoneal injections of 0.5 ml of serum from pemphigus patients bound and occasionally induced suprabasilar splitting in human oral mucosa, which had been transplanted onto athymic nude mice.
   b) Intraperitoneal injections of 50 to 100 mg/ml IgG purified from high titer sera of pemphigus patients consistently reproduced the disease clinically, histologically, and immunologically if given b.i.d. in doses of 5 to 10 mg IgG/g body weight to neonatal Balb/c mice. The induction of clinical lesions is dose-dependent as a function of IgG titer.

2. Pemphigoid
   a) IgG (50 μl) concentrated from serum of BP patients and injected into the cornea of New Zealand white rabbits induced lesions of the corneal epithelium that consistently reproduced the macroscopic, histologic, and immunologic aspects of pemphigoid blisters. The appearance of lesions was dose-dependent not as a direct function of the IgG titer, but rather of the ability of that IgG at the BMZ to bind complement.
   b) Hartley guinea pigs injected ID with 0.5 ml of either BF or sera from BP patients developed lesions that produce dermal-epidermal separation with a mixed perivascular infiltrate.
   c) Attempts at developing an adequate parenteral passive transfer model for BP have been unsuccessful to date, and more work is needed in this area to better establish the significance of circulating autoantibodies in the disease.

REFERENCES

1. Ablin RJ, Milgrom F, Kano K, et al: Pemphigus-like antibodies in patients with skin burns. *Vox Sang* 16:73–75, 1969.
2. Allansmith M, DeRamus A, Maurice D: The dynamics of IgG in the cornea. *Invest Ophthalmol Visual Sci* 18:947–955, 1979.
3. Anhalt GJ, Bahn CF, Labib RS, et al: Pathogenic effects of bullous autoantibodies on rabbit corneal epithelium. *J Clin Invest* 68:1097–1101, 1981.
4. Anhalt GJ, Labib RS, Vorhees JJ, et al: Induction of pemphigus in neonatal mice by passive transfer of IgG from patients with the disease. *N Engl J Med* 306:1189–1196, 1982.
5. Auspitz H: *System der hautkrankheiten.* Braunmuller, Vienna, 1881, pp 154–162.
6. Beutner EH, Chorzelski TP, Jarzabek M, et al: Studies in immunodermatology I. Passive induction of intraepidermal clefts in rabbits by transfer of sera from Brazilian pemphigus foliaceus patients. *Int Arch Allergy* 42:545–555, 1972.
7. Beutner EH, Jordon RE: Demonstration of skin autoantibodies in sera of pemphigus vulgaris patients by indirect immunofluorescent staining. *Proc Soc Exp Biol Med* 117:505–510, 1964.
8. Buschard K, Dabelsteen E, Bretlan P: A model for the study of autoimmune diseases applied to pemphigus: Transplants of human oral mucosa to athymic nude mice binds pemphigus antibodies *in vivo. J Invest Dermatol* 76:171–173, 1981.
9. Castro RM, Roscoe JT, Sampaio SAP: Brazilian pemphigus foliaceous in Ahmed AR (Ed): *Clinics in Dermatology, Pemphigus,* No. 2, Vol. 1, Lippincott, Philadelphia, 1983, pp 22–41.
10. Chorzelski TP, Beutner EH, Jarzabek M: Passive transfer of pemphigus to experimental animals. *Int Arch Allergy* 39:106, 1970.
11. Chorzelski TP, Jablonska S, Beutner EH: Pemphigoid. In Beutner EH, Chorzelski TP, Bean SF (Eds): *Immunopathology of the Skin,* ed. 2. Wiley, New York, 1979, p 246.
12. Cowen SJ, Anhalt GJ, Wicha MS, et al: Distribution of pemphigus and pemphigoid antigens, laminin and type IV collagen in corneal epithelium. *Invest Ophthalmol Vis Sci* 21:879–882, 1981.
13. Degos MMR, Touraine R, Belaich S, et al: Pemphigus chez unmalade traite par penicillamine pour maladie de Wilson. *Bull Soc Fr Derm Syphil* 76:751–753, 1969.
14. Diaz LA, Weiss HJ, Calvanico NJ: Phylogenetic studies with pemphigus and pemphigoid antibodies. *Acta Dermatol Venereol (Stockholm)* 59:537–540, 1979.
15. Emmerson RW, Wilson-Jones E: Eosinophilic spongiosis in pemphigus: A report of an unusual histological change in pemphigus. *Arch Dermatol* 97:252–257, 1968.
16. Fellner MJ, Fukujama K, Moshell A, et al: Intercellular antibodies in blood and epidermis: A histochemical study of IgG immunoglobulins in patients with late reactions to penicillins and their comparison with similar antibodies in patients with pemphigus vulgaris. *Br J Dermatol* 89:115–126, 1973.

17. Gammon WR, Lewis DM, Carlo JR, et al: Pemphigoid antibody mediated attachment of peripheral blood leukocytes at the dermal-epidermal junction of human skin. *J Invest Dermatol* 75:334–339, 1980.
18. Gange RW, Rhodes EL, Edwards CO, et al: Pemphigus induced by rifampin. *Br J Dermatol* 95:445–448, 1976.
19. Grab PJ, Inderbitzer TM: Pemphigus antigen and blood substances A and B. *J Invest Dermatol* 49:285–287, 1967.
20. Hashimoto K, Lever WF: An electron microscopic study on pemphigus vulgaris of the mouth and skin with special reference to the intercellular cement. *J Invest Dermatol* 48:540, 1967.
21. Holmes R, Black MM, Williamson DM, et al: Herpes gestationis and bullous pemphigoid: A disease spectrum. *Br J Dermatol* 103:535–541, 1980.
22. Holubar K, Chorzelski TP, Gauto M, et al: Studies in immunodermatology III. Induction of intraepithelial lesions in monkeys by intramucosal injections of pemphigus antibodies. *Int Arch Allergy* 44:631–643, 1973.
23. Jordon RE, Beutner EH, Witebski E, et al: Basement membrane zone antibodies in bullous pemphigoid. *JAMA* 200:751–756, 1967.
24. Jordon RE, Sams WM Jr, Beutner EH: Compelement immunofluorescent staining in bullous pemphigoid. *J Lab Clin Med* 74:548–556, 1969.
25. Katz A, Minta JO, Toole JWR, et al: Immunopathologic study of herpes gestationis in mother and infant. *Arch Dermatol* 113:1069–1072, 1977.
26. Lever WF: *Pemphigus and Pemphigoid.* Charles C Thomas, Springfield, IL, 1965, pp 15–72.
27. Lever WF, Shaumburg-Lever G: *Histopathology of the Skin.* Lippincott, Philadelphia, 1983, pp 70–73.
28. Lindenberg A: Quelques recherches tendant a etablir l'etiologie du pemphigus et du psoriasis. *Bull Soc Fr Dermatol Syphil* 44:1956–1961, 1937.
29. Naito K, Norioka S, Ogawa H. The pathogenic mechanisms of blister formation in bullous pemphigoid. *J Invest Dermatol* 79:303–306, 1982.
30. Petersen LL, Wuepper KD: Isolation and purification of the pemphigus vulgaris antigen from human epidermis. *J Clin Invest* 73:1113–1120, 1984.
31. Provost TT, Tomasi TB Jr: Immunopathology of bullous pemphigoid: Basement membrane deposition of IgE, alternative pathway components and fibrin. *Clin Exp Immunol* 18:193–200, 1974.
32. Roscoe JT, Diaz LA, Sampaio SAP, et al: Brazilian pemphigus foliaceus autoantibodies are pathogenic to BALB/c mice by passive transfer. *J Invest Dermatol* 85:538–541, 1985.
33. Sams WH, Gleich GJ: Failure to transfer bullous pemphigoid with serum from patients. *Proc Soc Exp Biol Med* 136:1027–1031, 1971.
34. Sams WM Jr, Jordon RE: Pemphigus antibodies: Their role in disease. *J Invest Dermatol* 56:474–478, 1971.
35. Sotto MN, Shimizu SH, Costa JM, et al: South American pemphigus foliaceus: Electron microscopy and immunoelectron localization of bound immunoglobulin in the skin and oral mucosa. *Br J Dermatol* 102:251–527, 1980.
36. Wintroub BW, Mihm MC Jr, Goetzl EJ, et al: Morphologic and functional evidence for release of mast cell products in bullous pemphigus. *N Engl J Med* 298:417–421, 1978.
37. Witebsky E, Rose NR, Terplan K, et al: Chronic thyroiditis and autoimmunization. *JAMA* 164:1439–1447, 1957.
38. Wood GW, Beutner EH, Chorzelski TP: Studies in Immunodermatology. II. Production of pemphigus-like lesions by intradermal injection of monkeys with Brazilian pemphigus foliaceus sera. *Int Arch Allergy* 42:556–564, 1972.

13
Pemphigus Antibodies: Reactions in Tissue Culture and Their Pathophysiology

Beno Michel
Mitchell S. Turner

INTRODUCTION

Pemphigus refers to an intraepidermal and intraepithelial blistering disease. The blister may occur in the stratum granulosum (e.g., pemphigus foliaceus and pemphigus erythematosus) or directly above the basal cell layer (e.g., pemphigus vulgaris and pemphigus vegetans). Acantholytic cells, representing keratinocytes that have lost their attachments to each other, are characteristically found within the blister cavity. Direct immunofluorescence (DIF) reveals the presence of immunoglobulin G (lgG) and, sometimes, also complement on the surface of keratinocytes. Circulating antiepidermal antibodies can be demonstrated by indirect immunofluorescence (IIF) in the sera of most patients with active pemphigus, and the titer generally correlates with the severity of the disease.

IMMUNOPATHOLOGY OF PEMPHIGUS

In 1964, Beutner and Jordan (3) demonstrated that sera from pemphigus patients contain antibodies that bind to the intercellular cement substance (ICS) of skin and mucous membranes. In 1965, Beutner et al. (4) utilized DIF on skin biopsy specimens from pemphigus patients to demonstrate the in vivo ICS binding of IgG. These fundamental observations raised the question: "Does the pemphigus antibody play a causal role in pemphigus acantholysis?"

The titer of circulating antiepidermal antibodies in the sera of most patients with active pemphigus has generally been found to correlate with the severity of the disease. In fact, the antibody often disappears with clinical remission and reappears upon clinical relapse. Such observations have made it quite tempting to assume an etiologic role for the pemphigus antibody. However, only specific laboratory evidence could have provided the necessary support for this rationale.

Sams et al. (20) transfused human pemphigus plasma by intravenous (IV) drip into monkeys, and antibody fixation occurred in the monkeys' skin. However, because subsequent acantholysis was not detected, there was reluctance in accepting a pathogenic role for the pemphigus antibody. In the ensuing years, Wood et al. (27) and Holubar et al. (13) reported additional passive transfer studies (Chap. 11). Using high titer pemphigus sera for repeated intracutaneous and intramucosal injections into monkeys, they demonstrated epithelial binding of the pemphigus antibodies and subsequent acantholysis. The pathology induced by pemphigus antibody transfer has been substantiated by additional studies (1) (see Chap. 12).

ORGAN CULTURE STUDIES

In 1974 and 1977, Michel and Ko (16,17) prepared organ cultures of normal human skin incubated with either control or pemphigus serum. The control serum did not yield immunoglobulin binding or acantholytic changes. The pemphigus antibody, on the other hand, did bind to the ICS, and this binding was detected by DIF staining within 6 hours. Significant suprabasilar separation also occurred, but only after 24 hours. Acantholytic cells were noted at 40 hours, and extensive acantholysis was seen at 72 hours (Fig. 1). The sequence of microscopic events provided key evidence for a pathogenic role of the pemphigus antibody in acantholysis. That antibody binding to the ICS does precede visible tissue destruction was further supported by electron microscopy (EM), which

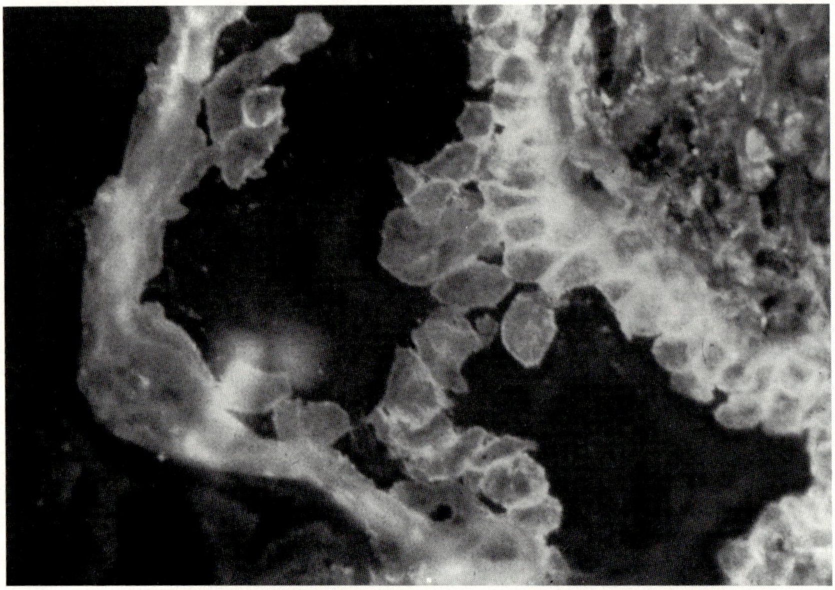

Figure 1. Direct IF for human IgG on 4 μm skin explant from a rhesus monkey that was cultured for 48 hours with serum from a pemphigus patient. The titer of the pemphigus antibodies was 80. The conjugate had a molar F/P ratio of 2:1 and an antibody protein content of 4.5 mg/ml or 16 U/ml, and was used at a concentration of 25 μg antibody protein/ml (i.e., a 1:180 dilution). Note acantholytic bulla with adherent epidermal cells on the floor and roof (120 x). (Photomicrograph from Ph.D. thesis of Walter Binder supplied by Ernst Beutner.)

detected no significant ultrastructural changes before 12 hours (14). *In vitro* EM findings were identical to those seen in the spontaneous disease. Deng et al. (10) and Barnett et al. (2) confirmed the conclusions of the above studies using monkey skin as the culture substrate.

Buschard et al. (7), using a unique method to study pemphigus, combined the techniques of tissue transplantation with that of passive transfer. After normal human mucosa was grafted to nude mice, pemphigus sera was injected intraperitoneally (IP) into the mice. Subsequent transplant acantholysis ensued.

In 1976, it was demonstrated that the IgG fraction from pemphigus serum is singly responsible for the tissue damage, and that complement is not required (21). Furthermore, it has become evident that the development of fluorescent and acantholytic changes in cultured skin explants is depends on pemphigus antibody concentration (Fig. 2) (5).

THE SEARCH FOR ACANTHOLYTIC ENZYMES

In 1959, Stoughton and Bagatell (25) concluded that cantharidine could induce acantholysis via a sulfhydryl-dependent enzyme produced by the skin. In 1978, Farb *et al.* (11) examined the possibility of an underlying enzymatic mechanism in P-IgG-induced acantholysis. The authors cultured radiolabeled neonatal mouse epidermal cells with either P-IgG or control IgG. After incubation for 8, 24, and 48 hours, the cells were washed and the supernatant evaluated for the amount of radioactivity. As suspected, significantly greater cell detachment occurred in the plates incubated with P-IgG than in those incubated with control IgG. Soybean trypsin inhibitor and α_2-macroglobulin inhibited the cell detachment in this system. This suggested that the actual loss of epidermal cell adhesion may be intimately related to a serine proteinase.

The possibility that P-IgG induces cell detachment by a cytotoxic mechanism was not supported by Farb et al., (11) since cells incubated with pemphigus serum showed no appreciable differences in either cell morphology or in radiolabeled amino acid incorporation into precipitable protein. These findings were in constrast to those obtained in

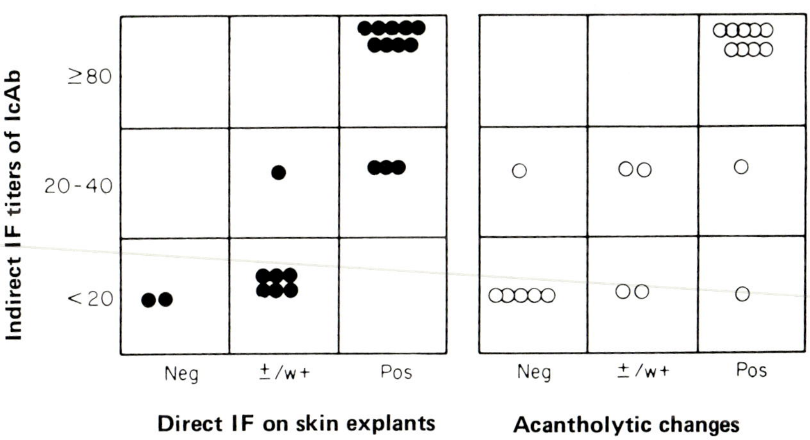

Figure 2. Correlation of IC antibody titers with DIF and acantholytic changes in cultured skin explants. From Binder, et. al. (5) with permission

the autoradiographic studies of Schiltz and Michel (21). They found that although basal cells remained viable, suprabasal cells had decreased uridine and amino acid incorporation into RNA and protein, respectively, and actual acantholytic cells incorporated neither of the precursors. Additional viability studies of cultured human keratinocytes (22) revealed that a pemphigus antibody titer exceeding 50 leads to: 1) Decreased accumulation of newly formed proteins by nearly 60%; 2) a shift of newly synthesized proteins from insoluble to soluble fractions; and 3) eventual death of 75% of the cells. It would then seem reasonable to explain the lack of cytotoxicity found in the study of Farb et al. as being due to the low titer (<10) of pemphigus antibody used. Schiltz and Michel did not propose cytotoxicity as a direct cause of epidermal acantholysis, but simply noted its occurrence in association with a high titer of pemphigus antibody.

While an enzymatic mechanism in pemphigus seemed very plausible, the isolation and characterization of an enzyme(s) was needed. In 1979, a non-IgG factor was recovered from a medium of human skin cultured with pemphigus antibodies (23). This "pemphigus acantholytic factor" appears to be a proteolytic enzyme with a pH optimum of 6.5. It is capable of causing acantholysis in organ culture. Since this protease does not manifest the pH optimum typical of cell organelle enzymes, it is not felt to be of lysosomal origin.

In recent years, plasminogen activator (PA) production has been noted to increase in the cell microenvironment under certain conditions. Hashimoto et al. (12) demonstrated that the binding of pemphigus autoantibody to human epidermal cells stimulates PA synthesis and secretion. The increased level of PA was not associated with release of lysosomal enzymes. The authors suggested that PA may be the sought after serine proteinase involved in pemphigus.

Singer and Lazarus (24) designed an experiment to ascertain if a direct link between plasminogen and acantholysis could be elucidated. They incubated normal skin explants with human plasminogen and/or P-IgG (affinity purified on protein A-Sepharose and plasminogen-free) from either pemphigus foliaceous or pemphigus vulgaris serum. No acantholysis was observed when the pemphigus foliaceous IgG (4 mg/ml) was used alone, or when the plasminogen (200 μg/ml) was used alone. However, simultaneous incubation of normal skin explants with both pemphigus foliaceous IgG and plasminogen, at the above concentrations, resulted in an upper epidermal acantholysis that was indistinguishable from lesional biopsy specimens.

Incubation of the tissue with only P-IgG (4 mg/ml) from pemphigus vulgaris patients could produce the histologic changes of pemphigus vulgaris. Although the addition of plasminogen (200 μg/ml) was not essential for the acantholysis to occur, it hastened the onset and increased the extent of suprabasilar acantholysis. Isserof and Rifkin (15) have demonstrated the presence of plasminogen in the basal layer of human epidermis. Such an endogenous plasminogen source may explain the acantholysis observed when pemphigus vulgaris IgG was used alone at a 4 mg/ml concentration. The acantholysis in the pemphigus foliaceous and pemphigus vulgaris experiments (24) could be inhibited by aprotinin or lima bean trypsin inhibitor, each of which inhibits plasmin but not PA.

Morioka et al. (18) inhibited IgG-induced acantholysis in organ culture by adding antiurokinase antibody. This antibody crossreacts with PA. The experiment thus suggested an important role for PA in the induction of acantholysis.

Based on their cumulative data, Hashimoto et al. (12) postulated the following autoimmune mechanism for pemphigus: "Binding of pemphigus autoantibody to the surface of human epidermal cells stimulates the production of plasminogen activator. In the presence of plasminogen, the increased levels of plasminogen activator result in an increased conversion of plasminogen to plasmin. Plasmin is then responsible for the loss of cellular adhesion, probably by degradation of cell surface molecules responsible for cell-cell adhesion within the epidermis."

In a study using Balb/c primary epidermal cell cultures (PECC), Woo et al. (26) found that P-IgG-induced cell detachment was not altered by a plasminogen-free growth media. Furthermore, when dexamethasone was added to growth media, it produced almost complete inhibition of plasminogen activity, but cell detachment was not affected. They concluded that cell detachment in growth media was independent of plasminogen activity. Cell detachment, however, was inhibited by $\alpha_2$macroglobulin, trasylol, soybean trypsin inhibitor, and pepstatin, indicating that proteinases are involved in the process of cell detachment.

The data presented in the various organ culture studies of Lazarus et al. provides convincing evidence for the role of PA in pemphigus acantholysis. The study of Woo et al. cast doubt on the need for plasminogen activator in cell detachment. The discrepancy may relate to the different organ culture systems used.

There appears to be little doubt that enzymes play a role in pemphigus acantholysis. The main issues to be resolved include the actual number of involved enzymes (i.e., PA, pemphigus acantholysis factor, or possibly others), the exact role played by each enzyme, and the way that such enzymes may be successfully inhibited for therapeutic gain.

PEMPHIGUS ANTIBODY INTERACTION WITH THE KERATINOCYTE PLASMA MEMBRANE

It has been shown that separated epidermal cells bind pemphigus antibodies (6,22). Therefore, the antigenic determinants are located on the keratinocyte's cell surface. In this regard, the ICS is best viewed merely as an extension of the cell surface. A new aspect of pemphigus research is to characterize the physical union of the pemphigus antibody with the keratinocyte's surface receptor extensions and to uncover the antibody's fate after this union.

Yaoita et al. (28), using freeze-fracture and electron spin resonance (ESR) techniques, studied the effect of pemphigus vulgaris antibodies on cultured keratinocyte plasma membranes. Freeze fracture demonstrated broken tight junctions and decreased size and number of desmosomes. ESR revealed increased membrane fluidity. It is of interest to note that one of the purified pemphigus antibody samples had no effect on the plasma membrane. This suggested that perhaps some pemphigus antibodies, and not others, directly affect the plasma membrane in the acantholytic process.

Citovsky et al. (8) observed a change over time in the fluorescence of guinea pig keratinocytes that were incubated with fluorescein-labeled P-IgG. The initial diffuse fluorescence of the cell surface gradually changed to microclustering, followed by internalization. The microclustering stage of the fluorescent complex was associated with a dramatic increase in cell death, suggesting that a correlation between antigen-antibody migration and cell death exists. Microclustering also occurred when the cells were incubated with fluorescein-labeled normal IgG, although without the onset of cell death. This suggests that a unique phenomenon occurs in pemphigus above and beyond migration and microclustering. In the same system, using (^{125}I)P-IgG and ferritin-conjugated IgG for autoradiographic and EM studies, internalization of P-IgG was demonstrated. Microtubule-disruptive drugs such as colchicine, theophylline, and theobromine inhibited cell surface migration of bound P-IgG and antibody-induced cell death in a similar dose-response fashion. Subsequently, Patel et al. (19) studied the fate of pemphigus-bound IgG in murine PECC. They showed that the bound P-IgG becomes clustered, internalized through surface pits into submembranous vesicles, and eventually fused with lysosomes.

Thus, new emphasis is being placed on the mechanism(s) by which the interaction between pemphigus antibody and the keratinocyte plasma membrane results in physical, biochemical, and molecular alterations in the skin.

CONCLUDING REMARKS

Since the initial work of Beutner and Jordan in 1964, considerable progress has been made in understanding the pathophysiology of pemphigus. The pemphigus antibody is now fully accepted as triggering the epidermal injury seen in pemphigus. Furthermore, it is becoming increasingly recognized that an enzymatic mechanism(s) is involved in pemphigus acantholysis. The exact nature and number of enzymes involved is still somewhat controversial, but will undoubtedly be elucidated within the foreseeable future. The exact sequence of biochemical events that occurs due to antibody binding of the keratinocyte to the enzyme's activation, release, and induction of acantholysis remains to be elaborated.

While the emphasis on this chapter has been on experimental models of pemphigus, the role of the host should be realized. It is already well appreciated, for example, that the quantitative serum antibody level produced by the host parallels disease severity. In addition, the spontaneous disease process also appears to be dependent upon "local" host factors. This may have been best illustrated by Cram (9). He reported a progressive increase of IgG deposits in previously unaltered skin of pemphigus patients when that skin was exposed to ultraviolet (UV) irradiation. The IgG binding became maximal at 24 hours, corresponding to a point in time when microscopic acantholysis appeared. Cram also reviewed a number of theories that might conceivably explain the observations. One such theory is that UV light alters the plasma-epidermal barrier, thereby allowing attainment of a specific local IgG threshold necessary for the induction of overt pathology. Alternatively, light may immunogenically stimulate epidermal cell antigens, thus resulting in enhanced antibody fixation. Regardless of what may actually facilitate IgG binding, the implication is that specific local alterations occurring in the natural host do affect the ultimate expression of the disease.

The most difficult issues that remain to be solved are: 1) The nature of the pemphigus surface receptor; 2) the role that this receptor plays in keratinocyte metabolism; 3) the reason(s) why certain people are prone to develop pemphigus; and 4) the optimal method(s) of treatment.

These questions provide opportunities for further research in the study of this chronic bullous disease.

REFERENCES

1. Anhalt GJ, Labib RS, Voorhees JJ, et al: Induction of pemphigus in neonatal mice by passive transfer of IgG from patients with the disease. *N Engl J Med* 306:1189–1196, 1982.
2. Barnett LM, Beutner EH, Chorzelski TP: Organ cultures studies of pemphigus antibodies II. Ultrastructural comparison between acantholytic changes *in vitro* and human pemphigus lesions. *J Invest Dermatol* 68:265–271, 1977.
3. Beutner EH, Jordan RE: Demonstration of skin antibodies in sera of pemphigus vulgaris in patients by indirect immunofluorescent staining. *Proc Soc Exp Biol Med* 117:505–610, 1964.

4. Beutner EH, Lever WF, Witebsky E, et al: Autoantibodies in pemphigus vulgaris. *JAMA* 192:682–688, 1965.
5. Binder WL, Beutner EH, Chorzelski TP: *In vitro* effects of pemphigus antibodies on skin. *Br J Dermatol* 99:39–42, 1978.
6. Brigden WD, Amos HE: The differential binding of antibody from the sera of patients with pemphigus and pemphigoid to isolated guinea-pig epidermal cells. *Br J Dermatol* 93:425–430, 1975.
7. Buschard K, Dabelsteen E, Bretlau P: A model for the study of autoimmune diseases applied to pemphigus: Transplants of human oral mucosa to athymic nude mice binds pemphigus antibodies *in vivo*. *J Invest Dermatol* 76:171–173, 1981.
8. Citovsky V, Naishtat S, Timberg R, et al: The cellular response of human and guinea pig keratinocytes to pemphigus IgG-cell death related to IgG-receptor surface migration and internalization. *J Invest Dermatol* 80:366, 1983.
9. Cram DL: Photo-induction of lesions in patients with pemphigus and bullous pemphigoid. In Beutner EH, et al. (Eds): *Immunopathology of the Skin*, Dowden, Hutchinson, Ross, Stroudsburg, PA, 1973, pp 44–54.
10. Deng JS, Beutner EH, Shu S, et al: Pemphigus antibody action on skin explants: Kinetics of acantholytic changes and stability of antigens in tissue cultures of normal monkey skin explants. *Arch Derm* 113:923–926, 1977.
11. Farbatol RM, Dykes R, Lazarus GS: Anti-epidermal cell surface pemphigus antibody detaches viable epidermal cells from culture plates by activation of proteinase. *Proc Natl Acad Sci (USA)* 75:459–463, 1978.
12. Hashimoto K, Shafran KM, Webber PS, et al: Anti-cell surface pemphigus autoantibody stimulates plasminogen activator activity of human epidermal cells: A mechanism for the loss of epidermal cohesion and blister formation. *J Exp Med* 157:259–272, 1983.
13. Holubar K, Chorzelski TP, Guato M, et al: Studies in immunodermatology: 3. Induction of intraepithelial lesions in monkey by intramucosal injection of pemphigus antibodies. *Int Arch Allergy Appl. Immunol.* 44:631–643, 1973.
14. Hu CH, Schiltz JR, Michel B: Pemphigus autoantibody induced *in vitro* suprabasilar acantholysis: A unique phenomenon of epidermal injury. *Am J Pathol* 90:345–362, 1978.
15. Isserof RR, Rifkin DB: Plasminogen is present in the basal layer of epidermis. *Clin Res* 30:605A, 1982.
16. Michel B, Ko CS: Effect of pemphigus and bullous pemphigoid sera and leukocytes on normal skin in organ culture: An *in vitro* model for the study of bullous disease. *J Invest Dermatol* 62:541, 1974 (abstract).
17. Michel B, Ko CS: An organ culture model for the study of pemphigus acantholysis. *Br J Dermatol* 96:295–302, 1977.
18. Morioka S, Jensen PJ, Lazarus GS: The role of plasminogen and plasminogen activator in acantholysis *in vitro*. *J Invest Dermatol* 82:399, 1984.
19. Patel HP, Diaz LA, Anhalt GJ, et al: Demonstration of pemphigus antibody-antigen (receptor) complexes on the cell surface of epidermal cells in culture and their internalization. *J Invest Dermatol* 82:428, 1984.
20. Sams WM Jr, Jordan RE: Pemphigus antibodies: Their role in disease. *J Invest Dermatol* 56:474–479, 1971.
21. Schiltz JR, Michel B: Production of epidermal acantholysis in normal human skin *in vitro* by the IgG fraction from pemphigus serum. *J Invest Dermatol* 67:254–260, 1976.
22. Schiltz JR, Michel B, Papay R: Pemphigus antibody interaction with human epidermal cells in culture. A proposed mechanism for pemphigus acantholysis. *J Clin Invest* 62:778–788, 1978.
23. Schiltz JR, Michel B, Papay R: Appearance of "Pemphigus Acantholysis Factor" in human skin cultured with pemphigus antibody. *J Invest Dermatol* 72:575–583, 1979.
24. Singer K, Lazarus G: Molecular aspects of the pathophysiology of pemphigus. *Clinics in Dermatology* 1, 106–121, 1983.
25. Stoughton RB, Bagatell F: The nature of cantharidin acantholysis. *J Invest Dermatol* 33:287–292, 1959.

26. Woo T, Barouski-Miller P, Gelehrter G, et al: Effector proteases and pemphigus antibody action. *J Invest Dermatol* 80:355, 1983.
27. Wood JW, Beutner EH, Chorzelski TP: Studies in immunodermatology 2. Production of pemphigus-like lesions by epidermal injection of monkeys with Brazilian pemphigus foliaceous serum. *Int Arch Allergy* 42:556–564, 1972.
28. Yaoita H, Kitajima Y, Kiyomi E, et al: Effect of IgG class pemphigus antibodies on keratinocyte plasma membrane. *J Invest Derm* 80:366, 1983.

14
Comparative Immunodermatology

Robert J. Seiler
Danny W. Scott
Robert M. Lewis

INTRODUCTION

The application of appropriate immunopathologic techniques to veterinary patient material has identified and allowed characterization of a group of naturally occurring, nonviral bullous skin diseases in domestic animal species; notably the dog, cat, horse, and goat. This progress in veterinary immunodermatology has been stimulated largely by the improved understanding of the human counterparts of these diseases (Chaps. 9 to 13, 15, 16, 30 and 36), and by the necessity for veterinary diagnosticians to explore in more detail the various refractory skin conditions confronting them. For the most part, the various diseases are rare, and there are only a few centers at which there is sufficient awareness and laboratory sophistication to make a definitive diagnosis. The center established at the New York State College of Veterinary Medicine (NYSCVM) has provided clinical and immunopathologic expertise for the past 8 years, so that the methodologies and diagnostics could be developed and standardized, and so that the clinical, serologic, histopathologic, and immunopathologic features of these diseases could be defined. The following discussion is derived largely from the experiences at this center. Several recent reviews in this field (1,2,4,5,12,22,24,26,31,32,34) describe the current approach to clinical diagnosis and therapy, and as well provide a complete pictorial documentation (often in color) of the immunopathologic manifestations of the various diseases. Hence, the information contained in this chapter represents an overview of both the current level of knowledge, the laboratory methods used, and certain experimental observations that have been made.

METHODS USED

Choice of Specimens

As with human bullous diseases and other biopsy procedures, the skin lesions submitted for examination should be truly representative of the condition. Serum is also collected from affected animals, and is tested by indirect immunofluorescent (IIF) methods. The microscopic processes of repair, or secondary infection and excoriation, may frequently be of sufficient magnitude to confuse or prevent definitive diagnosis. The most useful information comes from lesions at the early vesicular or bullous stages. In addition, areas of the lesion that demonstrate the junction of affected and normal skin should be chosen. The problem is complicated in veterinary patients, such as the dog, because the stratum spinosum is usually only two to five cell layers deep and, hence, vesicular changes occurring in this layer usually have a thin, fragile roof that ruptures easily. Animals also tend to further excoriate the lesions, leading to early ulceration of involved skin. Close observation by the owner or veterinarian is required to insure selection of an adequate biopsy sample. Since cosmetic factors are, for the most part, less important in veterinary patients, multiple biopy specimens are often possible. Once the lesion is collected, usually by circular skin punch under local anesthetic, the specimen is divided to allow for detailed immunopathologic and histopathologic examination. The optimum situation is to provide one face from a bilateral division of the lesion for each diagnostic technique. Our dermatologists usually place the excised lesion onto saline-moistened gauze for immediate delivery to the histology laboratory, where it is divided, with one half being snap frozen and the other half fixed in 10% neutral buffered formalin. Detailed descriptions of the freezing methods and alternative approaches will follow. Samples may also be submitted in Michel's transport medium for direct immunohistologic testing.

Freezing of Sections

The aim is to freeze the biopsy specimen instantly, thereby maintaining the normal cytoarchitecture. For this purpose, snap freezing is carried out in liquid isopentane, chilled to its freezing point in liquid nitrogen. The specimen, submersed in an aluminum foil capsule of cryomountant, is plunged into chilled isopentane. Care must be taken to maintain the appropriate orientation of the specimen throughout this procedure. Cryosections cut 2 to 4 μm in thickness may be collected on plain microscope slides or on those with inscribed wells. Once the sections are on the slide, they are left to air dry for 10 minutes at room temperature.

Immunopathologic Testing

The usual procedure outlined in Chapter 1 is followed for both direct, and indirect IF testing. Incubation times are regularly 30 minutes at room temperature in a humid chamber. Rinsing between incubations with reagents is for 3 × 10 min in phosphate-buffered (PBS). Appropriate controls for each test include a conjugate control, and negative and positive sera controls. For direct tests, a sample of normal skin from the patient is also included, if possible. Indirect serum IF tests are done on lip, tongue, or esophageal mucosae from normal individuals of the same species. After staining and rinsing, the specimen is finally mounted for ultraviolet (UV) viewing in PBS/glycerol or polyvinyl alcohol. Direct immunohistologic testing has been conducted on formalin-fixed, paraffin-embedded sections using both fluorescent antibody techniques and peroxidase-antiperoxidase (PAP) procedures. At this stage, the methods outlined below have not been fully validated, and further investigations are underway. When immunoperoxidase methods are used, subsequent dehydration and permanent mounting is done.

Experimental IF Technique for Paraffin Sections

1. Deparaffinize regular paraffin-embedded sections in xylene (5 minutes each).
2. Rehydrate (1 minute each) with ethanol (100%, 95%, 70%, 50%, D.H_20).
3. Incubate slides in 0.1% trypsin (type III Sigma, bovine pancreas) containing 0.1% $CaCl_2$ (adjust pH to 7.8, with 0.1 N NaOH) (37°C for 2 hours).
4. Wash with D.H_2O, then wash with PBS (2 × 10 minutes).
5. Apply unconjugated antiserum (e.g., rabbit antidog IgG) and incubate (2 hours at 37°C) in a humid chamber.
6. Wash 2 × 10 minutes, with PBS.
7. Incubate with fluorescent antiserum (e.g., goat antirabbit Ig) (30 minutes at 25°C) in a humid chamber.
8. Wash 2 × 10 minutes with PBS.
9. Mount in PBS/glycerol.

Experimental PAP Technique for Paraffin Sections

1-4. As above.

5. Incubate with 20% normal serum from same host as second antibody for 10 minutes (25°C) in a humid chamber. Shake off excess; do not wash.
6. Incubate with primary antibody for 1 to 4 hours at 37°C, or overnight at °C in a humid chamber.
7. Wash 2 × 10 minutes, with PBS.
8. Block endogenous peroxidase activity with fresh 0.5% H_2O_2 in methanol for 10 minutes.
9. Wash in PBS for 10 minutes.
10. Incubate with second antibody for 30 minutes (25°C) in a humid chamber.
11. Wash in PBS 2 × 10 minutes.
12. Incubate with PAP for 30 minutes (25°C) in a humid chamber.
13. Wash in PBS 3 × 10 minutes.
14. Wash in Tris/HCl, pH 7.6, for 5 minutes.
15. Incubate with 3.3-diaminobenzidene tetrahydrochloride (DAB) substrate (25°C).
16. Wash in H_2O for 5 minutes.
17. Counterstain (optional).
18. Dehydrate in ethanol—50%, 70%, 95%, 100%, then three changes of xylene.
19. Permanently mount by standard methods.

Reagents Used

For IF testing, a battery of appropriate antisera specific for each species is routinely used. These are antiwhole globulin, anti-β1C (complement factor 3), and for the dog, anti-IgG, lgM, and lgA. Antiwhole globulin antiserum is prepared in rabbits by immunization with triple ammonium sulfate-precipitated normal immunoglobulin fractions. This reagent serves as a general screening test for bound immunoglobulins in the test specimens. The other anti-immunoglobulin reagents are obtained from commercial suppliers. Fluorescent conjugates are prepared by methods outlined in a previous chapter, and purified by gel (Sephadex G-25) filtration chromatography. All conjugates are tested for specificity against the appropriate antigen by immunoelectrophoresis, and the activity is quantified by radial immunodiffusion. The molar fluorescein-to-protein (F/P) ratio is determined (Chap. 1), and only conjugates with a ratio of 1-1.5:1 are used. The concentration of specific antibody protein in the test reagents is routinely adjusted to 100 μg/ml.

Certain experiments have also been done using a protein A peroxidase (POPA) conjugate (35). The use of protein A for this and other immunologic procedures depends on the highly specific, "pseudoimmune" affinity of protein A for the Fc region of immunoglobulin. In both humans and dog, this specificity is directed mainly toward IgG and, to a lesser extent, toward IgM. POPA was prepared by the improved periodate method and purified by gel filtration. Typical preparations had an average molecular weight (M_w) of approximately 120,000 daltons. The efficacy of POPA was demonstrated in indirect tests on sera of human and canine patients with antinuclear, pemphigus, and bullous pemphigoid (BP) antibodies, as well as in dogs with antithyroid (antithyroglobulin and antimicrosomal) antibodies. Direct tests on the skin and kidney of dogs with pemphigus or glomerulonephritis were also done. In all cases, the appropriate controls were negative, and the staining patterns mirrored the appearance, sensitivity, and specificity seen with conventional IF. The concentration of protein A in the pooled conjugate was adjusted before storage to 100 μg/ml. Titrations of various POPA conjugates showed them to be generally useful at dilutions between 1:10 and 1:80 (equivalent to a protein A concentration in the conjugate of 2.5 to 10 μg/ml). A 1:40 dilution (protein A, 5 μg/ml) was usually found to combine most consistently maximum sensitivity with minimum background staining, and it was usually used in subsequent tests. Visualization of peroxidatic activity in stained tissue sections was achieved by incubation for 30 minutes (room temperature) in a fresh solution (0.5 mg/ml) of DAB in Tris HCl buffer (pH 7.6) containing 0.01% H_2O_2.

Results Using Michel's Solution

Generally the results of IF testing of samples submitted in Michel's solution have been found to be equivalent to those performed on fresh samples. In two studies comparing the two methods (3,17) for a variety of autoimmune and other dermatopathies in dog and horse, no false-positive or false-negative results were found. For the canine material, the samples were stored for 7 days before testing; while in the equine study, the results remained the same for samples stored for 8 months. Hence, this method appears to allow reliable preservation of speciments submitted to established testing centers from remote locations.

IMMUNOPATHOLOGIC FINDINGS

A total of 263 canine, 46 feline, 29 equine, 3 caprine, and 1 bovine biopsy specimens from animals with suspected immunopathologic skin conditions have been examined at the NYSCVM clinic according to a detailed clinicopathologic protocol, including IF testing. Of these, positive findings have been found in 88 cases, and the results are summarized in Table 1. Many of these cases have been referred specifically to this service; therefore, the results do not represent the probable prevalence of the various conditions in the general population.

Table 1. Summary of IF findings from animals with immunopathologic skin diseases examined at the NSYCVM

				DIF					IIF
Disease	*Species*	*No. of Animals*	*Distribution of fluorescence*	*Whole Ig*	*IgG*	*IgA*	*IgM*	*C3*	
Pemphigus									
Vulgaris									
	Can	11	ICS	11	11	0	0	0	0
	Fel	4	ICS	4	—	—	—	1	0
Foliaceus									
	Can	9	ICS	9	9	1	1	1	1(1:16)
	Fel	5	ICS	5	—	—	—	0	0
	Eq	9	ICS	7	—	—	—	0	5(1:10–1:8000)
	Cap	1	ICS	1	—	—	—	0	0
Erythematosus									
	Can	12	ICS	12	12	3	3	2	0
			BMZ	7	3	4	5	3	0
	Fel	1	ICS	1	—	—	—	1	0
			BMZ	1	—	—	—	1	0
B P									
	Can	7	BMZ	7	4	4	2	5	1 (1:2048)
			ICS	0	0	0	0	0	1 (1:2048)
	Eq	1	BMZ	0	—	—	—	—	1(1:80)
SLE									
	Can	11	BMZ	7	1	5	3	9	0
			ICS	2	1	2	0	0	0
			Dermal blood vessel walls	2	0	0	1	2	0
	Fel	1	BMZ	1	—	—	—	—	0
Discoid LE									
	Can	16	BMZ	16	7	5	8	12	0
			ICS	1	1	0	0	0	0
			Dermal blood vessel walls	0	0	0	0	1	0

DIF, direct IF test; IIF, indirect IF test; —, test not done.

Pemphigus

Pemphigus Vulgaris

Pemphigus vulgaris was the first autoimmune skin disease reported in domestic animals (7,38). No breed, age, or sex predilections have been established. Of 11 dogs studied, the breeds included: five mongrels, one collie, one Shetland sheepdog, one german shepherd, one great dane, one weimaraner, and one scottish terrier. Seven females and four males ranging in age from 2 to 7 years represented the patient group. In addition, four domestic short-haired cats were found to have the characteristic features of pemphigus vulgaris.

Pemphigus vulgaris is characterized clinically by symmetric vesiculo-bullous or ulcerative lesions that may affect the oral cavity, mucocutaneous junctions, skin, or any combination thereof. Onychomadesis may be seen, and pruritus or pain are variable. Histologically, the canine form of pemphigus vulgaris is characterized by suprabasilar acantholysis, with resultant suprabasilar cleft and blister formation (Fig. 1). The basal cells of the epidermis remain attached to the basement membrane, presenting a "tombstone" appearance. Hair follicles may be involved. Cellular infiltration of the underlying and adjacent dermis varies, ranging from minor perivascular accumulation of lymphocytes and plasma cells to wide bands of lymphocytes, plasma cells, and neutrophils beneath the basement membrane zone (BMZ).

Direct IF tests on affected skin revealed the consistent presence of host IgG in the intercellular (IC) spaces of stratified squamous epithelium (Fig. 2). Complement (C_3) was not demonstrated in the cases studied, nor was circulating autoantibody to intercellular ground substance (ICS) demonstrable by IIF techniques. These latter two negative findings are in contrast to what is usually reported in human pemphigus vulgaris. However, studies in humans have demonstrated that pemphigus antibodies may produce acantholysis without participation of complement (18), so that the absence of C_3 in skin lesions may not be a surprising finding (Chaps. 9 to 13). The reason for negative serum titers to pemphigus antigen in canine patients is unknown. It is conceivable that inappropriate substrate material is being used for testing. It is also possible that circulating antibody is quickly bound in vivo to appropriate antigen in the skin and mucous membranes, and therefore is removed from the circulation as rapidly as it is produced. Alternatively, the pathogenic mechanisms causing the lesion in dogs may be different from that in humans, although there is no experimental evidence to support this possibility.

Our limited experience with four cases of feline pemphigus vulgaris indicates that clinically it is a severe vesiculo-bullous disease that affects skin and mucous membranes. The histopathologic findings are similar to those in canine disease. All four affected cats had demonstrable host immunoglobulin in the IC space when examined by DIF. One of

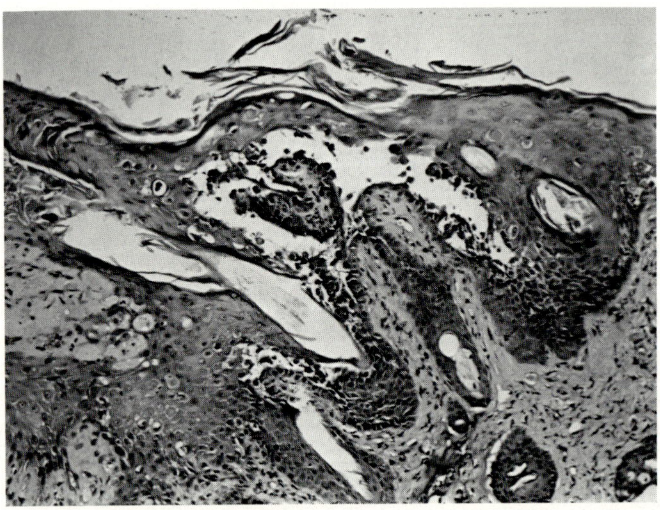

Figure 1. Histologic appearance of pemphigus vulgaris (feline). There is a suprabasilar cleft with basal epithelial cells remaining attached at the floor of the vesicle.

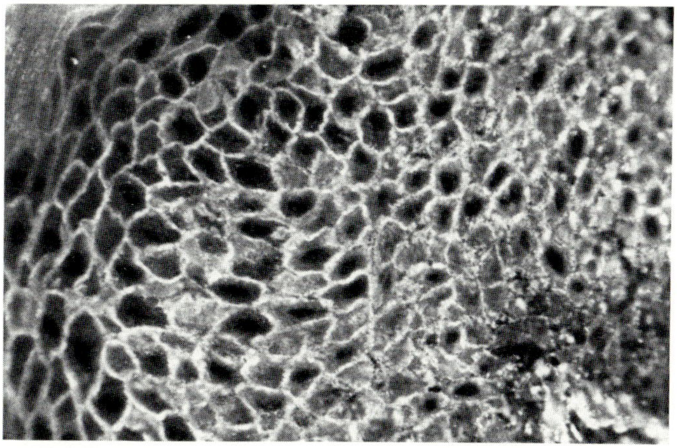

Figure 2. Positive DIF of the ICS in the skin of a dog with pemphigus vulgaris (anti-IgG conjugate).

the cats also had C_3 present in the IC space as well. Indirect fluorescent tests were negative in all four cases.

Pemphigus Foliaceus

Pemphigus foliaceus has been seem most commonly in dogs (5,6) and horses (8,13). Nine canine cases studied in our laboratory represented the following breeds: five mongrels, one beagle, one collie, one dachshund and one Shetland sheepdog. The patient group contained five females and four males, ranging in age from two to nine years. Seven equine cases occurred in horses 4 months to 10 years of age, with no breed or sex predilection. In addition, we have recognized pemphigus foliaceus in five domestic short-haired cats (14) 6 months to 11 years of age: (three male and two female), and also in a young female Nubian goat (28).

Pemphigus foliaceus is characterized clinically by symmetric vesiculo-bullous, pustular, or erosive dermatitis with pronounced crusting and scaling. It usually begins on the face and neck, eventually spreading to the entire body surface. Hair and nails may shed in association with severe lesions. Pain and pruritus vary, and oral lesions are rare. Microscopically, pemphigus foliaceus in each species is characterized by acantholysis and subsequent cleft and blister formation within the superficial epidermis, usually within the stratum granulosum (Fig. 3). Three important histologic features of this lesion are: 1) Involvement of hair follicles; 2) adherence of cells of the stratum granulosum to the roof of the blister; and 3) marked acantholysis. These three features of pemphigus foliaceus are important in distinguishing it from subcorneal pustular dermatitis and impetigo. The blister itself usually contains numerous eosinophils or neutrophils. Non specific epidermal changes include hyperkeratosis, parakeratosis, acanthosis, spongiosis, and leukocytic exocytosis. Dermal lesions include superficial congestion and perivascular accumulation of eosinophils, neutrophils, lymphocytes, and plasma cells.

In dogs, the immunopathologic findings are as described for canine pemphigus vulgaris, although IgM were demonstrable in one case and host IgA in another. Similarly, equine patients contained horse immunoglobulin in the IC spaces of affected epidermis. One dog had circulating antibody to ICS (titer 1:16), while IIF analysis of affected

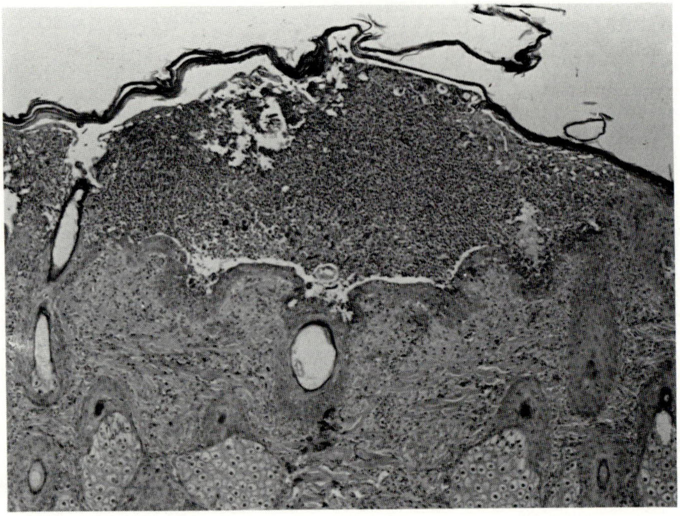

Figure 3. A subcorneal vesicle in the skin of a horse with pemphigus foliaceus. The vesicle is filled with acantholytic keratinocytes and polymorphonuclear inflammatory cells.

equine serum on normal horse tongue substrate revealed titers of circulating anti-ICS antibody of 1:10 to 1:8000. Affected skin from the feline patients and the goat contained host immunoglobulin in the IC spaces of the epidermis. Indirect IF testing was negative.

Pemphigus Erythematosus

Pemphigus erythematosus in humans is thought to be a benign variant of pemphigus foliaceus, which is localized to the head and neck. In animals (27), in addition to the usual gross and histopathologic features of pemphigus foliaceus, pemphigus erythematosus is characterized by the presence of positive DIF of both IC sustance and the BMZ, as well as the presence of circulating antinuclear antibody in some patients. Using these criteria, 12 canine cases of pemphigus erythematosus have been studied in our laboratory. Six mongrels, two beagles, two collies, one Labrador retriever, and one german shepherd constituted this patient group. They ranged in age from 1 to 12 years, and were more frequently male (8 of the 12). Pemphigus erythematosus was also recognized in an 8-year-old male American short-hair tabby cat.

The clinical and microscopic findings were similar to those of pemphigus foliaceus. Other prominent histopathologic findings seen in some of the lesions included spongiosis and hydropic degeneration of epithelial cells in the basal layer and stratum granulosum, focal epidermal necrosis, and severe lymphocytic and plasmacytic infiltration of the superficial dermis and rete ridges. Nonspecific changes included hyperkeratosis, parakeratosis, acanthosis, and subepidermal edema, congestion, and perivascular cellular infiltration. Immunopathologic findings included combinations of positive DIF results for host immune reactants in the ICS and the BMZ (Fig. 4). Three of the dogs had antinuclear antibody titers greater than 1:20. The multiple immunologic abnormalities in this patient group may be of value in future investigations concerning the possibility that pemphigus erythematosus may represent a disease in which pemphigus "overlaps" with cutaneous lupus erythematosus (LE).

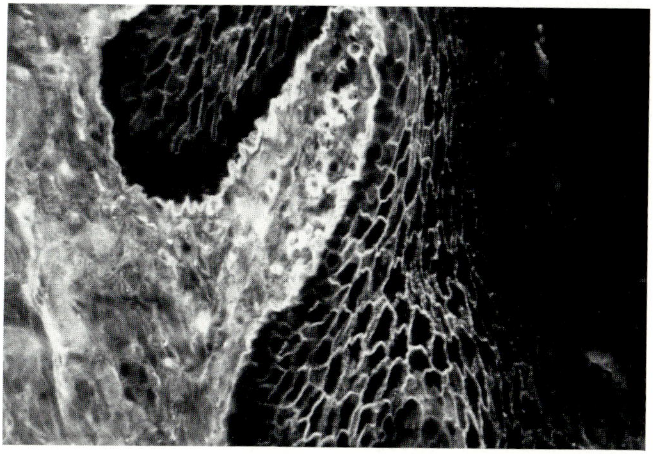

Figure 4. Pemphigus erythematosus in a dog showing positive IF of the ICS, and BMZ in the skin (anti-IgG conjugate).

Pemphigus Vegetans

Two dogs with manifestations suggestive of pemphigus vegetans have been seen (20,21), but results of IF tests are not available. A further dog is reported (19) to have had positive DIF of lesional skin. Histologically, the lesions are characterized by papillomatosis and intraepidermal abscesses composed primarily of eosinophils with few acantholytic keratinocytes. Dermal changes included congestion and perivascular accumulation of eosinophils, with fewer numbers of lymphocytes, plasma cells, and neutrophils.

Bullous Pemphigoid

Bullous pemphigoid (BP) has been reported as a canine disease (5,9). It is characterized by mucocutaneous vesiculo-bullous lesions that rapidly ulcerate. It is often difficult to distinguish BP from pemphigus vulgaris on the basis of clinical criteria; however, the histopathologic and IF findings are characteristically different. Seven dogs with BP have been studied in our laboratory. The breeds represented include two mongrels, one collie, one Shetland sheepdog, one dachshund, one cocker spaniel, and one great dane. Their ages ranged from 6 to 14 years, and the sex distribution was four female and three male. In addition, a similar condition has been seen in a horse. In this animal, DIF testing was negative, but there was a circulating antibody to the BMZ (titer 1:80).

Microscopically, canine BP is characterized by the formation of subepidermal blisters that may contain neutrophils, eosinophils, erythrocytes, and fibrin. Acantholysis is not a feature of the lesion, although focal spongiosis may occur adjacent to vesicles and ulcers. Dermal changes include scant-to-striking accumulations of lymphocytes, plasma cells, and occasionally neutrophils in the upper dermis, particularly subjacent to vesicles and ulcers. IF findings include the consistent presence of one or more host immunoglobulins (Fig. 5) and often complement components along the BMZ. The staining pattern is usually irregularly linear to granular in appearance. These DIF and IIF findings are similar to those reported in humans with BP (Chaps. 15 and 16). One of the

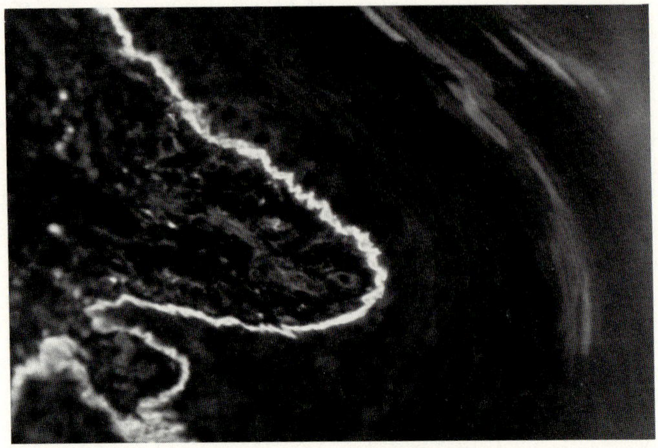

Figure 5. Direct IF of the lesion of BP in a dog. There is a dense linear band along the BMZ (anti-IgG conjugate).

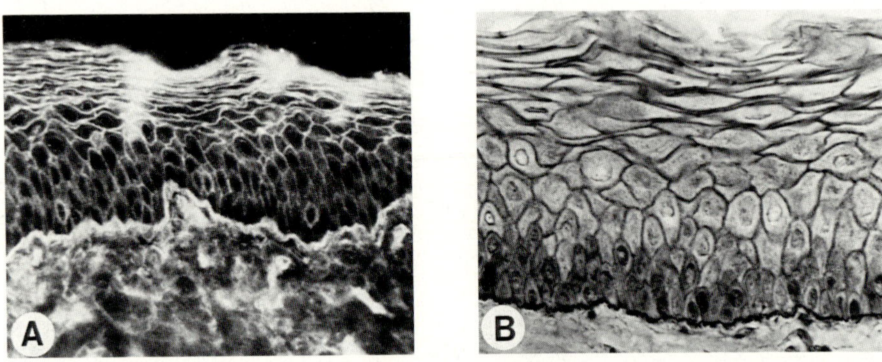

Figure 6. Indirect immunohistologic tests (using IF and POPA) of a serum (1:200) from a dog with BP tested on normal canine esophageal mucosa. A. FA control. B. POPA (1:40). Both tests show positive staining of the ICS and BMZ.

dogs studied had a high titer (1:2048) circulating antibody to basement membrane antigens by indirect immunohistologic testing (Fig. 6). This dog also had circulating antibodies present at the same high titer to epithelial IC substance; thus, the full extent of this disease is unknown.

Cutaneous Lupus Erythematosus

Systemic lupus erythematosus (SLE) was originally described as a spontaneous canine entity in 1965 (10). Since its initial recognition, other immunologic abnormalities in affected dogs, including those associated with dermal lesions, have been recorded (15,31). Dermal immunopathologic manifestations suggestive of cutaneous LE have also been described in a 9-year-old male cat (23).

Cutaneous LE in the dog presents with a variety of clinical features, including maculopapular, discoid, purpuric, urticarial, vesiculo-bullous, or seborrheic eruptions. To date, skin lesions have occurred during the course of the disease in approximately one of three canine patients. The affected dogs ranged in age from 2 months to 10 years, and seven males and four females have been seen. Affected breeds include five Shetland sheepdogs, two mongrels, one beagle, one English setter, one basenji, and one great dane. Microscopically, the lesions in cutaneous LE vary widely in association with the gross lesions. However, hydropic degeneration of basal epithelial cells has characterized the lesion in dogs. Subepidermal blisters may form in association with severe basal cell degeneration and resultant dermal-epidermal separation. In addition, subcorneal vesicles with neutrophils and acantholytic keratinocytes have also been observed. Other changes present include focal acanthosis, parakeratosis, spongiosis, leukocytic exocytosis, microvesicles and microabscesses, dermal congestion, and perivascular infiltrates of lymphocytes, plasma cells, and neutrophils.

IF studies of affected skin from dogs have demonstrated host immunoglobulin and/or host complement components present in the BMZ (Fig. 7) (see Chap. 30 for comparison with humans). The staining pattern is fine-to-coarse granular. All classes of immunoglobulin (IgG, IgM, and IgA) have been seen, although not usually in the same dog. Complement is detected at the BMZ in most biopsy specimens. Indirect IF testing has demonstrated antinuclear antibody (ANA) titers of 1:10 to 1:160 in most of the dogs and the cat, which have IF abnormalities in the skin (see Chaps. 2 and 31 for comparisons with human SLE). However, LE cell tests have been consistently negative in these dogs, while certain other dogs with the clinicopathologic features of SLE have had positive LE cell tests. To date, the specificity of host immunoglobulin deposits for single-stranded or double-stranded DNA has not been reported in the animal forms of this disease. A second group of dogs that usually have nasal dermatitis and immunopathologic changes similar to those dogs with SLE has been described as having a canine form of discoid lupus erythematosus (DLE) (32). This group had an age range of 1 to 9 years, 5 were male and 10 female. The breeds of affected dogs were three German

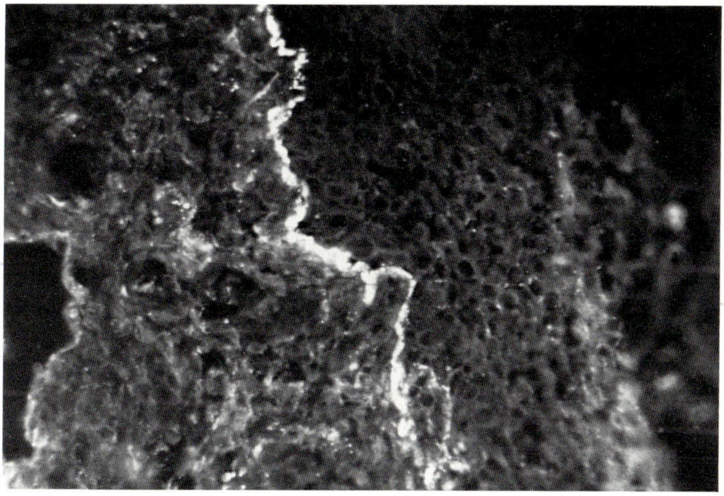

Figure 7. SLE in a dog showing positive IF of a band along the BMZ (anti-IgG conjugate).

shepherd dogs, two Shetland sheepdogs, one cross--bred Shetland sheepdog, three mongrels, two collies, one collie crossbreed, one Siberian husky, one samoyed, and one English pointer. In these dogs, there was no systemic involvement, LE tests were negative, and an ANA titer (1:20) was seen in only one dog. Linear IgA deposits at the BMZ are seen quite frequently in these dogs, and in a heterogeneous group that includes dogs with SLE, BP, and a unique subcorneal pustular dermatitis (25).

EXPERIMENTAL INVESTIGATIONS IN PEMPHIGUS

Since there were no previously reported investigations of pemphigus antigens from canine tissues, several experiments were carried out to study the specificity of human pemphigus sera to this antigen, and to establish some preliminary characteristics of canine pemphigus antigen (36,37). Investigations of the pathogenicity of canine pemphigus antibodies in vitro, or reciprocal studies of the specificity of canine pemphigus sera to human pemphigus antigen, have not been possible because of the previously mentioned lack of detectable antibodies in the circulation of canine patients.

Titrations of four human pemphigus sera on cryosections of the esophageal mucosa from 12 different dogs showed similar results to those seen using monkey esophagus (Chap. 3). The titers of these sera were 1:160 to 1:320, and the same titers were obtained by use of POPA reagents (Fig. 8) or conventional fluoresceinated antihuman IgG. Samples of 51 different human sera from patients without pemphigus were also tested on canine esophageal mucosa. Several of these sera contained pemphigus-like antibodies (PLA) in weak titers (1:20 to 1:40), as well as several other antibasal cell cytoplasmic and ANA. The same four human pemphigus sera were also treated on esophageal mucosa from rat, guinea pig, rabbit, green monkey, and baboon. The titers obtained on rat, guinea pig, and rabbit esophagus were generally less than the established titers determined using either canine, rabbit, monkey, or baboon mucosa.

Experiments were performed to establish some of the solubility and stability characteristics of canine pemphigus antigens by exposing standard sections of canine esophageal mucosa to a variety of potential solubilizing solutions prior to use of the sections in standard titrations of nonpemphigus sera. The methods used were similar to those previously described (16). These showed that the canine pemphigus antigen was remarkably and unexpectedly stable. A variety of aqueous and organic solvents had no effect for periods up to 10 minutes on the reactivity of the pemphigus antigen. Solvents used included 99.5% ethanol, 95% acetone, 95% ether, 1 M dimethylsulfoxide, 0.2% Triton X-100, and 10% neutral-buffered formalin. Prolonged exposure (up to 12 to 24 hours) to PBS or tris-acetate saline produced a gradual reduction in the antigen that was reactive with pemphigus foliaceus sera, but not that reactive with pemphigus vulgaris sera. The addition of $CaCl_2$ and dithiothreitol protected and restored the reactivity of the pemphigus foliaceus antigen, suggesting that the antigen may be temporally masked by the loss of the Ca^{2+} ions or the formation of intermolecular or intramolecular disulfide linkages. Exposure of sections to solutions containing dithiothreitol and $CaCl_2$ with a variety of added detergents (1%) showed that only Zwittergent and sodium dodecyl sulfate were capable of removing the reactivity of canine pemphigus antigen. Detergents such as Chaps, Deoxycholate, Nonidet NP-40, octyl-β-glucoside, Tween 20, Tween 80, and several others had no effect even if sections were exposed for 12 hours.

Attempts were then made to extract and purify pemphigus antigen from pooled canine esophageal mucosae. Frozen mucosa was ground to a fine powder and then washed several times in PBS. Pemphigus antigen resided in the insoluble sediment fractions from these washings, as was demonstrated by the ability of this sediment to

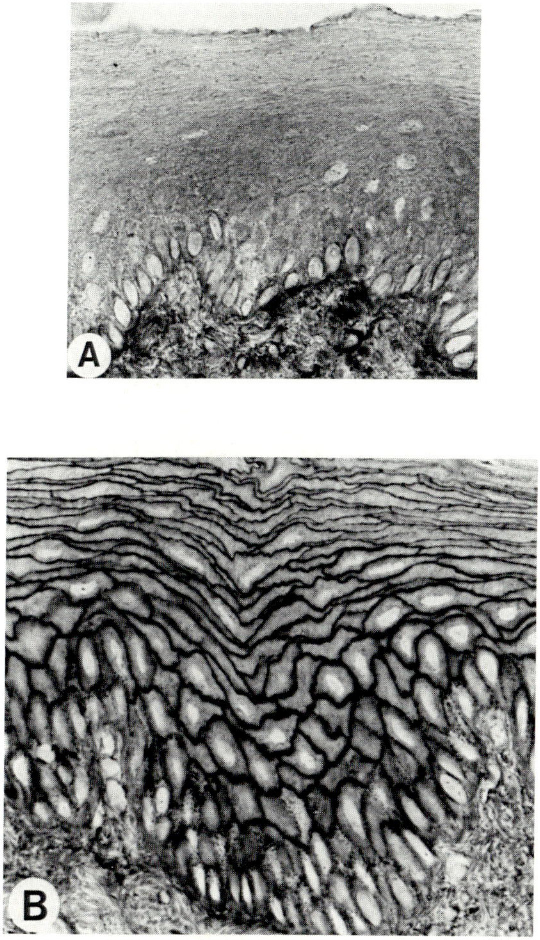

Figure 8. Examples of indirect immunohistologic tests of human pemphigus sera on canine esophagus using POPA. A. Normal human serum (1:10), negative staining. B. Pemphigus vulgaris serum (1:40), positive staining.

specifically absorb pemphigus antibody from pemphigus serum. Marked reduction in serum titer was produced by absorbing 200 μl of serum (diluted 1:40) with 10 to 20 mg of lyophilized sediment. Similar fractions prepared from pooled liver, kidney, and spleen did not absorb pemphigus antibody. Further attempts to isolate and purify the reactive antigen from lyophilized sediment in aqueous and detergent (especially Zwittergent) solutions were not successful.

A blocking method was also developed and used to determine serologic specificity of the human pemphigus sera being studied. For this test, $F(ab')_2$ fragments were prepared from each serum and used in reciprocal blocking of whole serum from the other patients. Since POPA would not detect tissue-bound $F(ab')_2$ fragments, even though these would bind and block the same antigenic determinants as whole immunoglobulin, positive blocking would be evidenced by the reduction of the titer of a second serum detected by POPA. Sera of the same specificity would show positive blocking in paired, reciprocal blocking tests, while sera with reactions of nonidentity would show no blocking in similar tests. The retention of reactivity in the $F(ab')_2$ fragments was verified by indirect tests using fluorescent antibody. Using this blocking method, it was found that a pair of pemphigus foliaceus sera had reactions of complete identity, and a pemphigus vulgaris serum had reactions of partial identity. A fourth serum had reactions of nonidentity with the other three. These differences in serologic specificity of the sera correlated with differences in the staining patterns (Fig. 9) observed (the two pemphigus foliaceus sera stained the ICS predominantly in the suprabasal layer with sparing of the basal cells, whereas the other two sera stained the ICS in the basal cell layer as well),

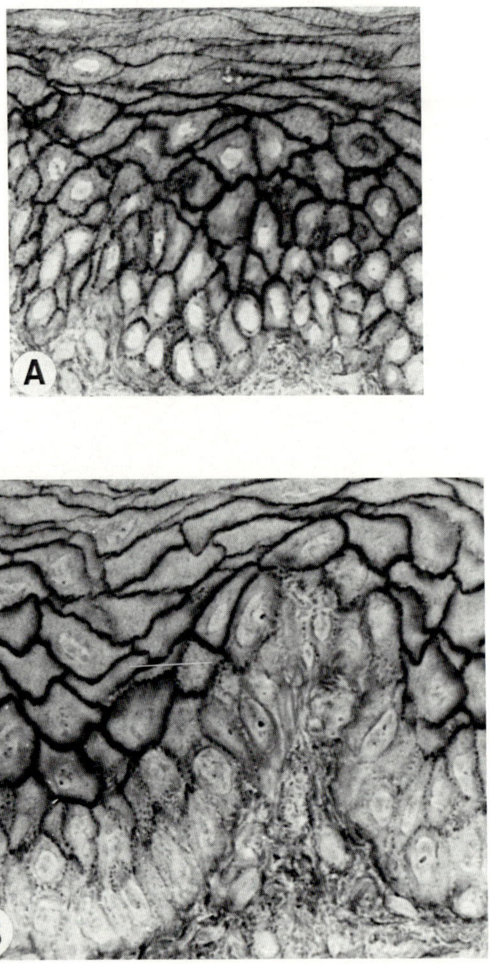

Figure 9. Contrasting staining pattern of human pemphigus sera on canine esophageal mucosa. A. Pemphigus vulgaris serum (1:40), ICS of basal epithelium stained. B. Pemphigus foliaceus serum (1:40), sparing of staining of basal epithelium.

and also with the physicochemical characteristics of the respective antigens determined in the previous experiments.

Preliminary studies of the responses of mice immunized with lyophilized esophageal sediment were done. The mice produced antiepidermal cell sera at low titers (1:20), which bound to both canine and murine esophageal mucosa in a pattern similar to that seen produced by pemphigus antibody. However, the POPA/F $(ab')_2$ blocking method showed lack of cross-reactivity between these murine antiepidermal cell sera and pemphigus antibody. Hence, these murine antisera were considered to represent PLA.

OTHER FINDINGS

We have encountered some false-positive test results during the examination of various canine tissues (29,30,33). In normal dogs, the planum of the nose and the footpad frequently have linear deposition of IgM at the basement membrane. In a study of the IF of the skin of normal dogs, granular deposits of IgM found in 5 of 11 footpads and 11 of 15 noses. Other immunoglobulin classes and complement were not seen. Hence, the use of only anti-IgM or polyvalent fluorescent antiserum may easily lead to misdiagnoses of BP or LE. Similar caution is required with equine biopsy specimens. In a series of horses examined (30 normal: 28 with various dermatologic diseases other than pemphigus, and 21 with nondermatologic disorders), two animals with dermatophilosis had diffuse deposits of immunoglobulin in the cutaneous ICS. The reason for the immunoglobulin depositions in these various animals is not known; however, we have had to reassess some of the earlier published findings for the immunopathologic conditions, so that the results tabulated herein represent the most accurate to date.

Circulating PLA, which are a problem for diagnosticians of human pemphigus, are rare in the sera of domestic animals. In the dog, only 1 of 100 animals tested had a circulating PLA at low titer (1:10). This dog had a dermatopathy due to generalized demidicosis, while the other dogs in this study were normal dogs (25), had other dermatologic diseases, or had nondermatologic diseases. A similar study of 75 feline sera (from 25 cats with dermatologic diseases, 25 with nondermatologic diseases, and 25 with no disease) failed to find any PLA. In the horse, however, 6 of 79 tested had PLA in the serum. Three were normal horses (titers, 1:40), two had dermatophilosis (titers, 1:10 and 1:80), and one had a systemic lymphoproliferative disease (titer, 1:320). These results suggest that "false-positive" IIF due to PLA is not likely in the dog and cat; but since the titers of true pemphigus sera are usually very low or negative, it will not be possible to differentiate the two on the basis of the titers. However, in the horse, the IIF test must be cautiously interpreted.

CONCLUSIONS

In general, the manifestations of the various veterinary immunodermatologic diseases are similar to those in humans; and the situation, at present, may be likened to that in human dermatology before the introduction of present-day diagnostic services. However, the state of the art is barely past the recognition phase, with little progress having been made to date in the use of these animal models as experimental subtrates for dermatologic research. The diagnostic procedures required in animals are also basically the same as in humans, with consistent results being obtained using standardized IF.

However, in many cases, immediate access to appropriate laboratory services is not available. In such situations, submission of samples in Michel's transport medium is a reliable alternative. There also occurs at most diagnostic laboratories a group of cases which have clinicopathologic findings suggestive of autoimmune disease, but for which only conventionally processed, paraffin-embedded samples are available. For these, the method using immunoperoxidase reagents appears to be suitable, but definitive experimental evidence is not yet available. In some situations, use of POPA may be appropriate, especially for screening purposes, since the same, relatively standardized reagent could be used on specimens from different species.

One of the most prominent points of difference between the human and animal immunodermatopathies occurs in pemphigus. In the dog and cat, almost invariably, the indirect immunohistologic pemphigus tests are negative, or insignificant titers are determined. The situation in the horse is different; in some cases, circulating pemphigus antibodies are present in high titer. Thus, it would appear that definite species differences occur in the immunobiology of equine and canine pemphigus foliaceus. To date, it has not been possible to perform tests of serum pathogenicity either in vitro or in vivo with canine or feline pemphigus or pemphigus-like sera. However, recently it has been shown that dog and horse pemphigus antibodies could induce acantholysis and binding of these antibodies in organ culture of skin (6a). No results are yet available regarding the potential experimental pathogenicity of equine pemphigus sera. Further differences between canine and human pemphigus are suggested by the preliminary data concerning canine pemphigus antigens. Although human pemphigus antibodies react with antigens in canine esophageal epithelium—and as such this source of antigenic substrate may find a more general use in pemphigus testing—the canine pemphigus antigens appear to be unexpectedly stable.

SLE and BP also have a similar clinicopathology to the human diseases. The variety of histopathologic lesions in canine and feline cutaneous LE mimics the diverse nature of the other systemic manifestations that occur in SLE. In a group of dogs in which there was a familial predisposition toward developing features of SLE (10), studies have shown that some of the serologic abnormalities could be transmitted to normal dogs and mice in cell-free extracts from affected dogs. This has been seen as implicating an infectious agent in the acquisition of the disease. Little experimental evidence pertaining to the pathogenesis of the canine lesions is available, but it is presumed to be related to deposition of immune complexes with resultant induction of inflammatory responses in affected tissues. In one dog with glomerulonephritis and SLE, there were antibodies to mammalian C-type viral, P-30 antigen in renal eluates, and detectable viral antigen on the surface of circulating lymphocytes (11). No evidence is available regarding the pathogenesis of the skin forms of animal LE or BP.

The rare and sporadic occurrence of each of these diseases described in animals usually does not provide opportunities better than those provided by human counterparts for systematic investigations of pathogenesis of therapeutic modalities. Also, apart from the situation in some forms of canine SLE, most of the diseases have not occurred with any apparent familial predisposition. However, extensive investigations of related individuals have generally not been performed. Nevertheless, should a familial predisposition be determined, it is logistically feasible to breed and maintain a colony of such animals for investigative purposes.

ACKNOWLEDGMENTS

The authors are grateful to Christina A. Smith for her expert technical assistance.

REFERENCES

1. Bennett D, Lauder IM, Kirkham D, et al: Bullous autoimmune skin disease in the dog: (1) Clinical and pathological assessment. *Vet Rec* 106:497, 1980.
2. Bennett D, Lauder IM, Kirkham D, et al: Bullous autoimmune skin disease in the dog: (2) Immunopathological assessment. *Vet Rec* 106:523, 1980.
3. Caciolo PL, Hurvitz AI, Nesbitt GH: Michel's medium as a preservative for immunofluorescent staining of cutaneous biopsy specimens in dogs and cats. *Am J Vet Res* 45:128, 1984.
4. Fukushima K; Pathogenesis of pemphigus vulgaris in dog and man—A review. *Can Vet J* 23:135, 1982.
5. Halliwell REW: Autoimmune disease in the dog. *Adv Vet Sci Comp Med* 22:221, 1978.
6. Halliwell REW, Goldschmidt MH: Pemphigus foliaceus in the canine: A case report and discussion. *J Am Animal Hosp Assoc* 13:431, 1977.

6a. Huang, JG: Canine and equine pemphigus: Serological studies, antigen extraction and characterization. Ph.D. Thesis, State University of New York at Buffalo, 1985, 233 pp.

7. Hurvitz AI, Feldman E: A disease in dogs resembling human pemphigus vulgaris: Case reports. *J Am Vet Med Assoc* 166:585, 1975.
8. Johnson ME, Scott DW, Manning TO, et al: Pemphigus foliaceus in the horse. *Equine Pract* 3:40, 1981.
9. Kunkle G, Goldschmidt MH, Halliwell REW: Bullous pemphigoid in a dog: A case report with immunofluorescent findings. *J Am Animal Hosp Assoc.* 14:52, 1978.
10. Lewis RM, Schwartz RS, Henry WB: Canine systemic lupus erythematosus. *Blood* 25:143, 1965.
11. Lewis RM: Evidence for a virus in canine systemic lupus erythematosus. In *Bayer-Symposium VI: Experimental Models of Chronic Inflammatory Diseases.* Springer-Verlag, New York, 1977, p 71.
12. Lewis RM, Scott DW: Spontaneous animal models for blistering disease. In Goldsmith LA (Ed): *The Biochemistry and Physiology of the Skin.* Oxford University Press, New York, Oxford, 1983, p 1056.
13. Manning TO, Scott DW, Rebhun WC, et al: Pemphigus-pemphigoid in a horse. *Equine Pract* 3:38, 1981.
14. Manning TO, Scott DW, Smith CA, et al: Pemphigus diseases in the feline: Seven case reports and discussion. *J Am Animal Hosp Assoc* 18:433, 1982.
15. Monier JC, Dardenne M, Rigal D, et al: Clinical and laboratory features of canine lupus syndromes. *Arthritis Rheum* 23:294, 1980.
16. Ogawa H, Taneda A, Morioka S: Characterization of pemphigus antigen. *J Invest Dermatol* 70:194, 1978.
17. Rosser EJ, Ihrke PJ, White SD, et al: The duration and quality of positive direct immunofluorescence in skin biopsies using Michel's fixative on a case of equine pemphigus foliaceus. *Equine Vet Sci* 3:14, 1983.
18. Schiltz JR: Pemphigus acantholysis: A unique immunological injury. *J Invest Dermatol* 74:359, 1980.
19. Schultz KT, Goldschmidt M: Pemphigus vegetans in a dog: A case report. *J Am Animal Hosp Assoc* 16:579, 1980.
20. Scott DW: Pemphigus vegetans in a dog. *Cornell Vet* 67:374, 1977.
21. Scott DW: Immunologic skin disorders in the dog and cat. *Vet Clin North Am* 8:641, 1978.
22. Scott DW: Pemphigus in domestic animals. *Clinics Dermatol* 1:141, 1983.
23. Scott DW, Haupt KH, Knowlton BF, et al: A glucocorticoid-responsive dermatitis in cats, resembling systemic lupus erythematosus in man. *J Am Animal Hosp Assoc* 15:157, 1979.
24. Scott DW, Lewis RM: Pemphigus and pemphigoid in dog and man: Comparative aspects. *J Am Acad Dermatol* 5:148, 1981.
25. Scott DW, Manning TO, Lewis RM: Linear IgA dermatoses in the dog: Bullous pemphigoid, discoid lupus erythematosus and a subcorneal pustular dermatitis. *Cornell Vet* 72:394, 1982.
26. Scott DW, Manning TO, Smith CA, et al: Observations on the immunopathology and therapy of canine pemphigus and pemphigoid. *J Am Vet Med Assoc* 180:48, 1982.

27. Scott DW, Miller WH, Lewis RM, et al: Pemphigus erythematosus in the dog and cat. *J Am Animal Hosp Assoc* 16:815, 1980.
28. Scott DW, Smith MC, Smith CA, et al: Pemphigus foliaceus in a goat. *Agri-Practice* 5:38–45, 1984.
29. Scott DW, Walton DK, Manning TO, et al: Pitfalls in immunofluorescence testing in canine dermatology. *Cornell Vet* 73:131, 1983.
20. Scott DW, Walton DK, Manning TO, et al: Pitfalls in immunofluorescence testing in dermatology. 2. Pemphigus-like antibodies in the cat, and direct immunofluorescence testing of normal dog nose and lip. *Cornell Vet* 73:275, 1983.
31. Scott DW, Walton DK, Manning TO, et al: Canine lupus erythematosus. 1. Systemic lupus erythematosus. *J Am Animal Hosp Assoc* 19:461, 1983.
32. Scott DW, Walton DK, Manning TO, et al: Canine lupus erythematosus. 2. Discoid lupus erythematosus. *J Am Animal Hosp Assoc* 19:481, 1983.
33. Scott DW, Walton DK, Smith CA, et al: Pitfalls in immunofluorescence testing in dermatology. 3. Pemphigus-like antibodies in the horse and direct immunofluorescence testing in equine dermatophilosis. *Cornell Vet* 74:305–311, 1984.
34. Scott DW, Wolfe MJ, Smith CA, et al: The comparative pathology of non-viral bullous skin diseases in domestic animals. *Vet Pathol* 17:257, 1980.
35. Seiler RJ: Staphylococcal protein A labeled with horseradish peroxidase for the immunohistologic diagnosis of canine autoimmune diseases. *Am J Vet Res* 44:195, 1983.
36. Seiler RJ: Interspecies reactivity of human pemphigus antibody with canine pemphigus antigen. Ph.D. Thesis, Cornell University, Ithaca, NY, 1984.
37. Seiler RJ, Huang J: Antigens of canine stratified squamous epithelium reactive with human pemphigus antibodies. *J Invest Dermatol* 80:379, 1983.
38. Stannard AA, Gribble DH, Baker BB: A mucocutaneous disease in the dog, resembling pemphigus vulgaris in man. *J Am Vet Med Assoc* 166:575, 1975.

Section IIB

PEMPHIGOID

15
The Immunopathology of Bullous Pemphigoid Antibodies

W. Ray Gammon

INTRODUCTION

Bullous pemphigoid (BP) is a chronic, self-limited, acquired blistering disease that affects older men and women of all races (1,37,46; Chap. 16). Cases occur sporadically, and there is no convincing evidence for a genetic predisposition. The disease is characterized clinically by a combination of steroid-responsive erythematous macules, papules, plaques, and vesicles, and large tense bullae and erosions. Lesions are usually generalized and often affect flexural and intertriginous skin. Mucous membranes (usually oral) are affected in 10 to 30% of cases. Lesions usually heal without scarring, but transient pigmentary changes and milia may occur. Several clinical variants have been reported (8). These include a "localized" variety in which lesions are confined either to the extensor surfaces of the lower extremities or head and neck region, an "erythematous" variety in which macular and palpable erythemas dominate the clinical picture, and a "vesicular" variant that clinically and histologically resembles dermatitis herpetiformis. A generalized bullous variety that heals with scars and atrophy has been reported, but these cases most likely are epidermolysis bullosa acquisita (EBA) (see Chap. 20).

The histology of BP is characterized by two consistent features: a subepidermal blister with a relatively intact epidermis, and dermal inflamation (38,47). Dermal inflammation may be relatively sparse or dense, and usually consists of a mixture of mononuclear cells (lymphocytes and monocytes) and granulocytes (eosinophils and neutrophils). Inflammatory cells are present around upper and middermal vessels, and are scattered in the mid- and upper dermis and at the basement membrane zone (BMZ). In most cases, eosinophils are abundant and outnumber neutrophils, but occasionally the reverse occurs. Occasionally, granulocytes are scarce and the infiltrate is composed almost entirely of a sparse accumulation of mononuclear cells. Careful studies of the sequential inflammatory features in evolving lesions have been reported, as well as studies correlating the histologic and clinical features (62). These reports have shown that histologic features are dynamic, and that specific findings depend on the morpho-

Supported in part by Grants 5-K04-AM00956-02 and 5-R01-AM30475-02 from the National Institutes of Health.

logic type and age of lesions sampled. Possibly other factors may affect inflammatory features and may account for the varying prominence of certain cell types.

Since the initial reports of circulating and tissue-bound anti-BMZ antibodies in BP, considerable information about the immunopathology of the disease has been obtained using several different techniques. These have included direct (DIF) and indirect (IIF) immunofluorescence (IF), complement-binding IF, immunoelectron microscopy (IEM), immunochemical methods, and methods for evaluating the functional immunologic properties of circulating and tissue-bound BP antibodies. These studies have been of critical value in providing immunologic diagnostic criteria for BP, differentiating it from other closely related bullous diseases and stimulating and directing most of the investigation into pathogenesis.

IMMUNOFLUORESCENCE STUDIES

Direct Immunofluorescence

Cutaneous deposits of IgG and complement were first resported in BP in the late 1960s (4,7,30,34). Since then, DIF has become a standard part of the evaluation of these patients and an important diagnostic study. The deposits are typically present in a fine linear (ribbon-like) pattern at the BMZ in clinically normal-appearing perilesional skin (Fig. 1). The pattern may be interrupted or granular in lesional skin (Fig. 2) (34). In tissue where there is epidermal-dermal separation, deposits may be absent or present in the blister roof or blister roof and base (60).

In general, immune deposits can be detected at any skin site in patients with generalized disease; however, in patients with localized lesions, deposits may be present only in skin near lesions. Since the characteristic linear pattern of fluorescence may be disturbed in lesional skin and deposits may be absent in skin distant from lesions, the optimal site for a biopsy procedure is clinically normal-appearing skin 1 to 2 cm away from a lesion. In a recent study, expression of BP antigen was found to be greatest in intertriginous skin. Therefore, the optimal site for obtaining a biopsy specimen may be perilesional skin in an intertriginous location (22).

Immune deposits in BP characteristically consist of IgG and complement (1,29). IgG deposits are present in 90 to 95% of cases and the third complement component (C3) has been detected in nearly 100% (see Chap. 16). IgG deposits are rarely present in the absence of C3. IgA, IgM, IgD, and IgE deposits have been reported (9,49); however, these immunoglobulin classes have been present in a minority of patients, always accompany IgG, and fluoresce less intensely than IgG. Complement components in addition to C3 are often present. They included components of the early classical pathway (C_1q, C4), the alternative pathway (factors B, D, and H), and the terminal pathway (C5 and C5b-C9 membrane attack complex) (5,33,39,48,49). In addition to IgG and complement, linear deposits of fibrin and platelet factor 4 have been detected (41,49). Current evidence suggests that IgG and C3 deposits disappear with remission (1,46).

Although linear IgG and C3 BMZ deposits are characteristic of BP, they are not specific. They are also characteristic of benign mucous membrane pemphigoid (cicatricial pemphigoid), herpes gestationis (HG), EBA, and what was reported in some patients as bullous eruption (BESLE) of systemic lupus erythematosus (SLE) (3,31,36,43). Currently, there is no reliable way of differentiating the deposits in BP from those in benign mucous membrane pemphigoid and HG. They can be distinguished from those in EBA and BESLE by direct IEM and double IF microscopic techniques (see Chap.

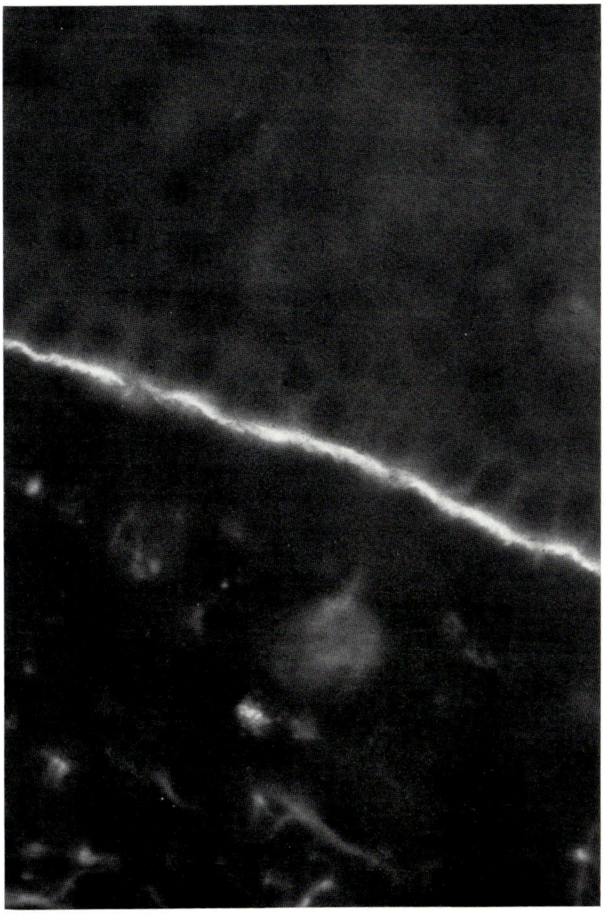

Figure 1. Photomicrograph showing direct IgG IF in perilesional BP skin. Note linear fluorescence at the BMZ (540x).

20) (21,27,43,64). Distinguishing the deposts in suspected cases of BP from those in EBA and BESLE may be necessary, since the cutaneous clinical, histologic, and DIF features may be indistinguishable (16).

Indirect Immunofluorescence

Anti-BMZ antibodies have been detected in the sera of 60 to 80% of patients with active BP (1,26,30). Circulating "BP antibodies" have been exclusively IgG, consist of all IgG subclasses, and both complement-binding and noncomplement-binding antibodies (32,33,51). They produce a fine linear pattern of fluorescence at the BMZ on a variety of stratified squamous epithelia, which is identical to the pattern observed by DIF in perilesional BP skin (6,10,35).

Although the average incidence of BP antibodies is about 70% using standard IIF,

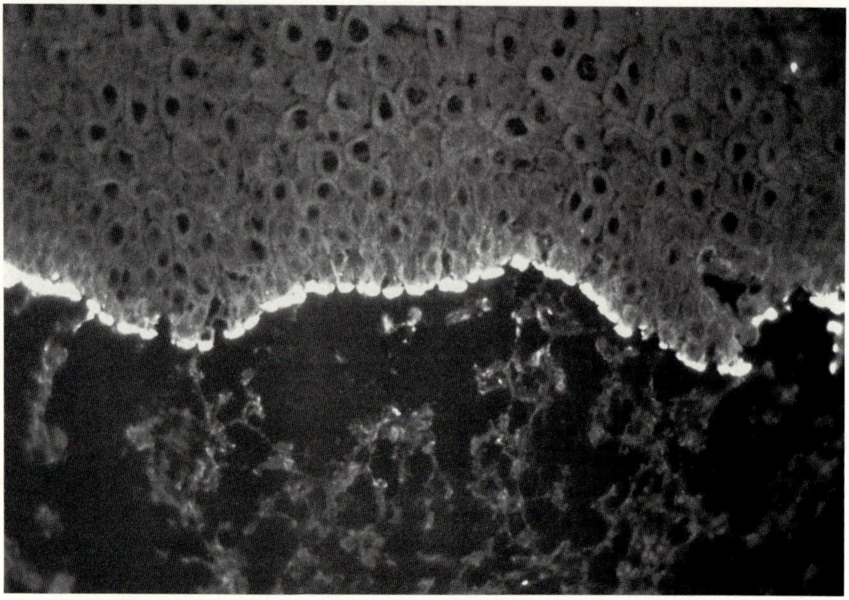

Figure 2. Photomicrograph showing direct IgG IF in lesional BP skin. Note discontinuous pattern of deposits at the blister roof (400x).

there is evidence that an even higher percentage of patients have BP antibodies in their sera. In some cases, the antibodies may be bound in circulating immune complexes (58). In one study, BP antibodies were detected in all four patients examined via IIF after treating serum with urea to dissociate complexes and separation of free BP antibody by gel filtration chromatography (24). In some cases, BP antibodies may be present in the circulation in too low a concentration to be detected by routine IIF, but may be detected by indirect complement-binding IF (40). An additional reason for failure to detect BP antibodies may be the choice of substrate. It has been shown that BP antibodies may show species, organ, intraorgan, and even individual specificities (6,35,65). Sera that have been negative on one substrate have been shown to be positive on another. Currently, the ideal substrate has not been determined. A variety of substrates have been used including monkey, guinea pig and rabbit lip, monkey and guinea pig esophagus, and skin from a variety of mammalian species including human. It has been suggested that monkey or guinea pig esophagus may approximate the ideal substrate, and these substrates have been commonly used. However, in a recent report comparing animal esophagus with human skin, BP antibodies were detected on human skin in 10% of sera that were negative on animal tissue (65). In our experience, human skin, particularly adult human skin from the flexural region of the thigh, is at least as good as animal tissue; it often gives titers of BP antibodies that are two to three doubling dilutions higher than on animal esophagus. The recent report showing that BP antigen may be maximally expressed in flexural regions of human skin would suggest that tissue from one of these sites may be the ideal substrate (22). Furthermore, the use of human tissue avoids the possibility of detecting heterologous anti-BMZ antibodies to animal skin, which could cause false-positive results.

IgG anti-BMZ antibodies are not specific for BP but also occur, usually at a lower frequency, in benign mucous membrane pemphigoid, HG, and EBA (3,31,64). There is currently no absolutely reliable method for distinguishing BP antibodies from those in benign mucous membrane pemphigoid and HG, but they can be differentiated from EBA antibodies by indirect IEM or more easily by IIF on skin separated through the lamina lucida by incubation in 1 M NaCl (see Chap. 20) (15,64). Although BP and HG antibodies cannot be differentiated by these methods, HG antibodies, unlike most BP antibodies, usually show complement-binding titers exceeding IgG titers (31). IgG anti-BMZ antibodies have occasionally been detected in burn patients and patients with other skin diseases, but are insufficiently common to be considered characteristic (59,61).

In general, BP antibodies do correlate with disease in the sense that when active disease is present, most patients have detectable antibodies, and with remission antibodies usually disappear from the circulation (1,30,46). In a small number of patients, a correlation between titer and disease activity or severity has been noted (35,44), but others have not found such a correlation (26,50). All reported attempts to correlate antibody titers with disease activity have examined only the correlation between activity and IgG titers, and none have examined a correlation between activity and complement-binding titers. Although there may be a correlation between antibody titers and disease activity in some patients, this does not appear to be a general phenomenon, and certainly is not as strong as in pemphigus.

Indirect Complement (C3) Binding Immunofluorescence

Complement-binding anti-BMZ antibodies can be detected by their ability to deposit complement at the BMZ in the presence of a complement source; for example, fresh serum (32). After incubating tissue with the antibody and complement source, deposition can be detected by staining for C3 or other components desposited at the BMZ. Using this method, it has been found that about 50% of BP patients have circulating complement-binding BP antibodies (29). Those antibodies are present in 70% of patients with detectable IgG BP antibodies. In general, complement-binding BP antibodies can be detected only in sera with positive indirect IgG IF, and titers of complement-binding antibodies are usually several doubling dilutions less than titers of IgG antibodies. Occasionally, complement-binding antibodies can be detected in sera that are negative by indirect IgG IF. For example, Millns et al. (40) found C3 binding activity in seven BP sera that were negative by routine indirect IgG IF. The presence of complement-binding activity in sera negative for IgG IF is similar to what has been described as the HG factor (Chap. 19), and is thought to be due to a potent complement-activating antibody that is present in insufficient concentration to be detected directly by IgG staining (31). Studies by Jordon et al. have shown that BP antibodies characteristically bind complement at the BMZ by activation of the classic pathway with amplification via the alternative pathway (33,40).

IMMUNOELECTRON MICROSCOPY

Direct IEM of BP skin using both ferritin and peroxidase/antiperoxidase (PAP) methods has shown that IgG and complement are deposited in a relatively homogeneous pattern in the lamina lucida between the basal cell plasma membrane and the lamina densa (Fig. 3) (27,52,53,60). The deposits are not preferentially concentrated at half-desmosomes (as has been suggested), but are contiguous with the basal cell plasma

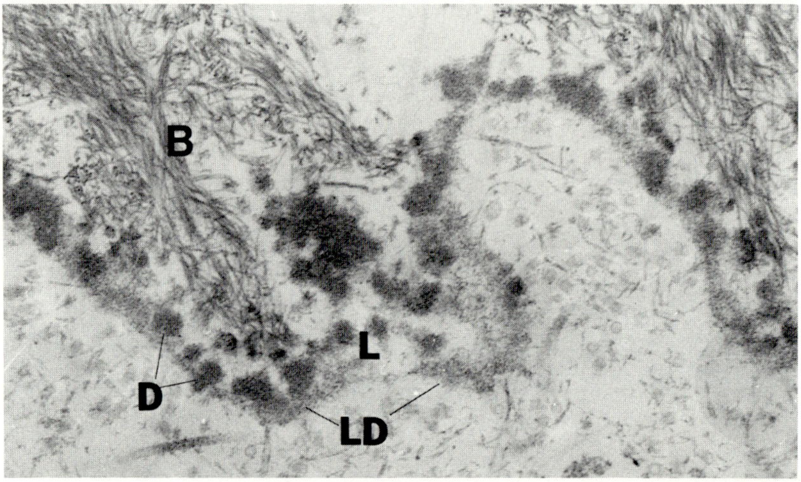

Figure 3. Immunoelectron micrograph of BP skin showing IgG deposits (D) in the lamina lucida (L) (LD, lamina densa; B, basal cell keratinocyte; 40,000x).

membrane. In specimens of skin with partial separation of dermis from epidermis, the deposits take on a more granular appearance and remain attached at the blister roof or the blister roof and base (60). The ultrastructural location of deposits in BP is identical to what has been described in benign mucous membrane pemphigoid and HG (14,28). Indirect IEM studies have shown that BP antibodies bind to the lamina lucida and are indistinguishable from deposits seen in BP skin using direct IEM (27,45).

Recently we reported a method in which antilamina lucida antibodies could be detected by IIF on 1 M NaCl separated skin (15; Table 2 in Chap. 20). This method obviates the need to perform indirect IEM to establish the presence of antilamina lucida antibodies, and has allowed us to easily examine large numbers of BP sera for antilamina lucida antibodies. We have now examined more than 90 of these sera and have shown that antilamina lucida antibodies are a uniform feature of the disease.

IMMUNOCHEMICAL STUDIES

Immunochemical studies have been used in recent years to identify and characterize the physicochemical properties of the antigen reactive with BP antibodies: BP antigen. Stanley et al. have reported the identification of BP antigen as a noncollagenous macromolecule composed of 220-kd subunits joined by disulfide bonds (56). These workers were able to immunoprecipitate radiolabeled antigen from cultured epidermal cell extracts, thus showing it to be synthesized in epidermal cells (55). They also showed that it was distinct from the lamina lucida glycoprotein, laminin, and from proteoglycan. More recently, Stanley et al. showed that an identical 220-kd glycoprotein could be extracted from intact skin, suggesting that the 220-kd moiety is a component of the lamina lucida and not just a precursor component synthesized by epidermal cells (57). In earlier studies, Diaz et al. reported recovery of a 30-kd glycoprotein from human skin that was able to absorb BP antibody as determined by blocking of BP antibody binding to the

BMZ (11). Rabbit antibodies to this material also reacted with an antigen in human saliva, urine, and extracts of esophagus. In another study, Diaz et al. reported recovery of an 18-kd glycoprotein (with a tendency to form higher molecular weight aggregates) from urine (13). The materials identified by Diaz et al. probably represented breakdown product of the 220-kd antigen identified by Stanley et al.

The variety of molecular weight structures identified as BP antigen(s), as well as other studies, suggest there may be some heterogeneity in the antigen. In one recent study, antibodies in a few BP sera seemed to be selective in binding to normal human skin from several different sources (65). We have noted differences in staining patterns of BP antibodies on normal human skin separated through the lamina lucida by 1 M NaCl. Most sera bind only to the epidermal side of the separation, but a few (about 10%) bind to both the epidermal and dermal sides of the separation (15). Although most, if not all, BP sera appear to have antibodies to a 220-kd lamina lucida glycoprotein, some may have antibodies to additional determinants.

The function of BP antigen has not been determined, but several lines of evidence suggest it may be important in dermal-epidermal adherence. These include its strategic location within the lamina lucida, its early appearance in the re-epithelialization of wounds (25,54), preliminary experiments suggesting that BP antibodies can interfere with epidermal cell-substrate adherence, and studies showing that the antigen is tightly bound to the attachment surface of the basal cell (12,23). In skin separated through the lamina lucida by thermal, chemical, and mechanical methods, the antigen separates with the epidermis (63).

FUNCTIONAL IMMUNOLOGIC STUDIES OF BP ANTIBODIES

Recently, bioassay methods called leukocyte attachment have been used for detecting and indirectly quantitating complement activation by in vivo-deposited BP complexes, and by complexes prepared by treating normal human skin with complement-binding BP antibodies (17,19). These methods have been of value in examining the functional properties of BP antibodies and in studies of interaction between BP antibodies, complement, leukocytes, and the BMZ.

Direct Leukocyte Attachment

The direct leukocyte attachment method (Table 1) has been used to detect and quantitate complement-activating immune complexes in BP skin, to compare complexes in BP skin with those in other diseases, and to compare complexes in lesional BP skin with those in nonlesional BP skin. In this method, skin is obtained from patients by 4 mm punch biopsy procedure under local xylocaine anesthesia, quick frozen in liquid nitrogen, mounted in embedding medium such as Ames OCT compound (Miles Laboratories, Elkhart, IN), and cut on a cryostat. Three to four 8 μm thick sections are cut and placed several millimeters apart in the center of gelatin-coated microscope slides. The sections are allowed to dry briefly on the slide at room temperature. A chamber is then constructed over the skin sections by covering the tissue slide with another microscope slide with two thicknesses of »88 vinyl tape (3-M Company, St. Paul, MN) attached to both ends. The tape prevents contact of the covering slide with tissue sections, and provides a chamber approximately 0.2 mm high and 0.3 ml in volume. The tissue slide and covering slide are taped or clamped together. The chamber is then injected (using a tuberculin syringe and 27-gauge needle) with 0.3 ml of 10×10^6 normal human periph-

Table 1. Leukocyte Attachment Methods

1. Place 3–4 6 μm thick cryostat sections of fresh-frozen skin in the center of gelatin-coated microscope slides and air dry briefly at 25°C. Store slides in a humid air atmosphere at 25°C between subsequent steps.
   a. If normal human skin is used, proceed to step 2.
   b. If skin already contains in vivo-deposited immune reactants, proceed to step 3.
2. Incubate normal human skin with 25–50 μl of heat-inactivated serum or IgG fraction containing complement-binding anti-BMZ antibody for 30 min at 4°C. Dilution of antibody can be made in any physiologic buffer. After incubation, rinse slides for 15 min at 25°C in 3 changes of PBS.
3. Remove excess moisture from slides by tissue blotting. Place 2 strips of vinyl tape at each end of another clean microscope slide. Position this slide over the tissue slide so that the tape prevents the two slides from making contact. Secure the two slides together by taping or clamping the ends (see Fig. 1 in Gammon et al. [16]).
4. Inject the chamber between the two slides with 0.3–0.4 ml of 10×10^6 freshly prepared normal human peripheral blood leukocytes suspended in Gey's Balanced Salt Solution—2% bovine serum albumin containing either 10% fresh normal human serum (complement source) or 10% heat-inactivated (56°C × 30 min) normal human serum (negative complement control). Injections should be made with a 2–5 ml syringe equipped with a 27- or 30-gauge needle.
5. Incubate chambers for a minimum of 30 min at 37°C in a humid air atmosphere.
6. Remove chambers and disassemble with care so as not to disturb skin sections. Gently immerse tissue slides in PBS. Rinse in several changes of PBS for 10–20 min.
7. Air-dry slides at 25°C for 30 min, fix tissue with 100% ethanol, and stain with H&E.

eral blood leukocytes and 10% fresh normal human serum in Geys Balanced Salt Solution (GBSS) containing 2% bovine serum albumin (Flow Laboratories, McLean, VA). Injection is performed carefully to avoid introducing air bubbles, and is continued until the chamber is filled. Controls used in these experiments generally include leukocytes suspended in heat-inactivated normal human serum (complement control), and skin that does not contain immune deposits at the BMZ (immune complex control). Once chambers are injected with leukocytes and serum, they are incubated at 37°C for 30 to 45 minutes in a humidified air environment. Chambers are then disassembled, washed free of serum and unattached cells by three 5-minute rinses in phosphate-buffered saline (PBS), dried at room temperature for 30 minutes, fixed in ethanol, and stained with hematoxylin and eosin (H&E). Leukocyte attachment in sections is quantitated by counting the number of leukocytes attached to the BMZ per millimeter of BMZ (Fig. 3). Counting is performed using a standard light microscope equipped with a linear micrometer eyepiece. A mean leukocyte attachment value is obtained for each biopsy specimen by counting leukocytes attached to the BMZ in two to three 1-mm portions of BMZ in each of three or four sections, and dividing by the number of 1-mm sections counted.

Using this method, we examined attachment in biopsy specimens of erythematous prebullous BP skin, specimens from adjacent normal-appearing skin obtained at the same time from the same patients, specimens of normal human skin, and specimens of lesional skin from patients with a number of skin diseases unassociated with BMZ immune deposits (19). In lesional BP skin—but not adjacent normal-appearing BP skin—normal skin, or skin from patients with other diseases, a significant degree of leukocyte attachment was observed. Evidence was obtained by control experiments that leukocyte attachment in lesional BP skin was due to complement-activating BP IgG immune complexes. Leukocyte attachment in lesional BP biopsy specimens was inhibited by substituting heat-inactivated serum for fresh serum, and by pretreating specimens with Fab_2 antibody against the Fc portion (complement-activating portion) of human IgG. This study showed that although there was no difference in the incidence or intensity of IgG and C3 IF in lesional and adjacent normal BP skin, lesional skin did demonstrate greater immune complex-mediated complement activation. These studies have provided evidence that BP immune deposits may play a role in inflammation and blister formation by showing that complement-activating complexes are present at the BMZ preceding the development of blisters.

Indirect Leukocyte Attachment

Indirect leukocyte attachment (Table 1) has been used to investigate the functional complement-activating properties of BP immune complexes formed with complement-binding BP antibodies, and to study the mechanism of leukocyte attachment, the pathway of BP antibody-mediated complement activation, and the interaction between complexes, leukocytes, and the BMZ. The method is similar to that used in direct leukocyte attachment with the following exceptions. Rather than tissue with in vivo-deposited complexes, fresh-frozen normal human skin is used. The skin is cut and placed on microscope slides, as previously described, and then treated with BP sera or IgG fractions diluted in PBS. Then 50 μl of diluted sera or IgG fraction is placed on each skin section, and slides are incubated at room temperature for 30 minutes in a humid environment. Slides are then rinsed for 15 minutes in three changes of PBS to remove excess serum, dried briefly at room temperature, and chambers are constructed and injected with normal human leukocytes and fresh serum in GBSS as previously described. Following a 30 to 45 minute incubation at 37°C, chambers are disassembled, rinsed in PBS, dried, fixed in ethanol, and stained with H&E. When complement-binding BP antibodies are used to sensitize sections, leukocytes attach to the BMZ as shown in Figure 4. The method is quantitated by counting cells attached per millimeter of

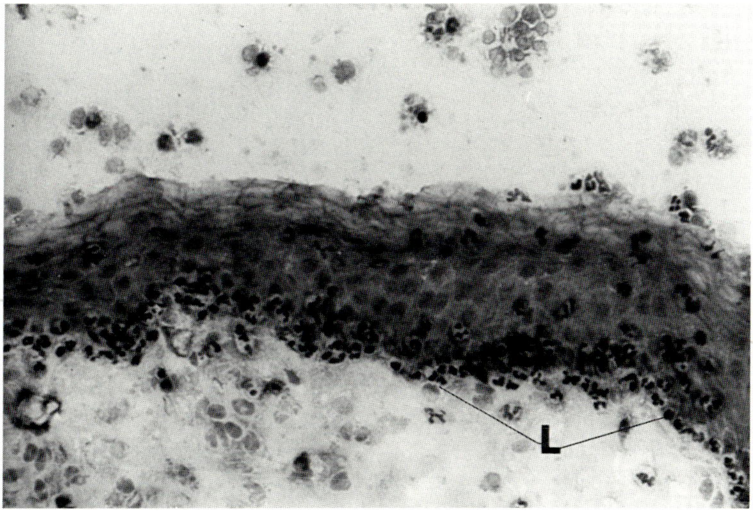

Figure 4. Photomicrograph of normal human skin section incubated with complement-binding BP antibody, serum complement, and normal human peripheral blood leukocytes. Note leukocytes (L) attached at the BMZ (250x)

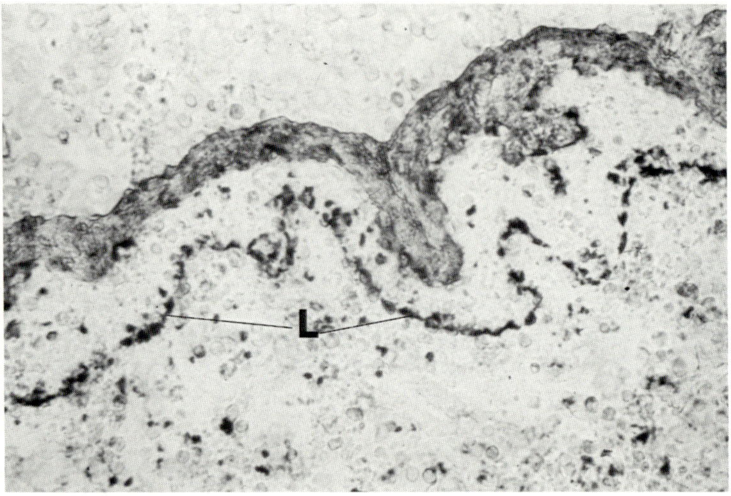

Figure 5. Photomicrograph of normal human skin section incubated with complement-binding BP antibody, serum complement, normal human peripheral blood leukocytes, and nitroblue tetrazolium. Note band of darkly stained leukocytes (L) along the BMZ. The dark stain is due to oxidation of nitroblue tetrazolium by activated leukocytes (250x).

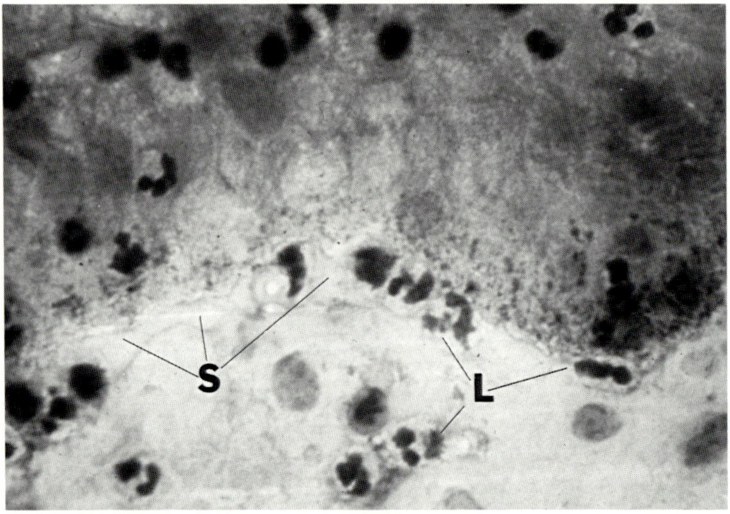

Figure 6. Photomicrograph of normal human skin section treated with complement-binding BP antibodies, serum complement, and normal human peripheral blood leukocytes (L). Note areas of separation (S) along the BMZ (450x).

BMZ. A requirement for complement-binding BP antibodies, fresh serum complement, and viable leukocytes in the reaction was shown with appropriate controls. Attachment was not observed when noncomplement-binding BP antibodies and BP sera without detectable antibodies were used to sensitize skin, when heat-inactivated human serum was substituted for fresh serum as a complement source, and when killed leukocytes were substituted for viable cells (17). Additional evidence supporting a requirement for complement included substituting fresh normal human serum with fresh serum deficient in C2, C4, C5, C7, or C8 (20). The reaction was blocked in the presence of C2, C4, or C5 deficient serum, but not C7 or C8 deficient serum.

In other experiments, it was shown that attachment required the directed migration of leukocytes to the BMZ (20). The presence of directed migration and a requirement for classic complement pathway components through C5 provided strong evidence that the mechanism responsible for leukocyte attachment was: 1) complement activation at the BMZ by complement-binding BP immune complexes; 2) production of C5-derived chemotactic activity; and 3) leukocyte migration to the BMZ in response to C5a chemotactic factor.

In additional experiments, it was shown that attachment correlates with the concentration of complement-binding BP antibody used to sensitize the BMZ. When antibodies were serially diluted, there was decreasing attachment with increasing dilutions of antibody, and a very close correlation was found between complement-binding titers and those titers that could mediate leukocyte attachment (18).

One of the major values of the indirect leukocyte attachment method is that it has provided a means of reproducing some of the inflammatory events that may be involved in the pathogenesis of immune complex-mediated BMZ injury. As previously noted, the method provides functional evidence that BP complexes can activate complement, generate chemotactic activity, and recruit leukocytes to the BMZ. In other experiments, it has been shown that leukocytes attached to the BMZ become activated and that prolonged incubation (60 to 120 minutes) of skin and leukocytes results in separation of the BMZ (Figs. 5 and 6) (19).

In Vivo Studies

Recently, additional evidence that complement-binding BP antibodies may be pathogenic was provided by in vivo passive transfer experiments in rabbits and guinea pigs (see Chap. 12). Anhalt et al. reported that injection of IgG fractions of BP sera containing BP antibodies into rabbit corneas caused binding of BP antibody and rabbit complement at the corneal epithelial basement membrane, inflammation in corneal stroma, separation of corneal epithelium from corneal stroma, and blistering (2). Corneal inflammation and separation depended on injection of complement-binding BP antibodies, and did not generally occur when noncomplement-binding antibodies were injected. These authors could not produce similar changes by intradermal injection in rabbit skin; however, Naito et al. recently reported that they could produce dermal inflammation and dermal-epidermal separation in guinea pigs by intraepidermal injection of BP sera containing complement-binding BP antibodies (42). Together, these experiments provide strong evidence supporting a role for complement-binding BP antibodies in the pathogenesis of the disease.

SUMMARY

Bullous pemphigoid antibodies and the antigens to which they are directed have been well characterized by DIF and IIF, direct and indirect IEM, and immunochemical methods. These studies have provided valuable information for the diagnosis and differential diagnosis of BP, and have significantly improved our understanding of normal and abnormal BMZ structure and function. The functional properties of BP antibodies have been characterized by indirect complement-binding IF, direct and indirect leukocyte attachment studies, and passive transfer experiments. These studies have provided considerable evidence supporting a role for BP antibodies, complement, and leukocytes in the pathogenesis of the disease. In addition, leukocyte attachment methods have provided an indirect means of quantitating complement activation by BP immune complexes. Additional studies and new approaches should help elucidate the precise mechanisms by which BP antibodies and complement contribute to inflammation in BP, and to what extent and how they interact with other inflammatory mediators.

More detailed analyses on the relation of clinical features to findings in routine immunopathologic studies of bullous pemphigoid and its variants appear in Chapter 16.

REFERENCES

1. Ahmed AR, Maize JC, Provost TT: Clinical and immunologic follow-up after successful therapy. *Arch Dermatol* 113:1043, 1977.
2. Anhalt GJ, Bahn CF, Labib RS, et al: Pathogenic effects of bullous pemphigoid antoantibodies in rabbit corneal epithelium. *J Clin Invest* 68:1097, 1981.
3. Bean SF: Cicatricial pemphigoid: Immunofluorescent studies. *Arch Dermatol* 110:552, 1974.
4. Beutner EH, Lever WF, Witebsky E, et al: Autoantibodies in pemphigus vulgaris. *JAMA* 192:682, 1965.
5. Carlo JR, Gammon WR, Sams WM Jr, et al: Demonstration of the complement regulating protein, Beta 1H, in skin biopsies from patients with bullous pemphigoid. *J Invest Dermatol* 73:551, 1979.
6. Chorzelski TP, Beutner EH: Factors contributing to occasional failures in the laboratory diagnosis of bullous pemphigoid by indirect immunofluorescence. *Br J Dermatol* 86:111, 1972.
7. Chorzelski TP, Cormane RH: The presence of complement "bound" in vivo in the skin of patients with pemphigoid. *Dermatologica* 137:134, 1968.
8. Chorzelski TP, Jablonska S, Beutner EH: Pemphigoid. In Beutner EH, Chorzelski TP, Bean SF (Eds): *Immunopathology of the Skin,* ed. 2. Wiley, New York, 1979, p 243.
9. Cormane RH, Gianetti A: IgD in various dermatoses, immunofluorescence studies. *Br J Dermatol* 84:523, 1971.
10. Cowen SJ, Anhalt GJ, Wicha MS, et al: Distribution of pemphigus and pemphigoid antigens, laminin and type 4 collagen in corneal epithelium. *Invest Ophthalmol Vis Sci* 21:879, 1981.
11. Diaz LA, Calvanico NJ, Tomasi TB Jr, et al: Bullous pemphigoid antigen: Isolation from normal human skin. *J Immunol* 118:455, 1977.
12. Diaz LA, Marcelo CL: Pemphigoid and pemphigus antigens in cultured epidermal cells. *Br J Dermatol* 98:631, 1978.
13. Diaz LA, Patel H, Calvanico NJ: Bullous pemphigoid antigen. II. Isolation from the urine of a patient. *J Immunol* 122:605, 1979.
14. Fine JD, Neises GR, Katz SI: Immunofluorescence and immunoelectron microscopic studies in cicatricial pemphigoid. *J Invest Dermatol* 82:39, 1984.
15. Gammon WR, Briggaman RA, Inman AO III, et al: Differentiating anti-lamina lucida and anti-sub-lamina densa anti-BMZ antibodies by indirect immunofluorescence on 1.0 M sodium chloride separated skin. *J Invest Dermatol* 82:139, 1984.
16. Gammon WR, Briggaman RA, Woodley DT, et al: Epidermolysis bullosa acquisita: A pemphigoid-like disease *J. Amer. Acad. Dermatol.* 11: 820–832, 1984.
17. Gammon WR, Lewis DM, Carlo JR, et al: Pemphigoid antibody mediated attachment of peripheral blood leukocytes at the dermal-epidermal junction of human skin. *J Invest Dermatol* 75:334, 1980.
18. Gammon WR, Merritt CC: A functional assay for complement activating antibodies to the cutaneous basement membrane zone. *Ann NY Acad Sci* 420:335–342, 1983.
19. Gammon WR, Merritt CC, Lewis DM, et al: Functional evidence for complement-activating immune complexes in the skin of patients with bullous pemphigoid. *J Invest Dermatol* 78:52, 1982.

20. Gammon WR, Merritt CC, Lewis DM, et al: Leukocyte chemotaxis to the dermal-epidermal junction of human skin mediated by pemphigoid antibody and complement: Mechanism of cell attachment in the in vitro leukocyte attachment method. *J Invest Dermatol* 76:514, 1981.
21. Gammon WR, Robinson T, Briggaman RA, et al: Double immunofluorescence microscopy: A method for localizing immune deposits in skin disease associated with linear basement membrane zone immunofluorescence. *J Invest Dermatol* 79:312, 1982.
22. Goldberg DJ, Bystryn JC: Regional variations in the expression of bullous pemphigoid antigen in human skin. *Clin Res* 31:568A, 1983.
23. Grekin PM, Levy GN, King AJ, et al: Some biochemical properties of pemphigoid antigen bound to the surface of dissociated epidermal cells. *J Invest Dermatol* 76:190, 1981.
24. Herrmann K, Lohrisch I, Bohme HJ, et al: Detection of antibodies after immune complex splitting in serum of patients with bullous pemphigoid and systemic lupus erythematosus. *Br J Dermatol* 99:635, 1978.
25. Hintner H, Fritsch PO, Foidart JM, et al: Expression of basement membrane zone antigens at the dermo-epibolic junction in organ cultures of human skin. *J Invest Dermatol* 74:200, 1980.
26. Hodge L, Marsden RA, Black MM, et al: Bullous pemphigoid: The frequency of mucosal involvement and concurrent malignancy related to indirect immunofluorescence findings. *Br J Dermatol* 105:65, 1981.
27. Holubar K, Wolff K, Konrad K, et al: Ultrastructural localization of immunoglobulins in bullous pemphigoid skin. *J Invest Dermatol* 64:220, 1975.
28. Honigsman H, Stingl G, Holubar K, et al: Herpes gestationis: Fine structural pattern of immunoglobulin deposits in the skin in vivo. *J Invest Dermatol* 66:389, 1976.
29. Jordon RE: Complement activation in bullous skin diseases. *J Invest Dermatol* 65:162, 1975.
30. Jordon RE, Beutner EH, Witebsky E, et al: Basement zone antibodies in bullous pemphigoid. *JAMA* 200:91, 1967.
31. Jordon RE, Heine KG, Tappeiner C, et al: The immunology of herpes gestationis: Immunofluorescence studies and characterization of "HG factor." *J Clin Invest* 57:1426, 1976.
32. Jordon RE, Sams WM Jr, Beutner EH; Complement immunofluorescent staining in bullous pemphigoid. *J Lab Clin Med* 74:548, 1969.
33. Jordon RE, Schroeter AL, Good RA, et al: The complement system in bullous pemphigoid. IV. Immunofluorescent evidence for both classical and alternate pathway activation. *Clin Immunol Immunopathol* 3:307, 1975.
34. Jordon RE, Triftshauser CT, Schroeter AL: Direct immunofluorescent studies of pemphigus and bullous pemphigoid. *Arch Dermatol* 103:486, 1971.
35. Katz SI, Halprin KM, Inderbitzin TM: The use of human skin for the detection of antiepithelial antibodies. *J Invest Dermatol* 53:390, 1969.
36. Kushniruk W: The immunopathology of epidermolysis bullous acquisita. *Can Med Assoc J* 108:1143, 1973.
37. Lever WF: *Pemphigus and Pemphigoid.* Charles C Thomas, Springfield IL, 1965, 266 pp.
38. Lever WF, Shaumburg-Lever G: *Histopathology of the Skin,* ed. 6. Lippincott, Philadelphia, 1983, p 113.
39. Dahl MV, Falk RJ, Carpenter R, et al: Deposition of the membrane attack complex of complement in bullous pemphigoid. *J Invest Dermatol* 82:132–135, 1984.
40. Millns JL, Meurer M, Jordon RE: The complement system in bullous pemphigoid. VI. C3 fixing activity in the absence of detectable antibody. *Clin Immunol Immunopathol* 13:475, 1979.
41. Mogavero HS Jr, Knauer KA: The presence of PF4 in bullous pemphigoid. *Clin Res* 31:265A, 1983.
42. Naito K, Morioka S, Ogawa H: The pathogenic mechanism of blister formation in bullous pemphigoid. *J Invest Dermatol* 79:303, 1982.
43. Olansky AJ, Briggaman RA, Gammon WR, et al: Bullous systemic lupus erythematosus. *J Am Acad Dermatol* 7:511, 1982.
44. Peck SM, Osserman KE, Weiner LB, et al: Studies in bullous diseases. Immunofluorescent serologic tests. *N Engl J Med* 279:951, 1968.
45. Pehamberger H, Gschnait F, Konrad K, et al: Bullous pemphigoid, herpes gestationis and

linear dermatitis herpetiformis: Circulating anti-basement membrane zone antibodies; in vitro studies. *J Invest Dermatol* 74:105, 1980.

46. Person JR, Rogers RS III: Bullous and cicatricial pemphigoid. Clinical, histopathologic and immunopathologic correlation. *Mayo Clin Proc* 52:54, 1977.
47. Pierard J, Whimster I: The histological diagnosis of dermatitis herpetiformis, bullous pemphigoid and erythema multiforme. *Br J Dermatol* 73:253, 1961.
48. Provost TT, Tomasi TB Jr: Evidence for complement activation via the alternate pathway in skin diseases. I. Herpes gestationis, systemic lupus erythematosus and bullous pemphigoid. *J Clin Invest* 52:1179, 1973.
49. Provost TT, Tomasi TB: Immunopathology of bullous pemphigoid: Basement membrane deposition of IgE, alternate pathway components and fibrin. *Clin Exp Immunol* 18:193, 1974.
50. Sams WM Jr, Jordon RE: Correlation of pemphigoid and pemphigus antibody titers with activity of disease. *Br J Dermatol* 84:7, 1971.
51. Sams WM Jr, Schur PH: Studies of the antibodies in pemphigoid and pemphigus. *J Lab Clin Med* 82:249, 1973.
52. Schaumburg-Lever G, Rule A, Schmidt-Ullrich B, et al: Ultrastructural localization of in vivo bound immunoglobulins in bullous pemphigoid—A preliminary report. *J Invest Dermatol* 64:47, 1975.
53. Schmidt-Ullrich B, Rule A, Schaumburg-Lever G, et al: Ultrastructural localization of in vivo-bound complement in bullous pemphigoid. *J Invest Dermatol* 65:217, 1975.
54. Stanley JR, Alverez OM, Bere EW, et al: Detection of basement membrane zone antigens during epidermal wound healing in pigs. *J Invest Dermatol* 77:240, 1981.
55. Stanley JR, Hawley-Nelson P, Yaar M, et al: Laminin and bullous pemphigoid antigen are distinct basement membrane proteins synthesized by epidermal cells. *J Invest Dermatol* 78:456, 1982.
56. Stanley JR, Hawley-Nelson P, Yuspa SH, et al: Characterization of bullous pemphigoid antigen: A unique basement membrane protein of stratified squamous epithelia. *Cell* 24:897, 1981.
57. Stanley JR, Woodley DT, Katz SI: Identification and partial characterization of pemphigoid antigen extracted from normal human skin. *J Invest Dermatol* 82:108, 1984.
58. Tappeiner G, Heine KG, Kahl JC, et al: C_1q binding sustances in pemphigus and bullous pemphigoid. Detection with a [^{131}I] C_1q binding assay. *Clin Exp Immunol* 28:40, 1977.
59. Thivolet J, Beyvin A, Andre D: Anticorps "pemphigus-like" et "pemphigoid-like" (pemphigus and pemphigoid-like antibodies). *Dermatologica* 140:310, 1970.
60. Trost TH, Steigleder GK, Bodeux E: Immunoelectron microscopical investigations with a new tracer: Peroxidase-labeled protein A: Application for detection of pemphigus and bullous pemphigoid antibodies. *J Invest Dermatol* 75:328, 1980.
61. Ullman S, Halberg P, Nielson R: Anti-basement membrane antibodies in sera from patients without bullous pemphigoid. *Acta Dermatol Venereol* 55:305, 1975.
62. Wintroub BU, Mihm MC Jr, Goetzl EJ, et al: Morphologic and functional evidence for release of mast cell products in bullous pemphigoid. *N Engl J Med* 298:417, 1978.
63. Woodley DT, Sauder D, Talley MJ, et al: Localization of basement membrane components after dermal-epidermal junction separation. *J Invest Dermatol* 81:149, 1983.
64. Yaoita H, Briggaman RA, Lawley TJ, et al: Epidermolysis bullous acquisita: Ultrastructural and immunological studies. *J Invest Dermatol* 76:288, 1981.
65. Zhu X-J, Bystryn J-C: Heterogeneity of pemphigoid antigens. *J Invest Dermatol* 80:16, 1983.

16
Bullous Pemphigoid: Relationship of Immunopathology to Clinical Findings

Tadeusz P. Chorzelski
Stefania Jablonska
Ernst H. Beutner

INTRODUCTION

Detection of anti-basement membrane zone (anti-BMZ) antibodies (Ab) as an immunologic marker of bullous pemphigoid (BP) (7) provided evidence that this disease is a distinct, immunologically mediated entity (35,44; Chap. 15). The immunofluorescence (IF) findings are presently accepted as a basic diagnostic criterion. With their wide use in dermatologic practice, it became increasingly evident that this disease is heterogeneous, and that some varieties could not have been recognized without IF tests. This holds true also for both pemphigus and some other subepidermal bullous diseases that may closely resemble each other and/or have such atypical appearance that the clinical diagnosis is not possible.

The rate of misdiagnosis in patients with bullous diseases referred to us for immunologic studies was as high as 17% (Table 1). The following examples illustrate how difficult the clinical diagnosis may be. Of two patients presenting features of erythema annulare centrifugum, one proved to be BP, and another pemphigus (see Chapter 10). Especially difficult may be the differentiation between BP and linear IgA bullous dermatosis (see below and Chaps. 22 and 23).

IMMUNOFLUORESCENCE FINDINGS IN CLINICAL VARIETIES OF BULLOUS PEMPHIGOID

There are several recognized clinical varieties of BP:

1. Bullous
2. Erythematous

3. Vesicular
4. Localized
5. Unclassified or atypical (e.g., nodular, erythrodermic, etc.)

The bullous form is the most common type of BP. A subset of cases with immunologic findings of pemphigoid and with cutaneous pemphigoid-like lesions associated with atrophy and scarring merits special attention. These cases need to be studied in terms of biopsy specimen findings with the methods described by Fine et al. (Chap. 21), and of the serum findings using the method of Gammon et al. (see Table 2 in Chap. 20). Cicatricial pemphigoid is discussed separately (see Chap. 17).

Bullous Type

Clinical features may be polymorphic with erythematous and urticarial lesions; but large, tense, sometimes hemorrhagic bullae, are prevalent (Fig. 1).

Table 1. Discrepancy Between the Tentative Clinical Diagnosis and the Final Diagnosis of Bullous Pemphigoid Based on IF Studies

Tentative clinical diagnosis (No. of cases)	*DIF BMZ immune deposits*	*IIF BMZ Ab*
Pemphigus (14)	14	10
DH (5)	5	4
IgA linear bullous dermatosus (4)	4	2
Erythema multiforme or erythema centrifugum annulare (6)	6	3
Total BP cases (170)	29/29 (100%)	19/29 (65.5%)
Misdiagnosed cases—29/170 (17%)		

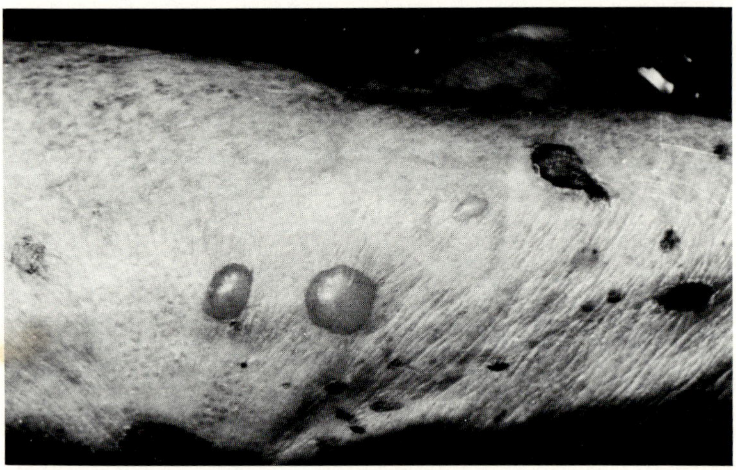

Figure 1. Case of bullous variety of pemphigoid. Large, tense bullae on erythematous, partially hemorrhagic skin and also on apparently normal skin. (With permission from Chorzelski et al. [14].)

Direct immunofluorescence (DIF) for IgG and/or complement is present in virtually all of our cases; and in a few of them, also IgA (Table 2). However, IgA is always accompanied by both IgG and usually complement (see below). Circulating anti-BMZ antibodies were found in 60% of cases.

The above-mentioned subset with atrophy and/or scarring differed from cicatricial pemphigoid by the prevalence of cutaneous involvement, whereas mucosal lesions were rare or absent. The cutaneous lesions were disseminated; some typical tense bullae regressed without atrophy, some leaving atrophy and/or scars (Table 3). The Brunsting-Perry variety may belong to this group, and its characteristic feature is a predilection for the scalp, neck, and face. This form of BP is often classified as cicatricial pemphigoid of the skin. As in other forms of pemphigoid, IgG and C3 are the most common DIF findings. In contrast to findings in cicatricial pemphigoid, in which IgA is a common component (see Chapter 17) in cutaneous form, it occurred only in 1 of 13 cases.

Table 2. Immunopathology of Clinical Varieties of Pemphigoid

Clinical type	*No. of cases*	*DIF (BMZ deposits)*			*IIF BMZ Ab (% positive)*
		IgG	*IgA*	*C*	
Bullous	106	98/105[a,c] (93%)	7/72 (10%)	69/71 (97%)	63/105[b] (60%)
Erythematous	34	23/34[c] (68%)	0/27 (0%)	24/26 (92%)	17/34 (50%)
Vesicular	19	17/19 (89%)	2/16 (13%)	18/18 (100%)	8/19 (42%)
Nonclassified	11	11/11 (100%)	1/11 (9%)	7/9 (78%)	3/11 (27%)
Total	170	149/169 (88%)	10/126 (8%)	118/124 (95%)	91/169 (54%)

[a]in one case only, IIF was performed.
[b]in one case only, DIF was performed.
[c]IgG deposits in the BMZ occur less frequently in the erythematous than bullous form of pemphigoid ($p < 0.0005$ by chi square analysis).

Table 3. Cutaneous BP with Atrophy and/or Scarring

Clinical varieties		*Total cases*	*DIF (BMZ deposits)*			*IIF BMZ Ab*
			IgG	*IgA*	*C3*	
Disseminated cutaneous	No mucosal involvement	2	2	0	2	2/2
	With mucosal involvement	4	3/4	1	2/3	1/4
Brunsting-Perry		6	6	0	6	1/5
Localized cicatricial		1	1	0	1	1/1
Total (% positive)		13	12 (92%)	1/13 (8%)	11/12 (92%)	5/12 (42%)

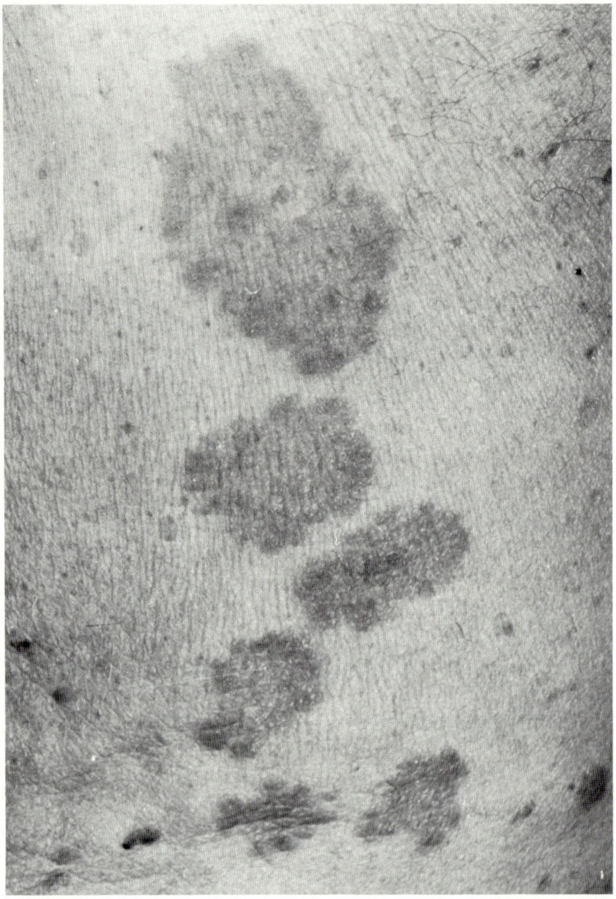

Figure 2. Case of erythematous variety of pemphigoid with no bullous lesions at the time of positive IF findings.

Erythematous Variety

The characteristic clinical features are erythematous, sometimes annular or serpiginous, plaques with no (Fig. 2) or isolated bullous lesions (Fig. 3). In the course of the disease, in some relapses, the clinical picture may change into the typical bullous form.

The frequency of IgG in skin deposits is lower in the erythematous form than in BP (see Table 2), but complement appeared more commonly as the only finding (see Table 4). Anti-BMZ antibodies were detected in about half of these cases, which is not significantly different from the bullous variety.

Vesicular Variety

The clinical picture often does not suggest BP and may resemble linear IgA bullous dermatosis (LABD) or dermatitis herpetiformis (DH), since the lesions are mainly vesicular and grouped, often in herpetiform arrangements (Fig. 4).

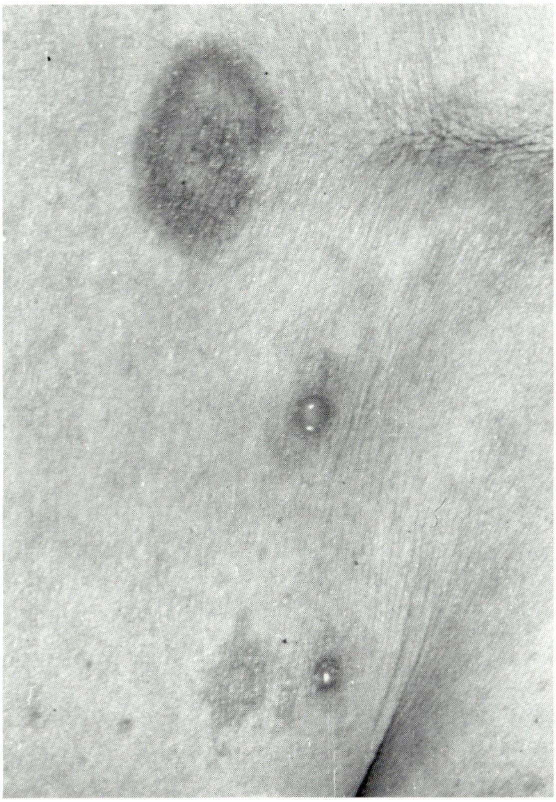

Figure 3. Case of erythematous variety of pemphigoid; vesicles are on a slightly erythematous base.

The main difference from DH is that there is no predilection for areas characteristically involved in the latter. The differentiation from LABD is especially difficult or impossible. This form was described by several authors (6,9,14,37).

IF findings are comparable to those of the bullous form of the disease (see Table 2). IgA was found in one case in combination with complement and IgG, and in one case it was accompanied by complement alone. This provides evidence that the vesicular variety belongs to the spectrum of BP.

Localized Variety

This designation is usually restricted to bullous eruption with a pretibial localization. It is more frequent in the older people (8,23,52). It is not possible to classify these cases without immunopathologic studies. Few cases have been found to be positive (3,25,45,56), and we currently have under study a patient with myasthenia gravis, in whom bullous lesions appeared on the legs after thymectomy, leaving areas of atrophy and scarring upon regression. Both DIF and indirect IF (IIF) were positive (see Table 3).

Table 4. Pemphigoid with In Vivo-Bound Complement as the Only DIF finding

Clinical type	*Total*	*IIF BMZ Ab positive*
Bullous	7/71 (10%)[a]	3/7 (43%)
Erythematous	11/26 (42%)[a]	5/11 (45%)
Vesicular	2/18 (11%)	0/2 (0)
Nonclassified	0/9 (0%)	0
Total (% positive)	20/124 (16%)	8/20 (40%)

[a]Complement occurs as the only IIF finding in the BMZ, more commonly in the erythematous than bullous form of pemphigoid (significant at $p < 0.0005$ by chi square analysis).

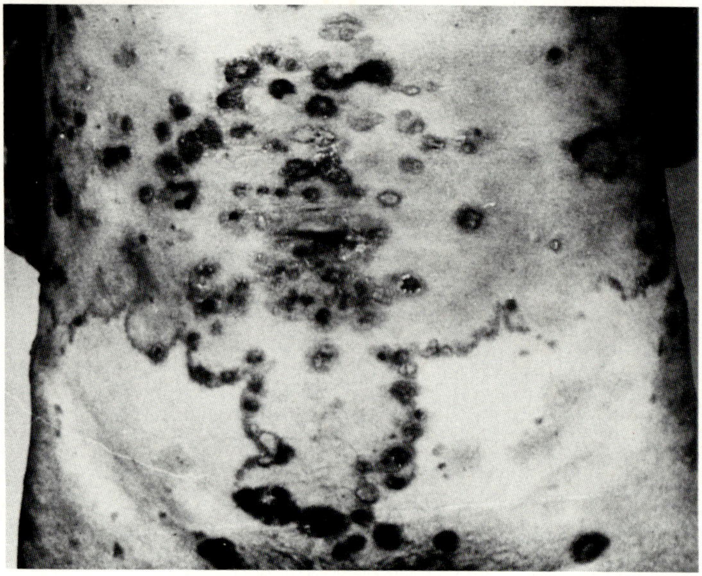

Figure 4. Case of vesicular form of pemphigoid with herpetiform arrangement of vesicles. (With permission from Chorzelski et al. [14].)

Atypical and Unclassified Varieties

This heterogeneous group comprises cases that are clinically atypical; for example, cases with nodular, erythrodermic, seborrhoic lesions and/or cases that are unclassified clinically (46,71,76,79). However, in most of these cases, the IF findings were comparable to the bullous form (see Tables 2 and 4), apparently with a lower percentage of cases with circulating BMZ antibodies (27% versus 60%) (see Table 2). The atypical cases also include some that need to be distingushed from LABD.

DIFFERENTIATION OF BULLOUS PEMPHIGOID FROM LINEAR IgA BULLOUS DERMATOSIS

The most difficult problem is the differentiation between atypical BP and LABD. In some cases, the IF findings are not decisive, especially if IgA in skin deposits is as intense as IgG. If circulating BMZ antibodies of the IgG class are detectable, the diagnosis of BP can be established (Table 5). If IgA is an additional component of lower intensity than IgG and complement, the cases can be classified as BP, even without circulating antibodies (Table 6). In some cases, IgA skin deposits are as strong as the other components; and despite this, clinical features are characteristic of BP (see Table 6, case SK). Classification of such cases on the basis of relative intensity of IgA and IgG deposits is arbitrary. However, the distinctions can frequently be made not only on the basis of serum findings (Table 5), but importantly, on the basis of complement deposits (Tables 5 and 6). Usually, complement is absent in LABD cases. Thus, if C3 is strongly positive, as in the cases listed in Table 6, the possibility of a diagnosis of BP should be considered even if IgA deposits in the BMZ are a bit stronger than IgG deposits (e.g., Table 6, case SJ). This interpretation is consistent with the corticosteroid responses of the five problem cases listed in Table 6.

Table 5. Problem Cases of BP/LABD Resolved by Demonstration of BMZ Antibodies

		Patients				
		JG[a]	*WO*	*MK*	*SD*[a]	*JM*
DIF	IgA	++	++	+++	+/++	+
	IgG	+	++	+++	+/+++	+
	C3	+	++	+++	+	+
IIF	Anti-BMZ Ab of IgG class titers	10,240	1280	40	40	20

[a]BP + Psoriasis.

Table 6. Problem cases of BP/LABD without Circulating BMZ Antibodies Resolved by Complement Reactions and Confirmed by Therapeutic Responses

		Patients				
		MK	*JK*	*SJ*	*AR*	*SK*
Clinical	Type DH	+	+	+	+	−
	Large tense bullae of BP type	+	−	+	−	+
DIF	IgA	±	+	+	±/+	+++
	IgG	+++	++	+/w	+++	+++
	C3	+++	+++	+++	+++	+++
IIF	Anti-BMZ IgG antibodies	0	0	0	0	0
Responses to sulfones		−	−	−	−	−
Responses to corticosteroids		+	+	+	+	+

Because of the importance of complement in atypical BP/LABD problem cases, it is advisable to do studies for the presence of various complement components of both classic and alternative pathways (i.e., C4, Clq, and properdin). If the activation is primarily through the classic pathway (deposition of C4, Clq), then the diagnosis of BP is most probable. On the other hand, if it is through the alternate pathway (deposition of properdin), then the diagnosis should be of LABD.

TITERS OF BMZ ANTIBODIES IN RELATION TO THE DISEASE ACTIVITY

There is no evident correlation, as in pemphigus, between the disease activity and titers of BMZ antibodies in pemphigoid. However, clinical remission is usually accompanied by disappearance of circulating BMZ antibodies, and relapse is accompanied by their reappearance. Sporadic cases have been described with unusual IF findings; that is, the presence of antibodies without BP (75). We have not seen cases of this type, but some relapses may be preceded by the appearance of circulating BMZ antibodies. Determination of the titers of BMZ antibodies, although of limited significance in evaluating activity of the disease (16,31,36), might be helpful for prediction of relapse and evaluation of the treatment. In cases in which the titers are persistently high, the prognosis should be cautious.

PEMPHIGOID PROVOKED BY VARIOUS FACTORS

Bullous lesions of the BP type with characteristic IF findings have been reported to develop following systemic therapy with different, nonrelated drugs: salicyl-azosulfapyridine (5), furosemide (26), penicillin (27), antidiabetic sulfonamides (30), and after external treatment with 5-fluorouracil (4) and benzyl-benzoate used for scabies (78). Several antipsoriatic compounds were reported to provoke BP; specifically anthralin (42,68) and salicylic ointment (42).

In our series, antiscabies treatment with benzyl benzoate was responsible for a majority of drug-induced BP cases. In one patient, BP lesions appeared after burns. In all cases, the changes were transient, with no relapse after regression. The immunopathologic pattern was characteristic of BP, with circulating BMZ antibodies present in two cases. In two of nine cases (one erythematous, and one vesicular type), complement was the only detectable component; and in one case of vesicular pemphigoid, complement was absent.

Of special interest is the fact that BP has been induced in patients with psoriasis either by Goeckerman regimen (2,53) or psoralen ultraviolet A (PUVA). Cases of bullous eruptions provoked by PUVA are reported in increasing numbers (1,29,58,68,74). These bullous lesions usually develop in an acral location, are not immunologically mediated, and are induced by phototoxic reaction, with characteristic "sunburn cells" at the epidermal-dermal junction (58). There are, however, cases with all clinical, histological, and immunological characteristics of BP; and in some cases, circulating BMZ antibodies have also been found (42,68). The mechanism of bulla formation is not clear. It has been well established that in patients with pemphigoid ultraviolet (UV) rays may produce immunohistochemical changes of the BP type (19). It is possible that a subclinical form of BP preexisted in those patients, and was precipitated by the therapy as hypothesized by Person and Rogers (53). Alternatively, destruction of basement membrane followed by release of BMZ anitgens could evoke, in predisposed individuals, an immunologic response. The induced forms of BP are usually transient, often localized, and generally disappear after discontinuation of administration of the provoking agent.

COEXISTENCE OF PEMPHIGOID WITH OTHER DISEASES

Pemphigoid has been reported to be associated with other immunologic disorders: rheumatoid arthritis (11,28,54,60), Hashimoto thyroiditis (10) or other thyroid disease (38), primary biliary cirrhosis (33), pemphigus (see Chap. 10), systemic lupus erythematosus (SLE) (see below), etc. Coexistence of various autoimmune diseases is presently well documented, but it is still not clear whether there is a common pathogenetic mechanism. Of special interest is the association of bullous eruption with SLE and lichen planus (LP), which occurs more frequently than with other disorders.

Bullous Disease Associated with SLE

Bullous and vesicular lesions associated with SLE—resembling BP, epidermolysis bullosa acquisita (EBA), DH, or LABD—are a matter of controversy (18,51,55; Chap. 8). These patients present with variable clinical pictures of the eruption. That is, many such patients exhibit vesicular and/or bullous eruption on the seemingly uninvolved skin and/or on an erythematous base, mainly in light-exposed areas and on the upper parts of the trunk. The histology, which is consistent with DH (that is, papillary microabscesses), is a frequent finding in these patients. They respond dramatically to treatment with sulfones (12,22,32,69). The severity of SLE does not parallel the activity of bullous eruption. Interpretation of findings in the skin may be very difficult due to the overlap of immune phenomena of SLE and a bullous disease. The patterns of immune deposits are granular, characteristic of SLE, linear as in BP, or a combination of these two. However, it should be stressed that linear homogeneous immune depositions may also occur in SLE without bullous eruption (40; Chap. 30), which makes the evaluation even more difficult. The deposits may be composed of all main immunoglobulin classes and complement, including IgA, which is more frequent than in SLE alone. In isolated cases, IgA may be a predominant component. Circulating anti-BMZ antibodies are usually undetectable, and in one such case, they were detected in tissue culture (43). This could be due to the interference by other antibodies. In tissue culture, the interfering antinuclear antibodies (ANA) are not reactive, and the BMZ antibodies may easily be visualized. It is probable that such rare cases represent a true coexistence of SLE and BP or EBA (see Chap. 20). The association of SLE with DH (47,73) has not been convincingly documented.

However, the majority of cases of vesicular bullous eruption in SLE patients cannot be classified as BP or DH. This is the reason why some authors consider such cases as vesiculo-bullous or bullous SLE (12,32,49).

The clinical features of DH and BP, histologic pattern of DH, dramatic response to sulfones, and a frequent presence of IgA in skin deposition may suggest a relationship with LABD. Contrary to BP, and consistent with LABD, there is usually no response to treatment with corticosteroids, even in high doses. Unlike in DH, the lesions are not as symmetric and not localized in typical areas, the pruritus is not as severe or absent, the eruption may regress without reappearance after withdrawal of sulfones, and linear IgA immune deposition does not persist in remission. Indeed, such cases have been described as IgA BP (69) or linear IgA dermatitis herpetiformis (synonymous with LABD) (72).

Case Histories

The complexity of this problem is illustrated by the following case histories. Diagnoses of SLE were based on the American Rheumatism Association criteria.

CASE 1. A 21-year-old white male had severe lupus nephritis confirmed by kidney biopsy, and anti-dDNA antibodies with titers of 160 to 640. Two years after the diagnosis of SLE, he developed a vesicular eruption in the light-exposed areas while receiving small doses of prednisone (20 mg). The increased dosage, up to 60 mg daily, did not control the skin rash.

Histologic studies revealed typical papillary microabscesses (Fig. 5). Direct IF studies showed granular IgG, IgM, and C3 at the dermal-epidermal junction (DEJ) in the light-exposed uninvolved skin, and around the vesicles there were granular IgG, IgM, C3, and linear IgA.

Circulating BMZ antibodies were not detected. Introduction of Dapsone, 100 mg daily, produced a dramatic response within 24 hours, and shortly after prednisone could be diminished to 15 mg. The remission lasted for several months, and only occasional single lesions appeared that were again controlled by Dapsone.

CASE 2. A 40-year-old white female had psoriasiform skin lesions of the subacute cutaneous lupus erythematosus (SCLE) type (Fig. 6), preceded by 9 years appearance of disseminated vesicular eruption both in the erythematous and seemingly normal skin. Histologic studies revealed a subepidermal bulla filled with polymorphonuclear leukocytes and fibrin. Direct IF of the uninvolved skin showed linear and granular deposition

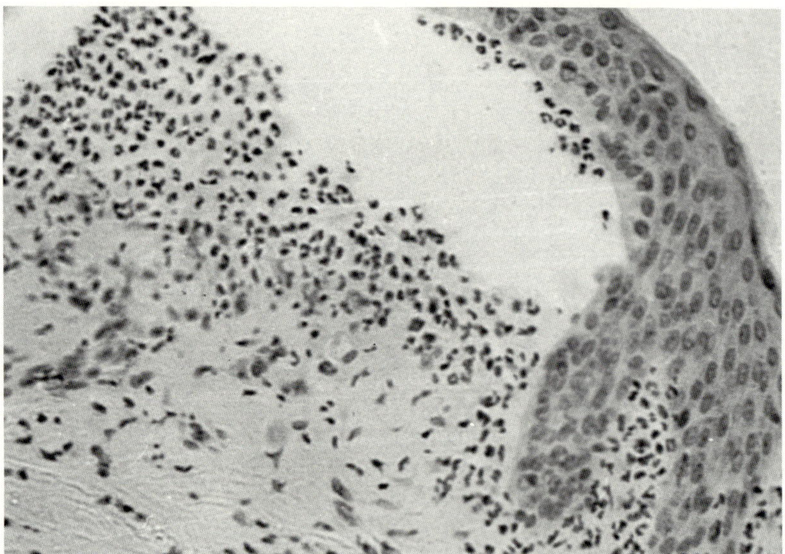

Figure 5. Case of SLE with a vesicular eruption. Histology shows papillary microabscess formation (400X).

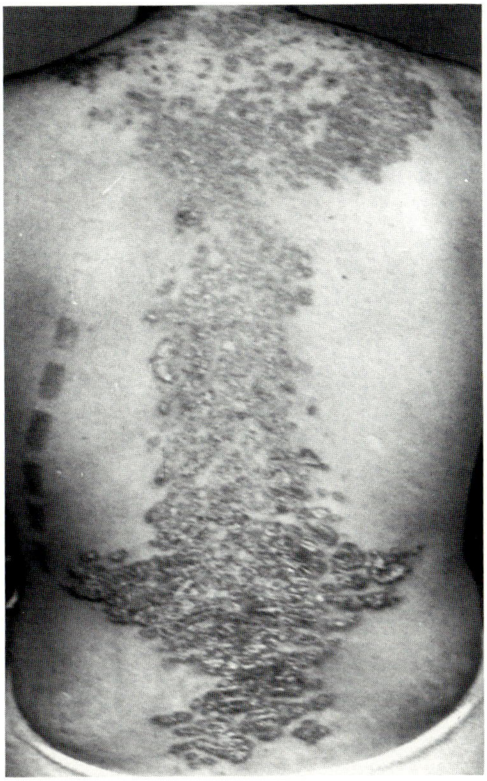

Figure 6. Case of subacute cutaneous LE with psoriasiform lesions and small vesicles.

of IgG, IgM, C3, and weak IgA (Fig. 7) at the BMZ. Direct IF of bullous and adjacent normal skin lesions revealed linear deposition of IgG, IgM, and C3 (Fig. 8). No circulating antibodies were detected. Vesicular lesions did not respond to treatment with prednisone, and again Dapsone produced a dramatic response. Sulfones had to be later disconinued because of severe adverse reaction, and the patient had several relapses.

Case 3. A 57-year-old male had disseminated discoid lupus erythematosus (DDLE) preceding vesicular and bullous rash by 6 years. Bullous eruption was pruritic and localized in light-exposed areas and on the trunk, in the discoid lesions, and in uninvolved skin. Histologic studies revealed subepidermal bulla. Direct IF of a skin biopsy specimen obtained from the edge of a bullae revealed IgG, IgM, and C3 primarily with a linear pattern. No IgA was present. Studies of the skin specimen from the LE type of lesion revealed IgG, IgM, and C3 deposits with a granular pattern. Direct IF studies of the uninvolved light-exposed skin was negative. No circulating BMZ and ANA were detected. There was a dramatic response of bullous lesions to dapsone (100 mg/day), with no immediate relapse after discontinuation of therapy. There were, however, several relapses during the course of the disease.

The first two cases represent the association of bullous eruption with SLE, while the third case shows that such lesions may also occur in DDLE without symptoms of SLE.

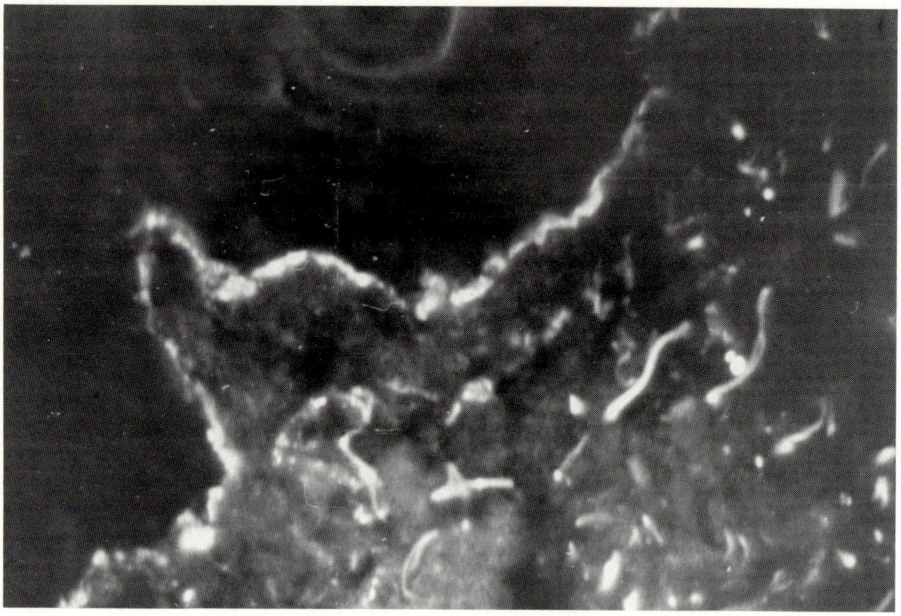

Figure 7. The same case as in Figure 5. Direct IF of normal skin, mostly granular IgG deposits at the dermal-epidermal junction.

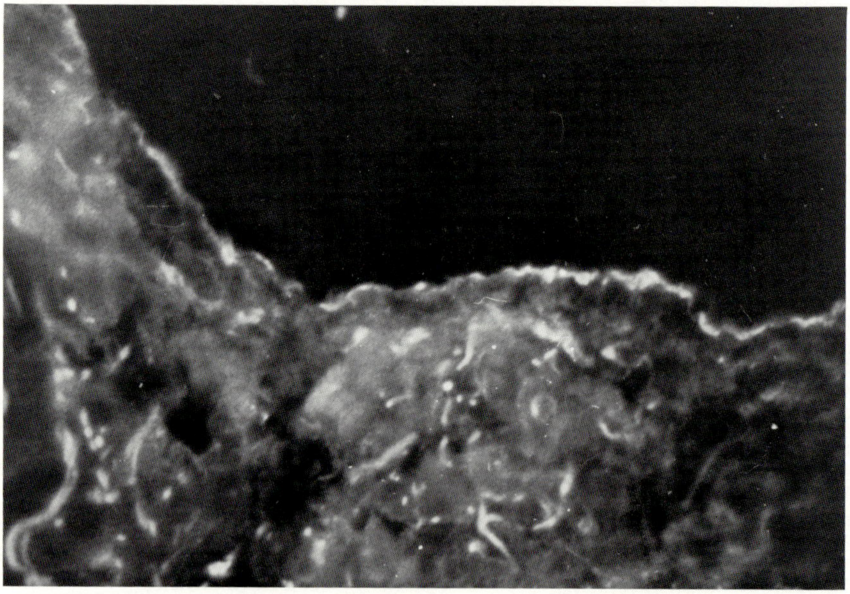

Figure 8. The same case as in Figure 6. Direct IF of normal skin adjacent to the vesicle. Linear and granular IgG deposits at the dermal-epidermal junction.

Classification of these cases as vesiculo-bullous SLE or coexistence of LABD-BP with LE remains to be determined. Despite some differences in histologic and IF findings (i.e., more or less similar to those in LABD or BP), these patients respond dramatically to sulfones, and this seems to be of basic practical importance.

Lichen Planus Associated with Bullous Eruption

Bullous rash associated with lichen planus (LP) may appear simultaneously with papular lesions of LP, or at any time during the course of the disease (34,65,66). In some cases of LP with bullous eruption, the latter was absent in recurrences of LP in the further course of the disease (48,62). Two forms of LP with bullae can be distinguished: one confined to the LP lesions, and other developing both on involved and seemingly normal skin.

The characteristic feature of the first variety is acral localization of the bullae arising on the confluent plaques of LP, often on the palms and soles. There are neither immunologic deposits at DEJ characteristic of BP nor circulating anti-BMZ antibodies, and the only immunologic marker is the presence of cytoid bodies. This form is often referred to as LP with bullae (61) or LP vesiculosus (63). The other form, referred to as LP pemphigoides (Figs. 9 and 10) has all clinical, histologic and immunologic characteristics of two diseases, and is regarded by some as a coexistence of LP and BP (34,57,66) and by others as a BP-like disease (62,65). Regardless, whether such bullous eruptions are called BP coexisting with LP or LP pemphigoides, a pathogenetic relation of these two is quite possible. The damage to the basement membrane in LP and the subsequent release of

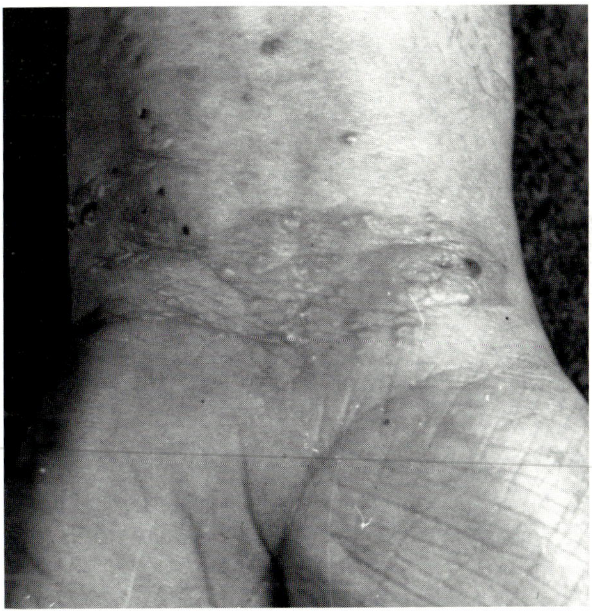

Figure 9. Case of LP associated with vesiculo-bullous eruption. Vesicles present in the lesions and on normal skin.

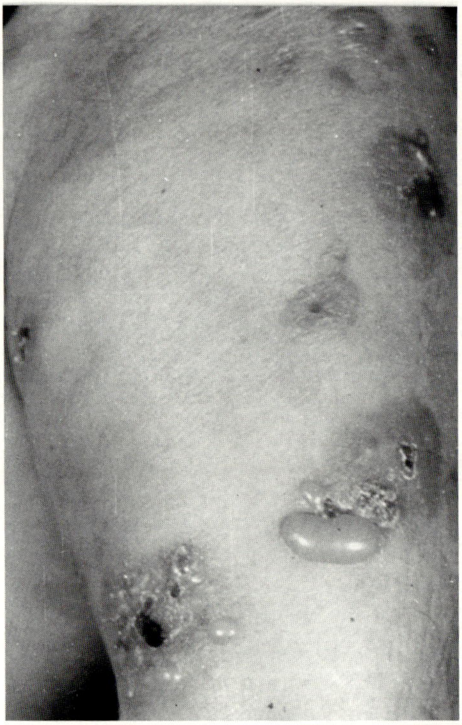

Figure 10. Case of lichen planus with bullous eruption around the lesions.

BMZ antigens may be the triggering mechanisms of antibody formation and the development of bullae, both in LP lesions and in the apparently normal skin. The presence of circulating anti-BMZ antibodies in some cases would favor such a hypothesis.

In our series, we also had cases of typical LP without bullae with linear IgG deposition at BMZ, as well as Ig bound to cytoid bodies (40). It is conceivable that in such cases, the anti-BMZ antibodies are formed, but, they are either devoid of pathogenic potential or are in amounts not sufficient to induce pathologic effect.

Bullous Pemphigoid and Malignancy

The association of pemphigoid with malignancy is still a matter of controversy. Although it is not certain whether BP may be classified as a paraneoplastic disorder, it appears that patients with pemphigoid are at higher risk for malignancy. In our recent series, tumors were detected in 20 of 148 (14%) BP cases. In 13 of these 20 cases, the tumor appeared before the onset of BP; and in seven, after or simultaneously with bullous lesions. This incidence of 14% is significantly higher ($p < 0.01$) than the frequency of cancer in the Polish population of a corresponding age and sex (17). No significant differences were found between the incidence of malignancies in BP patients, and matched controls in a series at the Mayo Clinic (67).

However, concurrent malignancy occurred in the Mayo Clinic group in 25% of seronegative versus 9% of seropositive BP patients (54), and in 23% of seropositive versus 4% of seronegative patients in the British group (36). In our studies, there was no evident association between the malignancy and the presence or absence of circulating BMZ antibodies (17). We believe that patients with BP, regardless of the serum findings, should be studied carefully for malignant tumors.

There is no association of BP with a specific type of neoplasia. It may accompany carcinomas of various organs: lung (59,59,80), breast (15,41), larynx (24), ovary (21), prostate (15,41,64,67), and metastatic skin cancer (39). The association of BP with lymphoma is less frequent than with carcinomas, and only isolated cases of different lymphomas and prelymphomas were reported (6,15,20,41,50).

The immunologic mechanism of BP associated with carcinomas is not clear. It is conceivable that BMZ antibodies are induced by antigens released from basement membranes of some epithelial tumors, as shown for bladder carcinoma (70). In the IF complement fixation tests, BMZ antibodies of the patient reacted both with the skin and the basement membrane of the tumor, whereas sera of other BP patients without associated carcinoma did not show such reactivity. However, experiments with mouse EHS sarcoma-producing basement membrane did not react with the tumor (77), but this could be due to species specificity of BMZ antibodies (13).

The causal relationship between BP and tumor is suggested by an improvement or disappearance of bullous lesions after surgery, and by a relapse of the disease concurrently with the recurrence of malignancy (15,41).

Causal relationship between BP and the tumor was questioned by some authors (21) due to the failure of the patient's own tumor cells to absorb BMZ antibody of the patient with BP and ovary carcinoma. However, tumor cells in this experiment did not proliferate in tissue culture, and thus the antigen could not be expressed. Further immunologic studies should be conducted on tissue culture of tumor cells with the use of autologus serum.

There are cases of BP-type bullous eruption associated with tumors and no detectable immunologic markers. We have followed the case of a 32-year-old woman with BP-type skin eruption that was resistant to any mode of treatment, including high dosages of corticosteroids. Repeated IF studies were negative for BMZ antibodies and in vivo-bound immune deposits at BMZ. The rash cleared completely without systemic or local treatment 24 to 48 hrs after a benign tumor of the ovary had been removed. The eruption never reappeared during 10 years of follow-up examinations. In this case, the causal relationship between bullous eruptions and the tumor is quite evident, but the mechanisms involved are entirely unknown.

SUMMARY

We would like to stress that pemphigoid represents a bullous disease with heterogeneous clinical manifestations including several subsets and clinically atypical forms. All forms can be identified by IF studies. There is no consensus on what mechanisms are involved in bullous eruption of the BP type associated with LE and LP; that is, a disease in which the dermal-epidermal junction undergoes destruction. Probably multiple mechanisms are operative. Also, the association of malignancy with BP is still somewhat controversial. However, we feel that all patients with BP should be checked for tumors.

REFERENCES

1. Abel EA, Bennett A: Bullous pemphigoid occurrence in psoriasis treated with psoralens plus long-wave ultraviolet radiation. *Arch Dermatol* 115:988, 1979.
2. Ahmed AR, Winkler NW: Psoriasis and bullous pemphigoid. *Arch Dermatol,* 113:845, 1977.
3. Ahmed AR, Maize JC, Provost TT: Bullous pemphigoid. Clinical and immunologic follow-up after successful therapy. *Arch Dermatol* 113:1043, 1977.
4. Bart BJ, Bean SF: Bullous pemphigoid following the topical use of fluorouracil. *Arch Dermatol* 102:457, 1970.
5. Bean SF, Good RA, Windhorst DB: Bullous pemphigoid in an 11-year-old boy. *Arch Dermatol* 102:205, 1970.
6. Bean SF, Michel B, Furey N: Vesicular pemphigoid. *Arch Dermatol* 112:1402–1404, 1976.
7. Beutner EH, Jordon RE: Demonstration of skin antibodies in sera of pemphigus vulgaris patients by indirect immunofluorescent staining. *Proc Soc Exp Biol Med* 117:505, 1964.
8. Björnberg A, Mobacken H: Recurrent bullous eruptions on the lower legs. *Acta Dermatol Venereol* 56:405, 1976.
9. Burnham TK, Nims LD: Case for diagnosis: Vesicular pemphigoid? Immunofluorescence microscopy studies. *Arch Dermatol,* 118:506, 1982.
10. Callen JP, McCall MW: Bullous pemphigoid and Hashimoto's thyroiditis. *J Am Acad Dermatol* 5:558, 1981.
11. Callen JP, Anderson TF, Chanda JJ, et al: Bullous pemphigoid and other disorders associated with autoimmune phenomena. *Arch Dermatol* 114:245, 1978.
12. Camisa C, Sharma HM: Vesiculobullous systemic lupus erythematosus. Report of two cases and a review of the literature. *J Am Acad Dermatol* 9:924–932, 1983.
13. Chorzelski TP, Beutner EH: Factors contributing to occasional failures in the laboratory diagnosis of bullous pemphigoid by indirect immunofluorescence. *Br J Dermatol* 86:111, 1972.
14. Chorzelski TP, Jabłońska S, Beutner EH: Pemphigoid. In Beutner EH, Chorzelski TP, Bean SF (Eds): *Immunopathology of the Skin,* ed. 2. Wiley, New York, 1979, pp 243–255.
15. Chorzelski TP, Jabłońska S, Błaszczyk M: Le rôle des rescherches immunopathologiques dans 1a différenciation des formes herpétiforme et pemphigoïde du syndrome de Duhring-Brocq. *Arch Belges Dermatol* 23:353, 1968.
16. Chorzelski TP, Jabłońska S, Błaszczyk M, et al: Autoantibodies in pemphigoid. *Dermatologica* 136:325–334, 1968.
17. Chorzelski TP, Jablonska S, Maciejowska E, et al: Coexistence of malignancies with bullous pemphigoid. *Arch Dermatol* 114:964, 1978.
18. Clayton CA, Burnham TK: Systemic lupus erythematosus and coexisting bullous pemphigoid: Immunofluorescent investigations. *J Am Acad Dermatol* 7:236, 1982.
19. Cram DL, Fukuyama K: The immunochemistry of ultraviolet-induced pemphigus and pemphigoid lesions. *Arch Dermatol* 106:819–824, 1972.
20. Cuni LJ, Grünwald H, Rosner F: Bullous pemphigoid in chronic lymphocytic leukemia with the demonstration of antibasement membrane antibodies. *Am J Med* 57:987–992, 1974.
21. Dahl MV, Ristow S: Bullous pemphigoid and ovarian cystadenocarcinoma. *Arch Dermatol* 114:903–905, 1978.
22. Davis MG, Marks R: Simultaneous systemic lupus erythematosus and dermatitis herpetiformis. *Arch Dermatol* 112:1292, 1976.
23. Eberhartinger C, Niebauer G: Zur Prognose und Therapie des Pemphigus vulgaris und Ahnlicher Erkrankungen. *Hautarzt* 12:503, 1961.
24. Ebner H, Spangler E: Untersuchungen über die Beziehung von bullose Pemphigoid und malignen Allgemeiner-krankungen. *Wien klin Wochenschr* 86:449–452, 1974.
25. Fellner MF, Enger P: Localized bullous pemphigoid resembling fixed-drug eruption. *NY State J Med* 79:1085, 1979.
26. Fellner MJ, Katz JH: Occurrence of bullous pemphigoid after furosemide therapy. *Arch Dermatol* 112:75, 1976.

27. Fincher DF, Dupree E, Bean SF: Bullous pemphigoid in childhood. Immunofluorescent studies. *Arch Dermatol* 103:88–90, 1971.
28. Gianini JM, Callen JP, Gruber GG: Bullous pemphigoid and rheumatoid arthritis. *J Am Acad Dermatol* 4:695, 1981.
29. Gissler K, Lischka G: PUVA-induziertes bullöses Pemphigoid bei Psoriasis vulgaris. *Akt Dermatol* 4:47, 1978.
30. Glander HJ, Barth J. Eine fixe bullöse Arzneimittelintoleranzreaktion unter dem klinischen und immunfluoreszenz-optischen Bild eines bullösen Pemphigoids. *Dermatol Monatschr* 161:455, 1975.
31. Gomes MA, Dambuyant C, Thivolet J, et al: Bullous pemphigoid: A correlative study of autoantibodies, circulating immune complexes and dermo-epidermal deposits. *Br J Dermatol* 107:43, 1982.
32. Hall RP, Lawley TJ, Smith HR, et al: Bullous eruption of systemic lupus erythematosus. Dramatic response to dapsone therapy. *Ann Intern Med* 97:165–170, 1982.
33. Hamilton DV, McKenzie AW: Bullous pemphigoid and primary billiary cirrhosis. *Br J Dermatol* 99:447, 1978.
34. Hinter H, Tappeiner G, Hönigsmann H, et al: Lichen planus and bullous pemphigoid. Acta Dermatol Venereol 59 (Suppl 85):77, 1979.
35. Hodge L, Black MM, Ramnarain N, et al: Indirect complement immunofluorescence in the immunopathological assessment of bullous pemphigoid, cicatricial pemphigoid, and herpes gestationis. *Clin Exp Dermatol* 3:61, 1978.
36. Hodge L, Marsden RA, Black MM, et al.: Bullous pemphigoid: The frequency of mucosal involvement and concurrent malignancy related to indirect immunofluorescence findings. *Br J Dermatol* 105:65–69, 1981.
37. Honeyman JF, Honeyman AR, de la Parra MA, et al: Polymorphic pemphigoid. *Arch Dermatol* 115:423–427, 1979.
38. How J, Bewsher PD, Stankler L: Bullous pemphigoid, polymyalgia rheumatica and thyroid disease. *Br J Dermatol* 103:201, 1980.
39. Ikai K, Imamura S, Ogino A, et al: Bullous pemphigoid and metastatic skin cancer. *Dermatologica* 156:55–58, 1978.
40. Jabłońska S, Chorzelski TP: Lupus erythematosus. In Fry L, Seah PP (Eds): *Immunological Aspects of Skin Disease.* Wiley, New York, 1974, pp 66–152.
41. Jabłlońska S, Chorzelski TP, Beutner EH, et al: Indications for skin and serum immunofluorescent studies in dermatology. In Beutner EH, Chorzelski TP, Bean SF, Jordon RE (Eds.); *Immunopathology of the Skin Labeled Antibody Studies.* Dowden Hutchinson & Ross, Stroudsburg, Pa, 1973, pp 1–24.
42. Koerber WA, Price NM, Watson W: Coexistent psoriasis and bullous pemphigoid: A report of six cases. *Arch Dermatol* 114:1643, 1978.
43. Kumar V, Binder WL, Schotland E, et al: Coexistence of bullous pemphigoid and systemic lupus erythematosus. *Arch Dermatol* 114:1187–1190, 1978.
44. Lever WF, Pemphigus. *Medicine* 32:1–123, 1953.
45. Levine N, Freilich A, Barland P: Localized pemphigoid simulating dyshidrosiform dermatitis. *Arch Dermatol* 115:320, 1979.
46. Massa MC, Connolly SM: Bullous pemphigoid with features of prurigo nodularis. *Arch Dermatol* 118:937, 1982.
47. Moncada B: Dermatitis herpetiformis in association with systemic lupus erythematosus. *Arch Dermatol* 109:723, 1974.
48. Mora RC, Nesbitt LT: Correspondence. *J Am Acad Dermatol* 10:290, 1984.
49. Olansky AJ, Briggaman RA, Gammon R, et al: Bullous systemic lupus erythematosus. *J Am Acad Dermatol* 7:511–520, 1982.
50. Parsons RL, Savin JA: Pemphigoid and malignancy. *Br J Cancer* 22:669–672, 1968.
51. Pedro SD, Dahl MV: Direct immunofluorescence of bullous systemic lupus erythematosus. *Arch Dermatol* 107:118, 1973.
52. Person JR: Hydrostatic bullae and pretibial pemphigoid. *Int J Dermatol* 22:237, 1983.

53. Person JR, Rogers RS: Bullous pemphigoid and psoriasis. Does subclinical bullous pemphigoid exist? *Br J Dermatol* 95:535, 1976.
54. Person JR, Rogers RS III: Bullous and cicatricial pemphigoid. Clinical, histopathologic and immunopathologic correlations. *Mayo Clin Proc* 52:54, 1977.
55. Penneys NS, Wiley HE: Herpetiform blisters in systemic lupus erythematosus. *Arch Dermatol* 115:1427, 1979.
56. Provost TT, Maize JC, Ahmed AR, et al: Unusual subepidermal bullous diseases with immunologic features of bullous pemphigoid. *Arch Dermatol* 115:156, 1979.
57. Rekant SI: Lichen planus and bullous pemphigoid. *Arch Dermatol* 12:1613, 1976.
58. Robinson JK, Baughman RD, Provost TT: Bullous pemphigoid induced by PUVA therapy. Is this the aetiology of the acral bullae produced during PUVA treatment? *Br J Dermatol* 99:709–713, 1978.
59. Rook AJ: A pemphigoid eruption associated with carcinoma of the bronchus. *Trans St Johns Hosp Dermatol Soc* 54:152–154, 1968.
60. Salo OP, Räsäsen JA: Pemphigoid and rheumatoid arthritis. *Ann Clin Res* 4:173–177, 1972.
61. Samman RD: Lichen planus and lichenoid eruption. In Rook A, Wilkinson DS, Ebling FJG (Eds): *Textbook of Dermatology*. Davis, Philadelphia, 1972, pp 1342–1343.
62. Saurat JH: Does the bullous eruption of lichen planus pemphigoides recur when the LP relapses? *J Am Acad Dermatol* 10:290, 1984.
63. Sauteyrand P, Pierini AM, Fernandez Bussy R, et al: Lichen planus pemphigoides: Entity or association? *Dermatologica* 162:414, 1981.
64. Skog E: Cutaneous manifestations associated with internal malignant tumours with particular reference to vesicular and bullous lesions. *Acta Dermatol Venereol* 44:114–117, 1964.
65. Sobel S, Miller R, Shatin H: Lichen planus pemphigoides. Immunofluorescence findings. *Arch Dermatol* 112:1280, 1976.
66. Stingl G, Holubar K: Coexistence of lichen planus and bullous pemphigoid. An immunopathological study. *Br J Dermatol* 93:313, 1975.
67. Stone SP, Schroeter AL: Bullous pemphigoid and associated malignant neoplasms. *Arch Dermatol* 111:991–994, 1975.
68. Stüttgen G, Bockendahl H, Remy W, et al: Psoriasis und bullöse Dermatosen. *Hautarzt* 29:134, 1978.
69. Szabo E, Husz S, Kovacs L: Coexistent atypical bullous pemphigoid and systemic lupus erythematosus. *Br J Dermatol* 104:71, 1981.
70. Tanaka T, Ogino A, Ogura K, et al: A case of bullous pemphigoid and transitional cell carcinoma of the bladder. Demonstration of circulating factor reactive with basement membrane zone of skin and of bladder carcinoma. *Arch Dermatol* 119:704, 1983.
71. Tappeiner G, Konrad K, Holubar K: Erythrodermic bullous pemphigoid. Report of a case. *J Am Acad Dermatol* 6:489, 1982.
72. Thaipisuttikul Y, Piamphongsant T, Suwanwela N: Coexistence of linear IgA dermatitis herpetiformis and systemic lupus erythematosus. *J Dermatol* 10:161, 1983.
73. Thomas JR, Su WPD: Concurrence of lupus erythematosus and dermatitis herpetiformis. A report of nine cases. *Arch Dermatol* 119:740, 1983.
74. Thomsen K, Schmidt H: PUVA-induced bullous pemphigoid. *Br J Dermatol* 95:568–569, 1976.
75. Ullman S, Malberg P, Nielsen R: Anti-basement membrane antibodies in sera from patients without bullous pemphigoid. *Acta Dermatol Venereol* 55:305, 1975.
76. Welke S: Das seborrhoische Pemphigoid (Schnyder). *Hautarzt* 31:18, 1980.
77. Wick G, Müller PU, Timpl R, et al: Studies on the immunology of basement membrane collagen using antibody to a tumor basement membrane. *Front Matrix Biol* 7:120–129, 1979.
78. Wranicz A, Czernielewski A: Pemphigoid provoked by Novoscabin? *Przeg Derm* 61:693, 1974.
79. Yung ChW, Soltani K, Lorincz AL: Pemphigoid nodularis. *J Am Acad Dermatol* 5:54, 1981.
80. Zinhsheim M, Gartmann H: Bulloses Pemphigoid und figurierte Erytheme als paraneoplastische Hautreaktion bei einem Bronchialkarzinom *Z Hautkr* 49:215–218, 1974.

17
Cicatricial Pemphigoid

Samuel F. Bean

INTRODUCTION

Cicatricial pemphigoid is a well-defined clinical and histologic entity that is characterized by blistering of mucous membranes, particularly the oral mucosa and conjunctiva. Skin involvement occurs in one-quarter to one-third of all cases. Histopathologically, the blister forms subepidermally.

The demonstration of immunoglobulins and complement components in a linear pattern at the basement membrane zone (BMZ) of the oral mucosa, conjunctiva, skin, and other tissues is now an established diagnostic test for cicatricial pemphigoid (Fig. 1) (1–4,11,13,14,25,27). C3 is the most commonly noted immunoreactant, but other immunoglobulins and complement components are found at the BMZ as well.

In a few cases, BMZ antibodies can be demonstrated in the sera using indirect immunofluorescence (IIF) (see Chaps. 8, 16, and 17).

BIOPSY FINDINGS (TABLES 1 AND 2)

Oral Mucosal Studies

Laskaris and Angeopoulis, in a recent study of oral mucosal specimens from 33 patients with cicatricial pemphigoid, reported IgG to be present in 32 patients (96.4%) (C3, 26; IgA, 9; IgM, 4; and fibrin, 13) (16). The control group in this study consisted of 21 healthy persons and 71 patients with various diseases. All were negative except for two patients with discoid lupus erythematosus (DLE) who showed granular staining with IgG and C3 at the BMZ. Daniels and White (7) examined 130 cases of oral disease, 33 of which were cicatricial pemphigoid, and found all to be positive for BMZ staining (IgG, 17; IgA, 10; IgM, 12; and C3, 32) without a false-positive being noted. These studies along with those of Rogers et al. (25), in which 123 oral mucosal specimens were examined without a false-positive being noted, confirms the specificity of direct immunofluorescence (DIF) in this disease when it occurs in the oral cavity.

Conjunctival Studies

In contrast to the initial study of conjunctival biopsy specimens in ocular cicatricial pemphigoid, in which we found only 4 of 20 patients to have BMZ staining of the conjunctiva (2), two recent reports in the ophthalmologic literature reported positive

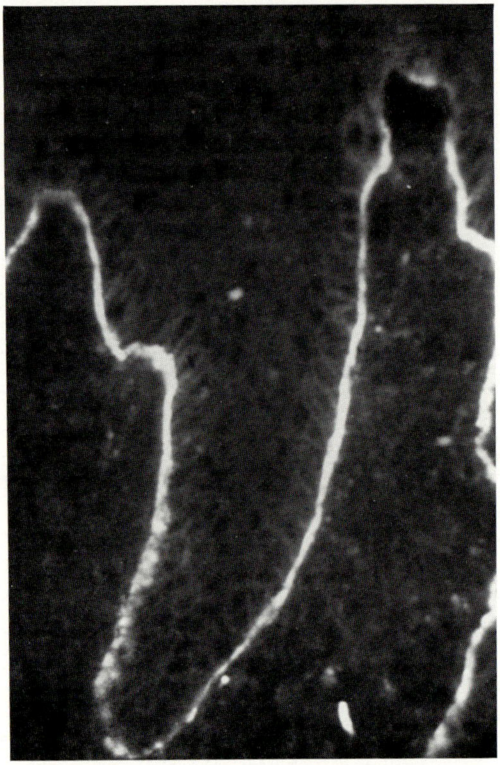

Figure 1. Continuous linear deposition of C3 at the BMZ of an oral mucosal biopsy specimen. (250x) (From [25] with permission of Williams & Wilkins.)

findings of 67 (20) and 84% (10). In the study by Mondino et al. (20), 8 of 12 patients were positive for immunoglobulins or complement components at the BMZ (IgG, 3; IgA, 2; IgM, 2; and C3, 4). They suggested that their higher percentage of positive specimens was the result of a more timely biopsy procedure and a more appropriate biopsy site. In addition to BMZ staining, the investigators noted intracellular immunoglobulin deposits in the conjunctival epithelia of six patients in this study. In the report by Foster et al. (10), 15 of 18 patients (84%) were positive for conjunctival BMZ staining (IgG, 14; IgA, 9; IgM, 2; and C3, 5). Interestingly, the six cases that were biopsied after immunosuppressive therapy were no longer positive.

SERUM FINDINGS

Circulating BMZ antibodies have rarely been demonstrated in the sera of persons with cicatricial pemphigoid when monkey esophagus and other often used sources of tissue were used as substrates. Antibodies were usually found in persons with widespread involvement, and the titers were low (1,6,8,24,27). These findings are in contrast to those of bullous pemphigoid (BP), in which 70 to 80% of the sera are positive for BMZ antibodies.

Table 1. Summary of Immunopathologic Observations of Cicatricial Pemphigoid Mucosal Lesions

	Linear BMZ pattern	
Antisera	No.	% positive
IgG	9/23	39
IgA	8/20	40
IgM	6/21	29
C3	17/21	81
Clq[a]	7/11	64
C4[a]	2/4	50
Factor B[a]	5/10	50
Properdin[a]	7/11	64
Fibrin	15/23	65
Positive BMZ pattern	19/23	83

From Rogers et al. (25) with permission of Williams & Wilkins.
[a]Modified IIF staining employed.

Table 2. Recent DIF Studies of Cicatricial Pemphigoid

		Immunoreactants					
Tissue	*No. of cases*	*IgG*	*IgA*	*IgM*	*C3*	*Fibrin*	*References*
	12	3	2	2	4		Mondino et al. (20)
Conjunctiva	18	14	9	2	5		Foster et al. (10)
	33	32	9	4	2	13	Laskaris and Angeopoulis (16)
Oral mucosa	33	17	10	12	32	ND[a]	Daniels and White (7)

[a]ND, not done.

Typical Reagents

The molar fluorescein-to-protein ratio (F/P) and antibody concentration of the conjugates and dilutions used are as follows: 1) IgG, F/P ratio 3.5, 1.9 mg Ab/ml, diluted to a concentration of 50 μg/ml; 2) IgM, F/P ratio 2.5, 0.3 mg Ab/ml, diluted to a concentration of 100 μg/ml; 3) BIC-globulin (C3), F/P ratio 3.1, 1.2 mg Ab/ml, diluted to 50 μg/ml; and 4) IgG, F/P ratio 2.8 mg Ab/ml diluted to a concentration of 100 μg/ml. Monkey esophagus served as a substrate tissue in the performance of the routine IIF test.

Basement Membrane Zone Antibodies

In 1974, using multiple animal and human substrate tissues, I found the sera of three persons with cicatricial pemphigoid to be positive for low titer BMZ antibodies (1). In 1981, Laskaris and Angeopoulis (16) demonstrated BMZ antibodies in 12 of 33 cases (36.4%) in titers of 1:10 to 1:40, using normal oral mucosa as a substrate tissue. These studies again suggested that antibody specificity may account, in part, for the low incidence of circulating BMZ antibodies in cicatricial pemphigoid. On the other hand, Fine et al. (9), in a recent report, found only one of eight patients with cicatricial pemphigoid to have a circulating BMZ antibody. Interestingly, this was an IgA antibody, and was detected using normal skin as a substrate. They tested all eight sera with normal human buccal mucosa from three different volunteers and found no specific binding along the BMZ. The difference in these studies is difficult to interpret, although it is clear that the use of IIF as a diagnostic test in cicatricial pemphigoid is not warranted.

Other Autoantibodies and Human Leukocyte Antigen (HLA) Studies
Antinuclear, thyroid, adrenal, pancreatic, and cytoplasmic and pemphigus-like antibodies (PLA) have been reported in persons with cicatricial pemphigoid (5,20). In addition, persons with cicatricial pemphigoid who have conjunctival involvement also have an increased incidence of HLA-B12 antigen (19), and about 50% have elevated IgA levels (2). The importance of these findings is not known at present.

RELATIONSHIP OF CICATRICIAL PEMPHIGOID TO OTHER BULLOUS DISEASES

Bullous Pemphigoid

A number of reports have documented the occurrence of a generalized cutaneous eruption clinically typical of bullous pemphigoid (BP) occurring in patients with cicatricial pemphigoid. I have seen three patients with cicatricial pemphigoid—two with oral involvement and another with conjunctival involvement—who had generalized cutaneous bullae. In one, there were multiple blisters, whereas in the other two, bullae were scattered and few in number. In one patient, the skin lesions preceded oral involvement by 1 year. The histopathology and immunofluorescence (IF) was typical of BP or cicatricial pemphigoid, and in one case there was a low-titer circulating BMZ antibody. These overlap cases, along with similar histopathologic changes, identical IF, and immunoelectron microscopy (IEM) (lamina lucida deposits) (9,23), suggest a relationship between BP and cicatricial pemphigoid (see Chaps. 15 and 16).

Brunsting-Perry Cicatricial Pemphigoid

This entity is characterized by tense single or grouped vesicles or bullae that occur on the scalp, face, and neck without mucosal lesions. Resolution of the lesions occurs with or without scarring or atrophy. The histopathology, IF and IEM changes are identical to those of cicatricial pemphigoid. (17,18,21). The concurrence of skin involvement typical of Brunsting-Perry cicatricial pemphigoid and mucosal lesions typical of cicatricial pemphigoid strengthen the concept that the two diseases are related. Most authorities now agree that Brunsting-Perry cicatricial pemphigoid is the cutaneous variant of cicatricial pemphigoid. Furthermore, our recent report of Brunsting-Perry cicatricial pemphigoid and BP occurring in the same patient suggests that a relationship exists between the three diseases as well (12). (See Chap. 16).

Desquamative Gingivitis

This is a reactive process of the gingival tissue characterized by vesiculo-bullous erosions and desquamation (see Chap. 18). Immunofluorescence in many of the cases shows BMZ staining identical to that of cicatricial pemphigoid. In a recent report, Rogers et al. (26) studied 41 cases of desquamative gingivitis, 37 of which were classified as cicatricial pemphigoid. suspects by histologic and IF criteria. Of these, 18 developed typical cicatricial pemphigoid. Although lichen planus (LP) and pemphigus vulgaris (PV) may also produce desquamative gingivitis, it seems evident that a number of patients with desquamative gingivitis represent a form fruste of cicatricial pemphigoid.

Epidermolysis Bullosa Acquisita (EBA)

This is a chronic blistering disease of unknown etiology that may sometimes be confused clinically and histologically with BP and cicatricial pemphigoid (see Chap. 20). In addition, the DIF findings are indistinquishable from BP and cicatricial pemphigoid, and in some cases of EBA, a circulating BMZ antibody may be detected. This had led to speculation that the three diseases might, in fact, be related. Recent studies, however, show that the immunoreactants in EBA are deposited below the basal lamina and not in the lamina lucida, as in cicatricial and pemphigoid and BP (22,23,28,30 Chap. 20).

Linear IgA Bullous Dermatosis (LABD)

Cases of cicatricial pemphogoid with IgA deposits at the BMZ in both adults (15) and children (20) were described recently. Also, in three of four children, circulating anti-BMZ antibodies of the IgA class were detected. The latter finding is consistent with the diagnosis of LABD. Interestingly, some but not all patients responded to sulfones, and there was no evidence of gluten-sensitive enteropathy; that is, the jejunal biopsy specimens were normal in the patients examined (29) (see Chaps. 22 and 23).

CONCLUSIONS

Recent studies have confirmed the usefulness of IF as a diagnostic aid in cicatricial pemphigoid and, in conjunction with IEM, have further defined the disease and its relationship to BP, Brunsting-Perry cicatricial pemphigoid, desquamative gingivitis, and EBA. These studies have also advanced our knowledge regarding insight into the pathophysiologic mechanisms responsible for the disease, and more importantly have aided development of a more rational approach to management of this difficult and frustrating disorder.

REFERENCES

1. Bean SF: Cicatricial pemphigoid: Immunofluorescent studies. *Arch Dermatol* 110:522, 1974.
2. Bean SF, Furey N, West C, et al: Ocular cicatricial pemphigoid (immunologic studies). *Trans Am Acad Ophthalmol Otolaryngol* 81:806, 1976.
3. Bean SF, Rogers RS III, Jordon RE, et al: Cicatricial pemphigoid. In Beutner EH, Chorzelski TP, Bean SF (Eds): *Immunopathology of the Skin,* ed. 2. Wiley, New York, 1979, p 257.
4. Bean SF, Waisman M, Michel B, et al: Cicatricial pemphigoid: Immunofluorescent studies. *Arch Dermatol* 106:195, 1972.
5. Cram DL, Griffith MR, Fukuyama K: Pemphigus-like antibodies in cicatricial pemphigoid. *Arch Dermatol* 109:235, 1974.
6. Dabelsteen E, Ullman S, Thomsen K, et al: Demonstration of basement membrane autoantibodies in patients with benign mucous membrane pemphigoid. *Acta Dermatovenereol* 54:189, 1974.

7. Daniels TE, Quandra-White C: Direct immunofluorescence in oral mucosal disease: A diagnostic analysis of 130 cases. *Oral Surg* 51:38, 1981.
8. Dantzig P: Circulating antibodies in cicatricial pemphigoid. *Arch Dermatol* 108:264, 1973.
9. Fine J, Neises GR, Katz SI: Immunofluorescence and immunoelectron microscopic studies in cicatricial pemphigoid. *J Invest Dermatol* 82:39, 1984.
10. Foster CS, Wilson LA, Ekins MA: Immunosuppressive therapy for progressive ocular cicatricial pemphigoid. *Ophthalmology* 89:340, 1982.
11. Griffith MR, Fukuyama K, Tuffanelli D, et al: Immunofluorescent studies in mucous membrane pemphigoid. *Arch Dermatol* 109:195, 1974.
12. Hanno R, Foster DR, Bean SF: Brunsting-Perry cicatricial pemphigoid associated with bullous pemphigoid. *J Am Acad Dermatol* 3:470, 1980.
13. Heydenreich G, From E, Deiderichsen H: Some unusual findings obtained by immunofluorescence method in bullous pemphigoid and benign mucous membrane pemphigoid. *Acta Dermatovenereol* 52:201, 1972.
14. Holubar K, Honigsmann H, Wolff K. Cicatricial pemphigoid. Immunofluorescence investigations. *Arch Dermatol* 108:50, 1973.
15. Kumar, V, Rogozinksi T, Yarbrough C, et al: A case of cicatricial pemphigoid or cicatricial linear IgA bullous dermatosis. *J Am Acad Dermatol* 2:327–331, 1980.
16. Laskaris G, Angelopoulis A: Cicatricial pemphigoid: Direct and indirect immunofluorescent studies. *Oral Surg* 51:48, 1981.
17. Michel B, Bean SF, Chorzelski TP, et al: Cicatricial pemphigoid of Brunsting-Perry. *Arch Dermatol* 113:1403, 1977.
18. Michel B: Localized chronic pemphigoid of Brunsting-Perry: Its relationship to bullous pemphigoid. In Beutner EH, Chorzelski TP, Bean SF (Eds): *Immunopathology of the Skin,* ed. 2. Wiley, New York, 1979, p 265.
19. Mondino BJ, Brown SL, Rabin BS: HLA antigens in ocular cicatricial pemphigoid. *Arch Ophthalmol* 97:479, 1979.
20. Mondino BJ, Ross AN, Rabin BS, et al: Autoimmune phenomenon in ocular cicatricial pemphigoid. *Am J Ophthalmol* 83:443, 1977.
21. Murata Y, Masahiro T, Kumano K: Localized chronic pemphigoid of Brunsting-Perry. Ultrastructural localization of IgG and complement components *Arch Dermatol* 119:921, 1983.
22. Nieboer C, Boorsma DM, Woerdeman MJ, et al: Epidermolysis bullosa acquisita: Immunofluorescence, electron microscopic and immunoelectron microscopic studies in four patients. *Br J Dermatol* 102:303, 1980.
23. Nieboer C, Boorsma DM, Woerdeman MJ: Immune electron microscopic findings in cicatricial pemphigoid: Their significance in relationship to epidermolysis bullosa acquisita. *Br J Dermatol* 106:419, 1982.
24. Person JR, Rogers RS III, Jordon RE. Cicatricial pemphigoid with circulating antibasement membrane antibodies: A report of three atypical cases. *Dermatologica* 154:90, 1977.
25. Rogers RS III, Perry HO, Bean SF, et al: Immunopathology of cicatricial pemphigoid: Studies of complement deposition. *J Invest Dermatol* 68:39–43, 1977.
26. Rogers RS III, Sheridan TJ, Nightingale SH: Desquamative gingivitis: Clinical, histopathologic, immunopathologic and therapeutic observations. *J Am Acad Dermatol* 7:729–735, 1982.
27. Tagami H, Inamura S: Benign mucous membrane pemphigoid: Demonstration of circulating and tissue-bound membrane antibodies. *Arch Dermatol* 109:711, 1974.
28. Wilson BD, Birnkrant AP, Beutner EH, et al: Epidermolysis bullosa acquisita: A clinical disorder of varied etiologies. *J Am Acad Dermatol* 3:280, 1980.
29. Wojnarowska F, Marsden RA, Bhagal B, et al: Childhood cicatricial pemphigoid with linear IgA deposits. *Clin Exp Dermatol* 9;402–415, 1984.
30. Yaoita H. Briggaman RA, Lawley TJ, et al: Epidermolysis bullosa acquisita: Ultrastructural and immunological studies. *J Invest Dermatol* 76:288, 1981.

18
Desquamative Gingivitis

Russell J. Nisengard
Roy S. Rogers III

INTRODUCTION

Desquamative gingivitis is a chronic gingival disease characterized by erythematous, erosive, vesiculo-bullous, and/or desquamative involvement of the free and attached gingivae (Fig. 1). In some cases, other mucosal surfaces and the skin may also be involved. Initially described by Tomes more than 100 years ago (23), the name "chronic diffuse desquamative gingivitis" was coined by Prinz (18) in 1932. While early reports suggested that desquamative gingivitis was a specific disease entity, Glickman (7), as early as 1953, speculated that it may represent a manifestation of several disease processes. Since then, histologic and immunologic findings have supported that it is a manifestation of several diseases and therefore has multiple etiologies. McCarthy et al. (13) and, more recently, Shklar (22) proposed a provisional classification based on etiologic considerations. This has been expanded by observations of others (3,5,14,20) and is summarized in Table 1. While many diseases or conditions have been associated with desquamative gingivitis, the majority of cases are dermatologic diseases, which account for approximately 75% of all cases. The most common dermatologic diseases are cicatricial pemphigoid and lichen planus (LP); which comprise over 95% of desquamative gingivitis with a dermatologic etiology (3,5,8,12,14,20). Other nondermatologic diseases associated with desquamative gingival lesions occur infrequently. Because of this, the balance of this chapter will focus on the immunopathology of desquamative gingival lesions associated with dermatoses.

Clinically, desquamative gingival lesions occur most frequently in females (Table 2). A summary of literature reports on 272 patients with desquamative gingivitis indicates approximately four of five (80%) are females (1,4,6,7,9,12–14,19,20,23). In these patients, lesions were localized to the gingivae in half the cases (91 of 182); and in the other half, lesions concurrently involved other intraoral and extraoral sites, including the buccal mucosa, palate, tongue, lips, skin, and conjunctiva (1,7,8,12,14,20,23). With time, lesions localized to the gingivae sometimes extended to sites other than the gingivae. While most patients are middle-aged, lesions occur in patients ranging from 7 to 78 years of age.

DIAGNOSIS

Until recently, the diagnosis of desquamative gingivitis was based solely on clinical and histologic criteria (Figs. 1 and 2). Frequently, neither parameter was sufficient to identify

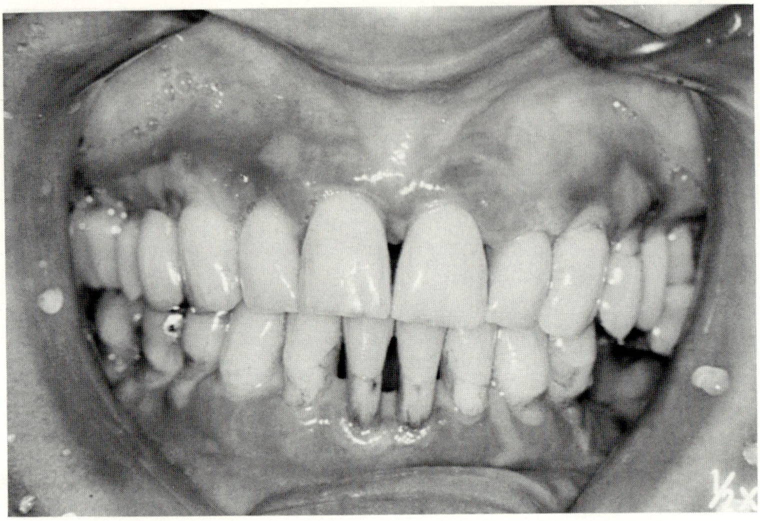

Figure 1. Desquamative gingivitis in a 70-year-old woman. Erythematous and erosive lesions were present for at least 1 year and localized to the buccal and lingual aspects of the free and attached gingiva. (Courtesy of Dr. S.L. Fischman.)

Table 1. Diseases Associated with Desquamative Gingival Lesions

I	Dermatoses
	Cicatricial pemphigoid
	Lichen planus
	Pemphigus
	Psoriasis
	Bullous pemphigoid
	Epidermolysis bullosa acquisita
	Contact stomatitis
II	Endocrine imbalance
	Estrogen deficiencies following oophorectomy and in post menopausal women
	Testosterone imbalance
	Hypothyroidism
III	Aging
IV	Abnormal response to bacterial plaque
V	Idiopathic
VI	Chronic infections
	Tuberculosis
	Chronic candidiasis
	Histoplasmosis

the underlying etiology. With the implementation of direct immunofluorescence (DIF) tests for examination of gingival biopsy specimens and indirect immunofluorescence (IIF) tests for examination of sera, an important third parameter—immunopathology—was added. Immunofluorescence (IF) has led to a more precise identification of the underlying etiology, and has permitted a dermatologic diagnosis to be made in a greater percentage of desquamative gingival lesions. DIF has proven to be an important parameter in diagnosis, since immune deposits can be identified not only in lesional gingival specimens, but also in perilesional and normal gingival specimens. This is of particular importance in the oral cavity, where vesiculo-bullous lesions quickly ulcerate, preventing proper interpretation of a lesional gingival biopsy specimen.

The DIF biopsy findings in 174 cases of desquamative gingivitis are summarized in Table 3 (1,9,12,14,20). A definitive diagnosis of cicatricial pemphigoid and pemphigus was made in 48.9% and 2.3% of the cases, respectively. IF findings suggestive of LP and psoriasis occurred in 23.6% and 0.6%, respectively. Negative findings were observed in 24.6% of the cases. Thus, on the basis of DIF, approximately one-half of the desquamative lesions are cicatricial pemphigoid, one-quarter are LP, one-quarter have no significant immunopathology. In addition, a small number are pemphigus and psoriasis.

SPECIMEN COLLECTION

Establishment of a dermatologic etiology for desquamative gingivitis by either light microscopy or DIF requires gingival biopsy specimens with intact epithelium. Desquamative gingival lesions, however, often exhibit epithelial separation as a consequence of

Table 2. Summary of Clinical Findings in Desquamative Gingivitis

Total no. of patients	272
No. of females	216 (79.4%)
No. of males	56 (20.6%)
Site of lesions	
Gingival lesions alone	91 (50%)
Gingival lesions plus intraoral and/or extraoral lesions	91 (50%)

Table 3. Summary of DIF Findings in Desquamative Gingivitis

Immunologic diagnosis[a]	*No. of patients*	*% of total*
Cicatricial pemphigoid[b]	85	48.9
Pemphigus	4	2.3
Lichen Planus[c]	41	23.6
Psoriasis[c]	1	0.6
Negative[d]	43	24.6
Total	174	

[a]Based on DIF findings in gingival biopsy specimens.
[b]Immunologic findings are diagnostic: Immune deposits along the BMZ in cicatricial pamphigoid and IC in pemphigus.
[c]Immunologic findings are suggestive, but not diagnostic: Large numbers of cytoid bodies and/or fibrin deposits along the BMZ in LP and immune deposits in the stratum corneum in the psoriasis form of psoriasis.
[d]No significant immune findings.

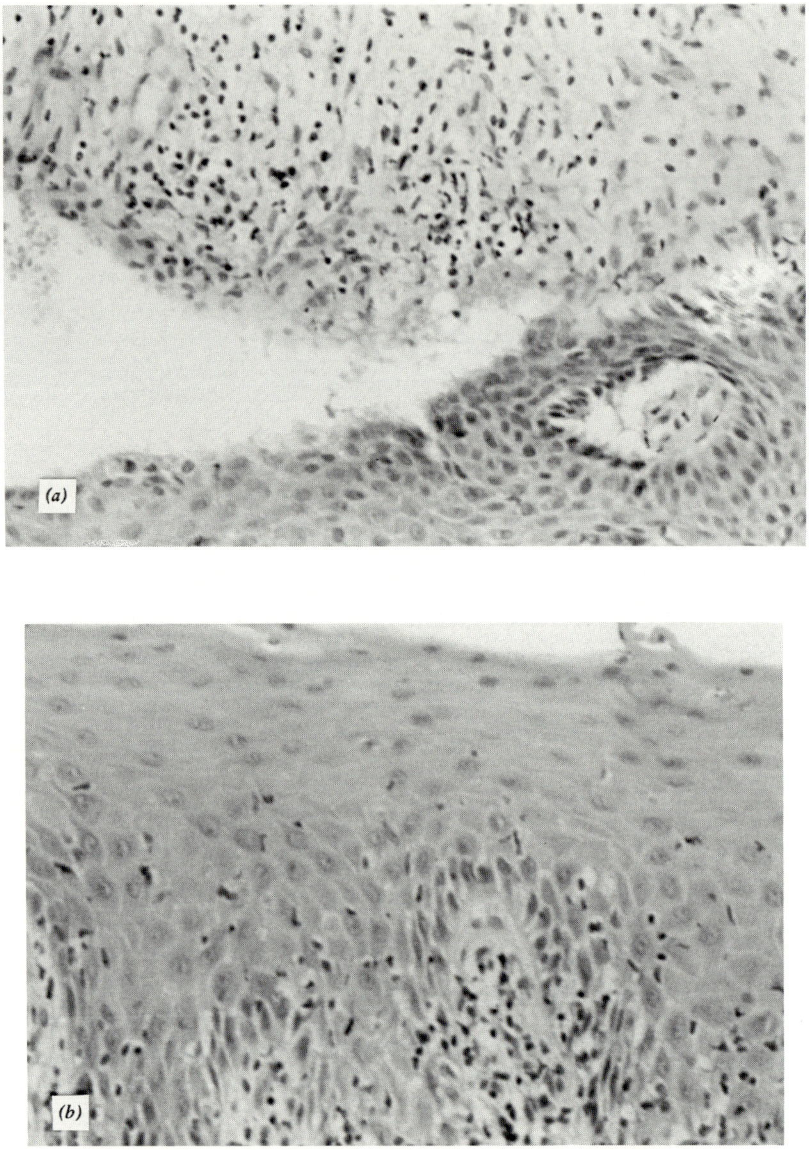

Figure 2. A. H&E-stained section from a perilesional gingival biopsy specimen revealing a subepithelial bulla consistent with cicatricial pemphigoid (400x). (Courtesy of Dr. S.L. Fischman.) B. H&E-stained section from a clinically normal gingival biopsy specimen revealing a chronic inflammatory infiltrate in the dermis (400x). (Courtesy of Dr. S.L. Fischman.)

disease or as a result of trauma from the biopsy collection. To minimize this problem, the biopsy site of choice for light microscopy and IF is perilesional rather than lesional. Past experience (14) indicates that clinically normal gingival biopsy specimens, even from other areas of the mouth (e.g., palatal gingival sites when lesions are limited to buccal gingiva of the mandible), have immune deposits similar to those observed in perilesional specimens, at least in cases of cicatricial pemphigoid and pemphigus. Because of this, for IF studies, a second biopsy of normal gingiva is often recommended (14,15) to ensure a specimen with intact epithelium.

The examination of sera from patients with desquamative gingivitis by IIF usually yields negative results except in patients with pemphigus and a small percent of patients with cicatricial pemphigoid (Table 4). Because of this, serum should not routinely be submitted for testing.

DESQUAMATIVE GINGIVAL LESIONS ASSOCIATED WITH CICATRICIAL PEMPHIGOID

Approximately 50% of the cases of desquamative gingivitis are associated with cicatricial pemphigoid. While conjunctival lesions caused by cicatricial pemphigoid can lead to blindness, a summary of data on the incidence of eye lesions in patients with desquamative gingivitis diagnosed as having cicatricial pemphigoid by DIF is only 10 of 96 patients (10.4%) (1,12,14,19,20). This appears to be lower than the 50 to 70% incidence of eye lesions in patients with cicatricial pemphigoid not reported to have desquamative gingival lesions (10,16). One explanation for this lower incidence of eye involvement in patients with desquamative lesions may be that they seek professional care earlier because of their sore mouths. Alternatively, they may represent a subset of cicatricial pemphigoid patients that does not manifest eye lesions as frequently (Chap. 17).

Histologically, the presence of a subepithelial blister is indicative of the pemphigoid group of diseases. Typically, intact epithelium is separated from the underlying lamina propria. The rete ridges are shortened, with minimal interdigitation of epithelium and lamina propria. Damage to basal cells may be noted, and fibrinous strands may traverse the blister cavity. The epithelium is otherwise intact. The lamina propria may contain both acute and chronic inflammatory cells depending on the age of the lesion. Round cells and plasma cells tend to dominate the infiltrate of established lesions. The vasculature is intact with no evidence for vasculitis. The supporting tissues may show some degenerative changes, especially in established lesions.

Immunologically, IF yields diagnostic findings in both gingival biopsy specimens and sera. In biopsy specimens, basement membrane zone (BMZ) deposits of IgG and C3 are most common (Fig. 3) (14). Sera from patients with desquamative gingivitis infrequently have IgG antibodies to the basement membrane, as identified by IIF. A summary of four reports indicates that only 6 of 61 (9.8%) sera from patients with immune deposits along the basement membrane have serum antibodies reactive with the base-

Table 4. Summary of IIF Findings in Desquamative Gingivitis

Immunologic Diagnosis[a]	*No. of patientsPositive (Total)*	*% positive*
Cicatricial pemphigoid	6/61	9.8
Pemphigus	3/3	100
Lichen planus, psoriasis, other	0/38	NSA[b]

[a]Immunologic diagnosis as determined by DIF examination of biopsy specimen.
[b]NSA, No specific antibodies detected by this method.

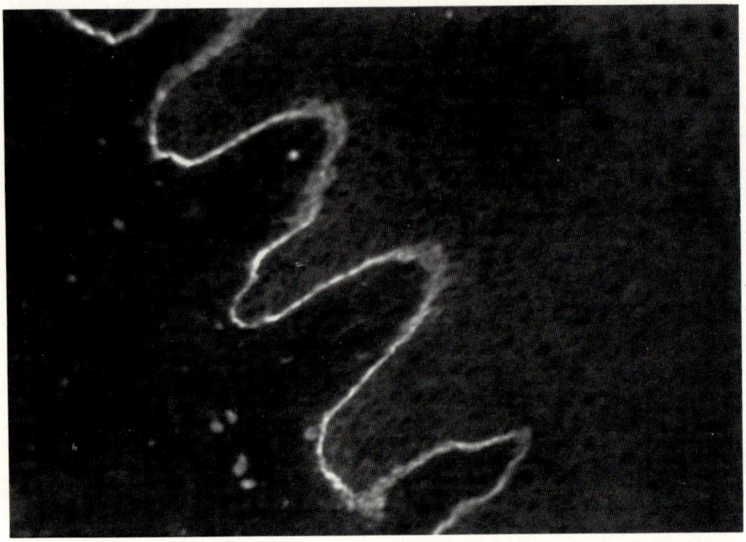

Figure 3. DIF for C3 on a section from a clinically normal biopsy specimen. C3 deposits along the basement membrane are consistent with cicatricial pemphigoid (400x).

ment membrane zone (Table 4) (8,12,14,19). Some studies of desquamative gingivitis have compared cases of cicatricial pemphigoid diagnosed by IF to those diagnosed by light microscopy (12,14,19,20). In general, DIF identifies more cases than light microscopy of cicatricial pemphigoid as the etiology of desquamative gingivitis. This slight but consistent difference probably occurs because BMZ immune deposits occur in perilesional and normal gingivae, where histologically there are only chronic inflammatory infiltrates and no vesicles or subepithelial bullae.

Treatment of localized oral pemphigoid is predicated on the degree of disability and the natural history of this form of desquamative gingivitis (20). Asymptomatic patients require only excellent oral hygiene to minimize bacterial plaque and careful dental care, including frequent thorough scaling and root planing. For those symptomatic patients with lesions limited to the gingivae, the applications of fluorinated corticosteroids two to three times each day, usually for a long period of time, may be sufficient to control the process. Some patients will undergo a spontaneous remission.

For those patients with moderate disability from their gingival disease or patients whose disease progresses to involve other oral mucosal or other mucosal surfaces, systemic therapy is indicated. Therapy should be commenced with dapsone following preliminary laboratory testing. A stepwise-increasing regimen of dapsone, including a dose of 25 mg/day for 3 days, 25 mg twice per day for 3 days, 25 mg three times per day for 3 days, and 50 mg twice per day for 7 days should be instituted. The dose is then increased to 125 mg/day for 7 days, and then to 150 mg/day thereafter. Blood counts are obtained weekly for 6 weeks. Most patients who will respond (85%) will do so within 6 to 12 weeks. Once control is established and maintained for 6 to 12 weeks, the dapsone may be tapered by 25 mg/week until the lowest dose effective in controlling the process is achieved. At times, the dapsone can be discontinued without exacerbation.

For those patients who do not respond to 150 mg/day of dapsone, sulfapyridine in a dose of 500 mg/day for 7 days, then twice per day for 7 days, and then three times per day thereafter may be used as primary therapy or added to the dapsone therapy.

Treatment may be supplemented with topical flourinated corticosteroids, and oral hygiene and dental care should be continued.

DESQUAMATIVE GINGIVAL LESIONS ASSOCIATED WITH PEMPHIGUS

Approximately 2% of cases of desquamative gingivitis are associated with pemphigus. All these patients also had skin involvement. While most pemphigus vulgaris (PV) cases develop intraorally at first (17,21), the gingiva does not appear to be a major intraoral site.

Histologically, acantholysis of epithelial cells with the resultant intraepithelial blister is indicative of pemphigus. The epithelium superficial to the acantholytic process is usually hyalinized and degenerated. Rounded squamous cells are noted free in the blister cavity. The base of the blister is lined with partially separated basal cells, which show some degenerative changes. The BMZ and lamina propria are intact and uninvolved, unless trauma or secondary infection have supervened. In this instance, an inflammatory cell infiltrate will be noted in the lamina propria. The vessels are spared involvement in typical cases.

Immunologically, desquamative gingivitis associated with pemphigus is identical to pemphigus involving any part of the body. DIF reveals intercellular (IC) deposits of IgG in the gingival epithelium, and IIF reveals IgG antibodies in sera reactive with the IC substance of squamous epithelium in most if not all specimens studied. In collecting the gingival biopsy specimen, care must be taken not to include crevicular or junctional epithelium from the wall of the gingival crevice or pocket that lines the tooth side of the gingivae, since this area can yield false-positive findings. In gingivitis and periodontitis, crevicular fluid containing IgG antibodies enters the gingival crevice through this epithelium; examination of epithelium from this area results in apparent IC immune deposits.

Treatment of the pemphigus variant of desquamative gingivitis is similar to the regimen for oral pemphigus, which is not limited to the gingivae. As the disease is very early in its evolutionary history, a prompt remission may be induced with early systemic therapy with corticosteroids. The reader is referred to Chapter 10 for details.

DESQUAMATIVE GINGIVITIS ASSOCIATED WITH LICHEN PLANUS

Approximately 25% of the cases of desquamative gingivitis are associated with lichen planus (LP). In particular, the erosive variant of LP could manifest as a desquamative gingival lesion.

Histologically, the presence of a band-like infiltrate below the BMZ is indicative of LP. Typically, intact epithelium overlies the inflammatory cell infiltrate. The basal cell layer shows damage with Civatte bodies above and below the BMZ, degeneration of the basal cells, invasion of the lower epithelium by chronic inflammatory cells, and a "sawtooth" interdigitation of the epithelium and lamina propria. Epithelial atrophy, thinning of the epithelial plate, separation of the epithelium from the lamina propria with loss of interdigitation, and a frank subepithelial blister may be noted in some patients. The lamina propria demonstrates a dense round cell inflammatory infiltrate abutting the BMZ and invading the epithelium. Civatte bodies and occasional acute inflammatory cells are admixed with this infiltrate, as is mild edema. The vessels and deeper lamina propria are usually spared.

Immunologically, desquamative gingivitis associated with LP is similar to LP elsewhere on the body. Gingival biopsy specimens reveal characteristic but not diagnostic findings, including cytoid bodies in the epidermis and dermis and fibrin (fibrinogen) deposits along the basement membrane.

Treatment of the LP variant of desquamative gingivitis is similar to the regimen used for the mild localized oral pemphigoid form of desquamative gingivitis.

DESQUAMATIVE GINGIVITIS ASSOCIATED WITH PSORIASIS

While only 1 of 174 cases of desquamative gingivitis was immunologically characterized as psoriasis (2,14), several clinical cases of psoriasis have been associated with desquamative gingivitis (3,5,11). The reported number of desquamative lesions associated with psoriasis may be less than actually occurs, since the immunopathology of psoriasis has only recently been identified (see Chap. 42).

Histologically, epithelial hyperplasia with a thickened stratum corneum, parakeratosis, hyperplasia of the stratum malpighi, and increased mitotic figures within the nuclei of the basal cell and epidermal microabscesses are indicative of psoriasis. Increased epithelial-lamina propria interdigitation may be noted. There is no blister formation and the vessels are uninvolved. The lamina propria contains a chronic inflammatory cell infiltrate that is scattered and diffuse. In acute lesions, polymorphonuclear leukocytes may be noted in the lamina propria and epithelium, but abscess formation is not noted.

Immunologically, desquamative gingival biopsy specimens reveal identical features with psoriasis of the skin; that is, antibodies and complement bound in vivo to the stratum corneum antigen.

Treatment of the psoriasiform variant of desquamative gingivitis is similar to the regimen used for the mild localized oral pemphigoid and LP variants of desquamative gingivitis.

CONCLUSIONS

It is now recognized that desquamative gingivitis is a clinical manifestation of several diseases. Most commonly, these include cicatricial pemphigoid, LP, and pemphigus. The diagnosis of the underlying etiology requires evaluation of clinical, histologic, and immunologic criteria. DIF examination of perilesional and/or normal gingival biopsy specimens now assumes prime importance in identification of dermatologic diseases.

REFERENCES

1. Barnett ML, Wittwer JW, Miller RL: Desquamative gingivitis in a 13 year-old male case report. *J Periodontol* 52:170, 1981.
2. Beutner EH, Nisengard RJ, Binder WL: Differentiation of autoantibodies to hidden and accessible antigens in oral mucosa. *J Dent Res* 56 (Special Issue B): B92, 1977.
3. Brayshaw HA, Orban B: Psoriasis gingivae. *J Periodontal* 24:156, 1953.
4. Chaiken BS: A treatment of desquamative gingivitis by the use of free gingival grafts. *Quintessence* 9:105, 1980.

5. DeGregori G, Pippen R, Davies E: Psoriasis of the gingiva and the tongue: Report of a case. *J Periodontol* 42:97, 1971.
6. Engel MD, Ray HG, Orban B: The pathogenesis of desquamative gingivitis: A disturbance of the connective tissue ground substance. *J Dent Res* 29:410, 1950.
7. Glickman I, Smulow JB: Chronic desquamative gingivitis: Its nature and treatment. *J Periodontol* 35:397, 1964.
8. Fine RM, Weathers DR: Desquamative gingivitis: A form of cicatricial pemphigoid? *Br J Dermatol* 102:393, 1980.
9. Forman L, Nally FF: Oral non-dystrophic bullous eruption mainly limited to the gingivae: A mechano bullous response. *Br J Dermatol* 96:111, 1977.
10. Hardy KM, Perry HO, Pingree GC, et al: Benign mucous membrane pemphigoid. *Arch Dermatol* 104:467, 1971.
11. Jones LE, Dolby AE: Desquamative gingivitis associated with psoriasis. *J Periodontol* 43:35, 1972.
12. Laskaris G, Demetriou N, Angelopoulos A: Immunofluorescent studies in desquamative gingivitis. *J Oral Pathol* 10:398, 1981.
13. McCarthy FP, McCarthy PL, Shklar G: Chronic desquamative gingivtis: A reconsideration. *Oral Surg* 13:1300, 1960.
14. Nisengard RJ, Neiders M: Desquamative lesions of the gingiva. *J Periodontol* 52:500, 1981.
15. Nisengard RJ, Alpert AM, Krestow V: Desquamative gingivitis: Immunologic findings. *J Periodontol* 49:27, 1978.
16. Person JR, Rogers RS III, Jordon RE: Cicatricial pemphigoid with circulating antibasement membrane antibodies. *Dermatologica* 154:90, 1977.
17. Pesanti S, Sharau Y, Kaufman E, et al: Pemphigus vulgaris: Incidence in Jews of different ethnic groups according to age, sex and initial lesion. *Oral Surg* 38:382, 1974.
18. Prinz H: Chronic diffuse desquamative gingivitis. *Dent Cosmos* 74:331, 1932.
19. Rogers RS III, Sheridan PJ, Jordon RE: Desquamative gingivitis. *Oral Surg* 42:316, 1976.
20. Rogers RS III, Sheridan PJ, Nightingale SH: Desquamative gingivitis: Clinical, histopathologic, immunopathologic and therapeutic observations. *J Am Acad Dermatol* 7:729, 1982.
21. Ryan JG: Pemphigus. *Arch Dermatol* 104:14, 1971.
22. Shklar G: Desquamative gingivitis and oral mucous membrane diseases. In Carranza F Jr (Ed): *Glickman's Clinical Periodontology*. Saunders, Philadelphia, 1984, p 164.
23. Zeskin DE, Zegarelli EF: Chronic desquamative gingivitis—a report of twelve cases. *Am J Orthod Oral Surg* 31:1, 1945.

19
Herpes Gestationis

N. Fred Eaglstein

Grant J. Anhalt

Harish P. Patel

Luis A. Diaz

INTRODUCTION

Herpes gestationis (HG) is a rare autoimmune disease that arises during pregnancy or the puerperium. The incidence of HG has been estimated to be from 1 in 10,000 deliveries (27) to 1 in 50,000 deliveries (36). The clinical hallmarks of HG are intense pruritus and a blistering skin eruption. The histopathology is characterized by a subepidermal split; and ultrastructurally, the blister forms as a result of disintegration of basal cells and the accumulation of fluid between basal cells and basal lamina (29). The immunopathologic features have been well characterized, and even though these features are similar to bullous pemphigoid (BP), subtle differences exist. The etiology of HG is unknown, but recent studies based on human leukocyte antigen (HLA) typing suggest that genetic factors may be involved (16,35). Although the linkage between pregnancy and the clinical manifestation of HG are not understood, recent evidence suggests that hormonally induced immune alterations may be important (6,16,26).

CLINICAL MANIFESTATIONS

Clinically, HG is characterized by intense pruritus, usually accompanied (but sometimes preceding) a polymorphous skin eruption. The lesions in HG usually begin as erythematous and edematous papules and plaques, followed by the formation of tense vesicles and bullae that break down to form erosions and crusts (Fig. 1). In rare instances, vesicles and bullae do not form, and these cases only show urticarial lesions (14,36). The erruption frequently begins around the umbilicus and spreads to involve the trunk and proximal extremeties. Additionally, the distal extremities, palms, soles, and occasionally the mucous membranes are affected (36).

This investigation was supported by U.S. Public Health Service Grants (R01-AM 32081, R01-AM 32599, R23-AM 32079, R23-AM 32490, and T32-AM 07324) from the National Institutes of Health and by a gift from the Estee Lauder Corporation.

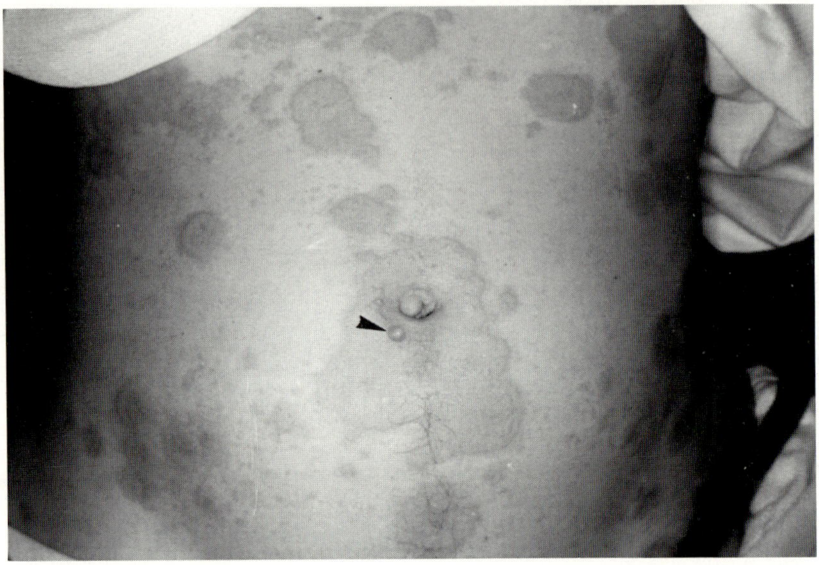

Figure 1. Herpes gestationis. Urticarial papules and plagues on the abdomen of a patient in the sixth month of pregnancy. Note the large periumbilical plague with central blister (arrow).

During the spread of the disease, new lesions may form adjacent to older lesions in a polycyclic pattern. As in BP, outbreaks may last from several days to weeks before a temporary remission ensues, often followed by another outbreak. Frequently, the disease flares within 12 to 48 hours of delivery (4,16,36).

Although HG commonly arises in the fifth or sixth months of pregnancy, cases may occur at any time from the first trimester to the postpartum period (4,13,14,18,36). The majority of patients recover within 3 months after delivery, although some cases persist for as long as 17 months postpartum (16). With the exception of a few cases (11,36), HG always recurs in subsequent pregnancies. The disease may recur in a mild form with each menses following delivery for several months to 1 year, and some patients experience recurrences when using oral contraceptives (11,14,16,18,30).

Infant morbidity and mortality have been studied by various investigators (5,23,28,36). Occasionally, infants born of affected mothers develop mild, transient urticarial or blistering lesions, which invariably resolve without therapy (5,23,36). In the series of Shornich et al. this occurred in two infants delivered to mothers with active HG. While there is general agreement in the literature regarding infant disease, the question of pregnancy-associated complications has been the subject of conflicting reports. In the series of Lawley et al. (28) (40 HG patients), there were nine premature deliveries (23%), three stillbirths (7.5%), and one spontaneous abortion (2.5%). Their data showed a rate of premature deliveries and stillbirths that was greater than the 5 to 10% premature birth rate and 1.3% stillbirth rate for the general population, but the rate of spontaneous abortion (2.5%) was not increased over the 10 to 15% rate found in the general population. On the other hand, in the series of Shornick etal. (36) (42 HG-associated pregnancies), there was one (2.5%) spontaneous abortion, three (7.5%) premature deliveries, and one (2.5%) stillbirth, none of which were increased over the expected rates in the general population.

IMMUNOPATHOLOGIC FEATURES

The perilesional and normal skin of patients with HG consistently demonstrate deposition of C_3 in a linear pattern along the basement membrane zone (BMZ) (Fig. 3) (13,14,16,18,19,22,24,31,36). In addition, direct immunofluorescence (DIF) shows linear BMZ deposition of IgG in 30 to 50% of cases (4,13,16,28,36). The number of patients with BMZ IgG may become more prevalent as more sensitive methods are used, such as a multistep horseradish peroxidase antihorseradish peroxidase technique. This may demonstrate BMZ IgG in cases where conventional DIF is negative (13,17). Other BMZ reactants possibly found by DIF are properdin, Clq, C_4, C_5, fibrin, and factor B (Table 1). Direct IF findings may persist from 6 months to 4 years following clinical remission of the disease (16). Similar DIF findings are also seen in the skin of neonates of affected mothers, regardless of whether or not the infant has HG lesions (5,23,24,32). Immunoelectron microscopy (IEM) reveals C3 deposition within the lamina lucida in a uniformly granular pattern (39). When present, IgG is also located in the lamina lucida, but tends to concentrate near the dermal side of the basal cell plasma membrane and hemidesmosomes (13,18).

In most cases, indirect immunofluorescence (IIF) fails to identify anti-BMZ antibodies in the serum of HG patients (4,16,22,24,31,36). Similarly, IIF is usually negative when umbilical cord sera from infants of affected mothers are tested (4,5,24). However, in 1973, Provost et al. (31) found that serum from HG patients contained a substance that could fix C_3 to the BMZ of normal human skin. He identified this substance by using the in vitro C_3 immunofluorescence (IF) technique described by Jordon et al (21). In this technique, normal human epidermis is incubated with heat-inactivated patient serum. Next, a source of complement is added (usually normal human or guinea pig serum). Following a period of incubation, fluorescein isothiocyanate (FITC) labeled anti-C_3 antisera is added. The resultant IF staining identifies C_3, which is fixed to the BMZ by the substance from the patient's sera. Other studies (4,24) showed that this complement-fixing substance was also present in cord serum from infants of affected HG patients. Provost termed this C_3-fixing substance from the serum of affected patients the "HG factor" (31).

After the initial report of the "HG factor" by Provost et al., other investigators focused their efforts on its identification (3,22,24). Jordon et al. (22) purified the IgG fraction of HG sera by ion exchange chromatography, and showed that the "HG factor" was retained within the purified IgG fraction. In another study, Katz et al. (15) determined that the C_3-fixing properties of HG sera could be abolished by preincubation of the serum with antihuman IgG. Furthermore, these studies demonstrated that the "HG factor" was sedimented on sucrose density gradients in the 7s region and chromatographed on gel filtration with IgG fractions. These experiments demonstrated that the "HG factor" had the sedimentation properties and molecular weight of IgG. Taken together, this data convincingly showed that the HG factor is a complement-fixing IgG directed against the BMZ. We assume that the reason routine IIF does not identify this anti-BMZ is because the concentration of circulating antibody is below the level of sensitivity of this technique.

HISTOLOGY AND ULTRASTRUCTURE

Light and electron microscopic changes appear after complement and IgG binding occurs in the BMZ. Light microscopic examination of hematoxylin- and eosin-stained

Table 1. Summary of DIF Studies in Herpes Gestationis (1973–1983)

References	*No. of cases*	*IgG*	C_3	*Properdin*	*Clq*	C_4	C_5	*Fibrin*	*Factor B*
Carruthers and Bleehan (4)	4	2	4	NT	NT	NT	NT	NT	NT
Harrington et al. (13)	11	5	7	NT	NT	0	NT	0	NT
Holmes et al. (16)	23	6	23	NR	NR	NR	NR	NR	NR
Jordon et al. (22)	9	1	9	9	4	NT	NT	NT	0
Katz et al. (24)	5	4	5	3	2	2	3	NT	3
Lawley et al. (28)	. 41	19	41	11	4	10	9	NR	NR
Provost and Tomasi (31)	2	0	2	1[a]	0[a]	NT	1[a]	NT	NT
Shornick et al. (36)	28	9	28	2[b]	1[b]	4[b]	NR	NR	NR

[a]One patient tested.
[b]No. of patients tested not reported.
NT, Not tested; NR Not reported.

sections exhibit a variety of histologic patterns, which reflect the polymorphous nature of this disease (Fig. 2). Urticarial lesions show a superficial and deep perivascular infiltrate composed of mononuclear cells, eosinophils, and occasionally neutrophils (14). Consistently, dermal papillary edema is found and may be intense (14) or mild (36). A characteristic feature found in the epidermis is focal necrosis of the basal cells, which is especially prominent at the dermal papillary tips (14). Keratinocyte necrosis and focal areas of spongiosis may also appear in the mid and lower levels of the epidermis. These generative epidermal changes are usually accompanied by exocytosis of eosinophils (29,36). Bullous lesions display intense degeneration of basal cells, with a resultant vesiculation at the dermal-epidermal junction (14,29). Scattered mononuclear cells and eosinophils commonly appear in the blister cavity.

Electron-microscopic (EM) studies of HG lesions have been thoroughly examined by various authors (13,29,40). In summary, these authors found that in normal skin and early erythematous lesions from HG patients, there were certain degenerative changes of intracytoplasmic organelles of the basal keratinocytes. This finding suggests that the earliest change in HG is within the basal cell. Urticarial lesions show further dissolution of basal cells, as well as focal destruction of the dermal side of the basal cell plasma membrane. As a result of these focal breaks on the dermal side of the basal cell plasma membrane, degenerated organelles from these cells can be seen within the slightly edematous-lamina lucida. Eventually, more advanced lesions exhibit complete liquefactive degeneration of the basal cells, accompanied by focal disruption of the basal lamina. Consequently, debris from degenerated basal cells now appears in the upper dermis. These latter changes are accompanied by inflammatory cell infiltration. These findings suggest that the earliest pathologic event in HG is basal cell degeneration, which subsequently results in subepidermal blister formation, followed by inflammatory cellular infiltration of the upper dermis.

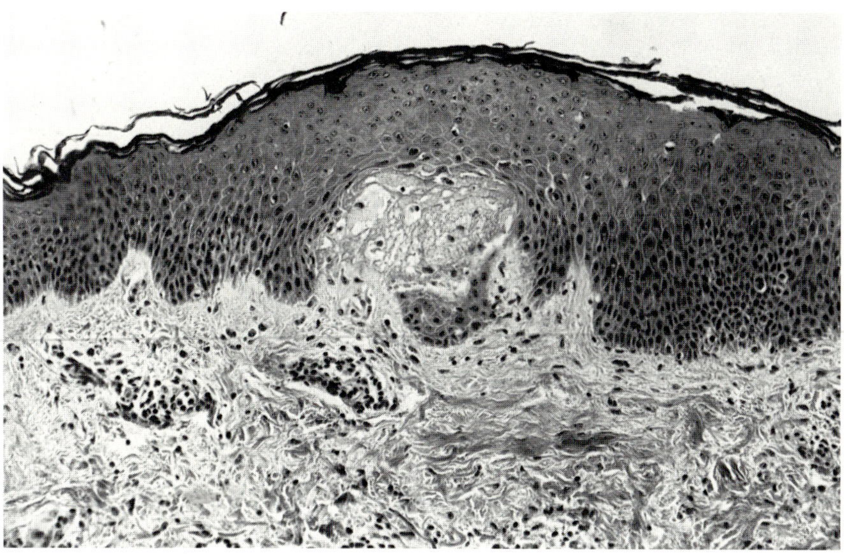

Figure 2. Biopsy specimen of an HG lesion showing early subepidermal vesicle formation. Note the basal cell layer degeneration occurring at the tip of a dermal papilla (H&E, original magnification, 100x).

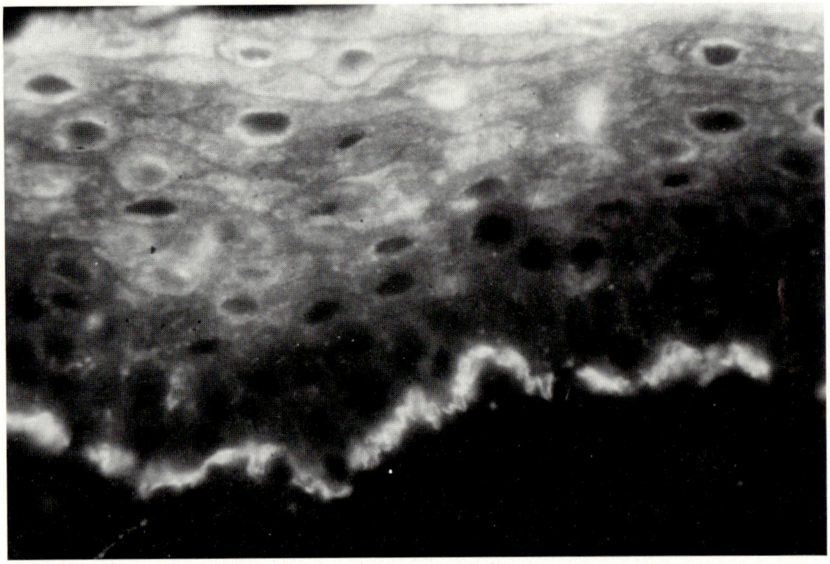

Figure 3. Direct IF of perilesional skin in a patient with HG. This shows the typical linear deposition of C3 in the BMZ (original magnification, 400x).

PATHOGENESIS

The role of circulating anti-BMZ antibodies and BMZ complement deposition in the pathogenesis of the disease is uncertain. Certainly, one may speculate that the "HG factor" is the result of humoral sensitization to foreign fetal antigens. The newly found antibodies subsequently cross-react with antigens of the BMZ. Ultimately, the binding of this antibody to BMZ antigens leads to complement activation generating an inflammatory response, and finally to clinical disease. However, this is merely supposition, as there is no direct proof that supports a pathogenic role of the "HG factor."

The mechanism by which complement activation occurs in HG has been studied in detail. Provost et al. (20) suggested that complement activation occurred via the alternate pathway because DIF often identified deposition of properdin and factor B in association with C_3. However, the frequent deposition of Clq and C_4 by the in vitro IF technique tends to favor complement activation by the classic pathway. The argument in favor of the classic complement pathway was reinforced by additional studies (3,22). These studies showed that if C_2-deficient human or guinea pig serum was used in place of normal human or guinea pig serum as a source of complement in the in vitro C_3 IF test, then HG serum failed to deposit C_3 along with BMZ. This finding demonstrated that early classic pathway components were required for complement fixation. The presence of alternate pathway components, properdin, and factor B along with C_3 is probably due to activation of the alternative pathway via the C_3b-positive feedback loop in which properdin binds to C_3b, stabilizing the C_3b-dependent C_3 convertase (10,33).

The recent study by Grimwood et al. (12) suggests another possible role for complement in the pathogenesis of HG. They found that the serum from a patient with HG contained a substance that had properties similar to the C_3 nephritic factor. This C_3 nephritic factor is an autoantibody of the IgG class directed against C_3b-dependent C_3

convertse and, like properdin, has a stabilizing effect. This factor may therefore play a role in the pathogenesis of HG by amplifying activation of the complement system. However, whether this is an isolated epiphenomenon or a prevalent feature of HG is unknown.

ETIOLOGY

The characteristic immunopathologic finding in HG supports the view that HG is an autoimmune disease. One feature suggesting that HG is an autoimmune disease is the tendency for it to occur in association with other autoimmune diseases, such as Graves disease, vitiligo, and alopecia areata (15,16). This increased tendency for more than one such disease to occur in the same patient is characteristic of a variety of autoimmune diseases, including BP (2,20) and pemphigus vulgaris (PV) (7). Another autoimmune-related feature in HG is the significantly increased incidence of HLA DR3, and also the combination of DR3 and DR4 (16,35). Increases in DR3 antigens are associated with a variety of autoimmune diseases such as dermatitis herpetiformis (DH), coeliac disease, Sjögren's syndrome, myasthenia gravis, and Graves' disease (37). Although the mechanistic link between these HLA antigens and autoimmunity is unknown, current thinking suggests that the genes encoding for these HLA antigens are in linkage disequilibrium with the immune response (IR) genes that confer a heightened state of immune responsiveness (37). Because of this heightened state of immunity, these patients tend to have an increased autoantibody production. It is therefore possible that the increase in anti-HLA antibodies found in the serum of HG patients, as recently reported by some authors (9,32,34), is a result of their genetically determined hyper-reactivity. Along this same line, the "HG factor" might also result from this increased state of immune responsiveness.

The causative role of pregnancy and the development of clinical manifestations of HG have not been elucidated; however, it is important to recognize that HG occurs only in association with pregnancy, menses, oral contraceptives (16), hydatidiform mole (8,39), or choriocarcinoma (38). All of these conditions have in common alterations of estrogen and progesterone levels. This hormonal disturbance may be taken as strong circumstantial evidence suggesting the link between hormonal alterations and expression of the disease. Recent studies show that estrogen has immunoenhancing properties (26), while progesterone has immunosuppressive properties (6). Based on these findings and the results of their own study of 25 HG patients, Holmes et al. (16) suggest that estrogen may be responsible for exacerbation of the disease, whereas progesterone has a modifying effect.

DIFFERENTIAL DIAGNOSIS

The vesicles and bullae found only in HG distinguish it from other pregnancy-related dermatoses, such as papular dermatitis of pregnancy, prurigo of pregnancy, and pruritic urticarial papules and plaques of pregnancy. However, in a minority of cases, typical blister formation does not occur (36). Therefore, this unusual variation of HG may be difficult to distinguish from urticaria or pruritic urticarial papules and plaques of pregnancy. In this situation, HG can be distinguished by DIF studies that are positive only in HG.

The occurrence of other bullous diseases arising in pregnancy, such as DH, erythema multiforme, or BP, may complicate the diagnosis of HG. Differentiating between DH and erythema multiforme is usually not difficult, especially when utilizing DIF. (25) (Chaps. 8 and 24). In erythema multiforme, DIF of early lesions shows immunoreactants within the walls of dermal vessels (25). Differentiation of HG from BP may be more difficult. BP may show identical cutaneous lesions, similar histology, and similar IF findings. A subtle histologic difference between HG and the inflammatory phase of BP is basal cell necrosis, which is not a characteristic feature of BP. Another difference between HG and BP are the DIF findings. In HG, DIF almost always shows C_3 deposition and less frequently deposition of IgG, properdin, Clq, C_4, and C_2; whereas in BP, DIF shows IgG deposition more frequently, as well as the deposition of C_3 and other complement components. The DIF findings are also different in these two diseases. In HG, IIF usually fails to identify anti-BMZ IgG; whereas in BP, IIF frequently demonstrates circulating anti-BMZ IgG (1).

Some differences in the ultrastructural localization of the immunoreactants have been reported. IEM in HG identifies C_3 in a uniform, granular pattern within the lamina lucida; whereas in BP, C_3 is concentrated near the dermal side of the basal cell plasma membrane and hemidesmosomes. In both HG and BP, IgG deposition is in a similar distribution. IgG is found within the lamina lucida and concentrated near the dermal side of the basal cell plasma membrane and hemidesmosomes. It is important to realize that the differences in the ultrastructural location of C_3 are subtle, and this is not a practical test for differentiating these diseases.

CONCLUSIONS

HG appears to be a disease that involves an aberrant immune response, possibly triggered by foreign antigens of fetal or placental origin. The recent studies that show an increased incidence of HLA antigen DR3 and the combination of DR3 and DR4 support the view that genetic factors are important for the acquisition of this disease. Furthermore, hormonal alterations also seem to be important, as evidenced by the occurrence of active disease during pregnancy, menses, or while taking oral contraceptives.

REFERENCES

1. Beutner EH, Chorzelski TP, Jordon RE: *Autosensitization in Pemphigus and Bullous Pemphigoid.* Charles C Thomas, Springfield, IL, 1970.
2. Callen JP, Anderson TF, Chanda JJ, et al: Bullous pemphigoid and other disorders associated with autoimmune phenomena. *Arch Dermatol* 114:245, 1978.
3. Carruthers JA, Black MM: Further studies in herpes gestationis. *Br J Dermatol* 95 (Supp 14):19, 1976.
4. Carruthers JA, Black MM, Ramnarain N: Immunological studies in herpes gestationis. *Br J Dermatol* 96:35, 1977.
5. Chorzelski TP, Jablonska S, Beutner EH, et al: Herpes gestationis with identical lesions in the newborn. *Arch Dermatol* 112:1129, 1976.
6. Clemens DE, Stiteri PK, Stites DP: Mechanisms of immunosuppression of progesterone on maternal lymphocyte activation during pregnancy. *J Immunol* 122:1978, 1979.
7. Diaz LA, Glamb RW, Silva S Jr: A syndrome of multiple immune autoreactivity. A breakdown in immune regulation. *Arch Dermatol* 116:77, 1980.
8. Dupont C: Herpes gestationis with hydatidiform mole. *Trans St Johns Hosp Dermatol Soc* 60:103, 1974.

9. Eberst E, Tongio MM, Eberst B, et al: Herpes gestationis and anti-HLA immunization *Br J Dermatol* 104:543, 1981.
10. Fearon DT, Austen KF: Properdin binding in C_3b and stabilization of the C_3b-dependent C_3 convertase. *J Exp Med* 142:856, 1975.
11. Gordon B: Herpes gestationis and the "pill." *Br Med J* 1:52, 1967.
12. Grimwood R, Arroyave CM, Weston WL, et al: *Arch Dermatol* 116:1045, 1980.
13. Harrington CI, Bleehen SS: Herpes gestationis: Immunopathological and ultrastructural studies. *Br J Dermatol* 100:389, 1979.
14. Hertz KC, Katz SI, Maize J, et al: Herpes gestationis: A clinicopathologic study. *Arch Dermatol* 112:1543, 1976.
15. Holmes RC, Black MM: Herpes gestationis: A possible association with autoimmune thyrotoxicosis (Graves' disease). *J Am Acad Dermatol* 3:474, 1980.
16. Holmes RC, Black MM, Jurecha W, et al: Clues to the/a etiology and pathogenesis of herpes gestationis. *Br J Dermatol* 109:131, 1983.
17. Holubar K, Konrad K, Singl G: Detection by immunoelectron microscopy of immunoglobulin G deposits in skin of immunofluorescence negative herpes gestationis. *Br J Dermatol* 96:569, 1977.
18. Honigsmann H, Stingl G, Holubar K, et al: Herpes gestationis: Fine structural pattern of immunoglobulin deposits in the skin in vivo. *J Invest Dermatol* 66:389, 1976.
19. Jablonska S, Chorzelski TP, Beutner EH, et al: Immunologic phenomena in herpes gestationis. *Arch Dermatol Forsch* 252:267, 1975.
20. Jordon RE, Muller SA, Hale WL, et al: Bullous pemphigoid associated with systemic lupus erythematosus. *Arch Dermatol* 99:17, 1969.
21. Jordon RE, Sams WM Jr, Beutner EH: Complement immunofluorescent staining in bullous pemphigoid. *J Lab Clin Med* 74:548, 1969.
22. Jordon RE, Heine KG, Tappeiner G, et al: The immunopathology of herpes gestationis. Immunofluorescence studies and characterization of "HG factor." *J Clin Invest* 57:1426, 1976.
23. Katz A, Minta JO, Toole JWP, et al: Immunopathologic study of herpes gestationis in mother and infant. *Arch Dermatol* 113:1069, 1977.
24. Katz SI, Hertz KC, Yaoita H: Herpes gestationis: Immunopathology and characterization of the HG factor. *J Clin Invest* 57:1434, 1976.
25. Kazmierowski JA, Weupper KD: Erythema multiforme: Immune complex vasculitis of the superficial cutaneous microvasculature. *J Invest Dermatol* 71:366, 1978.
26. Kenny JF, Pansburn PC, Trail G: Effect of estradiol on immune competence: In vivo and in vitro studies. *Infect Immunity* 13:448, 1976.
27. Kolodny RG: Herpes gestationis. A new assessment of incidence, diagnosis and fetal prognosis. *Am J Obstet Gynecol* 104:39, 1969.
28. Lawley TJ, Stinzl G, Katz SI, et al: Fetal and maternal risk factors in Herpes gestationis. *Arch Dermatol* 114:552, 1978.
29. Schaumburg-Lever G, Saffold OE, Orfanos CE, et al: Herpes gestationis. *Arch Dermatol* 107:888, 1973.
30. Lynch FW, Albrecht RJ: Hormonal factors in herpes gestationis. *Arch Dermatol* 93:446, 1966.
31. Provost TT, Tomasi TB Jr: Evidence for complement activation via the alternate pathway in skin diseases. 1. Herpes gestationis, systemic lupus erythematosus and bullous pemphigoid. *J Clin Invest* 52:1779, 1973.
32. Renula T, Karvonen J, Tiilikainen A, et al: Herpes gestationis: A high titre of anti-HLA-B8 antibody in mother and pemphigoid-like immunohistological findings in the mother and the child. *Br J Dermatol* 96:563, 1977.
33. Schreiber RD, Medicas RR, Golze O, et al: Porperdin and nephritic factor dependent C_3 convertases: Requirement of native C_3 for enzyme formation and the function of bound Cb as a properdin receptor. *J Exp Med* 142:760, 1976.
34. Shornick JK, Stastny P, Gilliam JN: Anti-HLA antibodies and paternal HLA typing in herpes gestationis. *Clin Res* 30:608A, 1982A.
35. Shornick JK, Stastny P, Gilliam JR: High frequency of histocompatibility antigens HLA-DR3 and DR4 in herpes gestationis. *J Clin Invest* 68:553, 1981.

36. Schornick JK, Bangert JL, Freeman RG, et al: Herpes gestationis: Clinical and histologic features of twenty-eight cases. *J Am Acad Dermatol* 8:214, 1983.
37. Svejgaard A, Morling U, Platz P, et al: HLA and disease associations with special references to mechanisms. *Transpl Proc* 13:193, 1981.
38. Tillman WG: Herpes gestationis with the hydatidiform mole and chorion epithelioma. *Br Med J* 1:1471, 1950.
39. Tindall JG, Rea TH, Shulman I, et al: Herpes gestationis in association with a hydatidiform mole. *Arch Dermatol* 117:510, 1981.
40. Yaoita M, Gullino M, Katz SI: Herpes gestationis. Ultrastructure and ultrastructural localization of in vivo bound complement. *J Invest Dermatol* 66:383, 1976.

Section IIC

MECHANO-BULLOUS DISEASES AND LINEAR IgA BULLOUS DERMATOSIS

20
Epidermolysis Bullosa Acquisita

W. Ray Gammon

B. Dale Wilson

Robert A. Briggaman

INTRODUCTION AND HISTORICAL PERSPECTIVE

Fox (19) recorded the first example of a blistering disease associated with increased skin fragility. Goldscheider (30) recognized its predilection to become hereditary. The term epidermolysis bullosa (EB) encompasses this group of patients. Elliot (16) recognized that some cases are not hereditary. Kablitz (37) first used the term epidermolysis bullosa acquisita (EBA) to distinguish those cases with an adult onset and a negative family history of EB.

By the early 1900s, several patients had been reported with skin lesions resembling EB, but with an adult onset and absence of a family history (16,19,20,37). At this time, the major controversy surrounding the disease was whether it was acquired or represented the late onset of an inherited form of EB (7,32,55). Similarly at this time, a number of cases were reported and characterized histologically by subepidermal blisters (2,4–6,8,17,32,35,36,44,52–56,60,61,64). It became apparent that the clinical and histologic features of EBA could develop in other acquired bullous diseases (17,44,53). This finding led to controversy over whether EBA was a distinctive disorder or both a nonspecific clinical pathologic reaction pattern and a manifestation of a heterogeneous group of diseases (44).

In 1971, Roenigk et al. reviewed previously published cases and reported three new ones. They concluded that EBA was a distinctive disease and proposed diagnostic criteria that included: 1) mild trauma producing bullae over joints of the hands, feet, elbows, and knees, and atrophic scars, milia, and nail dystrophy; 2) adult onset; 3) absence of a family history of EB; and 4) exclusion of all other bullous diseases (51). The clinical features proposed by these authors became the major hallmark of the disease and, until recently, the basis for diagnosis in most patients. In the 1970s, it was shown that EBA had immunologic features indistinguishable from those in the subepidermal bullous diseases, bullous pemphigoid (BP), and benign mucous membrane pem-

Supported in part by grants 5-K04-AM00956-02,, 5-R01-AM30475-02 and 5-R01-AM10546-18 from the National Institutes of Health.

phigoid (BMMP). These included linear deposits of IgG and complement (C) components at the basement membrane zone (BMZ) and circulating IgG anti-BMZ antibodies (3,28,31,38,41,49) (Chap. 8). These were accepted as additional feature of EBA, but prompted renewed controversy over whether EBA was distinct or a nonspecific reaction pattern (46). Several authors reported patients with BP and BMMP who developed clinical features of EBA, and one author claimed EBA and BMMP were the same disease (12,13).

In 1980, the immunoelectron microscopic (IEM) features of EBA were defined and shown to be different from those in BP and BMMP (10,22,23,45,65,66) (Chaps. 15 and 16). The IEM features were added to revised criteria for the diagnosis of EBA in 1981 (50,66). Those criteria included: 1) trauma-induced lesions with scarring and milia; 2) no family history; 3) subepidermal blisters histologically; 4) linear deposits of immunoglobulins at the BMZ by direct immunofluorescence (DIF); and 5) IgG deposits in the upper dermis below the basal lamina-anchoring fibril zone by IEM. Recently, the EBA antigen was also defined and shown to be distinct from BP antigen (65).

On the basis of patients defined by distinctive IEM and immunochemical features, it has recently become apparent that the classic clinical features of EBA may not be present initially, and that EBA may present with or develop clinical features of BP and BMMP (22,23). In view of these findings, suggested amended criteria for the diagnosis of EBA include: 1) a chronic acquired bullous disease, 2) a subepidermal blister, 3) linear deposits of IgG at the BMZ, and 4) IgG deposits in the upper dermis in the sublamina densa zone. Neither the age of onset nor the presence or absence of a family history of EB are pertinent to diagnosis, since the disease is now established as a distinctive immunologic entity. It is now clear that EBA is a pemphigoid-like disease with heterogeneous clinical manifestations, rather than a manifestation of a heterogeneous group of diseases.

INCIDENCE

Although the precise incidence of EBA is unknown, it is generally regarded as rare. Since it was originally described, only about 60 cases have been reported. Most have been single case reports. All but a few cases have been diagnosed on the basis of Roenigk's criteria, and not on the basis of distinctive IEM features. About half the cases have been evaluated by routine immunofluorescent (IF) tests, but less than 20 have been evaluated by IEM (10,13,23,45,66). Based on the relative number of reported cases of EBA, BP, and BMMP, it would appear that EBA is much less common than the other two diseases. However, recent evidence implying that some patients diagnosed as BP or BMMP probably had EBA suggests that the relative incidence is greater than the literature would indicate. In our own experience with bullous diseases in the past 8 years, we have seen approximately 70 cases of BP, 8 cases of EBA, and only 2 cases of BMMP, suggesting EBA may be more common than BMMP. Approximately 10% of patients with circulating IgG anti-BMZ antibodies diagnosed at our institution and one other medical center as BP (on the basis of routine clinical, histologic, and immunohistologic features) were found to have EBA (23). This would suggest that EBA may be approximately 1/10th to 1/20th as prevalent as BP.

CLINICAL FEATURES

The classic clinical features originally described in EBA mimic those in dominant dystrophic EB; they include extreme skin fragility, trauma-induced blisters and erosions, healing with scars and milia, absence of cutaneous inflammation (erythema, edema), a localization of lesions to extensor skin surfaces, dystrophic nails, mucous membrane lesions, and scarring alopecia (Fig. 1) (51). Extreme skin fragility, trauma-induced blisters and erosions, and healing with scars and milia are considered hallmarks of the disease, but numerous patients presenting without these features have been reported (5,8,14,18,20,22,47–49,55,64). Although most patients have had lesions localized to extensor skin surfaces, about one-third have had a more generalized process. Localization of blisters, erosions, scars, and milia over the dorsal hands resembling the distribution of lesions in porphyria cutanea tarda has been regarded as a characteristic feature, but has been reported in less than half the cases. Nail dystrophy, originally considered a characteristic feature, has been reported in less than half the patients. About 50% of cases have had erosions and scars affecting oral mucous membranes, and some have had lesions of laryngeal and esophageal mucosa (49). Esophageal stenosis may occur (14). Although scarring alopecia was initially listed as a distinctive feature of the disease, it has been relatively uncommon.

Recently, it has become aparent that patients may initially present with clinical features that closely resemble those in BP (22,23). These include a generalized bullous eruption, large tense bullae, involvement of flexural and intertriginous skin, spontaneous blisters, macular and plaque-like erythemas, blisters arising on erythematous skin, and healing of lesions without scars or milia (Fig. 2). Most of those patients have gone on to develop classic clinical features of EBA, but it is not yet clear that all do. Several patients

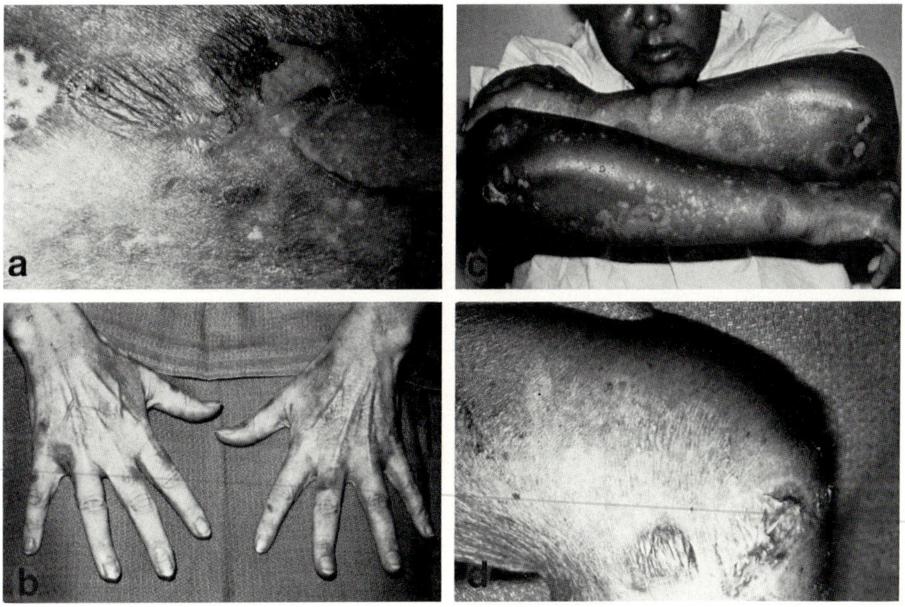

Figure 1. *Examples of classic clinical features in EBA.* A. A focal area of skin fragility showing healing with scar formation. B. Involvement of dorsal hands showing healing with scars and milia. These changes are indistinguishable from those seen in porphyria cutanea tarda. C. Involvement of extensor surfaces of the upper extremities. D. Skin fragility, scarring, and milia over the knee.

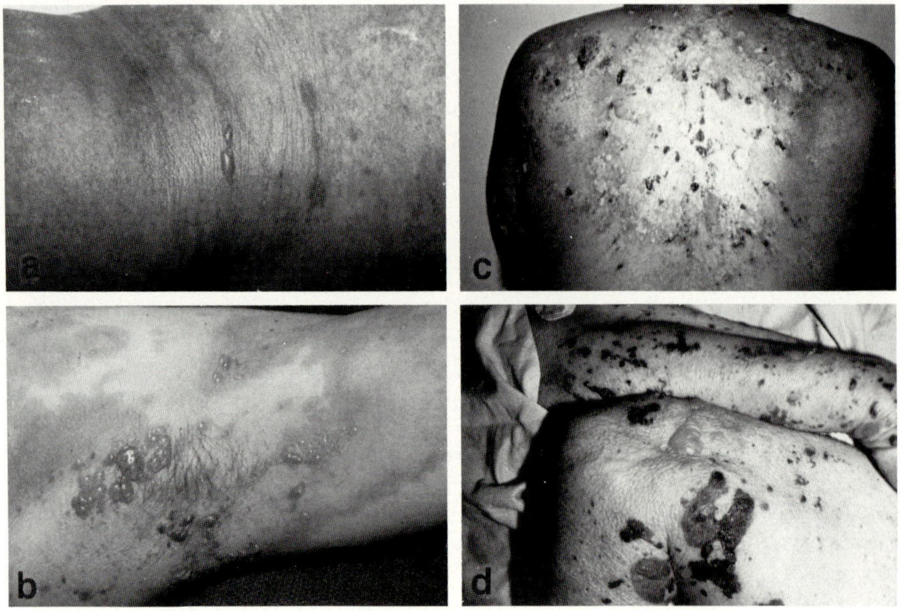

Figure 2. *Examples of EBA with classic features resembling those seen in BP.* A. Popliteal fossa showing macular erythematous lesions and small bullae. B. Axillae showing macular erythema, erythematous plaques, and vesicles arising on erythematous skin. C. Extensive erosions and bullae involving the back. D. Hemorrhagic and serous bullae over the upper and lower extremities.

have also been reported with clinical features that were considered distinctive for BMMP, including conjunctival inflammation and scarring and a localization of blisters and scars over the head and neck (12,22,23,49). Other patients have been reported who were initially thought to have clinical features of pemphigus, dermatitis herpetiformis (DH), erythema multiforme, toxic drug eruptions, and contact dermatitis (5,8,14,18,20,22,47–49,55,64). These reports suggest that the clinical features of EBA are highly variable, at least early in the disease.

Most patients with EBA have been over 50 years of age. Among 30 reported cases in which the age of onset was noted, the mean was 51 years with a range of 19 to 81 years (1,3,5,8–10,14,17,28,31,38–42,47,49,51,59,62,63,66). The sex incidence has been about equally divided, and members of all racial groups have been affected. In many cases, associated systemic diseases have been reported and have included Crohn's disease, systemic lupus erythematosus (SLE), hyperthyroidism, and others (40,50,51). The significance of most of these associations is not yet clear; however inflammatory bowel disease has been reported often (9,15,40,43,51). An additional characteristic clinical feature is the relative resistance to treatment with glucocorticosteroid, immunosuppressive, and cytotoxic agents, and with sulfones (14,31,41,45,51,66). Some patients have responded to prednisone or combination chemotherapy with prednisone and a cytotoxic agent (22,23,40,49). There are also cases of BP that present clinically with a relative resistance to treatment with a glucocorticosteroid alone or in combination with an immunosuppressive and sulfones (29).

HISTOPATHOLOGY

The histology of EBA is characterized by a subepidermal blister. The epidermis has been described as mildly acanthotic or atrophic, but is usually normal in appearance (28). Basal cell necrosis has been described in spontaneous lesions; but in experimentally induced (tape-stripped) lesions and many spontaneous lesions, this feature has not been present (51). Occasionally, intraepidermal and intradermal milia may be seen (51,63). In experimentally induced lesions, the dermis often appears relatively normal (66). In lesions arising on scarred skin, there is homogenization of upper dermal collagen, and usually either a sparse infiltrate of mononuclear cells around dermal papillary vessels or an absence of inflammation (51). Similar changes may be seen in lesions arising on nonerythematous and unscarred skin. In lesions arising on erythematous skin, dermal inflammation is often prominent and consists of a mixed infiltrate of mononuclear cells, neutrophils, and eosinophils (22,23). Neutrophils may be the predominant infiltrating cell (Fig. 3). Using special stains, the PAS-positive basement membrane has been reported as either split and adherent to the blister roof and floor or adherent just to the blister roof (40,41,51,63).

ELECTRON MICROSCOPY

Ultrastructural studies of spontaneous and tape-stripped lesions have shown that blisters typically form in the upper dermis, either just below the lamina densa or below the

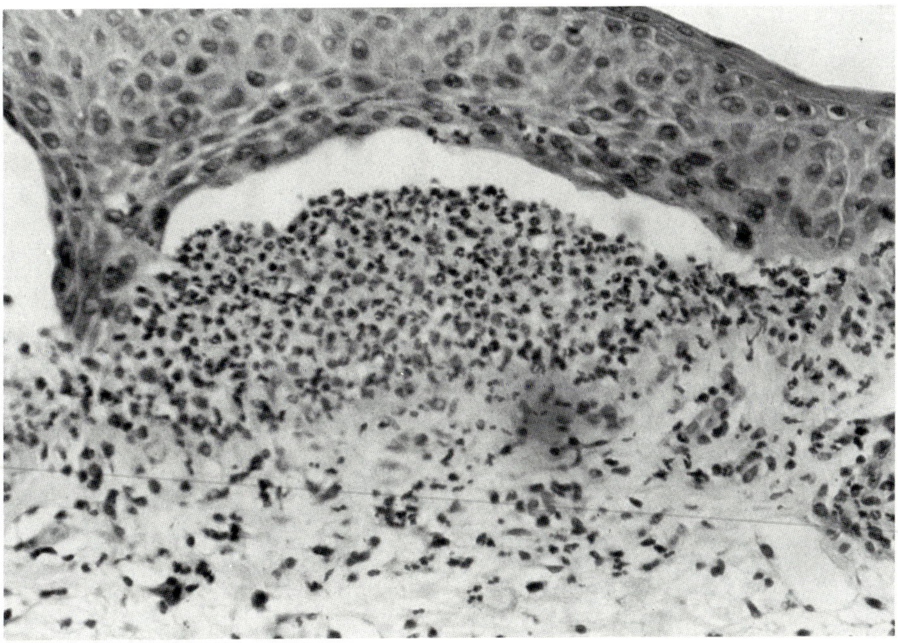

Figure 3. Routine histology of peribullous EBA skin showing subepidermal microvesicle and numerous polymorphonuclear granulocytes in the upper dermis and vesicle cavity (H&E stains, 450x).

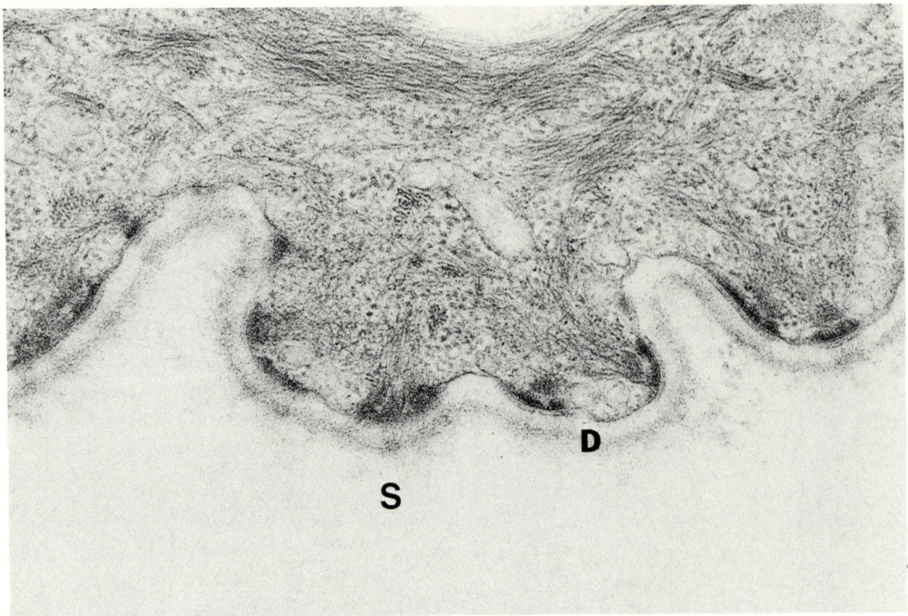

Figure 4. Electron microscopy of tape-stripped EBA skin showing separation (S) below the lamina densa (D) (75,000x).

lamina densa-anchoring fibril complex (28,45,66) (Fig. 4). Separation of the epidermis from the dermis through the lamina lucida has rarely been reported (12). The basal lamina is usually well preserved and usually attached to a relatively normal epidermis (66). Anchoring fibrils are usually reduced or absent in both spontaneous and experimentally induced lesions (66). In fully developed blisters, microfibrillar bundles, collagen, and elastic fibers are often reduced in number and difficult to identify (66). Amorphous deposits (probably representing immune deposits) in the sublamina densa zone are characteristic features, but have not been an invariable finding (63).

IMMUNOHISTOLOGY AND IMMUNOELECTRON MICROSCOPY

Direct IF of lesional and/or normal-appearing skin has been performed in about half the patients presenting with classic clinical features of EBA, and in a few of those presenting with clinical features of BP or BMMP (22,23,38,40,41,45,49,66) (Chaps. 8 and 15 to 17). Linear deposits of IgG at the BMZ have been detected in all cases (Fig. 5). C3 deposits have been reported in most cases, and factor B, factor P, C_{1q}, C5, and C4 have occasionally been observed (45). Linear deposits of IgA and IgM (usually of lesser staining intensity than IgG) have been present in a substantial number of patients, and they seem to occur more commonly than in BP (63). Although the IgG deposits observed by DIF are often more intensely stained and possibly wider than those in BP and BMMP, it is not possible to reliably differentiate them by using routine DIF. BP antigens have been demonstrated as having regional variations (29). Similarly, EBA

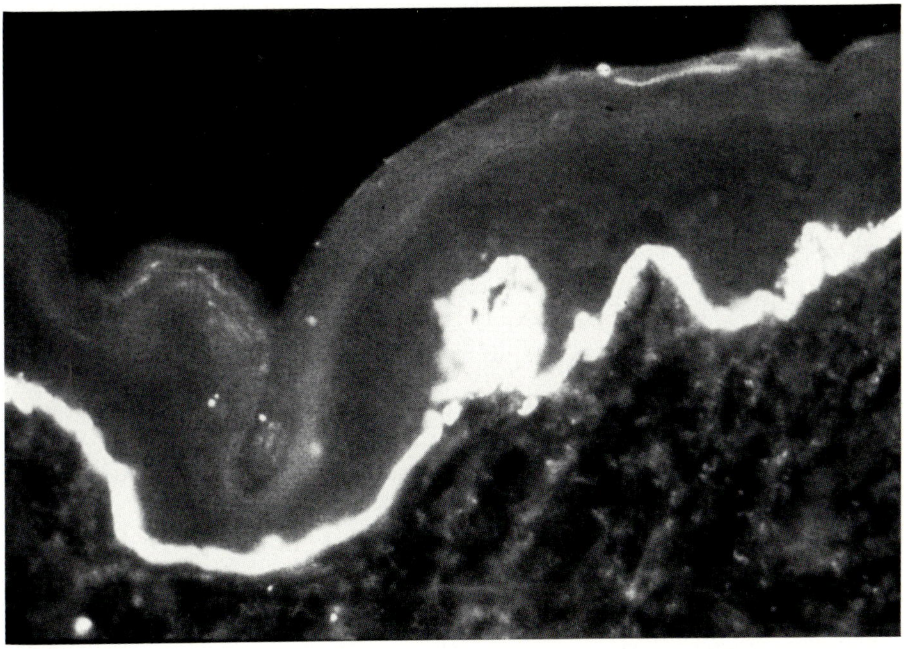

Figure 5. Direct IF of perilesional EBA skin showing linear deposits of IgG at the BMZ (450x).

antigens may also have a variable distribution. At present, a negative DIF test on a single specimen may not be conclusive to exclude the diagnosis of EBA.

Although the distribution of IgG deposits in EBA has not been well studied, it appears to be generalized. However, until this is more objectively established, it seems prudent to obtain biopsy specimens of uninvolved perilesional skin. One difficulty that may be encountered with punch biopsy procedures is loss of epidermis due to skin fragility. This can usually be avoided if special care and sharp punches are used. However, we have sometimes found it necessary to perform incisional procedures to overcome this problem.

EBA can also be differentiated from BP by studying the level of the split on the lesional skin biopsy specimen by indirect immunofluorescence (IIF) using fluoresceinated antilaminin and type IV collagen antibodies (see Chap. 21). Antilaminin and type IV collagen localize to the floor of the blister in specimens from BP patients compared to EBA, in which both of these antigens appear in the roof of the vesicle (32a).

Indirect IF tests in EBA have shown that circulating IgG anti-BMZ antibodies are present in about 25% of cases with classic clinical features. This incidence is greater than in BMMP (less than 10%), and is about one-third the incidence in BP (70 to 75%). In general, titers of anti-BMZ antibodies have been lower than in BP, and have ranged from 1:20 to 1:640. In a few cases, circulating EBA antibodies have been shown to bind C (C3) to the BMZ by the indirect complement-binding IF method (63). The pathway of C activation by these antibodies has not been well studied, but preliminary experiments from our laboratory suggest that both classic and alternate pathways are involved.

In a recent study of five patients with a BP-like presentation of EBA, we found incidences of IgG anti-BMZ antibodies of 80% and C3 binding anti-BMZ antibodies of 60% (23). This suggests that a high incidence of anti-BMZ antibodies in EBA patients with clinical features resembling BP may be similar to that reported in BP. It also suggests that the low incidence and relatively low titers reported in patients with classic features may be due to the fact that these cases have been studied late in their disease. Currently, there is no evidence for an association of titers of anti-BMZ antibodies with the disease activity in EBA.

Direct IEM has shown that IgG deposits in EBA are usually located in the upper dermis just below the lamina densa-anchoring fibril complex (Fig. 6) (45,66). In these cases, the anchoring fibril zone has been free of deposits. In some cases with a BP-like clinical appearance, the deposits appear to overlie the anchoring fibril zone and the lamina densa (Fig. 7) (23). In no case have deposits been restricted to the lamina densa. The reasons for this slight variation in location of deposits is not known; however, two lines of evidence suggest they are, in fact, variants and do not represent two different antigenic specificities. First, we have seen one patient with deposits in the sublamina densa-anchoring fibril zone by direct IEM. By indirect IEM on normal human skin, the antibodies in this patient produced deposits overlying the anchoring fibril zone and the lamina densa. Second, anti-BMZ antibodies from patients with deposits beneath the lamina densa-anchoring fibril zone appear to recognize the same antigen as those from patients with deposits overlying the anchoring fibril zone and lamina densa (Fig. 8).

IEM is particularly important in the diagnosis of EBA, since it is apparent that the histologic, immunohistologic, and even clinical features may be indistinguishable from those in BP and BMMP (23). Since the deposits in BP and BMMP are in the lamina lucida, IEM can reliably distinguish them from EBA (33,34). Since IEM is not a

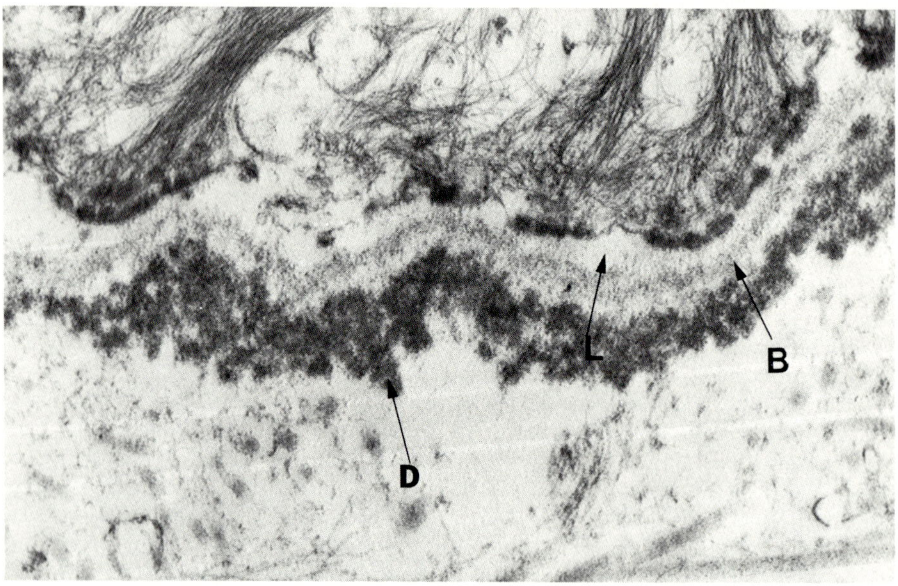

Figure 6. Direct IEM of EBA skin showing IgG deposits (D) beneath the lamina densa (B). No deposits are seen in the lamina lucida (L) (42,000x). (Reproduced with the permission of CV Mosby.)

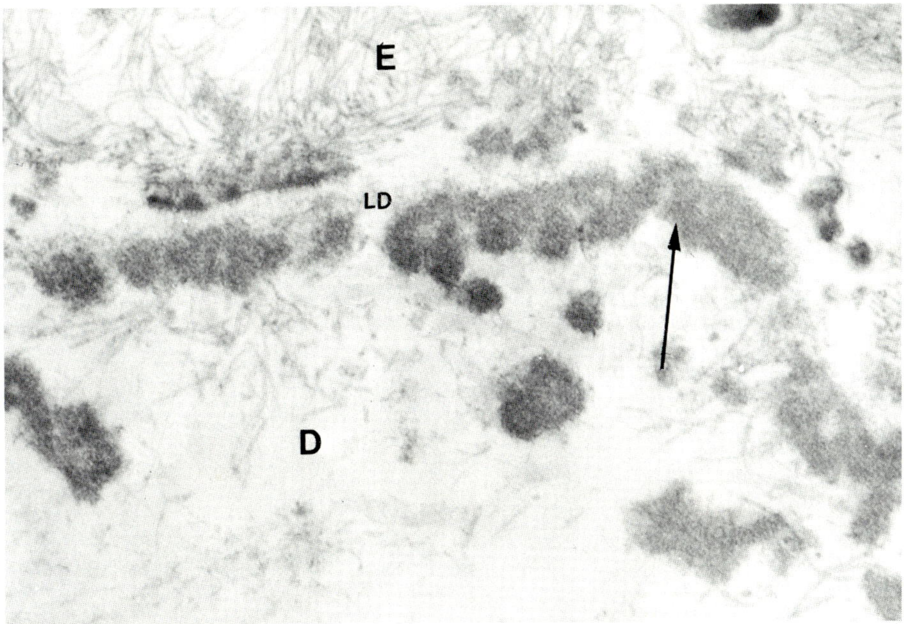

Figure 7. Direct IEM of EBA skin showing IgG deposits (arrow) in the upper dermis (D) and contiguous with the dermal aspect of the lamina densa (LD) (90,000x).

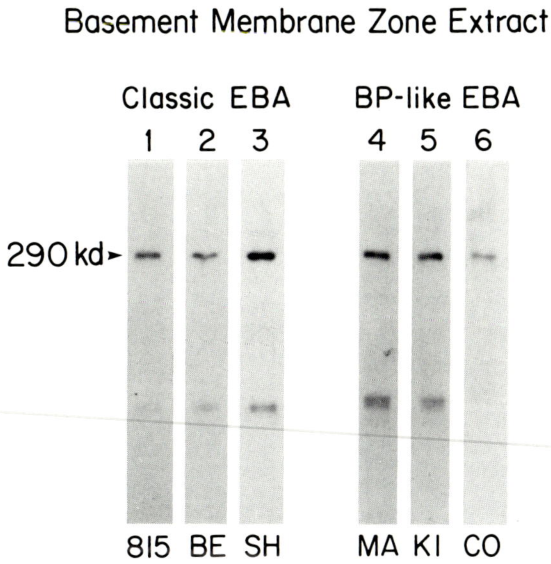

Figure 8. Immunoblots of dermal extract with six EBA sera showing IgG binding to 290 and 145 (lower band) kd proteins. Sera 1 to 3 were from patients with classic clinical features of EBA. Sera 4 to 6 were from patients with a BP-like clinical presentation. (Reproduced with permission of Dr. D.T. Woodley.)

procedure generally available for diagnosis, alternative methods for differentiating between lamina lucida and sublamina densa immune deposits have been sought. Recently, a double IF procedure for differentiating between lamina lucida and sublamina densa deposits in patients' skin was reported (27). The procedure is outlined in Table 1. In patients with circulating IgG anti-BMZ antibodies, the diagnosis can be made by standard IIF procedures using as substrate normal human skin separated through the lamina lucida by incubation in 1.0 M NaCl (Table 2) (21). Using this substrate, antilamina lucida antibodies bind to either the epidermal or both the epidermal and dermal sides of the separation, and antisublamina densa (EBA) antibodies bind only to the dermal side (Fig. 9). Using this substrate, we have examined over 80 BP and herpes gestationis (HG) sera containing antilamina lucida antibodies and 11 EBA sera containing antisublamina densa antibodies. We have never encountered antilamina lucida antibodies that stain only the dermal side of NaCl-separated skin. (Editors' note: See also Chap. 21 for

Table 1. Double IF Microscopy for Distinguishing Between Linear Lamina Lucida and Sublamina Densa IgG Deposits in Bullous Disease Skin

1. Air dry 6-mm thick cryostat sections of perilesional skin on glass microscope slides.
2. Incubate skin section for 30 min at 25°C with 50 ml of rhodamine isothiocyanide-conjugated antihuman IgG (dilution of conjugate determined by checkerboard titration). Rinse 3 × 5 min in PBS.
3. Incubate skin section for 15 min at 25°C with 50 ml of 50% heat-inactivated (56°C × 30 min) normal human serum diluted in PBS. Rinse 3 × 5 min in PBS.
4. Incubate skin sections for 30 min at 25°C with 50 ml of fluorescein isothiocyanide-conjugated BP IgG containing anti-BMZ antibodies (dilution of conjugate determined by checkerboard titration). Wash 3 × 5 min in PBS.
5. Coverslip tissue and read by fluorescence microscopy using fluorescein filters (Leitz barrier filter LP515, exciter filter BP450-490, and beam splitter PKP510). For more dependable interpretation, prepare control tissue with known lamina lucida and sublaminal densa deposits.
6. Lamina lucida IgG deposits show linear green fluorescence. Sublamina densa IgG deposits show contiguous linear green and yellow-orange fluorescence or yellow-orange fluorescence only.

From Gammon et al. (27).

Table 2. Preparation of 1.0 M NaCl Separated Skin for IIF Substrate

1. Obtain fresh cadaver or surgically excised human skin.
2. Keratome a 1–2 cm wide × 10 cm long strip of split-thickness skin using a Castroviejo keratome set at 0.4 mm.
3. Immerse split-thickness skin in 1 liter of 1.0 M NaCl at 4°C for 72–96 h. Exchange with fresh NaCl every 12 h.
4. Wash skin briefly in 0.01 M PBS, pH 7.2, and place skin dermis down on filter paper. Dislodge epidermis by gentle traction, but leave in place.
5. Cut skin into 4 mm × 15 mm strips with a razor blade and fold to form several thicknesses of split-thickness-separated skin.
6. Freeze separated skin at −70°C, mount in O.C.T. compound and cut 6–8 μm thick cryostat sections.
7. Place sections on gelatin- or ovalbumin-coated microscope slides and let dry. Proceed with standard IIF.

From Gammon et al. (21).

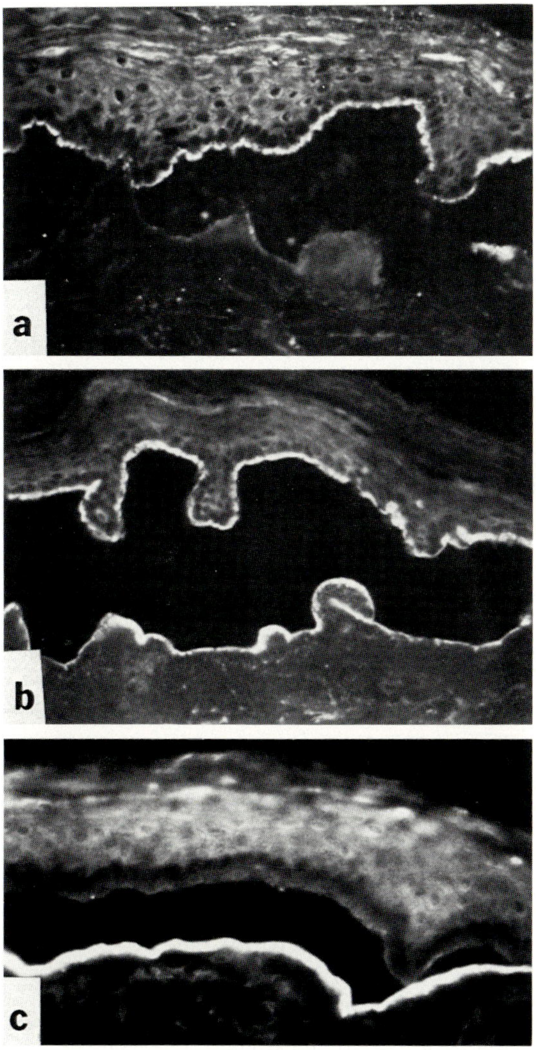

Figure 9. Indirect IgG IF of antilamina lucida (BP, HG) and antisublamina densa (EBA) anti-BMZ antibodies on 1.0 M Nacl-separated skin. A, B. Shown are the epidermal or combined epidermal and dermal staining patterns, respectively, seen with antilamina lucida antibodies. C. Dermal pattern seen with antisublamina densa antibodies.

a group of methods for determining the level of the split in subepidermal bulla and for differentiating EBA from BP.)

EPIDERMOLYSIS BULLOSA ACQUISITA ANTIGEN

Recent studies have reported the detection and partial characterization of EBA antigen in reduced extracts of normal human dermis (65). The antigen was identified by its reactivity with sera and eluates of EBA skin containing IgG anti-BMZ antibodies via polyacrylamide gel electrophoresis and immunoblot procedures. Using these methods, EBA antibodies appeared to react specifically with 290 kd and 145 kd proteins under reduced but not unreduced conditions (Fig. 8). This suggests that the molecule containing these antigens is of very high molecular weight, and that the 290 kd band may be a dimer consisting of 145 kd subunits. These bands were not identified by sera from patients with BP, DH, or pemphigus vulgaris (PV), or from normal individuals. They are distinct from the BMZ protein of 220 kd previously reported as the BP antigen and the 130 kd epidermal protein reported as PV antigen (57,58). EBA antigen appears to be distinct from other known BMZ and dermal components, including laminin, fibronectin, elastin, and types 1, 4, and 5 collagens. A monoclonal antibody to the EBA antigen has been reported. In preliminary experiments, the antigen has been localized to stratified squamous epithelia of several mammalian species. The function of EBA antigen and the cell responsible for its production are not known.

PATHOGENESIS OF EPIDERMOLYSIS BULLOSA ACQUISITA

The pathogenesis of EBA is unknown, but may be particularly complex and involve more than one mechanism. This is suggested by the fact that early in their course, patients may have an inflammatory disease both clinically and histologically (23). Later, they may have relatively little inflammation, but may have a significant defect in dermal-epidermal adherence. Thus, there is evidence suggesting both inflammatory and noninflammatory mechanisms in pathogenesis.

There is, of course, descriptive evidence suggesting that immunologic mechanisms may be involved. This includes the presence of linear deposits of IgG and C components at the BMZ and circulating IgG and complement-binding anti-BMZ antibodies (66). The ultrastructural site of blister formation (beneath the lamina densa) corresponds exactly to the site of immune deposits (66). These observations suggest that EBA antibody-mediated C activation may play a role in inflammatory lesions. In our experience, patients with inflammatory lesions have a high incidence of circulating IgG and C-binding anti-BMZ antibodies. In these cases, there appeared to be a correlation between titers of anti-BMZ antibodies and the presence of inflammatory skin lesions. We have seen several patients who presented with clinically and histologically inflamed lesions and relatively high titers (1:160 to 1:640) of anti-BMZ antibodies. As their disease became less inflammatory, the titers dropped significantly and have often become undetectable (unpublished observation). Another feature of inflammatory lesions that suggests C is involved is the presence of significant numbers of neutrophils in dermal infiltrates. These cells are characteristic of inflammatory reactions in which C-derived chemotactic factors are thought to play a role in leukocyte recruitment (11).

In recent studies, functional evidence has been obtained that EBA immune deposits may be involved in inflammation (Table 3). These studies showed that EBA immune complexes deposited in perilesional skin in vivo, and formed in vitro by treating normal human skin with C-binding EBA antibodies, are potent activators of C and can generate C-derived chemotactic activity capable of recruiting peripheral blood leukocytes to the BMZ (24). These studies were performed on cryostat sections of fresh-frozen skin using previously described leukocyte attachment methods (25,26). When compared to in vivo-deposited BP complexes or BP complexes formed by treating normal human skin with BP antibodies, EBA complexes were significantly more potent in recruiting leukocytes to the BMZ. In the same report, it was shown that leukocytes would migrate to the

Table 3. Pathogenesis of EBA Lesions

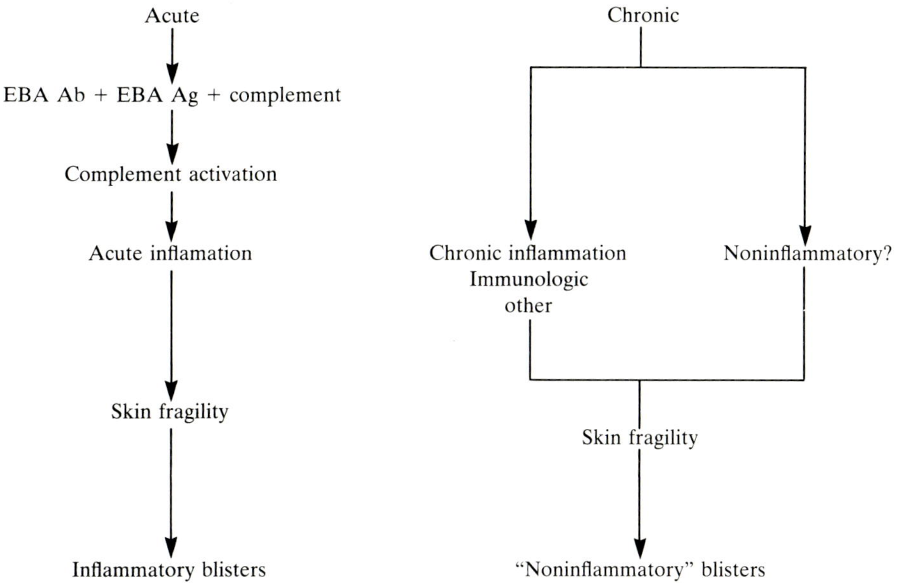

dermal-epidermal junction, and that dermal-epidermal separation would develop in intact viable skin treated with C-binding EBA antibodies, peripheral blood leukocytes, and serum C (24). BP antibodies did not mediate this reaction, even though C-binding titers were greater than those in EBA sera.

Although there is evidence for antibody and C involvement in acutely inflammed lesions, many lesions of EBA lack significant inflamation (Table 3). They are, however, characterized by extreme skin fragility and an apparent defect in dermal-epidermal adherence in the sublamina densa zone. This defect may be due to a decrease in anchoring fibrils, which may be deficient even in the normal-appearing skin of EBA (66). The cause for this decrease in anchoring fibrils is not known, but is probably an acquired phenomenon. It is conceivable that anchoring fibrils and other amorphous matrix molecules responsible for dermal-epidermal adherence are degraded by enzymatic activity. This could be due to a low-grade inflammatory reaction in dermis or to enzymes released from fibroblasts, epidermal cells, or other cells near the BMZ. A role for inflammatory cells in the pathogenesis of this defect cannot be excluded, since mononuclear cells are often present and since it is not possible to ascertain exactly when defective dermal-epidermal adherence develops. The defect in adherence certainly appears to be chronic, and could be due to inflammatory injury affecting strategic dermal adherence molecules that are slowly or poorly repaired.

ACKNOWLEDGMENTS

The authors wish to thank Dr. David T. Woodley for preparing Figure 8 and Mrs. Marlene E. Merzacco, Administrative Assistant for the Department of Dermatology, for preparing this manuscript.

REFERENCES

1. Almeyda J: Epidermolysis bullosa associated with neoplasm of the bronchus. *Br Dermatol* 87:70, 1972.
2. Beer WE, Cooke KB: Epidermolysis bullosa induced by penicillamine. *Br J Dermatol* 79:123, 1967.
3. Benedetto AR, Bergfeld WF, Guirgus M: Epidermolysis bullosa acquisita diagnosed by immunofluorescence and electron-microscopy. *J Invest Dermatol* 70:221, 1978 (abstract).
4. Black H: Acquired epidermolysis bullosa. *Aust J Dermatol* 6:181, 1962.
5. Bloom D: Epidermolysis due to sulfonamides. *NY State J Med* 53:1077, 1963.
6. Bloom RE: Acquired epidermolysis bullosa dystrophica. *Arch Dermatol* 85:130, 1962.
7. Bukovsky J: Ein Beitrag zur Lehre von der sogenannten epidermolysis bullosa hereditaria. *Arch Dermatol Syph* (*Woin Leipz*) 67:163, 1903.
8. Canizares O: Bullous dermatosis associated with hyperglobulinemia, proteinuria and plasmocytosis of bone marrow: Drug sensitivity reaction (?); multiple myeloma (?). *Arch Dermatol* 65:503, 1952.
9. Cheesbrough MJ, Kinmont POC: Epidermolysis bullosa acquisita and Crohn's disease. *Br J Dermatol* 99(Suppl 6):53, 1978.
10. Chorzelski T, Petrow L, Dabrowski J, et al: Epidermolysis bullosa acquisita (EBZ). *Hautartz* 32:487, 1981.
11. Cochran CG, Dixon FJ: Immune complex injury. In Samter M, et al. (Eds): *Immunological Disease.* Little, Brown, Boston, 1978, p 210.
12. Dahl MGC: Epidermolysis bullosa acquisita—a sign of cicatricial pemphigoid. *Br J Dermatol* 101:475, 1979.
13. Dahl MGC: Epidermolysis bullosa acquisita versus pemphigoid. *Acta Dermatol Vener* (*Stockholm*) 59:187. 1979.
14. Dotson AD, Raimer SS, Pursley W, et al: Systemic lupus erythematosus occurring in a patient with epidermolysis bullosa acquisita. *Arch Dermatol* 117:422, 1981.
15. Dupont A, Bourland A, Ponce R: Epidermolyse bullouse d'apparition tardive et de Crohn. *Bull Soc Fr Dermatol Syphilligr* 76:311, 1969.
16. Elliott GT: A contribution to the histopathology of epidermolysis bullosa (hereditaria). *NY State J Med* 71:585, 1900.
17. Epstein JH, Epstein NN, Greenlee M: Epidermolysis bullosa acquisita (tardive) and porphyria cutanea tarda. *Arch Dermatol* 80:713, 1959.
18. Fontaine A: Duhring dermatitis herpetiformis. *Acta Belg Arte Med Pharm Mil* 9:835, 1963.
19. Fox T: Notes on unusual or rare forms of skin disease. *Lancet* I:766, 1879.
20. Fox C: Pemphigus in a woman of nine years duration. *Br J Dermatol* 9:341, 1897.
21. Gammon WR, Briggaman RA, Inman AO III, et al: Differentiating antilamina lucida and anti-sublamina densa anti-BMZ antibodies by indirect immunofluorescence on 1.0M sodium chloride separated skin. *J Invest Dermatol*
22. Gammon WR, Briggaman RA, Wheeler CE: Epidermolysis bullosa acquisita presenting as an inflammatory bullous disease. *J Am Acad Dermatol* 7:382, 1982.
23. Gammon WR, Briggaman RA, Woodley DT, et al: EBA—a pemphigoid-like disease. *J Am Acad Dermatol* 11:820, 1984.
24. Gammon WR, Inman AO III, Wheeler CE Jr: Differences in complement-dependent chemotactic activity generated by bullous pemphigoid and epidermolysis bullosa acquisita immune complexes: Demonstration by leukocytic attachment and organ culture methods. *J Invest Dermatol* 83:57, 1984.
25. Gammon WR, Lewis DM, Carlo JR, et al: Pemphigoid antibody mediated attachment of peripheral blood leukocytes at the dermal-epidermal junction of human skin. *J Invest Dermatol* 75:334, 1980.
26. Gammon WR, Merritt CC, Lewis DM, et al: Functional evidence for complement-activating immune complexes in the skin of patients with bullous pemphigoid. *J Invest Dermatol* 78:52, 1982.
27. Gammon WR, Robinson T, Briggaman RA, et al: Double immunofluorescence microscopy:

A method for localizing immune deposits in skin disease associated with linear basement membrane zone immunofluorescence. *J Invest Dermatol* 79:312–317, 1982.

28. Gibbs RB, Minus HR: Epidermolysis bullosa acquisita with electron microscopic studies. *Arch Dermatol* 111:215, 1975.
29. Goldberg DJ, Bystryn JC: Regional variations in the experiment of BP antigen in the human skin. *J Invest Dermatol* 80:365, 1983 (abstract).
30. Goldscheider A: Hereditare Neigung zur Blasenbuildung. *Monatsh Prakt Dermatol* 1:163, 1882.
31. Goodwin P, Eady R: A case of ? epidermolysis bullosa. *Clin Exp Dermatol* 2:409, 1977.
32. Gorsky PP: Contribution a la caraderistique de l'epidermolyse bulleuse. *Ann Derm Syph (Paris)* 9:720, 1928.

32a. Hintner H, Stingl G, Schuler G, et al: Immunofluorescence mapping of antigenic determinants within the dermal-epidermal junction in mechanobullous diseases. *J Invest Dermatol* 76:113, 1981.

33. Holubar K, Wolff K, Konrad K, et al: Ultrastructural localization or immunoglobulin in bullous pemphigoid skin: Employment of a new peroxidase-antiperoxidase multistep method. *J Invest Dermatol* 64:220, 1975.
34. Honigsmann H, Stingl G, Holubar K, et al: Autoantibodies and immune complexes in immunodermatoses. Mapping of fine structural binding sites. *J Invest Dermatol* 66:263, 1976 (abstract).
35. Hundley JL, Smith DC: Epidermolysis bullosa acquisita. *Southern Med J* 34:364, 1941.
36. Johnson ML: Epidermolysis bullosa acquisita with esophageal cysts. *Proc Royal Soc Med* 670:1272, 1967.
37. Kablitz L: Ein Beitrog zur Frage der Epidermolysis Bullosa (Hereditary et Acquisita). *These Inaug Rostock Diss,* 1904.
38. Krivo JM, Miller F: Immunopathology of epidermolysis bullosa acquisita: Association with mixed cryoglobulinemia. *Arch Dermatol* 114:1218, 1978.
39. Kueppers F, Daniels F: Penicillamine-induced skin lesions in a patient with Wilson's disease. *Curtis* 4:35, 1969.
40. Kushniruk W: The immunopathology of epidermolysis bullosa acquisita. *Can Med J* 108:1143, 1973.
41. Livden JK, Nilsen R, Thunold S, et al: Epidermolysis bullosa acquisita and Crohn's disease. *Acta Dermatol Venereol (Stockholm)* 58:241, 1978.
42. Mascaro JM, Jorda E, Calop J: Epidermolysis ampollosa adquirida: Estudio imunopatológica y ultrastructural. *Med Cutan Iber Lat Am* 1:1, 1978.
43. Metz G, Metz J, Horst F: Epidermolysis bullosa acquisita Gei Morbus Crohn. *Hautarzt* 26:321, 1975.
44. Muller SA, Sams WM Jr, Dobson RL: Amyloidosis masquerading as epidermolysis bullosa acquisita. *Arch Dermatol* 99:739, 1969.
45. Nieboer C, Boorsma DM, Woerdeman MJ, et al: Epidermolysis bullosa acquisita: Immunofluorescence, electron microscopic and immunoelectron microscopic studies in four patients. *Br J Dermatol* 102:383, 1980.
46. Palestine RF, Kossard S, Dicken CH: Epidermolysis bullosa acquisita: A heterogeneous disease. *J Am Acad Dermatol* 5:1, 43, 1981.
47. Pass F, Dobson RL: Epidermolysis bullosa acquisita. *Arch Dermatol* 91:219, 1965.
48. Provost TT, Maize JC, Ahmed AR, et al: Unusual subepidermal bullous disease with immunologic features of bullous pemphigoid. *Arch Dermatol* 115:156, 1979.
49. Richter BJ, McNutt NS: The spectrum of epidermolysis bullosa acquisita. *Arch Dermatol* 115:1325, 1979.
50. Roenigk HH Jr, Pearson RW: Epidermolysis bullosa acquisita. *Arch Dermatol* 117:383, 1981
51. Roenigk HH Jr, Ryan JG, Bergfeld WF: Epidermolysis bullosa acquisita: Report of three cases and review of all published cases. *Arch Dermatol* 103:1, 1971.
52. Sasai Y, Fujuyama T: Histochemical study on the pathogenesis of epidermolysis bullosa acquisita. *Tohoku J Exp Med* 99:9, 1969.
53. Sams WM Jr, Smith JG Jr: Epidermolysis bullosa acquisita, dermal elastosis, amyloidosis. *Arch Dermatol* 90:137, 1964.

54. Sherry F, Dothridge MD: Case for diagnosis: Epidermolysis bullosa acquisita. *Proc Royal Soc Med* 55:409, 1962.
55. Siemens H: Zur klinischen und histologischen Kennthis einer richterblichen Form de Sog: Epidermolysis; Bullosa mechanica toxica ex usa arseni. *Arch Klin Exp Dermatol* 149:71, 1925.
56. Sneddon IB: Acquired localized epidermolysis bullosa. *Br J Dermatol* 81:389, 1969.
57. Stanley JR, Hawley-Nelson P, Yuspa SH, et al: Characterization of bullous pemphigoid antigen: A unique basement membrane protein of stratified squamous epithelia. *Cell* 24:897, 1981.
58. Stanley JR, Yaar M, Hawley-Nelson P, et al: Pemphigus antibodies identify a cell surface glycoprotein synthesized by human and mouse keratinocytes. *J Clin Invest* 70:281, 1982.
59. Tan R: Epidermolysis bullosa acquisita. *Br J Dermatol* 97 (Suppl 15):46, 1977.
60. Tolmach JA: Diagnosis: Epidermolysis bullosa acquisita (tardine)? *Arch Dermatol* 82:464, 1960.
61. Traub EF: Case for diagnosis: Acquired epidermolysis bullosa? Sun sensitivity eruption? Dermatitis herpetiformis? *Arch Dermatol* 82:139, 1960.
62. Trump DL, Allen H, Olson J, et al: Epidermolysis bullosa acquisita: Association with amyloidosis and multiple myleoma. *JAMA* 243:1461, 1980.
63. Wilson BD, Birnkrant AF, Beutner EH, et al: Epidermolysis bullosa acquisita: A clinical disorder of varied etiologies. *J Am Acad Dermatol* 3:280, 1980.
64. Wise F, Lautman MF: Epidermolysis bullosa beginning in adult life: The acquired form of the disease. *J Cut Dis* 33:441, 1915.
65. Woodley DT, Briggaman RA, O'Keefe EJ, et al: Identification of the epidermolysis bullosa acquisita antigen—a normal component of human skin basement membrane. *N Engl J Med* 310:1007, 1984.
66. Yaoita H, Briggman RA, Lawley TJ, et al: Epidermolysis bullosa acquisita: Ultrastructural and immunological studies. *J Invest Dermatol* 76:288, 1981.

21
Immunofluorescence Studies in Epidermolysis Bullosa Utilizing Polyclonal and Monoclonal Antibodies

Jo-David Fine
Helmut Hintner
Stephen I. Katz

INTRODUCTION

Epidermolysis bullosa (EB) is a heterogeneous disease characterized by marked skin fragility and blister formation following seemingly minor trauma to the skin; it is therefore referred to as a mechano-bullous disease (2). There are many distinct clinical forms of this disease, each having a specific mode of genetic transmission. As noted in Table 1, these diseases may be classified by determining ultrastructurally where cleavage and subsequent blister formation occurs within traumatized skin. Such classification is important for assessment of long-term prognosis, genetic counseling, and appropriate choice of therapy.

There are three forms of epidermolysis bullosa: EB simplex, junctional EB, and dystrophic EB. Direct immunofluorescence (DIF) of both involved and uninvolved skin is negative in each of these conditions. In contrast, in vivo-bound immunoreactants are detectable along the dermal-epidermal junction of perilesional skin from patients with acquired EB (26); this latter condition is discussed in detail in Chapter 20.

ULTRASTRUCTURE AND COMPOSITION OF THE SKIN BASEMENT MEMBRANE ZONE

In order to understand the rationale behind both immunofluorescence (IF) mapping and monoclonal antibody (MCA) studies in patients with EB, we must first briefly review the ultrastructure and biochemical composition of the basement membrane zone (BMZ)

Table 1. Classification of EB

Type of EB	*Level of skin cleavage*
Simplex	Intraepidermal
Junctional	Lamina lucida
Dystrophic	Sublamina densa

of human skin (Fig. 1) (15). Basement membrane delimits three areas within normal skin: the epidermis, dermal blood vessels, and dermal appendages. In epidermolysis bullosa, skin cleavage occurs at the level of or above the dermal-epidermal junction (epidermal BMZ); we will therefore confine our discussion to this particular structure. The dermal-epidermal junction, as defined by electron microscopy (EM), is composed of distinct structures: the basal cell plasma membrane, the lamina lucida, the lamina densa, and the sublamina densa zone containing anchoring fibrils (Fig. 1). The lamina lucida is a narrow linear, relatively electron-lucent area located just beneath and contiguous with the undersurface of the basal keratinocytes. Directly underneath the lamina lucida is a slightly wider, more electron-dense region known as the lamina densa (or basal lamina). Anchoring fibrils radiate down from the lamina densa into the underlying upper papillary dermis.

Several biochemical materials have now been ultrastructurally localized within the human dermal-epidermal junction. Bullous pemphigoid (BP) antigen, a glycoprotein of approximately 220 k molecular weight, is located exclusively within the lamina lucida contiguous with the overlying basal keratinocyte cell membrane (22,23). As a result, BP antigen is usually detectable on the roof of, rather than the base of, a mechanical suction blister induced on normal human skin. Another constituent of the lamina lucida is laminin, which is another high-weight glycoprotein (6). Although laminin is also located within the lamina lucida, antibodies to laminin bind primarily to the base of a mechanical suction blister. Laminin is also present within the basement membranes of dermal vessels and appendages. The lamina densa contains at least two distinct antigenic moieties: type IV collagen (27) and the antigen defined by KF-1 MCA (3). Type IV collagen is found in all basement membranes, while KF-1 antigen is restricted to the dermal-epidermal junction. In addition, AF-1 and AF-2 MCA define antigens within anchoring fibrils and, to a lesser extent, possibly also within the lower lamina densa (8). Finally, another recently defined dermal-epidermal junction component is the epidermolysis bullosa acquisita (EBA) antigen. This antigen has been detected within and immediately below the lamina densa of normal human skin by serum autoantibodies from EBA patients (25), whereas in vivo-bound immunoreactants in these patients are confined to the sublamina densa region (26).

ULTRASTRUCTURAL ABNORMALITIES IN EPIDERMOLYSIS BULLOSA

Each type of EB has characteristic EM findings. In EB simplex, skin cleavage occurs within the epidermis; by EM, cytolysis of basal or suprabasal keratinocytes can be seen (18,20). In junctional EB, skin cleavage occurs within the lamina lucida of the BMZ; the intact epidermis forms the roof, while the lamina densa remains attached to the dermis, forming the base of the lesional blister (1,11,13,17,19,21). An associated EM abnormality is the presence of either decreased numbers or abnormal appearance of hemidesmosomes. In dystrophic EB, blister formation occurs just beneath the lamina

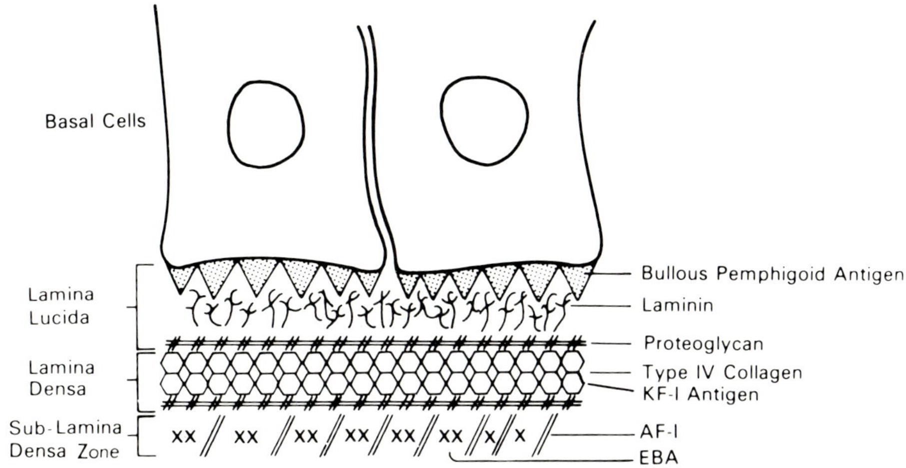

Figure 1. Schematic representation of the dermal-epidermal junction identifying the localization of the various components. (From Katz [15].)

densa (9,10,12,17). In addition, in the milder form of dystrophic EB, which is autosomal dominant in transmission, anchoring fibrils are reduced in number. In the more severe autosomal recessively transmitted form, anchoring fibrils are virtually absent.

IMMUNOFLUORESCENCE MAPPING STUDIES (14,24)

In the past, localization of the level of skin cleavage required EM, which is a costly and time-consuming technique available only in specially equipped laboratories. More recently, utilization of polyclonal and monoclonal antibodies directed against normal constituents of the dermal-epidermal junction by indirect immunofluorescence (IIF) has proven to be as accurate as EM in determining the level of cleavage within skin of EB patients (14,24). Antibodies employed in this technique are directed against BP antigen, laminin, and type IV collagen—substances shown to be in apparently normal amounts in skin from all patients with EB. This technique is referred to as IF mapping. There are several advantages of this technique over EM. First, the only specialized equipment needed is a fluorescence microscope. The only reagents required are antibodies to BP antigen, laminin, and type IV collagen (now available in several laboratories throughout the world), appropriate fluorescein-conjugated second-step antibodies, control sera, and buffer. IF mapping can be completed within a few hours, as opposed to the far more laborious EM. Furthermore, IF mapping can be performed at no greater expense than routine IIF.

In this technique, IIF is performed on cryostat-sectioned skin using BP sera and sheep sera containing antibodies to human laminin and type IV collagen. Simultaneously run controls are normal human serum and normal sheep serum, with each used at the same dilutions as corresponding positive antisera from the same species. Second-step antibodies utilized are fluorescein-conjugated goat anti-human IgG and fluorescein-conjugated rabbit anti-sheep IgG, respectively. All dilutions are performed in 0.0067 M phosphate-buffered saline (PBS), pH 7.4. Incubations are carried out for 30 minutes at room temperature within a humidified chamber. After each of the two incubation

Table 2. Antibody Binding Patterns in IF Mapping

	Location of antibody binding		
Type of EB	*BP*	*Laminin*	*Type IV collagen*
EB Simplex	Base	Base	Base
Junctional EB	Roof	Base	Base
Dystrophic EB	Roof	Roof	Roof

periods, the slides are washed three times for 5 minutes each in PBS. Coverslips are mounted with a 1:1 solution of glycerol in PBS, and each slide is then examined by fluorescence microscopy (see also Chap. 1).

Skin is obtained by a punch biopsy procedure from clinically normal-appearing skin from patients with EB; as control tissue, similar specimens of normal human skin are also obtained. We commonly obtain such specimens from the upper inner arm. If this site is inaccessible to a biopsy procedure, care must be taken to sample an area of the body known to adequately express the BP antigen (7). Usually, the circular motion of the punch biopsy procedure is sufficient to produce microscopic foci of skin separation. In those rare cases where no cleft is seen, a second biopsy specimen is obtained of normal-appearing skin following application of mild friction to the skin (i.e., by gently rubbing the site with a pencil eraser using a twisting motion). This latter maneuver will easily induce at least a microscopically detectable blister in EB skin; care must be taken, however, not to produce such a large blister that the roof is lost in subsequent processing.

Based upon our previous discussion of the biochemical composition of the human dermal-epidermal junction, it should be apparent that IF mapping permits ready determination of the level of cleavage in EB skin. Such localization is made by assessing whether the roof or base of the blister or cleft is stained by each of the three antisera. The resultant staining patterns, as depicted in Table 2, are diagnostic for simplex, junctional, and dystrophic forms of EB. For example, blisters in EB simplex are intraepidermal; therefore, antisera to all three of the basement membrane components bind to the base, but not the roof, of a newly induced blister (Fig. 1). In junctional EB, skin cleavage develops within the lamina lucida. As a result, BP serum binds to the roof, while antitype IV collagen antibodies bind to the blister base; antibodies to laminin usually bind to the base, although infrequently some roof staining may also be detected. Blisters form beneath the lamina densa in both forms of dystrophic EB. Therefore, all three of these basement membrane components are detectable on the blister roof.

MONOCLONAL ANTIBODY STUDIES

Three MCA have been created that appear to be useful reagents in studies of skin from patients with EB. These antibodies are named KF-1, AF-1, AF-2, and will be discussed separately.

KF-1

KF-1 is a murine MCA that was produced following immunization of a BALB/c mouse with viable human epidermal cells following trypsinization of the roof of a mechanical suction blister (3). This antibody defines a unique noncollagenous component of the lamina densa of the dermal-epidermal junction of primate-stratified squamous epithelium. In contrast to the other previously defined component of skin lamina densa, type IV collagen, KF-1 is not present within the basement membrane of dermal vasculature or appendages.

In a recently published study (4), we examined the binding of KF-1 to clinically normal-appearing skin of 25 patients with simplex (seven patients), junctional (five patients), or dystrophic EB (dominant, seven patients; recessive, six). In addition, we examined four obligate heterozygote carriers for recessive dystrophic EB and 51 normal human skin controls. Binding of KF-1 to EB skin was evaluated over a range of antibody dilutions known to result in strong binding to normal human skin. Binding of antibodies to type IV collagen, laminin, and BP antigen was tested simultaneously. Normal tissue staining was seen with the latter three antisera on each of the EB skins examined at all dilutions; however, KF-1 binding was normal only in skin of all patients with simplex and junctional EB. This latter finding is not unexpected, since skin cleavage occurs within the lower epidermis and lamina lucida, respectively, in these two forms of EB, whereas the antigen defined by KF-1 resides within the lamina densa. In contrast, KF-1 binding was abnormal in both dominant and recessive dystrophic EB skin. In dominant dystrophic EB, none of our seven specimens had normal binding of KF-1. In some, binding was seen at only low dilutions of the antibody; in others, KF-1 was bound to skin at all dilutions examined, although the degree of binding was both weaker and more diffuse than that observed in simultaneously run control human skin. KF-1 binding was also abnormal in each of six specimens of recessive dystrophic EB. In five of these tissues, no KF-1 binding was detectable; in one patient, weak binding was detectable only when undiluted or minimally diluted antibody was employed. This antigenic defect was a selective one within the lamina densa, since type IV collagen—another known component of the lamina densa—stained normally within the same tissue.

These findings suggest that clinically normal-appearing skin specimens from patients with dominant dystrophic EB contain reduced amounts of the lamina densa antigen defined by KF-1, while skin samples from patients with recessive dystrophic EB either lack or have only minute amounts of the KF-1 antigen present. Although these findings suggest a possible quantitative relationship between the degree of diminution of KF-1 antigen and type of dystrophic EB, there is insufficient data as yet to recommend the use of this antibody for routinely differentiating recessive from dominant forms of dystrophic EB.

Examination of skin from obligate heterozygote carriers for recessive dystrophic EB revealed KF-1 binding indistinguishable from skin of normal controls. Therefore, this antibody cannot be used to detect carriers of this disease.

As part of a study of the ontogeny of human skin basement membrane, we have found KF-1 antigen to be expressed as early as 16 weeks gestational age (5). Too few fetal specimens have as yet been examined to conclude that all normal fetuses have sufficient amounts of KF-1 antigen at this gestational age to be reproducibly detected by our present technique. However, should this prove to be the case, then KF-1 antibody may be potentially quite useful in screening fetuses at high risk for having recessive dystrophic EB by examining skin specimens obtained by fetoscopy.

AF-1 and AF-2

Two additional MCA, AF-1 and AF-2, have been utilized in studies of EB tissue (8). These murine antibodies were produced by immunization of mice with extracts from a cervical carcinoma cell line and human stratum corneum, respectively. By IIF, both antibodies have been shown to bind along the dermal-epidermal junction of normal human skin. Both antibodies are primate and stratified squamous epithelial specific. Both antibodies recognize antigens within anchoring fibrils and possibly also lower lamina densa.

Both of these antibodies bind normally to skin from patients with simplex and junctional forms of EB. Neither binds to skin from patients with recessive dystrophic EB. This latter finding is consistent with previous EM studies demonstrating absent anchoring fibrils in skin from patients with recessive dystrophic EB. In contrast to KF-1, however, neither AF-1 nor AF-2 binds abnormally to skin from patients with dominant dystrophic EB despite reduced numbers of anchoring fibrils in skin from such patients. Finally, neither of these antibodies binds to human fetal skin prior to 26 weeks gestational age (16). Therefore, although each may be useful in the diagnostic evaluation of patients with suspected recessive dystrophic EB, neither has potential application in the early prenatal diagnosis of this disease.

SUMMARY

Classification of patients having EB into simplex, junctional, and dystrophic forms is necessary for proper genetic counseling and appropriate choice of therapy. Recent advances in our understanding of the antigenic composition of skin basement membrane have led to the development of a simple but accurate technique—IF mapping—which permits ready classification of such patients. In addition, the application of MCA technology to skin research has resulted in the development of three MCA that define antigenic defects within the BMZ characteristic of patients with the dystrophic form of EB.

REFERENCES

1. Anton-Lamprecht I, Schnyder UW: Zur ultrastruktur der epidermolysen mit junktionaler blasenbildung. *Dermatologica* 159:377, 1979.
2. Bauer EA, Briggaman RA: The mechanobullous diseases (epidermolysis bullosa). In Fitzpatrick TB, Eisen AZ, Wolff K, et al. (Eds): *Dermatology in General Medicine.* McGraw-Hill, New York, 1979, p 334.
3. Breathnach SM, Fox PA, Neises GR, et al: A unique squamous epithelial basement membrane antigen defined by a monoclonal antibody (KF-1). *J Invest Dermatol* 80:392, 1983.
4. Fine JD, Breathnach SM, Hintner H, et al: KF-1 monoclonal antibody defines a specific basement membrane antigenic defect in dystrophic forms of epidermolysis bullosa. *J Invest Dermatol* 82:35, 1984.
5. Fine JD, Smith LT, Holbrook KA, et al: The appearance of four basement membrane zone antigens and fibronectin in developing human fetal skin. *J Invest Dermatol* 83:66, 1984.
6. Foidart J-M, Bere EW, Yaar M, et al: Distribution and immunoelectron microscopic localization of laminin, a non-collagenous basement membrane glycoprotein. *Lab Invest* 42:336, 1980.
7. Goldberg DJ, Sabolinski M, Bystryn J-C: Regional variation in the expression of bullous pemphigoid antigen and location of lesions in bullous pemphigoid. *J Invest Dermatol* 82:326, 1984.
8. Goldsmith LA, Briggaman RA: Monoclonal antibodies to anchoring fibrils for the diagnosis of epidermolysis bullosa. *J Invest Dermatol* 81:464, 1983.
9. Hashimoto I, Anton-Lamprecht I, Gedde-Dahl T Jr, et al: Ultrastructural studies in epidermolysis bullosa hereditaria: I. Dominant dystrophic type of Pasini. *Arch Dermatol Res* 252:167, 1975.

10. Hashimoto I, Gedde-Dahl T Jr, Schnyder UW, et al: Ultrastructural studies in epidermolysis bullosa hereditaria: II. Dominant dystrophic type of Cockayne and Touraine. *Arch Dermatol Res* 255:285, 1976.
11. Hashimoto I, Gedde-Dahl T Jr, Schnyder UW, et al: Ultrastructural studies in epidermolysis bullosa hereditaria: IV. Recessive dystrophic types with junctional blistering (infantile or Herlitz-Pearson type and adult type). *Arch Dermatol Res* 257:17, 1976.
12. Hashimoto I, Schnyder UW, Anton-Lamprecht I, et al: Ultrastructural studies in epidermolysis bullosa hereditaria: III. Recessive dystrophic types with dermolytic blistering (Hallopeau-Siemens types and inverse type). *Arch Dermatol Res* 256:137, 1976.
13. Hashimoto I, Schnyder UW, Anton-Lamprecht I: Epidermolysis bullosa hereditaria with junctional blistering in an adult. *Dermatologica* 152:72, 1976.
14. Hintner H, Stingl G, Schuler G, et al: Immunofluorescence mapping of antigenic determinants within the dermal-epidermal junction in mechanobullous diseases. *J Invest Dermatol* 76:113, 1981.
15. Katz SI: The epidermal basement membrane zone. *J Am Acad Dermatol* 11:1025,1984.
16. Lane AT, Helm KF, Goldsmith LA: Antigen development in human fetal skin. *J Invest Dermatol* 82:389, 1984. 1962.
18. Pearson RW: Epidermolysis bullosa, porphyria cutanea tarda, and erythema multiforme. In Zelickson AS (Ed): *Ultrastructure of Normal and Abnormal Skin.* Lea & Febiger, Philadelphia, 1967, p 320.
19. Pearson RW, Potter B, Strauss F: Epidermolysis bullosa hereditaria letalis: Clinical and histological manifestations and course of the disease. *Arch Dermatol* 109:349, 1974.
20. Pearson RW, Spargo B: Electron microscopic studies of dermal-epidermal separation in human skin. *J Invest Dermatol* 36:213, 1961.
21. Schachner L, Lazarus GS, Dembitzer H: Epidermolysis bullosa hereditaria letalis: Pathology, natural history, and therapy. *Br J Dermatol* 96:51, 1977.
22. Stanley JR, Hawley-Nelson P, Yuspa SH, et al: Characterization of bullous pemphigoid antigen: A unique basement membrane protein of stratified squamous epithelia. *Cell* 24:897, 1981.
23. Stanley JR, Woodley DT, Katz SI: Identification and partial characterization of pemphigoid antigen extracted from normal human skin. *J Invest Dermatol* 82:108, 1984.
24. Weber L, Krieg T, Muller PK, et al: Immunofluorescent localization of type IV collagen and laminin in human skin and its application in junctional zone pathology. *Br J Dermatol* 106:267, 1982.
25. Woodley, DT, Briggaman RA, O'Keefe EJ, et al: Identification of the skin basement-membrane autoantigen in epidermolysis bullosa acquisita. *N Engl J Med* 310:1007, 1984.
26. Yaoita H, Briggaman RA, Lawley TJ, et al: Epidermolysis bullosa acquisita: ultrastructural and immunological studies. *J Invest Dermatol* 76:288, 1981.
27. Yaoita H, Foidart J-M, Katz SI: Localization of the collagenous component in skin basement membrane. *J Invest Dermatol* 70:191, 1978.

22
Linear IgA Bullous Dermatosis

Tadeusz P. Chorzelski

Stefania Jablonska

Ernst H. Beutner

B. Dale Wilson

INTRODUCTION

The distinction of linear IgA bullous dermatosis (LABD) from dermatitis herpetiformis (DH) is of basic importance in terms of disease mechanisms, prognosis, and treatment (3,4). The detection of a gluten-sensitive enteropathy (GE) in DH that is indistinguishable from that of coeliac disease (9,13,14,16,29,30,35,40) was a breakthrough in the understanding of the pathomechanism of DH (see Chap. 25). As a consequence, a gluten-free diet (GFD) was introduced as a basic modality of treatment (12). Both gut involvement and skin rash in DH appear to be gluten-dependent (15, 26, Chapter 27).

The detection of IgA deposits in the skin of patients with DH provided a new diagnostic criterion (32). The immunofluorescence (IF) skin deposits have been widely accepted as the hallmark of the disease (5,11,18,20). However, recognition of at least two different IF patterns—granular (papillary) and linear (homogeneous) (Fig. 1)—was interpreted in divergent ways and led to much controversy (5). Indeed, one of the most important findings was that patients with linear IgA deposits in the skin usually do not have GE, or it is slight and significantly less frequent than in DH (see Chapter 25). Mobacken et al. (33) reported a low incidence (one of eight cases) whereas in the Multicenter Study (27), 7 of 29 cases were found to have some abnormalities in four of those gross morphologic changes. However, none of 34 cases with LABD had antigliadin antibodies (AGA), while 20 of 35 cases with papillary immune deposits had this antibody. We would like to stress that a newly detected marker of GE—an antibody of the IgA class, reactive with endomysium of smooth muscle (IgA-EmA)—was absent in all 26 of our cases with linear IgA pattern (6), and in all cases from other centers studied at the IF Testing Service (Chap. 27). Therefore, we believe that the IF pattern of immune deposits in the skin is of basic importance for diagnostic purposes, that is, differentiation between DH and LABD.

Supported in part by the Polish Academy of Science and in part by The IF Testing Service.

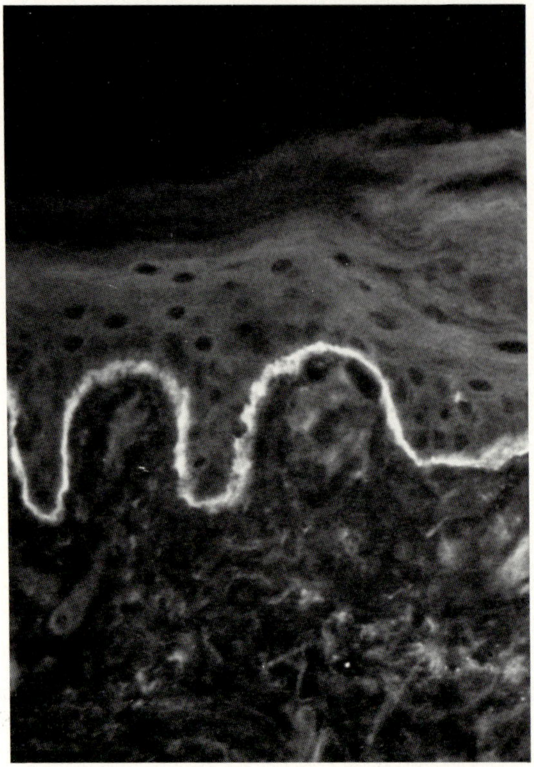

Figure 1. Direct IF with anti-IgA conjugate biopsy sections from the apparently normal skin of a patient with LABD. No linear IgA deposits at the BMZ.

This has also been presently recognized by others (25,27), who proposed the name "linear IgA disease of adults." Although the name is of no basic importance, we believe that the term "IgA disease" is too broad since there are other diseases (e.g., renal, vascular) associated with IgA deposits; whereas the designation "linear IgA bullous dermatosis" (LABD) specifies the cutaneous involvement and character of skin lesions.

MAJOR CHARACTERISTICS OF LINEAR IgA BULLOUS DERMATOSIS IN ADULTS COMPARED TO DERMATITIS HERPETIFORMIS AND BULLOUS PEMPHIGOID

Major characteristics of LABD, as compared with DH and bullous pemphigoid (BP), are presented in Table 1. Immunopathologic findings are diagnostic.

Clinical manifestations are variable. Subepidermal tense bullae are often indistinguishable from BP. Not infrequently, they appear in clusters (Figs. 2 and 3), in herpetiform arrangement (Fig. 4), on an erythematous base, and/or on the seemingly normal skin. The localization usually differs from that of DH. Bullous and vesicular lesions are often disseminated (Fig. 5) and not as symmetric as in DH. However, in some cases, clinical differentiation from DH may also be very difficult or impossible (Fig. 6). Cutaneous rash is usually accompanied by itching of varying intensity, sometimes as severe

Table 1. Major Characteristics of LABD in Adults

	LABD	*DH*	*BP*
Type of lesions	Small vesicles and large bullae	Papules and small vesicles	Large bullae and/or vesicles
Distribution of lesions	Usually no predilection	Typical areas	No predilection
Immunopathology			
Biopsy studies:			
Ig classes	IgA	IgA	IgG
site	at BMZ	under BMZ	at BMZ
pattern	linear	granular	linear
significance	diagnostic of LABD	diagnostic of DH	diagnostic of pemphigoid or EBA
C3 deposits	Usually (≈80%) negative	Usually (≈70%) negative	Linear at BMZ (>80%) diagnostic
Serum studies			
for BMZ Ab	rare IgA	No	IgG 60–70%
for IgA-EmA	No	50–70%	No
Histology	PMN micro-abscesses in dermal papillae or PMN and eosinophilic infiltrates in the dermis	PMN micro abscesses in dermal papillae	PMN and eosinophilic infiltrates
EM (bullae formation)	Lamina lucida or below lamina basalis	Below lamina basalis	Lamina lucida
IEM Ig deposits	Lamina lucida or below lamina basalis	Below lamina basalis	Lamina lucida
Gluten enteropathy	No or rare	Yes	No
HLA-B8	30–50%	85%	No specific association
Response to sulfones	Good	Dramatic	Usually no

as in DH. The duration of the disease is shorter than in DH, and not infrequently longer than in BP. However, in some cases, cutaneous lesions disappear within several months. When data are analyzed for age ranges, LABD patients are significantly younger than BP patients, although older than DH patients (41).

Histologic features are of the DH type with papillary polymorphonuclear leukocyte (PMN) microabscesses (Fig. 7) and of the BP type with subepidermal bullae (Fig. 8) and no microabscesses, but with infiltrates of both PMN and eosinophils. Often, there are prevailing features of one or the other in different biopsy specimens from the same patient and/or features of both in the same specimen.

Histologic differentiation between LABD and DH is, at times, very difficult and may even not be possible. However, with the use of a camera lucida technique, Smith et al. (37) found the number of papillary neutrophil microabscesses and the length of the

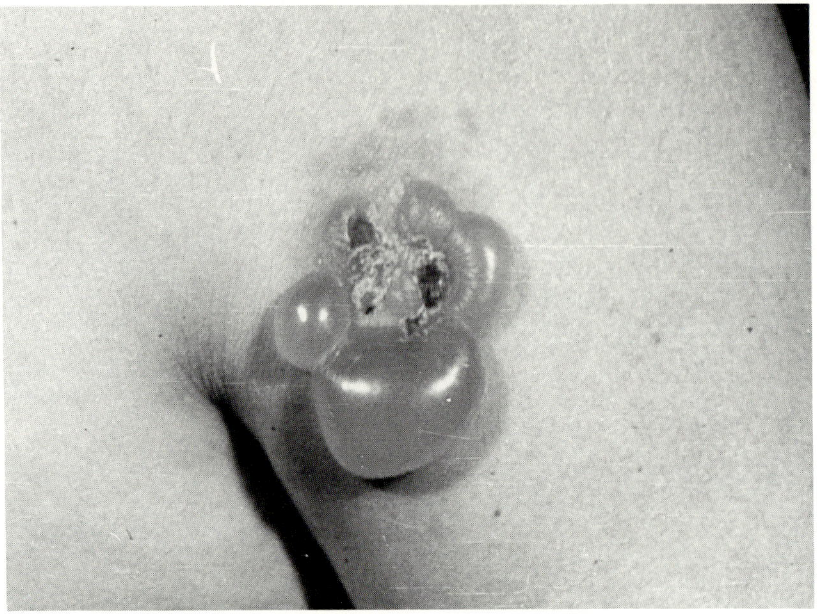

Figure 2. Tense bullae in a cluster.

epidermal basement membrane zone (BMZ) associated with them to be greater in DH than in LABD. On the other hand, the number of rete tips with neutrophils in basal vacuoles and the length of BMZ associated with them is greater in LABD than in DH. By using a probability model, they found that a correct histopathologic diagnosis can be made in almost all cases. Thus, careful histologic studies by Smith et al. (37) provided further support for the distinctiveness of LABD.

Electron microscopic (EM) studies of skin lesions of LABD revealed some features that are characteristic of DH and BP (i.e., fibrin deposition in the corium and separation of basal lamina beneath or in lamina lucida) (7).

Immunoelectron microscopic (IEM) studies have disclosed two sites of localization of immune deposits; notably in the lamina lucida as in BP and below the basal lamina as in DH (42), or in both (7) (see Chap. 23 for details). Direct immunofluorescence (DIF) has demonstrated antilamin and antitype IV collagen to be localized to the floor of the blister-like BP in some cases.

The course of LABD in adults is presented in Table 2. The mean duration of the disease was 4.2 years, and 8 of 24 patients followed for several years went into remission. This differs from the course of DH, since none of the adult cases in our series went into a lasting remission. In effect, LABD-like BP is a self-limiting disease.

THERAPY

It is a general agreement that the majority of patients with LABD respond to sulfones (10,19,20,28,33). However, some cases require very high dosages; therefore, we have proposed an alternative treatment modality: sulfones combined with prednisone, both

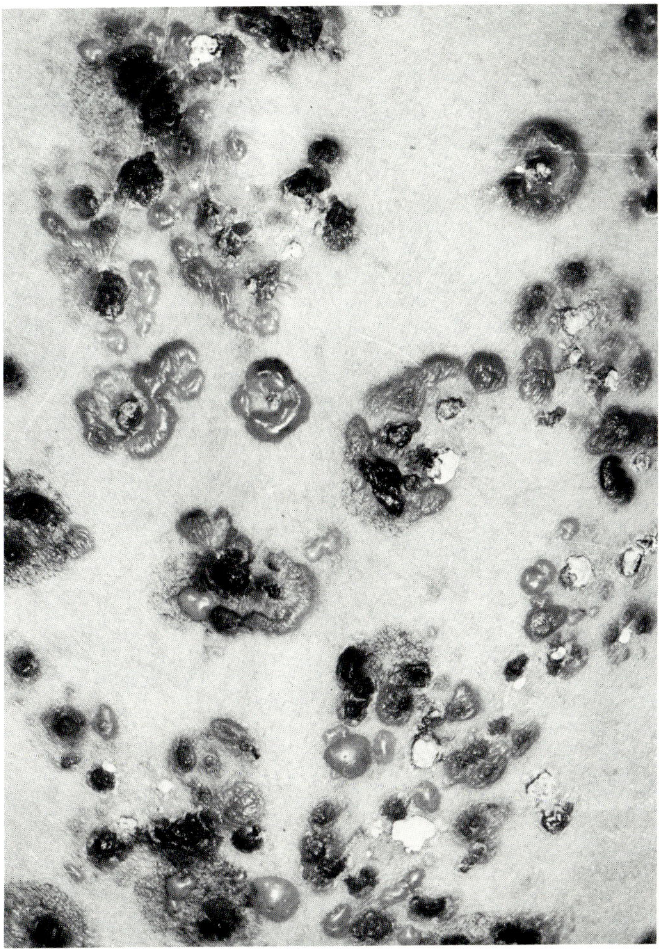

Figure 3. Numerous tense vesicles in herpetiformis arrangement and in clusters.

Table 2. LABD of Adult Patients in Remission[a]

	Patient	*Age (yr)*	*Duration of disease*	*Duration of remission*
1.	KK	39	8 mo	13 mo
2.	RR	79	15 mo	About 1 mo—exitus
3.	JK	54	10 yr	10 yr
4.	MK	20	6 yr	4.5 yr
5.	JM	60	4 yr	2 yr
6.	ESz	26	2 yr	5 yr
7.	JSz	66	2 yr	13 yr
8.	SSz	61	8 yr	7 yr—exitus
			Mean: 4.2 yr	Mean: 5.3 yr

[a]8 of 24 patients followed up for several years have been in remission.

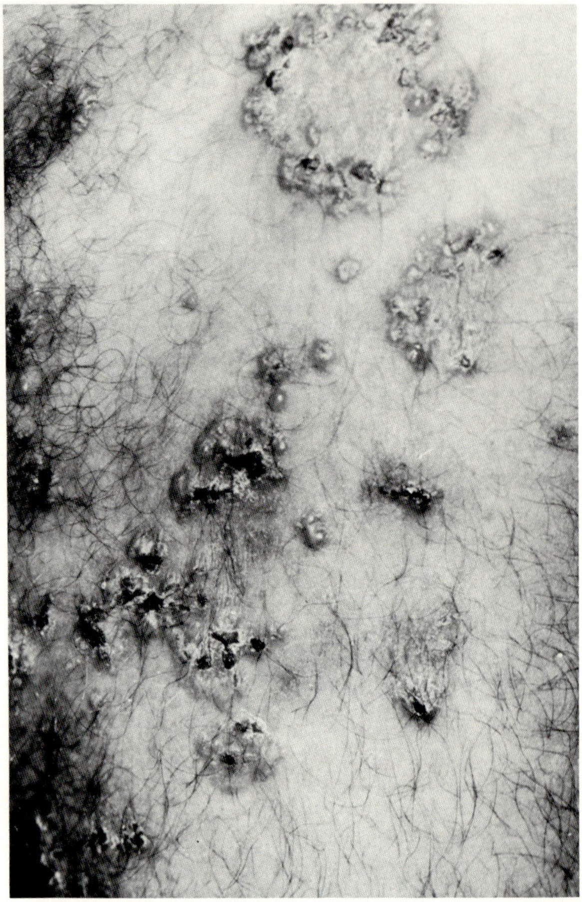

Figure 4. Small vesicles in herpetiformis arrangement.

in small doses. This has been confirmed by others (33,36,41). In addition, some patients have responded to corticosteroids, although most patients were treated with sulfones alone to determine the dose-response relationships.

In our series, the mean time of therapy for adults was 5 to 6 years; that is, significantly shorter than for patients with DH (Table 3). The patients who were in remission were followed for periods of up to 13 years, with no relapses. Our therapeutic results differ from those reported by Leonard et al. (see Chap. 23) who noticed remissions in 3 of 34 cases; while in our studies, 8 of 24 cases followed for several years went into remission. Our limited experience with GFD in two LABD patients was entirely unsuccessful; that is, without detectable affects on skin lesions.

LINEAR IgA BULLOUS DERMATOSIS OF CHILDHOOD

The so-called chronic bullous disease of childhood (CBDC) (for general review, see Chap. 23) is, in our opinion, a counterpart of LABD of adults (1,2).

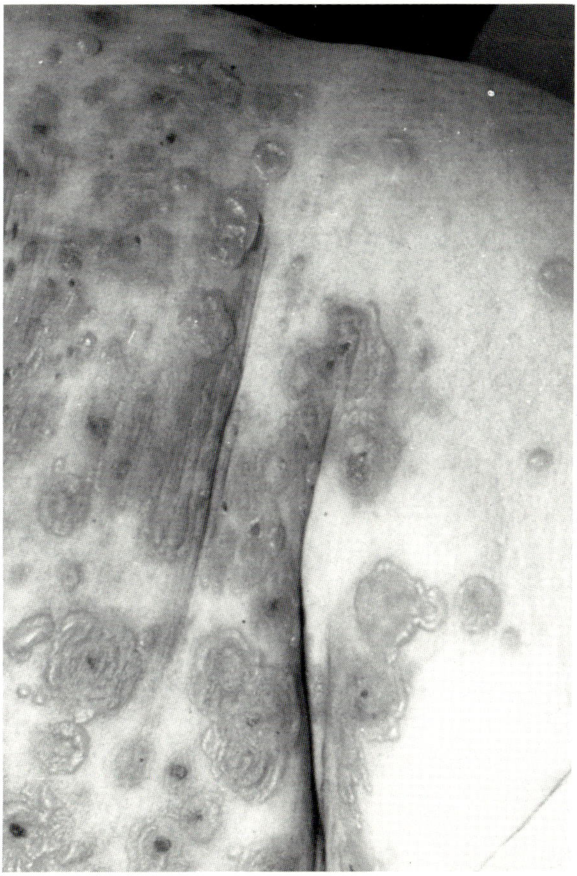

Figure 5. Widespread erythematosus and vesicular lesions: some grouping, some single vesicles localized on the normal skin.

Table 3. LABD of Adults: Duration of the Disease and Response to Treatment (36 Patients)

Duration of therapy (range)	10 mo to 14.5 yr (mean: 5.6 yr)
Treatment responses	Sulfones: 100–200 mg/day (17/27) or sulfapyridine 1. 5–3. 0 g/day
	Sulfones 100–25 mg/day + Prednisone 40–50 mg/day (15/15)
	Prednisone 100–300 mg/day (2/10)

There are slight clinical differences in localization of the lesions (27,31); that is, involvement in CBDC mainly of the pelvic region and lower extremities (Fig. 9), and often of the facial skin around the mouth. However, the character of cutaneous rash, histology, EM, immunopathology, IEM, and response to treatment are essentially the same. In both adults and children, there is no or very rare GE, and IgA-EmA was also

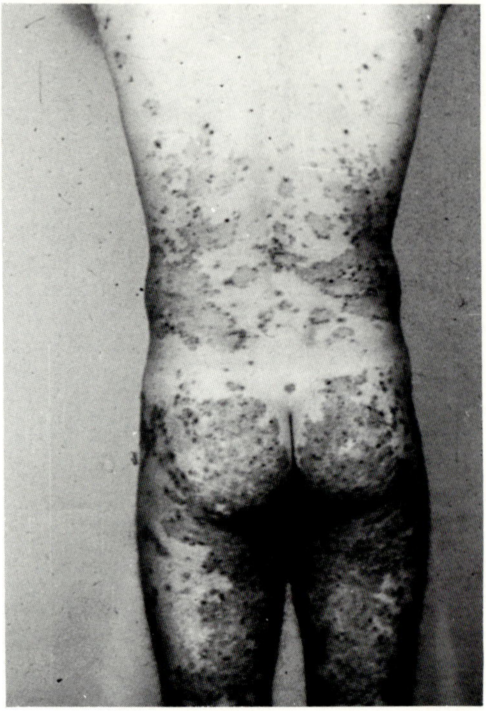

Figure 6. Symmetric distribution of herpetiform vesicular lesions as in DH.

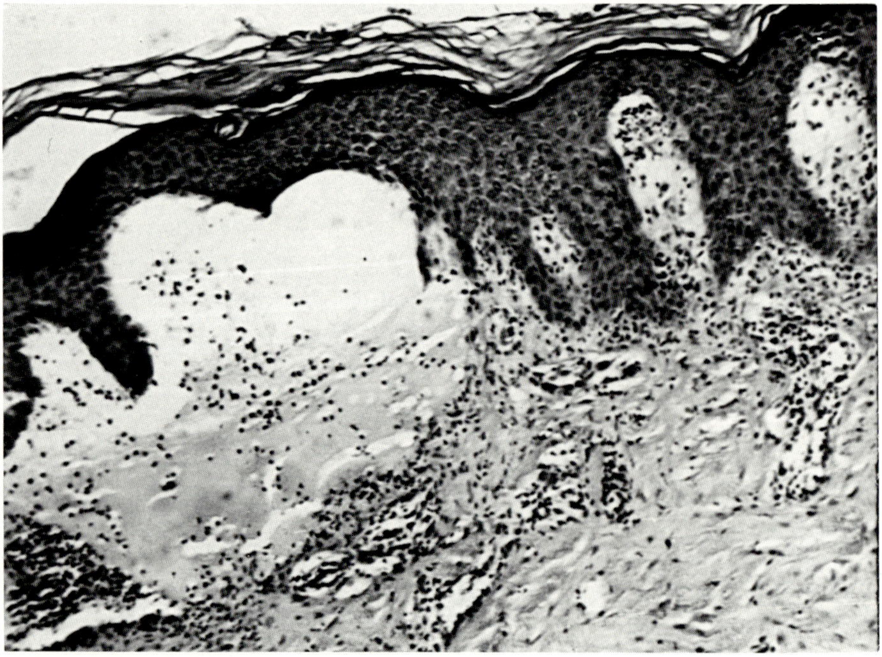

Figure 7. Histopathology from vesicular lesion. Note subepidermal bullae with microabscesses surrounding papillae.

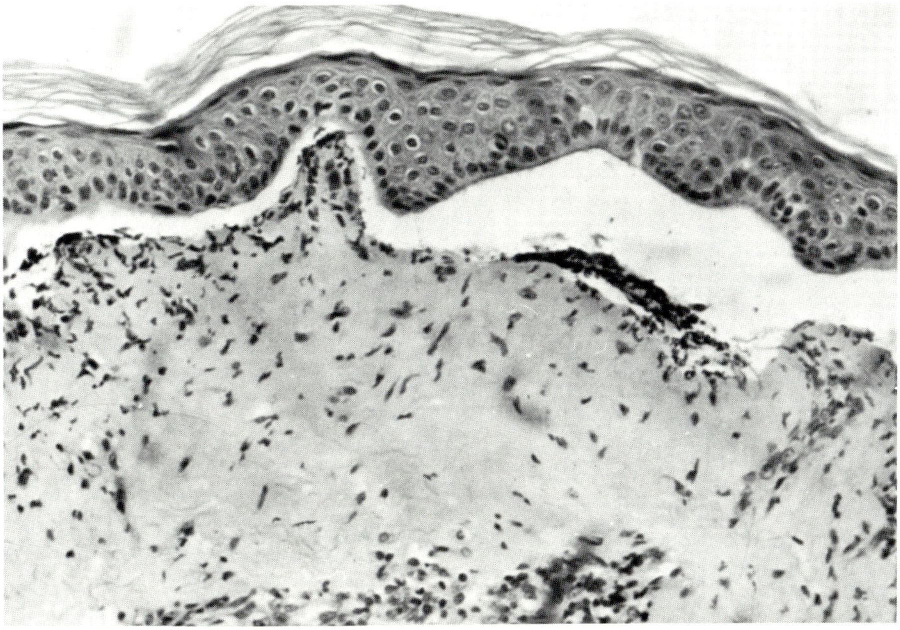

Figure 8. Histopathology of the bullae localized in apparently normal skin. Note subepidermal bullae without microabscesses.

not detected. Leonard et al. (27) have found circulating anti-BMZ antibodies (probably of the IgA class) in a majority of patients with CBDC, while in only 1 of 34 cases of LABD in adults. In our studies, the frequency of IgA BMZ antibodies was very low and comparable in both groups (1 of 8 in CBDC, and 1 of 26 in adults).

Direct IF studies of skin biopsy specimens of these patterns reveal the presence of IgA with or without the presence of other immunoglobulins (Ig). Marsden et al. (31) found only IgA and did not find IgG in skin of CBDC, which is contrary to the findings of Faber and van Joost (8) and to our experience.

In LABD of of childhood, we have found IgG in addition to IgA in 3 of 8 cases, and in 14 of 36 cases in LABD adults. Thus, also in this respect, there is no difference between the disease in children and in adults. Leonard et al. (27) report that CBDC, in contrast to LABD of adults, is a self-limiting disease. In their series, unlike in CBDC, only 3 of 34 adult patients went into remission. Similarly, in our series, remission occurred in 8 of 24 adult patients (see Table 2) and in 7 of 8 children followed for several months or years (Table 4). This difference is statistically significant. For children with LABD, the mean time of therapy was 4 to 5 years, while for adults, it was 4.2 years as indicated above. The follow-up period with no relapses was 6 months to 12.5 years. We do agree with Leonard et al. (see Chap. 23) that bullous disease with linear IgA deposits in children is a self-limiting disease, but it does not differ significantly from that of adults.

Two cases of LABD in children serve to illustrate treatment responses. One child, in whom the disease started at 2 years of age, responded dramatically to combined therapy, but is still not entirely controlled after 9 years. However, in contrast to DH, this 14-year-old boy is off treatment, and only rarely has a slight cutaneous rash; linear IgA

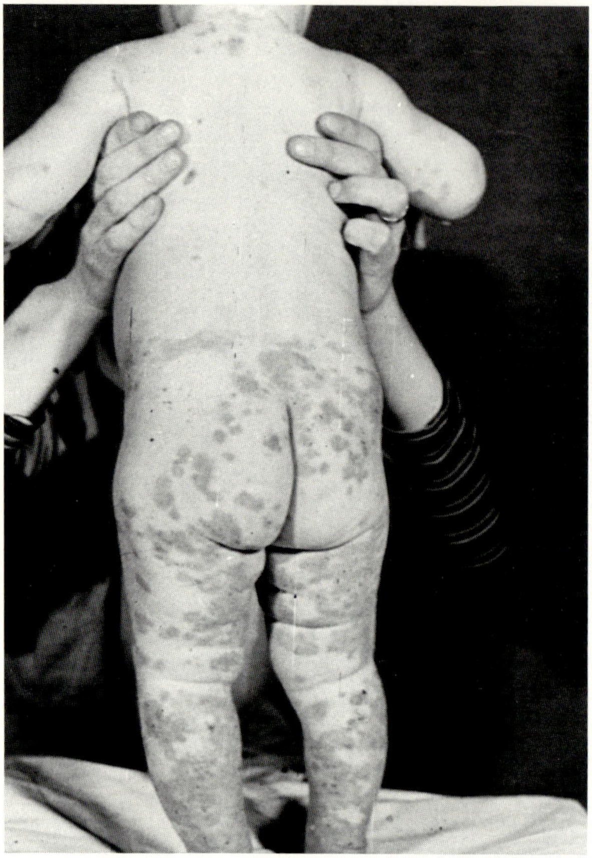

Figure 9. LABD in a child. Note erythematous and vesicular lesion localized in the buttocks and lower extremities.

deposits were still detectable 1 year ago. It is to be stressed that IgA skin deposits were found in another child 6 years after remission (see Table 4). Thus, also in this respect, LABD of childhood does not differ from LABD of adults.* In our limited experience with GFD in children with LABD, this therapy was unsuccessful, as in adults. As an example, we would like to mention a case of a 3.5-year-old boy diagnosed elsewhere as having DH who was put on a very strict GFD for 1 year with no effect. The diagnosis of LABD was established clinically and immunopathologically, and the diet was discontinued. When given 50 mg of Dapsone, combined with 10 mg of prednisone daily, a dramatic response was produced within 1 week. Since our results of combined treatment with sulfones and prednisone in small doses are very satisfactory (Table 3), we do not think that GFD should be recommended.

LABD occurs less frequently in children (3.1%) than in adults (8%). DH is the most frequent disease (14.5%) among these three entities in children, whereas BP prevails in adults (42.1%). However, according to Wilson et al. (41), LABD developed in a much younger group of patients as compared with BP.

*See also Chapter 23 for divergent views.

Table 4. LABD of Childhood: Patients in Remission[a]

	Patient	*Age at the onset of disease*	*Duration of disease*	*Duration of remission*	*Remarks*
1.	HM	3 yr	2 yr	5 yr	
2.	JR	10 mo	9–10 yr	6 yr	DIF-IgA ++/+++ in 6th year of remission
3.	JW	2 yr	9 yr	Very rare appearance of slight abortive rash	DIF 1 yr ago Weak IgA Weak IgA deposits
4.	MS	3 yr	3 yr	2 yr	
5.	AK	12 mo	1 yr	12.5 yr	
6.	AS	2 yr	6.5 yr	1 yr	
7.	MP	10 mo	3 yr	6 mo	
8.	RR	1 yr	2.5 yr Mean: 4.5 yr	7 mo	

[a]7 of 8 children followed up for several months or years have been in remission

Table 5. LABD in Children and Adults: Its Frequency as Compared with DH and BP in Two Populations-Poland and U.S.A.

	Children (age 14 yr or under)		*Adults (age 15 yr or older)*		*Totals*	
	Poland	*U.S.*	*Poland*	*U.S.*	*Poland*	*U.S.*
LABD	14 (3.2%)	1 (0.3%)	36 (8.0%)	26 (8.1%)	50 (11.2%)	27 (8.4%)
DH	65 (14.6%)	3 (0.9%)	132 (29.6%)	57 (17.8%)	197 (44.2%)	60 (18.7%)
BP	11 (2.5%)	2 (0.6%)	188 (42.1%)	232 (72.3%)	199 (44.6%)	234 (72.9%)
Totals	90 (20.1%)	6 (1.9%)	356 (79.8%)	315 (98.1%)	446	321

The response to treatment with sulfones was comparable in adults and in children, and we believe that it is not justified to control the disease with very high dosages of sulfones, either in adults or in children, when addition of small doses of corticosteroids allows the dose of sulfones to diminish considerably; thus, serious side effects can be avoided. Very much like Leonard et al. (see Chap. 23), we did not observe GE in cases of LABD of childhood; but in contrast to these authors, we have no GE in our studies of adults with LABD.

The rate of occurrence, in the United States and in Poland, of subepidermal bullous diseases in children as compared with adults is presented in Table 5. The relative frequency of each of the bullous diseases (LABD, DH, and BP) in children is 4- to 15-fold greater in Poland than in the United States. In adults, the relative frequency of LABD is about the same in the United States and Poland. But the relative frequency of DH is greater in Poland, while the relative frequency of BP is greater in the United States. The reason for this difference, which is highly significant ($p < 0.0001$, chi square = 32.85), is not clear. Among the possible explanations are genetic differences in the population, dietary differences in the form of different types of wheat proteins that could induce GE and the manner of collecting data. The Polish data came from a central referal clinic in Warsaw, which receives problem cases from all parts of the country. The U.S. data came from the IF Testing Service, which receives clinical material from physicians throughout the United States. It seems doubtful if the manner of collecting data can account for the highly significant differences between the relative U.S. and Polish frequencies of BP and DH. Such comparative studies merit further pursuit, since they may yield new insight into the underlying causes of the diseases.

In our opinion, there are no basic differences between LABD in adults and children, and we feel that there is no reason to consider them as separate entities.

COMMENTS

There is enough evidence for distinguishing LABD as a separate entity on the basis of clinical, histologic, and immunologic characteristics. Since this entity has features of both DH and BP, and in individual cases one or the other prevails, patients with LABD have been described as a subset of DH (23) or as a subset of BP (21,34).

Another differentiating feature is the dissociation of HLA-B8 in LABD (22). There are divergent findings in the frequency of HLA-B8: 30% in LABD by Lawley et al. (24) (i.e., comparable to that in normal individuals) and 56% in LABD versus over 80% in DH by Leonard et al. (see Chapter 24). Whatever may be the reason of this discrepancy, it is of special interest that in Japanese, in whom HLA-B8 is extremely rare, there are almost no cases of DH with papillary IgA deposits and GE. The Japanese cases, previously diagnosed as DH, proved to be LABD (17).

Even though immunopathologic studies have contributed enormously in classifying many atypical cases, which we now know belong to LABD, there are still cases that are difficult to classify. For example, we have observed a case that at one time had linear IgG and C3 and at another time had only IgA with a linear pattern.

Despite the description of certain cases with a coexistence of systemic lupus erythematosus (SLE) with pemphigoid, many authors have classified them as vesiculo-bullous or bullous SLE (see Chap. 8 and 16). Because the majority of this group of SLE patients exhibit atypical vesicular or bullous eruptions, it has been difficult to label them as BP, DH, or LABD. The IgA deposition in the skin of some of these reported cases is linear and not papillary granular, and the presence of papillary microabscesses and the dramatic response to sulfones may suggest the true coexistence of two well-defined autoimmune diseases: SLE and LABD (see Chap. 16). Examples of such coexistence is seen not only in our own case described above, but also in the literature (38); one such was also reported as a coexistence of SLE and linar IgA DH, and the authors stress that the latter is synonymous with LABD (39). Thus, LABD appears to be a heterogeneous disease, probably with several clinical variants.

REFERENCES

1. Bean SF, Furey NL, Chorzelski TP, et al: Childhood form of linear IgA bullous dermatosis (benign chronic bullous disease of childhood). Immunopathology of the skin, ed. 2. In Beutner EH, Chorzelski TP, Bean SF (Eds): Wiley, New York, 1979, pp 320–323.

2. Chorzelski TP, Jabłońska S: IgA linear dermatosis of childhood (chronic bullous disease of childhood). *Br J Dermatol* 101:535–542, 1979.
3. Chorzelski TP, Jabłońska S, Beutner EH: Adult form of linear IgA bullous dermatosis. In Beutner EH, Chorzelski TP, Bean SF (eds): *Immunopathology of the Skin* ed. 2. Wiley, New York, 1979, pp 315–319.
4. Chorzelski TP, Jabłońska S, Beutner EH, et al. Linear IgA bullous dermatosis. In Marks R, Christophers E (Eds) *The Epidermis in Disease.* MTP Press, Lancaster, UK, 1981, pp 577–584.
5. Chorzelski TP, Beutner EH, Jabłońska S, et al: Immunofluorescent studies in the diagnosis of dermatitis herpetiformis and its differentiation from bullous pemphigoid. *J Invest Dermatol* 56:373, 1971.
6. Chorzelski TP, Beutner EH, Sulej J, et al: IgA antiendomysium antibody. A new immunological marker of dermatitis herpetiformis and coeliac disease. *Br J Dermatol* 111:395–402, 1984.
7. Dąbrowski J, Jabłońska S, Chorzelski TP, et al: Electron microscopic studies in dermatitis herpetiformis in relation to the pattern of immune deposits in the skin. *Arch Dermatol Res* 259:213–224, 1977.
8. Faber WR, van Joost TH: Juvenile pemphigoid. *Br J Dermatol* 89:519, 1973.
9. Fry L: Dermatitis herpetiformis. In Beutner EH, Chorzelski TP, Bean SF (Eds): *Immunopathology of the Skin;* ed. 2. Wiley, New York, 1979, pp 283–301.
10. Fry L.: The treatment of dermatitis herpetiformis. *Clin Exp. Dermatol* 7:633–642, 1982.
11. Fry L, Seah PP: Dermatitis herpetiformis. An evaluation of diagnostic criteria. *Br J Dermatol* 90:137, 1974.
12. Fry L, McMinn RMH, Cowan JC, et al: Gluten-free diet and re-introduction of gluten in dermatitis herpetiformis. *Arch Dermatol* 100:129, 1969.
13. Fry L, Seah PP, Riches DJ, et al: Clearance of skin lesions in dermatitis herpetiformis after gluten withdrawal. *Lancet* 1:288–291, 1973.
14. Fry L, Kier P, McMinn RMH, et al: Small intestinal structure and function and haematological changes in dermatitis herpetiformis. *Lancet* 2:729, 1967.
15. Fry L, Leonard JN, Swain F, et al: Long term follow-up of dermatitis herpetiformis with and without dietary gluten withdrawal. *Br J Dermatol* 107:631–640, 1982.
16. Harrington CI, Read NW: Dermatitis herpetiformis: Effect of gluten-free diet on skin IgA and jejunal structure and function. *Br Med J* 1:872, 1977.
17. Hashimoto K, Miki Y, Nishioka K, et al: HLA antigens in dermatitis herpetiformis among Japanese. *J Dermatol* 7:289–291, 1980.
18. Holubar K, Doralt M, Eggerth G: Immunofluorescence patterns in dermatitis herpetiformis. Investigations on skin and intestinal mucosa. *Br J Dermatol* 85:505–510, 1971.
19. Jablońska S, Chorzelski TP: When and how to use sulfones in bullous diseases. *Int J Dermatol* 20:103–105, 1981.
20. Jablońska S, Chorzelski TP, Beutner EH, et al: Dermatitis herpetiformis and bullous pemphigoid. Intermediate and mixed forms. *Arch Dermatol* 112:45–48, 1976.
21. Jones RR, Goolamali SK: IgA bullous pemphigoid: A distinct blistering disorder. *Br J Dermatol* 102:719, 1980.
22. Katz SI: Dermatitis herpetiformis. The skin and the gut. *Ann Intern Med* 93:857, 1980.
23. Katz SI, Strober W: The pathogenesis of dermatitis herpetiformis. *J Invest Dermatol* 70:63, 1978.
24. Lawley TJ, Strober W, Yaoita H, et al: Small intestinal biopsies and HLA types in dermatitis herpetiformis patients with granular and linear IgA skin deposits. *J Invest Dermatol* 74:9–12, 1980.
25. Leonard JN, Haffenden GP, Unsworth DJ, et al: Evidence that the IgA in patients with linear IgA disease is qualitatively different from that of patients with dermatitis herpetiformis. *Br J Dermatol* 110:315–321, 1984.
26. Leonard J, Haffenden G, Tucker W, et al: Gluten challenge in dermatitis herpetiformis. *N Engl J Med* 309:816, 1983.
27. Leonard J, Haffendon GP, Ring NP, et al: Linear IgA disease in adults. *Br J Dermatol* 107:301–316, 1982.

28. Ljunghall K, Scheynius A, Jonsson J, et al: Gluten-free diet in patients with dermatitis herpetiformis. Effect on the occurrence of antibodies to reticulin and gluten. *Arch Dermatol* 119:970, 1983.
29. Marks J, Shuster S: Dermatitis herpetiformis. The role of gluten. *Arch Dermatol* 101:452–457, 1970.
30. Marks J, Shuster S, Watson AJ: Small bowel changes in dermatitis herpetiformis. *Lancet* 2:1280–1282, 1966.
31. Marsden RA, McKee PH, Bhogal B, et al: A study of benign chronic bullous dermatosis of childhood and comparison with dermatitis herpetiformis and bullous pemphigoid occurring in childhood. *Clin Exp Dermatol* 5–159–172, 1980.
32. Meer JB van der: Granular deposits of immunoglobulins in the skin of patients with dermatitis herpetiformis. An immunofluorescent study. *Br J Dermatol* 81:493–503, 1969.
33. Mobacken H, Kastrup W, Ljunghall K, et al: Linear IgA dermatosis: A study of ten adult patients. *Acta Dermatol Venereol* 63:123–128, 1983.
34. Provost TT, Maize JC, Ahmed RA, et al: Unusual subepidermal bullous diseases with immunologic features of bullous pemphigoid. *Arch Dermatol* 115:156–160, 1979.
35. Reunala T, Blomquist K, Tarpilla S, et al: Gluten free diet in dermatitis herpetiformis. *Br J Dermatol* 97:473, 1977.
36. Schiffner JH: Therapy of childhood linear IgA dermatitis herpetiformis. *J Am Acad Dermatol* 6:403, 1982.
37. Smith SB, Harrist TJ, Murphy GF, et al: Linear IgA bullous dermatosis dermatitis herpetiformis. *Arch Dermatol* 120:324–328, 1984.
38. Szabo E, Husz S, Kovacs L: Coexistent atypical bullous pemphigoid and systemic lupus erythematosus. *Br J Dermatol* 104:71, 1981.
39. Thaipisuttikul Y, Piamphongsant T, Suwanwela N: Coexistence of linear IgA dermatitis herpetiformis and systemic lupus erythematosus. *J Dermatol (Tokyo)* 10:161, 1983.
40. Weinstein WM: Latent celiac sprue. *Gastroenterology* 66:489, 1974.
41. Wilson D, Beutner EH, Kumar V, et al: Linear IgA bullous dermatosis: An immunologically defined disease. *Int. J. Dermatol.* 24:569–574, 1985
42. Yaoita H, Katz SI: Immunoelectronmicroscopic localization of IgA in skin of patients with dermatitis herpetiformis. *J Invest Dermatol* 67: 502–506, 1976.

23
Linear IgA Bullous Dermatosis in Adults—The St. Mary's View

Jonathan N. Leonard
Gerald P. Haffenden
Nicola P. Ring
Lionel Fry

INTRODUCTION

Linear IgA bullous dermatosis (LABD) may be defined as a rash characterized by spontaneous blistering and by the presence in uninvolved skin of a homogeneous linear deposit of IgA along the dermal-epidermal junction. We feel that there are good grounds for regarding LABD in adults as a distinct disease entity from benign chronic bullous dermatosis of childhood (CBDC) (10), dermatitis herpetiformis (DH), and bullous pemphigoid (BP).

FINDINGS IN LINEAR IgA BULLOUS DERMATOSIS

Clinical Features of LABD

By definition, LABD is characterized by the development of blisters. There is considerable variation in both the morphology and distribution of the lesions. Some patients present with excoriated papules over extensor surfaces and clinically resemble DH; a slightly larger number have large tense blisters in a distribution more suggestive of BP. The majority of patients, however, have a rash that is atypical for either of these diseases, and is hard to label clinically. Mucous membrane involvement is more common than in DH, with changes of oral ulceration and cicatrizing conjunctivitis indistinguishable clinically from that seen in cicatricial pemphigoid (8).

There is a 2:1 preedominance of females affected by LABD in contrast to the male predominance in DH. The incidence of spontaneous remission is only about 10%, which is much lower than in BP and benign CBDC, but similar to that of DH. When patients with LABD enter spontaneous remission, the IgA deposits can still be demonstrated in the skin.

Histology

No specific histologic features were found to be diagnostic for LABD (1).

Treatment

The majority of patients admitted to the multicenter study (5) responded well to therapy with Dapsone; doses on the order of 100 mg/day proved adequate. The addition of small amounts of corticosteroids was not found to be helpful in controlling the rash of those patients who were not very responsive to dapsone. We found that better control was achieved by using a combination of dapsone and sulfonamides such as sulfapyridine and sulfamethoxypyridazine.

Associated Disorders

Evidence of a coexisting enteropathy is an important issue in the classification of LABD among bullous dermatoses. In the multicenter study, 7 of 29 patients who underwent small intestinal biopsy procedure had a mucosal abnormality. However, only four had gross morphologic changes, as demonstrated through a dissecting microscope, and only one had any symptoms of celiac disease. Other series of patients with LABD showed a much lower incidence of enteropathy. Lawley et al. (4) found no case of enteropathy in six patients who were biopsied, and Chorzelski et al. (2) reported the incidence of jejunal abnormality to be low (see Chap. 22). In a recent study of 10 patients with LABD, Mobacken et al. (11) found only one of eight patients who were biopsied to have an abnormal jejunum. It is important to note that 5% of patients with DH had a normal small intestinal biopsy specimen, using the sensitive criteria described earlier; yet it is known that the rash will clear with a strict gluten-free diet (GFD) in these individuals (12). Therefore, absence of an enteropathy by itself in patients does not necessarily mean that gluten can be dismissed as the cause of the rash. The only way in which the issue can be resolved with certainty is to show a successful strict GFD controlling the rash and subsequent relapse on gluten challenge, or to show failure of any response of the rash to a strict GFD given for an adequate period of time. There are, as yet, no worthwhile data on the effect of GFD in patients with LABD.

LABD is too rare a disorder for there to be any valid epidemiologic studies on the incidence of malignancy. There do, however, seem to be some grounds for proposing that these patients are at risk. Five of 34 patients included in the multicenter study had a history of malignancy. Only one had a lymphoma, and at necropsy there was no evidence of bowel involvement (7).

IMMUNOLOGIC ABNORMALITIES IN THE SKIN

Immunofluorescent (IF) Findings

By definition, all patients with LABD have a homogeneous linear deposit of IgA along the dermal-epidermal junction of the uninvolved skin (Fig. 1). J-chain could not be

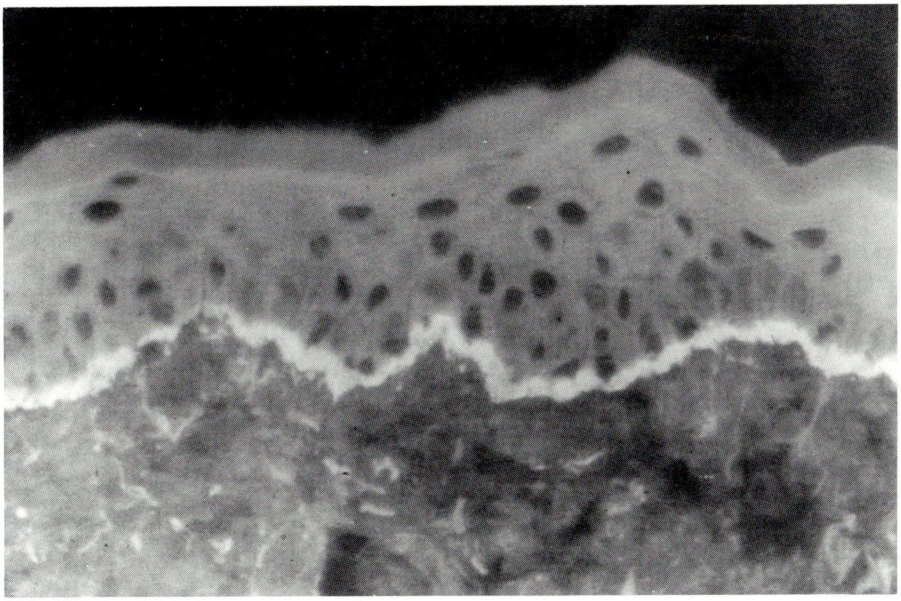

Figure 1. Direct IF of uninvolved skin showing the homogeneous-linear pattern of deposition of the IgA along the dermal-epidermal junction.

demonstrated in these deposits, which argues against a mucosal origin for the IgA (9). IgM and C3 were each found in about one-third of patients with LABD.

A major point of controversy arises when assessing the 30% of patients who had both IgA and IgG deposited in uninvolved skin. Most authorities consider that these patients should be classified as having BP, rather than LABD. The findings of the multicenter study, however, were unable to support this point of view. Using a number of parameters, it was not possible to distinguish between those patients who had IgA alone in the uninvolved skin and those with both IgA and IgG. The good response to treatment with sulfones suggests that, from the practical point of view, they should be considered as having LABD, rather than BP. (Editor's note: See Chap. 16 for examples of such problem cases.)

Immunoelectron Microscopic (IEM) Findings

Methods for Study

Fresh biopsy specimens of uninvolved skin were chopped into cubes no larger than 0.5 mm^3 to facilitate good penetration of the antibodies. IgA was demonstrated using a peroxidase-antiperoxidase (PAP) technique. After an initial wash in phosphate-buffered saline (PBS), the tissue was incubated sequentially in rabbit antihuman IgA, swine antirabbit immunoglobulin, and a PAP complex (Dako Reagents) for a minimum of 3 hours at room temperature with a wash in PBS after each incubation. The tissue was fixed in cacodylate-buffered gluteraldehyde after the final wash.

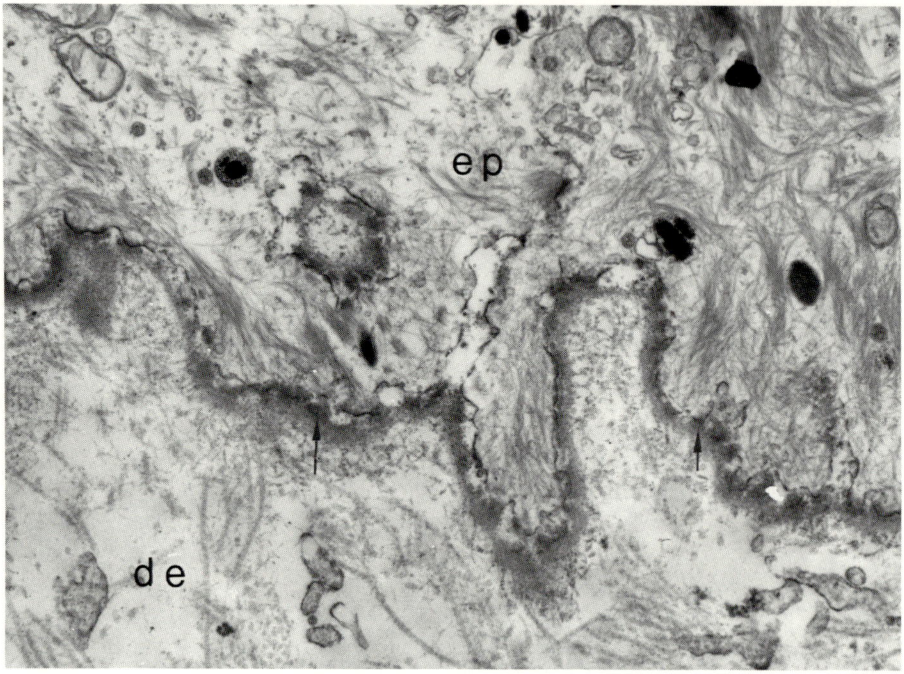

Figure 2. IEM showing the IgA deposits (arrowed) in the lamina lucida (de, dermis; ep, epidermis).

Peroxidase activity was demonstrated using 3'-3'-diaminobenzidine. Preincubation of the tissue for up to 30 minutes in the substrate before adding hydrogen peroxide was found to largely eliminate background staining.

Results

Two sites of localization of IgA were found as described in previous studies (3, 4, 6): 1) Finely granular deposits within the lamina lucida (Fig. 2); and 2) more coarsely granular deposits associated with anchoring fibrils just below the basal lamina (Figs. 3 to 6).

IEM was performed on the uninvolved skin from 14 patients with LABD; six had deposits within the lamina lucida, seven had deposits below the basal lamina associated with anchoring fibrils, and one patient had deposits in both sites. We were not able to predict the ulrastructural localization of the IgA from the IF appearances. It may be that there are two antigenic determinants involved—one in the lamina lucida that may be a glycoprotein, and one below the basal lamina that may be a collagen subtype.

IMMUNOLOGIC ABNORMALITIES IN THE SERUM

The incidence of circulating antibasement membrane zone antibodies (ABMZA) in the serum of patients with LABD was low in contrast to BP. However, there was a high incidence of antibodies directed against other nonorgan-specific targets, which implied a possible autoimmune basis for the disease.

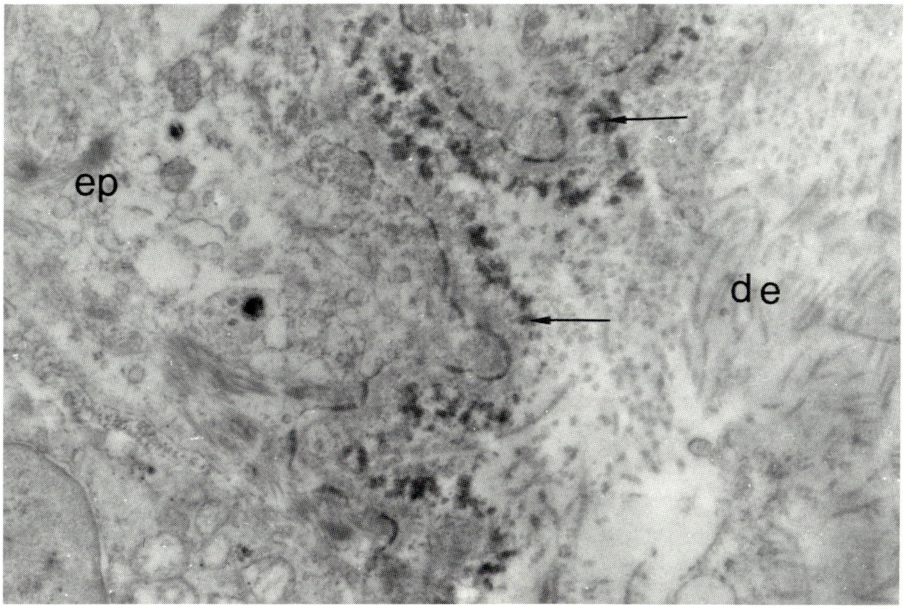

Figure 3. IEM showing the IgA deposits (arrowed) below the basal lamina in close proximity to the anchoring fibrils (de, dermis; ep, epidermis).

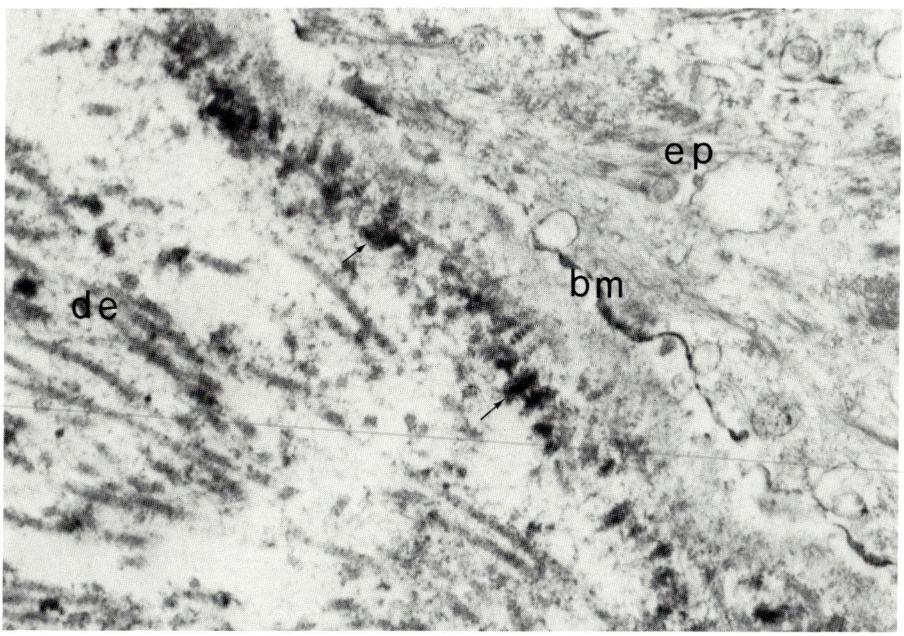

Figure 4. IEM showing the IgA deposits (arrowed) again in close association with anchoring fibrils (de, dermis; ep, epidermis; bm, basement membrane).

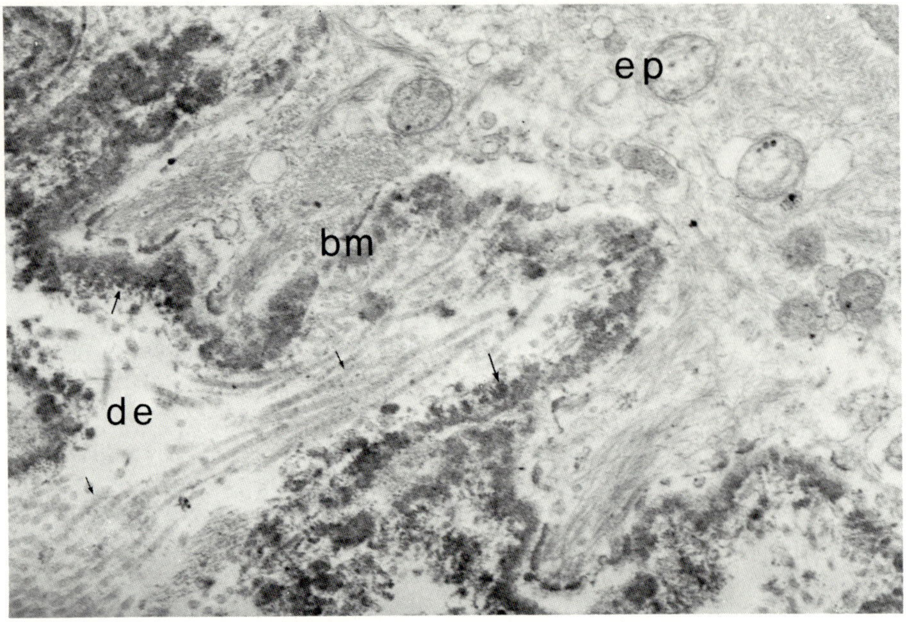

Figure 5. IEM showing a similar pattern of deposition to Figures 3 and 4, but with more electron-dense material giving a more linear appearance (large arrows). Note the absence of deposits on collagen fibers (small arrows) (de, dermis; ep, epidermis; bm, basement membrane).

IMMUNOGENETICS OF LINEAR IgA BULLOUS DERMATOSIS

There are only a few reports in the literature of the incidence of HLA-B8 in patients with LABD. Lawley et al. (4) found only 3 of 10 patients to have HLA-B8—a level not significantly different from the normal population. In the multicenter study, however, 56% of patients with LABD had HLA-B8, and this figure has been supported by the study of Mobacken et al. (11) in which five of nine patients had HLA-B8.

The finding that 56% of patients with LABD had HLA-B8 suggested that LABD may consist of two subgroups. One would have the same immunogenetic background as DH, with an incidence of HLA-B8 of over 80%, while the other would by immunogenetically distinct with an incidence of HLA-B8 equal to that of the normal population, bringing the overall incidence down to 56%.

DISCUSSION

LABD Versus DH

The major discriminants between these two groups were the clinical appearance, and the incidence of both enteropathy, and HLA-B8. Although the presence of enteropathy in some patients with LABD suggested that gluten may be the cause of the rash in a proportion of cases, it will take many years of study on the effects of glutten withdrawal

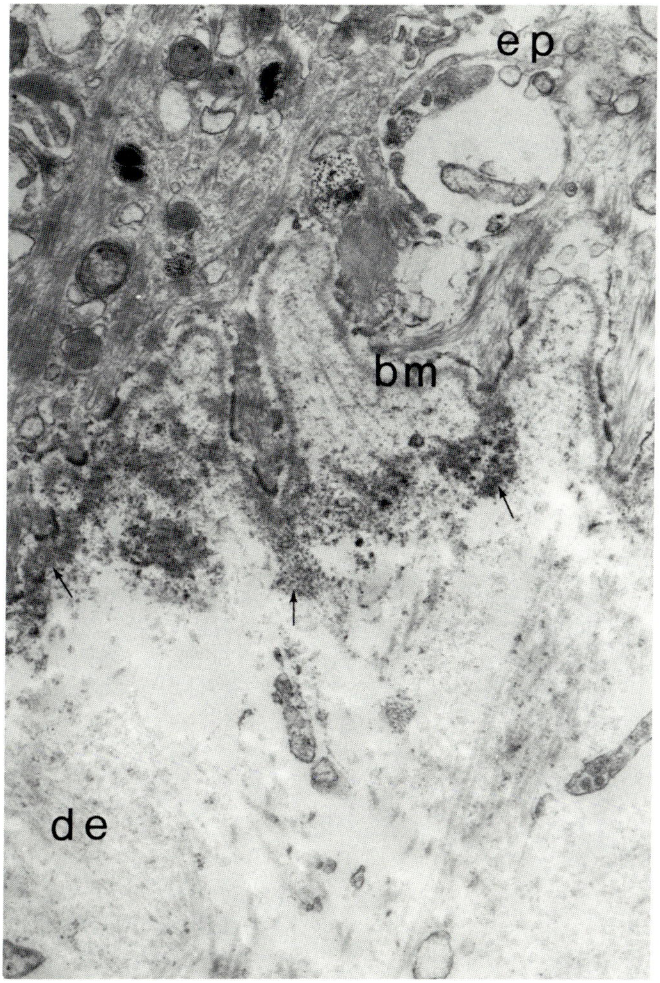

Figure 6. IEM showing a finely granular, electron-dense deposit below the basal lamina (arrows). Note that the deposit does not follow the line of the basement membrane and, in this case, does not appear to be associated with anchoring fibers (de, dermis; ep, epidermis; bm, basement membrane).

and challenge before the issue is resolved. Until the situation is clarified, we feel that the two disorders should be regarded as separate entities.

LABD Versus BP

The main findings that argued against the classification of LABD as a subgroup of BP were: 1) The younger age of onset; 2) the good response of the rash to sulfones; 3) the raised incidence of HLA-B8; 4) the presence of enteropathy in a quarter of those patients biopsied; and 5) the low incidence of circulating ABMZA in patients with

LABD. These arguments applied equally to the subgroup with IgA alone in uninvolved skin, and that with IgA and IgG deposited.

LABD versus benign CBDC

Comparison of findings of the multicenter study with those of Marsden et al. (10) showed the following features to distinguish LABD from benign CBDC: 1) The children presented with predominantly perioral and perineal lesions; while the adult picture was variable; 2) the children entered spontaneous remission as a rule, whereas this was unusual in adults—when the children entered spontaneous remission, the IgA was lost from the skin, while in the adults the IgA persisted; 3) none of the children had any evidence of enteropathy, while one-quarter of the adults had an enteropathy; 4) the majority of children had circulating ABMZA, but their presence was exceptional in the adult group; and 5) the incidence of HLA-B8 was higher in the children than in the adults.

CONCLUSIONS

The currently available evidence indicates that adults with LABD should be distinguished as a separate entity from DH, BP, and benign CBDC. However, there is evidence from the HLA typing and IEM microscopic studies to postulate the existence of at least two subgroups of LABD. Identification of subgroups will only become significant if it gives information about the pathogenesis of the disease and provides guidelines for treatment. Until such data are available, it is still important to identify patients with LABD, and to make the distinction from DH until conclusive evidence is available as to whether the rash in patients with LABD is gluten-dependent or not. This will avoid treating these patients unnecessarily with a GFD. The distinction of LABD from BP is important, because the rash of LABD is sulfone sensitive in the majority of patients and the unnecessary use of long-term systemic corticosteroids may be avoided.

ACKNOWLEDGMENTS

The data reported in this chapter come from a multicenter study reported in detail elsewhere (5). We would like to express our thanks to all those physicians who collaborated on that study. This section is entitled the "St. Mary's view" because not all of the collaborators necessarily share our interpretation of the available data.

REFERENCES

1. Blenkinsopp WK, Fry L, Haffenden GP, et al: Histology of linear IgA disease, dermatitis herpetiformis and bullous pemphigoid. *Am J Dermatopathol* 5:547, 1983.
2. Chorzelski TP, Jablonska S, Beutner EH: Adult form of linear IgA bullous dermatosis. In Beutner EH, Chorzelski TP, Bean SF (Eds): *Immunopathology of the Skin,* ed. 2. Wiley, New York, 1979, p 316.
3. Haffenden GP, Ring NP : Immuno-electron microscopy studies. In Kukita A, Seiji M (Eds): *Proceedings of the XVIth International Congress of Dermatology,* University of Tokyo Press, Tokyo, 1983, p 408.

4. Lawley TJ, Strober W, Yaoita H, et al: Small intestinal biopsies and HLA types in dermatitis herpetiformis patients with granular and linear IgA skin deposits. *J Invest Dermatol* 74:9, 1980.
5. Leonard JN, Haffenden GP, Ring NP, et al: Linear IgA disease in adults. *Br J Dermatol* 107:301, 1982.
6. Leonard JN, Haffenden GP, Ring N, et al: Ultrastructural localisation of IgA deposits in adult linear IgA disease. *J R Soc Med* 75:237, 1982.
7. Leonard JN, Tucker WFG, Fry JS, et al: Increased incidence of malignancy in dermatitis herpetiformis. *Br Med J* 286: 16, 1983.
8. Leonard JN, Wright P, Williams DM, et al: The relationship between linear IgA disease and benign mucous membrane pemphigoid. *Br J Dermatol* 110:307, 1984.
9. Leonard JN, Haffenden GP, Unsworth DJ, et al: Evidence that the IgA in linear IgA disease is qualitatively different from that in dermatitis herpetiformis. *Br J Dermatol* 110:315, 1984.
10. Marsden RA, McKee PH, Bhogal B, et al: A study of benign chronic bullous dermatosis of childhood and comparison with dermatitis herpetiformis and bullous pemphigoid occurring in childhood. *Clin Exp Dermatol* 5:159, 1980.
11. Mobacken H, Kastrup W, Ljunghall K, et al: Linear IgA dermatosis: A study of ten adult patients. *Acta Dermatol Venereol (Stockholm)* 63:123, 1983.
12. Reunala T, Blomquist K, Tarpilla S, et al: Gluten free diet in dermatitis herpetiformis. *Br J Dermatol* 97:473, 1977.

Section IID

Dermatitis Herpetiformis

24
Dermatitis Herpetiformis

Jonathan N. Leonard
Gerald P. Haffenden
Lionel Fry

INTRODUCTION

Dermatitis herpetiformis (DH) is an entity characterized clinically by urticarial lesions and blisters. Any part of the body may be involved, but the lesions are usually distributed symmetrically over the elbows, knees, upper back, and buttocks. The most common age of onset is in the third and fourth decades, but the disease may begin at any time in life after weening. For the majority of patients, the disease is lifelong, with varying periods of activity. In most series that have been reported, males are affected about twice as often as females.

The histology of an early lesion of DH shows collections of polymorphs in the dermal papillae. These are termed papillary microabscesses. Older lesions show subepidermal bulla formation, with a heavy polymorphonuclear infiltrate that may be difficult to differentiate from other subepidermal bullous dermatoses.

The rash of patients with DH is provoked by the application of iodides to the skin. It responds therapeutically to the administration of sulfone drugs and some sulfonamides (sulfapyridine and sulfamethoxypyridazine). For many years, the therapeutic response to these drugs was the major diagnostic criterion for the disease.

Over the past 20 years, a number of disorders have been found to be associated with DH, most notably celiac disease. Not only has it been shown that the majority of patients with DH have celiac disease of varying severity, but also that both the rash and the enteropathy respond to a strict gluten-free diet (GFD), and they relapse again on gluten challenge.

The application of immunologic techniques to the study of DH has added considerably to our knowledge of the disease. The initial observation was the presence of IgA in the uninvolved skin of patients with the disease; this has become the major diagnostic criterion for DH. Also, there is now good evidence for a genetic basis to the disease, as there is a high incidence of HLA-B8 and HLA-DR3 in affected individuals—a similar finding to that in celiac disease. Over recent years, the majority of research has been directed towards mechanisms by which the skin and intestinal lesions are linked in a pathophysiologic way, particularly with regard to humoral factors such as circulating antibodies and immune complexes. This chapter will review both the evidence for implicating gluten in the pathogenesis of DH and the contribution that immunologic techniques have made to our understanding of the disease.

CELIAC DISEASE AND DERMATITIS HERPETIFORMIS

Until 1966, DH was considered to be purely a skin disorder. Although some of the earlier descriptions of DH did mention ill health, loss of weight, and mental symptoms in patients, these were attributed to the effects of chronic skin irritation, which is a major feature of DH. In 1966 and 1967, there were three reports of a high prevalence of structural change of the upper small bowel mucosa in patients with DH; the changes resembled those found in idiopathic steatorrhoea (17,65,66,110). However, it was not until Fry et al. (20) reported their findings on small intestinal structure and function and hematologic changes in 12 patients with DH that gluten was suggested as being the cause of the disease. In addition to the enteropathy, the patients showed a high incidence of increased fecal fat excretion, reduced serum levels of folate and iron, and low serum IgM levels with evidence of splenic atrophy. The analogy was made with celiac disease where the enteropathy had been clearly shown to be caused by gluten (85).

Fry et al. provided further conclusive evidence of the association between DH and celiac disease when they showed an improvement in the small intestinal mucosa, a reduction in the fecal fat excretion, and restoration of normal serum levels of folate and iron on treatment with a GFD. On reintroduction of gluten into the diet, these changes were reversed, demonstrating the specificity of the pathogenic role of gluten in the disease (22,23).

Gluten is the protein fraction that remains after flour is washed free of starch (11,107). In a Western diet, the main sources of gluten are wheat, barley, and rye. The major constituents of wheat flour are summarized in Figure 1. There is now good evidence that the prolamine fraction of the cereal (gliadin in wheat) contains the causative agent in celiac disease.

The mechanism by which gluten causes the enteropathy in celiac disease is not known. Initial suggestions that it was due to a direct toxic effect of gluten are no longer accepted, and the disease is not thought to be immunologically mediated (15,69). Both humoral and cell-mediated mechanisms have been proposed, but neither entirely explains the observed phenomena. Nield (74) postulated that gluten rendered the enterocyte of the small intestine “foreign”, and thus initiated a localized graft versus host reaction. Marsh (69), in a recent review of immunologic mechanisms in celiac disease, implicated cell-mediated immunity culminating in mast cell degranulation in the pathogenesis of the lesion.

The incidence of enteropathy in patients with DH in the initial series was approximately 70% (17,20,95). However, further studies have shown that gluten-sensitive enteropathy (GE) occurs in all patients with DH, but to varying degrees. First, multiple biopsy specimens of the small intestine have shown the enteropathy to be patchy, so that if only one specimen had been obtained, it would have been possible to have missed a morphologically abnormal area of small intestine (5). When eight biopsy specimens were taken simultaneously from the upper small intestine, the incidence of morphologic abnormality rose to 95%. Second, Weinstein (112) was able to induce structural changes in a previously “normal-looking” small intestine by giving patients with DH an increased amount of gluten in the diet. This response to gluten loading does not generally occur in normal individuals, although there has been a recent report of its

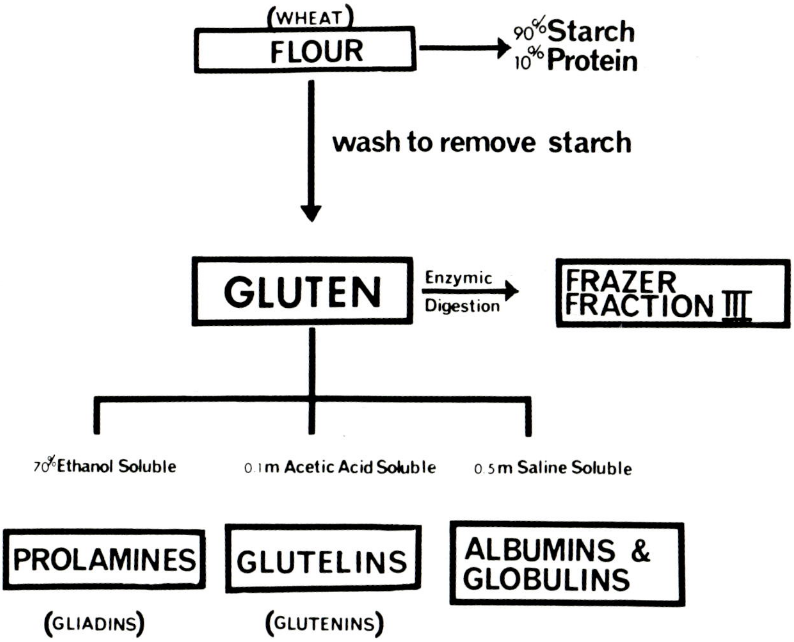

Figure 1. The composition of wheat flour.

occurrence in relatives of patients with celiac disease and in normal individuals with the histocompatibility antigen HLA-B8 (12). Third, it has been shown that regardless of the morphologic change in the small intestine, a histologic abnormality can be demonstrated in the majority of patients. The most useful abnormality is infiltration of the epithelium with lymphocytes, because this can be easily quantitated. The intraepithelial lymphocyte count is expressed as the number of lymphocytes per 1000 epithelial cells (24). There is also an increase in the number of lymphocytes in the lamina propria, but the cells here are more difficult to count reliably. The lymphocytes are presumably attracted to the mucosal surface as part of the immunologic response to gluten. Although the number of lymphocytes infiltrating the epithelium is increased in patients with DH, the predominance of T-suppressor cells seen in the normal gut is maintained (60).

It is possible that there is increased permeability of the small intestine to large molecules in patients with DH who have a morphologically normal small intestine. Recently described techniques using either probe molecules such as polyethylene glycol (44) or a ^{51}Cr-labeled absorption test (4) may help to demonstrate a physiologic abnormality in this group.

Effect of a GFD on the Rash of DH

It has now been established beyond all reasonable doubt that the skin lesions of DH are gluten sensitive. Within 2 years of the initial report of structural abnormality of the small intestine in DH, Fry et al. (21,22) described the effect on skin lesions of a 6-month trial of a GFD given to seven patients with DH. They found that two patients were able to stop taking dapsone, and another three showed a significant reduction in the dose of dapsone required to control the rash. There was a correlation between the fall in dapsone requirements and the improvement in small intestinal structure; that is, both the skin and intestinal lesions improved on the GFD. The same group of investigators showed that skin lesions of patients who had been on a GFD diet for 1 year and who required a significantly reduced dose of dapsone to control the rash or none at all, would reappear when gluten was added to the diet. Their dapsone had to be reintroduced or increased in dosage to suppress the rash. The intestinal abnormalities paralleled the dapsone requirements, in that there was a deterioration in the structure and function of the small intestine on reintroduction of the gluten. Fry et al. (22) therefore suggested that the skin lesions, as well as the intestinal lesions, were related to gluten, and that there was a direct relationship between the two. Nevertheless, a number of other reports (46,95,100,111) stated that the skin lesions did not improve with a GFD, and that the relationship between the skin and the small intestine was indirect. However, Fry et al. (23) stressed that the diet had to be strictly gluten-free to be successful, and had to be taken for many months before the rash could be controlled on diet alone. It was evident from the reports by Shuster et al. (95) and Weinstein et al. (111) that the diet had not been adhered to long enough to be effective, or that it had not been strict enough since the enteropathy was still present on further biopsy specimens while the patient was allegedly adhering to the diet (95). Support for Fry et al. (22) on the efficacy of a GFD in the treatment of DH has now come from many sources (19,36,39,47,62,68,81).

Fry et al. (29) reviewed their experience on the long-term follow-up of patients with DH with and without a GFD. There were 78 patients with DH included in the series, 42 of whom were treated with a GFD and 36 who had a normal diet and controlled their rash with drugs alone. Thirty (71%) of the 42 patients on the GFD were able to discontinue the drugs previously required to control the rash, compared with 5 (14%) of the 36 patients on a normal diet. The mean time taken to reduce drug requirements for patients on a GFD was 8 months (range, 4 to 30 months), and for stopping the drugs, 29 months (range 6 to 108 months). The incidence of macroscopic abnormality of the small intestine decreased from 69 to 15%, and there was also a significant reduction in the mean intraepithelial lymphocyte count. Conclusive evidence for the role of gluten in the causation of DH came from the study of Leonard et al. (57). They challenged 12 patients with DH whose rash had been controlled with a strict GFD for an average period of 7.6 years. The rash returned in 11 of the 12 patients after an average interval of 11.9 weeks from the start of the challenge. A biopsy specimen of the small intestinal mucosa obtained before the challenge and again at relapse of the rash showed a deterioration of the mucosa in 7 of 11 patients. The patient who failed to relapse on challenge probably represents the 14% of patients who enter spontaneous remission in DH (29). (Editor's note: See Chap. 27 for a review of findings of IgA-class endomysial antibodies in these 12 patients.)

The question still remains as to why all patients with DH do not respond to a GFD. Fry et al. (29) found that only 23 of the 42 patients who were on GFD were judged by the dietician to be strictly adhering to it. Twenty-two of these 23 patients were able to stop drugs completely, representing a success rate of 96% in this group. It should be noted that not all patients with celiac disease respond to a strict GFD, and the same may be true for DH. There have been reports that a milk-free diet in addition to a GFD may be necessary to control the rash in some patients with DH, but this remains to be substantiated (78). However, the most likely reason for failure of a GFD is that it has not been strictly maintained.

Increased Incidence of Malignancy in DH

Apart from gluten sensitivity, DH shares with celiac disease an increased risk for developing lymphomas (37,40,64,82). In a series of 109 patients presenting to St. Mary's Hospital, London, between 1969 and 1981, three developed a lymphoma (58). All three were described histologically as reticulum cell sarcomas. Only one of three lymphomas affected the small intestine; this lymphoma would now be classified as malignant histiocytosis of the small intestine (43). All three patients had morphologically abnormal small intestinal biopsy specimens at presentation of the rash. It is of interest to note, however, that two of the three patients had a normal jejunal lymphocytic infiltrate—an observation previously noted by Ferguson et al. (16) in the context of celiac disease complicated by lymphoma. It may therefore be that these patients have an abnormality in their immune response that eventually leads to the development of a lymphoma.

IMMUNOLOGIC ADVANCES

Immunologic Abnormalities in the Skin

The advent of immunofluorescence (IF) in the early 1960s gave dermatologists an invaluable tool for distinguishing between the blistering skin diseases. Beutner and Jordan (3) found immunoglobulins deposited in the intercellular (IC) spaces of the epidermis in pemphigus. The first report of immunoglobulins in the skin of patients with DH was that of Cormane (10), who found immunoglobulins in both the involved and uninvolved skin, although no mention was made of their class. In 1969, van der Meer (108) reported immunoglobulins in the uninvolved skin in 10 of 12 patients with a previous diagnosis of DH. The class of immunoglobulin was IgA, with IgG additionally present in a few patients. Van der Meer therefore showed that DH had an immunologic basis and one that was distinct from other bullous diseases. The presence of IgA in the dermal papillae of uninvolved skin in patients with DH is now the major laboratory criterion for the disease, and Fry and Seah (24) consider that the diagnosis should not be made without it.

Patterns of IgA Deposition

Chorzelski et al. (7) were the first to recognize the different sites of IgA deposition. They described two patterns of fluorescence: one in the dermal papillae and the other in a homogeneous line along the dermal-epidermal junction. Other groups of investigators have confirmed these initial findings (47,92), and that the papillary pattern is more common, accounting for 85 to 90% of patients. More recently, a third pattern of IgA deposition, termed granular-linear, was described (56,73). This consisted of a broken line of fluorescence along the dermal-epidermal junction. The three patterns of IgA deposition are described as presented below.

Papillary IgA Deposition. In this pattern, the IgA is predominantly deposited in the papillary dermis, although there may be extension up to the dermal-epidermal junction and down into the deeper dermis. The appearance may be granular, fibrillar, or clumped (Fig. 2). The IgA is thought to be bound to microfibrillar structures in the papillary dermis, and whether the appearance of the fluorescence is granular, fibrillar, or clumped depends on whether the fibrils have been sectioned transversely or longitudinally in the particular field being observed. It is not uncommon to have longitudinally

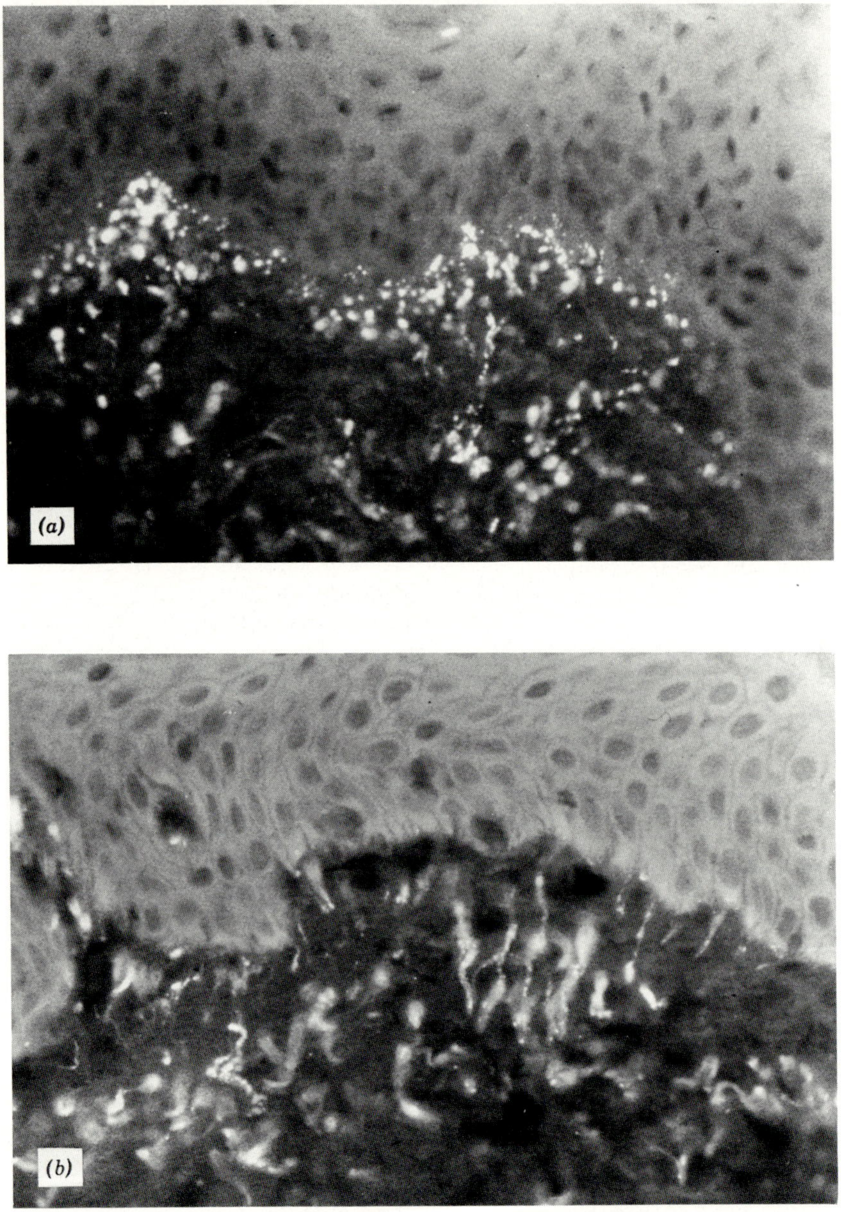

Figure 2. Patterns of papillary IgA deposition. A. Granular pattern. B. Fibrillar pattern. C. Clumped pattern. D. Granular, fibrillar, and clumped in the same biopsy specimen.

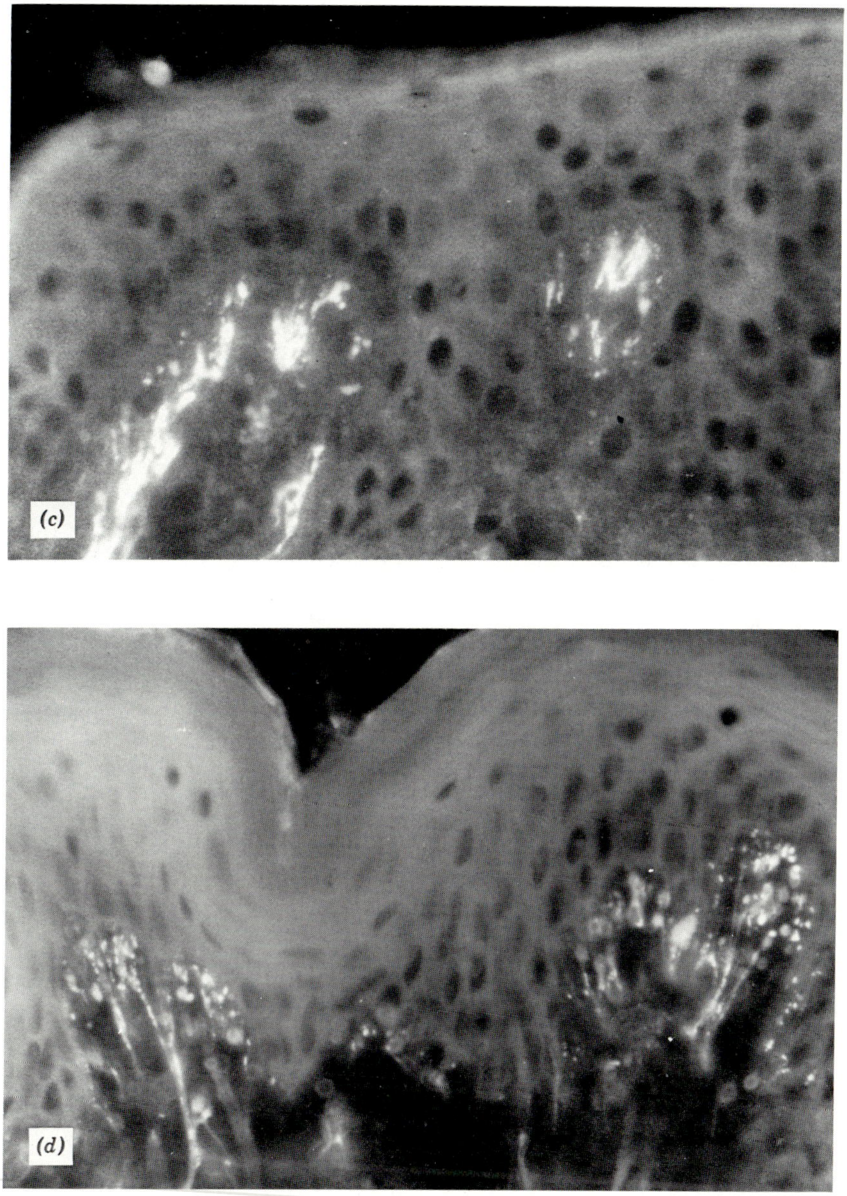

Figure 2 (continued)

(fibrillar) or horizontally (clumped or granular) sectioned fibrils in the same microscopic field. Rather than attach any pathophysiologic significance to these subgroups, it is simpler to describe them all as papillary.

HOMOGENEOUS-LINEAR IgA DEPOSITION. This pattern of deposition appears as a continuous line of fluorescence along the dermal-epidermal junction. There is no extension

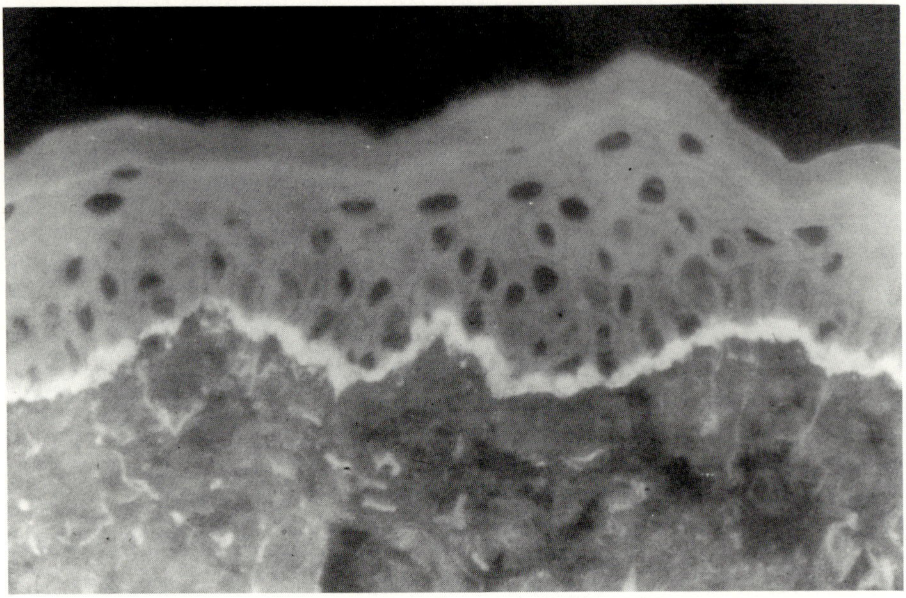

Figure 3. Homogeneous-linear deposition of IgA. A smooth unbroken line of fluorescence is seen along the dermal-epidermal junction.

into the papillary dermis (Fig. 3). The pattern is indistinguishable from that of bullous pemphigoid (BP).

GRANULAR-LINEAR IGA DEPOSITION. This pattern of deposition can be recognized by a broken line of fluorescence along the dermal-epidermal junction. It must be stressed that there is no extension into the papillary dermis (Fig. 4).

Consistency and Diagnostic Significance of the Patterns

Most investigative groups have found that the papillary and homogeneous linear patterns remain consistent in a given patient, both within a single biopsy specimen and between serial skin specimens obtained over a period of time and from different biopsy sites (32,47,48,62). There has been one isolated report (92) of both the papillary and homogeneous-linear pattern being found in the same biopsy specimen, but this is exceptional. The granular-linear pattern, however, is inconsistent. Both Mobacken et al. (73) and Leonard et al. (unpublished data) have found that on repeat skin biopsy specimens obtained over a period of time, the pattern of fluorescence no longer fulfills the criteria for the granular-linear type as it descends into the papillary dermis and becomes reclassified as papillary.

The current evidence indicates that patients with papillary IgA deposition should be classified as having DH. Those patients with the homogeneous-linear IgA pattern should be classified as having a separate disease termed linear IgA bullous dermatosis (LABD) by Chorzelski et al. (9). The reasons for regarding this as a distinct disease entity are reviewed elsewhere (Chap. 22 and 23). The granular-linear pattern is a rare finding. The inconsistency of the pattern on repeat biopsy procedure, and the fact that it only becomes papillary and never homogeneous-linear, indicates that these patients

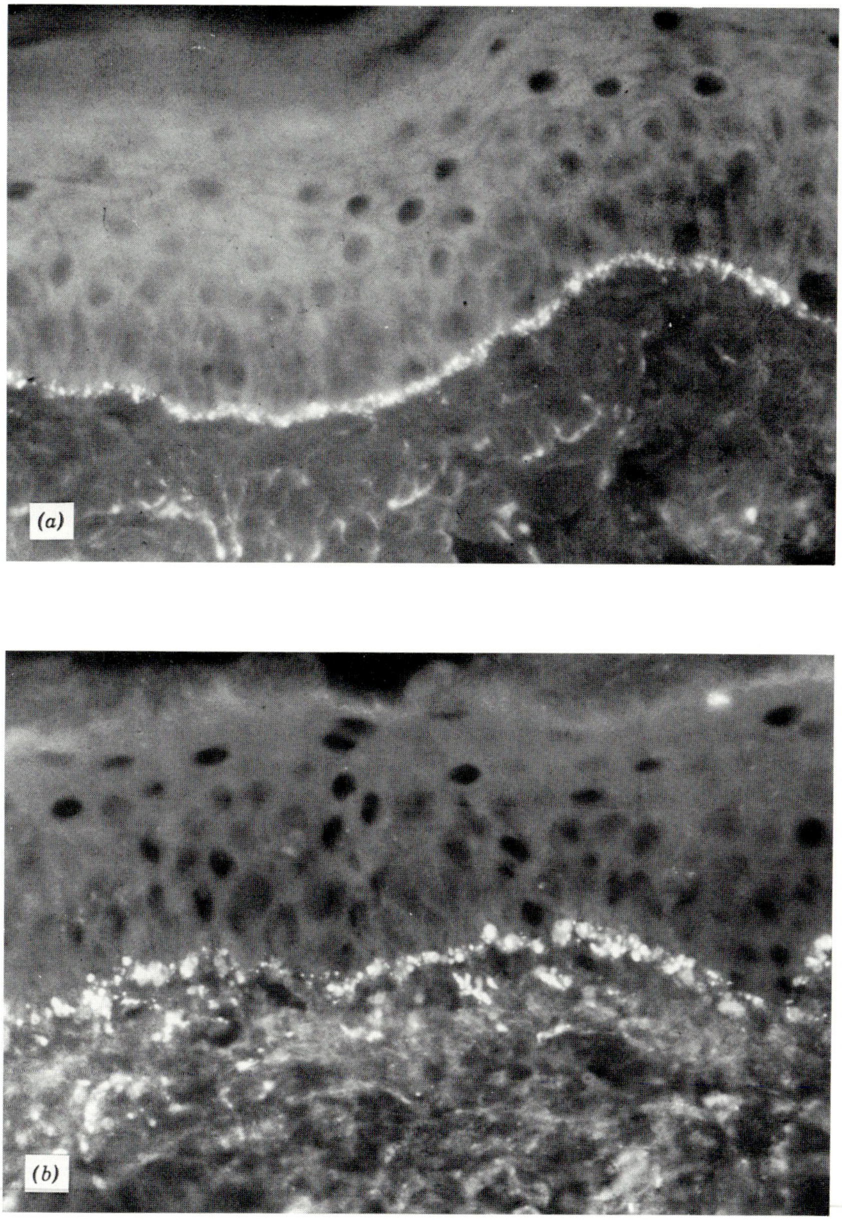

Figure 4. Granular-linear deposition of IgA. A. True granular-linear in which there is a broken line of fluorescence confined to the dermal-epidermal junction. B. High papillary deposition, which at first sight appears to be granular-linear, but may be distinguished by the presence of IgA in the papillary dermis.

form part of the papillary spectrum of IgA deposition and should be regarded as having DH. Distinction of the granular-linear pattern from the homogeneous-linear pattern is therefore of the greatest importance, and can only be done by careful examination of the section under high power.

Site of Attachment of the IgA

It is not known what structure the IgA is attached to in the skin of patients with DH. Initial studies by Seah (93), which compared the pattern of fluorescence with IgA antisera with that produced by silver stains, suggested that the IgA was bound to reticulin. More recent studies by immunoelectron microscopy (IEM) show the IgA to be bound within clumps in the dermal papillae, where they are closely associated either with anchoring fibrils (113) or with the microfibrillar component of elastic dermal microfibrillar bundles (96). Haffenden and Ring reported that the IgA was localized in large aggregates in the papillary dermis, and in small deposits lying in the bundles of collagen fibers (34).

Origin of the IgA

The association of DH with GE suggests that the IgA is of gut origin. This view is supported by recent work by Unsworth et al. (105), which showed that IgA in the skin of patients with DH contained J-chain and bound secretory component in vitro. The IgA was therefore predominantly dimeric and probably of mucosal origin. However, Hall et al. (35) using monoclonal antibodies (MCA) against IgA1 and IgA2, found a predominance of IgA1 which argued against a mucosal origin. These techniques are clearly at the limit of our current investigative capability and the results, although interesting, should be interpreted with caution at present.

How Specific is the Presence of Papillary IgA to the Diagnosis of DH?

The diagnostic value of IgA in the uninvolved skin of patients with DH was proposed by Fry and Seah (25) and supported by Chorzelski and Jablonska (8). It was questioned by Marks (67) and Ross et al. (84). Ross found that IgA was present in 4 of 15 patients with celiac disease, but it seems probable that these patients had latent DH. Seah et al. (89) studied the clinically normal skin of 22 patients with established celiac disease. Of the 22 patients, two were found to have immunoglobulin deposited in the skin. One patient had IgM and the other IgA in the papillary dermis. It was apparent on further study of the latter patient that she had had an itchy rash on the knees and elbows that had cleared on the GFD given for the celiac disease, suggesting that she had DH in addition.

Very occasionally, when the diagnosis of DH is suggested by the clinical features, response to sulfone therapy, and abnormal small intestinal mucosa, no IgA is found. In such instances, it is necessary to take serial sections through the skin biopsy specimen; if the result is still negative, a repeat biopsy procedure is needed. Seah and Fry (92), in a study of 50 patients, reported on two patients in whom the IgA was not found in the first biopsy specimen but was found in the second.

Ljunghall et al. (62), in reviewing the IF data from their laboratory, showed that none of the 1200 skin biopsy specimens obtained for other diagnostic purposes had papillary IgA, whereas 58 patients whose other criteria suggested DH had papillary desposits of IgA. Marks (67) argued that patients existed who clinically and histologically had DH and who showed a good response to sulfone drugs, but in whom it was not possible to demonstrate IgA in the skin. On the basis of one or two exceptional cases, they questioned the diagnostic validity of IgA deposits in DH. Fry et al. (28) reviewed the alternative diagnostic possibilities in patients with IgA-negative, dapsone-responsive dermatoses, and found that an alternative diagnosis could be made in nearly every instance; this was the same conclusion reached by Katz (47,48).

Which is the Best Site for a Skin Biopsy Procedure in DH?

Haffenden et al. (32) compared the intensity of IgA fluorescence in uninvolved skin biopsy specimens from three sites to try to determine which was the best for obtaining a specimen. They found no significant difference between the forearm, buttock, and thigh. Ljunghall et al. (62), however, found that the uninvolved skin from the buttock had a significantly higher intensity of IgA fluorescence than that of the forearm. Most patients prefer cosmetically to have skin taken from the buttocks rather than the forearm, and we have now made it our practice to obtain biopsy specimens from this site.

Effect of gluten on the Amount of IgA Fluorescence

Harrington and Read (36), in reporting their series of 10 patients with DH treated with GFD, found that two patients no longer required dapsone after 6 months on the diet, and that the IgA was no longer demonstrable in the skin biopsy specimens once the rash had been controlled by diet alone. Fry et al. (25) were not able to demonstrate such a rapid disappearance of the IgA, but did find that the amount of fluorescence was slowly reduced. It only disappeared from the skin in 4 of 23 patients who had been on a strict GFD for a minimum of 7 years (29). Similar findings were reported by Reunala (83), who found that 6 of 42 patients on a strict GFD lost the IgA from the skin, but only after a number of years. Another interesting observation is that IgA can still be demonstrated in the skin of patients who have entered spontaneous remission (56).

Leonard et al. (57) gluten challenged 12 patients with DH whose rash had been controlled with a strict GFD alone for a number of years. In three of these patients, IgA could no longer be demonstrated in the uninvolved skin at the time of challenge. However, the IgA deposits were demonstrated in all three patients 1 month after challenge, although one of them has not yet relapsed 3 years after the challenge commenced. In the remaining nine patients, there was no increase in the amount of the IgA fluorescence at the time of relapse of the rash compared with that prior to challenge.

Other Classes of Immunoglobulins in the skin in DH

Although all patients with DH have IgA deposition, IgG and IgM are occasionally found in addition. Chorzelski et al. (7) found IgG in six of their 19 patients and IgM in five. Seah and Fry (92) found IgG in two of their 78 biopsy specimens and IgM in seven. Of the nine patients who had IgG and/or IgM in addition to IgA, the pattern of immunoglobulin deposition was the same in eight. In the one biopsy specimen in which there was a difference, IgA was present in the homogeneous-linear pattern and IgM in the papillary. (This patient would no longer be classified as DH, but as LABD.) In the single biopsy specimen in which all three classes of immunoglobulin were found, IgA was present in the papillary pattern and IgG and IgM were present in the homogeneous-linear pattern. There appears to be no correlation between the presence of immunoglobulins other that IgA and any clinical or prognostic factors in patients with DH. Repeat biopsy specimens from a given patient with DH always show papillary IgA, but the other immunoglobulins may be present or absent. With the exception of the granular-linear pattern, the pattern of IgA deposition remains constant, while that of the other immunoreactants may change. This has led to the suggestion that the other immunoreactants seen in the uninvolved skin in patients with DH may represent secondary antibodies from damage to the basement membrane, or that they may simply represent the deposition of immune complexes of different classes with different affinity for the different structures of the basement membrane zone (BMZ) (27).

Complement in the Skin in DH

Van der Meer (108) found C3 component of complement in the uninvolved skin of patients with DH; this observation has since been substantiated by other groups of investigators (26,41,81). However, IgA is not thought to be able to activate complement by the classic pathway, and it had to be explained how complement came to be deposited in the absence of IgG or IgM. In 1971, it was shown that aggregated IgA was capable of activating complement by the alternate pathway (31). Seah et al. (91) reported on a detailed study of complement deposition, in relation to immunoglobulin deposition, in both the involved and uninvolved skin of patients with DH. These workers studied the deposits of C3 and C1q components of complement from 34 biopsy specimens obtained from 19 patients. IgA was present in all of these specimens, with IgG in three and IgM in nine. C3 was found in 16 (47%) of the specimens. The highest frequency was found in the subgroup of specimens obtained from an early lesion (eight of nine). However, C3 was also found in the uninvolved skin in three of nine patients whose rash was controlled with dapsone, and in three of eight patients whose rash was controlled with a GFD. C1q was present in only 3 of 34 biopsies; in one, IgG was present, and in two, IgM was present. These results were interpreted to imply that complement fixation in the skin of patients with DH occurred via the alternative pathway, as opposed to the classic pathway, and was due to the IgA. This view was supported by the work of Provost and Tomasi (79), who found evidence of alternative pathway activation in the skin of patients with DH. These studies demonstrated that complement is deposited in the skin in patients with DH and is likely to play some part in the pathogenesis of the skin lesion. In a recent evaluation of the influence of a GFD in DH (26), C3 component of complement was found in 12 of 18 patients who were on a normal diet and requiring dapsone to suppress their rash, but in only 3 of 19 patients whose rash was controlled by a strict GFD alone.

The concept that Dapsone acted by interference with the local activation of complement (72,79,99) is rendered less likely by the observation that C3 is present in two-thirds of patients whose rash is controlled by dapsone. Also, the dapsone concentrations required to suppress complement activation in vitro were many times higher than those likely to be present in vivo. An alternative explanation by Stendahl et al. (97), that dapsone acts by inhibition of polymorphonuclear enzymes, is an attractive one. However, polymorphonuclear infiltration is a feature of lesional skin in DH and not the uninvolved skin; it seems unlikely that this is the mode of action in this disease. A recent explanation proposed by Harvath et al. (38), that Dapsone inhibits the chemotaxis of polymorphs toward chemoattractants, overcomes both of these criticisms. It may be that there is constant low-grade, IgA-mediated activation of complement via the alternative pathway in the uninvolved skin of patients with DH that, for unknown reasons, can exceed the threshold of firing the complement cascade and produce lesions in certain sites. This threshold could be lowered by agents such as iodides, which are known to provoke blisters in patients with DH when applied to the uninvolved skin (1). Once chemotactic agents such as C5a are released into the skin, polymorphs are attracted into the upper dermis—a process that could be inhibited by dapsone (38). The polymorphs could then release enzymes into the upper dermis, which would lead to degradation of the components of the papillary dermis and dermal-epidermal junction, and lead to blister formation. The recent observation by Oikarinen et al. (75), that there are collagenases and elastases of polymorph origin in the blister fluid, is consistent with this suggestion. The reason that patients who are on a strict GFD do not produce skin lesions would be that there is less IgA in the skin to carry out the low-grade complement activation, and the threshold for firing the complement cascade would be relatively much higher. This hypothesis is supported by the lower incidence of C3 in the skin of patients on a GFD (26,62) and by the failure to induce lesions with locally applied potassium iodide in these individuals (33). This argument is clearly highly speculative and requires further experimental work to substantiate that of Harvath et al. (38) and Oikarinen et al. (75), as well as the development of methods for both eluting IgA from the skin of patients with DH to allow its characterization and investigating the role of iodides on complement activation.

Immunologic Abnormalities in the Serum

In the past, there have been many attempts to look for abnormalities in the serum levels of immunoglobulins in patients with DH. Although some abnormalities have been reported, they occur only in a minority of patients. Fry et al. (20) reported raised serum IgA levels in 1 of 12 patients studied, and also reported low serum IgM levels in one-third of patients with DH on a normal diet. These lower serum IgM levels, also reported by Fraser et al. (18), may be a manifestation of the lymphoreticular dysfunction that is known to occur in patients with DH (77) and celiac disease (70).

Auto-antibodies in DH

The methods for detection of relevant autoantibodies are given in Chapter 25. Here, we present an historic overview. Seah et al. (87) reported a high incidence of tissue-reactive autoantibodies in the serum of patients with DH. Gastric parietal cell antibodies, thyroid antibodies, and antinuclear antibodies (ANA) were particularly common. The incidence in DH was higher than that found in celiac disease, and Seah et al. (87) concluded that there was a more widespread immunologic disturbance in DH than in celiac disease.

Ljunghall et al. (59) found that autoantibodies were present in 29 of 43 patients with DH, and that 12 of these patients had more than one autoantibody. ANA were most commonly found. Zone et al. (117) found an increased prevalence of thyroid abnormalities in patients with DH. Of 50 patients studied, 2 were hyperthyroid, 5 were hypothyroid, 3 had thyroid nodules requiring thyroidectomy, and 5 had a symptomatic goiter. Thyroid autoantibodies (microsomal) were found in 38% of DH patients compared with 12% of age- and sex-matched but not human leukocyte antigens (HLA)-matched control subjects. Thyroglobulin autoantibodies were found in 12% of the patients.

Antireticulin Antibodies

In 1971, Seah et al. (88) described an autoantibody in the serum of children with celiac disease that was detected by indirect immunofluorescence (IIF) on a composite block of rat tissue. It appeared to be directed against a component of connective tissue. The staining was not abolished by pretreatment of the sections with collagenases, but was absorbed by treatment of the serum with adult human spleen reticulin. The pattern of staining was similar to that obtained with silver (90), and it was concluded that the antibody was directed against reticulin.

The incidence of antireticulin antibody in patients with DH is approximately 20% (53,90). The incidence is higher in adults with celiac disease—approximately 40% (2,53,90). The highest incidence of antireticulin antibodies is found in childhood celiac disease, where it is between 30 and 70% (6,90,102,109). Thus, the incidence of the antibody is related to the severity of GE, which is most severe in childhood celiac disease and least severe in DH. Lancaster-Smith et al. (53) confirmed this by studying a group of patients with DH and celiac disease. The more severe the enteropathy on a jejunal biopsy specimen, the higher the incidence of antireticulin antibody. The incidence of antibody is reduced in those patients on a GFD (53,90). It has been shown that in patients who have the antireticulin antibody present in their serum prior to a GFD, the titer of antibody gradually falls and eventually disappears from the serum (62,90).

The true significance of the antireticulin antibody has yet to be determined. The recent observation by Unsworth et al. (101) that gliadin binds in vitro to reticulin is of interest, particularly in view of the higher incidence of antireticulin antibody in patients with a severe enteropathy. It is possible that gluten in some way damages the reticulin of patients with GE and renders it immunogenic, leading to production of the antibody. Although IgA in the skin of patients with DH is thought to be attached to reticulin, there is little evidence for implicating the antireticulin antibody in the pathogenesis of the rash in the same way as, for example, the pemphigus antibody is held to be responsible. First, the incidence of antireticulin antibody is much higher in patients with celiac disease; and second, the majority of reports show the class antireticulin antibody to be IgG rather than IgA. An exception was the report of Ljunghall et al. who found that 12 of 15 positive sera had IgA-class antireticulin antibodies (59).

Antigliadin Antibodies

The associated GE has given rise to speculation that antibodies against gluten may play a pathogenic role in DH. Previous studies, however, have shown only 20% of patients with DH to have antigluten antibodies (13,42,52). In contrast, a recent study by Unsworth et al., using a newly developed IF technique (102) and a modification of the ELISA* technique, demonstrated antigliadin antibodies in 46% of patients with DH (104). Their presence correlated well with the severity of GE. Using similar techniques on the sera of patients with celiac disease, Unsworth et al. (103) found that all untreated children had antigliadin antibodies and that the titers fell on treatment with a GFD. Patients with GE, whether caused by celiac disease or in association with DH, tended to have antigliadin antibodies of both the IgA and IgG classes (51,71). It has been shown by the work of Salvilahti et al. (86) that the IgA-class antigliadin antibodies are the better indicator of GE, since the titers fall on a GFD in keeping with the clinical improvement of the patient, whereas the IgG-class antigliadin antibodies persist for longer time periods. The close relationship of IgA-class antigliadin antibodies in patients with GE and the fall in titer of these antibodies with a GFD (61,86,104) make their presence a useful screening test for GE in DH and a useful guide to response of the enteropathy, when present, to a strict GFD.

Antigliadin antibodies have not fulfilled their initial promise. The observation by Unsworth et al. (101), that gliadin was bound to reticulin, suggested that an immune complex consisting of gliadin and antigliadin antibodies of the IgA class might be produced in the small intestine and pass through the circulation to the skin, where it would bind to the reticulin through the gliadin. However, the inability to demonstrate gliadin in the skin of patients with DH and the finding that antigliadin antibodies are present in a higher incidence in patients with celiac disease make this suggestion untenable. Similarly, the possibility that antigliadin antibodies cross-react with reticulin in the papillary dermis of patients with DH seems unlikely. (Editor's note: See Chaps. 27 and 28 for reviews on IgA-class antiendomysial antibodies in DH and celiac disease.)

Circulating Immune Complexes

The regular finding of IgA and C3 in the skin of patients with DH has led to the suggestion that these individuals have circulating immune complexes (CIC) that give

*See list of abbreviations in the front of this book.

rise to the cutaneous deposition of immune reactants in the skin. CIC have been reported in a variable proportion of patients with DH, ranging in the majority of studies from 20 to 30% (47). Using the presently available sensitive assays, most investigators agree that about 20% of patients have immune complexes. Most of these assays are only able to detect IgG- and IgM-containing complexes. Zone et al. (115), however, described an IF assay for the detection of immune complexes of the IgA class and found them to be present in 30% of their patients.

Katz (48) described three methods to detect immune complexes: 1) the ^{125}I-Clq binding assay, which is able to detect IgG- or IgM-containing complexes; 2) the conventional Raji cell assay, which detected IgG-containing immune complexes; and 3) a modified Raji cell assay, which also detected IgA-containing immune complexes. They found the IgA-containing complexes to be present in 26% of patients with DH, whereas IgG- and IgM-containing complexes were found in only 13% of their patients. They also found that the presence of immune complexes did not correlate with disease activity or mode of treatment, and they concluded that the IgA-class immune complexes were not a primary factor in the pathogenesis of DH. Their test relied, however, on the ability of IgA to fix complement in the fluid phase, which is an assumption that may not be entirely valid.

The role of CIC in DH is uncertain. The main problem remains that there are as yet no entirely satisfactory methods for the detection of IgA-containing immune complexes. The finding of Lane et al. (54) that patients with DH and celiac disease have gluten in their sera, and the knowledge that these groups of patients have antigliadin antibodies, would indicate that such complexes should be present. Zone et al. (116) were able to induce complexes in patients with DH by feeding them with gluten. However, Yancey et al. (114) have demonstrated that gluten challenge does not influence the levels of CIC in patients with DH.

A failing of the current methods for detecting immune complexes is that they do not allow for detailed analysis of the components of the complex. Unsworth et al. (106) recently applied sucrose density centrifugation techniques to the demonstration of immune complexes in patients with DH and celiac disease, but the results were disappointing. Although there was evidence for complexes containing antigliadin antibody, these were present in no more than 30% of cases and usually were of the IgG class.

The current situation with immune complexes in DH is that there is no good evidence to implicate their role in the pathogenesis of the disease. It is worthwhile remembering at this stage that the clinical observations argue against an immune complex disorder; notably, that it takes an average of 28 months for the skin lesions to clear on a GFD and an average of 3 months to recur on gluten challenge.

THE IMMUNOGENETICS OF DERMATITIS HERPETIFORMIS

DH is extremely rare in patients who are not of Caucasian ancestry. The fact that genetic factors play a role in the pathogenesis of the disease was supported by the finding that DH, in common with celiac disease, is accompanied by a strikingly high incidence of certain histocompatibility antigens.

In the initial studies, 80% of patients with celiac disease, as diagnosed by findings of jejunal biopsy specimens, were shown to have HLA-B8, whereas only 20% of the control population had this antigen (14,98). In view of the similarity between celiac disease and DH, patients with DH were also examined for the presence of HLA-B8.

Initially, 58 to 78% of patients with DH were found to have HLA-B8 (30,46). When the presence of IgA in uninvolved skin became the diagnostic criterion for DH, the incidence of HLA-B8 rose to over 80% (80,94).

Pehamberger et al. (76) recently reported an increased incidence of another histocompatibility antigen—HLA–DR3—in patients with DH. The incidence of this antigen was found to be in excess of 90%—a finding similar to that in patients with celiac disease (50).

HLA-B8 and HLA-DR3 are coded by genes that are present on chromosome 6. Although the genes that manifest as HLA-B8 and HLA-DR3 on the lymphocyte surface do not actually code for the disease, they are thought to be closely linked to genes on the same chromosome that do and are split off with them during meiosis by the phenomenon of linkage disequilibrium. HLA-B8 and HLA-DR3 are found in a large number of diseases that are regarded as autoimmune in nature; therefore, it is of great interest that patients with DH have a raised incidence of tissue-reactive autoantibodies. On the other hand, the observation of Lawley et al. (55) that individuals with HLA-B8/DR3 have defective macrophage Fc-receptor function could fit in with the concept of immune complexes being responsible for the disease through their impaired clearance.

Katz (49), in a review of the immunogenetic factors relevant to DH, postulated a disease gene in linkage disequilibrium with HLA-B8 and DR3 that was one of two types. It could be either a gene controlling an antigen-nonspecific function that has an impact on a wide spectrum of immune responses, or a gene responsible for an antigen-specific abnormality of immune function with special relevance to the immune response to gluten. In support of the existence of such relatively unique disease genes is the finding of B-cell antigens, which are distinct from conventional HLA antigens, but nevertheless are coded for by genes on the major histocompatibility complex (63). In addition to the major histocompatibility complex, Kagnoff et al. (45) presented evidence that genes linked to the immunoglobulin heavy chain allotype locus of chromosome 14 may influence susceptibility to GE.

CONCLUSIONS

Over the past 15 years, several centers have studied DH in depth and confirmed the original observations that gluten is responsible for both the rash and the enteropathy of patients with DH, and that IgA in uninvolved skin is the best laboratory criterion for the disease. The finding that the IgA is dimeric would support the close immunologic association between the skin and the gut. Work on the immunogenetics of gluten sensitivity has confirmed the original finding that genetic factors play an important role in the pathogenesis of both celiac disease and DH. More recent work has indicated that the inheritance of DH is multifactorial, and it has given rise to optimism on possibility of finding why some patients develop DH while others only have GE.

The precise immunologic mechanisms by which gluten causes DH have thus far eluded current methods of investigation. CIC and antibodies have been demonstrated in the serum, but not in sufficiently high incidence to take credit for causing the disease. The answer clearly awaits the development and application of more powerful methods of immunologic investigation.

ACKNOWLEDGMENTS

We would like to express our thanks to all of the physicians who have referred patients with DH to our clinic at St. Mary's Hospital. We would also like to thank Professors

E.J. Holborow and R.M.H. McMinn for their long-standing collaboration in our research studies, and Professor H. Valdimarsson for his helpful discussions on the disease.

REFERENCES

1. Alexander JO'D: *Dermatitis Herpetiformis.* Saunders, London, UK, 1979, p 313.
2. Alp MH, Wright R: Auto-antibodies to reticulin in patients with idiopathic steatorrhoea, coeliac disease and Crohn's disease and their relationship to immunoglobulins and dietary antibodies. *Lancet* ii:82, 1971.
3. Beutner EH, Jordan RE: Demonstration of skin antibodies in sera of pemphigus vulgaris patients by indirect immunofluorescent staining. *Proc Soc Exp Biol Med* 117:505, 1964.
4. Bjarnasson I, Peters TJ, Veall N: A persistent defect in intestinal permeability in coeliac disease demonstrated by a ^{51}Cr-labelled EDTA absorption test. *Lancet* i:323, 1983.
5. Brow JR, Parker F, Weinstein WE, et al: The small intestinal mucosa in dermatitis herpetiformis: 2. Relationship of the small intestinal lesion to gluten. *Gastroenterology* 60:355, 1971.
6. Brown IL, Ferguson A, Carswell F, et al: Auto-antibodies in children with coeliac disease. *Clin Exp Immunol* 13:373, 1975.
7. Chorzelski TP, Beutner EH, Jablonska S, et al: Immunofluorescence studies in the diagnosis of dermatitis herpetiformis and its differentiation from bullous pemphigoid. *J Invest Dermatol* 56:373, 1971.
8. Chorzelski TP, Jablonska S: Diagnostic significance of the immunofluorescent pattern in dermatitis herpetiformis. *Int J Dermatol* 14:429, 1975.
9. Chorzelski TP, Jablonska S, Beutner EH. Adult form of linear IgA bullous dermatosis. In Beutner EH, Chorzelski TP, Bean SF (Eds): *Immunopathology of the Skin,* ed. 2. Wiley, New York, 1979, p 316.
10. Cormane RH: Immunofluorescent studies of the skin in lupus erythematosus and other diseases. *Pathol Eur* 2:170, 1967.
11. Dicke WK, Weijers HA, van der Kranier JH: An investigation into the injurious constituents of wheat in connection with their action on patients with celiac disease. *Acta Paediatr* 42:233, 1953.
12. Doherty M, Barry RE: Gluten induced mucosal changes in subjects without overt small bowel disease. *Lancet* i:517, 1981.
13. Eterman PK, Feltkamp TEW: Antibodies to gluten and reticulin in gastrointestinal disease. *Clin Exp Immunol* 31:92, 1978.
14. Falchuk ZM, Strober W: HLA antigens and adult coeliac disease. *Lancet* ii: 1310, 1972.
15. Falchuk ZM: Update on gluten sensitive enteropathy. *Am J Med* 67:1085, 1979.
16. Ferguson R, Asquith P, Cooke WT: The jejunal cellular infiltrate in coeliac disease complicated by lymphoma. *Gut* 15:458, 1974.
17. Fraser NG, Murray D, Alexander JO'D: Structure and function of the small intestine in dermatitis herpetiformis. *Br J Dermatol* 76:509, 1967.
18. Fraser NG, Dick HM, Crickson WB: Immunoglobulins in the skin in dermatitis herpetiformis and various other skin diseases. *Br J Dermatol* 71:89, 1969.
19. Frodin T, Gotthard R, Hed J, et al: Gluten free diet for dermatitis herpetiformis. The long term effect on cutaneous, immunological and jejunal manifestations. *Acta Dermatol Venereol (Stockholm)* 61:405, 1981.
20. Fry L, Kier P, McMinn RMH, et al: Small intestinal structure and function and haematological changes in dermatitis herpetiformis. *Lancet* ii:729, 1967.
21. Fry L, McMinn RMH, Cowan JD, et al: Effects of a gluten free diet on dermtological, intestinal and haematological manifestations of dermatitis herpetiformis. *Lancet* i:557, 1968.
22. Fry L, McMinn RMH, Cowan JD, et al: Gluten free diet and reintroduction of gluten in dermatitis herpetiformis. *Arch Dermatol* 100:129, 1969.
23. Fry L, Seah PP, Riches DJ, et al: Clearance of skin lesions in dermatitis herpetiformis after gluten withdrawal. *Lancet* i:228, 1973.

24. Fry L, Seah PP, Harper PG, et al: The small intestine in dermatitis herpetiformis. *J Clin Pathol* 27:817, 1974.
25. Fry L, Seah PP: Dermatitis herpetiformis. An evaluation of diagnostic criteria. *Br J Dermatol* 90:137, 1974.
26. Fry L, Haffenden G, Wojnarowska F, et al: IgA and C3 component of complement in the uninvolved skin in dermatitis herpetiformis after gluten withdrawal. *Br J Dermatol* 99:31, 1978.
27. Fry L: Dermatitis herpetiformis: Basic findings. In Beutner EH, Chorzelski TP, Bean SF (Eds): *Immunopathology of the Skin,* ed. 2. Wiley, New York, 1979, p 283.
28. Fry L, Walkden V, Wojnarowska F, et al: A comparison of IgA positive and IgA negative dapsone responsive dermatoses. *Br J Dermatol* 102:371, 1980.
29. Fry L, Leonard JN, Swain AF, et al: Long term follow-up of dermatitis herpetiformis with and without dietary gluten withdrawal. *Br J Dermatol* 107:631, 1982.
30. Gebherd RL, Katz SI, Marks JM, et al: HLA antigen type and small intestinal disease in dermatitis herpetiformis. *Lancet* ii:760, 1973.
31. Gotze O, Muller-Eberhard HJ: The C3 activator system. An alternative pathway of complement activation. *J Exp Med* 134(Suppl):905, 1971.
32. Haffenden GP, Wojnarowska F, Fry L: Comparison of immunoglobulin and complement deposition in multiple biopsies from the uninvolved skin in dermatitis herpetiformis. *Br J Dermatol* 101:39, 1979.
33. Haffenden GP, Blenkinsopp WK, Ring NP, et al: The potassium iodide patch test in dermatitis herpetiformis in relation to treatment with a gluten free diet and dapsone. *Br J Dermatol* 103:313, 1980.
34. Haffenden GP, Ring NP: Immuno-electron microscopy studies. In Kukita A, Seiji M (Eds): *Proceedings of the XVIth International Congress of Dermatology.* University of Tokyo Press, Tokyo, 1983, p. 408.
35. Hall RP, Nelson DL, Lawley TJ: Identification of IgA subclasses in the skin of patients with dermatitis herpetiformis. *J Invest Dermatol* 80:364, 1983 (abstract).
36. Harrington CI, Read NW: Dermatitis herpetiformis: Effect of gluten free diet on skin and jejunal structure and function. *Br Med J* i:872, 1977.
37. Harris OD, Cooke WT, Thompson H, et al: Malignancy in adult coeliac disease and idiopathic steatorrhoea, *Am J Med* 42:899, 1967.
38. Harvath L, Yancey KB, Katz SI: Selective inhibition of neutrophil chemotaxis by sulfones. *J Invest Dermatol* 80:321, 1983 (abstract).
39. Heading RC, Patterson WD, McClelland DBL, et al: Clinical response of dermatitis herpetiformis skin lesions to a gluten free diet. *Br J Dermatol* 94:509, 1976.
40. Holmes GKT, Stokes PL, Sorahan TM, et al: Coeliac disease, gluten free diet and malignancy. *Gut* 17:612, 1976.
41. Holubar K, Doralt M, Eggerth G: Immunofluorescent patterns in dermatitis herpetiformis. Investigations on skin and intestinal mucosa. *Br J Dermatol* 85:505, 1971.
42. Huff JC, Weston WL, Zirker DK: Wheat protein antibodies in dermatitis herpetiformis. *J Invest Dermatol* 73:570, 1979.
43. Isaacson P, Wright DH: Malignant histiocytosis of the small intestine: Its relationship to malabsorption and ulcerative jejunitis. *Hum Pathol* 9:661, 1978.
44. Jackson PG, Lessoff MH, Baker RWR, et al: Intestinal permeability in patients with eczema and food allergy. *Lancet* i:1285, 1981.
45. Kagnoff MK, Weiss JB, Brown RJ, et al: Immunoglobulin allotype markers in gluten sensitive enteropathy. *Lancet* i:952, 1983.
46. Katz SI, Falchuk ZM, Dahl MV, et al: HLA-A8. A genetic link between dermatitis herpetiformis and gluten sensitive enteropathy. *J Clin Invest* 51: 2997, 1972.
47. Katz SI, Strober W: The pathogenesis of dermatitis herpetiformis. *J Invest Dermatol* 70:63, 1978.
48. Katz SI. Dermatitis herpetiformis—the skin and the gut. *Ann Intern Med* 93:857, 1980.
49. Katz SI: Immunogenetics of dermatitis herpetiformis. In Kukita A, Seiji M (Eds): *Proceedings of the XVIth International Congress of Dermatology.* University of Tokyo Press, Tokyo, 1983, p 413.

50. Keuning JJ, Pena AS, van Leuven A, et al: HLA-Dw3 associated with coeliac disease. *Lancet* i:506, 1976.
51. Kieffer M, Barnetson R StC: Increased gliadin antibodies in dermatitis herpetiformis and pemphigoid. *Br J Dermatol* 108:673, 1983.
52. Kumar P, Ferguson A, Lancaster-Smith M, et al: Food antibodies in patients with dermatitis herpetiformis and adult coeliac disease—relationship to jejunal morphology. *Scand J Gastroenterol* 11:5, 1976.
53. Lancaster-Smith M, Kumar PJ, Clark ML, et al: Anti-reticulin antibodies in dermatitis herpetiformis and adult coeliac disease. Their relationship to a gluten free diet and jejunal morphology. *Br J Dermatol* 92:37, 1975.
54. Lane AF, Huff JC, Weston WL: Dectection of gluten in human sera by an enzyme linked immunoassay: Comparison of dermatitis herpetiformis and celiac disease patients with normal controls. *J Invest Dermatol* 79:186, 1982.
55. Lawley TJ, Hall RP, Fauci AS, et al: Defective Fc-receptor function associated with the HLA-B8/DRw3 haplotype. *N Engl J Med* 304:185, 1981.
56. Leonard JN, Haffenden GP, Ring NP, et al: Linear IgA disease in adults. *Br J Dermatol* 107:301, 1982.
57. Leonard JN, Haffenden GP, Tucker W, et al: Gluten challenge in dermatitis herpetiformis. *N Engl J Med* 308:816, 1983.
58. Leonard JN, Tucker WFG, Fry JS, et al: Increased incidence of malignancy in dermatitis herpetiformis. *Br Med J* 286:16, 1983.
59. Ljunghall K, Scheynius A, Forsum U: Circulating reticulin auto-antibodies of IgA class in dermatitis herpetiformis. *Br J Dermatol* 100:173, 1979.
60. Ljunghall K, Loof L, Forsum U: T lymphocyte subsets in the duodenal epithelium in dermatitis herpetiformis. *Acta Dermatol Venereol* (*Stockholm*) 62:485, 1982.
61. Ljunghall K, Scheynius A, Jonsson T, et al: Gluten free diet in patients with dermatitis herpetiformis. Effect on the occurrence of antibodies to reticulin and gluten. *Arch Dermatol* 119:970, 1983.
62. Ljunghall K, Tjerlund U: Dermatitis herpetiformis—effect of gluten restricted and gluten free diet on dapsone requirement and on IgA and C3 deposits in uninvolved skin. *Acta Dermatol Venereol* (*Stockholm*) 63:252, 1983.
63. Mann DL, Katz SI, Nelson DL, et al: Specific B-cell antigen associated with gluten sensitive enteropathy and dermatitis herpetiformis. *Lancet* i: 110, 1976.
64. Mansson T: Malignant disease in dermatitis herpetiformis. *Acta Dermatol Venereol* (*Stockholm*) 51:379, 1971.
65. Marks JM, Shuster S, Watson AJ: Small bowel changes in dermatitis herpetiformis. *Lancet* ii:1280, 1966.
66. Marks JM, Shuster S: Small intestinal mucosa in pemphigoid and sub-corneal pustular dermatosis. *Arch Dermatol* 100:136, 1969.
67. Marks JM: Dogma and dermatitis herpetiformis. *Clin Exp Dermatol* 2:189, 1977.
68. Marks R, Whittle MW: Results of treatment of dermatitis herpetiformis with a gluten free diet after one year. *Br Med J* ii:772, 1969.
69. Marsh MN: Immunocytes, enterocytes and the lamina propria: An immunopathological framework of coeliac disease. *J R Coll Physicians* (*London*) 17:205, 1983.
70. McCarthy CF, Fraser ID, Evans KT, et al: Lymphoreticular dysfunction in idiopathic steatorrhoea. *Gut* 7:140, 1966.
71. Menzell EJ, Pehamberger H, Holubar K: Demonstration of antibodies to wheat gliadin in dermatitis herpetiformis using ^{14}C-radioimmune assay. *Clin Immunol Immunopathol* 10:193, 1978.
72. Millikan LE, Conway FR: Effect of drugs on Pillemer pathway—dapsone. *J Invest Dermatol* 62:541, 1974 (abstract).
73. Mobacken H, Kastrup W, Ljunghall K, et al: Linear IgA dermatosis: A study of ten adult patients. *Acta Dermatol Venereol* (*Stockholm*) 63:123, 1983.
74. Nield GH: Coeliac disease: A graft versus host like reaction localised to the small bowel wall? *Lancet* i:811, 1981.
75. Oikarinen AI, Zone JJ, Ahmed R, et al: Demonstration of collagenase and elastase activities

in the blister fluids from bullous skin diseases. Comparison between dermatitis herpetiformis and bullous pemphigoid. *J Invest Dermatol* 81:261, 1983.

76. Pehamberger H, Holubar K, Mayr W. HLA-Dr_3 in dermatitis herpetiformis. *Br J Dermatol* 104:321, 1981.
77. Pettet JE, Hoffbrand AV, Seah PP, et al: Splenic atrophy in dermatitis herpetiformis. *Br Med J* 28:438, 1972.
78. Pock-Steen OC, Niorsson AM: Milk sensitivity in dermatitis herpetiformis. *Br J Dermatol* 83:614, 1970.
79. Provost TT, Tomasi TB: Evidence for activation of complement via the alternate pathway in skin diseases: 2. Dermatitis herpetiformis. *Clin Immunol Immunopathol* 3:178, 1974.
80. Reunala T, Salo OP, Tillikainen A, et al: Histocompatibility antigens and dermatitis herpetiformis with special reference to jejunal abnormalities and acetylator phenotype. *Br J Dermatol* 94:139, 1976.
81. Reunala T, Blomquist K, Tarpilla S, et al: Gluten free diet in dermatitis herpetiformis. *Br J Dermatol* 97:473, 1977.
82. Reunala T, Helin H, Kuokkanen K, et al: Lymphoma in dermatitis herpetiformis: Report on four cases. *Acta Dermatol Venereol* (*Stockholm*) 62:343, 1982.
83. Reunala T, Salo OP: Effects of long term gluten free diet in dermatitis herpetiformis. In Kukita A, Seiji M (Eds): *Proceedings of the XVIth International Congress of Dermatology.* University of Tokyo Press, Tokyo, 1983, p 411.
84. Ross IN, Thompson RA, Montgomery RD, et al: Immunoglobulin staining in the skin of patients with gastrointestinal disease. Specificity and significance of IgA deposition in dermatitis herpetiformis. In McNicholl B, McCarthy CF, Fottrell PF (Eds): *Perspectives in Coeliac Disease.* MTP Press, Lancaster, UK, 1978, p 217.
85. Rubin CE, Brandborg LL, Flick AL, et al: Studies of coeliac sprue III. The effects of repeated wheat instillation into the proximal jejunum of patients on a gluten free diet. *Gastroenterology* 43:621, 1962.
86. Savilahti E, Vilander M, Perkkio M, et al: IgA anti-gliadin antibodies—a marker of mucosal damage in childhood coeliac disease. *Lancet* i:320, 1983.
87. Seah PP, Fry L, Hoffbrand AV, et al: Tissue antibodies in dermatitis herpetiformis and adult coeliac disease. *Lancet* i:834, 1971.
88. Seah PP, Fry L, Rossiter MA, et al: Anti-reticulin antibodies in childhood coeliac disease. *Lancet* ii:681, 1971.
89. Seah PP, Fry L, Stewart JS, et al: Immunoglobulins in the skin in dermatitis herpetiformis and coeliac disease. *Lancet* i:611, 1972.
90. Seah PP, Fry L, Holborow EJ, et al: Anti-reticulin antibody: Incidence and diagnostic significance. *Gut* 14:311, 1973.
91. Seah PP, Fry L, Mazaheri MR, et al: Alternate pathway complement fixation by IgA in the skin in dermatitis herpetiformis. *Lancet* ii:175, 1973.
92. Seah PP, Fry L: Immunoglobulins in the skin in dermatitis herpetiformis and their relevance in diagnosis. *Br J Dermatol* 92:157, 1975.
93. Seah PP: Immunological studies in dermatitis herpetiformis. Doctoral Thesis, University of London, London, UK, 1975.
94. Seah PP, Fry L, Kearney JW, et al: A comparison of histocompatibility antigens in dermatitis herpetiformis and coeliac disease. *Br J Dermatol* 94:131, 1976.
95. Shuster S, Watson A, Marks JM: Coeliac syndrome in dermatitis herpetiformis. *Lancet* i:1101, 1968.
96. Stingl G, Honigsman H, Holubar K, et al: Ultrastructural localisation of immunoglobulins in the skin of patients with dermatitis herpetiformis. *J Invest Dermatol* 67:507, 1976.
97. Stendahl O, Molin L, Dahlgreen C, et al: The inhibition of polymorphonuclear leucocyte cytotoxicity in the treatment of dermatitis herpetiformis. *J Clin Invest* 62:214, 1978.
98. Stokes PJ, Asquith P, Holmes GKT, et al: Histocompatibility antigen associated with adult coeliac disease. *Lancet* ii:162, 1972.
99. Thompson DM, Souhami RL: Suppression of the Arthus reaction in the guinea pig by dapsone. *Proc R Soc Med* 68:273 1975 (abstract).

100. Trier JS: Dermatitis herpetiformis and coeliac sprue. *Gastroenterology* 60:468, 1971.

101. Unsworth DJ, Johnson GD, Haffenden GP, et al: Binding of wheat gliadin in vitro to reticulin in normal and dermatitis herpetiformis skin. *J Invest Dermatol* 7:88, 1981.

102. Unsworth DJ, Manuel PD, Walker-Smith JA, et al: A new immunofluorescent test for gluten sensitivity. *Arch Dis Child* 56:864, 1981.

103. Unsworth DJ, Kieffer M, Holbrow EJ, et al: IgA anti-gliadin antibodies in coeliac disease. *Clin Exp Immunol* 46:286, 1981.

104. Unsworth DJ, Leonard JN, McMinn RMH, et al: Anti-gliadin antibodies and small intestinal mucosal damage in dermatitis herpetiformis. *Br J Dermatol* 105:653, 1981.

105. Unsworth DJ, Payne AW, Leonard JN, et al: The IgA in dermatitis herpetiformis skin is dimeric. *Lancet* i:478, 1982.

106. Unsworth DJ, McCarthy D, Leonard JN, et al: Circulating gliadin-anti-gliadin immune complexes in dermatitis herpetiformis and coeliac disease. *Br J Dermatol* 109:690, 1983.

107. van der Kramer JH, Weijers HA: Coeliac disease—some experiments on the cause of the harmful effects of the gliadin. *Acta Paediatr* 44:465, 1955.

108. van der Meer JH: Granular deposits of immunoglobulins in the skin of patients with dermatitis herpetiformis—an immunofluorescent study. *Br J Dermatol* 81:493, 1969.

109. van Essen R, Savilahti E, Pelkonen P: Reticulin antibody in children with malabsorption. *Lancet* i:1157, 1972.

110. van Tongren JHM, van der Staak WJBM, Schilling PHM: Small bowel changes in dermatitis herpetiformis. *Dermatologica* 140:231, 1967.

111. Weinstein WB, Brow JR, Parker F, et al: The small intestinal mucosa in dermatitis herpetiformis: 2. Relationship of the small intestinal lesions to gluten. *Gastroenterology* 60:362, 1971.

112. Weinstein WM: Latent coeliac sprue. *Gastroenterology* 64:819, 1973 (abstract).

113. Yaoita H, Katz SI: Immuno-electron microscopic localisation of IgA in the skin of patients with dermatitis herpetiformis. *J Invest Dermatol* 67:502, 1976.

114. Yancey KB, Cason JC, Hall RP, et al: Dietary gluten challenge does not influence the levels of circulating immune complexes in patients with dermatitis herpetiformis. *J Invest Dermatol* 80:468, 1983.

115. Zone JJ, LaSalle BS, Provost TT: Circulating immune complexes of IgA type in dermatitis herpetiformis. *J Invest Dermatol* 75:152, 1980.

116. Zone JJ, LaSalle BS, Provost TT: Induction of IgA circulating immune complexes after wheat feeding in dermatitis herpetiformis patients. *J Invest Dermatol* 78:375, 1982.

117. Zone JJ, Cunningham MC: An increased prevalence of thyroid abnormalities in dermatitis herpetiformis patients. *J Invest Dermatol* 80:3631, 1983 (abstract).

25
Antireticulin and Antigliadin Antibodies in Dermatitis Herpetiformis and Celiac Disease

D.J. Unsworth

Jonathan N. Leonard

Lionel Fry

INTRODUCTION

Ever since the close association between dermatitis herpetiformis (DH) and gluten-sensitive enteropathy (GE) was recognized, the search has been continuing for a serologic factor that originated in the gut and circulated to the skin to cause the rash. The finding of IgA in the skin of patients with DH but not celiac disease supported this approach, and indicated that a target-specific autoantibody (as found in pemphigus and pemphigoid), or one that was directed against gluten and cross-reacted with structures in the papillary dermis, might be present in the serum.

Two circulating antibodies have previously been demonstrated in the serum of patients with DH and celiac disease. These are the R1 pattern antireticulin antibody and the antigliadin antibody (AGA). They are both found in patients with a severe GE for which their presence in the serum is a good marker. Recently, a third circulating antibody has been described in the serum of patients with GE whose titer appeared to be closely related to the severity of mucosal damage. The antibody was of the IgA class and reacted with the endomysium of smooth muscle—particularly that of monkey esophagus—and was termed the IgA antiendomysium antibody (see Chaps. 27 and 28). This chapter will describe the methods for the detection of all but the latter antibodies, and will discuss their significance in relation to the pathogenesis of the diseases in which they are found.

THE ANTIRETICULIN ANTIBODY

Background

The antireticulin antibody is detected by indirect immunofluorescence (IIF) on cryostat sections of reticulin-rich tissue. It was first described by Seah et al. (31) and thus termed because the pattern of reactivity closely resembled the tissue distribution of reticulin as stained histologically by silver impregnation methods (12). Reticulin is an antiquated histologic term and, even at present, the identity of the argyrophilic-connective tissue components is not known. Pras and Glynn (27) suggested that reticulin is composed, at least in part, of noncollagenous glycoproteins. Immunohistochemical studies have shown type I and type III collagens (42) and procollagens (25), fibronectin (34,42), and the noncollagenous reticulin component of Pras et al. (27,28) to be present in the areas stained by silver impregnation methods. However, recent studies (46) on the specificity of antireticulin antibodies have shown that they fail to react with collagen type III, noncollagenous-connective tissue or fibronectin. This suggests that the reactivity lies with other components of connective tissue yet to be identified.

Seah et al (31,33) reported an increased incidence of antireticulin antibodies in the sera of children and adults with celiac disease and DH. The association between antireticulin antibodies and active celiac disease has been confirmed by other groups (1,4,9,19,21,23,36,40,44,48). With the exception of Crohn's disease (1, 23, 33, 44), antireticulin antibodies are rarely found in diseases that do not have an associated GE. In DH, antireticulin antibodies tend to be found mostly in patients with severe villous atrophy (18,41). The overall results of the above studies put the incidence of circulating antireticulin antibodies at 35 to 100% in childhood celiac disease, 35 to 75% in adult celiac disease, 20 to 30% in adults with DH, and 15 to 25% in adults with Crohn's disease. The antireticulin antibody titer declines and eventually disappears on treatment with a strict gluten-free diet (GFD); in many cases, the titer reappears after gluten challenge (1,22,33). The antireticulin antibody is usually of the IgG or IgA class, although it has been suggested that antireticulin antibodies of the IgA class are specific for celiac disease (7,21,23).

Rizetto and Doniach (29) and Williamson et al. (48) described other antireticulin antibodies. These were directed against a range of intracellular and extracellular mesenchymal tissue antigens, and were present in sera from a variety of patient groups, including heroin addicts and patients with hiatal hernias, as well as patients with celiac disease and DH. With the exception of the R1 antibody (29), which is equivalent to the antireticulin antibody described by Seah et al. (31,33) and Alp and Wright (1), none of the other so-called antireticulin antibodies reacts selectively with reticulin; and, unlike the R1 antireticulin antibody, they do not give the complete reticulin pattern defined by silver staining.

The significance of the R1 antireticulin antibody is not yet clear, but several suggestions have been put forward. Ferguson et al. (11) considered that it was produced simply in response to dietary reticulin and played no part in the pathogenesis of GE. Seah et al. (32) suggested that an immunologic cross-reactivity might exist between gliadin and reticulin, but the evidence presented in support of this has been disputed by others who used a wide range of absorbants, including Fraser fraction III, whole gluten, and gliadin (1,4,23,43). Brown et al. (4) suggested that gluten protein might bind to reticulin, rendering it immunogenic. Unsworth et al. (38) provided evidence to support this by demonstrating that gliadins could bind selectively to reticulin in vitro.

Method for Detecting Antireticulin Antibodies

Antireticulin antibodies are detected by IIF, using defined techniques (3) on a substrate that is rich in reticulin. Cryostat sections cut from a composite block of rat kidney, liver, and stomach are used routinely.

The R1 pattern of staining is as follows: 1) In the kidney, the peritubular and pericapsular fibers are stained (Fig. 1A); 2) in the liver, adventitial fibers around the blood vessels and fine fibers in the parenchyma are stained (Fig. 1B); and 3) in the stomach, intergastric gland fibers and endomysium are stained (Fig. 1C). As the serum is diluted towards its endpoint, the fluorescence disappears first in the stomach, then in the liver, and finally in the kidney.

The R2 pattern of staining is seen as long strands of very thin and sharp fibers between the glands of the stomach mucosa. No staining is seen between the tubules or around the capsules of the kidney and the liver. The only staining that is seen is limited to short fibers around the blood vessels (Fig. 2).

Of the other reticulin patterns, Rs is the most common. This gives rise to staining around the sinusoids of the liver (Fig. 3).

Results

The Relationship Between the Type of Antireticulin Antibody and the Presence of GE (43)
The results of screening sera for the different types of antireticulin antibody as described above are shown in Table 1.

The results show that the R1 pattern of antireticulin antibody is associated with active GE in patients with celiac disease and DH. The R1 pattern of antireticulin antibody was not found in normal individuals. The other reticulin antibodies (R2,Rs) are found both in sera from patients with either DH or celiac disease and in sera from normal individuals. R1-type antireticulin antibodies are rarely found in other skin or gut diseases. They were found in 2 of 47 adults with Crohn's disease, none of 46 adults with ulcerative colitis, 1 of 29 adults with aphthous ulceration, none of 10 adults with bullous pemphigoid, (BP), none of 35 adults with linear IgA bullous dermatosis (LABD), none of 27 adults with pemphigus, 1 of 32 children with Crohn's disease, none of 12 children with ulcerative colitis, none of 5 children with BP, and none of 19 children with benign chronic bullous disease of childhood (BCBDC).

With very few exceptions, the titer of R1 antireticulin antibody in serum from patients with celiac disease and DH falls on treatment with a strict GFD. The R1 antireticulin antibody usually disappears within 4 to 8 weeks of starting the diet. The antireticulin antibody also reappears on gluten challenge in some instances. In children with celiac disease, for example, 1 of 15 patients was positive for antireticulin antibodies prior to challenge, compared with four patients postchallenge.

Discussion

The result presented in this section confirm the close association between the presence of circulating antireticulin antibodies of the R1 type and active GE as reported by other investigative groups (1,4,19,23,31,33,44). The presence of R1 antireticulin antibodies was found to be an excellent indicator of associated enteropathy, but the test failed as a good screening method because there were patients with biopsy-proven celiac disease who were negative for R1 antireticulin antibodies; that is, the incidence of false-negative

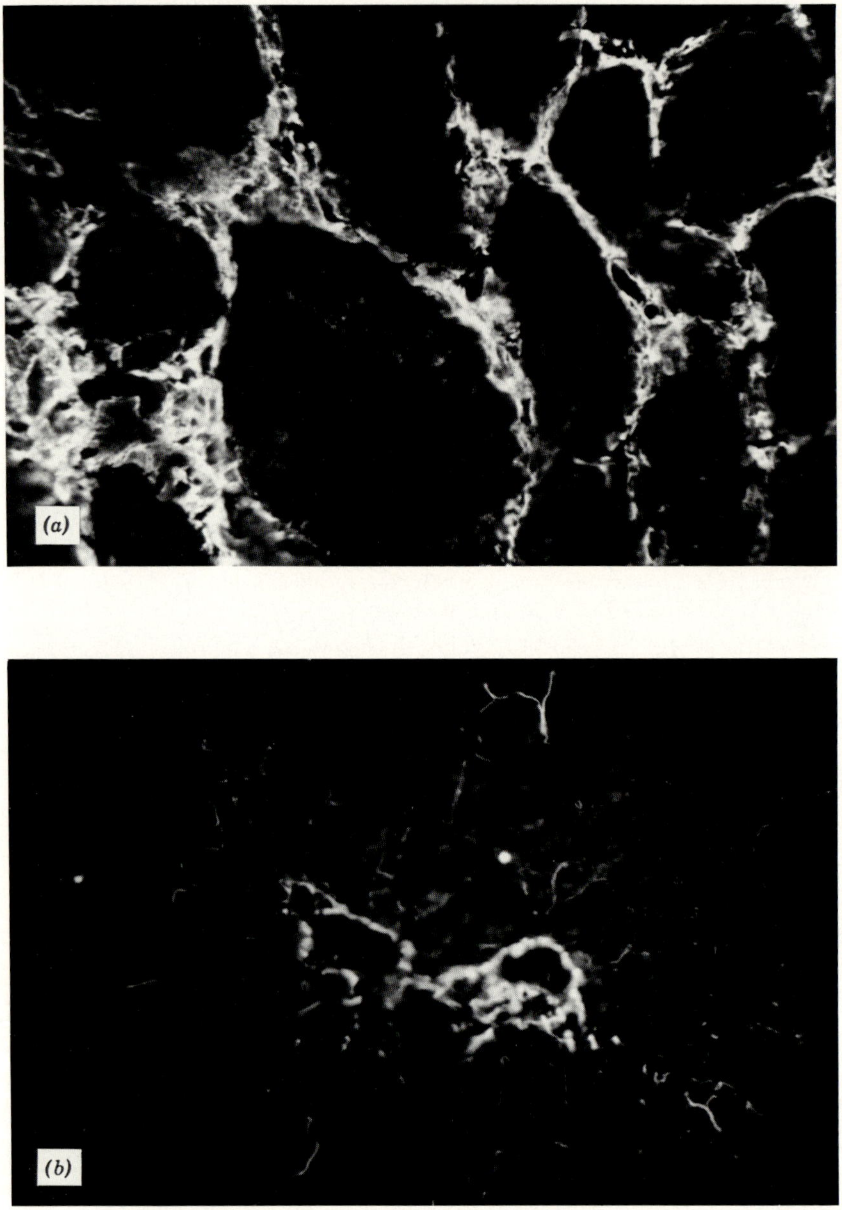

Figure 1. R1 pattern of antireticulin antibody staining. A. Kidney showing staining of peritubular and pericapsular fibers. B. Liver showing staining of adventitial fibers around the blood vessels and fine fibers in the parenchyma. C. Stomach showing staining of fibers between the gastric glands and of the endomysium.

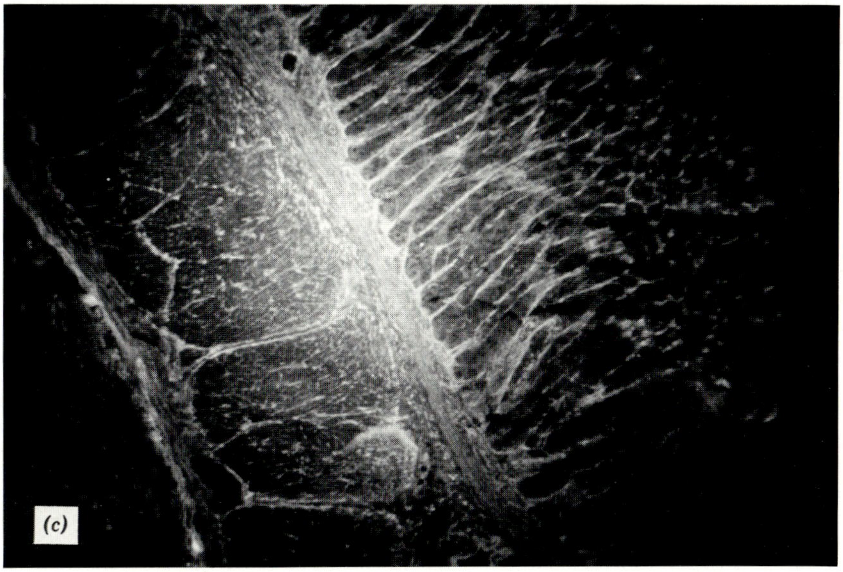

Figure 1 (continued)

Table 1. Relationship Between the Presence of Gluten Sensitivity and Type of Antireticulin Antibody.

Disease group	*Number of patients*	*R1* + ve	*R2* + ve	*Rs* + ve
Children: Normal diet				
Celiac disease	44	6	1	4
DH	17	2	0	0
Normal controls	18	0	2	1
Adults: Normal diet				
Celiac disease	31	7	3	4
DH	35	3	2	1
Normal controls	64	0	2	2

results was too high for an effective screening test. However, in our view the presence of R1 antireticulin antibodies justifies a small intestinal biopsy.

THE ANTIGLIADIN ANTIBODY (AGA)

What are Gluten and Gliadin?

Gluten is the protein moiety that remains after the removal of starch and water from defatted flour. Wheat gluten, which represents 10% by weight of flour, is composed of four main classes of proteins: albumins, globulins, gliadins, glutenins. These can be separated from one another on the basis of their differing solubilities in water, saline, 70% ethanol in water, and 0.1 M acetic acid, respectively (15), (Chap. 25). The gliadins

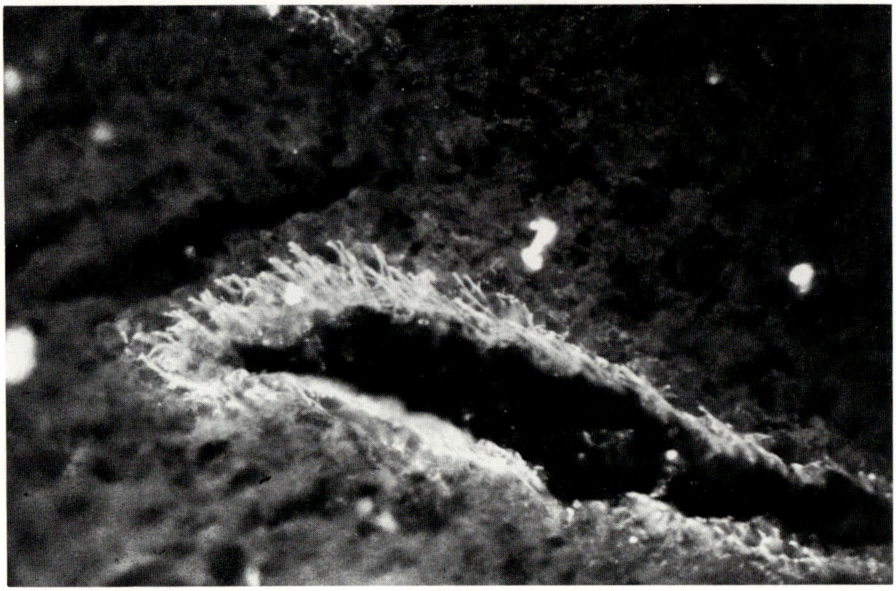

Figure 2. R2 pattern of antireticulin antibody staining in the liver, where it is limited to short fibers around the blood vessels.

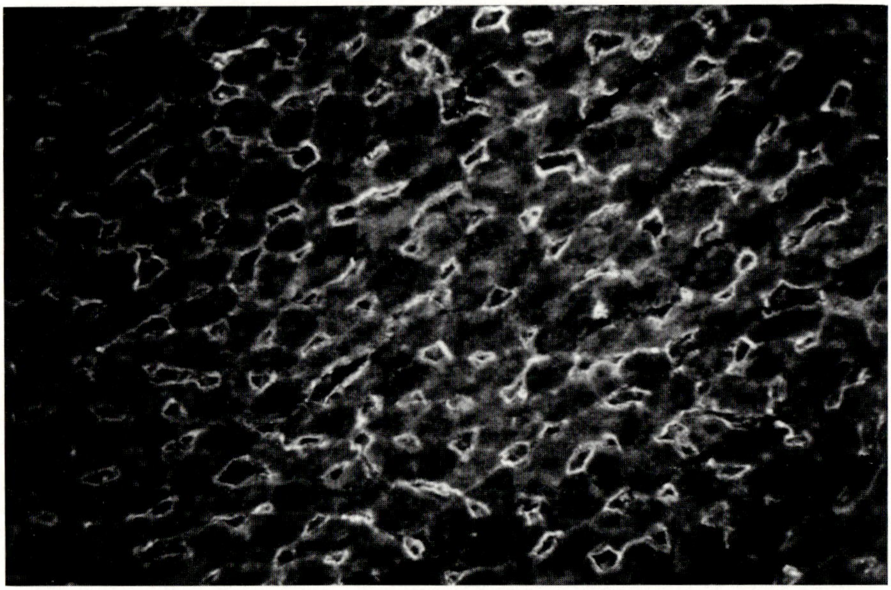

Figure 3. Rs pattern of antireticulin antibody staining in the liver, where it is limited to the sinusoids.

and glutenins are derived from the storage proteins of wheat endosperm, and are rich in glutamine and proline. The gliadin fraction is composed of 40 or more individual gliadins, with molecular weights ranging from 10,000 to 40,000. They may be separated from each other by ultracentrifugation (2) or by ion exchange chromatography (14,26). The identity of purified gliadins can be checked by starch gel electrophoresis or by polyacrylamide gel electrophoresis (6). Gliadins are grouped according to their electrophoretic mobility with the α−gliadins moving fastest, ahead of the β−, γ−, and ω−gliadins.

The Preparation of Crude Gliadin for AGA Tests

It has been shown that crude wheat gliadin extracts are just as good as purer extracts of gliadin in screening tests for gluten sensitivity (45). Crude gliadin is obtained from wheat flour by direct extraction with 70% ethanol in water (volume/volume) for 2 hours at room temperature, as described by Ewart (10).

The insoluble material is spun down at 900 g, and the supernatant is dialyzed with several changes against distilled water at 4°C. Precipitated material is discarded, and the water-soluble crude gliadin fraction is freeze dried. This crude gliadin fraction contains the expected range of α−, β−, γ−, and ω−gliadins as well as the minor wheat albumins, as demonstrated by polyacrylamide gel electrophoresis. It is always important to fully characterize any wheat protein prepared for use in screening tests.

Polyacrylamide Gel Electrophoresis. The method of Bushuk and Zillman (6) with minor modifications may be used with 5×10^{-3} M aluminum lactate (Prolabo Fance) buffered to pH 3.1. The gel recipe is given below.

> Acrylamide 12 g + N-methyl-bis-acrylamide 0.6 g + ascorbic acid 0.2 g + ferrous sulfate (90 g in 100 ml-distilled water) 10 ml + aluminum lactate (Prolabo) 0.5 g. Add lactic acid to pH 3.1 and distilled water to 200 ml.

The above mixture is prepared for each run and then chilled rapidly to about 1°C. Then 0.1 ml of 3% hydrogen peroxide is added as a catalyst and, after rapid mixing, the gel is poured into the cast as quickly as possible (at 4°C). The dimensions of the gel are 1 × 10 × 220 mm. Samples dissolved in 2×10^{-3} M aluminum lactate buffer, pH 3.1, are applied to the starting slots (10 mg in 20 μl).

We use an LKB multiphor flatbed electrophoresis set-up. The run is performed at a constant current of 20 mA (n/4 V cm^{-1}) for 3 hours (or 1 hour if fast-running albumins and globulins are being studied). The electrophoresis patterns are then fixed with 12% trichloroacetic acid and stained overnight with 0.25% Kanacid Blue in distilled water (5 ml of 12% trichloroacetic acid are added per 100 ml Kenacid Blue stain). Gels are destained for about 30 minutes with 12% trichloroacetic acid. The electrophoretic pattern given by gliadins from several different sources are shown in Figure 4.

Method for Detecting AGA

We use one of two methods in testing for the presence of AGA: IIF and the enzyme-linked immunosorbent assay (ELISA).

The IIF Test (40)

This test is based on the observation by Unsworth et al. (38) that wheat gliadin in aqueous solution binds extensively to reticulin fibers on cryostat sections of mammalian tissues in vitro.

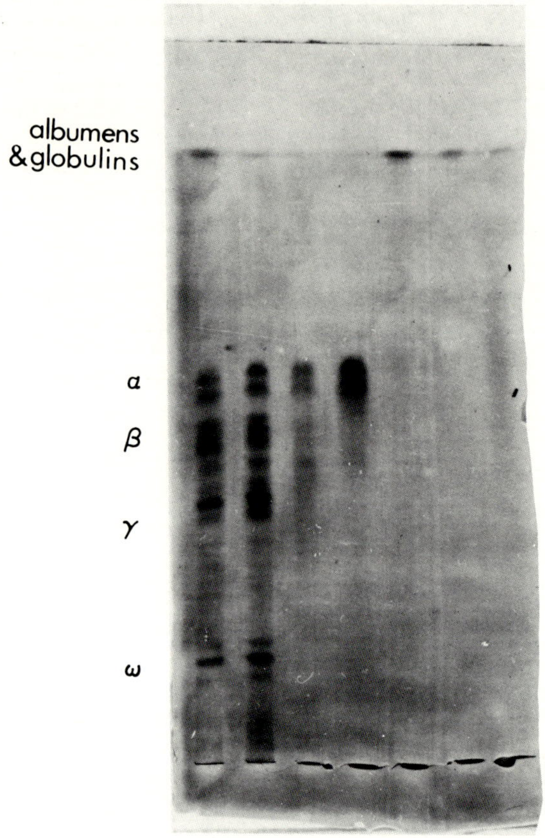

Figure 4. Polyacrylamide gel electrophoresis of seven standard wheat protein preparations. The wheat albumens and globulins run ahead of the gliadins as indicated. From left to right these were: 1) a crude extract of Flanders wheat flour; 2) a crude gliadin extract of Flanders wheat flour, but after repeated salt precipitation to remove contaminating albumins and globulins; 3) Flanders α-gliadins purified free of albumins, globulins, and γ- and ω- gliadins, but contaminated with β-gliadins; 4) α-gliadin; 5) Flanders wheat albumins and globulins removed from preparation (no. 1 above) by repeated salt precipitation; 6) wheat albumins and globulins extracted directly with saline; and 7) ethanol extract of a commercially available gluten-free product.

First, 6-μm thick cryostat sections of a composite block of rat liver, kidney, and stomach are allowed to dry in a forced draught for 1 hour. The sections are then incubated for 30 minutes with a solution of gliadin in distilled water (10^{-1} mg/ml) in a moist environment. The gliadin solution is then washed off the sections by immersion in a water bath containing phosphate-buffered saline (PBS), pH 7.2, for 30 minutes. The sections are then used to test dilutions of serum (1 in 10 and 1 in 40) by standard immunofluorescent (IF) techniques (3). Known positive sera are used as controls.

AGA-positive sera give a pattern of fluorescence on gliadin-pretreated sections that is indistinguishable from the R1 pattern of IF (29). Sera are scored as positive if the fluorescence is present at a dilution greater than 1 in 10.

In all cases, sera are tested on gliadin-pretreated and gliadin-nonpretreated sections in parallel. This is to prevent the inadvertent scoring of R1 antireticulin-positive sera as antigliadin positive. In our experience, sera in which both R1 antireticulin antibodies and AGA are present should be titered out to their respective endpoints. We have always found that the titer of the AGA is higher than that of the R1 antireticulin antibody. (We have cross-checked for the presence of AGA of lower titer using other methods of detection such as ELISA, to be described below.) Therefore, if antireticulin antibody activity (measured on a non-pretreated section) disappears on sequential titering before AGA activity (measured on a gliadin-pretreated section), the serum can be shown to contain both antibodies. Another point of difference is that the fluorescence of AGA disappears simultaneously from all three tissues on sequential titering, unlike the antireticulin antibody.

Positive AGA sera can be tested for class specificity by repeating the test on fresh gliadin-pretreated sections using class-specific antihuman antisera.

The ELISA Method

MATERIALS. The method used is basically the same as that described by Engvall and Perlman (8). The materials required for this test are as follows:

1. Micro-ELISA plates (Dynatech Ltd).
2. Horseradish peroxidase (HRP) conjugated antisera directed against polyvalent and class-specific human immunoglobulins. These antisera are used at working dilutions (usually between 1 in 100 and 1 in 1000) as determined by checkerboard titration.
3. HRP substrate—the HRP substrate is made up as follows:

   24.3 ml citric acid + 25.7 ml 0.2 M sodium phosphate + 50 ml distilled water + 34 mg O-phenylene-diamine (OPD) (Sigma chemicals) + 20 ml hydrogen peroxide (BDH Ltd). The substrate is light sensitive and must be prepared in a darkened bottle immediately before use.

4. PBS-Tween. This is prepared by mixing PBS with 0.05% Tween-20 (BDH Ltd). PBS-Tween is used to dilute all test sera and HRP-conjugated antisera, and for all working steps. Tween-20 is a detergent that prevents nonspecific binding of proteins to plastic plates. It is therefore never used in the antigen-binding step (see method below), but must be used thereafter in each step prior to the addition of substrate.

METHOD

Antigen-binding step. A solution of gliadin is made by dissolving it in 60% ethanol in water (volume/volume) to give a dilution of 20 μg/ml. Then 100 μl of this solution are added to each well on the ELISA plate. The plate is then incubated at 37°C for 2 hours, and then at 4°C for 14 hours.

Testing sera. The plate is washed twice with PBS-Tween to remove any excess gliadin. Patients' sera are then diluted in PBS-Tween to 1 in 1000, and 100 μl of this solution are added to each well. A known positive control must be added to each plate to quantitate the results. In addition, normal sera are used as controls. After 3 hours incubation at 37°C, the wells are washed three times with PBS-Tween. The wells are then incubated with HRP-labeled polyvalent sheep antihuman immunoglobulin for 3 hours, adding 100 μl to each well. The wells are again washed three times in PBS-Tween.

Then 100 μl of HRP substrate are added to each well and the plate is carefully observed. The end reaction depends upon the HRP-catalyzed breakdown of hydrogen peroxide producing superoxide, which acts upon OPD to produce a yellow reaction product. As soon as the known positive control is judged to have produced a satisfactory endpoint, the reaction is stopped in all wells by adding 4 M sulfuric acid (25 μl per well).

The optical densities are read at 492 nm in an ELISA reader (Dynatech Laboratories). Sera are judged to be positive if the optical densities of the reaction product are greater than 10% of the positive control. Sera are tested on gliadin-coated and uncoated (control) plates in parallel.

To find the class specificity of positive sera the test is repeated, substituting class-specific antihuman antiserum for the polyvalent antihuman HRP conjugate.

Results

Comparison of the IF and ELISA Methods (41)

Comparison of titers obtained on testing the same sera from adults with DH are shown in Figure 5. There was good interassay correlation. The ELISA test has the advantage over the IF method of not producing potentially false-positive results in patients with R1 antireticulin antibodies in their serum. This obviates the need for sequential dilution in screening these sera.

The Incidence of AGA in Patients with DH and Celiac Disease (39,41,43)

All 34 (100%) children with biopsy-proven celiac disease in one study were found to have AGA (39). In adults, the association was not quite as good, with only 27 of 31 (87%) patients having AGA. In DH, however, the incidence was lower, with AGA being found in only 6 of 13 (46%) children and 15 of 32 (42%) adults who were on a

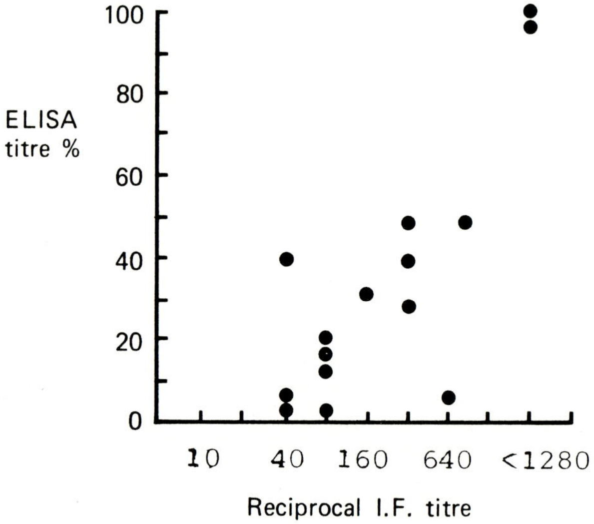

Figure 5. Comparison of titers obtained on testing the same sera from adults with DH for antigliadin antibodies by IF and ELISA.

normal diet. However, when the presence of AGA was correlated with the presence of GE in adults with DH, there was a good relationship between the severity of mucosal damage and the presence of AGA (41). There were no instances of a patient with a severely affected gut having negative antibody tests, and only one instance of a patient with a normal mucosa having positive titers of the antibody.

The Relationship of the Class of AGA to the presence of GE (43)
Sera from adult patients with celiac disease and DH on normal diets and GFD were tested by IF for the presence of AGA. Sera that were positive were retested using class-specific antisera. The results of these tests are summarized in Table 2.

With one exception, each of the positive sera contained AGA antibodies of the IgG class. Approximately half of the positive sera also contained AGA of the IgA class, and these patients had the most severe enteropathy. AGA of the IgM class were not found in any patient with DH, and were present in only two patients with celiac disease. Both of these patients were on a normal diet and, in both cases, AGA of the IgG and IgA classes were also present in the serum.

AGA in Diseases not Thought to be Related to Gluten Sensitivity (43)
The results of AGA screening in diseases that are not thought to be caused by gluten sensitivity are given in Table 3.

Table 2. Class of Antigliadin Antibody Found in Patients with Celiac Disease and DH

Disease group	*Number of patients*	*AGA*	*IgG*	*IgA*	*IgM*
Celiac disease					
Normal diet	31	27	26	12	2
Gluten-free diet	24	7	7	1	0
DH					
Normal diet	32	15	15	7	0
Gluten-free diet	14	0	0	0	0

Table 3. Antigliadin Antibodies in Diseases Not Thought to be Gluten-Sensitive

Disease group	*Number of patients*	*Number (%) positive*
Children		
Crohn's disease	32	14 (44)
Ulcerative colitis	12	1 (8)
BCBDC	19	0
BP	10	1 (10)
Adults		
Ulcerative colitis	46	2 (4)
Crohn's disease	47	8 (17)
BP	10	1 (10)
Cicatricial pemphigoid	27	6 (22)
Pemphigus	10	0
LABD	30	0

From Unsworth (.43)

The results show that the presence of AGA is not confined to patients with gluten-sensitive diseases. These results imply that their presence is secondary and not of primary importance in GE. It has been suggested that the presence of AGA is secondary to the presence of increased gut permeability due to gut damage. However, this cannot be the entire explanation, as they are not always found in children with enteropathies caused by agents other than gluten (e.g., cow's milk-sensitive enteropathy) (40). In the majority of instances of positive sera in these diseases, the class of antibody was IgG. The exception was in Crohn's disease, where over half of the sera that were positive had AGA of the IgA class in addition to IgG.

Effect of Gluten on the Presence of AGA in DH and Celiac Disease (20,42)
The titer of AGA in the sera of patients with celiac disease falls on treatment with a strict GFD. The AGA disappear, on the average, after 7 months in adults with celiac disease and after 5 months in children.

Sera from 15 children with celiac disease treated by GFD were tested for the presence of AGA pre- and postchallenge. Four patients were positive for AGA prechallenge compared with 14 postchallenge. Twelve adults with DH were similarly tested before and after gluten challenge. None of the patients was positive for AGA before challenge. At the time of relapse of the rash, however, five patients had AGA in the serum and, in all cases, these patients had abnormal jejunal biopsy specimens.

Discussion

The results of screening sera from adults and children with gut and skin diseases for AGA are in keeping with those of other investigative groups (9,13,16,22,24,35,36,37,47) that have used a variety of AGA detection methods. They found that a majority of adults and children with active celiac disease were positive for AGA, and that the AGA titer fell, eventually to zero, after some months on a GFD and rose again on gluten challenge. It was also shown that high-titer AGA were not exclusively associated with GE, but were also found in the sera of patients with other gastrointestinal diseases.

Other investigators, using a variety of methods, have also looked at the immunoglobulin class of AGA in patients with celiac disease and other gastrointestinal disorders (5,13,16,35). Their results were similar to those presented here, but because each group studied fewer patients, their results taken separately did not show the association between circulating AGA of the IgA class and active GE. In close agreement with the results reported here, the above investigators found AGA of the IgG class in all but one or two of the AGA positive sera that were studied, whether they were from patients with celiac disease or other gastrointestinal diseases. In contrast to the results presented here, IgM-class AGA were detected fairly frequently, although, in low titers. It may well be that the IF method is not good at detecting AGA antibodies of the IgM class.

Savilahti et al. (30) recently reported their findings in 31 children with celiac disease. They found IgA-class AGA to be a good marker for active GE. The titers fell rapidly when gluten was eliminated from the diet and rose again on reintroduction. IgG-class AGA, but not of the IgA class, were also found in children with diseases not thought to be gluten sensitive. They also found that the titer of IgA-class AGA fell rapidly in children with celiac disease with treatment on a strict GFD. The titers of IgG-class AGA, on the other hand, remained high even when the jejunal biopsy specimen had shown the mucosa to have returned to normal. However, it must be emphasized that even IgA-class AGA are not specific for GE. This has been shown in the results presented in this chapter, where they were found to be present in children with Crohn's disease, and also by a recent study (17) that clearly demonstrated the presence of AGA of the IgA class in patients with BP.

Despite the limitations mentioned in this chapter, AGA remains of real value in assisting in the diagnosis and management of children with celiac disease and DH (44). For example, the absence of AGA in a child's serum makes a diagnosis of celiac disease most unlikely, because all children with celiac disease were AGA positive. In those children tested who had DH, the presence of AGA was a good indicator of severe enteropathy. The presence of AGA, however, does not predict a diagnosis of celiac disease so accurately in adults; about 15% of adults with biopsy-proven celiac disease were negative on AGA testing. Nevertheless, the incidence of AGA of the IgA class in adults with diseases other than celiac disease was low. The presence of AGA, particularly of the IgA class, makes the probability of GE high and justifies obtaining a jejunal biopsy specimen.

As far as the management of patients with celiac disease and DH is concerned, a fall in the titers of circulating AGA would be consistent with a good response to a GFD, and would support the fact that the diet was being strictly adhered to. The titers would also help to judge the best time to repeat the jejunal biopsy procedure to confirm the improvement after gluten withdrawal.

The results of the two techniques described here showed a good correlation between them. There has also been work comparing the ELISA technique to the mixed, reverse solid-phase hemagglutination assay (Mrs PAH) (39,42) showing little interassay variability. Any of these methods can be used for routine screening of sera. The criticism that the presence of R1 antireticulin antibodies makes the IIF test for the detection of AGA difficult to interpret is not a serious one in practical terms. Sera should always be tested in parallel on gliadin-non-pretreated and gliadin-pretreated sections so that these sera can be identified. In any event, the presence of R1 antireticulin antibodies is a more specific marker than AGA for the presence of GE, and IIF, as described in this chapter, is a very effective screening test for this.

CONCLUSIONS

The diagnosis of GE can only be made with certainty by obtaining a jejunal biopsy specimen. It is necessary to show an abnormal mucosa while the patient is on a normal diet, improvement of the mucosa on a strict GFD, and subsequent relapse on gluten challenge. Jejunal biopsy is not a pleasant procedure, especially for a child, and any serologic factor that can be shown to be a reliable indicator of GE is of great value in the management of patients with suspected celiac disease. The data presented in this chapter, together with the results of other investigative groups, show the R1 antireticulin antibody and the IgA class AGA to be of value in predicting those individuals who should have a jejunal biopsy procedure, and also in monitoring their response to a GFD. However, the pathogenic significance of these antibodies is less clear, and the serologic factor responsible for the rash of DH has thus far eluded detection.

ACKNOWLEDGMENTS

We would like to thank Professor E.J. Holborow of The M.R.C. Immunology Group, The Bone and Joint Research Unit, London Hospital, for his contribution to the studies reported in this chapter. We would also like to thank all of the physicians who have sent us serum for the many collaborative studies summarized in this chapter. In particular, we would like to thank J.A. Walker-Smith, M.D., Professor of Pediatric Gastroenterology, and P Kumar, M.D., Senior Lecturer in Gastroenterology, St. Bartholomew's Hospital Medical School, London.

REFERENCES

1. Alp MH, Wright R: Auto-antibodies to reticulin in patients with idiopathic steatorrhoea, coeliac disease and Crohn's disease and their relation to immunoglobulins and dietary antibodies. *Lancet* ii:682, 1971.
2. Bernardin JE, Kasarda DD, Mecham DK: Preparation and characterisation of α-gliadin. *J Biol Chem* 242:445, 1967.
3. Beutner EH, Nisengard RJ, Kumar V: Defined immunofluorescence. Basic concepts and their application to clinical immunodermatology. In Beutner EH, Chorzelski TP, Bean SF (Eds): *Immunopathology of the Skin* Ed. 2. Wiley, New York, 1979, p 29.
4. Brown IL, Ferguson A, Carswell F, et al: Auto-antibodies in children with coeliac disease. *Clin Exp Immunol* 13:377, 1973.
5. Burgin Wolff A, Hernandez R, Just M et al: Immunofluorescent antibodies against gliadin: A screening test for coeliac disease. *Helv Paediatr Acta* 31:375, 1976.
6. Bushuk W, Zillman RA: Wheat cultivar identification by gliadin electrophoretograms. *Canadian J Plant Sci* 58:505, 1977.
7. Eade OE, Lloyd RS, Lang C, et al: IgA and IgG reticulin antibodies in coeliac and non-coeliac patients. *Gut* 18:991, 1977.
8. Engvall E, Perlman P: Enzyme linked immuno-sorbent assay—ELISA III. Quantitation of specific antibodies by enzyme labelled anti-immunoglobulins in coated tubes. *J Immunol* 109:129, 1972.
9. Eterman PK, Feltkamp TEW: Antibodies to gluten and reticulin in gastro-intestinal disease. *Clin Exp Immunol* 31:92, 1978.
10. Ewart JAD: Isolation of capel desprez gliadin. *J Sci Food Agri* 26:1021, 1975.
11. Ferguson A: Coeliac disease and gastro-intestinal food allergy. In Ferguson A, McSweeny RMN (Eds): *Immunological Aspects of the Liver and Gastro-intestinal Tract.* MTP Press, Lancaster, UK, 1976, p 178.
12. Gomori: Silver impregnation of reticulin in paraffin sections. *Am J Pathol* 13:993, 1937.
13. Huff WC, Weston WL, Zirker DK: Wheat protein antibodies in dermatitis herpetiformis. *J Invest Dermatol* 73:570, 1979.
14. Jos J, Charbonnier L, Mongerot JF, et al: Isolation and characterisation of the toxic fractions of wheat gliadin in coeliac disease. In McNichol B, McCarthy CF, Fotrell PF (Eds): *Perspectives in Coeliac Disease.* MTP Press, Lancaster, UK, 1978, p 75.
15. Kasarda DD, Bernardin JE, Nimmo CC: Wheat proteins. In Pomeranz Y (Ed): *Advances in Science and Technology,* vol. 1. American Association of Cereal Chemists, St. Paul, Min, 1976. chap. 4.
16. Kieffer M, Frazier PJ, Daniels NWR, et al: Serum antibodies (measured by Mrs Pah) to alcohol soluble gliadin in adult coeliac patients. *J Immunol Method* 42:129, 1981.
17. Kieffer M, Barnetson R, StC: Increased gliadin antibodies in dermatitis herpetiformis and pemphigoid. *Br J Dermatol* 108:673, 1983.
18. Kumar P, Ferguson A, Lancaster-Smith M, et al: Food antibodies in patients with dermatitis herpetiformis and adult coeliac disease—relationship to jejunal morphology. *Scan J Gastroenterol* 11:5, 1976.
19. Lancaster-Smith M, Kumar PJ, Clark ML, et al: Anti-reticulin antibodies in dermatitis herpetiformis and adult coeliac disease. Their relationship to a gluten free diet and jejunal morphology. *Br J Dermatol* 92:37, 1975.

20. Leonard JN, Haffenden GP, Tucker W, et al: Gluten challenge in dermatitis herpetiformis. *N Engl J Med* 308:816, 1983.
21. Ljunghall K, Scheynius A, Forsum U: Circulating anti-reticulin auto-antibodies of IgA class in dermatitis herpetiformis. *Br J Dermatol* 100:173, 1979.
22. Ljunghall K, Scheynius A, Jonsson T, et al: Gluten free diet in patients with dermatitis herpetiformis. Effect on the occurrence of antibodies to reticulin and gluten. *Arch Dermatol* 119:970, 1983.
23. Malgahaes AF, Peters TJ, Doe WF: Studies of the nature and significance of connective tissue antibodies in adult coeliac disease and adult Crohn's disease. *Gut* 15:234, 1974.
24. Menzell EJ, Pehamberger H, Holubar K: Demonstration of antibodies to wheat gliadin in dermatitis herpetiformis using the ^{14}C radio-immune assay. *Clin Immunol Immunopathol* 10:193, 1978.
25. Nowak H, Gay S, Wick G: Preparation and use in immunohistology of antibody specific for type I and type III collagen and procollagen. *J Immunol Meth* 12:117, 1976.
26. Patey AL, Evans FJ: Large scale preparation of gliadin proteins. *J Sci Food Agric* 24:1229, 1973.
27. Pras M, Glynn LE: Isolation of a non-collagenous reticulin component and its primary characteristics. *Br J Exp Pathol* 54:449, 1973.
28. Pras M, Johnson GD, Holborow EJ, et al: Antigenic properties of a non-collagenous reticulin component of normal connective tissue. *Immunology* 27:469, 1974.
29. Rizetto M, Doniach D: Types of reticulin antibodies detected in human sera by immunofluorescence. *J Clin Pathol* 26:841, 1973.
30. Salvilahti E, Viander M, Perkkio M, et al: IgA anti-gliadin antibodies—a marker of mucosal damage in childhood coeliac diseases. *Lancet* i:320, 1983.
31. Seah PP, Fry L, Rossiter MA, et al: Anti-reticulin antibodies in childhood coeliac disease. *Lancet* ii:681, 1971.
32. Seah PP, Fry L, Stewart JS, et al: Immunoglobulins in the skin in dermatitis herpetiformis and coeliac disease. *Lancet* i:611, 1972.
33. Seah PP, Fry L, Holborow EJ, et al: Anti-reticulin antibody: The incidence and diagnostic significance. *Gut* 14:311, 1973.
34. Stenman S, Valheri A: Distribution of a major connective tissue protein—fibronectin—in normal human tissue. *J Exp Med* 147:1054, 1978.
35. Stern M, Fischer K, Gruttner E: Immunofluorescent serum gliadin antibodies in children with coeliac disease and various malabsorptive disorders. *Eur J Paediatr* 130:155, 1979.
36. Stevens FM, Lloyd R, Egon-Mitchel B, et al: Reticulin antibodies in patients with coeliac disease and their relatives. *Gut* 16:598, 1975.
37. Taylor KB, Thompson DL, Truelove SC, et al: An immunological study of coeliac disease and idiopathic steatorrhoea. Serological reactions to gluten and egg proteins. *Br Med J* i:1727, 1961.
38. Unsworth DJ, Johnson GD, Haffenden GP, et al: Binding of wheat gliadin in vitro to reticulin in normal and dermatitis herpetiformis skin. *J Invest Dermatol* 7:88, 1981.
39. Unsworth DJ, Kieffer M, Holborow EJ, et al: IgA anti-gliadin antibodies in coeliac disease. *Clin Exp Immunol* 46:286, 1981.
40. Unsworth DJ, Manuel PD, Walker-Smith JA, et al: A new immunofluorescent test for gluten sensitivity. *Arch Dis Childhood* 56:864, 1981.
41. Unsworth DJ, Leonard JN, McMinn RMH, et al: Anti-gliadin antibodies and small intestinal mucosal damage in dermatitis herpetiformis. *Br J Dermatol* 105:653, 1981.
42. Unsworth DJ, Scott DL, Almond TJ, et al: Studies on reticulin I. *Br J Exp Pathol* 63:154, 1982.
43. Unsworth DJ: Humoral immunity in gluten sensitive enteropathy. Doctoral Thesis, University of London, London, UK, 1983.
44. Unsworth DJ, Walker-Smith JA, Holborow EJ: Gliadin and reticulin antibodies in childhood coeliac disease. *Lancet* i:874, 1983. (See also correction, *Lancet* i:1058, 1983)
45. Unsworth DJ, Holborow EJ, Kumar PJ, et al: Gliadin antibody levels in screening tests for coeliac disease. *Br Med J* 288:69, 1984.

46. Unsworth DJ, Scott DL, Walton KW, et al: Failure to demonstrate reactivity of anti-reticulin antibody with fibronectin, collagen type III or non-collagenous reticulin component. *Clin Exp Immunol* 57:609, 1984.

47. Varnio E, Kalimo K, Reunala T, et al: Circulating IgA and IgG antigliadin antibodies in dermatitis herpetiformis detected by the enzyme linked immunosorbent assay. *Arch Dermatol Res* 275:15, 1983.

48. Williamson N, Asquith P, Stokes PL, et al: Anticonnective tissue and other antitissue antibodies in the sera of patients with coeliac disease compared with the findings in a mixed hospital population. *J Clin Pathol* 29:484, 1976.

26
Uses of Antigliadin Antibody Tests

Jonathan N. Leonard
D.J. Unsworth
Lionel Fry

INTRODUCTION

In this chapter, we address ourselves to three groups of questions that were posed by the editors of this volume following their review of the preceding two chapters; notably:

1. Are antigliadin antibodies (AGA) specific for diagnosing celiac disease and dermatitis herpetiformis (DH)? What is the incidence of AGA in control subjects with gastrointestinal disorders other than celiac disease and in bullous disorders other than DH?
2. What is the relationship of AGA to histopathologic changes, gluten-free diet (GFD) and genetic factors? Specifically, can one replace histopathologic studies of gut biopsy specimens with tests for AGA? Can the level in serum be used as a marker to follow treatment responses? Is there an association between AGA levels and the genetic make-up of patients?
3. In view of the fact that various methods for detecting AGA give divergent results, as reported by many investigators, how can these differences be reduced or reconciled?

The following sections address these questions from our personal experience (9,10).

DIAGNOSTIC USE OF ANTIGLIADIN ANTIBODIES

Children and adults must be considered separately because the results are different among the age groups.

Children with Celiac Disease and DH

All children studied thus far with a firm diagnosis of celiac disease have had AGA in their serum. Approximately 15% of gastrointestinal disease control subjects are also positive. In children, therefore, the absence of AGA is useful in excluding a diagnosis of celiac disease, but the presence of AGA per se cannot prove it (Table 1) (6,8).

Table 1. Incidence of AGA in Children Under Investigation for Gastrointestinal Diseases

Disease groups	*No. studied*	*No. AGA positive*
Provisional celiac disease (untreated)	32	32 (100%)
Confirmed celiac disease (postgluten challenge)	34	34 (100%)
Celiac disease (provisional and confirmed) on GFD for 3 mo	54	21 (39%)
Transient gluten intolerance	15	7 (36%)
Cow's milk-sensitive enteropathy (untreated)	18	7 (39%)
Cow's milk-sensitive enteropathy (on milk-free diet)	12	1 (8%)
Multiple food protein intolerance	18	6 (33%)
Food allergy	7	1 (14%)
Crohn's disease	32	14 (44%)
Ulcerative colitis	12	1 (8%)
Toddler's diarrhea	34	3 (9%)
Gambian children	30	1 (3%)
Intractable diarrhea	12	0 (0%)
Postenteritis syndrome	11	1 (9%)
Miscellaneous gastrointestinal diseases	60	8 (13%)

Table 2. Incidence of AGA in Children Under Investigation for Skin Disease

Patients	*No. studied*	*No. AGA positive*
DH (normal diet)	13	6 (46%)
DH (GFD for over 3 mo)	4	2 (50%)
Pemphigus	5	0 (0%)
BCBDC	19	0 (0%)

Table 3. Incidence of AGA in Adults Under Investigation for Gastrointestinal Disease

Patients	*No. studied*	*No. AGA positive*
Celiac disease (normal diet)	31	27 (87%)
Celiac disease (GFD over 3 mo)	24	7 (29%)
Crohn's disease	47	8 (17%)
Ulcerative colitis	46	2 (4%)
Liver diseases	22	0 (0%)
Aphthous ulceration	29	4 (14%)
Miscellaneous gastrointestinal conditions	30	0 (0%)
Healthy adults (controls)	64	0 (0%)

AGA of the IgA class are more disease specific than those of the IgG or IgM class. With the exception of Crohn's disease (where they are present in 15% of positive sera), they were only found occasionally in disease controls subjects (9). However, IgA-class AGA are not found in all children with proven celiac disease—the remainder have IgG-class AGA, which are nonspecific. Thus, the IgG-class AGA are less specific for celiac disease of children, but provide a better screen as there are no false-negatives.

Forty-six percent of children with DH had AGA in the serum compared with none of 24 children with other bullous disorders (Table 2).

Adults with Celiac Disease and DH

Between 75 and 90% of adults with proven celiac disease have AGA. AGA are therefore not such a good screening test for potential celiacs as in children. Up to 17% of patients with other gastrointestinal disorders are positive (Table 3). The incidence of AGA in 64 healthy adult volunteers (laboratory staff) was zero.

Forty-seven percent of adults with DH have AGA in the serum. The AGA were found in highest incidence and highest titer in those patients with the most severe enteropathy. AGA were found in only a small number of patients with other skin diseases (Table 4). They were found particularly in patients with cicatricial pemphigoid (6 of 27) (4) and bullous pemphigoid (1 of 10) (9). (A higher incidence of AGA in other skin diseases has been reported by Kieffer and Barnetson [1].) Of the six patients with

Table 4. Incidence of AGA in Adults with Skin Disease

Disease group	*No. studied*	*No. AGA positive*
DH (normal diet)	32	15 (47%)
DH (On GFD for over 3 mo)	14	0 (0%)
Linear IgA bullous dermatosis	34	0 (0%)
BP	10	1 (10%)
Cicatricial pemphigoid	27	6 (22%)
Pemphigus	10	0 (0%)
Psoriasis	20	0 (0%)

cicatricial pemphigoid who had AGA-positive sera, five have had a jejunal biopsy procedure, but only one has had any macroscopic abnormality. In all six cases, the AGA were of the IgG class, which confirms the nonspecificity of this class of AGA. As yet, no adequate explanation has been given for their presence in diseases other than DH and celiac disease (see also data in Chap. 28).

RELATIONSHIP OF ANTIGLIADIN ANTIBODIES TO HISTOPATHOLOGY AND GFD

Histopathologic studies cannot be replaced by serologic tests for AGA. Although AGA provide a useful screen for whether a biopsy procedure is merited, no firm diagnosis can be made in the absence of a biopsy. It thus reduces the potential risk for unnecessary distress of patients, particularly children, by eliminating unnecessary jejunal biopsy procedures. It cannot replace the histopathologic studies of a biopsy specimen for confirmation of the diagnosis, as there are false-positives in children (e.g., Crohn's disease) and false-negatives (13% of our cases of celiac disease) in adults.

The presence of AGA is valuable for assessing the response to therapy. The IgA antibody disappears early in our experience—within 2 months of starting the diet. The IgG antibody persists longer—6 months to 1 year. Therefore, IgA-class AGA, when present at the outset of therapy with a GFD, are more sensitive markers for patient compliance (9,10). Other investigative groups have also found that the titers of AGA fall in response to a strict GFD. Savilahti et al. (5) have shown a sharp fall in the IgA-class AGA titers in children with celiac disease after 3 months on a diet, and there was a further decrease as the diet continued. Kieffer and Barnetson (3) found a significant fall in IgG-class AGA in adult patients with DH who kept to a GFD to such an extent that their dapsone requirements fell.

Our studies of the role of genetic markers has led us to the conclusion that there is no apparent relationship between HLA-B8 and an AGA titer (Fig. 1) or the presence of RI-type antireticulin antibodies.

ASSESSMENT OF METHODS FOR ANTIGLIADIN ANTIBODY DETECTION

A distinction must be drawn between published data over the past 4 to 5 years, in which the differences between groups are not all that great, and older reports where there was some disparity. A number of possible explanations account for this. Most importantly both the immunologic techniques and the preparation of gliadin available for use as a

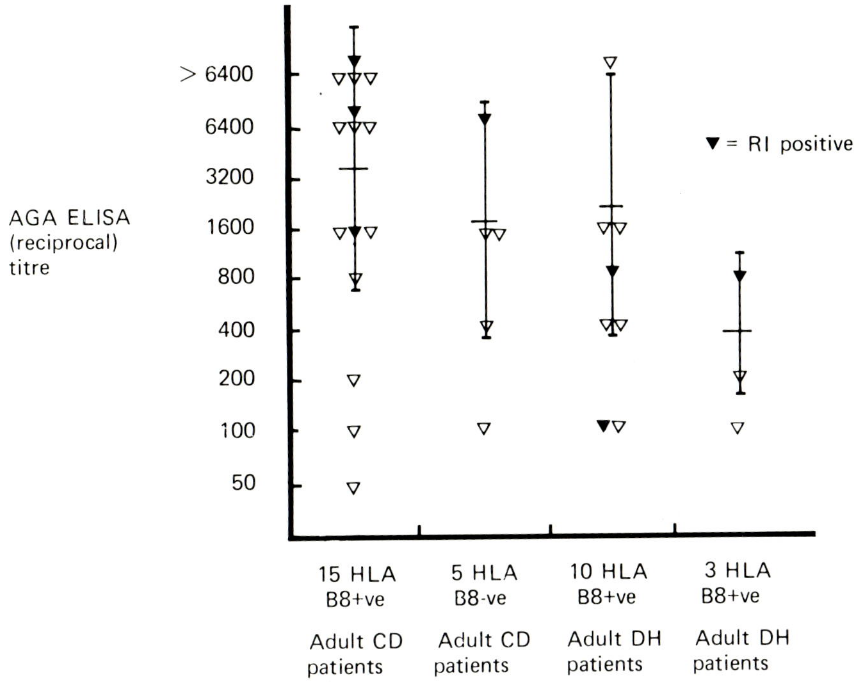

Figure 1 Possession of HLA B8 and hyper-responsiveness to gliadin.

substrate have improved, allowing for more sensitive assays and better reproducibility; that is, the tests are more easily standardized. The important distinction between the findings in children and adults with a gluten-sensitive enteropathy is now appreciated, and this removes a major source of inaccuracy when comparing studies. Also, there has been more awareness of the importance of class specificity for AGA.

In our own experience, we have published data comparing the immunofluorescent (IF) test and ELISA in adults with DH (7), and comparing the IF test and the mixed reverse solid-phase hemagglutination assay (Mrs PAH) in children with celiac disease (8). There has been very little interassay variability (for details of the Mrs PAH test, see [2]).

ACKNOWLEDGMENTS

The authors gratefully acknowledge the help in having some of the sera provided by J.A. Walker-Smith, M.D., St. Bartholomew's Hospital, London; P. Kumar, M.D., St. Bartholomew's Hospital, London; R.A. Marsden, M.D., St. Georges Hospital, London; and A. Ellis, M.D., Broadgreen Hospital, Liverpool.

REFERENCES

1. Kieffer M, Barnetson R StC: What is the role of gliadin in bullous pemphigoid? *Lancet* ii:806, 1981.

2. Kieffer M, Frazer PJ, Daniels NWR, et al: Serum antibodies (measured by Mrs PAH) to alcohol soluble gliadins in adult coeliac patients. *J Immunol Methods* 42:129, 1981.
3. Kieffer M, Barnetson R StC, Blackwell JN: Sequential studies of gliadin antibodies in patients with dermatitis herpetiformis. *Arch Dermatol Res* 276:74, 1984.
4. Leonard JN, Wright P, Williams DM, et al: The relationship between linear IgA disease and benign mucous membrane pemphigoid. *Br J Dermatol* 110:307, 1984.
5. Savilahti E, Vilander M, Perkkio M, et al: IgA antigliadin antibodies—a marker of mucosal damage in childhood coeliac disease. *Lancet* i:320, 1983.
6. Unsworth DJ, Manuel PD, Walker-Smith JA, et al: New immunofluorescent blood test for gluten sensitivity. *Arch Dis Childhood* 56:864, 1981.
7. Unsworth DJ, Leonard JN, McMinn RMH, et al: Anti-gliadin antibodies and small intestinal mucosal damage in dermatitis herpetiformis. *Br J Dermatol* 105:653, 1981.
8. Unsworth DJ, Kieffer M, Holborow EJ, et al: IgA antigliadin antibodies in coeliac disease. *Clin Exp Immunol* 46:286, 1981.
9. Unsworth DJ: Humoral immunity in gluten sensitive enteropathy. Doctoral Thesis, University of London, London, UK, 1982.
10. Unsworth DJ, Walker-Smith JA, Holborow EJ: Gliadin and reticulin antibodies in childhood coeliac disease. *Lancet* i:874, 1983 (see also correction, *Lancet* i:1058, 1983).

27
Antiendomysial Antibodies in Dermatitis Herpetiformis and Celiac Disease

Tadeusz P. Chorzelski
Stefania Jablonska
Ernst H. Beutner
Vijay Kumar
Jadwiga Sulej
Jonathan N. Leonard

INTRODUCTION

We have recently described a new type of IgA-class antibody to a component of smooth muscle (2,4–6). The reactive antigen appeared as a network of thin irregular lines around the sarcolemma of the individual smooth muscle myofibrils (Fig. 1). Silver impregnation (Belschowsky's method [11]) stained somewhat comparable structures (Fig. 2), suggesting that the antibody may be directed against the reticular component of the endomysium. Therefore, the term IgA-EmA or AEmA (IgA antiendomysial antibody) was introduced (5). The immunofluorescence (IF) pattern of IgA-EmA stands in sharp contrast with the homogeneous cytoplasmic staining of antismooth muscle antibody (ASMA) (Fig. 3).

IgA-EmA is best detected on monkey gastrointestinal tract tissue, while other organs, notably kidney and liver, are not reactive. This antibody can also be detected on the esophagus of other animals: cattle, calf, goat, guinea pig, but the titers are significantly lower and some are negative (6). Therefore, these substrates cannot be recommended for routine diagnostic purposes. In our preliminary studies, mouse and rat tissues were not reactive.

DETECTION OF IgA-CLASS ANTIENDOMYSIAL ANTIBODIES IN DERMATITIS HERPETIFORMIS AND CELIAC DISEASE

The presence of this antibody is related to gluten-sensitive enteropathy (GE) regardless of skin lesions (4,6). IgA-EmA was found in cases exclusively with granular IgA depos-

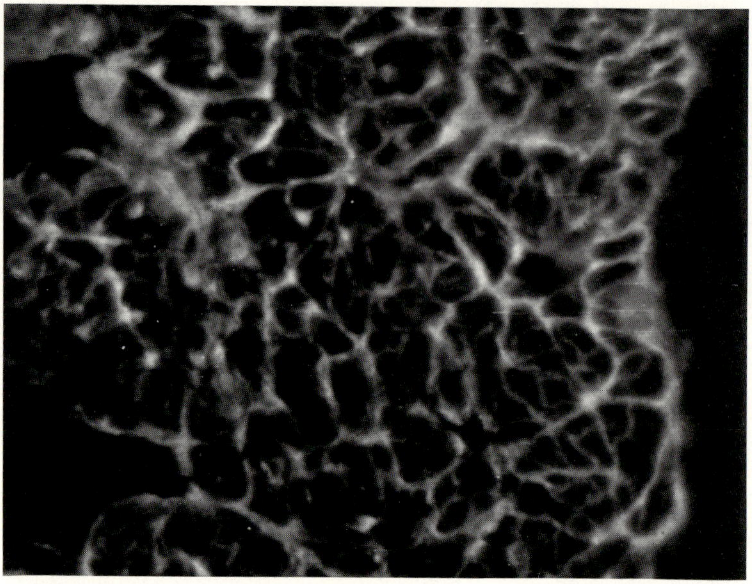

Figure 1. Indirect IF with DH serum containing IgA-EmA, with anti-IgA conjugate on sections of monkey esophagus. Note the reticulin-like pattern in smooth muscle.

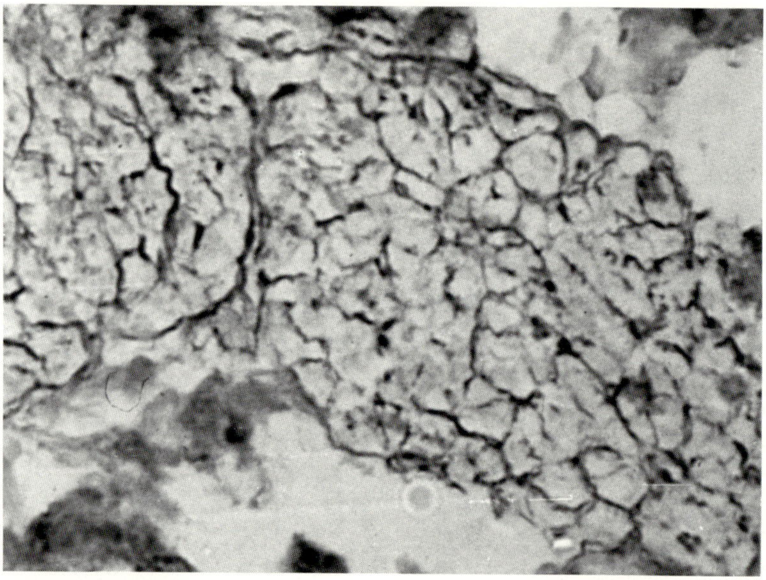

Figure 2. Silver impregnation (Belschowsky's method). Note reticulin-like pattern somewhat similar to that in Figure 1.

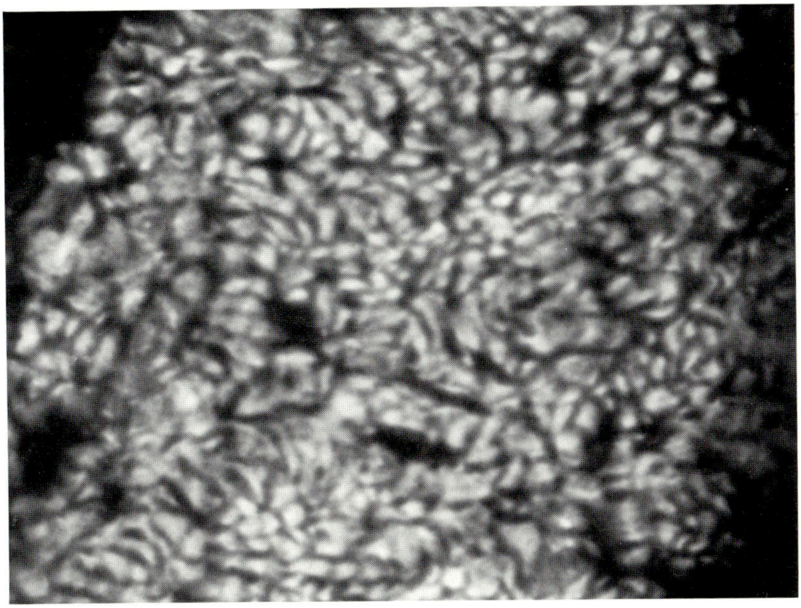

Figure 3. The same procedure as in Figure 1 with serum containing ASMA. Note cytoplasmic fluorescence in smooth muscle.

Table 1. IgA-EmA in DH, Celiac Disease, and Controls

Diagnoses	*IgA-EmA (positive/total)*	%
DH	75/104	72
Celiac disease	39/52	75
Crohn's disease	0/38	0
Ulcerative colitis	0/22	0
Milk enteropathy	0/4	0
Other gut diseases	0/109	0
Linear IgA bullous dermatosis	0/37	0
BP	0/17	0
Pemphigus	0/13	0
Other skin diseases	0/82	0
Normal subjects	0/14	0

Sera of patients with celiac disease were kindly provided by T. Zalewski, M.D. and A. Kapuscinska, M.D., Department of Pediatrics, Warsaw Academy of Medicine Warsaw, Poland.

its. It was not found in patients with linear IgA bullous dermatosis (LABD), other skin and gut diseases, nor in normal subjects (Table 1).

In dermatitis herpetiformis (DH), the overall frequency of positive results was 75 of 104 cases (72.1%) and in all (10 of 10) cases of jejunal mucosal atrophy of grades III and IV in our studies.

Table 2. Frequency of Detection of IgA-EmA in DH Sera Obtained from Different Centers

Center[a]	*No. pos/No. tested*[b]	% *positive*
A	75/104	72
B	8/11	73
C	17/33	52
D	3/4	75
E	4/4	100

[a]Center A: Warsaw Poland; author's clinic.
Coded sera were kindly provided by centers B, C, D, and E:
Center B: Leonard et al. (9).
Center C: S.I. Katz, M.D., Dermatology Branch, NIH, Bethesda, Maryland. (As noted in the text, 5 of the 17 cases with IgA-EmA that had titers of 5 or less were reported as "borderline" in this doubleblind study.)
Center D: S.F. Bean, M.D. Department of Dermatology University of Texas Medical School Houston, Texas
Center E: M. Meurer, M.D. Department of Dermatology Munich, West Germany
[b]DH cases not on gluten-free diets (1).

The 12 cases of DH that were controlled by GFD and challenged with gluten, according to the report of Leonard et al. (8), were re-examined in a double-blind study for IgA-EmA (9). The prechallenge sera were all negative for these antibodies; 1 month after challenge (before relapse), two of five cases examined had minimal titers of 2.5. At the time of relapse, 8 of 11 cases had IgA-EmA in titers ranging from 2.5 to 1280; the 12th case had no relapse and no detectable antibody.

In the patient who also manifested some deterioration in the jejunal mucosa, but who did not develop IgA-EmA in the serum, the change in morphologic appearance was only slight (grades I to II).

In 6 of the 12 cases, there was a progressive rise in the titer of IgA-EmA with time on gluten challenge, and also a correlation with the severity of GE.

In another double-blind study (Table 2) with Stephen Katz (1) from the National Institutes of Health, sera of 35 DH cases and 22 control subjects were examined; 14 of the DH sera had IgA-EmA titers of 10 or more, 3 had titers of 5 (called borderline in the study), and none of the 22 controls were positive. The controls include five cases with linear IgA deposits in the skin and five subjects with HLA B8-type histocompatibility antigens. Two of the 35 DH cases were on gluten free diets (GFD) (1).

In effect, the 8 of 11 (73%) IgA-EmA positives found in the relapsed DH cases of Leonard et al. (9) correspond to the 75 of 104 (72%) positives in the DH cases listed in Table 1, but not to the 17 of 35 (49%) positives found in Katz's study. Two of IgA-EmA negative cases in this study were on a GFD. In the three groups of patient materials, the overall frequency of IgA-EmA in titers of 2.5 or more in 102 positives of 150 DH cases examined is 68%.

In celiac disease (CD), the overall frequency of IgA-EmA is 75% (39 of 52) (Table 3). In florid CD, the IgA-EmA were found in 7 of 7 cases examined. These antibodies

Table 3. IgA-EmA in Various Stages of Celiac Disease

Treatment with GFD	*Positive/total*
Before GFD	7/7
After short GFD	2/5
After long GFD	0/10
After gluten challenge	9/9
Diet not observed	21/21

disappeared progressively on GFD; for example, before 3 months on GFD, two of five patients had IgA-EmA. These antibodies became undetectable in all cases examined (10 of 10) after 3 months on a GFD. Gluten challenge induced a reappearance of IgA-EmA in 9 of 9 cases (Table 2).

The titers of the antibody correlated positively with the flattening of the jejunal villi. IgA-EmA persisted in all 21 patients not observing the diet.

The antibody appears to be specific of GE, since the findings were negative in all 51 patients with other gut diseases, including ulcerative colitis, milk enteropathy, Crohn's disease, and others listed in Table 1. In the initial study (5), we reported our results on the unselected material available. This study included cases with tentative diagnoses of suspected celiac disease (positive results in 7 of 13 patients) and other gut diseases with no conclusive diagnosis (positive results in 3 of 11 patients). Re-evaluation of the series in the 2 years that followed has shown that positive findings occurred exclusively in patients who were subsequently shown to have CD, which was diagnosed according to the international criteria (10).

IgA-EmA was absent in 82 patients with other skin diseases and in all 51 patients with other gut disorders. Of special significance are negative results in all 26 cases of LABD studied in this series. This provides additional evidence that LABD is a distinct entity differing from DH (2,3) (Chap. 22, 23).

SIGNIFICANCE OF IgA-CLASS ANTIENDOMYSIAL ANTIBODIES

Case Report

The diagnostic significance of IgA-EmA may be best illustrated by the accidental finding of this antibody in a serum taken as a negative control. The patient was a 17-year-old girl with chronic urticaria that was unresponsive to any treatment, including large doses of corticosteroids. A biopsy specimen was obtained for IF studies. This gave negative results. The history revealed that the patient had CD in early childhood, and was treated for several years with GFD until all gastrointestinal symptoms regressed completely. Reintroduction of GFD at 17 years of age produced a dramatic disappearance of urticaria, and the girl was free of lesions, without other therapy. This would suggest that the patient had a latent CD (12), but this was not confirmed by a jejunal biopsy procedure due to the refusal of the patient. There was an acute but transitory relapse after she had eaten a candy containing flour (gluten challenge). In addition, cutaneous test with flour was positive (urticarial reaction), which indicates a gluten hypersensitivity. Thus, IgA-EmA IF-test disclosed a latent GE, with associated gluten skin hypersensitivity. The girl is still on a GFD and in full remission at present.

Practical Application of the IgA-EmA IF Test

In DH, the IgA-EmA IF test could be useful for diagnosing associated GE of grades III and IV, and especially for monitoring the response to GFD. Although in DH both skin rash and enteropathy are gluten-dependent, these two do not necessarily parallel each other (6). The patients with DH on GFD with negative IF tests for IgA-EmA may still have skin lesions, which not infrequently disappear only after 1 to 2 years on a strict diet (7).

This test can be recommended for diagnosis of CD and for monitoring response to GFD and gluten challenge. Due to the high sensitivity of the IgA-EmA IF test, it appears to be most suitable for controlling the strictness of GFD (Table 3). Since the antibody disappears and reappears earlier than morphologic changes of jejunal mucosa, the IgA-EmA IF test may be considered as an alternative to jejunal biopsy procedures in CD and DH.

REFERENCES

1. Beutner EH, Chorzelski TP, Kumar V, et al. Sensitivity and specificity of IgA class antiendomysial antibodies for dermatitis herpetiformis and findings relevant to their pathogenic significance. *J. Am. Acad. Dermatol* 15:464–473, 1986.
2. Chorzelski TP, Jablonska S, Beutner EH. Linear IgA dermatoses. In Beutner EH, Chorzelski TP, Bean SF (Eds): *Immunopathology of the Skin,* ed. 2. Wiley, New York, 1979, pp. 315–323.
3. Chorzelski TP, Jablonska S, Beutner EH, Linear IgA Bullous dermatosis. et al. In Marks R, Christophers E (Eds): *The Epidermis in Disease.* MTP Press, Lancaster, UK, 1981, pp 577–584.
4. Chorzelski TP, Sulej J, Kapuscinska A, et al: IgA class endomysium antibody. A specific immunological marker of celiac disease and dermatitis herpetiformis (abstract 47). In *XVIIth Annual Meeting of Paediatric, Gastroenterology and Nutrition.* Tampere, Finland, Abstract, 1984.
5. Chorzelski TP, Sulej J, Tchorzewska H, et al: IgA class endomysium antibodies in dermatitis herpetiformis and celiac disease. *Ann NY Acad Sci* 420:325–334, 1983.
6. Chorzelski TP, Beutner EH, Sulej J, et al: IgA antiendomysium antibody. A new immunological marker of dermatitis herpetiformis and celiac disease. *Br J Dermatol* 111:395–402, 1984.
7. Fry L, Riches DJ, Seah PP: Clearance of skin lesions in dermatitis herpetiformis after gluten withdrawal. *Lancet* 1:288, 1973.
8. Leonard J, Haffenden G, Tucker W, et al: Gluten challenge in dermatitis herpetiformis. *N. Engl J Med* 309:816, 1983.
9. Leonard JN, Chorzelski TP, Beutner EH, et al: IgA antiendomysial antibody detection in the serum of patients with dermatitis herpetiformis following gluten challenge. *Arch Dermatol Res* 277:349–351, 1985.
10. Meeuwisse GW: Diagnostic criteria in coeliac disease. *Acta Pediatr Scand* 59:461, 1970.
11. Unsworth DJ, Johnson GD, Haffenden G, et al: Binding of wheat gliadin in vitro to reticulin in normal and dermatitis herpetiformis skin. *J Invest Dermatol* 76:88, 1981.
12. Weinstein WM: Latent coeliac sprue. *Gastroenterology* 66:489, 1974.

28
Comparison of Disease Specificity of Antiendomysial and Antigliadin Antibodies

Vijay Kumar
Ernst H. Beutner
Aaron Lerner
Naresh Jain
Tadeusz P. Chorzelski

INTRODUCTION

Patients with celiac disease (CD) and dermatitis herpetiformis (DH) seem to have common biochemical and immunologic aberrations. As discussed in Chaps. 24 to 27, these patients have circulating antibodies to gliadin, reticulin, and endomysium of the smooth muscles. In this chapter, we will attempt to put in proper perspective the role of antigliadin and antiendomysial (EmA) antibodies from the point of view of their relative specificity and sensitivity.

METHODS

Detection of Antigliadin Antibodies

Antigliadin antibodies (AGA) were detected by the ELISA as well as by indirect immunofluorescence (IIF) methods (1–3). In brief, for the ELISA test, polystyrene microtiter plates (Immunon, Dynatech Labs, United States) were treated with 0.1% gluteraldehyde in 0.1 M carbonate, pH 9.6 buffer, for 2 hours and washed with distilled water. These gluteraldehyde-treated plates were then coated with 75μl of 1μg/ml of purified gliadin (Roth, West Germany) per well in 0.1 M carbonate buffer, pH 9.6. Upon incubation overnight at 4°C, the plates were washed in phosphate-buffered saline (PBS) with 0.05% Tween-20 (PBS-Tween). The unreacted sites were blocked by incubating with 100 μl of blocking solution (2% bovine serum albumin plus

2% glycine in PBS) for 2 hours at 37°C. After further washing, 75 μl of 1:25 dilution of the control's or patient's sera were added in the wells and incubated at 37°C for 1 hour. The plates were washed three times in PBS-Tween and further reacted with 75 μl of 1:100 dilution of biotinylated goat antihuman IgG (Vector Labs, United States). The plates were incubated at 37°C for 1 hour, washed three times in PBS-Tween, and further incubated with 75 μl of glucose oxidase-avidin reagent. Upon washing in PBS-Tween three times, the color was developed by adding 200 μl of substrate (1.5 mg/ml of 2.2-azino-di-[3-ethylbenzthiazoline sulphonic acid], 20 μg/ml of peroxidase, and 2 mg/ml of glucose in 0.1 M phosphate buffer pH 6.8), and incubating the plates at 37°C for 1 hour. The plates were read at 405 nm.

AGA were also detected by an IIF method similar to the one described by Unsworth et al. in Chap. 25, except that monkey esophagus sections were employed as described by Chorzelski et al. (4,5). Gliadin binds to the intercellular (IC) constituents of the mucosa and to the reticulin fibers of the smooth muscle bundles, as shown in Fig. 1. The tests were run by incubating the patient's sera at dilutions of 1:2.5 or higher on monkey esophagus sections treated with 0.1 mg/ml of gliadin in distilled water. Untreated sections served as controls for any false-positive staining due to pemphigus, pemphigus-like, or blood group antibodies (Chap. 3). The binding of AGA on tissue sections was determined with fluoresceinated goat antihuman IgG (molar F/P, 2.0 to 3.0) diluted to one-quarter of a unit of antibody.

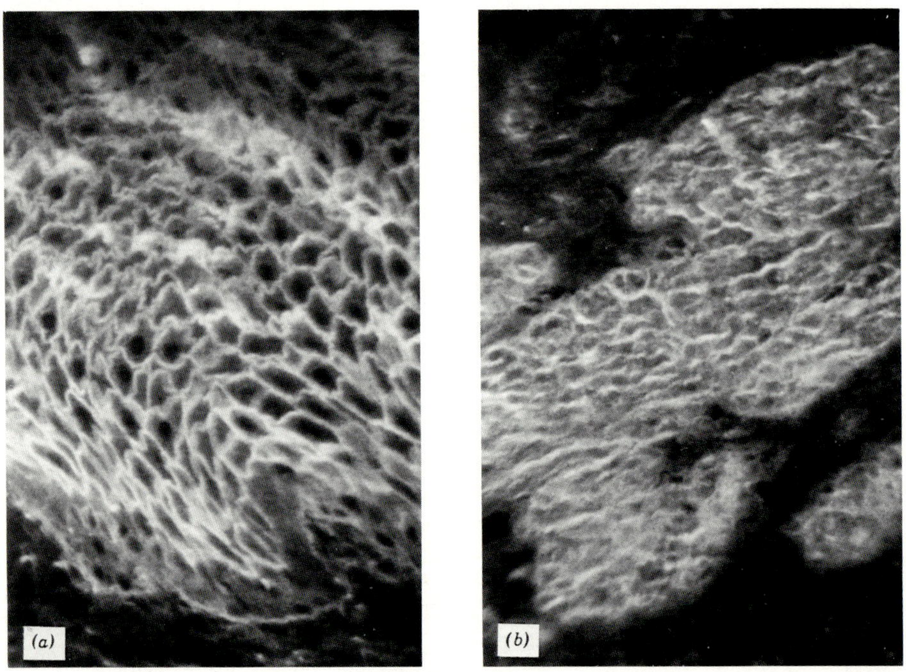

Figure 1. Detection of AGA on monkey esophagus sections by IIF. A. IC staining on gliadin-treated monkey esophagus mucosa. B. Muscularis mucosa staining seen only on gliadin-treated sections (112x).

Detection of IgA-Class Anti-EmA

EmA were detected by IF on monkey esophagus sections as described in Chap. 27. The sera were reacted at dilutions of 1:2.5 or greater. The detection of EmA was made by employing goat antihuman IgA conjugates (molar F/P, 2.0 to 3.0) diluted to one-quarter of an antibody unit.

COMPARISONS OF ANTIGLIADIN ANTIBODIES AND ANTIENDOMYSIAL ANTIBODIES

Frequency of AGA and EmA

There seem to be conflicting reports as to the incidence of AGA in patients with CD, DH, other gastrointestinal disorders, and even in normal healthy control subjects (5–16). These discrepant results might be due to either the type of gliadin used in the assay or the different levels of sensitivities of methods employed. We examined the sera of normal healthy control subjects for the presence of AGA and EmA. None of 90 normal sera tested were positive for EmA, whereas 25 of 90 were positive for IgG-class AGA. As shown in Table 1, the incidence tends to increase with age to approximately 39% by the sixth decade. There seems to be a general agreement that AGA are positive in almost all active cases of CD in children (see Chap. 26), and the incidence varied between 30 to 50% in other gastrointestinal disorders (Table 2). EmA were positive only in the sera of patients with CD and in none of the other disorders examined. There was no difference in the incidence of AGA in DH patients, as compared to pemphigus and pemphigoid. Similar results have also been reported by others (7,17). EmA, on the other hand, were specific for DH (Table 3). IgA-class AGA, on the other hand, were positive only in the sera of DH patients. The incidence, however, was only approximately 25%.

Effect of Gluten-Free Diet on AGA and EmA

There is a general agreement that levels of AGA fall on treatment with a gluten-free diet (GFD). As discussed by Unsworth et al. in Chap. 25, AGA disappears on a GFD in about 7 months in adults and about 5 months in children. However, they may not be negative in all patients, as 4 of 15 patients who were on a GFD had AGA; 14 of 15 became positive upon gluten challenge. Chorzelski et al. (Chap. 27) examined the levels

Table 1. Incidence of Gliadin and EmA in Normal Individuals with Relation to Age

Age	*Total no. of patients*	*No. positive*		*% positive*	
		AGA	*EmA*	*AGA*	*EmA*
11 + 4.25	17	3	0	17.6	0
29 + 7.37	42	10	0	23.7	0
57 + 5.31	18	7	0	38.8	0
75 + 6.89	14	5	0	35.5	0
Totals	91	25	0	27.4	0

AGA as detected by ELISA

Table 2. Frequency of AGA and Anti-EmA in Children with Various Gastrointestinal Disorders

	AGA				Anti-EmA	
	ELISA		IF			
Diagnosis	*No. pos.*	*% pos.*	*No. pos.*	*% pos.*	*No. pos.*	*% pos.*
Celiac disease (active)	3/3	100	3/3	100	18/18	100
(undifferentiated)	ND	—	18/27	69	31/48	65
Ulcerative colitis	4/7	57	2/7	29	0/7	0
Crohn's disease	20/32	63	9/25	36	0/25	0
Small bowel disease	3/4	75	2/4	50	0/4	0
Liver disorder	11/22	50	6/21	29	0/21	0
Miscellaneous[a]	8/25	32	8/24	33	0/24	0
Normals	2/17	12	2/15	13	0/15	0

[a]The miscellaneous group includes patients with abdominal pain, rectal bleeding, pancreatitis, dysphagia, duodenitis, GE reflex, and allergies

Table 3. Incidence of Antigliadin and Antiendomysial Antibodies in Various Bullous Disorders

	AGA				EmA	
	IgG		IgA			
Diagnosis	*No. pos. total*	*% pos.*	*No. pos. total*	*% pos.*	*No. pos. total*	*% pos.*
DH	20/23	87	5/23	22	38/48	76
LABD	ND	—	ND	—	0/15	0
Pemphigus	7/9	78	0/9	0	0/9	0
Pemphigoid	12/16	75	0/16	0	0/16	0

AGA as detected by ELISA.
ND, not done.

of EmA in the sera of CD patients before, during, and after a GFD. Seven of seven patients were positive for EmA during the active phase of the disease. Upon treatment with a GFD for less than 3 months, 3 of 5 patients became negative for EmA. Ten of 10 patients were negative when they were maintained on a GFD for longer than 3 months. In addition, gluten challenge caused the appearance of EmA in all cases studied. Most important, it was observed that the EmA disappeared before the mucosa became normal and reappeared before any pathologic changes of mucosa were observed. AGA, on the other hand, take a much longer time (6 to 7 months) to disappear on a GFD. However, parallel studies for both AGA and EmA need to be done to study their relationships to diet with time. There is general agreement in the literature that AGA levels may not completely disappear in patients who are on a GFD for a long time. This response has been associated with the genetic make-up of the patient. According to Mearin et al. (13), patients with DR3/DR7 or DR7/DR5 phenotypes had higher AGA titers when on a gluten diet than when they were on a GFD. However, children with DR3/DR3 phenotypes showed similar AGA titers regardless of diet. All cases examined to date for relationship of EmA titers to GFD or gluten challenge displayed titer fluctuations with diet changes. Studies relating the EmA titers to the HLA with diet need to be performed.

CONCLUSIONS

AGA and EmA are useful serologic markers of gut abnormalities in patients with CD and DH. AGA of the IgA class are more disease specific than those of the IgG class: however, they occur only in up to one-third of celiac patients. AGA of the IgG class, even though not disease specific, occur in all pediatric patients with active CD, 85 to 90% of adults with CD, and about half of patients with DH. Due to the diversity of disease association with positive AGA, they cannot be considered as a marker of CD. There is, however, a general agreement that when AGA are negative, it is very unlikely that the patient has CD, especially in children. Thus, methods of detecting AGA can be used in excluding rather than confirming the diagnosis. That AGA levels tend to fluctuate with disease activity seems to be true in many cases, but not in all, as shown by Mearin et al. (13). Hence, the levels of AGA must be interpreted with caution in assessing the response to therapy.

EmA are of the IgA class only, and are a marker of the underlying gut pathology in patients with CD and DH. These antibodies are found in 70 to 75% of CD and DH patients as a whole, and none in other disorders. EmA are positive in 100% of cases with active CD or DH with gut changes of types III and IV. In addition, the levels of EmA parallel the response to diet, and the changes in antibody levels precede the morphologic changes of the gut mucosa.

In summary, it appears that EmA may be related to the pathologic changes of the gut, whereas AGA are not.

REFERENCES

1. Barnes RMR, Barton PG, Doig JE, et al: Distribution of serum antibodies to wheat gliadin and bovine milk in atopic and non-atopic healthy adults. *J Clin Lab Immunol* 12:175–178, 1983.
2. Blazer S, Naveh Y, Berant M, et al: Serum IgG antibodies to gliadin in children with celiac disease as measured by an immunofluorescence method. *J Pediatr Gastroenterol Nutr* 3:205–209, 1984.
3. Burgin-Wolff A, Bertele RM, Berger R, et al: A reliable screening test for childhood celiac disease: Fluorescent immunosorbent test for gliadin antibodies. *J Pediatr* 102:655–660, 1983.
4. Chorzelski TP, Sulej J, Tchorzewska H, et al: IgA class endomysium antibodies in dermatitis herpetiformis and celiac disease. *Ann NY Acad Sci* 420:325–334, 1983.
5. Chorzelski TP, Beutner EH, Sulej J, et al: IgA antiendomysium antibody. A new immunological marker of dermatitis herpetiformis and celiac disease. *Br J Dermatol* 111:395–402, 1984.
6. Kieffer M, Barnetson RS: What is the role of gliadin in bullous pemphigoid? *Lancet* 2:806, 1981.
7. Kieffer M, Barnetson RS: Increased gliadin antibodies in dermatitis herpetiformis and pemphigoid. *Br J Dermatol* 108:673–678, 1983.
8. Kieffer M, Frazier PJ, Daniels NWR, et al: Serum antibodies (measured by Mrs PAH) to alcohol soluble gliadins in adult celiac patients. *J Immunol Methods* 42:129–136, 1981.
9. Kumar V, Beutner EH, Chorzelski TP: Distribution of monkey esophagus antigens reactive with IgA class antibodies in the sera of dermatitis herpetiformis patients. *Arch Dermatol Res* 276:293–296, 1984.

10. Kumar V, Beutner EH: Monkey esophagus: A unique antigenic substrate in immunodermatology. This volume-Chap. 3.
11. Kumar V, Jain N, Lerner A, et al: Comparative studies of different gliadin preparations in detecting anti-gliadin antibodies in celiacs. *J Pediatr Gastroenterol Nutri* 5:730–734, 1986.
12. Lane AT, Clark-Huff J, Zone JJ, et al: Class specific antibodies to gluten in dermatitis herpetiformis. *J Invest Dermatol* 80:402–405, 1983.
13. Mearin ML, Koninch CR, Biemond I, et al: Influence of specific factors on the serum levels of anti-gliadin antibodies in celiac disease. J Pediatr Gastroenterol Nutri 3:373–377, 1984.
14. O'Farrely L, Kelly J, Hebbins W, et al: Gliadin antibody levels: A serological test for celiac disease. *Br Med J* 286:2007–2010, 1983.
15. Signer E, Burgin-Wolff A, Berger R, et al: Antibodies to gliadin as a screening test for celiac disease. *Helv Pediatr Acta* 34:41–52, 1979.
16. Stern M, Fischer K, Gruttner R: Immunofluorescent serum gliadin antibodies in children with celiac disease and various malabsorptive disorders. *Eur J Pediatr* 130:155–164, 1979.
17. Unsworth DJ, Walker-Smith JA, Holborow EJ: Gliadin and reticulin antibodies in childhood celiac disease. *Lancet* 1:874–875, 1983.

Section III

CONNECTIVE TISSUE DISEASES

29
Comments on Clinical Significance of Immunologic Findings in Connective Tissue Diseases

Ernst H. Beutner

Tadeusz P. Chorzelski

Vijay Kumar

INTRODUCTION

The preceding section of this book on vesicular bullous diseases is divided into subsections, each with multiple chapters because the immunologic findings are clearly distinguishable for the various groups of diseases. In this section, the diverse connective tissue diseases are considered as a single group because the immunologic findings overlap extensively. Also, the clinical features of these diseases may leave extensive overlap.

Attention is focused in this introductory chapter, and in other chapters of this section, on those diagnostically relevant immunologic findings that are of value in dermatology services for differentiating systemic lupus erythematosus (SLE) and other connective tissue diseases from each other and other diseases.

Diagnostic Criteria for SLE in Dermatology Services

The revised criteria of the American Rheumatism Association (ARA) reported by Tan et al. in 1982 (9) deleted some of the criteria from those reported in 1971 (2), notably Raynaud's phenomenon and alopecia. Three immunologic criteria were added as indicated below.

To understand the significance of these criteria, we need to focus our attention on the controls used to generate them. The diagnostic specificity of the criteria listed in Table 1, and other criteria for diagnosis of SLE that were examined in the study of Tan et al. (9), are based on a control population from a rheumatology clinic. That is, the specificity data in this 1982 study (9) were based on 162 control patients with the following conditions: 95 rheumatoid arthritis (RA), 27 other joint diseases, 16 scleroderma, 6 dermatomyositis, and 18 other diseases (which included only one case of

Table 1. The 1982 Revised Criteria for Classification of SLE[a]

Criteria	*Definition*
1. Malar rash	Fixed erythema, flat or raised, over the malar eminences, tending to spare the nasolabial folds.
2. Discoid rash	Erythematous raised patches with adherent keratotic scaling and follicular plugging; atrophic scarring may occur in older lesions.
3. Photosensitivity	Skin rash as a result of unusual reaction to sunlight, by patient history or physician observation.
4. Oral ulcers	Oral or nasopharyngeal ulceration, usually painless, observed by a physician.
5. Arthritis	Nonerosive arthritis involving 2 or more peripheral joints, characterized by tenderness, swelling, or effusion.
6. Serositis	a. Pleuritis—convincing history of pleuritic pain or rub heard by a physician or evidence of pleural effusion; or b. Pericarditis—documented by ECG[b] or rub or evidence of pericardial effusion
7. Renal disorder	a. Persistent proteinuria greater than 0.5 g/day or greater than +3 if quantitation not performed; or b. Cellular casts—may be red blood cell, hemoglobin, granular, tubular, or mixed.
8. Neurologic disorder	a. Seizures—in the absence of offending drugs or known metabolic derangements; e.g., uremia, ketoacidosis, or electrolyte imbalance; or b. Psychosis—in the absence of offending drugs or known metabolic derangements; e.g., uremia, ketoacidosis, or electrolyte imbalance.
9. Hematologic disorder	a. Hemolytic anemia—with reticulocytosis; or b. Leukopenia—less than 4000/mm^3 total on 2 or more occasions; or c. Lymphopenia—less than 1500/mm^3 on 2 or more occasions or d. Thrombocytopenia—less than 100,000/mm^3 in the absence of offending drugs.
10. Immunologic disorder	a. Positive LE cell preparation; or b. Anti-DNA—antibody to native DNA in abnormal titer; or c. Anti-Sm—presence of antibody to Sm nuclear antigen; or d. False-positive serologic test for syphilis known to be positive for at least 6 mo and confirmed by *Treponema pallidum* immobilization of fluorescent treponemal antibody absorption test.

Table 1. *(Continued)*

Criteria	*Definition*
11. ANA	An abnormal titer of antinuclear antibody by IF or an equivalent assay at any point in time, and in the absence of drugs known to be associated with "drug-induced lupus" syndrome.

[a]The proposed classification is based on 11 criteria. For the purpose of identifying patients in clinical studies, a person shall be said to have SLE if any 4 or more of the 11 criteria are present, serially or simultaneously, during an interval of observation (Tan et al. [9]).
[b]ECG, electrocardiogram

discoid lupus erythematosus [DLE]). While such a population, which is made up largely (85%) of RA, scleroderma, and other joint diseases, is an appropriate control group for a rheumatology clinic, it is not an appropriate control population for a dermatology service. Clearly, the latter should include more cases of DLE as well as polymorphous light eruption cases and other skin diseases that dermatologists need to distinguish from SLE and not so many RA.

We can express the clinical significance of any of the criteria for the diagnosis of SLE (or any other disease) as follows (3):

$$\text{Sensitivity} = \frac{\text{no. of SLE cases that fulfill a criterion}}{\text{total no. of cases with SLE}}$$

$$\text{Specificity} = \frac{\text{no. of control cases negative for a criterion}}{\text{total no. of control cases}}$$

If SLE is the same disease regardless of whether patients are cared for by rheumatologists or dermatologists, then the sensitivity of each of the criteria should be comparable for the two specialties. While this may be true, it remains to be proven. The correct controls of diseases from which SLE needs to be distinguished by these two groups of specialists are, as indicated above, quite distinct. We must assume that the specificity of at least most, and probably all, of the criteria under consideration will be different. Thus, the discrimination of each of these criteria (which is based on their sensitivity and specificity) and, importantly, the selection of criteria for the two types of services may be expected to be different. These suggest that dermatologists need to consider not only the ARA criteria in the diagnosis of SLE (1,9), but also some criteria that were not evaluated with the ARA criteria either in 1971 (6) or in 1982 (9), notably:

1. Immunofluorescent (IF) band tests of lesional and normal skin biopsy specimens (see Chap. 30).
2. Serum studies for antibodies to Ro(SSA) and La(SSB) antigens as well as to ribonucleoprotein (RNP) antigen (see Chap. 33 to 35). The latter is considered to be a sign of SLE by some (7) and of mixed connective tissue disease (MCTD) by others (8)—a question that has not been resolved.
3. Raynaud's phenomenon, which was included in the 1971 (6) but excluded from the 1982 (9) ARA criteria, is considered to be of diagnostic value to dermatologists.

Until valid comparative studies in dermatology clinics are done on the sensitivity, specificity, and discrimination of the diversified criteria for the diagnosis of SLE, it will be necessary to use at least a combination of the ARA criteria listed in Table 1 and the above three criteria. Possibly other criteria deemed to be unacceptable by the ARA may also prove to be of diagnostic value to dermatologists.

Relevance of Immunologic Criteria in the Diagnosis of Connective Tissue Diseases

The value of immunologic studies in the diagnosis of SLE is evident from the revisions made in the ARA criteria in 1982 (9). These include the three immunologic criteria; notably tests for antibodies to double-stranded DNA (dDNA) and to Sm antigen (the 10th criterion), and the presence of antinuclear antibodies (ANA) (the 11th criterion). As indicated in Chapter 31, these immunologic criteria have been reported to have the highest discrimination (combined sensitivity and specificity) of any of the criteria (1,4,5). In light of the findings presented in Chapters 30 to 36, we may expect that tests for IF band and antibodies to Ro(SS-A), La(SS-B), and RNP will aid in discriminating SLE from DLE, or subsets of SLE and related diseases including neonatal SLE, MCTD (7,8), Sjögren's syndrome, and subacute cutaneous LE.

Similar comments can be made regarding progressive systemic sclerosis (PSS). The ARA criteria reported for PSS point to diffuse systemic sclerosis as the primary diagnostic criterion (6). However, these do not differentiate the so-called "CREST syndrome" (see Chap. 36 and 37), which has an immunologic marker, the anticentrome antibodies (ACA) from the form of PSS that have a less favorable prognosis. The latter have antibodies to Scl 70 antigen and ANA patterns other than ACA (see Chap. 37).

General Comments on Laboratory Methods

For direct IF (DIF) studies of skin or mucosal biopsy specimens, 4-μ frozen sections of specimens should be tested with conjugates monospecific for IgG, IgA, IgM, complement component C3, and fibrin. Other reagents can be used for special studies. Each of these reagents must have the proper conjugate characteristic, that is, 10% or more of the total protein should be antibody protein, the molar fluorescein-to-protein (F/P) ratio should be in the range of 1:3, and the dilution used for a DIF test should be adjusted to contain about 50 μg/ml antibody protein (see Chap. 1 on defined IF for details). Aside from these technical details, the key factors are the selection of the biopsy site (see next section) and the experience of the immunopathologist who makes the readings.

Serum studies for ANA or other relevant antibodies should be performed with the commercial kits when possible because these yield the greatest level of reproducibility as indicated by comparative studies. A key factor stressed in Chap. 2 is that there is no such thing as an ANA titer and pattern of a patient's serum except as ANA titer and pattern on a given substrate. While the best available reproducibility of titers and patterns are attained with commercial ANA kits, some yield greater precision than others. Some improvement in precision is achieved by performance evaluation programs instituted by some ANA kit manufacturers.

Clinicians requesting ANA or other diagnostic tests should: 1) request that methods be specified with reports on ANA and other serum studies; 2) request data on normal serum values; and 3) inquire if laboratories participate in any form of performance evaluation programs.

EXAMPLES OF THE USE OF IMMUNOLOGIC STUDIES FOR THE DIAGNOSIS OF CONNECTIVE TISSUE DISEASES

Biopsy specimens of normal and lesional skin for DIF studies should be taken from exposed areas, and either placed in transport medium for sending at room temperature or quick frozen (see Chap. 30). Such studies are indicated for SLE, DLE, and MCTD, and for certain cases of other connective tissue disease in which there may be an overlap syndrome. In typical cases of scleroderma, polymyositis and other connective tissue disease, biopsy studies by IF are of limited value, as indicated in Table 2.

Serum tests can be performed with approximately 3 to 5 ml samples. These can be sent to the laboratory at ambient temperature. Serum studies are of considerable diagnostic value for both exclusion and inclusion of the various connective tissue disease. Table 2 lists the most common connective tissue disease that are also discussed briefly in the following subsections. Others are considered in the following chapters of this section.

Systemic Lupus Erythematosus

Primary screening of patients with clinical signs suggestive of possible SLE is generally done with ANA tests.

Direct IF studies of lesional skin biopsy specimens are commonly used to rule out a diagnosis of SLE if an abnormal titer of ANA is found. The frequency of positive IF band test reactions due to Ig deposits in lesional skin in SLE was found to be 91% (42 of 46) in a recent survey performed by M. Blaszyczyk (personal communication). The findings were as follows in the 46 SLE cases examined:

	IgG	*IgM*	*IgA*	*IgG+IgM*	*IgG+IgA*	*IgM+IgA*	*IgG+IgM+IgA*	*C3*
No. positive	18	5	1	9	1	2	6	38
%	39	11	2	20	2	4	13	83

While negative findings help to rule out this diagnosis, other studies are needed since about 10% of proven SLE cases have negative IF band test reactions. A strongly positive reaction is highly suggestive but not strictly speaking diagnostic of SLE. However, IF band tests of normal skin can yield essentially diagnostic results, as indicated in Chapter 30. All cases of suspected SLE with a positive ANA should be examined for anti-dDNA antibodies and for antibodies to Sm, RNP, SS-A(Ro), and SS-B(La).

Tests for antibodies to Ro(SS-A) and La(SS-B) are also indicated in suspected cases of Sjögren's syndrome, neonatal SLE, ANA-negative SLE, subacute LE, and in certain other problem cases (see Chaps. 33 to 35).

Discoid lupus erythematosus

Serum and biopsy findings in LE may be summarized briefly as follows:

	Biopsy (IF band test)		*Serum studies*
Disease	*Lesional*	*Normal*	*ANA titers*
SLE	positive	positive	positive (≥160)
DLE	positive	negative	normal range

Table 2. Summary of the Diagnostic Significance of Serum and Skin Biopsy Findings in Common Connective Tissue Disease

Diseases	*Biopsy findings: Direct IF*	*Serum findings: Indirect IF and others*	*Relevance of IF and other findings*
Systemic LE[a]	IF band in normal skin (over 90% sun-exposed)	ANA elevated titers (about 95-99%) anti-dDNA (50%)	DIF and IIF usually diagnostic
MCTD	Nuclear IgG in epidermis; IF band in normal skin	Speckled ANA and anti-RNP antibodies	Serology and/or DIF of nuclei diagnostic for MCTD, SLE, or PSS
Discoid LE	IF band, mostly IgG, and C in lesional skin only	Essentially neg. ANA titers usually in normal range	IF band highly characteristic
PSS	Nucleolar IgG in few cases; some like MCTD,[a] most neg.	ANA (about 85%) speckled, etc. ACA in CREST	Limited value in typical PSS ACA of value in "CREST" IF of value in MCTD
Dermatomyositis	Skin-neg., muscle: Limited value	ANA usually positive	Limited value
Polymyositis	Skin-neg., muscle-neg.	ANA usually positive for Pm-1	Limited value

[a]If systemic LE or the overlap syndrome, MCTD are suspected, both serum and biopsy studies by IF afford useful diagnostic information.

Details of immunologic findings are given in Chapters 30 and 31. Histologic studies should be done in cases of suspected DLE.

Mixed Connective Tissue Disease

Serum tests that reveal ANA in high titers with speckled patterns are suggestive of possible antibodies to RNP. Antibodies to RNP are a sign of the overlap syndrome or MCTD (see Chap. 33).

IF findings of nuclear deposits of IgG on skin biopsy specimens occur in certain patients with antibodies to nuclear RNP. These appear most commonly in patients with MCTD or overlap syndrome cases. They may also occur in SLE and PSS, as indicated by the following data of Jablonska (personal communication).

	Nuclear IgG deposits		*Antibodies to RNP*
Diagnosis	*No. pos/No. cases*	*% pos.*	*No. pos/No. with nuclear IgG*
MCTD	4/11	36	3/4
SLE	4/83	5	1/4
PSS	8/24	33	2/8

(Note: PSS cases were selected on the basis of suspected overlap syndrome).

Progressive Systemic Sclerosis

Over 90% of PSS patients have significant ANA titers at some time. PSS may present initially as RA. ANA are frequently of a speckled or nucleolar pattern (see Chap. 37).

IF findings on skin biopsy specimens are usually negative in PSS, except in cases with the overlap syndrome. In cases of so-called inflammatory scleroderma, an IF band may be found (see MCTD for nuclear deposits).

Dermatomyositis and Polymyositis

Serum tests usually yield positive ANA in approximately 40 to 80% of patients, depending on the ANA substrate used. Antibodies to PM antigen are reported to be specific (see Chap. 33), although their frequency is low.

IF findings on skin biopsy specimens are usually negative. They are not indicated unless SLE is suspected. Muscle biopsy procedures for IF studies are also not indicated. If such studies are done, specimens at soft sites should be obtained. In suspected dermatomyositis, such specimens may show the presence of vascular immune deposits, particularly in children (about 80% are positive), but also in adults (about 45% positive). Such vascular deposits also occur in some SLE cases (about 35%), and sometimes in RA (about 20%), but less commonly in polymyositis (about 5%) and control muscle biopsy specimens (about 4%).

Histologic studies of skin are not diagnostic. However, histologic studies of muscle biopsy specimens are essentially diagnostic.

REFERENCES

1. Clough JD, Elrazak M, Calabrese LH, et al: Weighted criteria for the diagnosis of systemic lupus erythematosus. *Arch Intern Med* 144:281–285, 1984.
2. Cohen AS, Reynolds RE, Franklin EC, et al: Preliminary criteria for the classification of systemic lupus erythematosus. *Bull Rheum Dis* 21:643–648, 1971.

3. Griner PF, Mayewski RJ, Mushlin AI, et al: Selection and interpretation of diagnostic tests and procedures. *Ann Intern Med* 94:553–600, 1981.
4. Levin RE, Weinstein A, Peterson M, et al: A comparison of the sensitivity of the 1971 and 1982 American Rheumatism Association Criteria for the classification of systemic lupus erythematosus. *Arthritis Rheum* 27:530–538, 1984.
5. Manu P: Receiver operating characteristic curves of the revised criteria for the classification of systemic lupus erythematosus. *Arthritis Rheum* 26:1054–1055, 1983. (letter to the editor).
6. Masi AT, Rodnan GP, Medsger TA, et al: Preliminary criteria for the classification of systemic sclerosis (scleroderma). *Arthritis Rheum* 23:581–590, 1980.
7. Reichlin M: Three Views: Mixed connective tissue disease: Relation to other connective tissue diseases. In Beutner EH, Chorzelski TP, Bean SF (Eds) *Immunopathology of the Skin*, ed. 2. Wiley, New York, 1979, pp 330–331. (See also this volume, Chap. 33.)
8. Sharp GC: Three Views: Mixed connective tissue disease. In Beutner EH, Chorzelski TP, Bean SF (Eds): *Immunopathology of the Skin,* ed. 2. Wiley, New York, 1979, pp 328–329.
9. Tan EM, Cohen AS, Fries JF, et al: The 1982 revised criteria for the classification of systemic lupus erythematosus. *Arthritis Rheum* 25:1271–1277, 1982.

30
Direct Immunofluorescence in Lupus Erythematosus

Mark V. Dahl
James N. Gilliam

INTRODUCTION

Immunoglobulins and complement are deposited at the dermal-epidermal junction (DEJ) of skin of patients with lupus erythematosus (LE). Using direct immunofluorescence (DIF), these immunoreactants appear as a band that demarcates the dermis from the epidermis. The electron microscope (EM) shows these deposits in the most superficial layers of the dermis immediately subjacent to the epidermal basal cells (46).

HISTORY

In 1963, Burnham, et al. (10) applied fluorescein-labeled, antihuman gamma globulin to biopsy specimens of lesional skin of patients with systemic lupus erythematosus (SLE) and found a bright, well-demarcated band of immunoglobulins along the DEJ. Shortly thereafter, Cormane (15) demonstrated these immunoglobulins in normal skin of patients with SLE. These findings were quickly confirmed (30,39,49,50,51,53). The high degree of specificity and the fairly high degree of sensitivity associated with the presence of a band of gamma globulins at the DEJ stimulated dermatologists and others to utilize DIF examination of skin biopsy specimens as a diagnostic test for LE (lupus band test). Furthermore, since immunoglobulins were not found at the DEJ in normal skin of patients with discoid lupus erythematosus (DLE), but were present in the normal skin of patients with SLE, the "test" was also used to differentiate between these two disorders (52). Thus, if immunoglobulins were found at the DEJ of *normal* skin in a patient with DLE, then the patient probably had SLE with discoid skin lesions; the finding predicted a high incidence of antinuclear antibodies, elevated erythrocyte sedimentation rates (ESR), and decreases in total hemolytic complement levels. As fluorescein-labeled antibody to specific human immunoglobulins became commercially available, investigators began applying each of these sequentially to sections of biopsy specimens. Skin biopsy specimens were usually stained for the presence of IgG, IgM, IgA, C3 and fibrinogen, but some investigators also stained for IgE and various complement components. Over the

Dr. Gilliam died during the preparation of this manuscript.

years, the reagents improved. There was less nonspecific staining. The darker backgrounds increased sensitivity. Immunofluorescence (IF) microscopes also improved. Vertical field illuminators became commonplace. Because of these improvements, smaller amounts of immunoglobulins at the DEJ became detectable. The lupus band test gained sensitivity but lost specificity.

Because the reagents and equipment have changed over the past 20 years, it is difficult to compare results of studies done prior to 1975 with those done later.

Burnham coined the term "lupus band test" for DIF examination of skin of patients with suspected LE (7–9). The presence of immunoglobulins at the DEJ was recorded as a positive lupus band test, and their absence was recorded as a negative lupus band test. According to Burnham, the band test could be done on lesional skin, as well as on uninvolved skin. Others have felt that the term "lupus band test" should apply to uninvolved skin only (17). The presence of complement alone does not constitute a positive test (26).

COMPOSITION

The antibody specificity of immunoglobulins at the DEJ appears to be directed against both nuclear components and components of the basement membrane zone (BMZ). In addition to IgG, IgM, and IgA, the deposits may also contain IgD, IgE, Clq, C4, C3, C5, C8, C9, membrane attack complex, properdin, factor B, fibrin, and the regulator protein B1H (13,29,42,44,45).

Bands consist of one or more classes of immunoglobulins. Of 47 patients with SLE, Gilliam (23) found deposits of more than one immunoreactant in all but seven patients (Table 1).

The type of immunoglobulins present in deposits may relate to the types of antibodies to double-stranded DNA in serum. If the antibody is IgG, then the skin deposits are also usually IgG (often with IgM). If the antibody is IgM, then the skin deposits are also usually IgM (37).

The presence of IgG alone or in combination with other Ig and complement components in normal skin correlated with active disease. The presence of IgM alone indicates mild clinical disease (26). When both IgG and IgM are present, the disease activity is similar to patients with skin deposits of IgG alone.

Table 1. The Frequency Distribution of Subepidermal Immunoreactants in 47 Patients with SLE

Immunoglobulin	*No. of patients*
IgG	3
IgG + IgA	1
IgG + IgM	10
IgM	4
IgG + C3	6
IgM + C3	6
IgG + IgM + IgA	3
IgG + IgM + C3	10
IgG + IgM + IgA + C3	4
Total	47

PREVALENCE

The prevalence of immunoglobulins at the DEJ of patients with LE is determined, in part, by the age of the lesion, the morphology of the lesion, the activity of clinical disease, and topical or systemic treatment. The role of each of these factors will be discussed below. The prevalence is also dependent upon the criteria used for the diagnosis of SLE (47). It seems clear that patients with "many" criteria for LE very frequently have immunoglobulins at the DEJ, whereas those with ethereal findings more often have negative tests.

Tuffanelli (52) found that more than 90% of biopsy specimens of lesional skin from patients with SLE and DLE contained immunoglobulins at the DEJ, but most investigators have since found a lesser incidence. The overall prevalence is probably between 50 and 90% (9,36,40).

Blaszczyk's group (18) obtained biopsy skin lesions of patients with widespread DLE. Biopsy specimens were obtained from the face, sun-exposed nonfacial skin, and nonsun-exposed, nonfacial skin. Discoid lesions on the face almost always contained IgG or IgM (96%), while only about half of those on the body contained these deposits (48%). The incidence of a band in lesions on sun-exposed skin was more than twice as high (65%) as those on nonsun-exposed skin.

Prystowski and others in our group (43) found deposits at the DEJ of lesional skin in only 77% of patients with chronic cutaneous LE (DLE). Sontheimer et al. found lesional deposits at the DEJ in only 60% of patients with subacute cutaneous LE (49).

The prevalence of immunoglobulins at the DEJ in uninvolved skin is much less than the prevalence in involved skin. In patients with SLE, the prevalence is probably between 50 and 70% depending upon criteria for diagnosis (25), although much higher prevalences have been reported (3,35,38). Immunoglobulins are almost never seen in normal skin of patients with localized DLE.

The frequency of finding immunoglobulins at the DEJ in normal skin of patients with SLE is also dependent on the biopsy site. Sun-exposed normal skin seems more likely to have immunoglobulins at the DEJ junction than at the nonsun-cxposed skin.

Ahmed and Provost (1) studied biopsy specimens from 19 untreated patients with SLE. Bands of immunoglobulins were found at the DEJ of normal skin in 77% of patients if the specimen was obtained from the sun-exposed skin of the upper third of the extensor forearm. Only 37% of specimens from nonsun-exposed skin from the buttocks of these patients contained these bands.

We found that the overall prevalence of bands in normal skin of patients with SLE was 53%, and that bands disappeared in some patients treated with systemic prednisone and cyclophosphamide (Table 2) (23). Alcocer's group (2) found a prevalence rate of 68% using normal skin from the anterior forearm or inner arm. Boonpucknavig et al. (4) detected immunoglobulins at the DEJ in 92% of 38 patients with SLE by studying nonlesional, light-protected forearm skin. Stippled bands were especially common in patients with disease of less than 1 year.

The rate of epidermal turnover may be the factor that predisposes the skin of patients with LE to accumulate appreciable quantities of immunoglobulins at the DEJ. Sunlight may be one of many factors that increases epidermal turnover.

The prevalence of deposits is not universal. There are site-to-site variations even in skin with similar amounts of sun exposure (Table 3) (11). Concordance is better on sun-protected skin (27).

Table 2. Comparison of LBT-Negative and Positive Groups with Regard to Treatment

Treatment	*LBT-Neg. (N = 22) (%)*	*LBT-Pos. (N = 29) (%)*
Cytotoxic[a] drug and prednisone	27	52
Prednisone >40 mg (maximum daily dose)	50	10
Prednisone <40 mg (maximum daily dose)	18	34
No cytotoxic agent or prednisone	5	3

[a]Cytotoxic drug—usually cyclophosphamide; occasionally azathioprine or chlorambucil.

From Davis and Gilliam (20) with permission.

Table 3. Variability of Immunoglobulin Components and C3

		No. (%)		
Type of site	*≥1+ Specimen*	*2 Other + Specimens*	*1 Other +Specimen*	*0 Other + Specimen*
Sun exposed	IgG (n = 9)	3 (33)	5 (55)	1 (11)
	IgM (n = 14)	9 (64)	1 (7)	4 (29)
	IgA (n = 4)	2 (50)	1 (25)	1 (25)
	C3 (nc = 3)	1 (33)	0	2 (67)
Sun protected	IgG (n = 5)	4 (80)	0	1 (20)
	IgM (n = 10)	6 (60)	1 (10)	3 (30)
	IgA (n = 1)	0	1 (100)	0
	C3 (n = 2)	0	0	2 (100)

From Jacobs et al. (27), copyright, American Medical Association.

MORPHOLOGY AND TERMINOLOGY

There is no uniform descriptive terminology relating to the morphology of the deposits. Bands have been described as granular, linear, shaggy, fibrillar, homogeneous, thready, stippled, broad, segmental, focal, continuous, thick, or fine in character. We have arbitrarily chosen to consider several morphologic variants and define them here. The Task Force on Immunopathology of the American Academy of Dermatology is developing a uniform nomenclature that should help standardize reporting. This tentative new nomenclature will be discussed below in the section on "New Nomenclature."

Fibrillar Deposits

Fibrillar deposits appear as blurred and fuzzy deposits at the DEJ. Under the microscope, the deposits seem to be out of focus and fuzzy when compared to surrounding

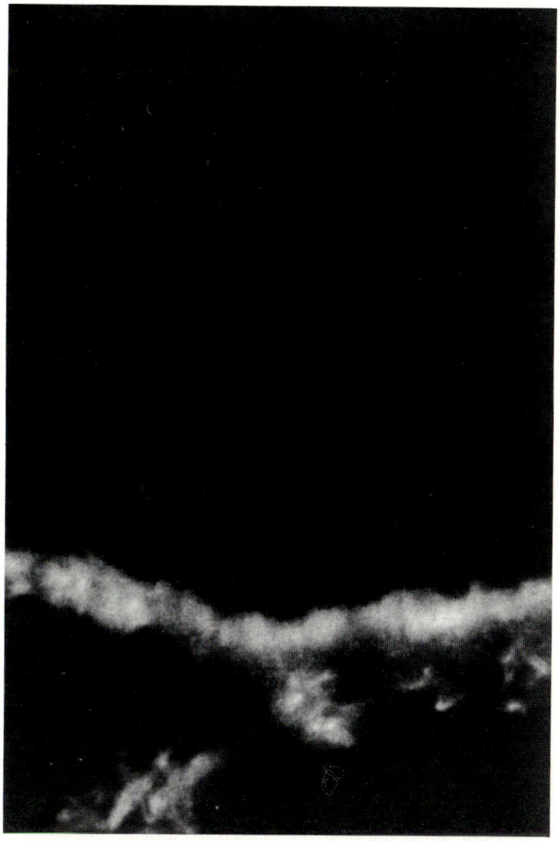

Figure 1 Fibrillar band. The band is broad and amorphous and appears "fuzzy" and out of focus. The new terminology would describe this as "thick linear deposits" (800x). (From Beutner and Kumar.)

tissue (Fig. 1). These bands are usually of uniform thickness and extend across the entire specimen. In many patients with DLE and SLE, this fibrillar band is bright and wide; but in other patients with LE or other disorders, the band is thinner and faint and merges step-by-step with the so-called fibrillar pseudobands that are an artifact (6). This pattern is brightest in chronic atrophic or hyperkeratotic lesions of DLE. A fainter variant of the fibrillar band has been called thready (7), because it consists of closely set threads or fibrils. It is seen in edematous plaques, erythematous patches, diffuse erythema, and normal skin of patients with systemic erythematosus.

Linear Band

A linear band has sharp, well-defined edges (Fig. 2). It is continuous and resembles a line drawn by a pencil that demarcates the DEJ. It is not as fuzzy or wide as a fibrillar band. Linear bands suggest the diagnosis of pemphigoid and are not usually seen in patients with LE.

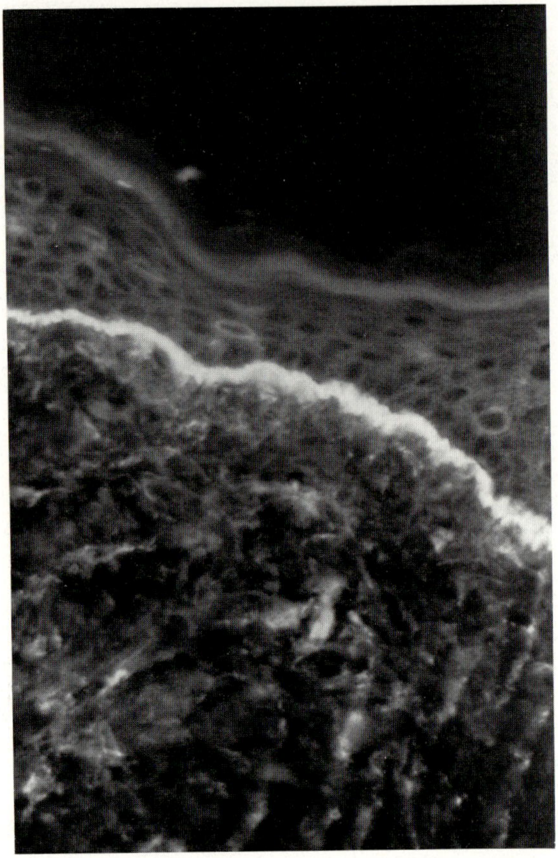

Figure 2. Linear band. A bright, continuous, thin, crisply demarcated band of immunoglobulins at the DEJ of the type found in BP. Such bands may also be seen occasionally in SLE, as shown in this patient. The new nomenclature would describe this as "thin linear deposits." (800x). (From Beutner and Kumar.)

Stippled Band

Stippled bands consist of particulate deposits of immunoglobulins at the DEJ (Fig. 3). These bands appear as brightly fluorescent specks at the DEJ and in the very most superficial dermis. A stippled band is frequently found in normal skin of patients with SLE. Stippled deposits also are found in involved skin. These are sometimes superimposed upon fibrillar bands.

It is not uncommon to see a few stipples of immunoglobulins along the DEJ not only in lesional skin and normal skin of patients with SLE, but also in skin from other patients. The pathologist must decide whether enough of these deposits are present to constitute a band of them. We use the term "stippled band" only when the deposits are dense enough to appear as a band if the eyes are somehow unfocused—a concentration of at least 20/rete peg.

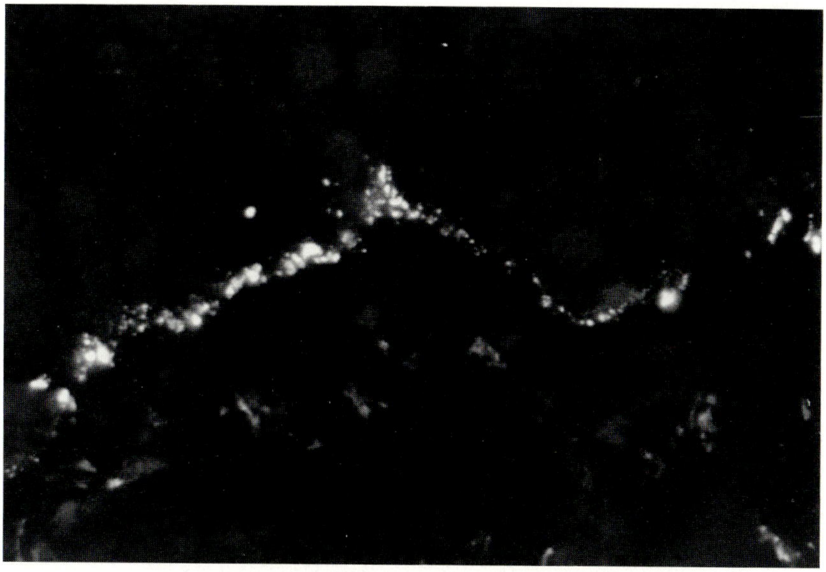

Figure 3. Stippled band. In this normal sun-exposed skin of an SLE patient, deposits of immunoglobulins (IgM) appear as discrete particles. The new nomenclature would describe this as "granular deposits" (300x). (From Beutner and Kumar.)

Shaggy Band

Large granules sometimes superimpose themselves on other large granules (Fig. 4). These appear to be "stacked up" so that they individually focus in different planes. This kind of band is seen mostly in lesional skin of patients with DLE, or SLE.

Fibrillar Pseudoband

A fibrillar pseudoband is an ill-defined faint glow of fluorescence at the DEJ (Fig. 5) (6). It is often associated imperceptably with background fluorescence in the dermis. It appears to be a band under low power, but under high power it becomes less apparent. Fibrillar pseudobands occur in skin that is edematous or in skin near dilated blood vessels, where the dermis is pressed against the DEJ so that the autofluorescence and nonspecific fluorescence of elastic tissue and other components mimic a band. This type of band is common in rosacea and telangiectatic skin. These bands are more likely to be seen in the dermal papillae than at the tips of the rete pegs. High contrast between dark epidermis and autofluorescent dermis may produce an optical illusion of a band, especially under low magnification.

Extent of bands

Focal Deposits

A focal deposit is not a morphologic type of band, but rather a band that does not extend across the entire specimen. Focal deposits are confined to a single small area of the biopsy specimen; for example, in lesions of vasculitis (Fig. 6).

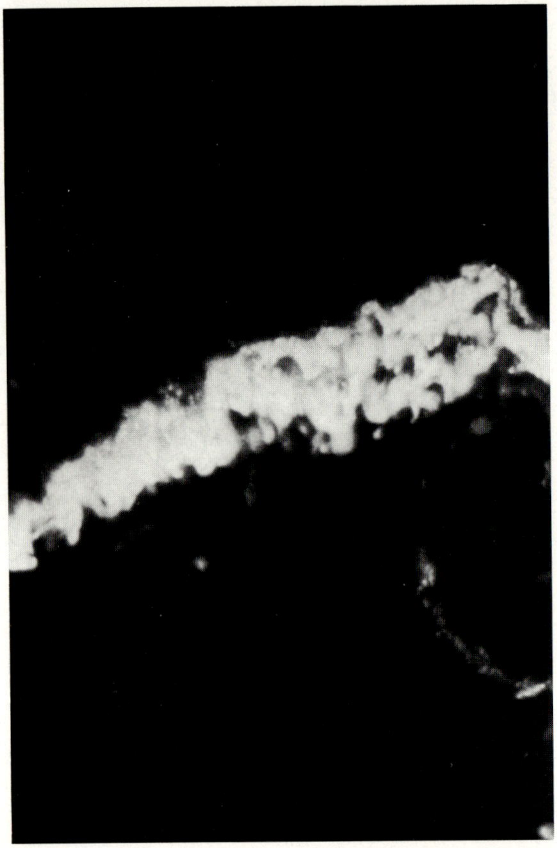

Figure 4. Lumpy, bumpy band. A very thick-appearing band of immunoglobulin deposits at the DEJ of lesional skin, such as illustrated here, strongly suggests DLE or SLE. The new nomenclature would describe this as "shaggy deposits" (300x).

Continuous Band

A continuous band, as the name implies, extends across the entire specimen. Figures 1 to 3 are examples of bands that were made up of continuous deposits.

Intermittent Bands

Intermittent bands demonstrate deposits of immunoglobulins segmentally, but not continuously across the entire specimen.

Ovoid Bodies

Ovoid bodies (cytoid bodies, hyaline bodies) appear at the DEJ in skin diseases with a lichenoid histology (Fig. 7). Even in lichen planus (LP), where these ovoid bodies litter the DEJ (32), we prefer not to describe them as constituting a band because the term "band" might be misinterpreted. Ovoid bodies are common in lesions of both SLE and DLE. They usually contain IgM and IgA and, to a lesser extent, IgG, complement, and fibrin.

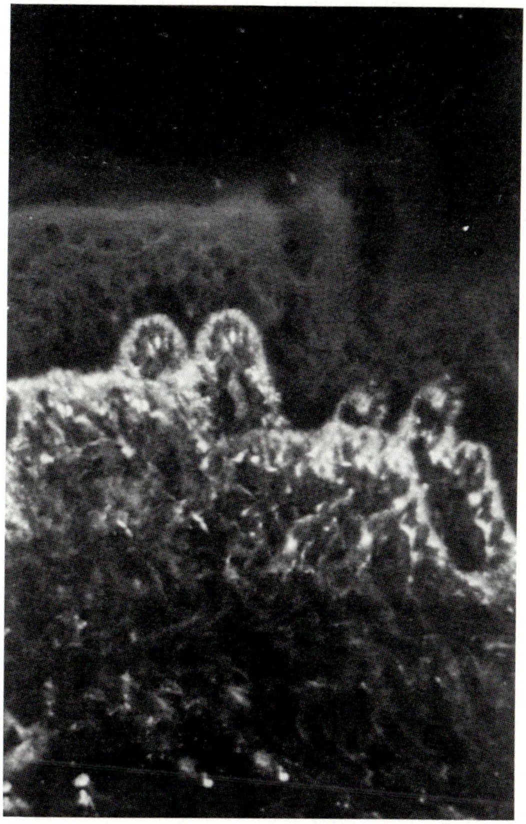

Figure 5. Fibrillar pseudoband. Fluorescent dermal fibers compacted against the DEJ give the appearance of a band of immunoglobulins (400x). As evident here, it is not always possible to be sure that small amounts of immunoreactants were not also present (160x). (From Beutner and Kumar.)

New Nomenclature

Despite the definitions given above, there is no universally accepted terminology for describing immune deposits at the DEJ. The Task Force on Immunopathology of the American Academy of Dermatology has tentatively adopted a new terminology in the hope of fostering standards. Whether or not this new system will prove to be any better than the old one remains to be seen. The new system does have the advantage in that it is descriptive rather than interpretive. Under this system, bands are linear, granular, or shaggy. Linear bands (e.g., Fig. 1) are continuous; granular bands are not. Shaggy bands are unique enough to warrant separate classification (Fig. 4). Linear bands are then subdivided into thin or thick. Thin linear bands are like those seen in bullous pemphigoid (BP), but also occasionally in LE (Fig. 2). Thick linear bands are wider (Fig. 1). Granular bands are subdivided into either coarse or fine, depending on whether they are large particles or small punctuate ones (Fig. 3). The type of band is then qualified as being continuous (present across the entire specimen) or intermittent

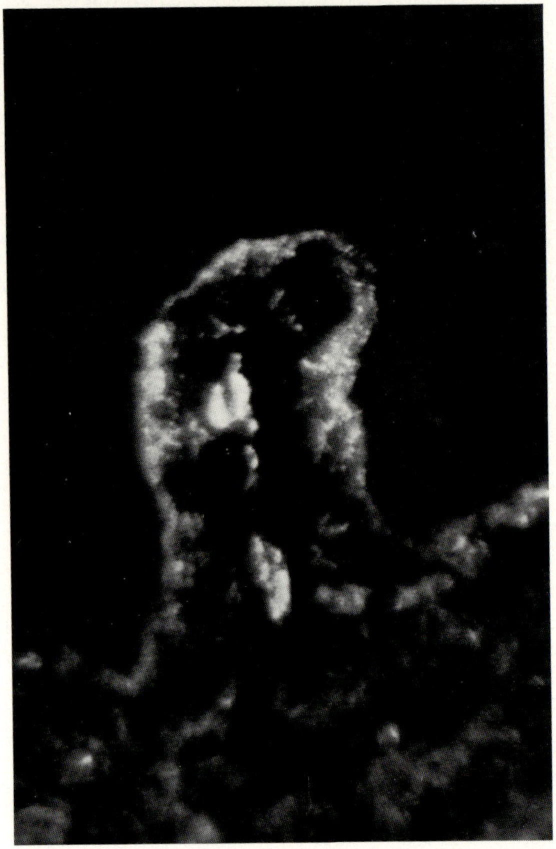

Figure 6. Focal stippled band. In this biopsy specimen of a vasculitis lesion, the deposits of IgM in the blood vessel are more intense than deposits along the DEJ. Sometimes, focal stippled bands are difficult to distinguish from fibrillar pseudobands. The new nomenclature would call this a "focal granular band" (300x). (From Beutner and Kumar.)

(focal or present in some areas but not others), and is also qualified by additional adjectives such as bright, moderately bright, or faint and sparse, moderately dense, or dense. Ovoid bodies are described by size, morphology, brightness, and location.

SENSITIVITY-SPECIFICITY

There is considerable debate about the sensitivity and specificity of the lupus band test.

Deposits of immunoglobulins have been found at the DEJ in *lesional* skin of patients with diseases other than LE. Some of these disorders are listed in Table 4. References to individual diseases can be found in other reviews (18,31). Deposits have been found in *normal* skin of patients with leukocytoclastic angiitis (31), progressive systemic sclerosis, dermatomyositis, rheumatoid arthritis (18,23), primary biliary cirrhosis (23), chronic active hepatitis, BP, herpes gestationis (HG), dermatitis herpetiformis (DH), and of

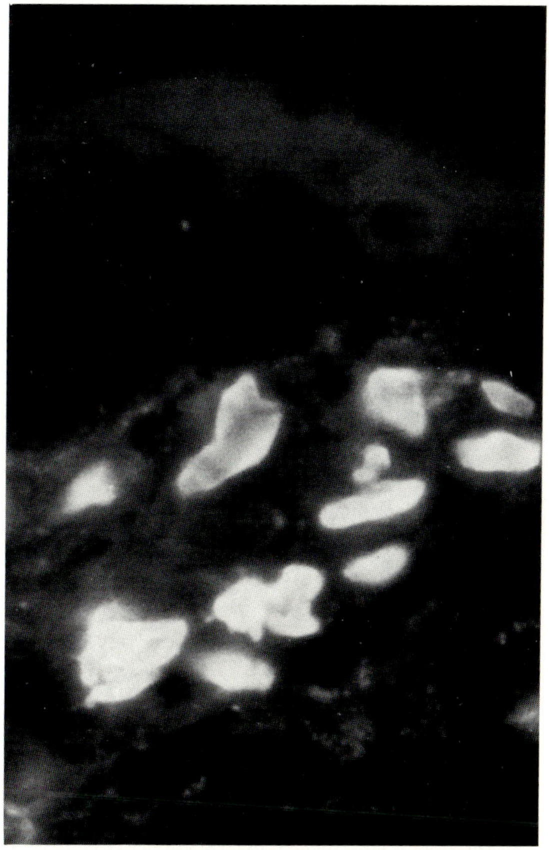

Figure 7. Dense deposits of immunoglobulin (IgM) on ovoid bodies in LP. Although ovoid bodies indicate a lichenoid reaction, their presence does not carry the same significance as other types of deposits in identifying LE (800x). (From Beutner and Kumar.)

course SLE including the drug-induced form (18,54). There are scattered reports of similar deposits in similar location in a variety of other disorders as well (31).

The most common immunoglobulin to be found at the DEJ of lesional skin is IgM, but the finding of IgM alone is also the least specific immunoglobulin suggesting LE (25). Most of the other diseases that have been associated with immunoglobulins at the DEJ have been associated with deposits of IgM there. Deposits of IgG are more specific for LE (99% in one study [25]), and the combined finding of IgM and IgG is common among patients with this disease.

The sensitivity of the test has already been discussed. In uninvolved skin, the test is fairly specific. Although bands have been found in patients with other disorders as discussed above, the incidence of bands among patients with disorders that could be confused with SLE is low. Provost evaluated normal skin of 700 biopsy specimens from the upper third of the extensor forearm and detected immunoglobulins at the DEJ in only four patients without connective tissue disease (CTD) (two had vasculitis, one chronic active hepatitis, and one an ill-defined heredity CTD). The incidence of "false-positive" lupus band tests on normal-appearing skin appears to be less than 1%.

Table 4. Diseases with Immunoglobulins at the DEJ in Lesional Skin

Systemic lupus erythematosus
Discoid lupus erythematosus
Subacute cutaneous lupus erythematosus
Bullous pemphigoid
Cicatricial pemphigoid
Herpes Gestationis
Dermatitis herpetiformis
Linear IgA bullous disease
Epidermolysis bullosa acquisita
Porphyria
Pemphigus erythematosus
Leukocytoclastic vasculitis
Facial telangiectasias
Rosacea
Polymorphic light eruption
Lichen planus
Jessner's lymphocytic infiltrate
Amyloidosis
Lepromatous leprosy
Sarcoidosis
Psoriasis
Pyoderma gangrenosum
Scabies
Pityriasis lichenoides
Granuloma faciale
Graft versus host disease
Granuloma annulare
Necrobiosis lipoidica
Mixed connective tissue disease
Progressive systemic sclerosis
Drug-induced lupus erythematosus
Phenobarbital-induced bullae

INTENSITY

There is no way to titer the quantity of immunoglobulins at the DEJ by DIF. However, the intensity of staining can be gauged qualitatively. Of diseases with deposits of immunoglobulins at the DEJ of normal skin, the deposits in SLE are the most intense if the bullous diseases are excluded. That is, the intensity of staining of immunoglobulins at the DEJ is usually weak for nonbullous skin diseases, except LE.

Sontheimer and Gilliam (48) showed that the intensity of fluorescence correlates to the titer of antibody to double-stranded DNA, which in turn correlates to disease activity. Therefore, bright bands imply active disease.

DYNAMICS

The process of deposition of immunoglobulins at the DEJ probably does not cause skin lesions. Bullous LE may be an exception (22). Many lupus patients without any skin disease have large amounts of immunoglobulins at the DEJ, whereas others with cutaneous involvement have no deposits in uninvolved skin. Furthermore, skin lesions can occur before immunoglobulins become apparent. This is illustrated by data from Blaczczyk et al. in Table 5. As patients are treated, the incidence of immunoglobulins at the DEJ decreases. For example, in a group of patients treated with prednisone and cyclophosphamide for 1 year, the incidence was only 12%; whereas in those treated with prednisone alone, the incidence was 76% (23). Treatment with azathioprine in 10 of 19 patients presented by Ojeda-Duran et al. (34) may explain why only 33% of their patients had immunoglobulins at the DEJ of volar forearm skin. However, treatment with topical corticosteroids and other treatments can also diminish the intensity of staining, and may cause immunoglobulin deposits to disappear entirely (14). The data of Blaszczyk et al. is presented in Table 6.

Patients with highly active SLE are more likely to have immunoglobulins at the DEJ than those whose disease is controlled or whose disease is in remission (18). Halberg et al. (25), for example, found bands in normal buttock skin in 91% of patients with active disease, but in only 33% of those with inactive disease. The lupus band test may convert from negative to positive or intensify during exacerbations. However, this correlation with disease activity is not particularly strong, so it is difficult to gauge the degree of clinical activity by the presence, absence, or intensity of staining of immunoglobulins at the DEJ. The presence of immunoglobulins at the DEJ does correlate with the presence of antibodies to double-stranded DNA, decreased complement levels, increased ESR, decreased lymphocyte counts, and other measures of clinical disease activity.

The presence of immunoglobulins at the DEJ also correlates with the presence of renal disease (5,8,21,32), although other studies have failed to demonstrate this relationship (4,12,25). It is clear that some patients without renal disease have immuno-

Table 5. Incidence of Bands Containing IgG or IgM in Lesions of DLE of Various Duration

Duration of the lesions	*No. of patients tested*	*No. with bands (%)*
Less than 1 mo	9	3 (33)
1–3 mo	36	20 (56)
3–6 mo	21	16 (76)
6–12 mo	22	16 (73)
More than 12 mo	124	102 (82)

From Blaszczyk et al., reproduced from *Arch Dermatol* 119:1012, 1983, copyright, American Medical Association.

Table 6. Immunoglobulin Deposits at the DEJ in Skin Lesions of DLE

	Frequency of band	
Status of lesion	*No. of patients*	*%*
Untreated	115/121	95
Untreated for 7–21 days prior to biopsy	22/31	71
Treated at time of biopsy	17/28	61

From Blaszczyk et al., reproduced from *Arch Dermatol* 119:1012, 1983, copyright, American Medical Association.

Table 7. Deposits in DEJ Compared With Other Variables Reflecting Disease Activity

	Active disease		Inactive disease		
Disease activity	*No. of patients*	*% of patients*[a]	*No. of patients*	*% of Patients*[a]	*t Test*
Deposits in DEJ (total)	49	91	39	33	$p<0.0005$
Deposits in DEJ (IgG)	49	30	39	5	$p<0.0005$
Deposits in DEJ (IgM)	49	80	39	33	$p<0.0005$
Deposits in DEJ (C3)	49	33	39	8	$p<0.002$
Subnormal serum C3 (<0.54 g/l)	35	62	36	19	$p<0.0005$
Subnormal serum C4 (<40 arbitrary units)	32	56	35	37	NS
Increased antidouble-stranded DNA concentration (>30% binding)	35	62	34	36	$p<0.02$
LE cells	38	74	34	47	$p<0.01$
Lymphopenia (<1,000/cu mm)	40	37	35	9	$p<0.005$
ESR>20 mm/h	47	72	37	51	$p<0.02$

[a]Percent with each abnormal finding.

From Halberg et al. (25), copyright, American Medical Association.

globulins in their skin, whereas some patients with renal disease may not. A skin biopsy specimen cannot substitute for a renal one if LE is suspected.

On the other hand, many studies do show a much higher incidence of renal disease among patients with immunoglobulins in uninvolved skin, especially when immunoglobulins in addition to or other than IgM are present. Even studies that have failed to show statistically significant associations usually show trends suggesting a positive correlation. When IgG is present in deposits of uninvolved skin, coexisting renal disease and immunoglobulin deposition is likely.

Several studies will be highlighted here. Noel et al. (33) found bands of immunoglobulins in 10 of 16 patients with nephritis. There was no relation with the presence of immunoglobulins and the morphologic type of glomerulitis. The combination of IgM deposits associated with Clq deposits had the highest degree of renal disease activity, but IgG deposits correlated best with lower serum C3 and C4 levels.

Grossman et al. (24) studied 26 patients with SLE; 78% of patients with renal disease had immunoglobulin deposits in light-protected skin, whereas only 41% of patients without renal disease had these deposits.

Provost et al. (41) found that 88% of untreated SLE patients with renal disease had deposits in extensor forearm skin. Although they studied 62 patients, only 22 had renal biopsy procedures, and 20 of these had renal disease. There were 36 patients who were assumed not to have renal disease since they did not have proteinuria nor elevated blood urea nitrogen or serum creatinine levels. Only 50% of these patients without renal disease had immunoglobulins at the DEJ. Three patients with renal disease did not have immunoglobulin deposits in skin.

Davis and Gilliam (20) found lupus nephropathy in 55% of patients with DEJ deposits in normal volar forearm skin, compared to an incidence of 23% in patients without DEJ deposits. Furthermore, the maximum serum creatinine was higher in the group with deposits. The 10-year survival was 95% if no deposits were present, but only 54% if deposits were detected.

Cunningham et al. (16) reported a patient with SLE and IgM deposits in skin who developed acute renal failure and skin deposits of IgG and IgA in addition to IgM.

Dantzig's group (19) studied skin from the lower back; 83% of patients with severe renal disease had a positive lupus band test, whereas only 18% of those with mild renal disease did.

Patients with LE and renal disease usually have very active systemic disease, and the correlation of renal disease with positive lupus band tests may relate more to the high activity in these patients than to the presence of renal disease per se.

Some investigators have suggested that biopsy specimens from nonsun-exposed skin are preferred to sun-exposed skin as predictors of renal disease because the degree of correlation of immunoglobulins in skin with immunoglobulins in kidney is greater.

CHOICE OF BIOPSY SITE

For reasons discussed above, there is no general consensus on the proper biopsy site. In order to aid the clinician, we offer some guidelines on where, how, and when to obtain a biopsy specimen. These guidelines reflect our biases.

In patients with DLE where IF is being used to confirm a diagnosis of lupus as opposed to some other disease, the biopsy specimen should be from involved skin, but preferably from skin that has not been aggressively treated with topical corticosteroids; 90% of patients with DLE have skin lesions containing immunoglobulin deposits at the DEJ.

In patients with DLE where one is trying to rule out the presence of SLE, a biopsy specimen should be from sun-exposed normal skin; for example, on the dorsal forearm or the deltoid area of the shoulder. Immunoglobulins are not found in normal skin of DLE patients. Since the prevalence of immunoglobulins in deltoid skin is twice that of buttock skin among SLE patients, the separation of these two diseases is more likely if the biopsy specimen is from the deltoid area or other sun-exposed site.

In patients with clinical or serologic findings suggestive of some sort of connective tissue disease where confirmation of disease is being sought, a biopsy procedure is best performed on normal sun-exposed skin such as the dorsal forearm or shoulder. Facial skin should be avoided, since false-positive tests in this location are more frequent.

In patients with known SLE where one is trying to gauge clinical disease activity, the correlation of disease activity with the positive band test is probably greater in nonsun-exposed skin. Therefore, a biopsy specimen is best obtained from a site such as the buttocks or proximal flexor forearm, but information gained from specimens of sun-exposed skin should also be considered.

In patients with marked actinic damage, a biopsy specimen should not be obtained from sun-exposed skin because the presence of fibrillar pseudobands is very high in these skin areas. In such patients with marked actinic damage, a biopsy specimen should be obtained from a site that is not clinically damaged or from unexposed skin such as the buttocks.

In deciding where to obtain a specimen, several other factors should be considered. Infection following a punch biopsy procedure seems to be more frequent on the lower legs, and seems especially likely over bony prominences on the dorsal hand. Since punch biopsy procedures do leave permanent scars, the cosmetic significance of a scar should be considered when selecting a biopsy site. The shoulder, upper chest, and angle of the jaw are prone to develop keloids if biopsy specimens are obtained from these sites in keloid-susceptible people.

BIOPSY PROCEDURE

The biopsy procedure itself is done in the same manner that specimens are obtained for ordinary pathologic examination. Usually 1% xylocaine without epinephrine is injected into the dermis. A 3 or 4 mm punch biopsy is used to excise a cylinder of skin tissue. Specimens less than 3 mm in diameter are not recommended because they are difficult to process, and because they provide inadequate material for the immunopathologist.

It is best to freeze the specimen in liquid nitrogen immediately following the procedure and to store the specimen in a liquid nitrogen or ultracool freezer until it can be processed. Some prefer to freeze the specimen in a liquid nitrogen and transfer it to dry ice until its eventual transfer to the freezer. Storage at −70° in special cold freezers is possible and usually satisfactory, provided the freezers are not self-defrosting. If liquid nitrogen is not available, specimens can be frozen with dry ice or placed in isopentane and frozen with dry ice.

If the patient is at great distance from the IF laboratory, it is often convenient to place the tissue specimen in a preservative medium especially designed for transport of such specimens to the laboratory. In this medium, the specimen can be mailed by regular first-class mail. When it is received at the laboratory, it must be washed before it can be snap-frozen. Experience has shown that the results of preservation using this special medium are good. Occasional false-negatives are encountered, but the morphology and findings usually correlate quite well with adjacent specimens processed by snap freezing and stored in regular manner.

PROBLEMS OF INTERPRETATION

The laboratory personnel will normally cut the specimen into 4-μm thick sections, and will stain sequential sections with fluorescein-labeled antihuman IgG, IgM, IgA, and C3. The immunopathologist will then examine the specimen and decide whether or not a band of immunoglobulins is present, and will categorize the band by morphology, continuity, and brightness. The findings are usually detailed in a descriptive report. The immunopathologist will also generally try to aid the clinician by giving an interpretation of the observed findings. Correlation with history and reason for obtaining the biopsy specimen are necessary. If the biopsy procedure was done for diagnosis, a listing of the clinical differential diagnoses by the clinician usually results in a more relevant interpretation.

The IF patterns of BP and DH are distinctive enough so that they should not usually confuse the experienced IF microscopist, particularly when clinical information suggesting a bullous disease is available. The exception here is with bullous LE, where linear bands containing IgG and IgA are frequent and suggest BP or linear IgA bullous dermatosis (LABD) (11,12).

The presence of IgM bands in involved skin of patients with various diseases is common, and therefore of little significance. The presence of multiple immunoglobulins, especially in large amounts, and multiple immunoglobulin classes suggests LE. When large amounts of many classes of immunoglobulins are found in normal skin, the diagnosis of SLE is strongly suggested.

Keeping this in mind then, the presence or absence of immunoglobulins at the DEJ should not automatically suggest or negate a clinical diagnosis of LE. The biopsy results must be interpreted in light of the clinical, histologic, and serologic features of the patient. The clinician should take note of whether or not large amounts of immunoglobulins were present and whether or not one or more immunoglobulin class was represented.

WHEN TO PERFORM A BIOPSY PROCEDURE

There are a number of situations where the lupus band test is especially useful. These are listed below:

1. To confirm a diagnosis of DLE or SLE.
2. To determine if the patient with discoid skin lesions and systemic illness has SLE.
3. To suggest a diagnosis of DLE or SLE in a patient with skin disease of varied morphology compatible with the diagnosis of LE. Of clinical diseases, the most common diagnostic problem is differentiating LE from LP. Other skin diseases such as psoriasis, scarring alopecia (28), polymorphic light eruption, bullous lupus erythematosus, dermatomyositis, inflamed actinic keratosis, and facial dermatitis are also among diagnostic challenges.
4. As an aid to gauging prognosis.

Several additional points may be made. Immunoglobulins can be found around the hair follicles of normal scalp in patients without LE. The presence of bands limited to hair follicles themselves is not as significant in the patient with scarring alopecia. On the other hand, the presence of complete bands along the skin in scarred areas or the presence of ovoid bodies in the dermis suggest the diagnosis of LE or LP (15–17).

False-positive lupus band tests are more common on the face. Because of this, results of facial biopsy procedures are especially difficult to interpret. Great heed should be paid to the morphology and the intensity of the band. Patients with telangiectasias, ruddy red faces, or rosacea very commonly have faint fibrillar continuous bands that are especially likely to be seen with antihuman IgM conjugates. Some of these bands are fibrillar pseudobands, but it is sometimes impossible to be sure.

SUMMARY

Lupus erythematosus is a disease associated with deposits of immunoglobulins at the DEJ of involved and uninvolved skin. Detection of these deposits by DIF can be helpful in the diagnosis of these diseases. Interpretation of results is not always a simple, straightforward, yes or no interpretation because stippled or intermittent deposits may be present, because the band may be faint and resemble a fibrillar pseudoband, or because aspects of treatment, age of lesions, or site of biopsy may influence the results. The clinician and immunopathologist must work together and communicate with each other in order to maximize the usefulness of IF testing.

REFERENCES

1. Ahmed AR, Provost TT: Incidence of a positive lupus band test using sun-exposed and unexposed skin. *Arch Dermatol* 115:228, 1979.
2. Alcocer J, Moreno J, Garcia-Torres R, et al: Immunofluorescent skin band test in the differential diagnosis of systemic lupus erythematosus. *J Rheumatol* 6:196, 1979.
3. Baart de la Faille-Kuyper EH, Cormane RH: The occurrence of certain serum factors in the dermal-epidermal junction and vessel walls of the skin in lupus erythematosus and other (skin) diseases. *Acta Dermatol Venereol* 48:578, 1968.
4. Boonpucknavig V, Boonpuckanavig S, Vuttivirojana O, et al: Immunofluorescent skin test for lupus erythematosus: A correlative study between frequency and patterns of skin test results, glomerular pathologic abnormalities and immunoglobulin findings. *Arch Pathol Lab Med* 101:350, 1977.
5. Bresnihan B, Hale GM, Bunn CC, et al: Immunoglobulin classes in skin basement membrane in systemic lupus erythematosus: Clinical significance and comparison with classes of serum anti-DNA antibodies. *Ann Rheum Dis* 38:351, 1979.
6. Burnham TK: The immunofluorescent "band" test for lupus erythematosus. *Br J Dermatol* 84:176, 1971.
7. Burnham TK, Fine G: The immunofluorescent "band" test for lupus erythematosus. I. Morphologic variations of the band of localized immunoglobulins at the dermal-epidermal junction in lupus erythematosus. *Arch Dermatol* 99:413, 1969.
8. Burnham TK, Fine G: The immunofluorescent "band" test for lupus erythematosus: III. Employing clinically normal skin. *Arch Dermatol* 103:24, 1971.
9. Burnham TK, Fine G, Neblett TR: Immunofluorescent "band" test for lupus erythematosus: II. Employing skin lesions. *Arch Dermatol* 102:42, 1970.
10. Burnham TK, Neblett TR, Fine G: The application of the fluorescent antibody technique to

the investigation of lupus erythematosus and various dermatoses. *J Invest Dermatol* 41:451, 1963.

11. Callerame ML, Condemi JJ: Variability of fluorescent band skin test studied by means of multiple-labeled biopsies from three autopsied SLE patients. *Arthritis Rheum* 19:792, 1976.
12. Caperton EM Jr, Bean SF, Dick FR: Immunofluorescent skin test in systemic lupus erythematosus: Lack of relationship with renal disease. *JAMA* 222:935, 1972.
13. Carlo JR, Rothfield NF, Ruddy S: Demonstration of Blh globulin together with C3 in the dermal epidermal function of patients with systemic lupus erythematosus. *Arthritis Rheum* 22:13, 1979.
14. Chorzelski TP, Jablonska S, Blaszczyk M: Immunopathologic investigations in lupus erythematosus. *J Invest Dermatol* 52:333, 1969.
15. Cormane RH: "Bound" globulin in the skin of patients with chronic discoid lupus erythematosus and systemic lupus erythematosus. *Lancet* 1:534, 1964.
16. Cunningham E, Provost T, Brentjens J, et al: Acute renal failure secondary to interstitial lupus nephritis associated with changing immunologic abnormalities. *Arch Intern Med* 138:1560, 1978.
17. Dahl MV: *Clinical Immunodermatology.* Year Book Medical Publishers, Chicago, 1981.
18. Dahl MV: Usefulness of direct immunofluorescence in patients with lupus erythematosus. *Arch Dermatol* 119:1010, 1983.
19. Dantzig PI, Mauro J, Rayhanzadeh S, et al: The significance of a positive cutaneous immunofluorescence test in systemic lupus erythematosus. *Br J Dermatol* 93:531, 1975.
20. Davis B, Gilliam JN: Prognostic significance of the lupus band test in systemic lupus erythematosus. A 10 year longitudinal study. *Arthritis Rheum* 25:57, 1982.
21. Deng J-S, Lin R-Y, Lu Y-C: Significance of in vivo-bound immunoglobulins and complement in the skin of systemic lupus erythematosus patients. *J Dermatol* 3:237, 1976.
22. Gammon WR, Briggaman RA, Inman AO, et al: Evidence suggesting a role for immune complex-mediated inflammation in the pathogenesis of bullous lesions of systemic lupus erythematosus. *J Invest Dermatol* 81:320, 1983.
23. Gilliam JN: The significance of cutaneous immunoglobulin deposits in lupus erythematosus and NZB/NZWF1 hybrid mice. *J Invest Dermatol* 65:154, 1975.
24. Grossman J, Callerame ML, Condemi JJ: Skin immunofluorescence studies on lupus erythematosus and other antinuclear antibody positive diseases. *Ann Intern Med* 80:496, 1974.
25. Halberg P, Ullman S, Jorgensen F: The lupus band test as a measure of disease activity in systemic lupus erythematosus. *Arch Dermatol* 118:572, 1982.
26. Harrist TJ, Mihm MC Jr: The specificity and clinical usefulness of the lupus band test. *Arthritis Rheum* 23:479, 1980.
27. Jacobs MI, Schned ES, Bystryn JC: Variability of the lupus band test. *Arch Dermatol* 119:883, 1983.
28. Jordon RE: Subtle clues to diagnosis by immunopathology: Scarring alopecia. *Am J Dermatopathol* 2:157, 1980.
29. Jordon RE, Schroeter AL, Winkelmann RK: Dermal epidermal deposition of complement components and properdin in systemic lupus erythematosus. *Br J Dermatol* 92:263, 1975.
30. Kalsbeek GL, Cormane RH: The occurrence of immunoglobulins in the dermo-epidermal junction of the skin in lupus erythematosus and related syndromes. *Dermatologica* 135:205, 1967.
31. Monroe EW: Lupus band test. *Arch Dermatol* 113:830, 1977.
32. Nesbitt LT, Gum OB: Direct cutaneous immunofluorescent test in lupus erythematosus. *South Med J* 66:991, 1973.
33. Noel L-H, Droz D, Rothfield NF: Clinical and serologic significance of cutaneous deposits of immunoglobulins, C3, and Clq in SLE patients with nephritis. *Clin Immunol Immunopathol* 10:381, 1978.
34. Ojeda-Duran S, Vargas-Rosendo R, Fernandez-Diez J: Skin immunofluorescence in patients with systemic lupus erythematosus, SLE: Relationship between the immunohistochemical pattern and systemic activity. *Arch Invest Med* 11:215, 1980.

35. O'Loughlin S, Schroeter AL, Jordon RE: A study of lupus erythematosus with particular reference to generalized discoid lupus. *Br J Dermatol* 99:1, 1978.
36. Pedro SD, Dahl MV: Direct immunofluorescence of bullous systemic lupus erythematosus. *Arch Dermatol* 107:118, 1973.
37. Pennebaker JB, Gilliam JN, Ziff M: Immunoglobulin classes of DNA binding activity in serum and skin in systemic lupus erythematosus. *J Clin Invest* 60:1331, 1977.
38. Percy J, Smyth CJ: The immunofluorescent skin test in systemic lupus erythematosus. *JAMA* 208:485, 1969.
39. Pohle EL, Tuffanelli D: Study of cutaneous lupus erythematosus by immunohistochemical methods. *Arch Dermatol* 97:520, 1968.
40. Provost TT: Lupus band test. *Int J Dermatol* 20:475, 1981.
41. Provost TT, Andres G, Maddison PJ, et al: Lupus band test in untreated SLE patients: Correlation of immunoglobulin deposition in the skin of the extensor forearm with clinical renal disease and serologic abnormalities. *J Invest Dermatol* 74:407, 1980.
42. Provost TT, Tomasi TB Jr: Evidence for complement activation via the alternate pathway in skin diseases. I. Herpes gestationis, bullous pemphigoid and lupus erythematosus. *J Clin Invest* 52:1779, 1973.
43. Prystowski SD, Herndon JH, Gilliam JN: Chronic cutaneous lupus erythematosus (DLE): A clinical and laboratory investigation of 80 patients. *Medicine* 55:183, 1975.
44. Rothfield N, Ross HA, Minta JO, et al: Glomerular and dermal deposition of properdin in systemic lupus erythematosus. *N Engl J Med* 287:681, 1972.
45. Schrager MA, Rothfield NF: Clinical significance of serum properdin levels and properdin deposition in the dermal-epidermal junction in systemic lupus erythematosus. *J Clin Invest* 57:212, 1976.
46. Schreiner E, Wolff K: Systemic lupus erythematosus: Electron microscopic localization of in vivo bound globulins at the dermal-epidermal junction. *J Invest Dermatol* 55:325, 1970.
47. Sharp GC, Anderson PC: Current concepts in the classification of connective tissue diseases. *J Am Acad Dermatol* 2:269, 1980.
48. Sontheimer RD, Gilliam JN: A reappraisal of the relationship between subepidermal immunoglobulin deposits and DNA antibodies in systemic lupus erythematosus. A study using crithidea lucilae immunofluorescence anti DNA assay. *J Invest Dermatol* 2:29, 1979.
49. Sontheimer RD, Thomas JR, Gilliam JN: Subacute cutaneous lupus erythematosus. A cutaneous marker for a distinct LE subset. *Arch Dermatol* 115:1409–1415, 1979.
50. Tan EM, Kunkel HG: An immunofluorescent study of the skin lesions in systemic lupus erythematosus. *Arthritis Rheum* 9:37, 1966.
51. Ten Have-Opbroek AAW: Demonstration of immunoglobulins and complement in the skin of patients with lupus erythematosus. *Acta Dermatol Venereol* 46:68, 1966.
52. Tuffanelli DL: Cutaneous immunopathology: Recent observations. *J Invest Dermatol* 65:143, 1975.
53. Tuffanelli DL, Kay D, Fukuyama K: Dermal-epidermal junction in lupus erythematosus. *Arch Dermatol* 99:652, 1969.
54. Ullman S, Wilk A, Kobaysi T, et al: Drug-induced lupus erythematosus syndrome. *Acta Dermatol Venereol* 54:387, 1974.

31
The Biochemical Nature of Nuclear Antigens Reactive with Antinuclear Antibodies

Georg Reimer

Roger Cornell

Eng M. Tan

INTRODUCTION

Serum antinuclear antibodies (ANA) are a hallmark of patients with systemic autoimmune diseases. The diseases dealt with in this chapter comprise different entities with multiorgan involvement of variable severity and prognosis. Systemic lupus erythematosus (SLE) is the classic multisystem autoimmune disease in which ANA almost invariably occur. The other diseases in this group include mixed connective tissue disease (MCTD), progressive systemic sclerosis (scleroderma), dermatomyositis, polymyositis, Sjögren's syndrome, and rheumatoid arthritis (RA). Skin involvement can occur in any of these autoimmune diseases, but it is most frequently encountered in scleroderma, dermatomyositis, and SLE.

The clinician is often confronted with patients who have either minimal symptoms or features of more than one well-defined autoimmune disease occurring at the same time or subsequently. An accurate clinical diagnosis can thus be difficult and may require more elaborate laboratory investigations.

The incidence of serum ANA is very high in many of the systemic autoimmune diseases also referred to in the literature as systemic rheumatic or connective tissue diseases. In recent years, clinicians have increasingly made use of ANA as markers for the diagnosis and management of certain of these diseases. ANA are presently an integrated part of diagnostic laboratory tests. In basic research, analysis of reactive nuclear antigens using the advanced technologies of immunobiology, immunochemistry,

Supported by NIH Grants AM30263 and AI10386.

cell biology, and molecular biology has led to a better understanding of the nature of the nuclear antigens involved. In addition, studies using ANA as probes in molecular biology have begun to clarify functions of nuclear and cytoplasmic macromolecules in cell regulation.

The first and second sections of this chapter deal with immunologic specificities and profiles of ANA in systemic autoimmune diseases. The macromolecular identity, significance, and function of some of the soluble nuclear antigens are presented and discussed in the third section.

IMMUNOLOGIC SPECIFICITIES OF ANTINUCLEAR ANTIBODIES

Antibodies to nuclear antigens in systemic autoimmune diseases have been detected in the sera of patients using a variety of immunologic methods. Indirect immunofluorescence (IIF), using either frozen tissue sections or more recently tissue culture cell lines as the substrate, is still the initial screening test in most diagnostic laboratories (9,11). Immunodiffusion methods, passive hemagglutination, radioimmunoassays, and enzyme-linked solid phase immunoassays form part of the battery of immunologic tests to dissect and identify immunologic specificities of ANA (22,29,44,57,59). Most recently, immunoprecipitation procedures using radiolabeled cell extracts followed by gel electrophoresis have been successfully applied to the identification of nuclear antigens reactive with ANA at a macromolecular level (18,31,36,37). The latter techniques, however, are not readily available at a practical level, and are thus mainly used in basic research.

It is feasible to divide ANA into different groups to provide a more systematic classification. Table 1 gives a list of ANA that react with DNA, RNA, and histones. Anti-DNA antibodies can be classified according to their reactivities with double- or single-stranded DNA. The first class of these antibodies binds to antigenic determinants that reside only on double-stranded DNA. There is no cross-reaction with single-stranded DNA (4,20). These antibodies are present in rare cases in SLE. The second class of antibodies to DNA cross-reacts with antigenic determinants shared by double- and single-stranded DNA (4,10,28,66,68). These antibodies probably recognize the de-

Table 1. Antinuclear Antibodies to DNA, RNA, and Histones

	Reactive antigen	*Disease association*
1.	Double-stranded DNA only	SLE (rare cases)
2.	Double/single-stranded DNA with shared antigenic determinants	SLE (70–80%)
3.	Single-stranded DNA only. Antigenic determinants related to purine and pyrimidine bases	SLE, other autoimmune diseases and nonautoimmune diseases
4.	Left-handed Z-DNA	SLE (90% cases)
5.	Double/single-stranded RNA	SLE (rare cases)
6.	Histones H1, H2A, H2B, H3, H4, H2A-H2B, and H3-H4 complexes	Drug-induced LE (95–100%) and SLE (80%), rheumatoid arthritis (15–20%), and SLE

oxyribose-phosphate backbone of DNA. There is evidence that a single strand of the deoxyribose-phosphate backbone is not sufficient for antigenicity. Folding back of a single-stranded DNA to form a secondary helical structure may create the antigenic determinant recognized by antibodies reactive with both double- and single-stranded DNA (63). The size of the reactive DNA fragments, however, appear to be 40 to 50 base pairs with a wide range (48). The prevalence of these antibodies in SLE sera varies with the activity and the type of organ involvement. In patients with active nephritis, the prevalence may approach 70 to 80%. The third type of anti-DNA antibodies reacts only with single-stranded DNA (28,61,66,68). The antigenic determinants are related to purines and pyrimidines on single-stranded DNA. These antibodies will not react with double-stranded DNA, since the bases here are buried within the helix and are sterically less accessible. The clinical association of these antibodies includes a variety of autoimmune diseases with no clear-cut prevalence for one entity. Recently, naturally occurring antibodies to left-handed Z-DNA have been demonstrated in sera of SLE patients (30). Antibodies to single- and double-stranded RNA also have been identified in SLE (15,28). Antibodies to single-stranded RNA appear to be involved in immune complex nephritis of rare cases with SLE (3).

Antibodies to histones that form the major nuclear protein of chromatin in eukaryotic cells have been shown to react with all the major classes, that is, H1, H2A, H2B, H3, and H4 (19,23,62). In addition, complexes of H2A-H2B and H3-H4 appear to have unique antigenic determinants that are recognized by certain antibodies. These antigenic determinants do not appear to be present on the individual histone subclasses (51,57). Histones have been reported to be the target of autoantibodies in up to 80% of SLE patients (23,57,58). Antihistone antibodies can be induced by drugs such as procainamide and hydralazine in laboratory animals (72). A high incidence of antibodies to histones are present in patients who are given these drugs, and are a major serologic feature of drug-induced lupus erythematosus (LE) (19,23,62). The mechanism of autoantibody generation by procainamide or hydralazine has not been elucidated. However, studies have shown that hydralazine has a high binding affinity to DNA-histone (nucleoprotein); as a result, the nucleoprotein-drug complex renders the histone moiety of nucleoprotein more resistant to tryptic digestion (67). Persistence of the putative antigen due to impaired metabolic degradation may again enhance its immunogenicity. Further research in this area may provide more information on the pathogenesis of autoantibody production in systemic autoimmune disease in general.

Indirect IF using tissue culture cells as the substrate has revealed three different nucleolar staining patterns. These staining patterns are associated with scleroderma or scleroderma-like syndromes, of which Raynaud's phenomenon is a major feature (5,48,69). Table 2 presents a list of antibodies to nucleolar antigens. Certain sera that

Table 2. Antinuclear Antibodies to Nucleolar Antigens

Reactive antigen	*Disease association*
Homogenous nucleolar IF pattern	
1. 4S-6S nucleolus-specific RNA, possible U3RNA	Scleroderma and scleroderma-like overlap syndromes associated with Raynaud's phenomenon
2. Clumpy and speckled nucleolar IF pattern (antigen unidentified)	

give homogeneous immunofluorescent (IF) patterns of nucleoli have been shown by immunodiffusion to precipitate with a low molecular weight 4S-6S nucleolus-specific RNA (41,49). It is conceivable that this antibody may be identical with antinucleolar sera that precipitate U3-RNA of ^{32}P-labeled cellular extracts (55). The macromolecular nature of the other two nucleolar antigens that give a clumpy and a speckled IF pattern is thus far unknown.

The other major class of ANA in systemic autoimmune diseases is characterized by reactivities with soluble, nonhistone nuclear proteins and RNA-protein complexes. Most of these acidic proteins are readily extractable in physiologic buffers, and can be detected by immunodiffusion methods using the appropriate antigen extracts and reference sera. Precipitin antibodies to soluble nuclear antigens have become of increasing importance in the differential diagnosis of systemic autoimmune diseases, since some of these autoantibodies are restricted to certain disease entities. The marker antibodies are those against Sm antigen for SLE, Scl-70 for scleroderma, and kinetochore antigens for the CREST subset of scleroderma (70). Antibody to Sm can be detected by classic immunologic methods such as immunodiffusion, passive hemagglutination, and counterimmunoelectrophoresis (29,44,65). The Sm antigen was the first soluble nuclear antigen to be described (65). Antibody to Scl-70 has been shown to react with a 70-kd basic nuclear protein closely associated with chromatin (14). Anticentromere antibody recognizes protein antigens closely related and tightly bound to the kinetochore of chromosomes (8,43). The exact nature of these proteins is not yet known. The kinetochore antigens are not extractable without loss of antigenicity, and thus no immunoprecipitin system for the detection of anticentromere antibody exists. However, this antibody gives a characteristic IF staining pattern in dividing cells (43).

Antibodies with a wider distribution include anti-nRNP, SS-A/Ro, and SS-B/La antibodies. Antibody to nRNP precipitates an extractable nuclear antigen that is associated with Sm in a complex now generally referred to as extractable nuclear antigen (ENA) (38,47,60). The nRNP antigen in this complex has been shown to be RNase sensitive, whereas Sm antigen has been found to be resistant to RNase digestion (47,60,65). Anti-nRNP antibodies are present in high titer in the sera of patients with MCTD. Antibody to SS-A/Ro and SS-B/La give precipitin lines with antigens extracted from Wil-2 cells—a human B-cell lymphoblastoid line (1). Anti-SS-A/Ro and anti-SS-B/La antibody have a high incidence in Sjögren's syndrome. Antibody to SS-B/La is also present in patients with SLE, whereas antibody to SS-A/Ro has been found to be related to subacute cutaneous lupus erythematosus (SCLE) and neonatal lupus erythematosus (NLE) (17,21,39).

An interesting antibody, insofar as its reactivity is restricted to proliferating cells, is present in 3% of SLE patients. The reactive antigen has been termed proliferating cell nuclear antigen (PCNA). PCNA is not restricted to cell type, but it appears to be present in all proliferating cells (42,64). The Ma antigen reactive with sera from some SLE patients is distinct from Sm, n-RNP, SS-A/Ro, and SS-B/La antigen, as shown by various immunodiffusion, IF, and physicochemical studies (75). Antigen-antibody systems found in dermatomyositis and polymyositis include Jo-1, PM-1, Mi-1, and Ku antigens (40,45,46,53,76). Antibody to Jo-1 seems to be specific for polymyositis, whereas at least Mi-1 has been shown to occur also in SLE (71).

Antibody to rheumatoid arthritis-associated nuclear antigen (RANA) is present in patients with RA. It is not restricted to RA patients, but it occurs in higher frequency, and the titer in RA is clearly higher than in other diseases and in normal subjects. This antigen is different from other soluble nuclear antigens since it is induced by Epstein-Barr virus (EBV), and is therefore only present in EBV-infected cells (2). Table 3 gives

Table 3. Antinuclear Antibodies to Soluble Nuclear Proteins and RNA-Protein Complexes

	Reactive antigen	*Disease association*
1.	Sm (12–35K proteins with U-RNA)	SLE (30–40%): Marker antibody
2.	nRNP (68K protein with U1-RNA)	MCTD (95–100%): Also in SLE, scleroderma, and other systemic autoimmune diseases at lower frequency and titer
3.	SS-A/Ro (55K protein with RNA)	Sjogren's syndrome (60–70%), SLE (30–40%)
4.	SS-B/La (45K phosphoprotein with RNA pol III transcript)	Sjogren's syndrome (50–60%), SLE (10–15%)
5.	Scl-70 (70K basic protein)	Sclerderma (15–20%): Marker antibody
6.	Centromere/kinetochore (protein antigens)	CREST-syndrome (70–90%). Marker antibody
7.	RANA (rheumatoid arthritis-associated nuclear antigen	Rheumatoid arthritis (90-95%)
8.	Ma antigen	SLE (20%)
9.	PCNA (proliferating cell nuclear antigen	SLE (5–10%)
10.	PM-1	Polymyositis/scleroderma overlap (87%), dermatomyositis (17%)
11.	Mi-1	Dermatomyositis (11%)
12.	Jo-1 (50K protein) (histidyl-tRNA synthetrase)	Polymyositis (31%)
13.	Ku	Polymyositis/scleroderma (55%)

a list of relevant antigen-antibody systems reactive with soluble nuclear antigens, the disease associations, and prevalence.

PROFILES OF ANTINUCLEAR ANTIBODIES

With the exception of the marker antibodies, it has become apparent that no single immunologic test can provide satisfactory data for the differential diagnosis of systemic autoimmune diseases. Instead, profiles of ANA specificities have proved to provide more valuable diagnostic information to the clinician than individual tests. In SLE, the profile of ANA is characterized by multiplicity of autoantibodies to nuclear antigens, with each ANA present in different frequency. In MCTD and drug-induced LE, the profiles of ANA are less complex. Antibody to ribonucleoprotein (RNP) and histones, respectively, are almost the only ANA present. On the other hand, antibody to Sm is exclusively confined to SLE sera and hence is a specific diagnostic marker of the disease. Antidouble-stranded DNA antibodies are also characteristic of SLE, and generally do not occur in other autoimmune diseases. Antibody to nRNP is present in MCTD, SLE, scleroderma, and Sjögren's syndrome, with a prevalence of almost 100% in MCTD. Antibody to SS-A/Ro and SS-B/La frequently occur in Sjögren's syndrome, but are also present in SLE. Antibody to Scl-70 is again restricted to scleroderma, whereas antikinetochore (centromere) antibodies are specific for the CREST syndrome. By contrast, antisingle-stranded DNA antibodies reveal little diagnostic significance, since they are present in most autoimmune diseases. Figure 1 shows the profiles of ANA encountered in four diseases discussed in this section.

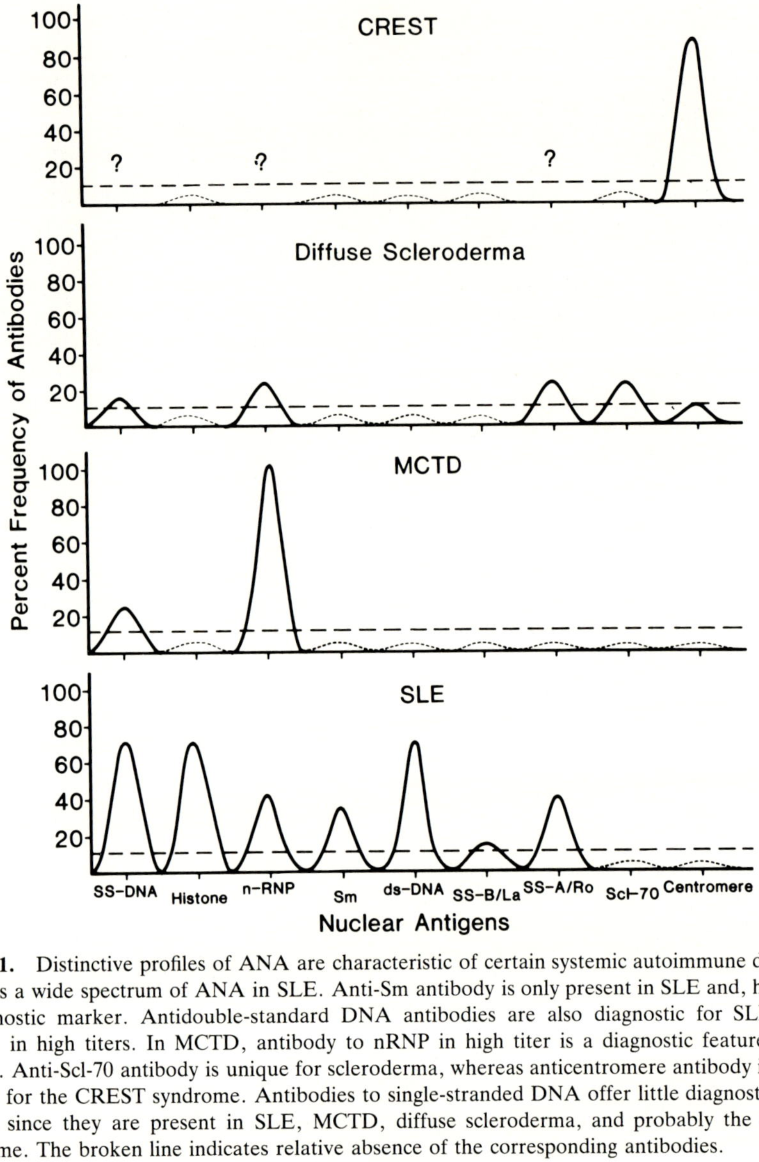

Figure 1. Distinctive profiles of ANA are characteristic of certain systemic autoimmune diseases. There is a wide spectrum of ANA in SLE. Anti-Sm antibody is only present in SLE and, hence, is a diagnostic marker. Antidouble-standard DNA antibodies are also diagnostic for SLE when present in high titers. In MCTD, antibody to nRNP in high titer is a diagnostic feature of the disease. Anti-Scl-70 antibody is unique for scleroderma, whereas anticentromere antibody is highly specific for the CREST syndrome. Antibodies to single-stranded DNA offer little diagnostic information since they are present in SLE, MCTD, diffuse scleroderma, and probably the CREST syndrome. The broken line indicates relative absence of the corresponding antibodies.

MACROMOLECULAR CHARACTERIZATION OF SOLUBLE NUCLEAR ANTIGENS REACTIVE WITH ANTINUCLEAR ANTIBODIES

A better understanding of the major precipitin antigens encountered in systemic autoimmune diseases at a macromolecular level has emerged by applying more advanced techniques of biochemistry and molecular biology in this area of research. These techniques have included *Staphylococcus aureus* protein A-facilitated immunoprecipitation of ^{32}P- and ^{35}S-labeled cellular extracts followed by sodium dodecyl sulfate polyacrylamide gel electrophoresis (SDS-PAGE) (18,25,31,37). In addition, other laboratories have been using immunoblotting techniques; that is, transfer of electrophoretically separated cell proteins to nitrocellulose paper, and probing with the respective antibody preparations (6,12,73,74). Further characterization of nuclear antigens have been performed by enzyme digestion, such as trypsin and RNAse pretreatment of the antigens (16,43,47,60,65).

Some of the better known antigens that have been recently characterized on a macromolecular level include nRNP, Sm, SS-A/Ro, and SS-B/La. Antibodies to nRNP and Sm from patient sera, as well as monoclonal anti-Sm and-nRNP antibody derived from spleen cells of MRL-mice, have been used in attempts to determine the structure and function of nRNP and Sm antigen (6,31,33). Using immunoprecipitation techniques, it has been shown that antibodies to nRNP and Sm bind to small nuclear (sn) RNPs. Small nuclear RNPs are complexes of snRNA and protein. These snRNPs are highly conserved throughout evolution. Although their presence has been familiar to molecular biologists for some time, little is known about their function in macromolecular cell regulation. The RNA components of snRNPs consist of uridine-rich RNA, which is different from messenger (m)-RNA, transfer (t)-RNA, or ribosomal (r)-RNA. Antibody to nRNP reacts with an snRNP particle containing U1-RNA, whereas antibody to Sm precipitates five small RNA; that is, U2, U4, U5, and U6 in addition to U1-RNA (31). Figure 2 shows the snRNAs of ^{32}P-labeled Hela cell extracts immunoprecipitated by antibody to Sm and nRNP. Interestingly, the U1 RNA has a sequence that is complementary to common splice junction sequences of newly transcribed RNA, leading to the interpretation that U1 snRNP may be involved in RNA splicing (32,56). One hypothesis of the splicing mechanism suggests that genomic DNA-containing introns are transcribed into heterogeneous nuclear (hn)RNA in the nucleus. The U1 snRNP aligns with the splice junction at the end of the intron, and splices the intron from hnRNA to form m-RNA. Translation of m-RNA into protein then takes place in the cytoplasm. In addition to precipitation of U1, U2, U4, U5, and U6 RNA, antibodies to Sm and nRNP bring down small nuclear proteins that are associated with these RNAs (16,31,33,37). It can be demonstrated that the protein moiety of Sm and nRNP reveals antigenicity, since pretreatment of the cellular extract with RNase did not affect immunoprecipitation of the proteins, except for a 35k protein recognized by anti-Sm and anti-nRNP antibody (16). There is still controversy as to the identity of the protein components that constitute Sm and nRNP antigens. The numbers of protein bands for Sm by SDS-PAGE or immunoblotting techniques reported by different investigators range from seven or eight (16,31) to two or four (12,77), and the molecular weight ranges from 12 to 35K. The explanation for these differences may be limited proteolysis during isolation procedures of the antigenic material, which vary in different laboratories. In addition, species variation of Sm also appears to account for differences in this molecule (7,13). Perhaps more important, human sera used as reagents are rarely monospecific, and the different results obtained may reflect the presence of multiple antibodies in the sera. Careful studies such as sequential absorptions to remove contaminating antibodies have rarely been done (12). A U1-specific polypeptide of 68K has recently been identified by immunoblotting as the target of anti-nRNP antibodies (27,77). It has been suggested that the low molecular weight proteins commonly seen by SDS-PAGE of nRNP immunoprecipitates may be breakdown products of this 68K protein. In addition, anti-nRNP-containing MCTD sera recognize a 70K nuclear matrix protein devoid of RNA (24) and, hence, are different from the 70K polypeptide recognized by an anti-(U1)nRNP monoclonal antibody by immunoblotting (6).

Other autoantibodies in autoimmune diseases reactive with RNA-protein complexes

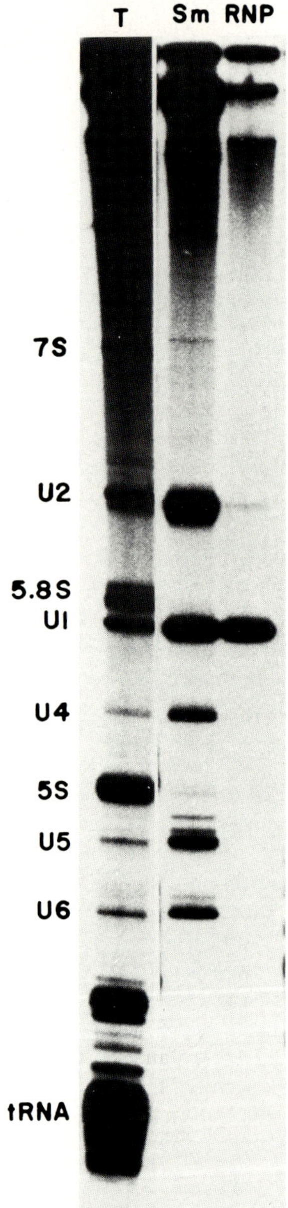

Figure 2. Small RNAs of the small nuclear ribonucleoprotein particles immunoprecipitated by antibody to Sm and nRNP antigen. HeLa cells were labeled with ^{32}P, and the soluble extract of these cells were immunoprecipitated with anti-Sm (lane 2) and anti-nRNP (lane 3) antibodies. The total RNA of cell extract is displayed in lane 1 of this SDS-urea polyacrylamide gel electrophoresis. Anti-Sm precipitated five species of RNAs (U1, U2, U4, U5, and U6), whereas anti-nRNP antibody precipitated only U1-RNA.

include antibodies to SS-B/La and SS-A/Ro antigen. These antigens have also recently been better characterized on a macromolecular level. The small RNAs of SS-B/La and SS-A/Ro, which are complexed to protein (35), have been shown to consist mainly of RNA polymerase III products (26,52). Recent experiments have indicated that SS-B/La protein antigen participates in the maturation of RNA polymerase III transcripts (18,26,54). In addition, SS-B/La protein particle also binds to adenovirus-associated RNA (VA RNA) (18) and EBV-associated RNA (34). This finding may indicate the implication of these viruses in diseases in which this antibody is present. Molecular weight studies of the protein component of SS-B/La antigen have revealed a 45K polypeptide that is phosphorylated (18,50). The SS-A/Ro antigen was shown to have a molecular weight of 55K (73).

More recently, an RNA-associated 50K polypeptide antigen present in about 30% of patients with myositis, called Jo-1, has been identified as histidyl t-RNA synthetase, with the RNA component being t-RNA^{His} (36). It has been hypothesized that a virus may be involved in myositis, carrying a histidine residue attached to its RNA. This complex may bind to histidyl t-RNA synthetase, rendering it immunogenic, which may lead to generation of antibody to t-RNA synthetase itself.

The interaction of cellular proteins with altered or nonself nucleic acid fragments can be regarded as a possible mechanism to induce autoimmunity. These nucleic acid fragments could well be of viral origin, rendering cellular proteins immunogenic. This hypothetical mechanism can be applied to certain RNA-protein antigens. In general, however, most of the soluble nuclear antigens remain poorly understood in terms of structure and function at a macromolecular level despite chromatographic and molecular weight data obtained thus far.

CONCLUSIONS

Antinuclear antibodies are useful tools in the diagnosis and management of patients with systemic autoimmune diseases. Intensive immunologic studies have emerged in the characterization of a variety of distinct ANA subsets. Clinical studies have shown that ANA reactive with Sm, Scl-70, and centromere antigens are highly specific for defined disease entities. Anti-Sm, Scl-70, and centromere antibodies now serve as markers for SLE, scleroderma, and the CREST syndrome, respectively. In addition, characteristic profiles of ANA have been established, facilitating the diagnosis of certain autoimmune diseases.

A great deal of work in the basic research of ANA has been performed in different laboratories, with the emphasis on identifying the macromolecular nature of reactive antigens. The antigens recognized by anti-DNA and antihistone antibodies have been characterized in great detail. However, nonhistone-soluble nuclear antigens, as a rule, remain poorly understood in terms of structure and function at a molecular level, with the exception of Jo-1, Sm, and nRNP. The latter two antigens appear to play a role in the splicing mechanism of heterogeneous nuclear RNA. Jo-1 antigen seems to be identical with histidyl t-RNA synthetase.

By learning more about the macromolecular nature and function of soluble nuclear antigens reactive with ANA, it is conceivable that questions as to why abundant, highly conserved nuclear proteins become immunogenic may be answered more satisfactorily. An answer to these questions may shed light on etiologic factors involved in eliciting an autoimmune response.

REFERENCES

1. Alspaugh MA, Tan EM: Antibodies to cellular antigens in Sjogren's syndrome. *J Clin Invest* 55:1067, 1975
2. Alspaugh MA, Jensen FC, Rabin H, et al: Lymphocytes transformed by Epstein-Barr virus. Induction of nuclear antigen reactive with antibody in rheumatoid arthritis. *J Exp Med* 147:1018, 1978.
3. Andres GA, Accinni L, Beiser SM, et al: Localization of fluorescein-labeled antinucleoside antibodies in glomeruli of patients with active systemic lupus erythematosus nephritis. *J Clin Invest* 49:2106, 1970.
4. Arana R, Seligmann M: Antibodies to native and denatured deoxyribonucleic acid in systemic lupus erythematosus. *J Clin Invest* 46:1867, 1967.
5. Bernstein RM, Steigerwald JC, Tan EM: Association of antinuclear and antinucleolar antibodies in progressive systemic sclerosis. *Clin Exp Immunol* 48:43, 1982.
6. Billings PB, Allen RW, Jensen FC, et al: Anti-RNP monoclonal antibodies derived from mouse strain with lupus-like autoimmunity. *J Immunol* 128:1176, 1982.
7. Billings PB, Hoch SO: Isolation of intact Sm/RNP antigens from rabbit thymus. *J Immunol* 131:347, 1983.
8. Brenner S, Pepper D, Bern MW, et al: Kinetochore structure, duplication and distribution in mammalian cells: Analysis by human autoantibodies from scleroderma. *J Cell Biol* 91:95, 1981.
9. Burnham TK, Bank PW: Antinuclear antibodies. I. Patterns of nuclear immunofluorescence. *J Invest Dermatol* 62:526, 1974.
10. Cohen SA, Hughes GRV, Noel GL, et al: Character of anti-DNA antibodies in systemic lupus erythematosus. *Clin Exp Immunol* 8:551, 1971.
11. Cleymaet JE, Nakamura RM: Indirect immunofluorescent antinuclear antibody test: Comparison of sensitivity and specificity of different substrates. *Am J Clin Pathol* 58:338, 1972.
12. Conner GE, Nelson D, Wisniewolski R, et al: Protein antigens of the RNA-protein complexes detected by anti-Sm and anti-RNP antibodies found in serum of patients with systemic lupus erythematosus and related disorders. *J Exp Med* 156:1475, 1982.
13. Dang H, Fischbach M, Lerner E, et al: Molecular and antigenic nature of isolated Sm. *J Immunol* 130:2782, 1983.
14. Douvas AS, Achten M, Tan EM: Identification of a nuclear protein (Scl-70) as a unique target of human antinuclear antibodies in scleroderma. *J Biol Chem* 254:10514, 1979.
15. Eilat D, Steinberg AD, Schechter AN: The reaction of SLE antibodies with native and single-stranded RNA: Radioimmunoassay and binding specificities. *J Immunol* 120:555, 1978.
16. Fisher DE, Conner GE, Reeves WM, et al: Synthesis and assembly of human small nuclear ribonucleoproteins generated by cell-free translation. *Proc Natl Acad Sci USA* 80:6356, 1983.
17. Franco HL, Weston WL, Peebles C, et al: Autoantibodies directed against sicca syndrome antigens in the neonatal lupus syndrome. *J Am Acad Dermatol* 4:67, 1981.
18. Francoeur AM, Mathews MB: Interaction between VA RNA and the lupus antigen La: Formation of a ribonucleoprotein particle *in vitro*. *Proc Natl Acad Sci USA* 79:6772, 1982.
19. Fritzler MJ, Tan EM: Antibodies to histones in drug-induced and idiopathic lupus erythematosus. *J Clin Invest* 62:560, 1978.
20. Gilliam A, Land D, LoSpalluto JJ: Antibodies to double-stranded DNA: Purification and characterization of binding specificities. *J Immunol* 125:84, 1980.
21. Gilliam JM, Sontheimer RD: Distinctive cutaneous subsets in the spectrum of lupus erythematosus. *J Am Acad Dermatol* 4:471, 1981.
22. Ginsberg B, Keiser H: A millipore filter assay for antibodies to native DNA in sera of patients with systemic lupus erythematosus. *Arthritis Rheum* 16:199, 1973.
23. Gioud M, Aitkaci M, Monier JC: Histone antibodies in systemic lupus erythematosus. *Arthritis Rheum* 25:404, 1982.
24. Habets WJ, DeRooji DJ, Salden MH, et al: Antibodies against distinct nuclear matrix proteins are characteristic for mixed connective tissue disease. *Clin Exp Immunol* 54:265, 1983.

25. Hardin JA, Rahn DR, Shen C, et al: Antibodies from patients with connective tissue disease bind specific subsets of cellular RNA-protein peptides. *J Clin Invest* 70:141, 1982.
26. Hendrick JP, Wolin SL, Rinke J, et al: Ro small cytoplasmic ribonucleoproteins are a subclass of La ribonucleoprotein: Further characterization of the Ro and La small ribonucleoproteins from uninfected mammalian cells. *Mol Cell Biol* 1:1138, 1981.
27. Hinterberger M, Pettersson I, Steitz JA: Isolation of small nuclear ribonucleoproteins containing U1, U2, U4, U5 and U6 RNAs. *J Biol Chem* 258:2604, 1983.
28. Koffler D, Carr RI, Agnello V, et al: Antibodies to polynucleotides in human sera: Antigenic specificity and relation to disease. *J Exp Med* 134:294, 1971.
29. Kurata N, Tan EM: Identification of antibodies to nucleic acidic antigens by counterimmunoelectrophoresis (CIE). *Arthritis Rheum* 19:574, 1976.
30. Lafer EM, Vall RPC, Moller A, et al: Z-DNA-specific antibodies in human systemic lupus erythematosus. *J Clin Invest* 71:1176, 1983.
31. Lerner MR, Steitz JA: Antibodies to small nuclear RNAs complexed with proteins are produced by patients with systemic lupus erythematosus. *Proc Natl Acad Sci USA* 76:5495, 1979.
32. Lerner MR, Boyle JA, Mount SM, et al: Are snRNPs involved in splicing? *Nature* 283:220, 1980.
33. Lerner EA, Lerner MR, Janeway CA Jr, et al: Monoclonal antibodies to nucleic acid containing cellular constituents: Probes for molecular biology and autoimmune diseases. *Proc Natl Acad Sci USA* 78:2737, 1981.
34. Lerner MR, Andrews NC, Miller G, et al: Two small RNAs encoded by Epstein-Barr virus and complexed with protein are precipitated by antinuclear antibodies from patients with systemic lupus erythematosus. *Proc Natl Acad Sci USA* 78:805, 1981.
35. Lerner MR, Boyle JA, Hardin JA, et al: Two novel classes of small ribonucleoproteins detected by antibodies associated with lupus erythematosus. *Science* 211:400, 1981.
36. Mathews MB, Bernstein RM: Myositis autoantibody inhibits histidyl t-RNA synthetase: A model for autoimmunity. *Nature* 304:177, 1983.
37. Matter L, Schopfer K, Wilheim JA, et al: Molecular characterization of ribonucleoprotein antigens bound to antinuclear antibodies. *Arthritis Rheum* 25:1278, 1982.
38. Mattioli M, Reichlin M: Physical association of two nuclear antigens and mutual occurrence of their antibodies: The relationship of the Sm and RNA protein (Mo) system in SLE sera. *J Immunol* 110:1318, 1973.
39. Mattioli M, Reichlin M: Heterogeneity of RNA protein antigens reactive with sera of patients with systemic lupus erythematosus. *Arthritis Rheum* 6:189, 1979.
40. Minori T, Akizuki I, Yamagata M, et al: Characterization of a high molecular weight acidic nuclear protein recognized by autoantibodies in sera from patients with polymyositis-scleroderma overlap. *J Clin Invest* 68:611, 1981.
41. Miyawaki S, Ritchie RF: Nucleolar antigen specific for antinucleolar antibody in the sera of patients with systemic rheumatic diseases. *Arthritis Rheum* 16:726, 1973.
42. Miyachi K, Fritzler MJ, Tan EM: Autoantibodies to a nuclear antigen in proliferating cells. *J Immunol* 121:2228, 1978.
43. Moroi Y, Peebles C, Fritzler MJ, et al: Autoantibody to centromere (kinetochore) in scleroderma sera. *Proc Natl Acad Sci USA* 77:1627, 1980.
44. Nakamura RM, Peebles C, Tan EM: Microhemagglutination test for detection of antibodies to nuclear Sm and ribonucleoprotein antigens in systemic lupus erythematosus and related diseases. *Am J Clin Pathol* 70:800, 1978.
45. Nishikai M, Reichlin M: Purification and characterization of a nuclear non-histone basic protein (Mi-1) which reacts with anti-immunoglobulin sera and the sera of patients with dermatomyositis. *Mol Immunol* 17:1129, 1980.
46. Nishikai M, Reichlin M: Heterogeneity of precipitating antibodies in polymyositis and dermatomyositis. *Arthritis Rheum* 23:881, 1980.
47. Northway JP, Tan EM: Differentiation of antinuclear antibodies giving speckled staining patterns in immunofluorescence. *Clin Immunol Immunopathol* 1:140, 1972.
48. Papalian M, Lafer E, Wong R, et al: Reaction of systemic lupus erythematosus antinative

DNA antibodies with native DNA fragments from 20 to 1200 base pairs. *J Clin Invest* 65:469, 1980.

49. Pinnas JL, Northway JD, Tan EM: Antinucleolar antibodies in human sera. *J Immunol* 111:996, 1973.
50. Pizer LI, Deng J-S, Stenberg M, et al: Characterization of a phosphoprotein associated with the SS-B/La nuclear antigen in adenovirus-infected and uninfected KB-cells. *Mol Cell Biol* 3:1235, 1983.
51. Portanova JP, Rubin RL, Joslin FG, et al: Reactivity of anti-histone antibodies induced by procainamide and hydralazine. *Clin Immunol Immunopathol* 25:67, 1982.
52. Reddy R, Henning D, Tan EM, et al: Identification of a La protein binding site in RNA polymerase III transcript (4.5 RNA). *J Biol Chem* 258:8352, 1983.
53. Reichlin M, Mattioli M: Description of a serological reaction characteristic of polymyositis. *Clin Immunol Immunopathol* 5:12, 1976.
54. Rinke J, Steitz JA: Precursor molecules of both human ribosomal RNAs are bound by a cellular protein reactive with anti-La antibodies. *Cell* 29:169, 1982.
55. Ro-Choi TS, Busch H: Low-molecular-weight nuclear RNA's In Busch, H (Ed): *The Cell Nucleus,* vol. 3. Academic Pres, New York, 1972, pp 152–208.
56. Rogers J, Wall R: A mechanism for RNA splicing. *Proc Natl Acad Sci USA* 77:1877, 1980.
57. Rubin RL, Joslin FG, Tan EM: Specificity of anti-histone antibodies in systemic lupus erythematosus. *Arthritis Rheum* 25:779, 1982.
58. Rubin RL, Joslin FG, Tan EM: An improved ELISA for anti-native DNA by elimination of interference by anti-histone antibodies. *J Immunol Meth* 63:359, 1983.
59. Schur PH, DeAngelis D, Jackson JM: Immunological detection of nucleic acids and antibodies to nucleic acids and nuclear antigens by counterimmunoelectrophoresis. *Clin Exp Immunol* 17:209, 1974.
60. Sharp GC, Irvin WS, Tan EM, et al: Mixed connective tissue disease: An apparently distinct rheumatic disease syndrome associated with a specific antibody to an extractable nuclear antigen (ENA). *Am J Med* 52:148, 1972.
61. Stollar BD, Levine L, Lehrer HI, et al: The antigenic determinants of denatured DNA reactive with lupus erythematosus serum. *Proc Natl Acad Sci USA* 48:874, 1962.
62. Stollar BD: Reaction of systemic lupus erythematosus sera with histone fractions and histone-DNA complexes. *Arthritis Rheum* 14:485, 1971.
63. Stollar BD, Papalian M: Secondary structure in denatured DNA is responsible for its reaction with antinative DNA antibodies of systemic lupus erythematosus sera. *J Clin Invest* 66:210, 1980.
64. Takasaki Y, Deng J-S, Tan EM: A nuclear antigen associated with cell proliferation and blast transformation. Its distribution in synchronized cells. *J Exp Med* 154:1899, 1981.
65. Tan EM, Kunkel HG: Characteristics of a soluble nuclear antigen precipitating with sera of patients with systemic lupus erythematosus. *J Immunol* 96:464, 1966.
66. Tan EM, Schur PH, Carr RI, et al: Deoxyribonucleic acid (DNA) and antibodies to DNA in serum of patients with systemic lupus erythematosus. *J Clin Invest* 45:1732, 1966.
67. Tan EM: Drug-induced lupus erythematosus. *Fed Proc* 33:1894, 1974.
68. Tan EM, Natali PG: Comparative study of antibodies to native and denatured DNA. *J Immunol* 104:902, 1970.
69. Tan EM, Rodnan GP, Garcia J, et al: Diversity of antinuclear antibodies in progressive systemic sclerosis. *Arthritis Rheum* 23:617, 1980.
70. Tan EM: Autoantibodies to nuclear antigens (ANA): Their immunobiology and medicine. *Adv Immunol* 33:167, 1982.
71. Targoff IN, Raghu G, Reichlin M: Antibodies to Mi-1 in SLE: Relationship to other precipitins and reaction with bovine immunoglobulin. *Clin Exp Immunol* 53:76, 1983.
72. Ten Veen JH, Feltkamp TEW: Studies on drug induced lupus erythematosus in mice. I. Drug induced antinuclear antibodies (ANA). *Clin Exp Immunol* 11:265, 1972.
73. Venables PJW, Smith PR, Maini RN: Purification and characterization of Sjogren's syndrome A and B antigens. *Clin Exp Immunol* 54:731, 1983.

74. White PJ, Gardner WD, Hoch SO: Identification of the immunologically active components of Sm and RNP antigens. *Proc Natl Acad Sci USA* 78:626, 1981.
75. Winn DM, Wolfe JF, Harmon D, et al: Characterization of a distinct nuclear acidic protein antigen (Ma) and clinical findings in systemic erythematosus patients with Ma antibodies. *J Clin Invest* 64:820, 1979.
76. Wolfe JF, Adelstein E, Sharp GC: Antinuclear antibody with distinct specificity for polymyositis. *J Clin Invest* 59:176, 1977.
77. Wooley JC, Zuckerberg LR, Chung S: Polypeptide components of small nuclear ribonucleoprotein. *Proc Natl Acad Sci USA* 80:5208, 1983.

32
Extractable Nuclear Antigens: Preparation, Standardization, and Method for Detecting Anti-ENA Antibodies

Jau-Shyong Deng

Vijay Kumar

PREPARATION OF EXTRACTABLE NUCLEAR ANTIGENS AND THE SCREENING OF ANTIBODIES IN SERA OF PATIENTS WITH VARIOUS DISEASES

Extractable nuclear antigens (ENA) refer to those antigens present either in whole cell or isolated nuclei that can be extracted and are soluble in phosphate-buffered saline (PBS). Some ENA of diagnostic significance are RNP, Sm, SS-A/Ro, SS-B/La, PCNA, JO-1, Pm-1, and Ma (57).

The distribution and concentration of ENA varies, and is dependent upon the source and type of tissue. RNP, Sm, and SS-B/La antigens are present in various tissues from different species of animals such as rabbit, mouse, guinea pig, calf, and human tissue. On the other hand, SS-A/Ro is primarily present in tissue from human, dog, and calf (25). In addition to the distribution of these antigens in various tissues, the concentration and ratio of these antigens vary. For example, one may think that one source of tissue extract such as that from calf thymus, which contains RNP, Sm, SS-A/Ro, and SS-B/La antigens, can be used for detecting antibodies to these antigens. Even though the above is true, due to varying concentrations of these antigens to the extract, it is not recommended to use a single source for all of these antigens. We have found that calf thymus is a good source of RNP, Sm, and SS-B/La antigen, but not of SS-A/Ro (Table 1). The concentration of SS-A/Ro antigen in calf thymus is about fivefold less than the concentrations of RNP, Sm, and SS-B/La.

Table 1. General Characteristics of Extractable Nuclear Antigens

Antibody specificity	*Recommended source of antigen*	*Localization*	*RNA components*	*Major protein components*
Anti-RNP	Calf thymus or Rabbit thymus	Nuclear	U1	65K, 30K 70K, 30K
Anti-Sm	Calf thymus Rabbit thymus	Nuclear	U1 U2 U4 U5 U6	16K, 13K 13K
Anti-La(SS-B)	Calf thymus Rabbit thymus Monkey liver Human spleen	Nuclear	La 4.5	43K, 47K
Anti-Ro(SS-A)	Monkey liver Human spleen (calf thymus)[a]	Nuclear	Mouse y1–y2 Human y1–y5	60K

[a]The concentration of Ro antigen in calf thymus is much lower than other tissues.

The methods for detecting anti-ENA antibodies are primarily gel precipitation and hemagglutination (9,20,31,51,54,57,59,65). The hemagglutination method involves coating erythrocytes with the calf or rabbit thymus extract. A positive agglutination with the patient's sera indicates the presence of ribonucleoprotein (RNP) and Sm antibodies, which are differentiated from each other by their agglutination behavior on antigen-coated erythrocytes upon ribonuclease treatment. A positive hemagglutination before and after ribonuclease treatment indicates Sm antibodies, and abolition of agglutination upon ribonuclease treatment indicates the presence of RNP antibodies. However, the antigen employed in the hemagglutination method is a crude preparation containing not only RNP and Sm, but also many other antigens against which autoantibodies have been found in connective tissue disease. The presence of such other antigen-antibody systems limits the reliability of the hemagglutination method in detecting RNP and Sm antibodies. In addition, such an assay system fails to detect multiple antibodies that are frequently found in SLE patients.

The gel precipitation method, even though less sensitive than hemagglutination, allows distinguishing anti-ENA antibodies directed against various ENA antigens by use of the prototype reference sera. Because of the simplicity and ease of identifying anti-ENA antibodies, the gel precipitation method is described in detail.

Preparation of ENA

Extracts containing RNP, Sm, SS-A/Ro, and SS-B/La antigens can be obtained either from acetone powder obtained commercially or from tissues obtained from a slaughterhouse or commercially.

Preparation of Extract From Acetone Powder

Acetone powders of either calf or rabbit thymus (Pel Freeze Biologicals, Rogers, AR) can be utilized as a source of RNP, Sm, and SS-B/La antigens: 1) For the extraction of these antigens, weigh certain amount of the acetone powder to which is then added PBS containing 0.1 mM phenylmethyl sulfonylfluoride (PMSF) and 1 mM mercaptoethanol (1 ml PBS/100 mg of acetone powder). 2) Stir the mixture in cold room for at least 6 hours or overnight. 3) Centrifuge the mixture at 800 g for 20 minutes at 4°C to get rid of large clumps. Aliquot the supernatant in small amounts and store frozen at −70°C. The extract is stable for about 1 year if kept at −70°C.

Preparation of Tissue Extracts

Calf thymus can be obtained either from Pel Freeze Biologicals (Rogers, AR) or from a slaughterhouse. The extract can be prepared as follows.

Thaw calf thymus while it is cold, and cut into small pieces with scissors or a sharp knife. Rinse the tissue in cold PBS to get rid of most of the blood.

Add two volumes of cold PBS containing 0.1 mM PMSF and 1 mM mercaptoethanol to 1 volume by weight of calf thymus, and homogenize the tissue in baring blender for 3 minutes; stir the homogenate for 2 to 4 hours at 4°C.

Pass the suspension through three layers of cheesecloth and discard the clumps of connective tissue.

Centrifuge the suspension at 10,000 g for 20 minutes and collect the supernatant. Concentrate the supernatant 10-fold in an Amicon concentrator. Divide the ENA preparation into small aliquots and keep frozen at −70°C. The extract is stable for 1 year if kept frozen.

Similarly, an extract of human spleen or monkey liver can be obtained. This extract contains Sm, SS-A/Ro, and SS-B/La activity, but is poor in RNP activity.

If extract from tissue culture cells such as WiL2 cells, HeLa cells, or HEp-2 cells is used for screening the presence of Sm, RNP, SS-B/La, or SS-A/Ro antibodies, the techniques are basically the same. Equal volumes of extraction solution and packed cells are mixed together and then subjected to ultrasonication in order to disrupt the cells and solubilize the cellular materials. After centrifugation at 35,000 rpm (Beckman ultracentrifuge, SW-40 rotor) for 30 minutes, the supernatant is collected and used as the antigenic material (5).

Preparation of Immunodiffusion Plates

Weigh a sufficient amount of agarose to prepare 1% agarose solution in PBS, allowing 7 ml of gel per plate (Falcon, 60 x 15 mm). Weigh sodium azide to prepare a final concentration of 0.1% of sodium azide and add to the agarose powder. Add PBS to the desired final volume. Heat it until agarose dissolves completely (in a water bath). Place the approximate number of plates on a paper towel on the countertop. The toweling is used to prevent scratching the bottom of the plates. Add 7 ml of the warm agarose solution into each plate. Place the lids on the plates once the agarose has sufficiently solidified, and store upside down in a refrigerator.

Detection of Anti-ENA Antibodies

Screening Procedure

Punch the gel with template of the type and dimensions as shown in Figure 1 shortly before use. Label plates for proper identification, and place a mark at well 1. To one set of plate add approximately 60 μl of neat serum or its dilutions to peripheral wells 1 to 6 and 100 μl of rabbit thymus extract or calf thymus extract to the central well. To the other add human spleen or monkey liver in the center well rather than the thymus extract. Allow the plates to remain at room temperature and observe the reaction after 24 hours for the presence of precipitin lines. The plates are read against a black back-

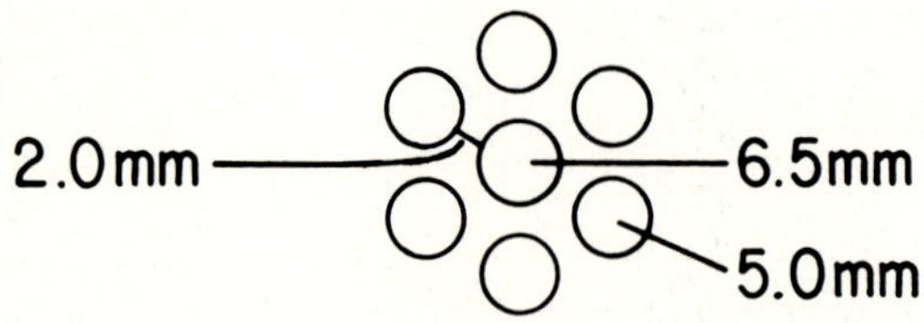

Figure 1. Template depicting well sizes and distances between wells employed in punching gel plates.

ground, using a fluorescent lamp. Record the results or photograph the plates for a permanent record. Test one or two control sera each time the tests are performed.

Identification Procedure

Prepare appropriate dilutions of the prototype sera, as determined by previous testing, and of the patient serum samples. If the patient serum gives precipitin lines against rabbit thymus extract, set up the identification plates using Sm, RNP, and SS-B/La prototype sera. If the patient dilutions give precipitin line against monkey liver or human spleen extract only, set up the identification plates using SS-A/Ro prototype only. If the patient serum gives precipitin line(s) against thymus and spleen/liver extracts, set up the identification plates using Sm, RNP, SS-B/La, and SS-A/Ro prototype sera. Place approximately 60 μl of the appropriate sample dilutions in each peripheral well as in the screening procedures. For identification purposes, the prototype serum samples are usually placed in wells 1, 3, and 5, with patients' samples being placed in wells 2, 4, and 6. Allow the reactants to diffuse at room temperature and read at 24 hours. (We have noted that 24-hour reading is optimal.) Record results or photograph for a permanent record. As the protein content and, more importantly, the antigen content varies due to differences of the tissue employed and methods of extracting the antigens, it is very important to determine the suitability and the appropriate use dilution of these extracts (see the third main section in this chapter).

Interpretation

ENA preparations contain not only RNP, Sm, SS-A/Ro, and SS-B/La antigens, but also other antigens. Thus, these extracts may detect precipitin lines other than ENA (RNP, Sm, SS-A/Ro, and SS-B/La) antibodies. These lines will not form lines of identity with the prototype sera. The appearance of the line of identity with the corresponding prototype sera confirms the presence of either RNP, Sm, SS-B/Ro, or SS-B/La antibodies. As shown in Figure 2, serum from patient 1 has anti-RNP antibodies and patient 2 has both anti-RNP and anti-Sm antibodies. This is due to serum from patient 1 giving a line of identity with prototype sera positive for anti-RNP antibodies. Patient 2 showed two precipitin lines with the calf thymus extract. One of the two lines gave a line of identity with anti-RNP control sera, whereas the other showed a line of identity with anti-Sm prototype sera. Patient 3 was negative for anti-RNP or anti-Sm antibodies.

BIOCHEMICAL AND MOLECULAR CHARACTERISTICS OF THE NUCLEAR ANTIGENS: Sm, RNP, SS-B/La, AND SS-A/Ro.

In the previous section, methods for preparing the extractable cellular antigens and for screening for the presence of the four different precipitin antibodies (anti-Sm, RNP,

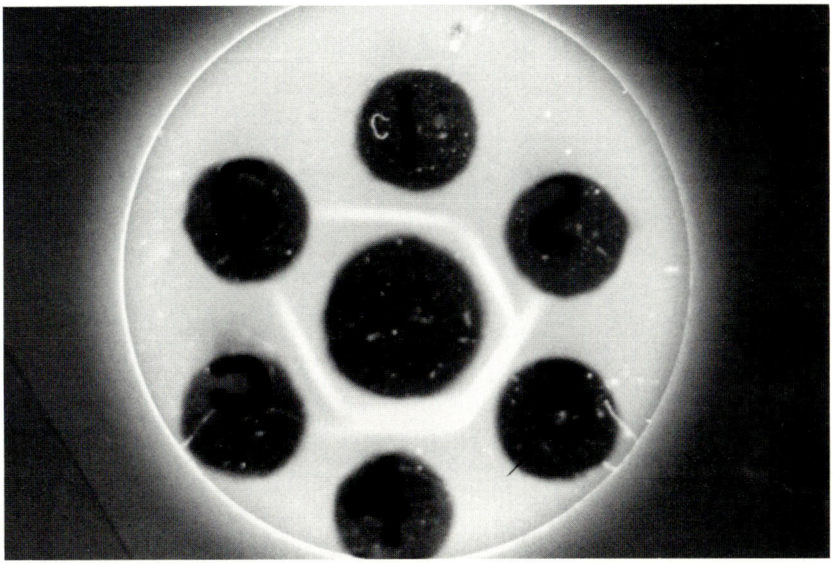

Figure 2. Typing of antibodies present in the sera of SLE patients by immunodiffusion. The central well contains calf thymus antigen preparation. Peripheral wells contain either the patient sera or prototype anti-RNP and anti-Sm sera. Well 1, anti-RNP; well 2, patient 1; well 3, anti-Sm; well 4, patient 2; well 5, anti-RNP; and well 6, patient 3.

SS-B/La, and SS-A/Ro) were described. In this section, some biochemical and molecular characteristics of these four antigens from WiL2 cell extract will be discussed.

Historically, anti-Sm antibody was identified in patients with systemic lupus erythematosus (SLE) by Tan and Kunkel in 1966 (58); it was later found to be a characteristic marker for this disease. RNP antibodies were reported subsequently by several investigators, and they were found in patients with various diseases, including SLE, discoid lupus erythematosus (DLE), scleroderma, rheumatoid arthritis (RA), Sjögren's syndrome, mixed connective tissue disease (MCTD), and others (23,29,39,40,42,43,47,52,53). Sera containing antibodies to Sm or RNP gave speckled nuclear staining, indicating the presence of these two antigens in cell nuclei. RNP was very sensitive to RNase and trypsin, while Sm was resistant to RNase and partially sensitive to trypsin (42).

In 1962, Anderson et al. demonstrated the precipitating antibodies in patients with Sjögren's syndrome, SLE, and RA (6). One of the precipitating antibodies they found could be similar to what was described later as Ro by Clark et al. (12); and the other was possibly, La as described by Mattioli and Reichlin in 1974 (41). In 1969, Clark et al. (12) reported finding a serum antibody reacting with a cytoplasmic antigen extracted from human tissues obtained at autopsy, and the antigen was named Ro. It was present in spleen, liver, kidney, and lymph node, and was also present in dog spleen. It was presumed to be cytoplasmic because it was present in the cytoplasmic fraction of homogenized cells; attempts to localize it, however, in the cytoplasm by immunofluorescence (IF) were unsuccessful (12). At that time, Ro antigen was found to be resistant to proteolytic enzyme digestion such as trypsin, pepsin, and chymotrypsin, or to DNase and RNase. Following this, Mattioli and Reichlin reported the findings of Ro antibodies and other precipitin antibodies to a soluble cytoplasmic RNA protein antigen La from patients with SLE. They found La antigen was sensitive to trypsin and RNase, and was present in the cytoplasmic fraction of homogenized calf thymus, but absent from the nuclear fraction (41). In 1975, Alspaugh and Tan (5) described the presence of three precipitin lines by double immunodiffusion using both sera from patients with Sjögren's syndrome and cellular extract of WiL2 cells as the antigenic sources. The corresponding antigens were called SS-A, SS-B, and SS-C (5).

In a subsequent study, it was demonstrated that sera with anti-SS-A and anti-SS-B showed positive nuclear fluorescent staining. Anti-SS-B sera showed nuclear staining on human WiL2 cell substrate and mouse kidney sections, but anti-SS-A was positive only on human WiL2 cells. The antigenicity of SS-A and SS-B was sensitive to trypsin, but resistant to RNase and DNase (4). Even though different precipitin antibodies were demonstrated in patients with various connective tissue diseases by different groups of investigators, it was finally demonstrated—in an interlaboratory study by Alspaugh and Maddison—that the Ro and SS-A antigens were immunologically identical by double immunodiffusion analysis, using several different sera and antigens prepared from different tissues. Similarly, the La and SS-B antigens were also found to be immunologically identical (3). Although the Ro and La antigens were originally thought to be cytoplasmic antigens, more recent evidences suggest the possibility that both antigens may be predominantly nuclear in location.

In 1977, Akizuki et al. prepared extracts from nuclei of calf thymus, calf liver, and rat liver, and showed the presence of a nuclear antigen (Ha), which precipitated with antibody present in sera of patients with Sjögren's syndrome and SLE (1,2). The antigen was localized by indirect immunofluorescence (IIF) in the nuclei of rat and mouse liver and kidney using antibody isolated from immune precipitates. The Ha antigen was found to be immunologically identical to SS-B, and the antigenicity was sensitive to trypsin, but not to DNase or RNase.

The cellular extract from WiL2 cells was used primarily in the following studies. WiL2 cell line is a line of continuously growing human diploid B lymphocytes originally obtained from the spleen of a patient with hereditary spherocytosis (37). The cells were maintained in suspension culture on a gyratory shaker. The culture medium consisted of MEM (Flow Laboratory, Inglewood, CA) supplemented with 2 mM glutamine, vitamins, nonessential amino acids, sodium pyruvate, 100 U/ml penicillin, 100 μg/ml streptomycin, and 10% fetal calf serum (Flow Laboratory, CA). The cells were seeded at a concentration of 2×10^5/ml, and were normally subcultured every 3 to 4 days. The cells were collected by centrifuging the cell suspension at 1000 rpm for 5 minutes. After harvesting, the cells were washed twice in cold PBS. Equal volume of cold extraction solution, as described in the previous section, was added to the packed cell pellet. The cells were disrupted by extensive sonication at 4°C; and the supernatant, after clarification by centrifugation at 100,000 g for 30 minutes, was collected as the source of antigen (cellular extract). The cell extract thus obtained was then subjected to the enzyme susceptibility test, temperature resistance test, and further characterization of the four different cellular antigens (Sm, RNP, SS-B/La, and SS-A/Ro).

Figure 3 depicts the immunodiffusion analysis with saline extract of WiL2 cells in the center well, and in sera containing antibodies to Sm, RNP, SS-B/La, and SS-A/Ro in the peripheral well. The saline extract contains multiple cellular antigens, including cytoplasmic and nuclear materials. On immunodiffusion analysis, Sm and RNP precipitin lines give spur formation, but may sometimes intersect each other (7,42). These two precipitin lines definitely cross over the precipitin lines of SS-B/La and SS-A/Ro. Similarly, the SS-A/Ro precipitin line crosses over the SS-B/La precipitin line, and sometimes gives spur formation as well. The spur formation between Sm and RNP has been

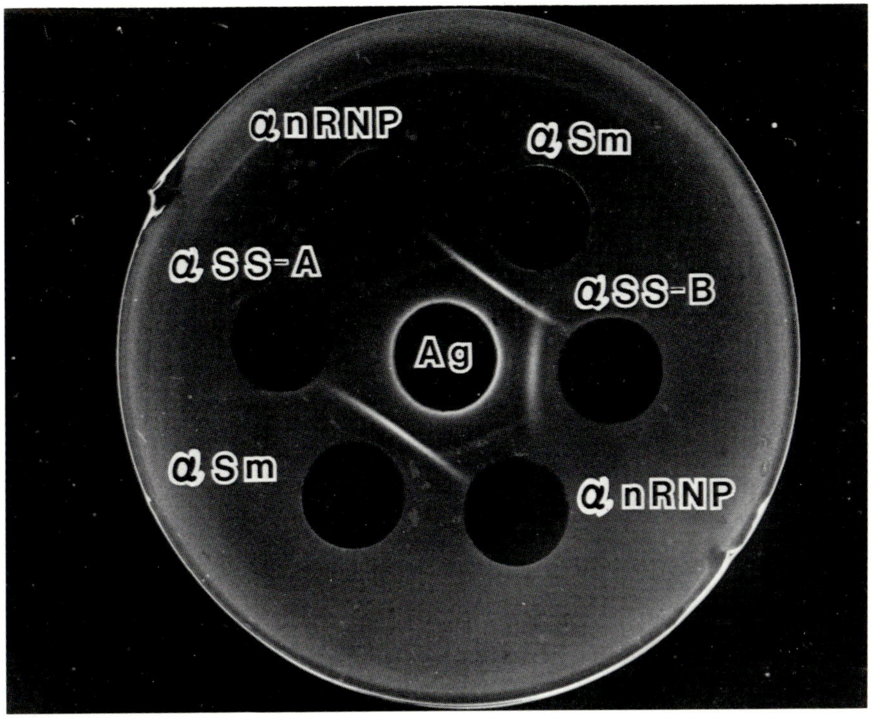

Figure 3. Immunodiffusion analysis of the four different cellular antigen-antibody systems: anti-Sm, anti-RNP, anti-SS-B/La, and anti-SS-A/Ro. The central well contains the WiL2 cell extract as the antigenic material. The peripheral wells contain the sera with different antibodies: anti-Sm, anti-RNP, anti-SS-B/La, and anti-SS-A/Ro.

explained as partial identity of the RNP to Sm. Recent evidences have indicated that most RNP particles are complexed with Sm, whereas there are free Sm molecules without accompanying RNP (40,42). Recently, SS-A/Ro molecules have been found hidden in some SS-B/La particles. Some free SS-B/La molecules are also found in the cellular extract (15,27). These might also explain the spur formation between SS-B/La and SS-A/Ro precipitin lines.

Biochemical studies have been done to differentiate these four different cellular antigens. The stability and susceptibility to several enzymes are listed in Table 2. Only Sm is stable at 56°C for 1 hour. This indicates that Sm is more stable than the other three antigens. The antigenicity of the four cellular antigens remains intact at room temperature for 4 days. Among these four antigens, RNP is the most sensitive to pH. It is stable only at pH 7.0 to 9.0. SS-B/La and SS-A/Ro are stable at pH 3.0 to 9.0 while Sm is stable at pH 3.0 to 11.0. All four of these antigens are resistant to DNase (100 μg/ml). RNP is very susceptible to RNase (100 μg/ml), while the other three antigens are resistant. Sm is partially sensitive to trypsin (1 μg/ml), and the rest of the three are sensitive to trypsin (1 μg/ml). All four antigens are acidic in nature and migrate electrophoretically to anode and react with the specific antibodies in counter immunoelectrophoresis.

These four acidic, nonhistone, cellular antigens can be partially differentiated according to different purification procedures. Table 3 shows the distribution of the four

Table 2. Stability and Susceptibility of ENA to Enzymes

	Loss of antigenic activity upon treatment with			*Temperature*		
	Trypsin	*RNase*	*DNase*	*4 days*	*56°C, 1 h*	*at pH*
nRNP	++[a]	++	−[a]	−	++	7–9
Sm	+/−[a]	−	−	−	−	3–11
SS-A/Ro	+[a]	−	−	−	+	3–9
SS-B/La	+	−	−	−	+	3–9

[a]+, sensitive; ++, very sensitive;
−, resistant; +/−, partly sensitive.

Table 3. Antigenicity of Sm, nRNP, SS-B/La, and SS-A/Ro in Ammonium Sulfate-precipitated Fractions From WiL2 Cell Extract

	Percent of ammonium sulfate-saturated solution			
Antigen	*0–30*	*30–50*	*50–66*	*66–100*
nRNP	++[a]	+	−[b]	−
Sm	+	++	−	−
SS-B/La	−	++	++	+
SS-A/Ro	−	++	+	−

[a]Positive antigenicity.
[b]Negative antigenicity.

antigens in different fractions obtained from sequential ammonium sulfate precipitation. RNP is present primarily in fractions precipitated by 0 to 50% saturated ammonium sulfate solution, while Sm is present in fractions precipitated by 0 to 66% saturated ammonium sulfate solution. SS-A/Ro and SS-B/La are present in fractions by 30 to 66% saturated ammonium sulfate solution. In this way, RNP and Sm are present in fraction precipitated by 30% saturated ammonium sulfate solution, and are not contaminated by SS-B/La and SS-A/Ro antigens. SS-B/La is also present in leftover fraction. This indicates physically that there is some free SS-B/La antigen in the cellular extract.

Figure 4 depicts both the G-200 gel filtration profile of fractions precipitated with 30 to 66% saturated ammonium sulfate solution and the distribution of the four antigens. In G-200 gel filtration, Sm is present in fractions of wider range. The RNP is also present in fractions containing Sm activity (42). This raises the possibility that there is some physical association between RNP and Sm molecules (40,42). This is further confirmed by immunoprecipitation experiments, and will be discussed later (36). SS-A/Ro and SS-B/La antigens can be separated from Sm and nRNP antigens. SS-B/La is found in fractions with or without accompanying SS-A/Ro antigenic activity (15).

These four antigens bind to DEAE ion exchange column, and can then be eluted from the column with NaCl gradient. As indicated before by Northway and Tan (42) in 1972, Sm can be eluted from the column with 0.1 to 0.35 M NaCl, the same is true for RNP with 0.2 to 0.35 N NaCl. This suggests that Sm antigens are more heterogeneous, and can be dissociated from the ion exchange cellulose with a wider range of salt concentration.

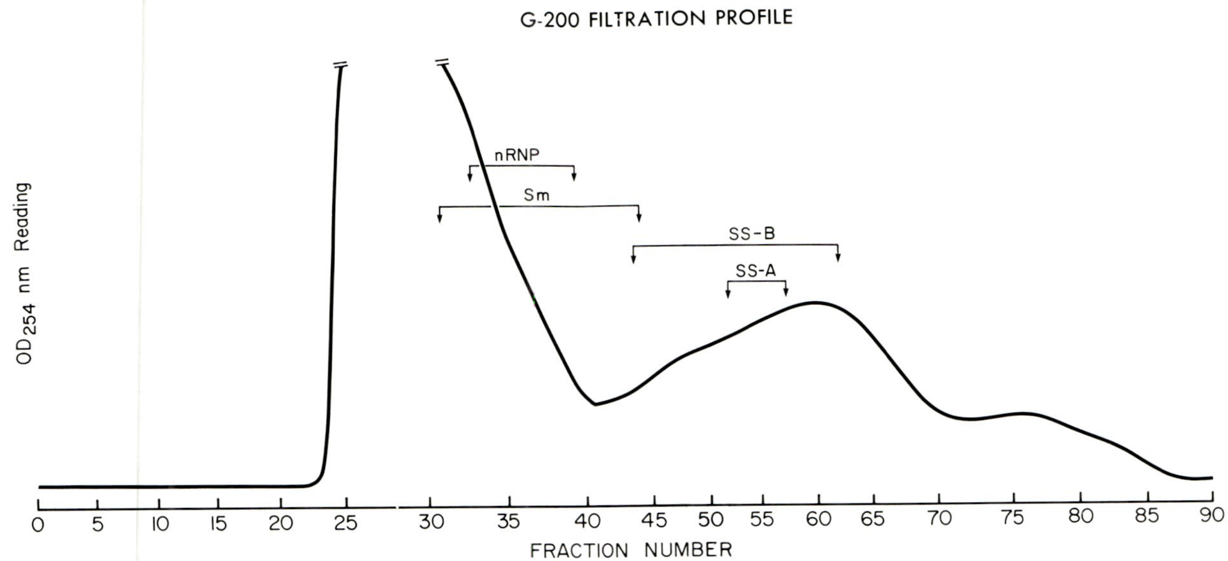

Figure 4. G-200 gel filtration profile and the distribution of the Sm, RNP, SS-B/La, and SS-A/Ro antigens in different fractions. The starting material is the precipitate obtained with 30 to 66% saturated ammonium sulfate precipitation. The gel column is 90 × 2.6 cm. RNP antigen is present in fractions having Sm activity. Sm and RNP antigens are present in fractions without accompanying SS-B/La and SS-A/Ro activities. Sm and SS-B/La are present in fractions of a wider range than those for RNP and SS-A/Ro.

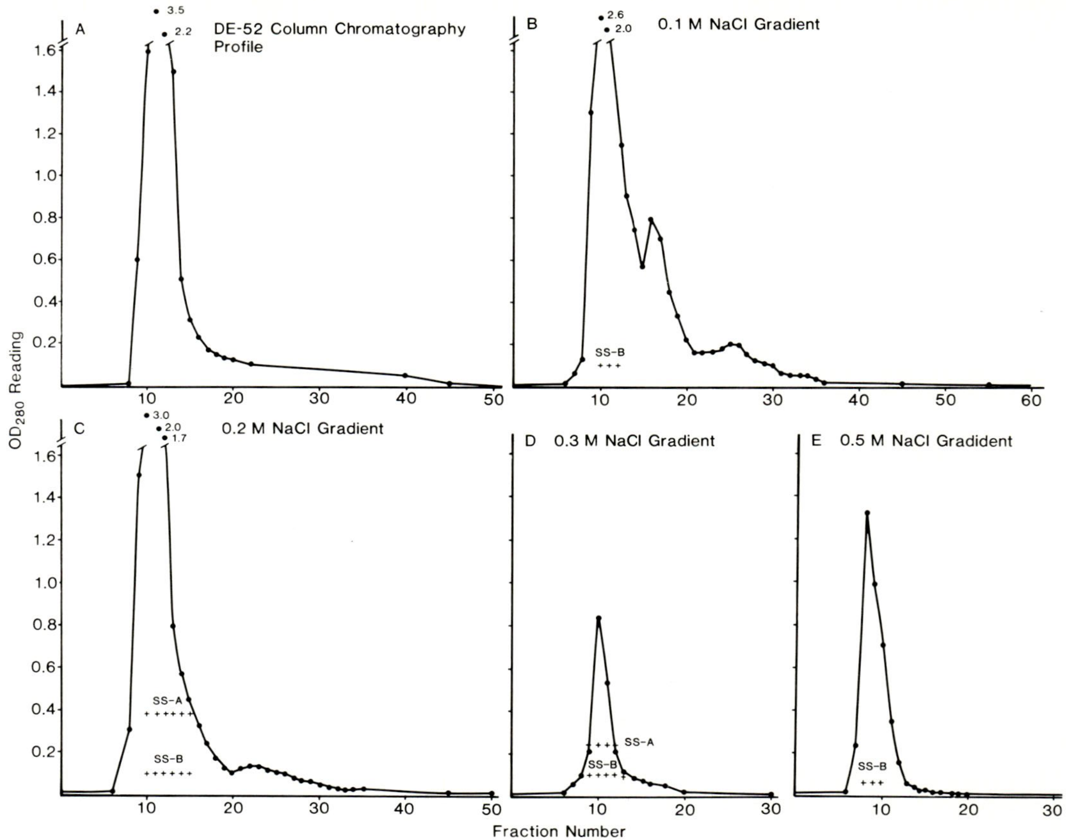

Figure 5. DE-52 ion exchange chromatography profile with phosphate buffer, 0.01 M, pH 8.0. The starting material is obtained from the second peak fractions of the G-200 gel filtration column. The proteins were eluted initially with (A) 500 ml of phosphate buffer with 0.1 M NaCl gradient, then (B) 500 ml of phosphate buffer with 0.2 M NaCl gradient, then (C) 500 ml phosphate buffer with 0.3 M NaCl gradient, and finally (D) 500 ml phosphate buffer with 0.5 M NaCl gradient. As seen in the elution profile, SS-B/La and SS-A/Ro activities were present in fractions eluted with 0.2 and 0.3 M NaCl gradients. However, some SS-B/La activity was also present in fractions eluted with 0.1 and 0.5 M NaCl gradients.

SS-B/La can also be separated from SS-A/Ro on DEAE ion exchange chromatography, as shown in Figure 5. SS-B/La antigen can be dissociated from the DEAE ion exchange column with 0.1 to 0.5 M NaCl gradients, while SS-A/Ro is only detected in eluates of 0.2 and 0.3 M NaCl gradients. The simultaneous occurrence of SS-B/La and SS-A/Ro in the same fractions from the ion exchange column chromatography suggests that there is a certain physical association between SS-B/La and SS-A/Ro antigenic molecules. This observed phenomenon is similar to that observed between Sm and RNP (40,42). The physical interactions between these antigens perhaps explain the coexistence of the autoantibodies; that is, anti-Sm with anti-RNP and anti-SS-B/La with anti-SS-A/Ro in some patients with connective tissue disease.

Lerner and Steitz used the autoantibodies as tools, and applied to the field of molecular cell biology (36). They labeled cells with ^{32}p-phosphoric acid or ^{35}S-methionine and then analyzed the nuclear antigens associated with small cellular RNAs and polypeptides. They identified some small cellular RNAs that were associated with certain distinct cellular antigenic molecules, and have opened an area of research that provides new insights into our understanding of autoimmune diseases and also cellular metabolism and cellular organelles, which was not known before (27,33,34,36). Tissue culture cells such as WiL2 cells (Fig. 6A) or KB cells (Fig. 6B) were labeled with ^{32}p-phosphoric acid. The ^{32}p-labeled cell extract was used to react with an appropriate amount of the autoantibody containing sera (anti-Sm, anti-nRNP, anti-SS-B/La, or anti-SS-A/Ro). The particles carrying the antigens interacted with the antibodies, and formed immune complexes that were subsequently absorbed onto the protein A-carrying staphylococci (pansorbin, Calbiochem, La Jolla, CA). After extensive washing, the whole immune complexes were eluted from the staphylococci. The cellular antigens associated with RNAs were then analyzed on a 10% acrylamide-urea gel electrophoresis. The associated RNA profiles were shown in Figures 6A and 6B. Figure 6A is obtained from WiL2 cell extract, and Figure 6B is from KB cell extract. Sm is associated with U1, U2, U4, U5, and U6 RNAs (lane 3), while RNP is only with U1 RNA (lane 4). These RNAs belong to the small nuclear RNAs described earlier by several groups of investigators (26,45,62). Lerner and Steitz showed that the nucleotide sequence of U1 RNA had a high degree of homology with nucleotide sequences across splice junction of Hn RNA, and proposed that U1 RNP may play a role in the processing of HnRNA to messenger RNA (35).

It has also been shown that the antibody (anti-RNP) does inhibit the splicing of the RNAs in an in vitro system that transcribes mature mRNA from the adenovirus genome (66). The small RNAs precipitated by anti-Sm and anti-RNP antisera were very similar in both gel profiles and nucleotide fingerprints when cells from different animal species were used, suggesting that these RNAs were highly conserved in different species through the course of evolution. Soon after this, Hendrick et al. reported that anti-SS-B/La and anti-SS-A/Ro sera could precipitate other unidentified cellular RNAs (27). As shown in Figure 6, lane 1, SS-B/La antigen is found to be associated with several RNAs, and two of the RNAs are similar to 5S and 4.5S RNAs (27,33,34). In addition, adenovirus VA RNA (34) and Epstein-Barr virus (EBV) encoded RNAs (EBER) (33) (as seen in lane 1 of Fig. 6A) were also precipitated by anti-SS-B/La antibodies, but not by other autoantibodies, from adenovirus infected cells or EBV transformed cells, respectively. Using a similar approach, they identified SS-A/Ro associated RNAs, as seen in lane 2 of Figure 6 (27,34). The small cellular RNAs precipitated by anti-SS-B/La or anti-SS-A/Ro are different from those RNAs precipitated by anti-Sm or anti-RNP; and they are also different between mouse and human cells (27,33,34). From mouse Ehrlich ascites cells, anti-SS-B/La precipitated both 4.5 S RNAs (24,27,33,49) and a species 5S rRNA-like molecules (27,33,34). The latter was also precipitated from human cells (HeLa cells, KB

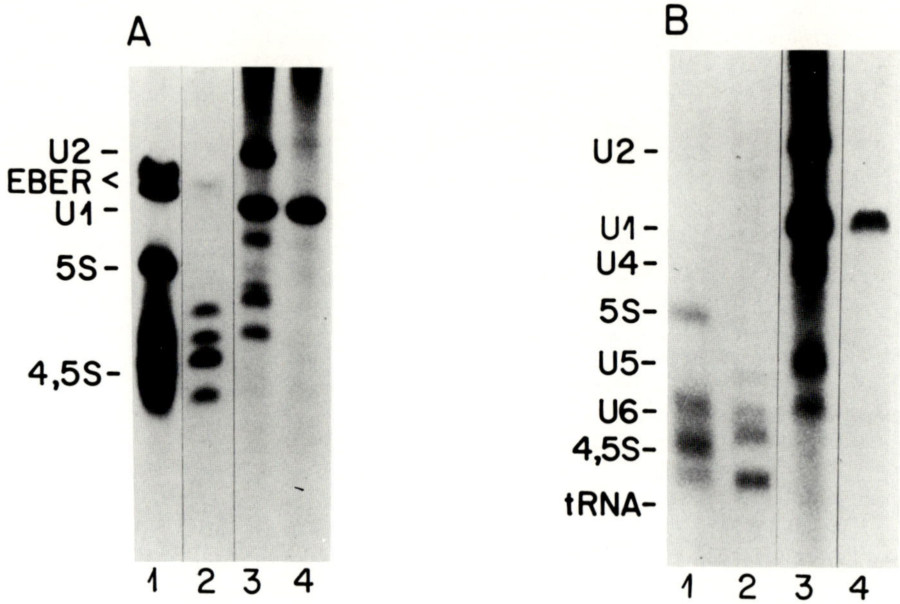

Figure 6. Cellular antigen-associated RNA profiles obtained from immunoprecipitation experiments. A. Obtained from ^{32}P-labeled WiL2 cell extract. B. Obtained from ^{32}P-labeled KB cell extract. Monospecific serum was added to cell extract and incubated at 4°C for 15 minutes, and then protein A-bearing staphylococci (Pansorbin, Calbiochem., La Jolla, California) was added. After another 15 minutes of incubation at 4°C, the whole staphylococci were washed extensively with the washing solution containing 50 mM tris, 150 mM NaCl (pH 7.5), 0.5% NP-40, and 0.5% sodium deoxycholate. The immune complexes were eluted from the staphylococci at 60°C for 10 minutes in 50 μl of 50 mM tris (pH 8.0), 3% SDS, 10% glycerol. To prepare RNA, the immune complexes were treated with 10 μl of proteinase K (Boehringer Mannheim Corp), 1 mg/ml for 30 minutes at 37°C, mixed with 50 μl of formamide, and boiled for 2 minutes. Bromophenol blue was added to 0.001%, and the samples were subjected to electrophoresis on a 24-cm, 10% acrylamide gel (24:1 acrylamide: bisacrylamide) containing 7 M urea and Tris-borate-EDTA, pH 8.2 (89 mM Tris, 89 mM boric acid, 2.5 mM EDTA) at 200 V for 15 hours. Radioactive RNA was detected by autoradiography. Lane 1: SS-B/La-associated RNAs; lane 2: SS-A/Ro-associated RNAs; lane 3: Sm-associated RNAs; and lane 4: RNP-associated RNA.

cells, and lymphoblastoid cells) (27,33,34,44), but the 4.5 S RNA species were not. In human cells, 5S RNA and three other small RNAs were precipitated by anti-SS-B/La sera, and were called ha, hb, and hy5 RNAs by Hendrick et al. (27). In the mouse system, meanwhile, 5 S, 4.5 S, ma, and mb RNAs were precipitated by anti-SS-B/La sera (27,34).

Similarly, two small RNAs called mY1 and mY2 RNAs were precipitated from mouse Ehrlich ascites cells by anti-SS-A/Ro sera (34). In human cells, hy1, hy2, hy4 and hy5 RNA were precipitated by anti-SS-A/Ro sera, as shown in lane 2 of Figure 6 (15,27,34); hy5 RNA can also be precipitated by anti-SS-B/La sera (34). Using sequential immunoprecipitation analysis, Sm antigen was found to be associated with RNP antigen; similarly, SS-B/La was found with SS-A/Ro (15,27). However, there are free Sm (40,42) and SS-B/La (15). These suggest there are at least four groups of RNP

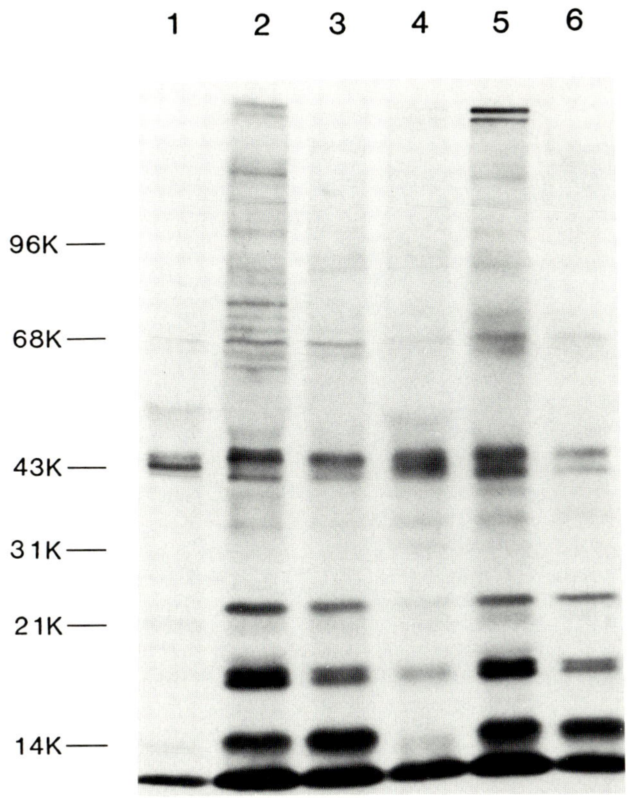

Figure 7. Cellular antigen-associated peptide profiles from ^{35}S-methionine-labeled WiL2 cell extract. The immunoprecipitin procedures were similar to those described in Figure 6. The immune complexes dissociated from staphylococci were treated with 10 μl of RNase A, 1 mg/ml, for 30 minutes at 37°C, and then boiled for 2 minutes in sample buffer (80 mM Tris-HCl, pH 6.8, 10% glycerol, 3% SDS, and 3% beta-mercaptoethanol). Electrophoresis was carried out in a 10% acrylamide slab gel. After electrophoresis, dried gels were subjected to autoradiography on Kodak XRP-5 film. Lanes 1 and 4: SS-B/La peptide profile, with a specific 43 Kd peptide noted; lanes 2 and 5: Sm peptide profile; and lanes 3 and 6: RNP peptide profile. Sm and RNP were found to be associated with at least six common peptides.

particles associated with the autoantibodies present in patients with various connective tissue disease. The first group is Sm and nRNP; the second is free Sm; the third is free SS-B/La; and the fourth is both SS-B/La and SS-A/Ro.

Since the antigenicity of Sm, SS-B/La, and SS-A/Ro is protein, but not RNAs, it is reasonable to predict that specific antibodies could also precipitate specific peptides. Using similar immunoprecipitation analysis, specific antibodies precipitate specific peptides, as shown in Figure 7 (36,44). When ^{35}S-methionine-labeled cell extract was used as the antigenic source, anti-SS-B/La react with a 43K peptide (lanes 1 and 4, Fig. 7), while anti-Sm (lanes 2 and 5, Fig. 7) and anti-RNP (lanes 3 and 6, Fig. 7) precipitate six common peptides of molecular weights ranging from 10 to 50K. However, there was no specific peptide recognized by anti-SS-A/Ro sera. In the past several years, there are several reports concerning the peptides of these four different cellular antigens. There

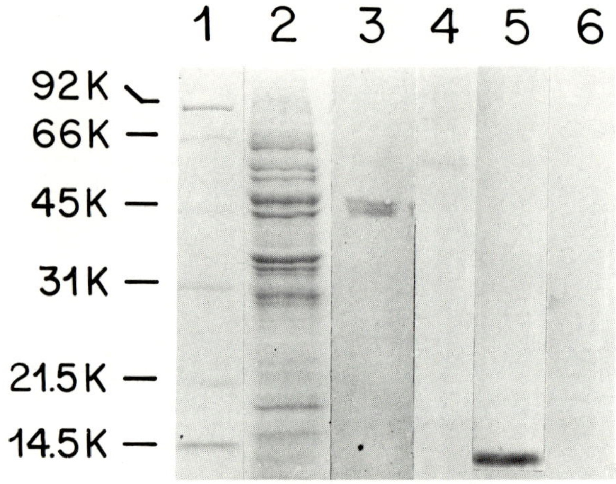

Figure 8. Protein profile of WiL2 cell extract on SDS-10% acrylamide gel electrophoresis and the immunoblot profiles for the four different cellular antigens. WiL2 cell extract was subjected to 10% acrylamide gel electrophoresis and then transferred to nitrocellulose paper (Western blotting). After blotting, strips of nitrocellulose papers were cut and soaked in a dilution of monospecific serum containing anti-Sm, anti-RNP, anti-SS-B/La, or anti-SS-A/Ro antibodies for several hours. After washing in solution containing 50 mM Tris-HCl, 150 mM NaCl, 0.25% gelatin, and 0.1% NP-40, the strips of papers were soaked in dilution of HRP-labeled goat anti-human IgG antiserum for 4 hours. After washing the nitrocellulose paper strips were incubated in 50 mM Tris-HCl (pH 7.5) solution containing 0.2 mg/ml diaminobenzidine and 0.01% H_2O_2 for color development. The presence of a band indicated the location of the specific antigen-antibody interaction. Lane 1: molecular weight standard; lane 2: WiL2 cell extract protein profile; lane 3: a 43–45 Kd peptide picked up by anti-SS-B/La antibody; lane 4: a peptide of 55–60 Kd reacted with anti-SS-A/Ro antibody; lane 5: a peptide of molecular weight less than 14 Kd was recognized by anti-Sm antibody; and lane 6: no specific peptide recognized by anti-RNP antibody.

are controversies about the exact antigenic peptides of these antigens. Using immunoprecipitation analysis, anti-Sm and anti-RNP antibodies precipitated several common peptides, as shown in Figure 7 (13,28,36). Using a different approach, several common peptides could similarly be eluted from the anti-Sm and anti-RNP affinity columns (18,19,22,55,56,63). Most of these studies did agree that the peptides of molecular weight ranging from 13 to 35K were frequently found in RNP particles carrying the antigens of Sm and RNP. These studies also indicate the complexity of the RNP particles. Since the development of the immunoblot technique, it is easy to pinpoint the peptide that is responsible for the antigenicity (10,60). In this way, several peptides of different molecular weights were recognized by the anti-Sm antibodies. One of these is a 13K peptide as seen in Figure 8, lane 5 (17,64). Several other smaller peptides were also recognized as described by other investigators (13). As far as RNP antigen is concerned, there was no specific peptide recognized by anti-RNP antibodies in immunoblot analysis, as seen in Figure 8, lane 6 (13). However, other peptides such as 30K, 40K, and 70K were detected (17,64). The controversial reports concerning the antigenic peptides for Sm and RNP may indeed reflect the heterogeneity of the antibodies present in patients with various connective tissue disease. In lieu of the recent progress—especially the purification of U1, U2, and other U series RNAs, and also the use of more different serum samples obtained from different patients—it turns out that differ-

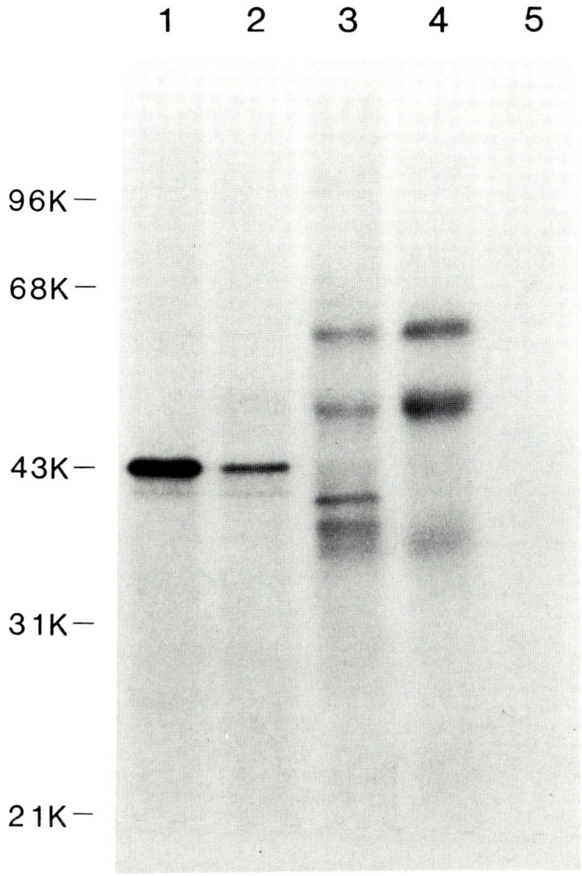

Figure 9. Phosphoprotein profiles for the four cellular antigens. ^{32}P-labeled WiL2 cell extract was used to study the cellular antigen-associated phosphoproteins. The immunoprecipitation was carried out exactly the same as in Figure 7. Lane 1: SS-B/La; lane 2: SS-A/Ro; lane 3: Sm; lane 4: RNP; and lane 5: normal human serum control. SS-B/La and SS-A/Ro were associated with two common phosphoproteins, and the major one was the 43 Kd peptide. Sm and RNP shared three common phosphoproteins.

ent RNP particles contain different peptides, in addition to several common peptides (28). Thus far, U1 RNP is thought to contain U1 RNA and seven to nine peptides. One of them is 70K peptide, which could be the marker protein for U1 RNP. U2 RNP is composed of U2 RNA, and possibly six peptides. Five of them are common to the U1 RNP peptides, having a molecular weight ranging from 10 to 35K (Steitz, personal communication). RNP particles of Sm and RNP also contain phosphoproteins, as shown in Figure 9. Anti-Sm (lane 3) and anti-RNP (lane 4) sera precipitated three common phosphoproteins of molecular weights ranging from 35 to 65K (44). Additionally, anti-Sm sera precipitated one specific phosphoprotein of 40K molecular weight (see Fig. 9, lane 3). In similar analysis, anti-SS-B/La and anti-SS-A/Ro sera precipitated two phosphoproteins, as shown in Figure 9 lane 1 (for anti-SS-B/La) and lane 2 (for anti-SS-A/Ro) (44). The 43K one is the major one. Using immunoblot analysis, the 43K peptide was recognized by anti-SS-B/La antibodies as seen in Figure 8, lane 3. This 43K peptide seemed to be similar to what was described earlier by other investigators who claimed the molecular weight of SS-B/La peptide was 43 to 50K (1,21,38,44,48). The SS-B/La peptide is labile and subjected to spontaneous degradation to smaller peptides such as 30K (15), which is similar to what was described previously by Mattioli and Reichlin (41). The instability of the SS-B/La antigen could explain the different molecular weights of SS-B/La antigen obtained from different antigenic sources (1,41,61). It has been shown that SS-B/La antigen binds several cellular RNAs, as seen in Figure 6, lane 1 (27,33,34,44), adenovirus-associated RNAs (VA RNA) (34,44,50), and EBV-coded RNAs (EBER) (33,50). Recently, the leader RNA of vesicular stomatitis virus was also found to be associated with La antigen (32). Using anti-SS-B/La antibodies as tools, Rosa et al. demonstrated that EBER showed striking similarities to VA RNA (50). SS-B/La proteins bind to the terminal nucleotides of VA RNA, but not to the stem structure (21) and the 3' end of 4.5 I RNA (46). Moreover, some precursors of 5S rRNA and of certain tRNAs are also found to be associated with SS-B/La protein transiently (48). This suggests that newly synthesized 5S RNA molecules are associated with SS-B/La protein, and that the SS-B/La protein might play an essential role in the synthesis or maturation of certain RNAs, especially the transcripts of RNA polymerase III (48). This finding might explain the presence of SS-B/La antigen in the nucleus of cells at late G_1 to early S phase of cell cycle (16). Anti-SS-B/La antibodies frequently coexist with anti-SS-A/Ro antibodies (41). Anti-SS-A/Ro antibodies also precipitate certain smaller cellular RNAs, as seen in Figure 6, lane 2 (33,34). The SS-A/Ro-associated RNAs were found to be hidden in the SS-B/La RNP particles described by Hendrick et al. (27). This could not rule out, however, the possibility that it is due to the contamination of the anti-SS-B/La antibodies in the serum used in that particular assay with anti SS-A/Ro antibodies.

In the sequential immunoprecipitation and phosphoprotein analyses, both anti-SS-A/Ro and antiSS-B/La antibodies precipitated a phosphoprotein of 43K molecular weight. Anti-SS-B/La antibodies could inhibit the precipitation of 43K peptide by anti-SS-A-/Ro antibodies, but anti-SS-A/Ro antibodies could not abolish the precipitation of 43K peptide by anti-SS-B/La antibodies. These findings plus the biochemical characteristics of anti-SS-B/La and SS-A/Ro antigens indicate that there is free SS-B/La antigen without accompanying SS-A/Ro antigen, while there is no free SS-A/Ro antigen. SS-A/Ro antigen is present in RNP particles also carrying SS-B/La antigen. The amount of SS-A/Ro antigen in cells is much less than that of SS-B/La. The antigenic peptide for SS-A/Ro is a peptide of 60K (as seen in Fig. 8, lane 4) that may possibly not contain methionine and phosphoamino acids. SS-A/Ro antigen is present predominantly in nuclei (14). This observation is confirmed by a monoclonal antiSS-A/Ro antibody (11).

STANDARDIZATION OF GEL PRECIPITATION TESTS FOR ANTIBODIES TO Sm AND RNP

The gel precipitation method is simpler to perform; but if not properly standardized, it may give us divergent results. The various reasons of such divergent results in the gel precipitation method are: 1) The size of the wells and the distance of the peripheral wells from the central well, 2) the concentration and thickness of agarose, and 3) the antigenic composition of the antigenic preparation (8,30).

The template employed for punching wells into the agarose is critical; greater distances reduce the sensitivity of detection, especially of weak reactions, and smaller distances affect the resolution and readability of the test system. We studied the effect of different templates on the sensitivity of detecting anti-RNP and anti-Sm antibodies. The template distances that give consistent and most suitable test results are depicted in Figure 1. The center antigen well of this template has a diameter of 6.5 mm, and the peripheral serum wells are 5 mm in diameter. The distance from the center to the peripheral wells is 2 mm.

In the literature, 0.6% agarose has been recommended; however, we have found that 1 to 1.2% agarose give sharper precipitin lines than 0.6% agarose concentration. We also found that the volume of agarose is critical in the detection of anti-ENA antibodies. A fill volume of 7 ml of agarose per Falcon dish (60 × 15 mm, Becton Dickinson, CA) was found to yield higher antibody titers. In addition, we also examined the effect of temperature and time on anti-ENA antibodies detection. We found that incubation of the agarose plates at room temperature for 24 hours gave optimum results, and that incubation either at 4°C or a higher temperatures and for prolonged periods was not necessary.

As mentioned earlier, the amount of protein present in ENA extracts is dependent on the source and type of tissue and experimental conditions employed in extraction, and that the amount of protein of these extracts is a poor indication of the antigenic activity of these extracts (30). It is a well-known fact that ENAs are present in various tissues from different species of animals, and that distribution and concentration of these antigens vary depending on the tissue employed in extraction of these antigens. In addition, different methods of ENA preparation along with different substrates may yield preparations of varying antigen potencies. Because of such a wide selection of antigen substrates and varying methods of antigen isolation, there is a strong need to standardize the ENA preparation to provide reproducible results. This could be achieved by chessboard titration of the type shown in Table 4. By performing many such titrations during the past several years, we have found that for RNP and Sm, the optimum working antigen dilution is one to two dilutions above the antigen endpoint titer.

Thus, in summary, to obtain reproducible results we recommend the following.

1. The central antigen well is 6.5 mm in diameter, peripheral wells are 5 mm, and the distance between central and peripheral well is 2 mm.

Table 4. Standardization of Extractable Nuclear Antigen (RNP and Sm) Preparation by Chessboard Titration

		Antigen dilution			
Serum dilution	*Undiluted*	*1:2*	*1:4*	*1:8*	*1:16*
Undiluted	+	+	+	+	−
1:2	+	+	+	+	−
1:4	+	+	+	+	−
1:8	+	+	+	+	−
1:16	−	+	+	+	−
1:32	−	−	−	+	−
1:64	−	−	−	−	−
		↑ Use dilution		↑ Antigen endpoint	

2. One percent agarose in order to provide sharp precipitin lines.
3. The fill volume for the central well should be 100 μl; and for peripheral wells, 60 μl. This could be achieved by adding 7 ml of 1% agarose in Falcon (Becton, Dickinson, CA) plates.
4. The working antigen dilution should be one or two doubling dilutions above the endpoint titer, as revealed by two-dimensional chessboard titrations.

ACKNOWLEDGMENTS

The authors deeply appreciate the support and encouragement of E.M. Tan, J.N. Gilliam, and E.H. Beutner. The excellent secretarial assistance of Sonya Patridge and Veronica Sanfilippo is also appreciated.

REFERENCES

1. Akizuki M, Boehm-Truitt MJ, Kassan SS, et al: Purification of an acidic nuclear protein antigen and demonstration of its antibodies in subsets of patients with sicca syndrome. *J Immunol* 119:932–938, 1977.
2. Akizuki M, Powers R Jr, Holman HR: A soluble acidic protein of the cell nucleus which reacts with serum from patients with systemic lupus erythematosus and Sjögren's syndrome. *J Clin Invest* 59:264–272, 1977.
3. Alspaugh MA, Maddison P: Resolution of the identity of certain antigen-antibody systems in systemic lupus erythematosus and Sjogren's syndrome: An interlaboratory collaboration. *Arthritis Rheum* 22:796–798, 1979.
4. Alspaugh MA, Talal N, Tan EM: Differentiation and characterization of autoantibodies and their antigens in Sjogren's syndrome. *Arthritis Rheum* 19:216–222, 1976.
5. Alspaugh MA, Tan EM: Antibodies to cellular antigens in Sjogren's syndrome. *J Clin Invest* 55:1067–1073, 1975.
6. Anderson JR, Gray KG, Beck JS, et al: Precipitating autoantibodies in the connective tissue diseases. *Ann Rheum Dis* 21:360–369, 1962.
7. Barque JP, Yeni P, Perandeau L, et al: Nuclear ribonucleoproteins recognized by human antinuclear antibodies in retrovirus-infected cells. *Biochem Biophys Res Commun* 99:284–291, 1981.
8. Binder WL, Gockel S, Rippe D, et al: Standardization and performance characteristics of a double diffusion test for autoantibodies to Sm and RNP. *ASM Ann Meeting*, 1984, p 72, (abstract).
9. Bresnihan B, Bunne C, Snaith ML, et al: Anti-ribonucleoprotein antibodies in connective tissue disease: Estimation by counterimmunoelectrophoresis. *Br Med J* 1:610–611, 1977.
10. Burnette WN: "Western blotting": Electrophoretic transfer of proteins from sodium dodecylsulfate-polyacrylamide gels to unmodified nitrocellulose and radiographic detection with antibody and radioiodinated protein A. *Anal Biochem* 112:195–203, 1981.
11. Chang JY, Deng JS, Sontheimer RD, et al: A monoclonal anti-SS-A/Ro antibody binds to human but not murine cell nuclei. *Clin Res* 31:920A, 1983 (abstract).
12. Clark G, Reichlin M, Tomasi TB: Characterization of a soluble cytoplasmic antigen reactive with sera from patients with systemic lupus erythematosus. *J Immunol* 102:117–122, 1969.
13. Conner GE, Nelson D, Wisniewolski R, et al: Protein antigens of the RNA-protein complexes detected by anti-Sm and anti-RNP antibodies found in serum of patients with systemic lupus erythematosus and related disorders. *J Exp Med* 156:1475–1485, 1982.
14. Deng JS, Sontheimer RD, Gilliam JN: Characterization of the relationship between SS-A/Ro antibody (abs), antinuclear antibodies (ANA) and subacute cutaneous lupus erythematosus (SCLE). *Clin Res* 31:262A, 1983 (abstract).

15. Deng JS, Sontheimer RD, Gilliam JN: Molecular characteristics of SS-B/La and SS-A/Ro cellular antigens. *J Invest Dermatol* 84:86–90, 1985.
16. Deng JS, Takasaki Y, Tan EM: Nonhistone nuclear antigens reactive with autoantibodies. Immunofluorescent studies of distribution in synchronized cells. *J Cell Biol* 91:654–660, 1981.
17. Douvas AS: Autoantibodies occurring in two different rheumatic diseases react with the same nuclear ribonucleoprotein particle. *Proc Natl Acad Sci USA* 79:5401–5405, 1982.
18. Douvas AS, Stumph WE, Reyes P, et al: Isolation and characterization of nuclear ribonucleoprotein complexes using human antinuclear ribonucleoprotein antibodies. *J Biol Chem* 254:3608–3616, 1979.
19. Eisenberg RA, Klapper DG, Cohen PL: The polypeptide structure of the SM and RNP nuclear antigens. *Mol Immunol* 20:187–195, 1983.
20. Farber SJ, Bole GG: Antibodies to components of extractable nuclear antigen. *Arch Intern Med* 136:425–431, 1976.
21. Francoeur AM, Mathews MB: Interaction between VA-RNA and the lupus antigen La: formation of a ribonucleoprotein particles in vitro. *Proc Natl Acad Sci USA* 79:6772–6776, 1982.
22. Gibbons JJ Jr, Augustynek D, Tsai CC, et al: Characterization of RNP and Sm ribonucleoprotein nuclear antigens. *Mol Immunol* 19:765–777, 1982.
23. Grennan DM, Bunn C, Hughes GRV, et al: Frequency and clinical significance of antibodies to ribonucleoprotein in SLE and other connective tissue disease subgroups. *Ann Rheum Disease* 36:442–447, 1977.
24. Harada F, Kato N: Nucleotide sequences of 4.5S RNAs associated with poly (A)-containing RNAs of mouse and hamster cells. *Nucl Acid Res* 8:1273–1285, 1980.
25. Harmon CE, Deng JS, Peebles CL, et al: The importance of tissue substrate in the SS-A/Ro antigen-antibody system. *Arthritis Rheum* 27:166–173, 1984.
26. Hellung-Larson P. Frederiksen S: Occurrence and properties of low molecular weight RNA components from cells at different taxonomic levels. *Comp Biochem Physiol* 58B: 273–281, 1977.
27. Hendrick JP, Wollin SL, Rinke J, et al: Ro small cytoplasmic ribonucleoproteins are a subclass of La ribonucleoproteins: Further characterization of the Ro and La small ribonucleoproteins from infected mammalian cells. *Mol Cell Biol* 1:1138–1149, 1981.
28. Kinlaw CS, Dusing-Swartz SK, Berget SM: Human U1 and U2 nuclear ribonucleoproteins contain common and unique polypeptides. *Mol Cell Biol* 2:1159–1166, 1982.
29. Koffler D, Carr R, Agnello V, et al: Antibodies to polynucleotides in human sera: Antigenic specificity and relation to diseases. *J Exp Med* 134:294–312, 1971.
30. Kumar V, Beutner EH, Dabski K, et al: A standardized method of detecting antibodies to extractable nuclear antigens (RNP and Sm) by gel precipitation. *J Clin Lab Immunol* 15:163–166, 1984.
31. Kurata N, Tan EM: Identification of antibodies to nuclear acidic antigens by counterimmunoelectrophoresis. *Arthritis Rheum* 19:574–580, 1976.
32. Kurilla MG, Keene JD: The leader RNA of vesicular stomatitis virus is bound by a cellular protein reactive with anti-La lupus antibodies. *Cell* 34:837–845, 1983.
33. Lerner MR, Andrews NC, Miller G, et al: Two small RNAs encoded by Epstein-Barr virus and complexed with protein are precipitated by antibodies from patients with systemic lupus erythematosus. *Proc Natl Acad Sci USA* 78:805–809, 1981.
34. Lerner MR, Boyle JA, Hardin JA, et al: Two novel classes of small ribonucleoproteins detected by antibodies associated with lupus erythematosus. *Science* 211:400–402, 1981.
35. Lerner MR, Boyle JA, Mount SM, et al: Are snRNPs involved in splicing? *Nature* (*London*) 283:220–224, 1980.
36. Lerner MR, Steitz JA: Antibodies to small nuclear RNAs complexed with proteins are produced by patients with systemic lupus erythematosus. *Proc Natl Acad Sci USA* 76:5495–5499, 1979.
37. Levy JA, Violainen M, Defendi V: Human lymphoblastoid lines from lymph node and spleen. *Cancer* 22:517–524, 1968.
38. Matter L, Schopfer K, Wilheim JA, et al: Molecular characterization of ribonucleoprotein antigens bound by antinuclear antibodies. *Arthritis Rheum* 25:1278–1283, 1982.

39. Mattioli M, Reichlin M: Characterization of a soluble nuclear ribonucleoprotein antigen reactive with SLE sera. *J Immunol* 107:1281–1290, 1971.
40. Mattioli M, Reichlin M: Physical association of two nuclear antigens and mutual occurrence of their antibodies: The relationship of the Sm and RNA protein (Mo) systems in SLE sera. *J Immunol* 110:1318–1324, 1973.
41. Mattioli M, Reichlin M: Heterogeneity of RNA protein antigens reactive with sera of patients with systemic lupus erythematosus. Description of a cytoplasmic nonribosomal antigen. *Arthritis Rheum* 17:421–429, 1974.
42. Northway JD, Tan EM: Differentiation of antinuclear antibodies giving speckled nuclear patterns in immunofluorescence. *Clin Immunol Immunopathol* 1:140–154, 1972.
43. Notman DD, Kurata N, Tan EM: Profiles of antinuclear antibodies in systemic rheumatic diseases. *Ann Intern Med* 83:464–469, 1975.
44. Pizer LI, Deng JS, Stenberg RM, et al: Characterization of a phosphoprotein associated with the SS-B/La nuclear antigen in adenovirus infected and uninfected KB cells. *Mol Cell Biol* 3:1235–1245, 1983.
45. Reddy R, Busch H: U snRNAs of nuclear snRNPs. In Bush, H (Ed): *The Cell Nucleus,* vol. 8. Academic Press, New York, 1981, pp 261–306.
46. Reddy R, Henning D, Tan EM, et al: Identification of a La protein binding site in a RNA polymerase III transcript (4.5 I RNA). *J Biol Chem* 258:8352–8356, 1983.
47. Reichlin M, Mattioli M: Correlation of a precipitin reaction to a RNA protein antigen and a low prevalence of a nephritis in patients with systemic lupus erythematosus. *N Engl J Med* 286:908–911, 1972.
48. Rinke J, Steitz JA: Precursor molecules of both human 5S ribosomal RNA and transfer RNAs are bound by a cellular protein reactive with anti-La lupus antibodies. *Cell* 29:149–159, 1982.
49. Ro-Choi TS, Reddy R, Herring D, et al: Nucleotide sequence of 4.5S ribonucleic acid of Novikoff hepatoma cell nuclei. *J Biol Chem* 247:3205–3222, 1972.
50. Rosa MD, Bottlieb E, Lerner MR, et al: Striking similarities are exhibited by two small Epstein-Barr virus-encoded ribonucleic acids and the adenovirus-associated ribonucleic acids VA1 and VAII. *Mol Cell Biol* 1:785–796, 1981.
51. Schaefen JL, Schrohenloher RE: Quantitation of antibodies to extractable nuclear antigens (ENA) by hemagglutination: A useful modification. *Arthritis Rheum* 22:557–558, 1979.
52. Sharp GC, Irvin WS, Lerogue RL, et al: Association of autoantibodies to different nuclear antigens with clinical patterns of rheumatic disease and responsiveness to therapy. *J Clin Invest* 50:750–759, 1971.
53. Sharp GC, Irvin WS, Tan EM, et al: Mixed connective tissue disease—an apparently distinct rheumatic disease syndrome associated with a specific antibody to an extractable nuclear antigen (ENA). *Am J Med* 52:148–159, 1972.
54. Struckmann J, Manthorpe R, Bendixen G: Anti-ENA antibody in serum determined by ELISA-technique. Description of method and recommended procedure. *Allergy* 36:397–403, 1981.
55. Takano M, Agris PF, Sharp GC: Purification and biochemical characterization of nuclear ribonucleoprotein antigen using purified antibody from serum of a patient with mixed connective tissue disease. *J Clin Invest* 65:1449–1456, 1980.
56. Takano M, Golden SS, Sharp GC, et al: Molecular relationships between two nuclear antigens, ribonucleoprotein and Sm: Purification of active antigens and their biochemical characterization. *Biochemistry* 20:5929–5936, 1981.
57. Tan EM: Autoantibodies to nuclear antigens (ANA): Their immunobiology and medicine. In Kunkel HG, Dixon FJ (Eds): *Advances in Immunology,* Academic Press, New York, vol. 33. 1982, pp 167–240.
58. Tan EM, Kunkel HG: Characterization of a soluble nuclear antigen precipitating with sera of patients with systemic lupus erythematosus. *J Immunol* 96:464–471, 1966.
59. Tan EM, Peebles C: Quantitation of antibodies to Sm antigen and nuclear ribonucleoprotein by hemagglutination. In Rose NR, Friedman H (Eds): *Manual of Clinical Immunology.* American Society for Microbiology Press Washington DC, 1980, chap. 116, pp 866–870.
60. Towbin H, Staehelin T, Gordon J: Electrophoretic transfer of proteins from polyacrylamide

gels to nitrocellulose sheets: Procedures and some applications. *Proc Natl Acad Sci USA* 76:4350–4354, 1979.

61. Venables PJW, Charles PJ, Buchanan RRC, et al: Quantitation and detection of isotypes of anti-SS-B antibodies by ELISA and Farr assays using affinity purified antigens. *Arthritis Rheum* 26:146–155, 1983.
62. Weinberg RA, Penman S: Small molecular weight monodispose nuclear RNA. *J Mol Biol* 38:289–304, 1968.
63. White PJ, Gardner WD, Hoch SO: Identification of the immunogenically active components of Sm and RNP antigens. *Proc Natl Acad Sci USA* 78:626–630, 1981.
64. White PJ, Hoch SO: Definition of the antigenic polypeptides in the Sm and RNP ribonucleoprotein complexes. *Biochem Biophys Res* Comm 102:365–371, 1981.
65. Whittingham S: A solid phase radioimmunoassay for detection of antibodies to extractable nuclear antigens. *J Immunol Methods* 61:73–81, 1983.
66. Yang VW, Lerner MR, Steitz JA, et al: A small nuclear ribonucleoprotein is required for splicing of adenoviral early RNA sequences. *Proc Natl Acad Sci USA* 78:1371–1375, 1981.

33
Antibodies to Extractable Nuclear Antigens: Clinical Significance

Morris Reichlin
John B. Harley

INTRODUCTION

Antibodies to ENA are best defined by precipitin reactions in double diffusion experiments between autoantibody-containing sera from patients with rheumatic diseases and soluble extracts from animal or human tissue. The term ENA (extractable nuclear antigens) has now been superseded by knowledge of the precise molecular nature of the reactive antigens. In addition, the diagnostic specificity of these reactions has extended far beyond their original application to patients with systemic lupus erythematosus (SLE). There are specific precipitin reactions that have now been defined not only for SLE, but also for the diseases polymyositis and scleroderma (progressive systemic sclerosis [PSS]). In this chapter, current knowledge about the systems that are characteristic of SLE and polymyositis will be reviewed. Newer approaches for the detection and study of these systems will also be presented.

PRECIPITATING ANTIBODIES CHARACTERISTIC OF SLE PATIENTS: ANTIBODIES TO SM AND nRNP

Precipitating antibodies to soluble antigens occur with appreciable frequency to four antigens. These are the nRNP, Sm, Ro/SSA, and La/SSB antigens. As antibodies to these antigens tend to occur in pairs, the nuclear pair Sm and nRNP will be discussed first.

The Sm and nRNP antigens are nuclear in origin, and recent work has shed much light on their structure. Early characterization of the Sm antigen showed it to be periodate sensitive, but trypsin, RNase, or DNase did not affect its antigenicity in precipitin reactions (37). The ability of the nRNP antigen to precipitate (18) or to coat cells for a hemagglutination reaction (32,33) was ablated by either RNase or trypsin. The frequent, nonrandom mutual occurrence of antibodies to Sm and nRNP was noted (28), and their molecular association was demonstrated by immunochemical methods (20).

These early studies (20) and, later, more elegant immunoaffinity studies have shown that Sm and nRNP antigenic determinants exist in a molecular complex, and that there exists a molecular form of Sm free of nRNP (11,35).

Two major advances have enhanced the understanding of the antigenic structure of these antigens. One is the work of Lerner and Steitz, who characterized the RNA components of RNA-protein particles, which carry the Sm and nRNP epitopes (15). The second development was the application of the "immunoblot" or Western blot technique, as well as other quantitative analyses (elution from SDS polyacrylamide gels) of the antigenicity of the protein components of the Sm and nRNP particles (11,14,35,36).

The picture that emerges is that the particle bound by anti-nRNP is composed of an RNA component designated U1 that is complexed to at least seven proteins varying in molecular weight from 12 to 65K, and the Sm particle is composed of the same seven proteins as well as U1, U2, U4, U5, and U6 RNAs containing 196, 171, 145, 120, and 95 nucleotides, respectively. As already mentioned, there is a smaller antigenic version of the Sm particle lacking RNA, but having several small protein bands and a total molecular weight (Mw) of 70K. Precipitation reactions of nRNP with its antibody require the whole particle—both RNA and protein. Protein alone is sufficient for the precipitation of Sm with anti-Sm. Takano et al. (35) have shown direct binding of protein components of Mw 65K and 30K with anti-nRNP, and of 30K and 13K to anti-Sm. Douvas finds nRNP antigenicity to be associated with a 30K protein and Sm antigenicity to be related to a 13K protein by the immunoblot technique (15). Differences in elution conditions (3 M KSCN versus 0.01 M HCl) may account for some of the differences in antigenicity noted by these two groups. There is no evidence for the direct binding of RNA to either antibody. Studies designed to detect antibodies specific for the whole particle have not yet been reported. The antigenic epitopes for both Sm and nRNP may only be represented on protein molecules, but more work is necessary to settle this issue. Recently, a hybridoma-producing anti-Sm was formed by fusion of spleen cells from an autoimmune MRL/1 mouse, with an appropriate myeloma cell line (14). This mouse monoclonal antibody (MCA) precipitates the same RNA protein particle, as does the human antibody; the immunoblot technique indicates that the MCA bind a 26K protein. Further data on biochemical characteristics of RNP and Sm appear in Chapter 32.

The clinical significance of antibodies to nRNP and Sm has received much attention, and only a brief summary of that information will be presented. There is agreement among investigators in this area that antibodies to the Sm antigen are highly specific for SLE patients, and serve as marker antibodies for lupus patients. There are patients, however, with anti-Sm who do not fulfill criteria for SLE. Only long-term follow-up of such patients will reveal the ultimate diagnostic specificity of anti-Sm in this population. No characteristic clinical features are apparent for this group of patients, although there are reports that the nephritis of such patients is mild and follows a benign course (25,40). It has also been reported that antibodies to Sm are associated with central nervous system involvement when it occurs as an isolated clinical manifestation of the disease (39). A recent report provides evidence for fluctuation of anti-Sm levels with disease activity, suggesting both participation in immune complex disease and use as a possible indicator of clinical activity in some patients (7).

The presence of antibodies to nRNP as the sole precipitin system, demonstrated by the Ouchterlony technique, identifies a subset of lupus patients with a low frequency of antibodies to DNA and a low frequency of clinically apparent renal disease (29,32,33). Patients with anti-nRNP in their sera develop nephritis only when antibodies of other specificities are present, notably anti-DNA antibodies (16,24). We have also noted that nephritis occurs not only when anti-nRNP antibodies are associated with anti-DNA antibodies, but also when antibodies to Sm or Ro/SSA are concurrently present.

Much attention has centered on a group of patients with overlapping features of SLE, PSS, and polymyositis who have been designated as mixed connective tissue disease (MCTD) patients by Sharp et al. (32,33). These patients all possess antibodies to nRNP in their sera and, like other patients with anti-nRNP antibodies who lack overlapping features, have a low frequency of antibodies to DNA and a low frequency of nephritis.

Two reports of immune complex nephropathy in patients with MCTD and anti-nRNP antibodies have appeared (9,12), but in neither report were antibodies to Ro/SSA or ssDNA sought in the sera of the nephritic patients. Both of these systems have been shown to participate in immune complex nephritis, and occur in 10 to 15% of patients with anti-nRNP antibodies. Special tests are required for their detection, and unless specifically sought, they are easily overlooked.

MCTD patients present with very heterogeneous clinical features, which is a point noted in the initial description and re-emphasized in the follow-up of the original 25 patients (22). The only uniform finding in these patients is, by definition, the presence of antibodies to nRNP. No immunologic, clinical, genetic, or biochemical characteristics have yet been described that give this syndrome a definition. The finding(s) that will distinguish MCTD from its component connective tissue diseases (SLE, myositis, and PSS) awaits recognition.

ANTIBODIES TO Ro/SSA AND La/SSB/Ha

Antibodies to the soluble antigens Ro and La were originally described in patients with SLE and Sjögren's syndrome (10,19). Both antigens were thought to be cytoplasmic, since they were quantitatively recovered from the cytoplasmic fraction of cells prepared in strong sucrose solutions. Moreover, specifically purified antibodies to the Ro antigen stained predominantly the cytoplasm of KB cells (a human tissue culture line), thymocytes, and Wil_2 cells (a lymphoblastoid B cell line), while specifically purified antibodies to La stained both the nucleus and cytoplasm of these cells (Maddison and Reichlin, unpublished data).

Alspaugh and Tan described two nuclear antigens extracted from Wil_2 cells, termed SSA and SSB, that precipitated with sera of patients with Sjögren's syndrome (5). Akizuki et al. described a soluble nuclear antigen termed HA, which precipitated with the sera of patients with SLE-Sjögren's syndrome overlap (1). Interlaboratory exchange of sera and antigen extracts have clearly shown that Ro and SSA (on the one hand) and La, SSB, and Ha (on the other) are antigenically identical. Problems still remain about the cellular localization of Ro/SSA and La/SSB/Ha, but it is now known that these antigens are both RNA protein conjugates (13). While all RNA is synthesized in the nucleus, much of the cellular RNA eventually resides in the cytoplasm. Some of the confusion about the cellular localization of these antigens might result from differences in the location of the antigen at different stages of the cell cycle. Examination of the cellular location of such antigens during different phases of the cell cycle, employing monospecific specifically purified antibodies or MCA, should provide definitive answers to these questions.

La/SSB/Ha from all sources is both trypsin sensitive and RNase sensitive only under certain circumstances. Ro/SSA is trypsin sensitive only when derived from Wil_2 cells,

Table 1. Antigens Reactive with SLE Sera

Antigen	*Chemical Nature of Antigen*	*Subunit characteristics of antigen*
Sm	RNA protein	U1, U2, U4, U5, and U6 RNAs plus 7 proteins from 12–65K
nRNP	RNA protein	U1 RNA and 7 proteins from 12–65K
Ro/SSA	RNA protein	RNAs (85–112 bases) complexed to 60K protein; native particle approximately 100K.
La/SSB	RNA protein	Heterogeneous RNAs (80–160 bases) complexed to 50K protein; native particle approximately 70–90K.

and it is not RNase sensitive. In neither case does isolated RNA have antigenic activity, and the consensus is that the antigenic epitopes in both instances are on protein subunits of the RNA protein conjugates. The antigenicity for Ro/SSA resides in a 60K polypeptide, while that for the La/SSB antigen resides in a 50K polypeptide. Chemical and subunit characterization of these antigens, which are targets of autoimmune attack in SLE patients, are detailed in Table 1.

The clinical specificity of antibodies to these antigens in North American populations is that they occur principally in two diseases: SLE and Sjögren's syndrome. Antibodies to Ro/SSA occur in 25 to 40% of unselected SLE patients when the assay utilized is the relatively insensitive agar diffusion method. Antibodies to La/SSB/Ha occur in 10 to 15% of SLE patients, all of whom also have antibodies to Ro/SSA in their sera. There is considerable variation in the reported frequency of these antibodies in the sera of patients with Sjögren's syndrome. Anti-Ro/SSA has been reported in 40 to 70% of primary Sjögren's syndrome, and in 10 to 40% of patients with the sicca complex and rheumatoid arthritis (RA) (2–5).

Using sensitive, recently developed ELISA tests for anti-Ro/SSA, we have found that the incidence of anti-Ro/SSA in both primary and secondary Sjögren's syndrome is about 90% (Harley and Reichlin, unpublished data).

Of considerable interest is the vastly different frequency of occurrence of anti-Ro/SSA in Japanese patients with connective tissue disease. The frequency of occurrence in SLE is 58%, while the frequencies in RA, scleroderma, polymyositis, and undifferentiated connective tissue disease are 24%, 29%, 15%, and 45%, respectively (42). These frequencies are much higher than those exhibited by North American patients with these same diseases; this difference is not explained by a more frequent occurrence of Sjögren's syndrome in the Japanese patients. Analysis of this difference in anti-Ro/SSA frequency in Japanese versus North American patients with connective tissue disease should yield important clues to the genesis and regulation of this specific immune response.

A number of interesting clinical phenomena have emerged that are associated with the presence of anti-Ro/SSA in SLE patients. These are listed in Table 2.

ANA-positive anti-Ro/SSA SLE patients are not clinically distinguishable from SLE patients without these antibodies, except for a high frequency of rheumatoid factors that occur in 75 to 80% of these patients. As already mentioned, antibodies to Ro/SSA occur in 63% of patients with clinical SLE but with negative ANA tests on cryostat sections of rodent liver or kidney sections. On the other hand, within the ANA-positive subset of SLE patients who have anti-Ro/SSA, important clinical and serologic differ-

Table 2. Clinical and Serologic Phenomena Associated with Anti-Ro/SSA in SLE Patients

1. Rheumatoid factor occurs in 80% of patients with anti-Ro antibodies.
2. SLE patients with anti-Ro/SSA antibodies have a high frequency of nephritis while those with both anti-Ro/SSA and anti-La/SSB antibodies have a low frequency of nephritis.
3. Anti-Ro/SSA antibodies occur in 62% of "ANA-negative SLE" patients.
4. Anti-Ro/SSA antibodies occur in 63% of SCLE patients.
5. Increased frequency of DR2 and DR3 antigens occur in SLE patients with anti-Ro/SSA antibodies.
6. 85% of homozygous C2-deficient patients with SLE picture have anti-Ro/SSA antibodies. No other precipitins are demonstrable.
7. Anti-Ro/SSA and/or anti-La/SSB antibodies occur almost invariably in neonatal SLE. No other precipitin is found.

ences distinguish patients who produce anti-Ro/SSA alone from those who produce both anti-Ro/SSA and anti-La/SSB (38).

There is a great similarity in nonrenal findings in these two groups of patients, but a striking difference in the frequency and severity of renal disease. Thus, 16 of 30 (52%) anti-Ro/SSA patients had one or more of the following three findings: 1) a serum creatinine greater than 3.0 mg%; 2) proteinuria exceeding 1.5 grams in 24 hours; and 3) cellular casts in the urine. Only 2 of 23 (9%) of the anti-Ro/SSA and anti-La/SSB patients had such evidence for nephritis. The serologic correlation of this difference in renal disease was a 77% incidence of anti-DNA antibodies in the anti-Ro/SSA antibody-positive group and a 30% incidence of such antibodies in the anti-Ro/SSA and anti-La/SSB antibody-positive group. Details of the titers and specificities of these antibodies to DNA have been published, but the titers of both anti-dsDNA and anti-ssDNA were higher in the anti-Ro/SSA antibody-positive group than in the patients who had both anti-Ro/SSA and anti-La/SSB antibodies in their sera (38).

Recently, a subset of lupus patients with a characteristic nonscarring dermatitis designated subacute lupus erythematosus (SCLE) has been described (34). The skin disease is intermediate in severity, between the acute erythematous eruption of SLE and the chronic indolent scarring lesions of discoid lupus erythematosus (DLE). The patients exhibit a wide distribution of lesions, with the face, arms, and trunk being affected. Seventy percent of these patients are ANA positive on KB cells, and they have a mild systemic illness very similar in character to that described in the so called ANA-negative SLE patients (17). The common factor shared by the ANA-negative SLE patients and the SCLE patients that may relate to their mild disease and the low frequency of nephritis is the low frequency of antibodies to dsDNA.

It has also been reported that 73% of these SCLE patients are DR3 positive, a great increase above the control frequency of 24% for this particular HLA antigen (34). These patients' sera have recently been examined for the presence of antibodies to soluble cellular antigens, and it has been found that 62% have antibodies to Ro/SSA and/or La/SSB antigens (34). As mentioned previously, 25 to 40% of SLE patients and only 3% of DLE patients have anti-Ro/SSA antibodies in their sera. In a recent report by Bell and Maddison, an even tighter linkage between antibodies to Ro/SSA and the HLA-antigen DR3 has been demonstrated (8). In their SLE population, all of the anti-Ro/SSA antibody-positive patients (10/10) were positive for the DR3 antigen. The frequency of DR3 in their control populations was 26%. These data suggest that a set of genetic determinants in the major histocompatibility complex (MHC) are associated with the production of anti-Ro/SSA antibodies.

Further data supporting a genetic influence on anti-Ro/SSA antibody production comes from a study of patients with homozygous C2 deficiency. The genes for C2 are known to reside in the MHC on chromosome 6. Antibodies to Ro/SSA were detected in 10 of 20 such C2-deficient sera, and it was the only precipitin detected. Interestingly, none of these patients produced anti-La/SSB antibodies; their sera contained only antibodies to Ro/SSA. Of even greater interest is that of 12 of these patients with an SLE picture, nine possessed anti-Ro/SSA antibodies; the remaining anti-Ro/SSA antibody-positive patient had DLE. Therefore, all 10 of the homozygous C2-deficient, anti-Ro/SSA antibody-positive patients were symptomatic (26).

As it is known that all homozygous C2-deficient patients studied thus far carry the DR2 antigen, it appears that antibodies to Ro/SSA can be associated with either the DR2 or DR3 antigens.

It has long been known that in children who develop neonatal SLE, the major clinical features are dermatitis and complete heart block. Recent studies show that antibodies to Ro/SSA and, to a lesser extent, La/SSB have been found in almost every child and mother examined in this clinical setting (31). The dermatitis and anti-Ro/SSA disappear with the same time course, suggesting the possible participation of the anti-Ro/SSA antibodies in the pathogenesis of the dermal lesion. Some of the mothers have not been clinically ill, and the anti-Ro/SSA and anti-La/SSB antibodies have been demonstrated in their sera in the course of evaluating the clinical and serologic status of the children. Chapter 35 describes in further detail this association of antibodies to Ro/SSA with dermatitis and complete heart block.

POLYMYOSITIS

Although it has long been known that 30 to 40% of patients with polymyositis have positive antinuclear antibodies (ANA), no particular antibody specificities have been associated with this disorder until recently. A number of antigen-antibody reactions have now been described that show specificity for this disorder; in addition, studies on tissue culture cells (HEp-2) with sera from myositis patients detect ANA in 86% of those patients (Reichlin, unpublished data).

The first ANA characteristic for this disorder was detected by a complement-fixing antibody to a nuclear antigen Mi, which occurred in 60% of dermatomyositis (DM) patients and a smaller proportion of polymyositis (PM) patients (30). Soon thereafter, a precipitating antibody to a nuclear antigen, designated PM_1 was described by Wolfe et al., and it was said to be present in 60% of PM patients (41). It is now recognized that no single precipitin reaction using both crude extracts and patient sera is present, in more than 30% of PM sera, and that the system originally designated PM_1 was a collection of precipitins—one of which (PM_1) occurred in a subset of PM patients, at least half of whom had an overlap of PSS and PM. This system has been renamed the PM-Scl system, is probably of nucleolar antigen, and occurs in 8 to 10% of unselected PM patients (27).

The most frequently found precipitating antibody in PM patients is designated Jo_1 and it occurs in 30% of idiopathic PM and less than 10% of DM patients (23). This antibody is not found in SLE, RA, or PSS patients' sera. The antigen is an acidic molecule of Mw 150K. There are genetic factors influencing production of these antibodies, since 67% of patients with anti-Jo_1 carry the DR3 antigen on their Ia-positive cells, while only 25% of nonanti-Jo_1 myositis patients possess the DR3 antigen (6). The antigen is poorly represented in mouse liver and kidney sections; negative ANA tests

Table 3. Antigens Reactive with Polymyositis Sera

Antigen	*Chemical nature of antigen*	*Cellular localization of antigen*
Jo_1	Protein that has enzyme activity, histidyl tRNA synthetase; reactive protein subunit, 50K	Cytoplasmic; native antigen approximately 150K
Mi_2	Mw 50, 58K protein	Nuclear
PM-Scl	Protein, Mw unknown	Nucleolar
nRNP	U1 RNA and 7 proteins from 12–65K	Nuclear

are the rule on these substrates. On tissue culture cells, a cytoplasmic pattern of immunofluorescence (IF) is frequently seen in association with this antibody.

Several other precipitating antibodies are seen in myositis patients, but are generally seen in overlap patients. Thus, anti-nRNP is seen in the majority of patients with SLE-myositis; the previously mentioned PM_1 or PM-Scl is seen in PSS-myositis patients in North America, and a system designated Ku (which is seen in PSS-myositis) has thus far been found only in Japanese patients (21). Exchange of reagents has established the independent identities of the nRNP, PM-Scl (PM_1), and Ku systems. Although the Ku antigen is nuclear, it is not represented in mouse tissue, and ANA tests are positive only on bovine or human tissues.

There is clearly great heterogeneity in the ANA characteristic of PM and DM, and an aggregate of antigens represented in crude extracts of tissue form precipitates with 60% of these sera. PM-Scl (PM_1), nRNP, and Jo_1 are major systems occurring in 10 to 30% of PM patients, but a number of other minor reactions constitute the total spectrum of antigens toward which antibodies are demonstrable (27). Of the remaining 40% of sera that do not form precipitates with tissue extracts, fewer than 10% are ANA positive on cryostat sections of rodent liver or kidney. About 80% of such sera, however, do bind to HEp-2 cells. The patterns seen are nuclear, cytoplasmic, and nucleolar. While none of these patterns are specific for the myositis syndromes, they illustrate the heterogeneity that exists among these antibodies. In addition, it is notable that almost all the patients exhibit some autoantibody. These findings also re-emphasize the capacity of the human tissue culture lines to detect autoantibodies not demonstrate on cryostat sections of rodent tissues. The chemical nature and cellular localization of the most frequent antigenic targets for autoantibody formation in myositis patients are listed in Table 3.

REFERENCES

1. Akizuki M, Powers R, Holman HR: A soluble acidic protein of the cell nucleus which reacts with serum from patients with systemic lupus erythematosus and Sjögren's syndrome. *J Clin Invest* 59:254, 1977.
2. Alexander EL, Hirsch TJ, Arnett FC, et al: Ro (SSA) and La (SSB) antibodies in the clinical spectrum of Sjögren's syndrome. *J Rheumatol* 9:239, 1982.
3. Alspaugh MA, Buchanan WW, Whaley K: Precipitating antibodies to cellular antigens in Sjögren's syndrome, rheumatoid arthritis, and other organ and nonorgan specific diseases. *Ann Rheum Dis* 37:244, 1978.

4. Alspaugh MA, Talal U, Tan EM: Differentiation and characterization of autoantibodies and their antigens in Sjögren's syndrome. *Arthritis Rheum* 19:216, 1976.
5. Alspaugh MA, Tan EM: Antibodies to cellular antigens in Sjögren's syndrome. *J Clin Invest* 55:1067, 1975.
6. Arnett FC, Hirsch TJ, Nishikai M, et al: The Jo_1 antibody system. Clinical and immunogenetic associations in myositis. *J Rheumatol* 8:925, 1981.
7. Barada FA Jr, Andrews BS, Davis JA IV, et al: Antibodies to Sm in patients with systemic lupus erythematosus. *Arthritis Rheum* 24:1236, 1981.
8. Bell DA, Maddison PJ: Serologic subsets in SLE: An examination of autoantibodies in relationship to clinical features of disease and HLA antigens. *Arthritis Rheum* 23:1268, 1980.
9. Bennett RM, Spongo BH: Immune complex nephropathy in mixed connective tissue disease. *Am J Med* 63:534, 1977.
10. Clark G, Reichlin M, Tomasi TB: Characterization of a soluble cytoplasmic antigen reactive with sera from patients with systemic lupus erythematosus. *J Immunol* 102:117, 1968.
11. Douvas AS: Autoantibodies occurring in two different rheumatic diseases react with the same ribonucleoprotein particle. *Proc Natl Acad Sci USA* 79:5401, 1982.
12. Fuller TJ, Richman AV, Auerbach D, et al: Immune complex glomerulonephritis in a patient with mixed connective tissue disease. *Am J Med* 62:761, 1977.
13. Lerner MR, Boyle JA, Hardin JA, et al: Two novel classes of small RNA proteins detected by antibodies associated with lupus erythematosus. *Science* 211:400, 1981.
14. Lerner EA, Lerner MR, Janeway CA Jr, et al: Monoclonal antibodies to nucleic acid-containing cellular constituents: Probes for molecular biology and autoimmune disease. *Proc Natl Acad Sci USA* 78:2737, 1981.
15. Lerner MR, Steitz JA: Antibodies to small nuclear RNAs complexed with proteins are produced by patients with systemic lupus erythematosus. *Proc Natl Acad Sci USA* 76:5495, 1979.
16. Maddison PJ, Mogavero H, Reichlin M: Patterns of clinical disease associated with antibodies to nuclear ribonucleoprotein. *J Rheumatol* 5:407, 1978.
17. Maddison PJ, Provost TT, Reichlin M: ANA-negative SLE. *Medicine* 60:87, 1981.
18. Mattioli M, Reichlin M: Characterization of a soluble nuclear ribonucleoprotein antigen reactive with LE sera. *J Immunol* 197:1281, 1971.
19. Mattioli M, Reichlin M: Heterogeneity of RNA protein antigens reactive with sera of patients with systemic lupus erythematosus. *Arthritis Rheum* 17:421, 1974.
20. Mattioli M, Reichlin M: Physical association of two nuclear antigens and mutual occurrence of their antibodies: The relationship of the Sm and RNA protein (Mo) systems in SLE sera. *J Immunol* 110:1318, 1973.
21. Mimori T, Akizuki M, Yamagata H, et al: Characterization of a high molecular weight acidic nuclear protein recognized by autoantibodies in sera from patients with polymyositis-scleroderma overlap. *J Clin Invest* 68:611, 1981.
22. Nimelstein SH, Brody S, McShane D, et al: Mixed connective tissue disease: A subsequent evaluation of the original 25 patients. *Medicine* 59:239, 1980.
23. Nishikai M, Reichlin M: Heterogeneity of precipitating antibodies in polymyositis and dermatomyositis. Characterization of the Jo_1 antibody system. *Arthritis Rheum* 23:881, 1980.
24. Parker MD: Ribonucleoprotein antibodies: Frequency and clinical significance in systemic lupus erythematosus, scleroderma, and mixed connective tissue disease. *J Lab Clin Med* 82:769, 1973.
25. Powers R, Akizuki M, Boehm-Truitt MJ, et al: Substantial purification of the Sm antigen and association of high titer antibody to Sm with a clinical subset of systemic lupus erythematosus. *Arthritis Rheum* 20:131, 1977 (abstract).
26. Provost TT, Arnett FC, Reichlin M: Homozygous C2 deficiency, lupus erythematosus, and anti-Ro/SSA antibodies. *Arthritis Rheum* 26:1279, 1983.
27. Reichlin M, Maddison PJ, Targoff I, et al: Antibodies to a nuclear/nucleolar antigen in patients with polymyositis overlap syndromes. *J Lab Clin Immunol* 4:40, 1983.
28. Reichlin M, Mattioli M: Antigens and antibodies characteristic of systemic lupus erythematosus. *Bull Rheum Dis* 24:756, 1974.
29. Reichlin M, Mattioli M: Correlation of a precipitin reaction to an RNA protein antigen and a

low prevalence of nephritis in patients with systemic lupus erythematosus. *N Engl J Med* 286:908, 1972.

30. Reichlin M, Mattioli M: Description of a serological reaction characteristic of polymyositis. *Clin Immunol Immunopathol* 5:12, 1976.
31. Scott JS, Maddison PJ, Taylor PV, et al: Connective tissue disease, antibodies to ribonucleoprotein and congenital heart block. *N Engl J Med* 309:209, 1983.
32. Sharp GC, Irvin WS, Ian EM, et al: Mixed connective tissue disease—an apparently distinct rheumatic disease syndrome associated with a specific antibody to an extractable nuclear antigen (ENA). *Am J Med* 52:148, 1972.
33. Sharp GC, Irvin WS, Laroque Velez C, et al: Association of autoantibodies to different nuclear antigens with clinical patterns of rheumatic disease and responsiveness to therapy. *J Clin Invest* 50:350, 1971.
34. Sontheimer RD, Maddison PJ, Reichlin M, et al: Serologic and HLA associations in subacute cutaneous lupus erythematosus, a clinical subset of lupus erythematosus. *Ann Intern Med* 97:664, 1982.
35. Takano M, Agris PF, Sharp GC: Purification and biochemical characterization of nuclear ribonucleoprotein antigen using purified antibody from serum of a patient with mixed connective tissue disease. *J Clin Invest* 65:1449, 1980.
36. Takano M, Golden SS, Sharp GC, et al: Molecular relationship between two nuclear antigens, ribonucleoprotein and Sm: Purification of active antigens and their biochemical characterization. *Biochemistry* 21:5929, 1981.
37. Tan EM, Kunkel HG: Characteristics of a soluble nuclear antigen precipitating with the sera of patients with systemic lupus erythematosus. *J Immunol* 96:464, 1966.
38. Wasicek CA, Reichlin M: Clinical and serological differences between systemic lupus erythematosus patients with antibodies to Ro versus patients with antibodies to Ro and La. *J Clin Invest* 69:385, 1982.
39. Winfield JB, Brunner CM, Koffler D: Serologic studies in patients with systemic lupus erythematosus and central nervous system dysfunction. *Arthritis Rheum* 21:289, 1978.
40. Winn DM, Wolfe JR, Lindberg DA, et al: Identification of a clinical subset of systemic lupus erythematosus by antibodies to the Sm antigen. *Arthritis Rheum* 22:1334, 1979.
41. Wolfe JF, Adelstein E, Sharp GC: Antinuclear antibody with distinct specificity for polymyositis. *J Clin Invest* 59:176, 1977.
42. Yamagata H: The antibodies to the SS-A antigen in patients with connective tissue disease. *Keio Igaku* 58:381, 1981 (in Japanese).

34
Sjögren's Syndrome

Elaine L. Alexander
Rodolfo Molina
Thomas T. Provost

INTRODUCTION

Cutaneous lesions, which are often a reflection of inflammatory vascular disease (IVD), are seen in approximately 25% of patients with primary Sjögren's syndrome (SS) (22). The two most common clinical presentations are palpable purpura, often of the lower extremities, and chronic urticaria (10). Two main histopathologic types of IVD have been observed (10): mononuclear inflammatory vascular disease (MIVD) and neutrophilic inflammatory vascular disease (NIVD), which is indistinguishable from leukocytoclastic vasculitis (LCA). Patients with these two histopathologic forms of vasculitis differ in their seroreactivity with respect to rheumatoid factor and antibodies to Ro (SS-A). SS patients with NIVD are seropositive, while patients with MIVD are generally seronegative (41).

This chapter will stress the importance of the recognition of these SS patients with cutaneous vasculitis, because these patients also frequently develop peripheral and central nervous system dysfunction (5–7,9,11). Furthermore, it is especially important for dermatologists to recognize this group of SS patients, because in our experience the cutaneous vasculitic lesions frequently antedate the onset of nervous system disease.

GLANDULAR FEATURES OF SJÖGREN'S SYNDROME

The first patient with purported primary SS, described by Mikulicz in 1882, was a 42-year-old farmer with bilateral parotid and lacrimal gland enlargement, the pathology of which revealed extensive small cell infiltration of the interstitial connective tissue and atrophy of the acinar parenchyma (40). In 1933, Henrik Sjögren, a Swedish ophthalmologist, described keratoconjunctivitis sicca (KCS) in the clinical setting that was later to bear his name (51).

Patients who are symptomatic for the sicca complex have xerophthalmia ("dry eyes"), xerostomia ("dry mouth"), and often recurrent or persistent salivary gland

This work was supported by U.S Public Health Service grants (R01 AM 25650 and HL 30748) from the National Institutes of Health, by a Kroc Foundation Grant, and by a gift from the Noxell Corporation.

enlargement. Unlike other rheumatic disorders, such as systemic lupus erythematosus (SLE), rheumatoid arthritis (RA), or progressive systemic sclerosis (PSS), there are no established criteria for the diagnosis of SS. Several systems, however, have been proposed (22,50,55,59). The most stringent system requires the presence of both KCS and a positive minor salivary gland biopsy procedure (55), unless there is an associated connective tissue or lymphoproliferative disorder. In our own experience, particularly with the recent advent and use of methycellulose eye drops, a significant number of patients with classic primary SS (including extraglandular features) do not have frank KCS. Furthermore, the severity of systemic manifestations is not correlated with the severity of ocular involvement. Thus, to establish the diagnosis of primary SS, we require the patient to have two of the three following symptoms: xerophthalmia, xerostomia, or recurrent/persistent salivary gland enlargement; additionally, the patient should have either KCS or a positive minor salivary gland biopsy procedure.

SS can occur alone (i.e. primary SS), or in association with another connective tissue disease such as SLE, RA, PSS, or mixed connective tissue disease (MCTD (i.e., secondary SS) (2,3,23,45). The incidence of primary SS is unknown. It is stated that SS is the second most common connective tissue disease (58), with RA being the first. From our experience over the past several years at a tertiary referral center (The Johns Hopkins Medical Institutions), SS is probably at least as common as RA, and it is the most under-recognized rheumatic disorder. In the vast majority of cases, the diagnosis had not been considered or established prior to referral. This experience is very similar to that of others (50,58).

SS, as with other rheumatic disorders, occurs predominantly in women. Although, it is most common in middle-aged and elderly women, this disorder is being recognized increasingly in young women and children. Although, prevalence data are not available, the female-to-male sex ratio appears to be approximately 9:1 (58). Recently, we have described a group of 36 men with primary SS (42). While the clinical manifestations of this group of men were similar to a comparable group of women with primary SS (and included systemic complications such as vasculitis and nervous system disease), the men tended to be seronegative, particularly with respect to rheumatoid factor and antibodies to Ro (SS-A).

Elicitation of the symptoms of the sicca complex requires a specific and detailed review of systems such as those utilized at the National Institutes of Health (44,45). The symptoms can be subtle and are often insidious in development; thus, patients may have come to accept their symptoms as a normal variant. For example, while patients seldom volunteer that their eyes are dry or they cannot cry, they do complain of a foreign body sensation, grittiness, burning, or matting. They may be observed to have blephorospasm and to rub their eyes frequently. Furthermore, not all patients with KCS are symptomatic. In one large study, ocular sicca symptoms were present in only two-thirds to three-quarters of the patients (7).

Xerophthalmia is evaluated by several methods (50,58). The Schirmer's test assesses tear production by measuring the rate of wetting of a piece of filter paper placed under the lower eyelid. Less than 5 mm of filter paper moistening in a 5-minute period is considered abnormal in an anesthetized eye. Tear breakup time less than 30 seconds is abnormal. The rose bengal dye test and/or slit lamp examination is required to establish the presence of KCS. Following installation of the dye, a slit lamp is generally employed to examine the cornea for the characteristic punctate or filamentous keratitic lesions (class III or IV of Holms).

The solicitation of the symptoms of xerostomia also requires careful questioning. It is not adequate to ask the patient if his mouth is dry. Instead, the patient must be queried about how much fluid of what type he or she drinks per day. Do they get up in the night to get a drink of water or do they have a glass of water at their bedside? Do they have difficulty swallowing? Do they wash their food down with liquids? Can they chew and swallow several crackers without drinking fluid? Does the patient suck on ice, hard candy, lozenges, or chew gum frequently? Has the patient experienced an acceleration of dental caries or pyorrhea? Were the teeth extracted at an early age?

The physical examination provides clues to the presence of xerostomia. Absence of or a diminished salivary pool beneath the frenulum of the tongue, stomatitis, chelosis, red tongue, or poor oral hygiene with absent or carious teeth are clues to the diagnosis. A number of diagnostic tests have been proposed to evaluate xerostomia (50,58). Sialography, in which a contrast dye is injected into Stenson's duct, demonstrates a characteristic ectasia of the small salivary ducts in some patients with SS. In addition, 99m Tc scintigrams of the salivary glands show abnormalities of isotope uptake. The most diagnostically specific technique for demonstrating alteration of salivary gland structure in SS, however, is a minor salivary gland biopsy procedure. A biopsy procedure of the major salivary glands (i.e., parotid and/or submandibular) is contraindicated because of potential injury to the facial nerve or fistula formation. An excisional procedure of a major salivary gland is recommended only when a malignancy is suspected. A minor salivary gland procedure, however, is a minor one with a low risk of potential complications. Following local anesthesia, a small incision is made at the inner aspect of the lip proximal to the vermillion border. The minor salivary glands appear as small white lobules that can be excised. Optimally, four individual glands (approximately 4 mm^2 of tissue) should be removed to obtain a representative sample. The small incision can then be closed with an absorbable suture that does not require removal. An ice pack should be placed on the lip to minimize swelling and to promote hemostasis.

Histologically, SS patients demonstrate infiltration of the minor salivary glands with mononuclear cells (predominantly lymphocytes [T cells and foci of B cells] and plasma cells) (1,15). Characteristically, the infiltrate surrounds the salivary gland ducts and extends into the acinar tissue. With severe inflammation, there is a subsequent loss of secretory epithelium and a generalized replacement of the gland with fibrous tissue. The extent of the inflammatory infiltrate can be graded by quantitating the number of focal aggregates containing more than 50 mononuclear cells, and then employing either the Greenspan et al. or Tarplay et al. classifications (class III or IV) (27,57).

SYSTEMIC MANIFESTATIONS OF PRIMARY SJÖGREN'S SYNDROME

During the past 20 years, it has been recognized increasingly that primary SS patients can manifest a spectrum of systemic (extraglandular) manifestations (53,56). In our own experience, we have been impressed by the frequency of IVD (i.e., vasculitis) (7,8,41) and nervous system involvement (5–7,9,11). In this section, we will review the systemic complications of SS and emphasize our recent observations on vasculitis and nervous system disease.

Respiratory System

Dryness of the mucous membranes of the nasopharynx and upper respiratory tract (tracheobronchiolitis) commonly causes a dry nonproductive cough, and predisposes to chronic sinusitis, bronchitis, and pneumonia. Primary involvement of the pulmonary parenchyma is a frequent complication of primary SS. The most common presentation is restrictive pulmonary disease, with decreased helium lung volumes and diffusing capacity associated with interstitial infiltrates on chest radiography (58). These changes are secondary to interstitial pneumonitis and fibrosis. A second, less well recognized form of pulmonary disease in SS is a necrotizing bronchioalveolitis, resulting in obstructive pulmonary disease (47). We have seen several patients in whom the rapid onset of severe obstructive and restrictive pulmonary disease has been either the presenting sign or a major component of primary SS.

Gastrointestinal Disease

A number of reports have been published indicating that acute pancreatitis and chronic relapsing pancreatitis appear to occur with increased frequency in patients with SS. Pancreatic function in SS patients, as measured by impaired volume and bicarbonate responses to secretin and pancreozymin, can be impaired, and serum pancreatic amylase levels may be elevated (58).

There is an increased prevalence of autoimmune liver disease (chronic active hepatitis and primary biliary cirrhosis) in SS patients. Increased levels of antimitochondrial antibodies have been detected among SS patients. One study reports 5 of 80 SS patients had clinical manifestations of primary biliary cirrhosis (50). Conversely, in a series of patients with primary biliary cirrhosis, one-third to one-half had SS. One recent study described classic SS, biliary cirrhosis, and antibodies to Ro (SS-A) (48).

Renal Disease

Several types of renal disease occur in primary SS (58). The most common disorders are defects in renal tubular function resulting in renal tubular acidosis, which may be either overt or subclinical with an inability to excrete an acid urine following a standard acid load. Serious complications of renal tubular acidosis, such as hypokalemia, nephrocalcinosis, and osteomalacia, have been described. A histopathology of the kidneys of patients with SS and renal tubular acidosis demonstrates mononuclear inflammatory interstitial infiltrates.

A second, much less frequent renal complication of SS, is acute or chronic glomerulonephritis. This type of disease process is often associated with the presence of immunoglobulin and complement in the diseased glomeruli demonstrated by immunofluorescence (IF), as well as by the presence of hypocomplementemia. Some of these patients have developed cryoglobulinemia as their glomerulonephritis emerged. Antibodies to Ro(SS-A) have been demonstrated to be enriched in the kidneys of SLE patients with renal vasculitis (35), although their role in pathogenesis is unknown.

Other Extraglandular Features

Another common extraglandular manifestation of SS is a transient, migratory, nonerosive, nondeforming polyarthritis (in contradistinction to the symmetric, additive, erosive, deforming polyarthritis of RA). We have observed several patients, however, with this pattern of polyarthritis for many years who also developed nodules that resembled rheumatoid nodules both clinically and histopathologically.

Inflammatory muscle disease (myositis) is not an uncommon manifestation of SS (25). In addition to the more common proximal myopathy, we have seen several cases with a predominant distal distribution. The disease is often insidious and more chronic than primary polymyositis or dermatomyositis, and it may result in considerable fibrosis. The creatinine phosphokinase (CPK) may be only mildly elevated and, in some cases, normal. Mild focal myopathic changes may be seen in electromyographic studies. A muscle biopsy specimen, however, shows diffuse or focal inflammatory infiltrates and fibrosis. Inclusion bodies may be present. We have been impressed by the number of patients who have concomitant inflammatory vascular disease (predominantly mononulear in histopathologic type) within muscle. These patients also often have simultaneous protean nervous system dysfunction.

Neither the incidence nor frequency of malignant lympho-proliferative disorders in SS is known. A transition from benign polyclonal lymphoid hyperplasia to either malignant lymphoma (usually of the non-Hodgkin's B-cell type) or lymphocarcinoma has been described (16,56,61). Primary SS patients and RA patients with SS have approximately a 43-fold increased risk of developing a malignancy (31).

AUTOIMMUNE ASSOCIATIONS

In the SS patient population, autoimmune thyroid disease is a common association, and it has been reported in 10 to 15% of patients (29). Autoimmune thyroiditis (of the Hashimoto's type) may occur alone or, less commonly, as a sequelae to antecedent hyperthyroidism (Grave's disease). This is another end-organ manifestation of SS that is insidious in onset and, thus, not appreciated by the patient, family, or physician. Frequently, there are anti-thyroid antibodies (antithyroglobulin or antimicrosomal) without overt thyroid dysfunction. There are case reports suggesting an association of SS with myasthenia gravis.

NERVOUS SYSTEM DISEASE

Since our initial report of central nervous system (CNS) involvement in primary SS (5), we have now seen over 50 patients at our institution with primary SS and CNS disease unattributable to other etiologies (i.e., hypertension, atherosclerosis, diabetes mellitus). The spectrum of neurologic dysfunction spans the entire neuroaxis and involves both the brain and spinal cord. The neurologic manifestations of a group of 30 SS patients with active CNS disease are presented in Table 1. The manifestations are often multifocal, and the patients are at risk for multiple events that can occur over time. Focal

Table 1. Neurologic Manifestations of Patients with Central Nervous System (CNS) Sjögren's Syndrome

		No. of patients (%) (N=30)
CNS		30 (100)
Brain[a]		23 (77)
Focal	16	
Diffuse	17	
Spinal cord		11 (37)
Peripheral nervous system		12 (40)

[a]Many patients had more than one neurologic event.

cerebral neurologic dysfunction is common and includes hemipareses, hemisensory deficits, brain stem dysfunction (cerebellar ataxia, internuclear ophthalmoplegia, horizontal jerk nystagmus), seizure disorders (particularly focal motor and temporal lobe), movement disorders (extrapyramidal syndromes, essential tremor, chorea), and optic neuritis.

Diffuse cerebral involvement also has been observed and includes acute encephalopathy and aseptic meningoencephalitis, which are often recurrent. In addition to focal and diffuse neurologic dysfunction, we also have been impressed with the occurrence of significant, progressive cognitive dysfunction in relatively young individuals, and also the frequent occurrence of neuropsychiatric disturbances in patients with primary SS. In a group of 40 SS patients seen by our division and evaluated by a psychiatrist, the majority were felt to have a significant psychiatric disturbances on clinical grounds; many had an abnormal Minnesota multiphasic personality inventory, showing hysteria, psychosomatization, and depression.

Spinal cord involvement is seen in approximately one-third of our patients with CNS involvement. We have observed Brown Sequard syndrome, transverse myelitis (often recurrent), chronic progressive myelopathy, and neurogenic bladder.

Concomitant peripheral nervous system involvement is seen in 40% of SS patients with CNS dysfunction. Manifestations have included sensory and motor polyneuropathies, mononeuritis multiplex, carpal tunnel syndrome, and cranial neuropathies. Previous studies have estimated that approximately 10% of SS patients have a peripheral neuropathy (19), and there may be a predilection for trigeminal neuropathy in SS (28).

Cerebral spinal fluid (CSF) analyses in patients with SS and active CNS disease may provide important clues to disease immunopathogenesis. We initially observed CSF abnormalities in a small group of patients with recurrent aseptic meningoencephalitis (6). These included hypoglycorrachia, mild elevation of protein and IgG concentrations, and increased IgG indices (indicative of intrathecal synthesis of IgG). Agarose gel electrophoresis showed one or more oligoclonal bands that migrated in the region of IgG. CSF pleocytosis was associated with an increased number of plasma cells and lymphoblastoid cells (activated lymphocytes) on cytologic examination.

Subsequently, we have expanded our studies on the CSF to include 30 patients with SS and active CNS disease (SS_A) and 20 SS patients without CNS disease (SS_{IA}). These findings are summarized in Table 2. There was a statistically significant difference between SS_A and SS_{IA} patients with regard to the following parameters: total protein, CSF IgG, CSF/serum IgG, and IgG index. In addition, 25 of 29 (87%) SS_A patients had one or more oligoclonal bands ($p = 0.00001$), which were present in only 3 of 18 (17%) SS_{IA} patients (all of whom had a remote history of CNS involvement). The CSF/serum albumin ratio was normal in all but one patient, indicating the preservation of blood brain barrier integrity. CSF pleocytosis ($p = 0.002$) in SS_A was associated with the presence on cytologic examination of lymphoblastoid (activated lymphocytes) and plasma cells ($p = 0.0001$) in SS_A. Thus, several lines of evidence suggest that intrathecal synthesis of IgG is associated with the entry of immunocompetent cells into the CNS of SS patients with active CNS disease. Furthermore, these studies emphasize that both the clinical presentations and CSF analyses of SS_A patients can closely resemble another autoimmune CNS disorder; that is, multiple sclerosis.

There is a striking association between CNS disease and the presence of concomitant peripheral inflammatory vascular disease. Of 30 SS_A patients, 13 (40%) had biopsy-documented vasculitis (skin, nerve, or muscle). This observation suggests that a similar vasculitic involvement of cerebral blood vessels may be involved in the immunopathogenesis of CNS disease in SS. Other investigators have proposed that vasculitis may play a pathophysiologic role in the peripheral neuropathy seen in association with SS. Kal-

Table 2. Cerebrospinal Fluid (CSF) Analysis in Primary Sjögren's Syndrome

	No. (%) positive		
	SS_A (n = 30)	SS_{IA} (n = 20)	p Value[a]
Total protein (>45 mg/dl)	16 (53)	1 (5)	0.001
CSF IgG (>6 mg/dl)	13 (43)	2 (10)	0.005
CSF IgG (>14%) serum	11 (37)	2 (10)	0.04
IgG index (≥0.7)	21 (70)	4 (20)	0.004
Oligoclonal banding	25/29 (87)	3/18 (17)	0.00001
CSF Albumin (>10 × 10^3) serum	1	0	NS
Pleocytosis (>5 cells/mm^3)	15 (50)	1 (5)	0.002
Cytology (Plasma and lymphoblastoid cells)	18 (60)	0/19 (—)	0.0001

[a]Fisher's exact two-tailed test.
SS_A, Sjögren's syndrome with active CNS disease.
SS_{IA}, Sjögren's syndrome with inactive CNS disease.
NS = Not significant

treider and Talal (28) reported that of 10 patients with peripheral neuropathy, 9 had biopsy-documented vasculitis. One of these patients had seizures, and on autopsy examination had diffuse cerebral vasculitis.

Over the last several years, we have gained considerable experience regarding the treatment of patients with SS who have CNS involvement. Initially, we were cautious about recommending immunosuppressive therapy, because at least some patients we first evaluated had transient, reversible neurologic deficits. With increasing experience, however, our views have been modified. Neurologic deficits tended to recur over time and often progressed. In some cases, previously transient deficits eventually became fixed. Most patients responded clinically to moderate-dose corticosteroid therapy, with a complete or partial inprovement in neurologic dysfunction. Several patients required the addition of an immunosuppressive agent (cyclophosphamide) for stabilization of neurologic dysfunction.

We are beginning to accumulate data suggesting that CSF analyses may be helpful in managing patients with SS. Fourteen SS patients had more than one CSF analysis. Of 10 patients treated with corticosteroids, all had a decrease in IgG index. Five of nine of these patients also had a decrease in the number of oligoclonal bands; in the remainder, the intensity of band (s) decreased. One such patient initially had five oligoclonal bands; on subsequent analysis, the number of bands decreased to four and then to three. This is unlike the case in multiple sclerosis, where the oligoclonal banding pattern is not altered with therapy. We now recommend a course of moderate-dose corticosteroid therapy for major neurologic dysfunction, and suggest that CSF parameters (particularly the IgG index and oligoclonal banding pattern) be monitored serially. If disease is not stabilized, the addition of an immunosuppressive agent is recommended.

CUTANEOUS INFLAMMATORY VASCULAR DISEASE

Cutaneous vasculitis is a frequent complication of SS. We recently have analyzed 45 patients with SS with biopsy-documented vasculitis, 41 of whom had cutaneous lesions

Table 3. Cutaneous Manifestations of Sjögren's Syndrome Patients with Inflammatory Vascular Disease of Two Histopathologic Prototypes

	No. of patients (%)		
Cutaneous manifestations	*NIVD (n = 25)*	*MIVD (n = 16)*	*Total (n = 41)*
Purpura	12 (48)	4 (25)	16 (39)
Urticaria	7 (28)	4 (25)	11 (27)
Erythematous lesions	4 (16)	7 (44)	11 (27)
Subcutaneous nodules	2 (8)	1 (6)	3 (7)

NIVD, Neutrophilic inflammatory vascular disease.
MIVD, Mononuclear inflammatory vascular disease.

(Table 3). The common cutaneous manifestations are palpable purpura (usually lower extremity), urticaria (chronic), erythema multiforme, erythema nodosum, and diffuse erythematous macules.

Benign hypergammaglobulinemic purpura of Waldenström has been observed previously by several authors to occur in a minority of patients with SS (32,54,59). It has been estimated that 20 to 30% of patients with benign hypergammaglobulinemic purpura will subsequently develop SS (55).

Our studies also indicate that purpuric lesions of the lower extremities in SS are sometimes accompanied by the presence of a mixed cryoglobulinemia. Based upon our preliminary observations, we believe that unrecognized SS patients composed a significant proportion of the patients previously described by Meltzer and Franklin as having mixed cryoglobulinemia (38,39).

Two main histopathologic types of IVD have been observed: neutrophilic (NIVD) and mononuclear (predominantly lymphocytic) (MIVD). Clinically, one cannot distinguish the histopathologic type from the appearance of the gross cutaneous lesion (i.e., both purpuric and urticarial lesions may be secondary to either NIVD or MIVD). Phenotypically, the clinical expression of these two distinct inflammatory vasculopathies appears to be an ischemic process leading, in extreme forms, to ulceration and, in its more benign forms, to purpura or urticaria (Figures 1 and 2).

The two histopathologic forms of IVD are associated with different serologic profiles (Table 4) (41). Patients with NIVD tend to be seropositive for hyperglobulinemia (p = 0.01), rheumatoid factor (p = 0.002), and antibodies to Ro (SS-A) (p = 0.00006). In contrast, patients with MIVD tend to be seronegative. Sixteen (60%) of 27 patients with NIVD had both rheumatoid factor and antibodies to Ro (SS-A), while none with MIVD had these autoantibodies (p = 0.000016). In addition, when hypocomplementemia was present in one SS patient population, it was observed almost exclusively in NIVD, rather than MIVD (Table 4).

The role of circulating immune complexes in the development of vasculitis in SS is not known. As in other studies of cutaneous vasculitis (34), immunoglobulin and complement deposition have been observed by IF in only a minority of our SS patients, suggesting possible alternative mechanisms of vascular injury.

Patients with NIVD had significantly lower mean total hemolytic complement (CH50) levels (25.2 ± 11.6 units) than patients with MIVD (33.4 ± 10.1 units) p =0.03, 2-tailed test (Table 4). The proportion of NIVD patients with abnormal values (12/24 [50%]) was also higher than for MIVD patients (2/16 [13%]) (p = 0.03, Fisher's exact p

Table 4. Inflammatory Vascular Disease in Sjögren's Syndrome Serologic/Histopathologic Correlates

	No. patients (%) (n = 45)			
	Glob[a]	*RF*[b]	*Ro (SS-A)/LA (SS-B)*[c]	*Hypocomplementemia*[d]
NIVD[e] (*n* = 27)	14 (52)	18 (67)	20 (74)/12 (44)	12/24 (50)
MIVD[f] (*n = 18)*	2 (11)	3 (17)	2 (11)/2 (11)	2/16 (13)
p value	0.01	0.002	0.00006/0.036	0.03

[a]Glob, Serum globulin concentrations > 4 g/dl.
[b]RF, Rheumatoid factor by latex fixation ≥ 1:80.
[c]Antibodies to Ro (SS-A) and La (SS-B).
[d]CH_{50} < 25 units.
[e]NIVD, Neutrophilic inflammatory vascular disease.
[f]MIVD, Mononuclear inflammatory vascular disease.
p Value obtained by using the two-tailed Fisher's exact text.

value). There were no differences between the two groups in the mean C3 or C4 concentrations (C3:NIVD [110.6 ± 51.6 mg/dl], MIVD [122.8 ± 49.1 mg/dl]; C4:NIVD [22.1 ± 15.7 mg/dl] MIVD [23.6 ± 10.2 mg/dl]), nor in the proportion of individuals with abnormal values (C3:NIVD, 6/23 [26%]; MIVD, 2/23 [9%]; C4:NIVD, 12/23 [53%]; MIVD, 8/23 [35%]. Of the 13 patients with decreased CH50 levels who also had C3 and C4 determinations, 11 (85%) had decreased C4 and 8 (62%) had decreased C3.

Evidence for two histopathologic types of cutaneous vasculitis has been presented by others. Soter et al., (52) in a series of 14 patients with necrotizing vasculitis, described four SS patients with lower extremity palpable purpura. Likewise, urticaria-like lesions have been associated with both types of histopathology. (43).

The following case is an example of a patient with SS in whom urticaria-like vasculitic lesions and progressive pulmonary disease were prominent features. The patient was a 50-year-old white woman who 1 year prior to evaluation noted the development of nonpruritic, urticaria-like lesions involving the trunk and extremities that persisted for days. A biopsy specimen of an urticaria-like lesion revealed (NIVD). Serologic evaluation showed hypergammaglobulinemia, a significantly elevated rheumatoid factor titer, antibodies to Ro (SS-A), and hypocomplementemia. A presumptive diagnosis of hypocomplementemic, urticaria-like vasculitis was made.

Concomitantly, the patient, who had never smoked or been exposed to environmental toxins, developed severe dyspnea on exertion and a rapidly progressive decline in pulmonary function (both restrictive and obstructive defects). An open lung biopsy procedure demonstrated interstitial inflammatory infiltrates composed predominantly of mononuclear cells (lymphocytes and plasma cells), and patchy interstitial fibrosis. In addition, an intense mononuclear infiltrate surrounded the terminal bronchi. Because of the severe, rapidly progressive pulmonary disease, the patient was treated with cyclophosphamide (1.5 mg/kg). On this regimen, the urticaria-like lesions of vasculitis disappeared and the pulmonary function tests stabilized. Therapy was continued for 18 months. Two years following the gradual withdrawal of therapy, there is no evidence of vasculitis or the progression of pulmonary disease as judged by serial pulmonary func-

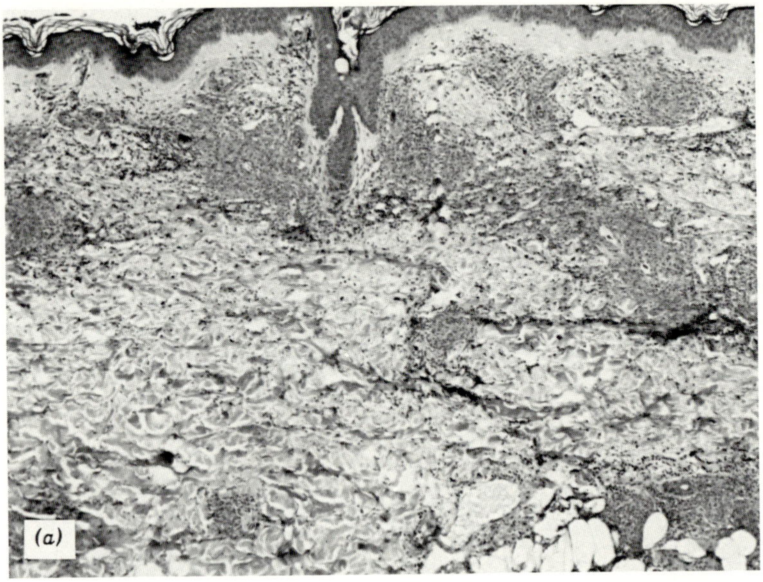

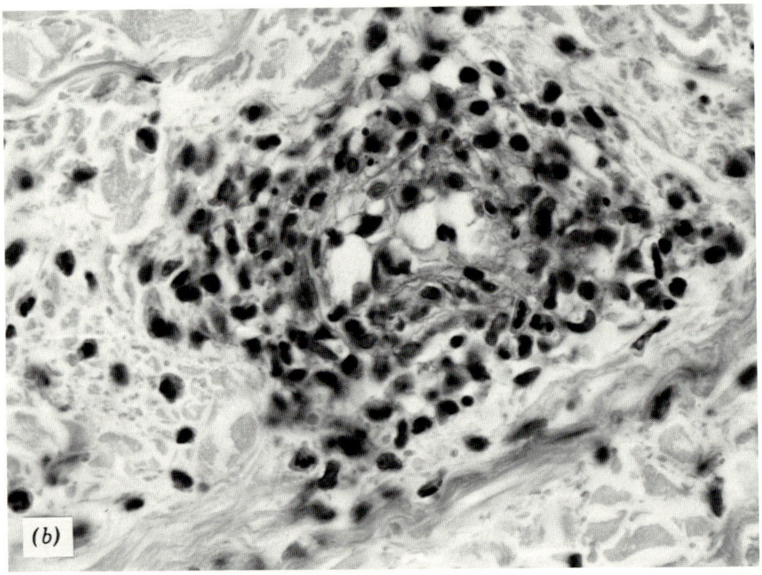

Figure 1. A. Skin biopsy specimen from a patient with cutaneous vasculitis. The papillary and reticular dermis are infiltrated by inflammatory cells that surround and, in some cases, invade vessel walls (60X). B and C. NIVD (mild and more severe) in patients with lower extremity papable purpura and hyperglobulinemia B., 340X; C., 325X). D. Mononuclear infiltrate in a patient with lower extremity palpable purpura and hyperglobulinemia (425X).

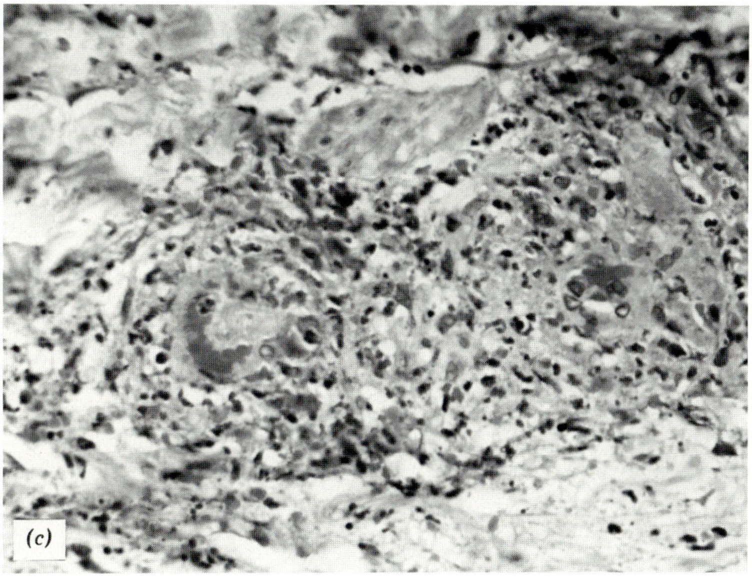

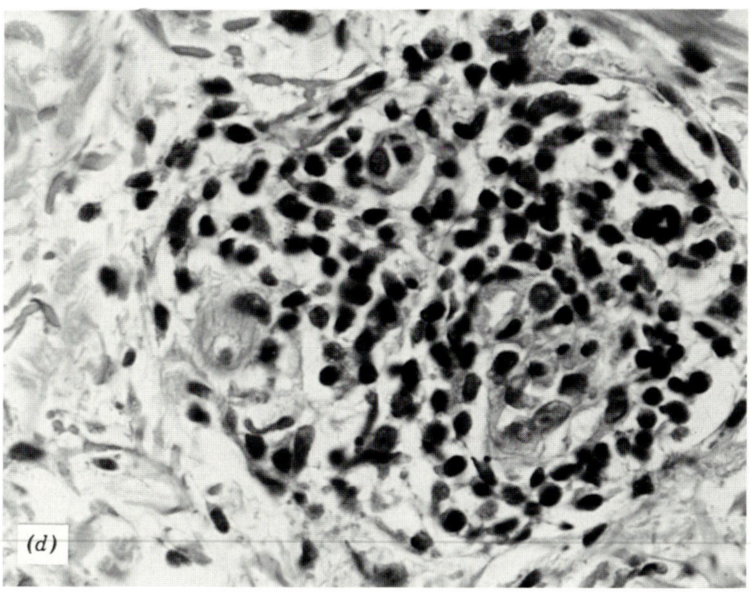

tion tests. The patient, however, continues to demonstrate the presence of the Ro (SS-A) antibody.

This case illustrates several features of primary SS. Extraglandular manifestations (in this case, interstitial fibrosis and urticaria-like vasculitic lesions) may antedate the diagnosis of SS. In this case, the diagnosis of SS was not considered and established until the

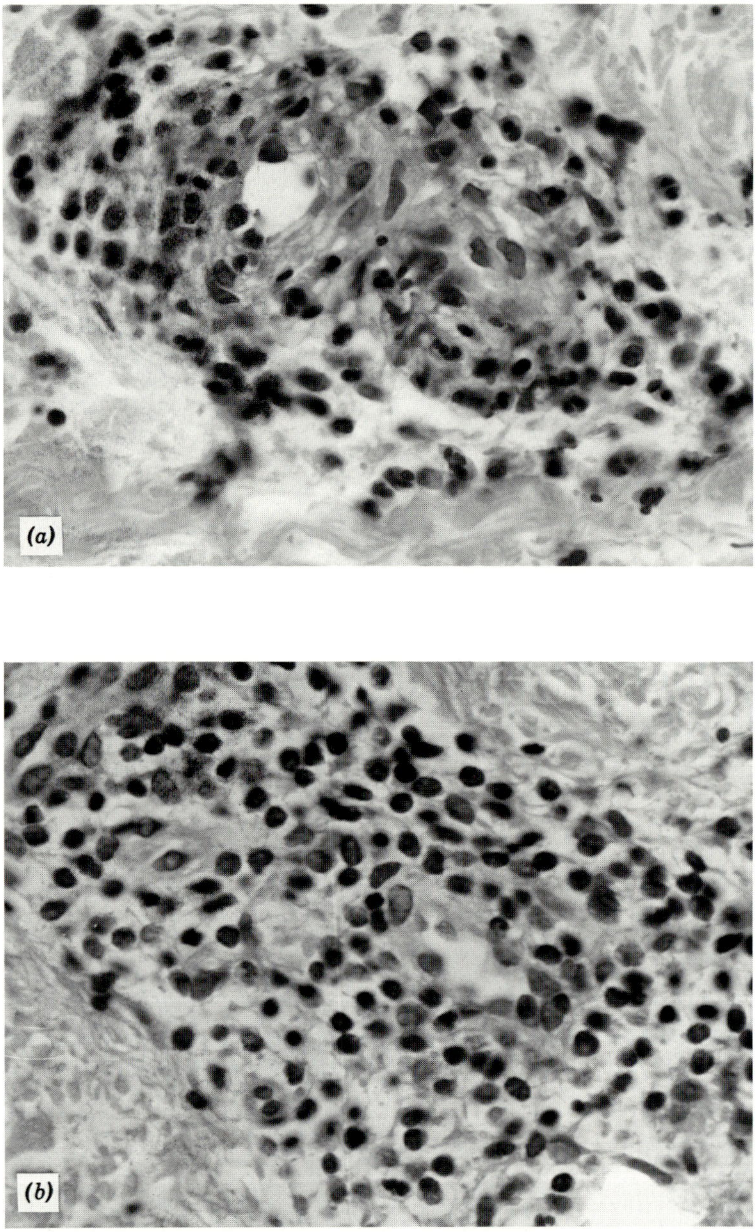

Figure 2. A. NIVD with chronic urticaria and hypocomplementemia (650X.) B. MIVD in a patient with chronic urticaria and normocomplementemia (600X). C. MIVD in a patient with indurated erythematous skin lesions (115X). D. Necrotizing panniculitis and NIVD in a patient with erythema nodosum (300X).

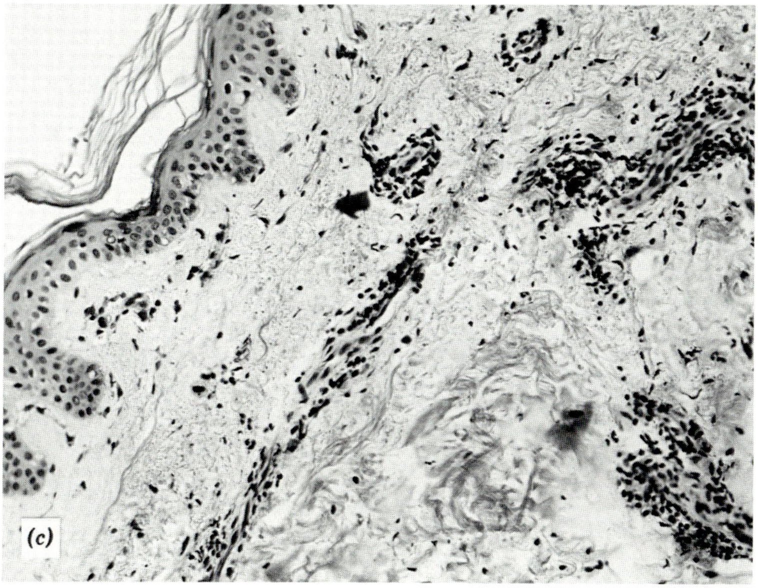

(c)

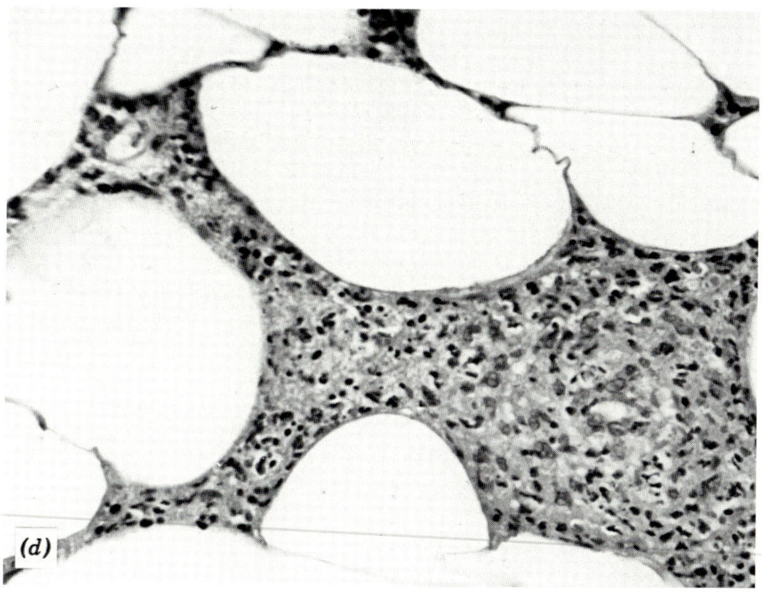

(d)

lung biopsy specimen demonstrated the characteristic peribronchiolar and interstitial mononuclear infiltrates often associated with SS (47), and the serologic studies suggested the presence of an underlying connective tissue disease. In retrospect, the patient had xerophthalmia and xerostomia for many years.

SEROLOGIC FEATURES IN SJÖGREN'S SYNDROME

A variety of different autoantibodies have been found to occur in SS. These include IgM and IgG rheumatoid factors, antinuclear antibodies (ANA), and antibodies to smooth muscle, mitochondria, salivary gland duct, thyroglobulin, microsomes, and parietal cells. In addition, serum immune complexes have been detected by the Raji and Clq ginding assays and, although occurring in the presence of IgG rheumatoid factor, they do not possess rheumatoid factor activity (26,33).

Precipitin antibodies are frequently detected in patients with SS. Anderson et al., in 1961, described precipitating antibodies in 31% (9/29) of patients with SS (17). Two distinct autoantibodies were demonstrated. They were designated SjD (SS reference serum patient DON) and SjT (SS reference serum patient TRA). Subsequent examinations revealed that 13 of 42 (31%) patients with SS possessed SjD antibodies and 8 (19%) had SjT antibodies (18,20).

Subsequently, Clark et al. (24) and Mattioli and Reichlin (37) described antibodies against the cytoplasmic macromolecule termed Ro and La (each after the surname of the patient in whom these antibodies were first described). The Ro antibody system has been shown to be identical to the SS-A antibody system described by Alspaugh et al. (13,14), and La is identical to the SS-B and Ha antibody systems (30). It is highly likely, although unproven, that the SjD antibody system described by Anderson et al. (17), is identical to the Ro (SS-A) antibody system, and that the SjT antibody is identical to the La (SS-B, Ha) antibody.

The Ro (SS-A) and La (SS-B) autoantibodies occur frequently in SS (7,12,36,60). The Ro (SS-A) antibody, detected by gel double diffusion, occurs in approximately 40 to 47% of patients with SS. The La (SS-B) antibody prevalence is much more variable, being reported in 10 to 80% of patients (7,30,44). It has recently been reported by some observers that these antibody systems occur almost exclusively in patients with SS alone. These observations led to the suggestion that these autoantibodies were diagnostic markers that would effectively serve to differentiate SS alone from SS accompanying RA. Our studies, however, have definitely established that these autoantibodies occur in all forms of SS; that is, primary SS and SS accompanying other rheumatic diseases such as SLE, RA, PSS, and dermatomyositis (Table 5) (7,8).

Our studies, however, have demonstrated that the Ro-positive SS patients, in sharp contrast to the Ro-negative SS patients, have a statistically significant increased preva-

Table 5. Autoantibodies to Ro (SS-A) and La (SS-B) in Various Clinical Groups of Sjögren's Syndrome

Group	*No.*	*Ro (SSA)*	*La (SSB)*
SS	30	15 (50%)	7 (23%)
SS_{RA}	18	7 (39%)	1 (6%)
SS_{SLE}	12	7 (58%)	2 (17%)
SS_{PSS}	10	2 (20%)	0 (—)
SS_{CTD}	5	2 (40%)	2 (40%)
Totai	75	33 (44%)	12 (16%)

From Alexander et al. (8).

RA, Rheumatoid arthritis; SLE, Systemic lupus erythematosus;

PSS, progressive systemic sclerosis; CTD, other connective tissue disease (overlap or undifferentiated syndromes).

Table 6. Sjögren's Syndrome Patients: Clinical and Laboratory Association with Antibodies to Ro (SS-A)

	No. of patients		
Feature	*Ro-(SS-A) positive (n = 33)*	*Ro-(SS-A) negative (n = 42)*	*p* Value
Clinical			
Vasculitis	24	4	0.0005
Salivary gland enlargement	26	15	0.0005
Lymphadenopathy	19	4	0.0005
Purpura	12	1	0.0005
Hematologic			
Anemia	19	6	0.0005
Leukopenia	14	3	0.001
Thrombocytopenia	7	1	0.025
Serologic			
Hypergammaglobulinemia	21	8	0.0005
Rheumatoid factor	29	17	0.0005
Antinuclear antibody	31	10	0.0005
Cryoglobulinemia	7/13	0/22	0.001
Hypocomplementemia	11	2	0.005

From Alexander et al. (7).

lence of vasculitis, salivary gland enlargement, lymphadenopathy, and purpura (Table 6) (7,8). In addition, these Ro-positive patients have a statistically significant increased prevalence of cytopenia. Serologically, the Ro-positive SS patients, in sharp contrast to the Ro-negative patients, demonstrated hypergammaglobulinemia, rheumatoid factor activity, antinuclear antibodies, cryoglobulinemia, and hypocomplementemia.

Thus, the presence of the Ro (SS-A) antibody appears to define a subset of patients with SS who have systemic clinical manifestations, including NIVD, hematologic abnormalities, and serologic hyper-reactivity. In addition, the Ro-positive patients in our study closely resemble those SS patients, classified clinically by Strand and Talal (53), as having extraglandular complications. The features of our Ro-positive patients with vasculitis are similar to SS patients with extraglandular manifestations (lymphadenopathy, purpura, leukopenia, and vasculitis) who may develop lymphoid neoplasms (16,56,61). In a study by Talal et al. (56), 54% of their SS patients with extraglandular manifestations and a lymphoproliferative disease had vasculitis, while only 22% of the SS patients without lymphoproliferative disease had vasculitis. Thus far, six of our SS patients have developed lymphoproliferative disorders (angioimmunoblastic lymphadenopathy with dysproteinemia or lymphoma). We believe, based on our data and that of Talal et al. (56,61), that our Ro-positive patients with vasculitis are the SS patients who may be at risk for developing malignant, predominantly B-cell lymphoproliferative disorders.

HLA STUDIES IN SJÖGREN'S SYNDROME

HLA-DW3 (DR3) has been reported in increased frequency (compared with race-matched controls) in primary but not secondary SS (46,60). Another B-cell alloantigen,

MT_2 (HLA-DRw52) (49), however, has been observed in increased frequency in both primary as well as secondary SS (46,60). A correlation between HLA-DW (DR) specificities and autoantibody expression has been observed in connective tissue disease (4,21). HLA-DR3 has been associated with the presence of antibodies to Ro (SS-A) in patients with SLE (4). A similar association has been reported recently in patients with SS (60). Among HLA-DR3-negative SS patients, HLA-DR2 also correlated with the presence of anti-Ro (SS-A) antibodies. Thus, the expression of autoantibodies to Ro (SS-A) is strongly linked to the B-cell alloantigens HLA-DR2 and HLA-DR3.

In summary, these studies suggest that HLA-DRw52 is the strongest MHC determinant associated with either primary or secondary SS, and that HLA-DR2/DR3 may, in part, be playing roles as permissive antigens for modulation of immunoreactivity.

REFERENCES

1. Adamson TC, Fox R, Frisman DM, et al: Immunohistologic analysis of lymphoid infiltrates in primary Sjögren's syndrome using monoclonal antibodies. *J Immunol* 130:203–208, 1983.
2. Alarcon-Segovia D: Symptomatic Sjögren's syndrome of mixed connective tissue disease. *J Rheum* 3:191–195, 1976.
3. Alarcon-Segovia D, Ibanz G, Velazquez-Forero F, et al: Sjögren's syndrome in systemic lupus erythematosus: Clinical and sub-clinical manifestations. *Ann Intern Med* 80:577–583, 1974.
4. Ahearn JM, Provost TT, Dorsch CA, et al: Interrelationship of HLA-DR, MB and MT phenotypes. Autoantibody expression and clinical features in systemic lupus erythematosus (SLE). *Arthritis Rheum* 25:1031–1040, 1982.
5. Alexander GE, Provost TT, Stevens MB, et al: Sjögren's syndrome: Central nervous system manifestations. *Neurology* 31:1391–1396, 1981.
6. Alexander EL, Alexander GE: Aseptic mengoencephalitis in primary Sjögren's syndrome. *Neurology* 43:593–598, 1983.
7. Alexander EL, Arnett FC, Provost TT, et al: Sjögren's syndrome: Association of Anti-Ro(SSA) antibodies with vasculitis, immunologic abnormalities, and serologic hyperreactivity. *Ann Intern Med* 98:155–159, 1983.
8. Alexander EL, Hirsch TJ, Arnett FC, et al: Ro(SSA) and LA(SSB) antibodies in the clinical spectrum of Sjögren's syndrome. *J Rheum* 9:239–246, 1982.
9. Alexander EL, Kraft C, Dorsch CA, et al: Necrotizing arteritis and spinal subarachnoid hemorrhage in Sjögren's syndrome. *Ann Neurol* 11:632–635, 1982.
10. Alexander EL, Provost TT: Cutaneous manifestations of primary Sjögren's syndrome: A reflection of vasculitis and association with anti-Ro(SSA) antibodies. *J Inv Dermatol* 80:386–391, 1983.
11. Alexander EL, Provost TT, Stevens MB, et al: Neurologic complications of primary Sjögren's syndrome. *Medicine* 61:247–257, 1981.
12. Alspaugh MA, Buchanan WW, Whaley K: Precipitating antibodies to cellular antigens in Sjögren's syndrome, rheumatoid arthritis and other organ and non-organ specific autoimmune diseases. *Ann Rheum Dis* 37:244–246, 1978.
13. Alspaugh MA, Maddison P.: Resolution of the identity of certain antigen antibody systems in systemic lupus erythematosus and Sjögren's syndrome: An interlaboratory collaboration. *Arthritis Rheum* 22:796–798, 1979.
14. Alspaugh MA, Talal N, Tan EM: Differentiation and characterization of autoantibodies and their antigens in Sjögren's syndrome. *Arthritis Rheum* 19:216–222, 1976.
15. Anderson LG, Cummings NA, Asofsky R, et al: Salivary gland immunoglobulin and rheumatoid factor synthesis in Sjögren's syndrome: Natural history and response to treatment. *Am J Med* 53:456–463, 1972.
16. Anderson LG, Talal N: The spectrum of benign malignant lymphoproliferation in Sjögren's syndrome. *Clin Exp Immunol* 9:199–221, 1971.
17. Anderson JR, Gray KG, Beck JS: Precipitating autoantibodies in Sjögren's syndrome. *Lancet* II:456–458, 1961.

18. Anderson JR, Gray KG, Beck JS: Precipitating autoantibodies in the connective tissue diseases. *Ann Rheum Dis* 21:316–372, 1962.
19. Attwood W, Poser CN: Neurologic complications of Sjögren's syndrome. *Neurology* (*Mineap*) 11:1034–1041, 1961.
20. Beck JS, Anderson JR, Lock KJ: Antinuclear and precipitating autoantibodies in Sjögren's syndrome. *Ann Rheum Dis* 24:16–32, 1965.
21. Bell DA, Maddison PJ: Serologic subsets in systemic lupus erythematosus: An examination of autoantibodies in relationship to clinical features of disease and HLA antigen. *Arthritis Rheum* 23:1268–1273, 1980.
22. Bloch KJ, Buchanan WW, Wohl MJ, et al: Sjögren's syndrome: A clinical pathological and serological study of 62 cases. *Medicine* 44:187–231, 1965.
23. Cipoletti JF, Buckingham RB, Barnes EL, et al: Sjögren's syndrome and progressive systemic sclerosis. *Ann Intern Med* 87:535–541, 1977.
24. Clark G, Reichlin M, Tomasi TB: Characterization of a soluble cytoplasmic antigen reactive with sera from patients with systemic lupus erythematosus. *J Immunol* 102:117–121, 1969.
25. Denko CW, Old JW: Myopathy in the sicca syndrome (Sjögren's syndrome). *Am J Clin Pathol* 51:631–637, 1969.
26. Fischbach M, Char D, Christensen M, et al: Immune complexes in Sjögren's syndrome. *Arthritis Rheum* 23:791–795, 1980.
27. Greenspan JS, Daniels TE, Talal N, et al: Histopathology of Sjögren's syndrome and labial salivary gland biopsies. *Oral Pathol* 37:217–221, 1974.
28. Kaltreider HB, Talal, N: The neuropathy of Sjögren's syndrome: Trigemo nerve involvement *Ann Intern Med* 70:751–761, 1969.
29. Karsh J, Pavlides N, Weintraub BD, et al: Thyroid disease in Sjögren's syndrome. *Arthritis Rheum* 23:1326–1329, 1980.
30. Kassan SS, Akizuki M, Steinberg AD, et al: Antibody to a soluble acidic nuclear antigen in Sjögren's syndrome. *Am J Med* 63:328–335, 1977.
31. Kassan SL, Terry TL, Moutsopoulos HM, et al: Increased risk of lymphoma in sicca syndrome. *Ann Intern Med* 89:888–892, 1978.
32. Kyle RA, Gleich GA, Bayrd ED, et al: Benign hypergammaglobulinemic purpura of Waldenstrom. *Medicine* 50:113–123, 1971.
33. Lawley TJ, Moutsopoulos HM, Katz SI; Demonstration of circulating immune complexes in Sjögren's syndrome. *J Immunol* 123:1382–1387, 1979.
34. Mackel SE, Tappeiner G, Brumfield H, et al: Circulating immune complexes in cutaneous vasculitis: Vasculitis detection with Clq and monoclonal rheumatoid factor. *J Clin Invest* 64:1652–1660, 1979.
35. Maddison PJ, Reichlin M: Deposition of autoantibodies to a soluble cytoplamic antigen in the kidneys of patients with systemic lupus erythematosus. *Archritis Rheum* 22:858–862, 1979.
36. Martinez-Lavin M, Vaughan JH, Tan EM: Autoantibodies and the spectrum of Sjögren's syndrome. *Ann Intern Med* 91:185–190, 1979.
37. Mattioli M, Reichlin M: Heterogeneity of RNA protein antigens reactive with sera of patients with systemic lupus erythematosus. Description of a cytoplasmic, Non-ribosomal antigen. *Arthritis Rheum* 17:421–425, 1974.
38. Meltzer M. Franklin EC: Cryoglobulinemia—a study of twenty-nine patients: I. IgG and IgM cryoglobulins and factors affecting cryo precipitability. *Am J Med* 40:828, 1966.
39. Meltzer M, et al: Cryogloblinemia—a clinical and laboratory study II: Cryoglobulins with rheumatoid factor activity. *Am J Med* 40:837, 1966.
40. Mikulicz J: Discussion at Verein for Wissenschaftliche Heilkunde zu Kongaberg. *Berl Klin Wchschr* 25:759, 1888.
41. Molina R, Provost TT, Alexander EL: Two histopathologic types of inflammatory vascular disease (IVD) in Sjögren's syndrome (SS): Differential association with seroreactivity to rheumatoid factor (RF) and antibodies to Ro (SS-A). *J Invest Dermatol* 82:428, 1984.
42. Molina R, Provost TT, Alexander EL: Sjögren's syndrome in men. *Arthritis Rheum* 26 (suppl):832, 1983.
43. Monroe EW, Schulz CI, Maize JC, et al: Vasculitis in chronic urticaria: An immunopathologic study. *J Invest Dermatol* 76:103–107, 1981.

44. Moutsopoulos HM, Chused TM, Mann DE, et al: Sjögren's syndrome (sicca syndrome): Current Issues. *Ann Intern Med* 92:212–226, 1980.
45. Moutsopoulos HM, Klippel JH, Pavlidis N, et al: Correlative histologic and serologic findings of sicca syndrome in patients with systemic lupus erythematosus. *Arthritis Rheum* 23:36–40, 1980.
46. Moutsopoulos HM, Mann EL, Johnson AH, et al: Genetic differences between primary and secondary sicca syndrome. *N Engl J Med* 301:761–763, 1979.
47. Newball HH, Brahim SA: Chronic obstructive airway disease in patients with Sjögren's syndrome. *Am Rev Resp Dis* 115:295–304, 1977.
48. Penner E, Reichlin M: Primary biliary cirrhosis associated with Sjögren's syndrome: Evidence for circulating and tissue deposited Ro/anti-Ro immune complexes. *Arthritis Rheum* 25:1250–1253, 1982.
49. Reinersten GL, Klippel JH, Johnson AH, et al: B lymphocyte alloantigens associated with systemic lupus erythematosus. *N Engl J Med* 299:515–518, 1978.
50. Shearn M: *Sjögren's Syndrome.* Saunders, Philadelphia, 1971.
51. Sjögren H: Zur Kenntnis Derm Keratoconjunctivitis Sicca (keratitis filiformis bei hypunfunktion der tranendrusen). *Acta Ophthalmol* 11:1–151, 1933.
52. Soter NA, Mihm MC, Gigli I, et al: Two distinct cellular patterns in cutaneous necrotizing angiitis. *J Invest Dermatol* 66:344–350, 1976.
53. Strand V, Talal N: Advances in the diagnosis and concept of Sjögren's syndrome (Autoimmune Exocrinopathy). *Bull Rheum Dis* 30:1046–1052, 1980.
54. Strauss WG: Purpura hyperglobulinemia of Waldenstrom. *N Engl J Med* 260:857–860, 1959.
55. Talal N: Sjögren's syndrome. *Bull Rheum Dis* 16:404–407, 1966.
56. Talal N, Sokoloff L, Barth WF: Extrasalivary lymphoid abnormalities in Sjögren's syndrome (reticulum cell sarcoma, psuedolymphoma, macroglobulinemia). *Am J Med* 43:50–63, 1967
57. Tarpley TM, Anderson LG, White CL: Minor salivary gland involvement and Sjögren's. *Oral Surg* 37:64–74, 1974.
58. Whaley K, Buchanan WW: Sjögren's syndrome and associated diseases. In Parker C (Ed): *Clinical Immunology,* vol. 1. Saunders, Philadelphia, 1980, pp 632–666.
59. Whaley K, Webb J, McAvoy BA, et al: Sjögren's Syndrome II. Clinical associations and immunological phenomena. *Quart J Med* 42:513–548, 1973.
60. Wilson RW, Provost TT, Bias WB, et al: Sjögren's Syndrome: Influence of multiple HLA D-region alloantigens on clinical and serologic expressions. *Arthr Rheum* 27: 1245–1253, 1984.
61. Zulman J, Jaffe R, Talal N: Evidence that the monoclonal lymphoma of Sjögren's syndrome is a monoclonal B-cell neoplasm. *N Engl J Med* 299:1215–1220, 1978.

35
Neonatal Lupus Erythematosus

Rosemarie M. Watson
Thomas T. Provost

INTRODUCTION

An inflammatory disorder manifesting the clinical, serologic, and histologic features of lupus erythematosus (LE) has recently been reported with increased frequency in newborns. This syndrome, called neonatal lupus erythematosus (NLE), was originally described by McCuistion and Schoch in 1954 (32). These investigators described a 6-week-old boy who, at birth, demonstrated on the scalp and face discrete erythematous macules varying from 0.5 to 3.0 cm in diameter. Scaling, follicular plugging, and atrophy were present. Histologic examination revealed typical features of LE. The dermatitis disappeared by 5 months of age, leaving a trace of atrophy at sites of previous involvement. The mother was asymptomatic during the pregnancy, but subsequently developed systemic lupus erythematosus (SLE) 11 months postpartum.

This case illustrates well the dynamic nature of the cutaneous lesions in NLE, and is similar to the subsequent reports of NLE.

In addition to cutaneous lesions, it is now evident that complete heart block (60) is a major clinical feature of the NLE syndrome. NLE infants also frequently show manifestations of systemic disease, specifically hepatosplenomegaly, lymphadenopathy, pneumonitis, leukopenia, thrombocytopenia, and a Coombs positive hemolytic anemia. These systemic features, however, are mild, and these infants generally do not satisfy the American Rheumatism Association's criteria for the diagnosis of SLE.

Approximately 100 cases of NLE presenting with prominent cutaneous features have been documented. Only 21 of these infants and their mothers, however, have thorough serologic evaluation (reported herein). This entity is most certainly under-recognized for several reasons: 1) The transient nature of the skin lesions in the neonate, especially in the absence of maternal disease, often precludes histologic investigation of the infant's lesions; 2) the fact that cardiac conduction defects are an integral and often sole manifestation of NLE has only recently been described; and, 3) the Ro(SSA) antibodies, the

This work was supported by U.S Public Health Service grants R01 AM28412, R01 AM25650, K04 AM00524, and T32 AM07324 from the National Institutes of Health, and by a gift from the Noxell Corporation.

most valuable and often the only serologic finding are not detected by routine fluorescent antinuclear antibody (ANA) analysis, and may thus go unrecognized.

As with adult SLE, NLE has demonstrated a propensity for clinical heterogeneity, allowing for classification into two distinct clinical subgroups. These include neonatal infants with:

1. Lupus skin lesions with or without other manifestations (noncardiac).
2. Cardiac conduction defects with or without cutaneous lesions.

CLINICAL FEATURES

Previous reports suggested a greater incidence of NLE among females. A preponderance of females was more noticeable in those infants with cutaneous disease than in those with congenital heart block (CHB). However, when the cases from our own series (males, seven; females, three) are added to those NLE patients recently reported, no sexual predominance is noted (57).

Cutaneous Lesions

The lupus lesions most frequently occur on the head or scalp, with a predilection for the periorbital region (Fig. 1). These lesions have also been described on the ears, neck, trunk, buttocks, and limbs, but generally remain confined to light-exposed areas. Characteristic lesions appear as circumscribed, annular, erythematous macules or plaques,

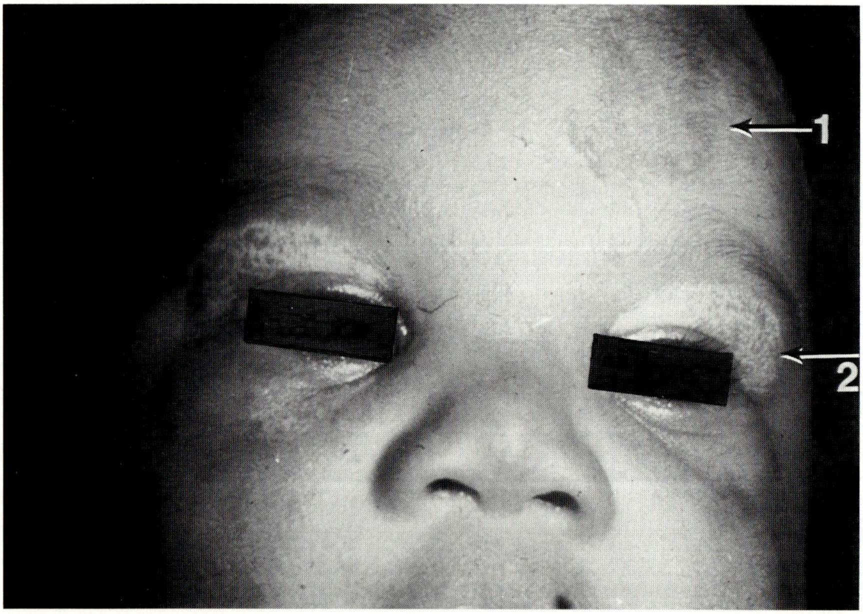

Figure 1. 1. Annular erythematous cutaneous lesion on forehead of infant with NLE. 2. Mottled periorbital hypopigmentation was the presenting feature at 10 days of age in this infant.

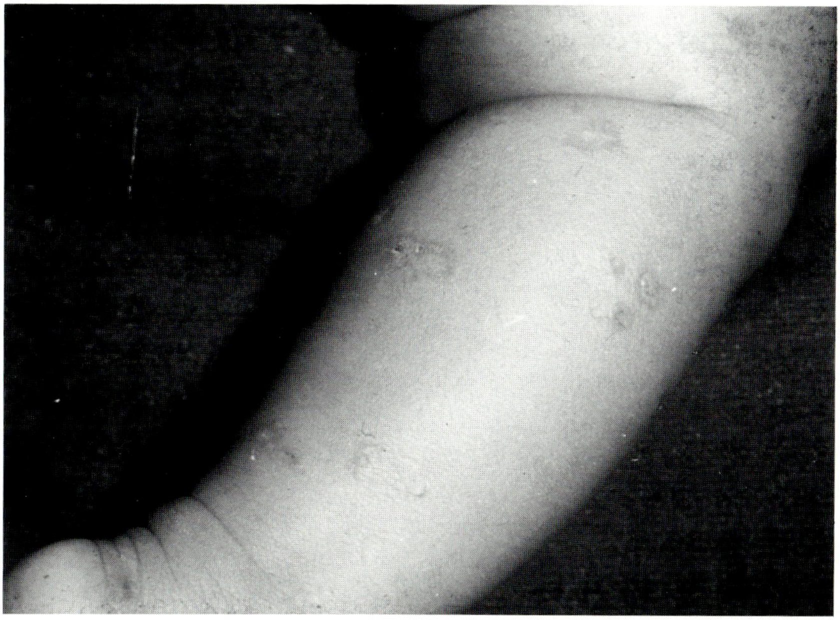

Figure 2. Discrete annular lesions on infant's leg with minimal elevation, scaling, and hyperpigmentation.

and may occasionally demonstrate confluency, thus forming annular, polycyclic lesions (Fig. 2). Scaling and atrophy are generally uncommon. Follicular plugging and telangiectasia are also not prominent features. Purpura or petechiae may precede development of lesions, and may be the cutaneous expression of a concomitant autoimmune thrombocytopenia. Lesions may continue to appear for some time after birth. Prior exposure to sunlight has, in some instances, been noted to percede the onset of these lesions (Table 1). Indeed, in some cases, a sunburn has been documented prior to the onset of lesions (2,58). The presence of cutaneous disease at birth in some infants, however, indicates that ultraviolet (UV) light is not always a prerequisite for the emergence of these cutaneous lupus lesions. Although the skin lesions in the majority of cases disappear within 6 months, leaving minimal or no scarring, occasionally resolution is delayed (see Table 1); subtle changes in pigmentation may be detected for much longer periods.

Differential diagnosis of cutaneous NLE lesions includes eczema, psoriasis, erythema multiforme, and the genodermatoses that display photosensitivity; that is, Blooms syndrome, Rothmund Thomson syndrome, Cockayne syndrome, and congenital ectodermal dysplasia.

Biopsy specimens of cutaneous lesions of neonatal LE commonly demonstrate characteristic features of adult lupus (Figs. 3 and 4). Hyperkeratosis, epidermal atrophy, at times striking liquefaction degeneration of the basal layer, edema with splitting of collagen bundles, vascular ectasia, and a patchy dermal infiltrate composed of lymphocytes and histiocytes surrounding blood vessels and adnexa are frequently described. Occasionally, however, the pathology in some infants is not typical. Our experience is detailed in Table 1.

Table 1. Clinical and Histopathologic Findings in 10 NLE[a] Infants

				Clinical features					Skin biopsy		
Patient no.	*Sex*	*Race*	*Age at onset of Rash (wk)*	*Sites of involvement*	*Photosen-sitivity*	*cutaneous findings*	*Course*	*Systemic features*	*H&E*	*DIF*	*EKG*
1	M	W	8	Face, arms legs	+	Butterfly rash papules, plaques central atrophy scale, hyperpig-mentation	Resolution at 15 mo	None	Consistent with LE	ND	Normal
2	M	B	4	Face, neck, thighs	–	Annular plaques dusky center, erythematosus papules on neck	Resolution at 1 yr	None	Consistent with LE	ND	Normal
3	M	W	8	Arm	–	Erythematous papules	Unchanged at 4 mo	None	ND	ND	CHB, RBBB, ventricular rate, 90
4	F	W	7	Scalp, face	+	Papules and plaques, central atrophy, adherent scale, telangiec-tasia, hypopig-mentation	Resolving at 6 mo	None	ND	ND	Normal

5	F	B	1.5	Scalp, face ears, trunk, extremities	–	Annular erythematous papules, central hypopigmentation, peripheral scale	Resolution at 5 mo residual pigmentary change	Transient abnormal liver function	Suggestive of LE	Negative	Normal
6	M	W	16	Scalp	–	Erythema and edema	Complete resolution at 7 mo	None	Suggestive of LE	ND	ND
7	M	W	4	Scalp & face (perioribal & forehead)	–	Confluent macules with annular lesions at periphery, scale present	Complete resolution at 5 mo	Pneumonitis, hemolytic anemia	Consistent with LE	ND ND	Normal
8	M	W	2	Face, spread to trunk and limbs at 7 wk	–	Annular scaling lesions, central atrophy, hypopigmentation	Resolving at 3 mo	Abnormal liver function	Nonspecific changes	IgG at dermal-epidermal junction	Normal
9	M	B	4	Scalp, face, trunk, limbs	–	Annular macules, papules, and plaques, central clearing, hyperpigmentation	Resolution at 4 mo and hyperpigmentation	None	Consistent with LE	ND	Normal
10	F	H	Present at birth	Trunk	Unknown	Confluent erythematous lesions with scaly center	Unknown, lost to follow-up	None	Consistent with LE	ND	ND

[a]NLE, Neonatal lupus erythematosus.
[b]CHB & RBBB, Congenital heart block and right bundle branch block.
ND-Not done; M-male; F-female; W-white; B-black; H-Hispanic
From Watson, et al. (57).

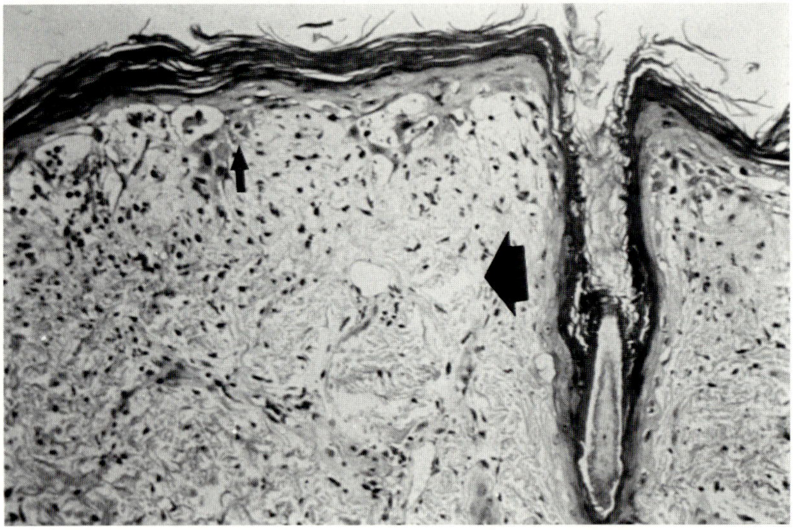

Figure 3. Histology of NLE lesion demonstrating hyperkeratosis, patulous follicle, epidermal atrophy, basal vacuolization, dermal edema, and mononuclear infiltrate. Thin arrow, epidermis; thick arrow; dermis (H&E).

Direct immunofluorescence (DIF) of biopsied lesions may infrequently demonstrate granular deposits of IgG, IgM, and C3 at the dermal-epidermal junction (DEJ). It should be noted that negative immunofluorescence (IF) does not preclude a diagnosis of NLE, as these cutaneous lesions may not be of adequate age to demonstrate positive findings. In addition, certain features of the characteristic skin lesions of NLE are most compatible with subacute cutaneous LE (SCLE). This distinctive cutaneous lupus subset demonstrates positive lesional IF findings in only 60% of patients (48).

Congenital Heart Block

The other major finding in NLE is (CHB). In approximately 50% of cases, isolated CHB is the only manifestation of NLE. On occasions, conduction defects other than CHB have also been described. These include Wenckebach phenomenon and bundle branch block (18,50). Bradycardia is frequently detected in utero.

In approximately 25% of infants with CHB, there is an associated structural congenital heart disease. Transposition of the great vessels, patent ductus arteriosus, atrial and ventricular septal defects, anomalous venous drainage, and mitral insufficiency are the most common abnormalities reported (13). In addition, the limited autopsy information available indicates these infants with CHB also frequently demonstrate extensive endocardial fibroelastosis (10,13,21,28).

The first major work demonstrating the association of connective tissue disease connective tissue disease with CHB was only reported recently by McCue et al. in 1977 (31). These investigators reported 22 children with CHB, and found that 63% were the offspring of mothers with clinical or laboratory evidence of connective tissue disease (primarily SLE). A review of the literature by the authors revealed five previous case reports of CHB in infants of mothers with SLE.

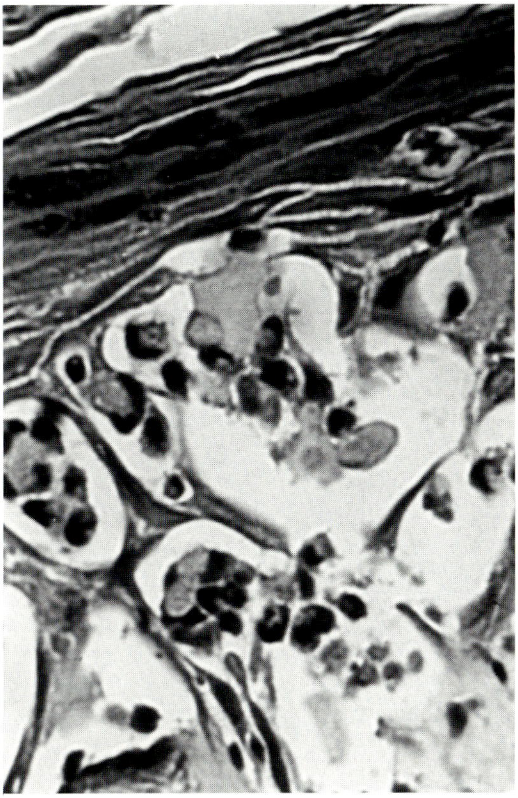

Figure 4. Higher magnification of epidermis in Figure 3 demonstrating liquefaction degeneration of the basal layer.

Subsequently, there have been several reports documenting the association of CHB with maternal connective tissue disease, most commonly SLE (10,13,19,45). Chameides et al. reported six babies with CHB and maternal connective tissue disease (10). Esscher and Scott described 27 cases of CHB, and reviewed the reports of 40 additional CHB patients (13). They found one-third of the mothers who delivered babies with isolated CHB had or subsequently developed connective tissue disease. Of the mothers with connective tissue disease, 38% had SLE, 16% had rheumatoid arthritis (RA), 25% had undifferentiated connective tissue disease, and 20% had only positive connective tissue disease serology.

Hematology

Hematologic abnormalities including hemolytic anemia, leukopenia, and thrombocytopenia occur in 15% of NLE infants. These abnormalities are seldom of clinical significance. Red blood cell, white blood cell, and platelet indices usually spontaneously return to normal. An immune pathogenesis resulting from transplacental passage of maternal antibody is likely in these infants. Indeed, in one case, thrombocytopenia was manifest in the mother, and neonate and antiplatelet antibodies were found in both

(38). Hypersplenism may also contribute to the hematologic abnormalities. Occasionally, corticosteroids are required to treat an infant's severe thrombocytopenia, and the beneficial therapeutic response is usually immediate (37).

Only two reported neonates with an LE-like syndrome did not have either cutaneous LE or CHB (39,47). In one case, maternal SLE was associated with hemolytic anemia, leukopenia, and thrombocytopenia in the newborn infant. The other infant had a Coombs positive hemolytic anemia and a positive LE preparation.

Serology

McCuistion and Schoch first suggested the possibility of an NLE transmittable etiologic agent passing from mother via the placenta to the child, and they implicated the LE factor (32). The LE factor is an IgG antibody and can cross the placenta. It is highly unlikely, however, that the LE Factor is of pathogenetic importance in neonatal lupus because clinically normal infants of SLE mothers have been shown to possess the LE factor during the neonatal period.(5,6,53)

ANA are also frequently detected in asymptomatic infants of SLE mothers (3). However, neither the LE factor nor ANA are universally present in NLE. The ANA is positive in less than 50% of NLE cases. Rheumatoid arthritis precipitin (RAP) and rheumatoid factor (RF) have been described occasionally in both mothers and affected babies.(18,55) RF was present in 7 of 10 mothers, but in none of the infants in our own series (57). RF has been described in the neonatal period in NLE, and it has also been shown to develop at 8 months of age in one infant (42). Since RF detected by Latex and Rose-Waaler methods is predominantly an IgM antibody and IgM does not cross the placenta, the RF in all probability originated in the infant in these isolated cases. The finding of RF in 70% of our Ro(SSA)-positive mothers was not surprising as an association of the Ro(SSA) antibody with RF has already been documented (1,30).

In contrast to the ANA, RF, and LE factor recent studies show that the Ro(SSA) antibody, which is an antibody against the RNA macromolecule, is present in virtually all NLE infants and their mothers. This association was first recognized by Franco et al. (18) in 1981, and was confirmed by Kephart et al. (24) and Miyagawa et al. (34). Thus far, our and other investigators' data indicate that all of the approximately 21 NLE infants tested possess LA(SSB) and/or Ro(SSA) antibodies (see Tables 2 and 3). All of the mothers have the Ro(SSA) antibody. The transient presence of the antibody in the infant correlates well with clinical disease; the majority of infants by 6 months of age are free of lupus skin disease and are serologically negative.

Of perhaps the greatest importance in this regard is the recent observation by Scott et al. of a strong correlation between isolated CHB and the Ro(SSA) antibodies in the maternal serum, regardless of the presence of maternal signs or symptoms of connective tissue disease (45). Seventy-five percent of the asymptomatic mothers of CHB infants had anti-Ro(SSA) antibody. Ro(SSA) antibody was not present in any infant tested after 6 months of age, again suggesting maternal transplacental transfer of the antibody (Fig. 5). Lee et al. reported 9 of 11 mothers of isolated CHB infants to be positive for Ro(SSA) antibody; all five neonates available for testing were also Ro(SSA) positive (25). Thus far, 64 of 73 mothers of infants with either cutaneous lesions and/or the isolated CHB variant of NLE are positive for the Ro(SSA) antibody; 32 of 34 of the infants tested are Ro(SSA) positive (24,25,29,34,45,57,58). Of the two infants who did not have Ro(SSA) antibody, one had the La(SSB) antibody (45,58). It is probable that detectable concentrations of the Ro(SSA) antibody were present in these infants at a time other than when serum was drawn. Other studies indicate that the Ro(SSA)

Table 2. Serologic Findings in 10 NLE[a] Infants and Their Mothers

	Infant				Mother			
Patient No.	*ANA (Mouse liver Substrate)*	*Ro(SSA) Antibody*	*La(SSA) Antibody*	*Rheumatoid factor (Lx, latex fixation Rw, rose waaler)*	*ANA (Mouse Liver Substrate)*	*Ro(SSA) Antibody*	*La(SSB) Antibody*	*Rheumatoid factor (Lx, latex fixation Rw, rose waaler)*
1	Negative	Positive	Negative	Negative	Negative	Positive	Negative	Lx, Positive, 1:320 Rw, Positive, 1:2560
2	Negative	Positive	Positive	Negative	Negative	Positive	Positive	Lx, Positive, 1:160 Rw, Positive, 1:80
3	Negative	Positive	Negative	Negative	Negative	Positive	Negative	Lx, Positive, 1:640 Rw, Positive, 1:160
4	Negative	Positive	Positive	Negative	Positive ≥160 (Speck)	Positive	Positive	Lx, Positive, 1:80 Rw, Positive, 1:40
5	Negative	Positive	Negative	Negative	Negative	Positive	Positive	Lx, Negative Rw, Negative
6	Negative	Positive	Negative	Negative	Negative	Positive	Negative	Lx, Positive, 1:40 Rw, Positive, 1:40
7	Positive (1:40)	Positive	Positive	Negative	Positive ≥160 (Speck)	Positive	Positive	Lx, Positive, 1:40 Rw, Positive, 1:80
8	Negative	Positive	Positive	Negative	Positive 1:640 (Speck)	Positive	Positive	Lx, Positive, 1:160 Rw, Positive, 1:40
9	Positive 1:20 (Speck)	Positive	Positive	Negative	Positive ≥160 (Speck)	Positive	Positive	Lx, Negative Rw, Negative
10	Positive 1:20 (Speck)	Positive	Positive	Negative	Positive ≥160 (Speck)	Positive	Positive	Lx, Negative Rw, Negative

[a]NLE, Neonatal lupus erythematosus.
From Watson et al. (57).

Table 3. Summary of Neonatal Lupus Infants with Documented Serology: Review of the Literature

		Infant					*Mother*	
Case	*Race*	*Sex*	*Clinical features*	*ANA*	*Ro(SSA) antibody*	*La(SSB) antibody*	*Clinical features*	*Source*
1	B	F	Lupus dermatitis	+	+	–	Asymptomatic	Weston et al. (58)
2	W	F	Lupus dermatitis, congenital heart block	+	+	+	Asymptomatic	
3	H	F	Lupus dermatitis	+	–	+	Asymptomatic	
4	B	M	Congenital heart block	+	+	–	Dry mouth	
5	W	F	Lupus dermatitis	–	+	–	Asymptomatic	
6	W	F	Lupus dermatitis	+	+	–	Sjögren's syndrome	

7	B	F	Congenital heart block	+	+	–	SLE	
8	W	F	Lupus dermatitis	+	+	–	Dry mouth	
9	Or	M	Lupus dermatitis	–	+	+	SLE	Miyagawa et al. (34)
10	Or	M	Lupus dermatitis	–	+	+	SLE	Miyagawa et al. (34)
11	W	F	Lupus dermatitis, congenital heart block	+	+	+	Photosensitivity, alopecia, sicca symtoms, (approx. 1 yr post partum)	Lockshin et al. (29)

Case report by Kephart et al. (24) is included in our own series, case number 5 (Table 2).
B-Black; W-White; H-Hispanic; Or-Oriental; M-male; F-female; SLE, systemic lupus erythematosus.
Case report by Kephart et al. (24) is included in our own series, case number 5 (Table 2).

antibody is almost always present when La(SSB) antibodies are detected, but may be in such low concentrations as to escape detection by gel double precipitation techniques.

The frequency of the La(SSB) antibody in NLE infant/mother pairs is noteworthy. Thus far, the La(SSB) antibody has been detected in 18 of 29 NLE infants. La(SSB) antibody was found in 6 of 10 infants and in 7 of 10 mothers in our own NLE series (Table 2). In Scott's NLE CHB series, La(SSB) antibody was present in 17 of 34 mothers and 6 of 8 infants (45). The significance of this finding is currently unknown.

Unindentified precipitin antibodies have been occasionally detected by gel double diffusion techniques in NLE infants, but nRNP and/or Sm antibodies are absent. There is also only one report of DNA antibody being described in an infant with NLE (12).

These data strongly suggest that nDNA, Sm, and nRNP antibodies are not important in the pathogenesis of NLE. Thus, the Ro(SSA) antibody may be regarded as a serologic marker for NLE. In fact, in view of our present data, we believe failure to find the Ro(SSA) antibody in a newborn with suspected cutaneous lupus or CHB, or in the mother, constitutes strong evidence against the diagnosis of NLE.

PATHOGENESIS

Significance of Ro(SSA) Antibody

The findings of the Ro(SSA) antibody in almost all NLE infants in whom the antibody has been sought suggests a pathogenetic role. However, in view of the development of knowledge concerning antibody-mediated effects in other neonatal forms of autoimmune disease (e.g., thyroid disease), it is possible that a closely related, unidentified antibody is at fault. For example, in neonatal hyperthyroidism, long-acting thyroid stimulator (LATS) was first suspected as the cause of excessive thyroid stimulation; later, LATS protector, a closely related antibody, was found to be responsible (46,52). Indeed, the Ro(SSA) antibody may be an epiphenomenon. In favor of an epiphenomenon is the fact that we have documented at least six instances where mothers known to be Ro(SSA) positive during their pregnancy produced asymptomatic babies. In addition, a retrospective review of the pregnancy history of 50 Ro(SSA)-positive women who produced 61 living children detected only one case of NLE (55).

Another piece of evidence cautioning against a direct cause-and-effect role for the Ro(SSA) antibody is the variability in disease expression of CHB. Despite the same maternal influences, disease expression can vary considerably in the infants involved. For example, Scott et al. (45) reported dizygous twins—one with CHB and one with no abnormality.

Role of Ultraviolet Light (UV)

It has been historically recognized that UV light initiates or exacerbates the development of some of the cutaneous lesions of NLE. (2,58) The precise mechanism and the role, if any, of the Ro(SSA) antibody, however, are unclear. It has been demonstrated in vitro that UV irradiation of human epidermal cells in tissue culture may lead to the expression of the Ro(SSA) antigen. Following sublethal UVB irradiation, epidermal keratinocytes demonstrate Ro(SSA) antigen in the cytoplasm, and then along the epidermal keratinocyte cell surface (27). This observation may provide a possible pathophysiologic role for the UV light in this condition.

The putative antigen may be generated only in areas limited to UV light exposure.

This may, in turn, explain why these infants have their disease limited primarily to sun-exposed areas.

Possible Immune Mechanisms

If the Ro(SSA) antibody is of pathophysiologic significance in the etiology of the cutaneous lupus lesion, the question that remains is: "How is this mediated?" Thus far, typing the infiltrate in chronic cutaneous lupus, including Ro-positive subacute cutaneous lupus lesions, has demonstrated that T cells predominate (51). Other recent studies indicate that the Ro(SSA) antibody may be capable of affecting antibody-dependent cellular cytotoxicity in which mononuclear or T cells actually become the effector cells (40). Much more work, however, must be done in this promising area in order to ascribe a definite immunologic mechanism for the Ro(SSA) antibody in the pathogenesis of NLE lesions.

HLA Studies

Immunogenetic studies have demonstrated a statistically significant increase frequency of the HLA DR2 and/or DR3 antigens in patients with SLE and Sjögren's syndrome (9,43,44). In addition, DR2 and/or DR3 phenotypes have been strongly associated with the expression of the Ro(SSA) antibody (1). A striking concordance of SCLE (a condition manifesting identical cutaneous lesions to those of NLE), anti Ro(SSA) antibody, and the DR3 phenotype has been demonstrated by Sontheimer et al. (49). HLA typing of six families of NLE infants, performed by Lee et al. (26), showed a statistically significant increased incidence of DR3 phenotypes in the mothers, but not in affected infants—a finding in accord with previous data by Lockshin et al. (29). Thus, in striking contrast to the mothers, no HLA association was noted in the NLE infants. Of further interest is the unusual frequency of HLA B8 and DR3 in mothers, but not children, with the CHB variant of the NLE syndrome (54).

We have recently had the opportunity to extend these studies by investigating the HLA phenotypes of 11 additional families with NLE infants. (57) The mothers of these patients demonstrated a statistically significant increased prevalence of HLA A1, B8, DR3, MB2, and MT2 phenotypes (Table 4). The antigens HLA, B8, MB2, and MT2 are known to be in linkage disequilibrium with HLA DR3. MB and MT are alleles for B-cell alloantigens that reside in or near the HLA DR region. It has been proposed that these two alleles are more strongly associated with autoimmune disease than are gene products of the HLA DR locus. However, because these alloantigens are more prevalent in the general population than HLA DR3, definitive conclusions regarding their relative significance cannot be drawn at this time.

In order to investigate a differential genetic predisposition between affected and unaffected mother/infant pairs, we compared our results with the HLA phenotypes of six families where a Ro(SSA)-positive mother gave birth to a clinically normal infant (Table 5). By contrast, these Ro-positive mothers with normal infants had increased frequencies of the HLA DR2 and MB1/MT1 phenotypes. Why infants of DR2-positive mothers might be protected from developing NLE is unclear.

These data suggest that infants of Ro(SSA)-positive mothers bearing HLA A1, B8, DR3, MB2, and MT2 phenotypes are at increased risk for developing NLE, which is in sharp contrast to neonates of Ro(SSA)-positive mothers having DR2 and MB1/MT1 phenotypes. Our results support the hypothesis that whereas HLA DR2 and DR3

Table 4. HLA Phenotypes in Mothers of Neonatal Lupus Infants

Mother of Patient	*Race*	*HLA Loci* *A*	*B*	*DR*	*Source*
IIIb.	W	2,w24	8,w60	3,6	Lockshin et al. (29)
1	W	1,3	8,7		Barber et al. (2)
2	W	1	8		Barber et al. (2)
4	W	11,w23	7,w35		Barber et al. (2)
5	–	1,25	8,18		Barber et al. (2)
1	B	19,28	8,45	3,9	Lee et al. (26)
2	Mexican American	1,32	8,38	6,8	Lee et al. (26)
3	W	1,33	8,14	3,7	Lee et al. (26)
4	W	1,2	8,7	3,2	Lee et al. (26)
5	W	1,2	8,62	3,4	Lee et al. (26)
6	W	1,29	8,60	3,6	Lee et al. (26)
1	W	2,29	51,44w4	2,7	Watson[a] et al (57)
2	B	1,26	8,18,w6	3	Watson[a] et al (57)
3	W	1,2	8,44w4, w6	3,6	Watson[a] et al (57)
4	W	2,28	7,53w4, w6	3,5	Watson[a] et al (57)
5	B	2,26	8,17, w4w6	6,7	Watson[a] et al (57)
6	W	1,11	8,35	3,1	Watson[a] et al (57)
7	W	1,3	8,7, w6	3,6	Watson[a] et al (57)
8	B	1,33	8,51	2,5	Watson[a] et al (57)
9	W	1,23	8, w6	3,6	Watson[a] et al (57)
10,11	W	2,29	8, w6	3,4	Watson[a] et al (57)
12	W	1,24	7, w4w6	3,2	Watson[a] et al (57)

[a]Mothers of patients 1 to 6 correspond to mothers of patients 1–4, 9, and 6, respectively, in Table 2.
W-white; B-black.

phenotypes are indeed associated with Ro(SSA) antibody formation, the clinical manifestations of lupus (in this instance, the lupus skin disease in infants) are not under direct genetic control (57).

Etiology of CHB

The association of CHB and neonatal LE is of considerable interest. CHB is a rare clinical entity with an incidence of 1 in 20,000 live births (33). The occurrence of CHB in adults with SLE is also rare, but it has been documented (4,35). Plant and Steven, in 1945, described the first case of CHB in an infant born to a mother with SLE (41).

Lev et al. reported nine autopsies on infants with CHB; all had fibroelastosis, and some had calcification in the most distal part of atrial musculature (28). Death in all of these infants probably resulted from extensive myocardial fibrotic damage. Carter et al. (7) demonstrated evidence of lesions in three different areas of the conductive system.

Table 5. HLA Phenotypes in Ro(SSA) Positive Mothers with Clinically Normal Neonates

		HLA loci		
Case	*Race*	*A*	*B*	*DR*
1	W	1,24	8,53, w4, w6	3,8
2	W	2,25	62, 18, w4, w6	2,3
3	W	2, 3	51, 7, w4, w6	2
4	W	25	18, w6	2
5	W	1,3	7, 8	2,3
6	W	25	18, w4, w6	2

From Watson et al. (57).

In some cases, a myocardial connection between the atrial conduction tissue and the atrioventricular (AV) node was absent, and the node was entrapped in excessive fibrous tissue; in others, the AV node was absent, or there was evidence of degeneration of a previously developed nodal structure. A third group demonstrated lesions in the AV bundle.

A review of the reported numbers of isolated CHB by Winkler et al. revealed that 9 of 14 displayed multiple involvement (CHB) among siblings without involvement in any other generation, suggesting a maternal factor in the etiology (59). Chameides (10) documented three mothers with two involved siblings, and Wright et al. (59) reported one mother who had three CHB infants. Many mothers with NLE infants have also given birth to normal siblings. Hull et al. reported a mother with two normal children followed by one with discoid skin lesions, and then one with CHB and hepatosplenomegaly who died.(21)

There are two possible explanations for the pathology of CHB in NLE. These are:

1. Cardiac injury is occurring during heart development.
2. Cardiac injury is due to destruction and fibrosis—the result of an inflammatory process.

The AV node originates separately from the bundle of His during the third and fourth week of gestation, and it subsequently joins the latter. IgG antibodies are known to cross the placenta as early as 12 weeks of gestation. Thus, injury at this stage is possible, and is supported by the frequent occurrence of structural heart defects found in association with CHB. However, in favor of a degenerative process is that the majority of antibodies cross the placenta in the third trimester. It is conceivable that the Ro(SSA) or another antibody may cause an inflammatory response that leads to myocardial damage and replacement of the conduction system by fibrosis. Another point in favor of a degenerative process is that the autopsy findings in CHB patients with adult SLE or other connective tissue disease are similar to those in NLE.(4,35) The presence of incomplete block in some infants may also be explained by a limited inflammatory response. Finally, the report that an SLE woman had two CHB children and two apparently healthy children with incomplete right bundle branch block also provides support for an inflammatory process theory (5).

The question arises as to why the mother, generally with higher titers of Ro(SSA) antibodies than her affected infant, does not develop cardiac damage. Perhaps the antigens to which the antibodies are directed are exposed only during heart embryogenesis.

MATERNAL FEATURES

Initially, most cases of NLE were reported in infants of mothers with SLE or Sjögren's syndrome. It has now become clear that the majority of mothers are asymptomatic (60%). Eight of 10 mothers in our own series were asymptomatic (57). Photosensitive eruptions have been noticed in some mothers, but the majority of these photosensitive problems occurred in the absence of specific cutaneous findings. Interestingly, no cardiac conduction defects have been reported in the mothers. As previously mentioned, mothers who have one child with NLE may be at significant risk for having a second affected child.

Of the mothers that do have disease, SLE is the most common; Sjögren's syndrome, RA, and undifferentiated connective tissue disease have also been documented. It is very provocative to realize that Ro(SSA)-positive Sjögren's syndrome mothers are giving birth to NLE infants. From a biological point of view, this fact suggests that Sjögren's syndrome and SLE may be more closely related diseases than has been previously recognized. Of those mothers with clinical disease, approximately 20% become manifest shortly after pregnancy (within 1 year). Of great interest is a recent report of a mother developing SLE 16 years after the birth of an NLE infant (23).

FETAL WASTAGE

The reported incidence of spontaneous abortion and stillbirths in LE varies from 7 to 40%; some report increased fetal wastage in women before the onset of symptomatic SLE (14,15,17). Increased fetal wastage in SLE has been attributed to renal disease and hypertension in the past, but many reports since then show that the mortality is still increased in the absence of these factors (8,11). A tendency of increased fetal wastage may also be included in the spectrum of NLE. Indeed, Harticainen-Sorri and Karla (20) reported a woman with SLE who had nine previous spontaneous abortions. At the beginning of her 10th pregnancy, a high titer of ANA was noted, treatment with prednisone was initiated, and the pregnancy was uncomplicated. The newborn infant had CHB.

To evaluate the suggestion that fetal wastage may be increased in mothers of NLE infants, we performed a retrospective evaluation of obstetric histories of 50 women known to possess the Ro(SSA) antibody (age range 15 to 50 years) and compared the results with those of 47 women possessing nRNP antibodies (56). Anti-DNA antibodies and Sm antibodies were absent in both groups. Whereas no significant difference in fetal wastage was detected in either group overall, when adjustment for race was made within the group previously diagnosed as having SLE, there was a significant increase in fetal wastage in Ro(SSA)-positive women. Of interest is the fact that only one Ro(SSA)-positive woman had an infant with documented NLE. One potential conclusion from this study is that the Ro(SSA) antibody per se is unlikely to be the sole factor in the etiology of increased fetal wastage in SLE. Further studies of a large number of mothers of NLE infants will be necessary before definitive statements regarding their relative risk for fetal wastage can be fully determined.

PROGNOSIS

The prognosis of NLE in the absence of CHB is excellent, with the clinical and serologic features disappearing by 1 year of age. The presence of CHB seems to change the

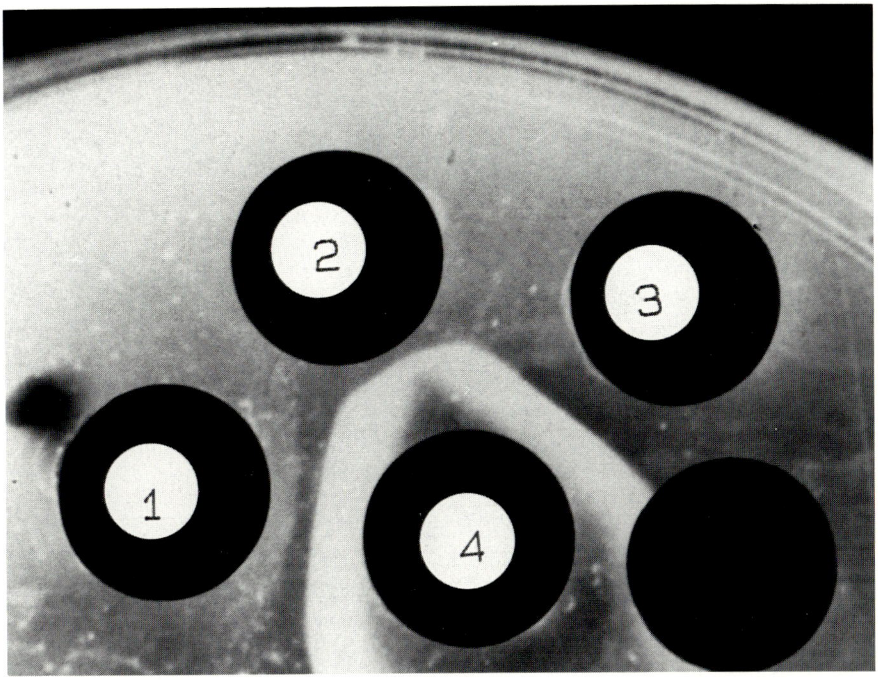

Figure 5. Demonstration of Ro(SSA) antibody in NLE mother and infant by immunodiffusion. Well 1: Mother's serum; well 2: Ro (SSA) positive control serum; well 3: Infant's serum; well 4 (center well): Human spleen extract.

mortality from 0 to 30%. This is mainly due to the presence of other cardiac defects and associated cardiomyopathy. Death in the CHB variant of NLE may be sudden or follow prolonged congestive heart failure. Fatal Stokes Adams attacks have been described (36). At the other end of the spectrum, McCue et al. (31) reported one untreated CHB child who had two normal pregnancies of her own without untoward effects.

LONG-TERM FOLLOW-UP

There are two reports of NLE progressing to adult LE, and there is one report of RA developing in the fourth year (13,16,22).

MANAGEMENT

Infants with cutaneous disease should avoid direct exposure to UV light. In fact, all infants of mothers known to possess Ro(SSA) antibody should avoid direct sun exposure during the first 6 months of life because UV light may trigger the disease. Topical steroids (e.g., 1% hydrocortisone cream q.i.d.) are effective therapeutic measures, but the NLE lesions may disappear spontaneously.

Detection of CHB as early as possible is recommended by employing ultrasound and fetal monitoring at women at risk for having an infant with NLE. Complete heart block usually needs no immediate treatment, but babies with profound bradycardia and poor cardiac output require pacemaker insertion.

SUMMARY

NLE is an inflammatory disorder of neonates characterized by transient cutaneous lesions and/or CHB. The cutaneous lesions usually heal without scarring, but healing may be delayed for many months in occasional cases. In contrast to the previous suggestion of a female predominance, the incidence of this disorder appears to be equally distributed in both sexes. Photosensitivity is being recognized as a component of this syndrome. Of note is the fact that a large proportion of this maternal population are asymptomatic, although their potential risk for developing connective tissue disease in the future remains to be determined. Moreover, this maternal group may exhibit a tendency to fetal wastage.

Of considerable interest is the observation that La(SSB) and/or Ro(SSA) antibody is/are almost universally present in the sera of the neonatal lupus mothers and their infants. While it is tempting to speculate a pathogenetic role for the Ro(SSA) antibody system in NLE, it appears that the relationship is not simply one of cause and effect. Whatever the relationship of the serologic and clinical features of NLE, screening of infants with isolated CHB and/or cutaneous lesions suggestive of LE, and their mothers, for the presence of Ro(SSA) antibody is strongly recommended.

Recognition of the protean manifestations of this complex disorder, by obstetricians, pediatricians, cardiologists, and dermatologists will undoubtedly lead to increased detection of NLE and will afford the opportunity to elucidate the etiology of this syndrome.

ACKNOWLEDGMENT

We thank Ms. Katey Courtney and Ms. Denise Fritter for their excellent secretarial assistance.

REFERENCES

1. Ahearn JM, Provost TT, Dorsch CA, et al: Interrelationships of HLA-DR, MB and MT phenotypes: Autoantibody expression and Clinical features in systemic lupus erythematosus. *Arthritis Rheum* 25:1031–1040, 1982.
2. Barber KA, Jackson R: Neonatal lupus erythematosus: Five new cases with HLA typing. *Can Med Assoc J* 129:139–141, 1983.
3. Beck JS, Oakley CL, Rowell NR: Transplacental passage of antinuclear antibody. *Arch Dermatol* 93:656–663, 1966.
4. Becker JH: Systemic lupus erythematosus causing heart block. *Wisconsin Med J* 64:396–400, 1965.
5. Bouziane N, et al: Lupus érythématosus chez le nouveau-né un cas de transmission placentaire du facteur LE. *Ann Pediatr* 38:557, 1965.
6. Bridge RG, Foley FE: Placental transmission of the lupus erythematosus factor. *Am J Med Sci* 227:1–8, 1954.
7. Carter JB, Blieden LC, Edwards, JE: Congenital heart block, anatomic correlations and review of the literature. *Arch Pathol* 97:51–57, 1974.
8. Cederquist LL, Markatz IR, Litwin SD: Fetal immunoglobulin synthesis following maternal immunosuppression. *Am J Obstet Gynecol* 129:687–690, 1977.

9. Celada A, Barras C, Benzonana G, et al: Increased frequency of HLA-DRw3 in systemic lupus erythematosus (C). *Tissue Antigens* 15:283–288, 1980.
10. Chameides L. Truex RC, Vetter V, et al: Association of maternal lupus erythematosus with congenital complete heart block. *N Engl J Med* 297:1204–1207, 1977.
11. Coté CJ, Meuwissen HJ, Pickering RF: Effects on the neonate of prednisone and azathioprine administered to the mother during pregnancy. *J Pediatr* 85:324–328, 1974.
12. Draznin TH, Esterly NB, Furey NL, et al: Neonatal lupus erythematosus. *J Am Acad Dermatol* 1:437–442, 1979.
13. Esscher E, Scott JS: Congenital heart block and maternal systemic lupus erythematosus. *B Med J* 1:1235–1238, 1979.
14. Estes D, Larson DL: Systemic lupus erythematosus and pregnancy. *Clin Obstet Gynecol* 8:307–321, 1965.
15. Fine LG, Barnett EU, Donovitch GM, et al: Systemic lupus erythematosus in pregnancy. *Ann Intern Med* 94:667–677, 1981.
16. Fox RJ Jr, McCuistion CH, Schoch EP Jr: Systemic lupus erythematosus: Association with previous neonatal lupus. *Arch Dermatol* 115:340, 1979.
17. Fraga A, Mintz G, Orozco J, et al: Sterility and fertility rates, fetal wastage and maternal mortality in systemic lupus erythematosus. *J Rheum* 1:293–298, 1974.
18. Franco HL, Weston WL, Peebles C, et al: Autoantibodies directed against sicca syndrome antigens in the neonatal lupus syndrome. *J Am Acad Dermatol* 4:67, 1981.
19. Hardy JD, Solomon S, Banwell GS, et al: Congenital complete heart block in the newborn associated with maternal systemic lupus erythematosus and other connective tissue disorders. *Arch Dis Child* 54:7–13, 1979.
20. Hartikainen-Sorri AL, Kaila J: Systemic lupus erythematosus and habitual abortion: Case report. *Br J Obstet Gynaecol* 87:729–731, 1980.
21. Hull D, Binns BAO, Joyce D: Congenital heart block and widespread fibrosis due to maternal lupus erythematosus. *Arch Dis Child* 41:688, 1966.
22. Jackson R, Gulliver M: Neonatal lupus erythematosus progressing into systemic lupus erythematosus. *Br J Dermatol* 101:81–86, 1979.
23. Kasinath BS, Katz AI: Delayed maternal lupus after delivery of offspring with complete heart block. *Arch Intern Med* 142:2317, 1982.
24. Kephart DC, Hood AF, Provost TT: Neonatal lupus erythematosus: New serologic findings. *J Invest Dermatol* 77:331–333, 1981.
25. Lee LA, Reed BR, Harmon C, et al: Autoantibodies to SS-A/Ro in congenital heart block *Arthritis Rheum* 20(4)(Suppl):S24 1983 (abstract).
26. Lee LA, Bias WB, Arnett FC, et al: Immunogenetics of the neonatal lupus syndrome. *Ann Intern Med* 99:592–596, 1983.
27. LeFeber WP, Norris DA, Weston WL, et al: Induction of nuclear antigen expession in human keratinocytes by ultraviolet light (UVL). *Clin Res* 31:148A, 1983 (abstract).
28. Lev M, Silverman J, Fitzmaurice FM, et al: Lack of connection between the atria and the more peripheral conduction system in congenital atrioventricular block. *Am J Cardiol* 27:481, 1971.
29. Lockshin MD, Gibofsky A, Peebles CL, et al: Neonatal lupus erythematosus with heart block: Family study of a patient with anti SSA and SSB antibodies. *Arthritis Rheum* 26:210–213, 1983.
30. Maddison PJ, Provost TT, Reichlin M: Serological findings in patients "ANA-negative" systemic lupus erythematosus. *Medicine* 60:87–94, 1981.
31. McCue CM, Mantakas ME, Tinglstad JB, et al: Congenital heart block in newborns of mothers with connective tissue disease. *Circulation* 56:82–90, 1977.
32. McCuistion CH, Schoch EP: Possible discoid lupus erythematosus in newborn infant. *Arch Dermatol Syph* 70:782–785, 1954.
33. Michaelsson M, Engle MA: Congenital complete heart block: An international study of the natural history. *Cardiovasc Clin* 4:85–101, 1972.
34. Miyagawa S, Kitamura W, Yoshioka J, et al: Placental transfer of anticytoplasmic antibodies in annular erythema of newborns *Arch Dermatol* 117:569–572, 1981
35. Moffett GR Jr: Complete atrioventricular dissociation with Stokes Adams attacks due to disseminated lupus erythematosus: Report of a case. *Ann Intern Med* 63:508–511, 1965.

36. Molthan ME, Miller RA, Hastreiter AR, et al: Congenital heart block with fatal Adams-Stokes attacks in childhood. *Pediatrics* 30:32–41, 1962.
37. Motoya B, Horino K, Fukui J: Neonatal lupus erythematosus: A case report and a review of the literature. *Acta Paediatr JN* 75:171, 1971.
38. Nathan DJ, Snapper I: Simultaneous transfer of factors responsible for LE cell formation and thrombocytopenia. *Am J Med* 25:647–653, 1958.
39. Nice CM Jr: Congenital disseminated lupus erythematosus. *Am J Roentgenol* 88:585–587, 1962.
40. Norris DA, Ryan SR, Fritz KA, et al: The role of RNP, SM and SSA specific antisera from patients with lupus erythematosus in inducing antibody dependent cellular cytotoxicity (ADCC) of ribonucleoprotein-coated targets. *Clin Res* 30:264a, 1982 (abstract).
41. Plant RK, Steven RA: Complete A-V block in a fetus: Case report. *Am Heart J* 30:615–618, 1945.
42. Reed WB, May SB, Tuffanelli DL: Discoid lupus erythematosus in a newborn. *Archatol Derm* 96:64–66, 1967.
43. Reinersten JL, Klippel JH, Johnson AH, et al: B lymphocyte alloantigens associated with sytemic lupus erythematosus. *N Engl J Med* 299:515–518, 1978.
44. Scherak O, Smolen JS, Mayr WR: HLA-DRW3 and systemic lupus erythematosus. *Arthritis Rheum* 23:954–957, 1980.
45. Scott JS, Maddison PJ, Taylor PV, et al: Connective tissue disease, antibodies to ribonucleoprotein and congenital heart block. *N Engl J Med* 309:209–212, 1983.
46. Scott JS: Immunological diseases occurring in pregnancy. In Sakamoto S, Tojo S, Nakayma T (Eds): *Gynecology and Obstetrics, Proceeding of the IX World Congress of Gynecology and Obstetrics. Tokyo, Oct 25–31, 1979.* Excerpta Medica, Amsterdam, 1980, p 225–231.
47. Siep M: Systemic lupus erythematosus in pregnancy with hemolytic anemia, leukopenia and thrombocytopenia in the mother and her newborn infant. *Arch Dis Child* 35:364–366, 1960.
48. Sontheimer RD, Gilliam JN: Subacute cutaneous lupus erythematosus, a cutaneous marker for a distinct lupus erythematosus subset. *Arch Dermatol* 115:1409–1415, 1979.
49. Sontheimer RD, Stastny P. Gilliam JN: Human histocompatibility antigen associations in subacute cutaneous lupus erythematosus. *J Clin Invest* 67:312–316, 1981.
50. Stephenson O, Cleland WP, Hallidie-Smith K: Congenital complete heart block and persistent ductus arteriosus associated with maternal systemic lupus erythematosus. *Br Heart J* 46:104–106, 1981.
51. Synkowski DR, Provost TT: Characterization of the inflammatory infiltrate in lupus erythematosus lesions using monoclonal antibodies. *J Rheum* 10:920–924, 1983.
52. Thomson JA, Dirmikis SM, Murro DS, et al: Neonatal hyperthyroidism and long-acting thyroid stimulator protector. *Br Med J* 2:36, 1975.
53. Toumtis A, et al: Clinical and serological observations in patients with rheumatoid arthritis and their relatives. *J Pediatr* 62:463, 1963.
54. Vasquez-Rodriguez JJ, Garcia-Seoane J, Gial-Aguado, et al: Complete heart block and the HLA system *Ann Intern Med* 96:126, 1982 (letter).
55. Vonderheid EC, Koblenzer PJ, et al: Neonatal lupus erythematosus: Report of four cases with review of the literature. *Arch Dermatol* 112:698–705, 1976.
56. Watson RM, Braunstein BL, Watson AJ, Hochberg MC: Fetal wastage in women with anti-Ro(SS-A) antibody. *J Rheumatol* 13(1):90–94, 1986.
57. Watson RM, Lane AT, Barnett NK, et al: Neonatal lupus erythematosus: A clinical, serological and immunogenetic study with review of the literature. *Medicine* 63(6):362–378, 1984.
58. Weston WL, Harmon C, Peebles C, et al: A serological marker for neonatal lupus erythematosus. *Br J Dermatol* 107:377–382, 1982.
59. Winkler RB, Nora AH, Nora JJ: Familial congenital complete heart block and maternal systemic lupus erythematosus. *Circulation* 56:1103–1107, 1977.
60. Wright FS, Adams P, Anderson RC: Congenital atrioventricular heart block. *A J Dis Child* 98:72–79, 1959.

36
Antinuclear Antibodies: The Clinical Significance of Nuclear Immunofluorescent Patterns

Thomas K. Burnham

INTRODUCTION

The nuclear immunofluorescent (IF) patterns have been found to have considerable diagnostic and prognostic significance in evaluating patients suspected of having a connective tissue disease. Specific nuclear IF patterns not only can confirm clinical diagnoses of certain connective tissue diseases (5,6), but also serve as markers for different subsets and various distinctive clinical presentations within these diseases. (18,21)

DIAGNOSTIC SIGNIFICANCE

The shrunken peripheral and peripheral general patterns (Fig.1) confirm a clinical diagnosis of systemic lupus erythematosus (SLE) (5,15). Anti-DNA antibodies and kidney involvement are frequently associated with these patterns (6). On serum dilution and during clinical remission, the peripheral patterns sequentially convert from shrunken peripheral to peripheral to homogeneous (Fig. 2) (5). Only a homogeneous titer of 160 or greater is significant for one of the connective tissue diseases. Dermatomyositis, however, is essentially ruled out by a general homogeneous titer of 160 or greater (12). Such significant homogeneous titers are also not found in discoid lupus erythematosus (DLE).

The thready pattern (5) reactive with the nuclear membrane-associated antigen (17) confirms a diagnosis of SLE. It is also seen occasionally in scleroderma, but not in rheumatoid arthritis (RA). (5) This pattern is one of the "particulate" patterns (8) because it shows stained particles, whereas the peripheral and homogeneous patterns do not and comprise the "nonparticulate" system (8). Antibodies to extractable nuclear antigen (ENA) Sm are considerably more frequently associated with the thready pattern than with the other particulate patterns (21). The nucleolar (2) and true speckled-anti-centromere (Fig. 3 and 4) particulate patterns (10,20) confirm a diagnosis of scleroderma and are not found in lupus erythematosus (LE) (10).

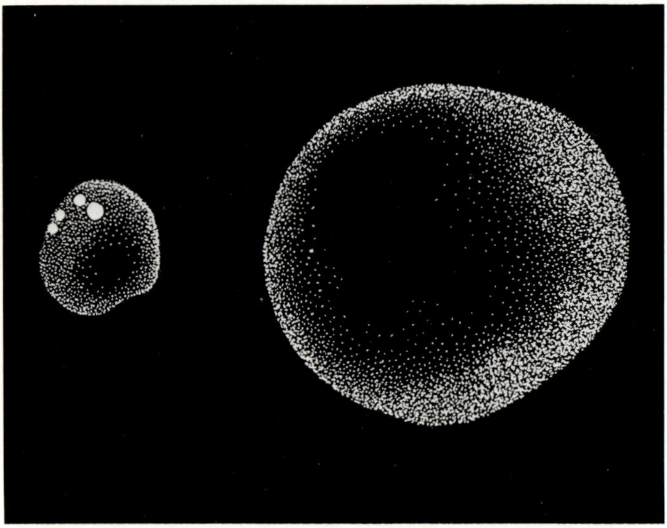

Figure 1. Diagrams of the shrunken peripheral general (left) and peripheral general (right) patterns. The shrunken peripheral nucleus is about one-third the size of the peripheral nucleus. Note the small round clumps inside and at the edge of the shrunken peripheral nucleus.

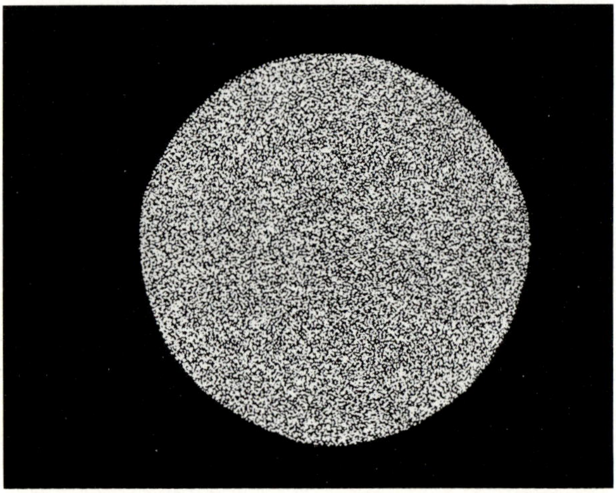

Figure 2. Diagram of homogeneous general fluorescence. Diffuse nuclear fluorescence is demonstrated in one nucleus.

The nonparticulate leukocyte-specific antinuclear antibody (LSANA) (13,14), like the general nonparticulate system, is comprised of shrunken peripheral, peripheral, and homogeneous fluorescence (Fig. 5). This antibody reacts only with granulocytic nuclei, and is demonstrated on human spleen imprints by brighter fluorescence of the granulocytic nuclei than is seen in the majority of nuclei. LSANA is found most frequently in RA and Felty's syndrome, but can be seen in LE usually associated with a particulate pattern. The Pronestyl-induced, SLE-like syndrome (16) and, rarely, scleroderma also show this pattern. Only a homogeneous titer of 640 or greater is significant for SLE or RA. A consistently negative test employing a human substrate containing granulocytes virtually excludes the diagnosis of SLE in a patient who has active disease and is not and has not been on immunosuppressants at the time of the test. Internal malignancy must also be considered with a consistently positive test if other causes for this have been ruled out. (4,5)

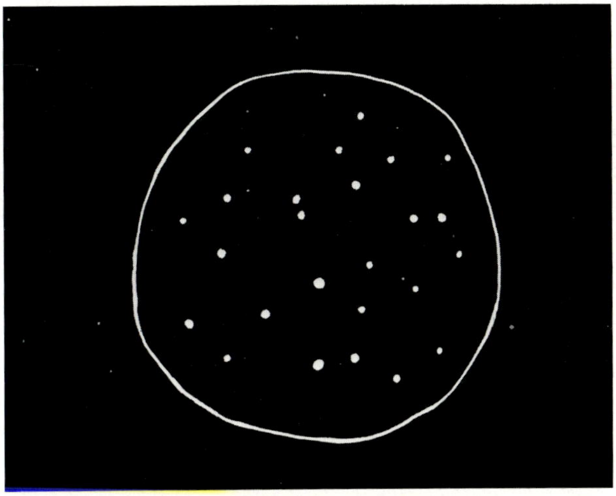

Figure 3. Drawing of true speckles. Multiple round, evenly distributed "pepper dots" are present in the outlined nucleus. This particulate pattern should be differentiated from the "other particulate" patterns.

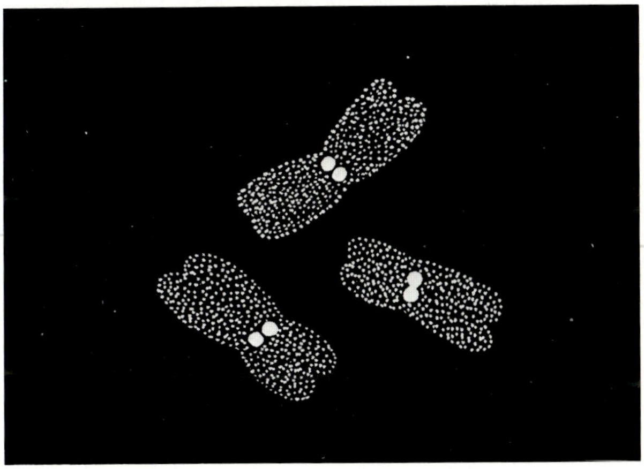

Figure 4. Illustration of centromere (kinetochore) fluorescence produced by sera showing the true speckled ANA pattern. Chromosome spread with two small, round fluorescent structures in each of three pairs of chromosomes at the sites of the kinetochores is illustrated.

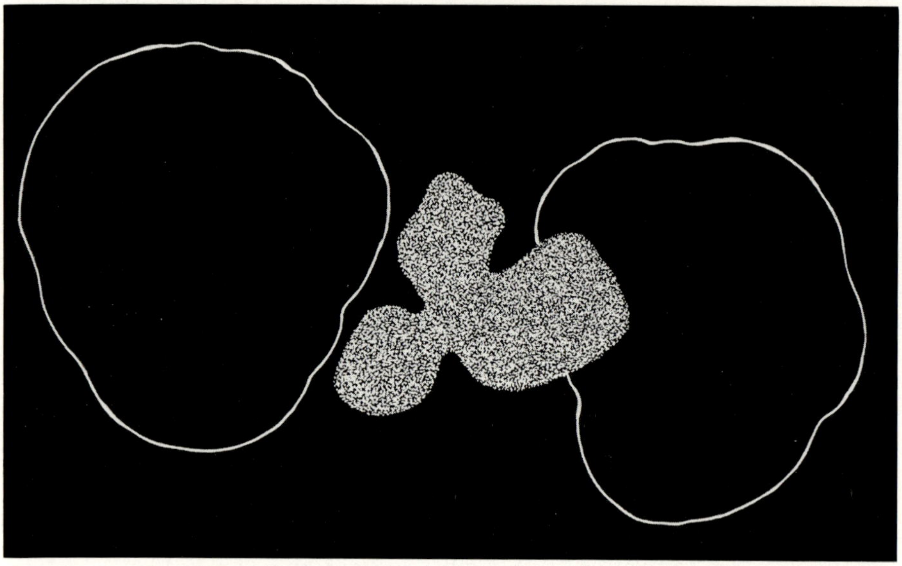

Figure 5. Drawing of homogeneous leukocyte-specific ANA. Strong homogeneous fluorescence of one granulocytic nucleus is demonstrated, while the adjacent nongranulocytic nuclei are negative.

PROGNOSTIC SIGNIFICANCE

Autoantibody profiles consisting of ANA results and other autoantibody test results are not only immunologic markers for the different connective tissue diseases, but also for specific clinical subsets and different clinical presentations within them.

Lupus Erythematosus

The autoantibody profile of the peripheral general ANA patterns (Fig. 1), along with significantly positive results for IgG anti-DNA antibodies, is a marker for severe systemic disease with kidney involvement (21). On the other hand, the profile of the large speckle-like thready pattern (Fig. 6) without anti-DNA or anti-ENA antibodies is a marker for a benign LE subset (21). These patients only have generalized skin lesions with or without joint involvement. A serum exchange with Robert E. Jordon, M.D. (unpublished data) has shown that this pattern is closely associated with anti-Ro antibodies, although these antibodies are possibly not identical.

The thready pattern when seen in SLE patients with renal involvement, has been found to be a marker for a benign subset of renal SLE. Less impairment of renal function is found in these patients, who tend to have membranous glomerulonephritis (1). The significance of these ANA has also been discussed in Chapter 31.

Scleroderma

The true speckled-anticentromere (Figs. 3 and 4) pattern is an immunologic marker for a benign clinical subset of scleroderma (10,18) (see also Chap. 37). Only acrosclerosis,

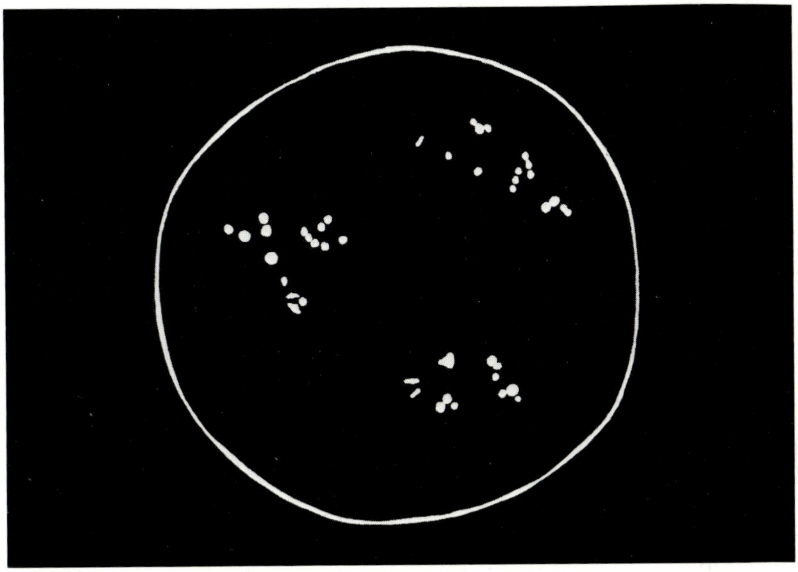

Figure 6. Illustration of large speckle-like threads. This pattern is a particulate pattern classified as "other particulate" by the simplified classification. Note the asymmetric distribution of groups of small round and thread-like structures. (From Burnham [8]).

Raynaud's phenomenon, esophageal dysmotility, and calcinosis are generally seen in this group. Recent studies of apparent Raynaud's disease patients with this pattern (19) appear to confirm the earlier studies (7) that these patients probably have subclinical benign scleroderma.

The thready pattern is associated with pulmonary involvement, while nucleolar fluorescence is a marker for diffuse skin involvement (18). Paradoxically negative ANA test results are associated with the most severe scleroderma, including renal failure.

NUCLEAR SUBSTRATES

A number of different nuclear substrates with various degrees of sensitivity have been used (12,24). Mouse liver sections used by Provost et al. (22) are not as sensitive for certain ANA patterns as human spleen imprints and human tumor cell lines (24). The so-called "ANA-negative SLE" patients (22) are ANA negative on mouse liver sections, but are frequently positive on human substrates (24). Provost's (22) ANA-negative SLE patients clinically resemble both the more benign patients in Sontheimer's et al. subacute cutaneous LE (SCLE) group (21,23) and the patients in our benign LE subset with the large speckle-like thready (SLT) ANA pattern (21). All of these patients have a tendency for benign disease, skin lesions, and a high incidence of photosensitivity. Anti-Ro antibodies were frequently found in Provost's (22) and Sontheimer's (23) patients and, as mentioned, are also closely associated with the SLT-ANA pattern. Provost's patients were ANA negative because the less sensitive mouse liver sections were used (21), whereas we used human spleen imprints (21). Sontheimer et al. also used human tissues in the form of the KB and HEp-2 tumor cell lines (24).

The nuclear substrate employed should not only be human, but should contain enough granulocytes to demonstrate the LSANA pattern (14). Blood smears and human spleen imprints have enough granulocytes; however, we prefer human spleen imprints as they demonstrate the different nuclear IF patterns more distinctly than do other substrates.

ANA TITERS

In evaluating the significance of ANA titers, it is essential to evaluate the nonparticulate peripheral homogeneous and particulate systems (8) separately. The nonparticulate system is closely associated with disease activity. In spontaneous- or immunosuppressant-induced remission, just as with serum dilution, the peripheral patterns convert to the homogeneous ones with a gradual fall in titers, and sometimes even with a total loss of the homogeneous patterns. Conversely, the particulate patterns do not demonstrate such a close association with changes in disease activity and tend to persist in remission, even though there is also some frequent fall in titers (11). Titers of particulate patterns such as the thready pattern tend to be higher than those of the nonparticulates, and are not critical for diagnostic purposes. (24)

METHODS

Staining Procedure

The indirect fluorescent antibody technique should be employed as described previously (5,9). The conjugate characteristics should be as defined by Beutner et al. (3) regardless of whether the substrate is HEp-2 cells, KB cells, or human spleen imprints. Positive control sera demonstrating the various patterns and negative controls should be tested with every procedure. In addition, unstained slides and slides stained only with both the conjugate and 0.5% aqueous fluorescein isothiocyanate should be examined to avoid mistakes in interpretation due to autofluorescence and/or nonspecific fluorescence. Furthermore, before actually employing a new lot number of substrate or a new spleen, all the controls should be tested to ensure that the substrate to be employed is able to show all the desired patterns adequately.

Microscopic Examination

Adequate magnification is essential for proper pattern identification. Slides should be examined under oil immersion with a final magnification of at least 950x. If too low a magnification (250x or less) is employed, the various particulate patterns resemble each other and cannot be individually identified (12). This has been responsible in the past for many of these particulate patterns being mistakenly called "speckled," instead of reserving the term "speckles" for the true speckled-anticentromere pattern. We use a 95x fluorite oil immersion objective with 10x oculars (5), giving 950x magnification. Furthermore, we do not use coverslips, thereby avoiding extra glass surfaces that could defract light.

SUMMARY

The clinical significance of either ANA patterns alone or autoantibody profiles comprised of both ANA results and the presence or absence of other antibodies, such as anti-ENA and anti-DNA antibodies, are both of diagnostic and prognostic value. Certain profiles will not only confirm a clinical diagnosis of SLE or scleroderma, but will also serve as immunologic markers for different clinical subsets and various distinctive clinical features within these diseases. Profiles of the peripheral general ANA patterns along with significant levels of IgG anti-DNA antibodies both confirm a diagnosis of SLE and also serve as markers for SLE kidney involvement. Conversely, the profile of the large SLT ANA pattern without anti-ENA or anti-DNA antibodies is a marker for a benign LE subset. Similarly, the true speckled-anticentromere ANA pattern not only confirms a diagnosis of scleroderma, but is also a marker for a benign acrosclerotic subset of this disease. Strict attention to details, however, both regarding the staining procedure and microscopic morphology, is essential to realize the full diagnostic and prognostic potential of these procedures.

ACKNOWLEDGMENTS

I wish to thank Robert H. Mohr, Director of the Medical Arts Department at Henry Ford Hospital for his accurate drawings.

Technical assistance was given by Gizella D. Baker, B.S.; the late Paula W. Bank, M.S.; Mary K. Cohen, B.S.; Sameera T. Pirzada, B.Sc., and Caryle A. Spence, H.T.

This research was supported in part by the James and Lynelle Holden Fund, Detroit.

REFERENCES

1. Akbar S, Tello Al, Luvira U, et al: Significance of antinuclear antibody (ANA) immunofluorescent patterns and titers in systemic lupus erythematosus nephritis. 1986 (in preparation).
2. Beck JS: Autoantibodies to cell nuclei. *Scot Med J* 8:373–388, 1963.
3. Beutner EH, Nisengard RJ, Kumar V: Defined immunofluorescence: Basic concepts and their application to clinical immunodermatology. In Beutner EH, Chorzelski TP, Bean SF (Eds): *Immunopathology of the Skin,* ed. 2. Wiley, New York, 1979, pp 29–75.
4. Burnham TK: Antinuclear antibodies in patients with malignancies. *Lancet* 2:436–437, 1972.
5. Burnham TK, Bank PW: Antinuclear antibodies: I. Patterns of nuclear immunofluorescence. *J Invest Dermatol* 62:526–534, 1974.
6. Burnham TK: Antinuclear antibodies: II. The prognostic significance of nuclear immunofluorescent patterns in lupus erythematosus. *Arch Dermatol* 111:203–207, 1975.
7. Burnham TK: Linear morphea (discussion). *Arch Dermatol* 114: 1565, 1978.
8. Burnham TK: Antinuclear antibodies: A simplified classification of the nuclear immunofluorescent patterns. *Arch Dermatol* 114:1343–1344, 1978.
9. Burnham TK: Antinuclear antibodies: Significance of nuclear staining patterns. In Beutner EH, Chorzelski TP, Bean SF, et al (Eds): *Immunopathology: Labeled Antibody Studies.* Dowden, Hutchinson & Ross, Stroudsberg, PA, 1973, pp 379–393.
10. Burnham TK, Kleinsmith DM: The "true speckled" antinuclear antibody (ANA) pattern: Its tumultuous history. *Sem Arthritis Rheum* 13:155–159, 1983.
11. Burnham TK: Antinuclear antibodies (ANA): How useful is the ANA test today? *J Int Dermtaol* 24:41–44, 1985.
12. Burnham TK: Indirect immunofluorescence. Antinuclear Antibodies (ANA): The diagnostic

and prognostic significance of the nuclear immunofluorescent patterns. In Stone J (Ed): *Dermatologic Allergy and Immunology,* St. Louis, CV Mosby, 1985, pp 279–286.

13. Faber V, Elling P, Norup G, et al: An antinuclear factor specific for leukocytes. *Lancet* 2:344–345, 1964.
14. Faber V, Elling P: Leukocyte-specific antinuclear factors in patients with Felty's syndrome, rheumatoid arthritis, systemic lupus erythematosus and other diseases. *Acta Med Scand* 179:257–267, 1966.
15. Gonzalez EN, Rothfield NF: Immunoglobulin class of pattern of nuclear fluorescence in systemic lupus erythematosus. *N Engl J Med* 274:1334–1338, 1966.
16. Gorsulowsky DC, Pank PW, Goldberg DA, et al: Antinuclear antibodies as indicators for the procainamide-induced SLE-like syndrome and its clinical presentations. *J. Am. Acad. Dermatol.* 12:245–253, 1985.
17. Heinzerling RH, Burnham TK, Belviso HM, et al: Characterization of a nuclear membrane-associated antigen reactive with autoantibodies producing the thready ANA pattern. *J Invest Dermatol* 72:209–210, 1979 (abstract).
18. Kleinsmith DM, Heinzerling RH, Burnham TK: Antinuclear antibodies as immunologic markers for a benign subset and different clinical characteristics of scleroderma. *Arch Dermatol* 118:882–885, 1982.
19. Kleinsmith DM, Burnham TK: Prognostic significance of antinuclear antibody results in patients with Raynaud's phenomenon. Presented as a poster-type exhibit at the annual meeting of the American Rheumatism Association, Minneapolis, MN, June 9, 1984 (in preparation).
20. Moroi Y, Peebles C, Fritzler MJ, et al: Autoantibody to centromere (kinetochore) in scleroderma sera. *Proc Natl Acad Sci USA* 77:1627–1631, 1980.
21. Pelachyk JM, Heinzerling RH, Burnham TK: Serologic profiles as immunologic markers for different clinical presentations of lupus erythematosus. *Sem Arthritis Rheum* 12:382–389, 1983.
22. Provost TT, Reichlin M: Antinuclear antibody-negative systemic lupus erythematosus. I. Anti-Ro (SSA) and anti-La (SSB) antibodies. *J Am Acad Dermatol* 4:84–89, 1981.
23. Sontheimer RD, Thomas JR, Gilliam JN: Subacute cutaneous lupus erythematosus. A cutaneous marker for a distinct lupus erythematosus subset. *Arch Dermatol* 115:1409–1415, 1979.
24. Sontheimer RD, Deng JS, Gilliam JN: Antinuclear and anticytoplasmic antibodies. Concepts and misconceptions *J Am Acad Dermatol* 9:335–343, 1983.

37
Clinical Significance of Laboratory Findings in Scleroderma

Stefania Jablonska
Maria Jarzabek-Chorzelska
Maria Blaszczyk
Ernst H. Beutner
Tadeusz P. Chorzelski

INTRODUCTION

Systemic sclerosis is a chronic inflammatory disease characterized by vascular changes, fibrotic changes, and several immune abnormalities. Fibrosis involves the skin and/or internal organs. In some cases, skin fibrosis is absent or very slight, and is confined exclusively to the hands. However, also in these cases, the fibrotic process is usually systemic and of the same type as in other forms of scleroderma. In the cutaneous forms (i.e., morphea, linear scleroderma, and subcutaneous varieties), the increased collagen deposition is a typical finding in the skin and subcutaneous tissue. However, also in some cutaneous forms, the changes are primarily atrophic (atrophoderma Pasini-Pierini), as in early acrosclerosis. Cutaneous scleroderma differs from the systemic forms of the disease by the absence of visceral involvement and Raynaud's phenomenon. These are both characteristic symptoms of systemic sclerosis regardless of the clinical form. Also, immune disturbances are much more pronounced in the systemic forms of the disease, although circulating antinuclear antibodies (ANA) and immune deposits in the skin were also reported in some cutaneous forms of scleroderma (see the following text). The morphology and pathology of cutaneous indurations are similar (54,55). There are cases that are intermediate between the cutaneous and systemic varieties (54). Chronic graft-versus-host disease (GVHD) following allogenic bone marrow transplantation mimics scleroderma. Diffuse cutaneous and subcutaneous sclerosis, hyperpigmentation, and depigmentation, as well as articular contractures, are comparable with those of generalized morphea (117,120,131). The histopathologic pattern of GVHD is fairly characteristic.

This work was supported, in part, by grant 10.5 of the Polish Academy of Sciences and the United States Schleroderma Foundation.

Besides vacuolization of the epidermal basal cells and lymphocytic infiltrations at the basement membrane as main features of GVHD, there are lymphocytic infiltrates around the blood vessels, skin appendages, and small nerves in the reticular dermis and pronounced fibrosis in the dermis and subcutis (115). Deposition of IgM at the dermal-epidermal junction and IgM and complement in the skin vessels was noticed by some investigators (120). Abnormal humoral responses may or may not be present (115,120,128), since the basic abnormality is thought to be an increase in suppressor T-cell number (37) and an increase in monocytes (130). Chronic GVHD in experimental animals appears to be a suitable model for scleroderma (60).

ABNORMALITIES OF CELL-MEDIATED IMMUNITY IN SCLERODERMA

Abnormal cell-mediated immune (CMI) responses have been noted by several investigators. The patients with progressive systemic sclerosis (PSS) showed a significantly greater degree of leukocyte migration inhibition than normal controls with the use of autologous lymphocytes and other antigens (48). A deficiency of T lymphocytes (49) and impaired lymphocyte reactivity to mitogens (47,50,107) correlated with the extent of visceral involvement. Other CMI abnormalities include abnormal, autologous mixed lymphocyte responses (83), decreased natural killer cell activity, and antibody-dependent lymphocyte cytotoxicity (140). However, the lymphocyte transformation response to mitogens was reported to be normal by other investigators (10,138). Depression of immune responses is due to immunoregulatory T-cell imbalance and decreased number of T lymphocytes (10,44).

T-suppressor cells, as measured by T-lymphocyte Fc receptors for IgM and IgG or by monoclonal antibody (MCA) assays, were found to be decreased by some investigators (27,51,70), but normal by others (2,74,111). The relationship of T-cell subpopulations (i.e., T-helper and T-suppressor cells as defined by MCA OKT4 and OKT8, respectively) is not yet fully clarified (24). Regardless of the OKT4/OKT8 ratio, which was found to be either elevated or normal, an excess helper function was well documented (51,73,83). These cells are mainly responsible for lymphokine generation and altered, hyperactive B-cell function.

Divergent findings of decreased (44) or increased T-helper (73,83) and T-suppressor cells (27,44,70) might be due to sampling of the patients; that is, different varieties of PSS and various degrees of severity of the disease. Systemic sclerosis is not a homogeneous group, and the CMI responses differ with the type and extent of cutaneous and visceral involvement.

ROLE OF MONOCYTES-MACROPHAGES

Interactions among lymphocytes and macrophages appear to play an important role in the pathogenesis of scleroderma, both for vascular involvement and for fibroblast proliferation. Activated monocyte-macrophage cells are found to secrete large quantities of proteases (28), and those appear to be, in a great part, responsible for endothelial injury in scleroderma (62,63). A macrophage-derived factor, fibronectin, which attracts fibroblasts, modulates fibroblast functions; monocyte-derived interleukin I appears to be a regulator of fibroblast proliferation (109).

Activated monocytes release monokines, which concurrently with lymphokines activate CMI reactions in vivo. Monocytes and macrophages in scleroderma spontaneously release fibroblast growth factor (75). A macrophage-released factor was shown to induce collagen synthesis by cultured lung fibroblasts from idiopathic pulmonary fibrosis (14). However, the supernatant of the adherent mononuclear cells (monocytes and adherent lymphocytes) also contain fibroblast growth-inhibiting factor (74,111). Thus, these are factors that stimulate and inhibit fibroblast growth (106,132).

INTERACTIONS OF LYMPHOCYTES AND MONOCYTES IN SCLERODERMA

Inflammatory infiltrates composed of T lymphocytes and monocytes are a characteristic finding in early sclerodermatous skin, that precedes fibrosis (33). Lymphocytes from patients with scleroderma were shown to produce soluble factors that enhance collagen accumulation (22). The activated T-helper lymphocytes from patients with scleroderma (73) are able to generate lymphokines either spontaneously (97) or as a response to normal cutaneous antigens (72) and/or collagen (123).

IMMUNOLOGICALLY MEDIATED VASCULAR INVOLVEMENT

Monokines and lymphokines released by activated monocytes and lymphocytes are also mediators of angiogenesis in GVH reactions (7) that are presumed to be involved in the pathogenesis of scleroderma (60). Abnormalities of the microvasculature appear to be a basic event in the pathogenesis of the disease. In all forms of systemic sclerosis, Raynaud's phenomenon is a prominent symptom with a characteristic capillaroscopic pattern of enlarged, gigantic loops with uneven, distorted outlines and stasis in the central portion. Progressively, the Raynaud's loops disappear, and the involutionary capillaries become almost not visible (scleroderma loops), with capillary loss in some areas (34,79).

The endothelial damage may be induced by the action of serum proteases. These were shown to be present in some scleroderma patients (62). They could exert a toxic effect on the endothelial cells in vitro (64,78). The presence of increased concentrations of factor VIII, von Willebrand factor, and its activity may be the underlying cause of endothelial damage (63). It is doubtful whether this endothelial injury is caused by specific antibodies eluted from circulating lymphocytes (30). The latter appear to be a result rather than a cause of endothelial injury. Regardless of the initial causative agent, endothelial injury appears to precede sclerosis.

Mononuclear cells, which produce angiogenic factors, are involved in the repair mechanism. Normally, endothelial injury is followed by a rapid replacement via proliferation of a new endothelium. This process is related to the angiogenic factors (141). If the mechanisms responsible for the production of angiogenic factors are disturbed, repair of the endothelium is delayed. The test that allows assessment of the effect of CMI responses on microvasculature is the lymphocyte-induced angiogenic (LIA) assay introduced by Auerbach et al. (8,116). This test shows the capability of peripheral blood lymphocyte to induce new blood vessel formation in a local graft-versus-host reaction (GVHR) in the mouse skin. Intradermal injections of incompatible human lymphocytes into X-ray-immunosuppressed mice evoke new blood vessel formation at the injection site. The number of newly formed blood vessels that is assessed by morphologic criteria is mainly dependent on the dose and immunocompetence of the injected cells. The lymphocytes from patients with systemic scleroderma—both acrosclerosis and diffuse scleroderma—showed a significant decrease in angiogenic capability, as compared with lymphocytes from healthy individuals (67). This reflects the decreased CMI responses, and might be important for the pathomechanism of the disease. Injury to the endothelium, possibly by serum factors (64) or other factors (e.g., inflammatory cells and their products), are normally repaired by the renewing population of endothelial cells (36). If the mechanisms responsible for production of angiogenic factors are disturbed, repair of the endothelium is delayed and the capillary loops undergo regression, as shown for corneal capillaries (9). Depression of CMI leads to a defect of LIA (67), which might be responsible for the capillary loss characteristic of systemic sclerosis (56,57,79–81).

Depressed LIA in acrosclerosis, diffuse scleroderma, and intermediate forms reflects vascular abnormalities affecting chiefly the microvasculature and small arteries in all varieties of systemic sclerosis. However, it was unexpected that the decrease in LIA was similar in CREST, with telangiectasia as a most characteristic symptom, and in diffuse scleroderma with prevailing fibrosis and inflammatory changes.

Sera of patients with early acrosclerosis including CREST, in contrast to sera from patients with diffuse scleroderma and long-lasting severe acrosclerosis, were shown to enhance markedly the angiogenic capability of normal human mononuclear cells. This LIA-enhancing activity of the serum did not correlate with the titers and types of ANA nor with the presence of circulating immune complexes (CIC) (78). The nature of the enhancing factors is not known. They could be lymphokines or monokines, or low-density lipoproteins (LDL), which may have an immunoregulatory function in systemic sclerosis (40) and/or serum protease which, in lower concentrations, might have a stimulatory effect on the endothelium.

Interestingly, the disappearance of the enhancing effects of sera from patients with severe long-lasting acrosclerosis, which was transitional to diffuse scleroderma, was parallel to the slowly developing CMI defect in these cases. In diffuse scleroderma, both a decrease in the number of T cells and a low response to dinitrochlorobenzene (DNCB) sensitization were found to be present almost at onset of the disease, and were related to its progression, to cutaneous sclerosis, and to visceral involvement. In the acrosclerostic variety, the CMI defect was related to duration of the disease. That is, it appeared several (9 to 14) years after the onset of indurations when at least three main systemic systems (heart, lung, and gastrointestinal tract) as well as skin were involved.[43]

IMMUNOLOGICALLY INDUCED FIBROSIS

The varying degrees of fibrosis in patients with systemic sclerosis were found to be related to the extent of CMI abnormalities. The early inflammatory infiltrates, which are composed of activated lymphocytes and monocytes and macrophages (35), are most pronounced in the lower dermis and subcutis. These cells release lymphokines and monokines that may be responsible for the increased collagen synthesis and fibrosis. The antigenic stimulus for this inflammatory reaction is unknown. A presumption that the vascular injury induces a release of the basement membrane antigens, specifically type IV collagen, was based on the presence of IgG-class antibodies to this type of collagen in the serum of scleroderma patients (76).

Autoantibodies to type IV collagen, laminin, and other constituents of basement membrane were suggested to be a primary immune phenomenon responsible for the generation of inflammatory reaction, and later for CMI responses (100). That is, these antibodies were thought to induce continuous endothelial injury. Thus, vascular damage, lymphocyte and monocyte and macrophage activation and their interactions, followed by an increased collagen production, all appear to be the most important steps in the immune mechanisms in systemic sclerosis.

DIVERSITY OF ANTIBODIES IN SYSTEMIC SCLEROSIS

Deranged humoral immune responses are present in almost all cases of systemic sclerosis. Circulating ANA are nearly as frequently demonstrated as in systemic lupus erythematosus (SLE) (see Chaps. 31 and 35). Some of the nuclear antigens reactive with various autoantibodies have been isolated, thus providing a basis to characterize disease by the detection of autoantibodies against defined nuclear and cytoplasmic antigens.

ANTINUCLEAR ANTIBODIES

The frequency of ANA detection depends mainly on the technique used (see Chap. 2) and on sampling of the patients. The percentage of positive results is extremely variable, from 48% in the early reports (61) to 96% with the use of HEp-2 tissue culture cell substrate (126).

SIGNIFICANCE OF THE SUBSTRATE FOR ANTINUCLEAR ANTIBODY DETECTION IN SCLERODERMA

The comparison of different substrates used for the indirect immunofluorescence (IIF) reaction revealed the lowest percentage of positive results (61%) on rat liver and the highest (about 95%) on monkey esophagus (15). However, some sera do not react with monkey esophagus, but are reactive with rat or mouse liver and mouse kidney. Some antibodies fail altogether to react on tissue sections, and can be detected exclusively on tissue culture cells (126). Thus, the most suitable substrate for detection of ANA in systemic sclerosis are human cell line HEp-2 cells or KB cells. HEp-2 proved to be the substrate of choice among the eight antigenic substrates in IIF tests in CREST sera (13). As indicated in Chapter 2, the highest levels of precision in ANA determinations on HEp-2 cells (or any other substrate) can now be attained by use of well-standardized commercial kits. While HEp-2 cells are now accepted as the substrate of choice for ANA studies, at least in systemic sclerosis the foundation for our present understanding of ANA in this disease rests on earlier studies using tissue sections.

FREQUENCY OF ANTINUCLEAR ANTIBODIES IN SYSTEMIC SCLEROSIS

The frequency of positive ANA findings on tissue sections is presented in Table 1. In a series of 298 patients followed for several years, no difference was detected between acrosclerosis and diffuse scleroderma (60 versus 64%) if single studies were performed. However, when immunofluorescence (IF) studies were repeated, the frequency of ANA-positive tests increased considerably, to 80 and 94%, respectively. This indicates that patients with systemic sclerosis usually have demonstrable ANA at one time or another in the course of the disease. In 20% of the patients with acrosclerosis, ANA were not detectable on tissue sections. (The question of anticentromere antibodies in this group is considered later in this chapter.) The intermediate form comprises cases

Table 1. Frequency of ANA in Systemic Sclerosis

			Determination			
	Total		Single		Repeated	
Variety of systemic sclerosis	*No. tested*	*No. positive (%)*	*Total No. tested*	*No. positive (%)*	*Total No. tested*	*No. positive (%)*
Diffuse scleroderma	78	66 (84.6)	25	16 (64)	53	50 (94.3)
Intermediate form	31	31 (100)	10	10 (100)	21	21 (100)
Acroscleroderma	189	136 (71.9)	78	47 (60.2)	111	89 (80.1)
Total	298	233 (78.1)	113	73 (64.6)	185	160 (86.4)

Table 2. ANA Titers in Systemic Scleroderma

		ANA titer[a]				
Variety of systemic sclerosis	*No. of cases*	*40–80 (%)*	*160–320 (%)*	*640–1280 (%)*	*2560–5120 (%)*	*>5120 (%)*
Acroscleroderma	136	32 (23.5)	55 (40.4)	32 (23.5)	15 (11)	2
Diffuse scleroderma	66	8 (12.1)	21 (31.8)	26 (39.3)	9 (13.6)	2
Intermediate form	31	6 (19.3)	8 (25.8)	10 (32.2)	7 (22.5)	
Total	233	46 (19.7)	84 (36.0)	68 (29.1)	31 (13.3)	4 (1.7)

[a]Tests on monkey esophagus. ANA nonreactive at a dilution of 1:40 were considered to be negative.

with symptoms of both acrosclerosis and diffuse scleroderma. The patients predominantly have vascular changes with proximal and central indurations. These cases usually start as acrosclerosis, but after 9 to 14 years, they manifest a more severe systemic involvement. These patients were found to have very low CMI responses (43).

The titers of ANA do not show an evident correlation with the type of systemic sclerosis, although higher titers (640 to 5120) appear to be somewhat more frequent in diffuse and intermediate forms in more than half of the cases versus one-third of acrosclerosis cases (Table 2). However, both low and very high titers may be found in all varieties of systemic sclerosis. Most commonly, titers are in the range of 160 to 1280. It should be stressed that the titers may vary widely at various stages of the disease, but usually do not correlate with the extent and severity of visceral involvement.

ANA PATTERNS AND ANTICENTROMERE ANTIBODIES

Burnham was the first to repeatedly stress the diagnostic significance of the true speckled pattern for scleroderma (17–20; see Chap. 36). Using the tumor or spleen imprints for IIF tests, he noticed different particulate patterns, which were reported by other investigators as speckles. The pattern designated by him as "true speckles," and recognized as a marker for Raynaud's disease and abortive acrosclerosis (18,20,71), proved to be identical with the pattern that was characteristic of autoantibody to chromosomal centromere (kinetochore) for which the term anticentromere antibody (ACA) was coined (87,88,126). This pattern was shown to be a specific marker for an abortive form of scleroderma (23,38,88,121,126,129). Only in isolated cases was this antibody reported to also occur in other connective tissue diseases; for example, SLE, mixed connective tissue disease (MCTD) (38), and lupus panniculitis (129).

CREST SYNDROME AND ANTICENTROMERE ANTIBODIES

CREST is a benign variant of systemic scleroderma characterized by a longevity of the disease, prevalence in females, pronounced Raynaud's phenomenon, telangiectasia, and calcinosis, with only limited sclerosis or indurative edema confined to the fingers (139).

In the first description of the relation of ACA to CREST syndrome by Tan et al. (126), ACA was found in 57% of patients with CREST and in only 8% of patients with diffuse scleroderma. Almost the same proportion was reported by Catoggio et al. (23). Kallenberg et al. (65), using human fetal fibroblast monolayers as a substrate, detected, ACA in 70% (7 of 10) of patients with CREST, in 18% (7 of 40) of patients with scleroderma, and in seven patients with Raynaud's phenomenon without evident symptoms of connective tissue disease. It should be emphasized that the distinction between the CREST type of acrosclerosis and the more severe forms of the disease may be difficult in some cases, and the diagnosis is rather arbitrary.

There are no generally recognized criteria for the classification of acrosclerosis and CREST (127). This is probably the reason why the frequency of ACA in acrosclerosis varies from 40% to 98% (38,65,129).

According to the preliminary criteria for the classification of systemic sclerosis: "CREST is a form of systemic sclerosis with prominent calcinosis as well as a Raynaud's phenomenon, esophageal dysfunction, limited involvement of the skin (often confined to the fingers or face), and telangiectasia. Precise definition of full spectrum of systemic sclerosis and its recognized subgroups will require further elucidation of etiology and pathogenesis" (124). Steen et al. (121) reported a 49% incidence of ACA in CREST syndrome patients, which is a frequency similar to our own findings (48%) listed in Table 3. Their ACA-positive and ACA-negative cases had comparable cutaneous involvement in degree and extent. Specifically, in 20% of their CREST syndrome cases both with and without ACA, the skin thickening extended to the forearm and face. These investigators suggest "that a definition of the CREST syndrome should not arbitrarily exclude patients with sclerodermatous skin changes in the extremities extending beyond the digits." Thus, the difference in results reported by various authors probably lies primarily in the definition of terms.

The clinical conditions listed in Table 3 constitute an apparent continuum ranging from Raynaud's disease, in which there are no clinical signs of scleroderma, to diffuse systemic sclerosis type with widespread cutaneous and systemic changes. The cases of so-called "idiopathic" Raynaud's disease that have ACA (about 7% in our cases) are the ones at risk; that is, cases that may be expected to develop CREST syndrome. The presence of distorted, gigantic capillaries with enlarged central portions may be the earliest marker of a possible transition into CREST. Two subsets of patients with clinical features of CREST syndrome can be distinguished. That is, those with ACA may be expected to continue a clinical course with minimal cutaneous involvement, and those without ACA may or may not go on to develop a more severe form of acrosclero-

Table 3. Frequency of ACA in Systemic Scleroderma and Idiopathic Raynaud's Disease

Clinical diagnoses	*No. Of cases*	*ACA positive*	
		No.	*%*
Raynaud's disease	54	4	7
Acrosclerosis			
Cases with indurative edema or induration confined to the digits[a]	44	21	48
Cases with pronounced sclerodactyly, contractures, and immobilization of fingers (grip)	40	0	0
Intermediate form (i.e., cases intermediate between severe acrosclerosis and diffuse scleroderma)	10	0	0
Diffuse scleroderma (i.e., cases with induration extending beyond the wrist to the upper extremities, trunk, and face)	30	0	0

[a]Such cases are referred to as CREST syndrome in the literature. CREST-Calcinosis, Raynaud's phenomenon, esophageal immotility, sclerodactyly, telangiectasis.

sis with contractures and immobilization of fingers (26). As further data on the relation of serum antibodies to clinical features become available, we may expect better recognition of prognostic prospects and subsets of the disease.

While there is general agreement on the association of CREST syndrome with ACA, there are divergent findings on the extent of systemic involvement. Some authors report findings of only minimal renal and other visceral involvement (38,65,71,84,129), although severe pulmonary hypertension and other complications may occur (104). Also, other visceral involvement is comparable, and the heart and lungs were found to be involved even in a higher percentage of ACA-positive than ACA-negative cases (26). We have also observed a patient with CREST syndrome and pulmonary hypertension, as reported by Salerni et al. (108).

ACA also appears to be a marker of developing scleroderma in patients with primary biliary cirrhosis. All 10 cases in a 10-patient study of primary biliary cirrhosis, who were positive for ACA, had features of CREST; that is, Raynaud's phenomenon, calcinosis, and telangiectasia (12). The presence of ACA in primary biliary cirrhosis was also noticed by Tuffanelli et al. (129). In our series, a female patient with both primary biliary cirrhosis and positive ACA had some features of CREST.

ANTIBODY TO Scl-70

Scl-70 is another antibody specific for scleroderma that is detectable by immunodiffusion (126). This is a basic nonhistone protein localized on the chromosomes of the cells in mitosis (32; see Chap. 33). In IF tests on HEp-2, it produces diffuse fine, dense

Table 4. Antibodies to Scl-70

Clinical diagnosis	*No. of cases*	*Scl-70 positive*	
		No.	*%*
Diffuse scleroderma	24	10	42
Intermediate form	12	9	75
Acrosclerosis including CREST syndrome[a]	48	17	35
Total	84	36	43

[a]None of the sera with Scl-70 contained ACA.

speckles. In our studies (Table 4), this antibody was found in 42% of patients with diffuse scleroderma, in 75% with the intermediate form, and in 35% with acroscleroderma. Thus, Scl-70, which is believed to be characteristic for diffuse scleroderma, has been detected in both diffuse variety and acroscleroderma, but not in abortive, ACA-positive CREST variety with slight, if any, cutaneous involvement.

ANTICENTRIOLE ANTIBODY

This antibody binds specifically to the antigens located in the centrioles of both cultured cells and human peripheral leukocytes (89). It is detectable by IF as a pair of dots in the cytoplasm of an interphase cell, or as a single spot adjacent to the nucleus. There are few reports on the presence of this antibody in the sera of patients with scleroderma or Raynaud's disease with some features of early scleroderma (89,95,129). McCarty et al. (85) detected an autoantibody against the mitotic-spindle apparatus in sera from patients with some rheumatic diseases, but this antibody differed from ACA (89).

NUCLEOLAR PATTERN

The nucleolar pattern, associated with antibody directed against nucleolar RNA (102), is highly characteristic of systemic scleroderma, but it is not disease specific. It often appears in combination with other particulate patterns; that is, with the large speckles or diffuse dense, fine speckles of Burnham. This latter is not infrequently mistaken for homogeneous staining. According to Burnham (71; Chap. 36), this staining pattern is associated with diffuse cutaneous involvement and Raynaud's phenomenon.

OTHER NUCLEAR PATTERNS

Other particulate patterns of Burnham, as well as the fine diffuse and large speckles described by Tan et al. (126), were not found to be associated with any particular clinical characteristics. The thready pattern was associated with pulmonary involvement in scleroderma patients (71), and ANA-negative tests were found in the most severe cases, including patients with renal failure.

ANA IN LOCALIZED SCLERODERMA

The percentage of positive ANA findings reported for some cases of localized scleroderma are quite variable, which is probably related to different substrates used for the test and sampling of patients. Burnham et al. (21) reported frequencies of 39% with the use of human tumor imprint technique. Recent studies on HeLa cells by Takehara et al. (125) compared results obtained on HeLa cells and mouse kidney sections. In tests with HeLa cells, ANA were demonstrated in 73% of sera from patients with localized scleroderma, in 50% of patients with morphea, in 67% of cases with linear scleroderma, and in 100% of the generalized morphea cases. On mouse kidney substrate, their results were positive with 50% of the sera. Thus, the findings of various investigators vary from 18% (91) or 48% (11) positive results to 100% (125). This variation is clearly related to both the substrate and sampling of patients. Regarding the latter, some forms such as linear scleroderma are frequently positive, while other forms, such as subcutaneous morphea, are usually negative.

In our own studies of 64 cases with monkey esophagus sections (Table 5), 29% of all of localized scleroderma patients were positive for ANA. The same frequency of ANA was found in generalized morphea. ANA were detected in linear scleroderma in 45% of cases. The frequency of detection was higher in children with localized scleroderma than in adults. No other autoantibodies were demonstrated in sera from patients with localized scleroderma.

ANTIBODIES TO RNA AND TO POLYURIDYLIC ACID IN SYSTEMIC SCLEROSIS

Antibodies to RNA were demonstrated in sera from all patients with scleroderma, and in 50% of sera from patients with SLE (1). Anti-RNA antibodies in scleroderma were uracil specific and reactive with polyuridylic acid, whereas RNA antibodies found in SLE were heterogeneous and not directed to uracil. A high level of serum antibody that reacted with polyuridylic acid was reported to be suggestive of active diffuse scleroderma (46). However, the serum factor reactive with synthetic polyribonucleotides, including polyuridylic acid, was found to be associated with LDL, and not with immunoglobulins. LDL were shown to have an immunoregulatory activity modulating specifically the E-rosette function of human lymphocytes (25).

Table 5. Frequency of ANA in Localized Scleroderma

Localized scleroderma	*No. of cases*	*ANA positive ≥40 (% pos.)*
Linear scleroderma	20	9 (45)
Generalized morphea	14	4 (29)
Symmetric morphea	5	1
Scleroderma fasciitis	2	2
Subcutaneous morphea	8	0
Other forms	15	3
Total	64	19 (29)

Although precipitin reactions with polyribonucleotides are not due to specific antibodies, a high percentage of positive results in systemic scleroderma is of interest because of the immunoregulatory role of serum LDL.

ANTIBODIES TO COLLAGEN

Antibodies to collagen were presumed to play a role in the pathogenesis of rheumatic diseases (122); for example, in the CMI responses to collagen in systemic scleroderma (123). Antibodies to type I (interstitial) and type IV (basement membrane) collagens were detected using the enzyme-linked immunosorbent assay (ELISA), and their levels were found to correlate positively with pulmonary involvement (76).

Since capillaries and arterioles are believed to be a primary site of injury in scleroderma, destruction of the endothelium and basement membrane may induce immune reactions to type IV collagen. Inflammatory cells and their mediators may be responsible for immune responses to type I collagen.

The role of these antibodies in scleroderma remains to be elucidated. Also, autoantibodies to fibroblasts have been reported to occur in scleroderma (16). With the use of IIF and viable fibroblasts in monolayer cultures as a substrate, these antibodies show cell membrane staining. The significance of this finding is not clear.

ANTIRIBONUCLEOPROTEIN ANTIBODIES

Antibody to nuclear ribonucleoprotein (RNP) is a characteristic serologic marker for collagen diseases. Most patients with MCTD have high titers of these antibodies, as detected by hemagglutination and immunodiffusion tests (113). RNP antibody, although highly characteristic of MCTD, is not disease specific; it appears in a high percentage of cases of SLE (see Chaps. 31 and 33), most commonly, in association with other antibodies to nuclear or cytoplasmic components. RNP antibodies were also found in some patients with systemic scleroderma: in 4 of 22 patients of Northway and Tan (92), and in 2 of 18 patients of Parker (96). However, they were not detected in any of the five patients studied by Williamson et al. (135), probably due to the small number of cases examined. Presence of RNP antibodies in scleroderma was reported to be associated with some symptoms less characteristic of the disease; for example, hemolytic anemia (96). Recognition of RNP-positive scleroderma subset has some practical significance, since the patients usually respond to steroid therapy, which otherwise is usually not indicated in systemic sclerosis.

The frequency of RNP antibodies in systemic sclerosis, as compared with other collagen diseases, is shown in Table 6. In our series, RNP antibody was found in severe acrosclerosis or in the transitional form, and in diffuse scleroderma. The incidence was lower than in SLE. However, there are patients with classic features of MCTD and no RNP antibodies; conversely, RNP antibodies may be a finding in other collagen diseases.

The incidence of IgG nuclear staining is significantly higher in MCTD and systemic sclerosis than in SLE. The speckled pattern of in vivo nuclear staining is highly characteristic of MCTD, and is present in 50% (133), 75% (42) or even 94% of cases with this diagnosis (66). In patients with systemic sclerosis, the pattern of nuclear deposits may also appear to be homogeneous, very much as the dense, fine speckled pattern of

Table 6. Frequency of RNP Antibodies and Incidence of IgG Nuclear Staining of Epidermal Cells in Collagen Diseases

	Frequency of RNP antibodies		*Incidence of IgG nuclear staining in epidermal cells by DIF*		
Collagen diseases	*No. of cases positive/ No. of cases tested*	*%*	*No. of cases positive/ No. of cases tested*	*%*	*ANA titers of RNP-positive sera*
Systemic sclerosis	11/188	(5.8)	10/46	(21.2)	160–10,240
SLE	32/178	(17.9)	18/162	(11.1)	160–2560
MCTD	12/16	(75)	7/15	(46.4)	1280–20,480

Table 7. Presence of Antibodies to Extractable Nuclear (*ENA*) and Ro/La Antigens and Deposition of Immunoglobulins at the Dermal-Epidermal Junction (*DEJ*) in Cases with Epidermal Nuclear Staining

Antigens (ENA) for precipitin tests	*No. of cases with given clinical conditions*		
	Systemic scleroderma (10)	*SLE (14)*	*MCTD (7)*
RNP	5	3	5
RNP + Sm	0	3	0
Sm	0	1	0
Sm + Ro	0	1	0
La	0	0	1
Unidentified	2	1	1
IF band tests (DEJ deposits of Ig) in the uninvolved skin	0	12	2

circulating ANA is frequently mistaken in tissue sections for homogeneous staining. The nucleolar pattern of staining in epidermal cells in direct immunofluorescence (DIF) studies of systemic sclerosis is rather an infrequent finding (66,99). This is consistent with our own findings.

There is still controversy as to whether ANA can penetrate into the keratinocytes in vivo; that is, whether nuclear epidermal staining is a true in vivo phenomenon, as shown by some investigators (3,39,53,66,114) and denied by others (42,52,99).

We found antibodies to extractable nuclear antigens (ENA) in most paitients with nuclear deposits: 7 of 10 in systemic scleroderma, 9 of 14 in SLE, and in all 7 patients classified as MCTD (Table 7). Whether the failures to find anti-RNP antibodies in all cases with nuclear IgG deposits is a question of technique remains to be determined. There was no correlation between the presence of antibodies to ENA and the deposition of immunoglobulins at the dermal-epidermal junction (DEJ). DEJ deposits were not detected in our cases of systemic sclerosis with RNP antibodies, but they were almost a constant finding in patients with SLE, as seen in Table 7. Also, a not infrequent discrepancy between the patterns and classes of immunoglobulins fixed in the epidermis and circulating ANA favors a true in vivo phenomenon; that is, although circulating ANA were of the IgM class in a proportion of cases, only IgG is bound in vivo in normal skin (66). This is compatible with experimental data, since only IgG anti-RNP antibodies were found to be capable of penetrating living cells (39,114). The presence of IgG nuclear deposits in clinically uninvolved skin indicates that they do not induce detectable pathologic changes (6).

Detection of RNP and nuclear epidermal deposits in patients with systemic sclerosis is not infrequently associated with symptoms rather characteristic of MCTD: fever, anemia, lymphadenopathy, severe myositis, polyarthritis, etc. However, a comparison of cases with RNP that are recognized as scleroderma showed some differences from cases classified as MCTD. The latter present with more severe myositis, more pronounced hematologic abnormalities, and less prominent visceral involvement.

ANTIBODIES TO RO AND LA ANTIGENS

The Ro antigen was originally described as a cytoplasmic acidic glycoprotein, and La as a cytoplasmic nonribosomal antigen (82). These antigens were found to be identical with soluble antigens identified by Alspaugh and Tan (5), respectively, as SS-A and SS-B (4). Anti-Ro antibodies were demonstrated mainly in SLE (110), and both anti-Ro and anti-La were found in Sjögren's syndrome (5,77). They are detected in cases of systemic sclerosis associated with this syndrome (93).

CIRCULATING IMMUNE COMPLEXES

Circulating immune complexes (CIC) were reported to be present in a proportion of patients with systemic sclerosis (31,98,112). However, some investigators using a ^{131}I-Clq binding assay, failed to detect them in a small series of patients (94,118), even in a patient with clinical evidence of renal involvement (94). Comparison of results obtained with various assays have shown that the Raji cell assay is the most sensitive (72% results), and Clq binding assay is the less sensitive one (24%). Agarose gel electrophoresis, as described by Kelly et al. (69), was positive in 52% of cases. Only 18% of sera were negative with all three assays (112). In this study, levels of IgG, ANA, and rheumatoid factor were all increased in CIC-positive patients. The Raji assay was most often abnormal in patients with diffuse scleroderma, whereas Clq binding assay showed comparable levels of immune complexes, both in diffuse scleroderma and in CREST syndrome. The findings of CIC correlated positively with serum rheumatoid factor and pulmonary involvement.

Our study was performed using an immunoelectrophoretic method described by Swierczynska et al. (124a); that is, polyethylene glycol (PEG) precipitation procedure followed by immunoelectrophoretic analysis of the sediment. This method allows the detection of CIC composed of antibodies of all immunoglobulin classes.

As shown in Table 8, 59% of sera tested were found to be positive for CIC. Sera from patients with diffuse scleroderma and acrosclerosis did not differ in the frequency of CIC findings. However, the highest incidence of positive results was in patients with an intermediate form of the disease.

As indicated in Table 9, there was no significant difference in the frequency of ANA in sera positive versus those that were negative for CIC (Table 9). However, approximate mean titers of ANA were somewhat higher in sera positive for CIC. RNP, Ro, La, and/or unidentified ENA autoantibodies were present in 37.5% of sera positive for CIC, while none were detected in sera negative for CIC. Anti-ssDNA antibodies,

Table 8. Occurrence of Immune Complexes in Patients with Various Types of Systemic Sclerosis

Varieties of systemic sclerosis	*No. of patients*	*Positive for immune complexes*	
		No.	*%*
Diffuse scleroderma	10	5	50
Intermediate form	5	4	80
Acrosclerosis	26	15	58
Total	41	24	59

Table 9. Comparison of the Presence of CIC, ANA and Other Autoantibodies in Patients with Systemic Sclerosis

Results of PEG sediment studies for CIC	*No. of samples studied*	*No. of samples positive for antibodies to*					
		ANA (titers)	*Native DNA (CLT)*[c]	*Denatured DNA (CIE)*[b]	*RNP*	*Sm*	*Ro/La and/or unidentified*
Positive	24	16 (66%) (40–1280; mean,640)	0	24	1	0	8
Negative	17	10 (about 59%) (40–640; mean, 160)	0	15	0	0	0
Total	41	26 (63.4%)	0	39 (95.1%)	1 (2.4%)	0	8 (19.5%)

[a]CLT, *Crithidia luciliae* test.
[b]CIE, counterimmunoelectrophoresis.

detected by counterimmunoelectrophoresis, were found in all CIC-positive sera and in 15 of 17 CIC-negative sera.

The pathogenic significance of immune complexes for visceral involvement, especially renal and pulmonary disturbances, is not known. However, a high incidence of their detection and their association with other serologic abnormalities are suggestive of a possible role in vascular damage.

IMMUNOPATHOLOGIC FINDINGS IN SCLERODERMA

DIF Findings in the Skin

DIF studies performed in the skin of patients with systemic sclerosis (58,68,103) generally failed to disclose immune deposits at the DEJ or in the dermal vasculature. Only some apparently nonspecific staining is found in telangiectatic areas (59). Winkelmann et al. (136,137) described mesenchymal or inflammatory scleroderma cases with some features of myositis or SLE; that is, with overlapping symptoms. In these patients, IF studies of the involved, sun-exposed skin demonstrated IgM immune deposits at the DEJ or vascular deposits, or both. Cases of scleroderma with overlap features were characterized by hypergammaglobulinemia, high titers of ANA (which were frequently of a speckled pattern), rheumatoid factor, elevated muscle enzyme levels, and positive LE cell test. These patients ususally gave favorable respoonse to steroids. DIF was proposed as the best method for identifying this variety of systemic scleroderma (29). In our experience, most cases of systemic sclerosis are negative on DIF, but some cases with features overlapping those of SLE are positive (5 of 66 lesional biopsy specimens in our series). On the other hand, Reimer et al. (101) reported granular IgM deposition in light-exposed skin of systemic sclerosis patients in 18 of 30 patients, and granular deposits in vessels in five of these cases. Deposition of IgG, IgM, and C3, as well as vascular deposits, were reported in vasculitis cases associated with systemic sclerosis (119).

Direct IF findings of nuclear IgG deposits are reviewed in the preceding section regarding anti-RNP antibodies.

Immunopathologic Studies of the Skin in Localized Scleroderma

Nishikawa (90) reported IgM deposition at the DEJ of lesional skin in 6 of 12 cases of morphea; at least two were of the linear scleroderma type. Immunoelectron microscopy performed in one case showed IgM deposition beneath the basal lamina, as in LE.

With the use of antihuman renal glomerulus antisera, the major immunopathologic finding in both localized and systemic sclerosis was intercollagenous staining for connective tissue antigens in the reticular layer of the dermis (105). This finding was interpreted as a collagen neogenesis.

Immunopathologic findings in the Visceral Organs and Muscle

Deposition of IgG immunoglobulins and complement and/or fibrin in arterioles and glomeruli of some scleroderma patients with renal involvement was interpreted as a nonimmunologic phenomenon. Immune deposits were reported to be present in renal vascular lesions (41,45) and in pulmonary hypertension associated with CREST (108).

IgM deposits were primarily demonstrated in the vessel walls of interstitial muscle tissue (134), and IgG deposits and complement, in a linear pattern, at the sarcolemma or subsarcolemmal zone (86). Vascular IgM deposition in the muscles of scleroderma patients is not such a common finding, as in childhood dermatomyositis (134).

REFERENCES

1. Alarcon-Segovia D, Fishbein E: Immunochemical characterization of the anti-RNA antibodies found in scleroderma and systemic lupus erythematosus. I. Differences in reactivity with Poly (U) and Poly (A) Poly (U) *J Immunol 115*:28, 1975.
2. Alarcon-Segovia D, Palacios R, DeKasep GI: Human postthymic precursor cells in health and disease. VII. Immunoregulatory circuits of the peripheral blood mononuclear cells from patients with progressive systemic sclerosis. *J Clin Lab Immunol* 5:143, 1981.
3. Alarcon-Segovia D, Ruiz-Argquelles A, Fishbein E: Antibody to ribonucleoprotein penetrates live human mononuclear cells through Fc receptors. *Nature* 271:67, 1978.
4. Alspaugh MA, Maddison P: Resolution of the identity of certain antigen-antibody systems in systemic lupus erythematosus and Sjögren's syndrome: An interlaboratory collaboration. *Arthritis Rheum* 22:796–798 1979.
5. Alspaugh MA, Tan EM: Antibodies to cellular antigens in Sjögren's syndrome. *J Clin Invest* 55:1067, 1975.
6. Anderson I, Andersen P, Elling P, et al: Epidermal nuclear immunoglobulin deposits in some connective tissue diseases: Correlation with ENA antibodies. *Ann Rheum Dis* 42:163, 1983.
7. Auerbach R: Angiogenesis-inducing factors: A review. In Pick E (Ed): *Lymphokines,* vol. 4. Academic Press, New York, 1981, pp 69–88.
8. Auerbach R, Sidky YA: Nature of the stimulus leading to lymphocyte induced angiogenesis. *J Immunol* 123:751, 1979.
9. Ausprunk DH, Felterman K, Folkman J: The sequence of events in the regression of corneal capillaries. *Lab Invest* 38:284, 1978.
10. Baron M, Keyston EC, Gladman DD, et al: Lymphocyte subpopulations and reactivity to mitogens in patients with scleroderma. *Clin Exp Immunol* 46:70, 1981.
11. Barthelmes H: Das Verhalten der antinukleären Faktoren bei Sklerodermie. *Dermatol Machr* 161:536, 1975.
12. Bernstein RM, Callender ME, Neuberger JM, et al: Anticentromere antibody in primary biliary cirrhosis. *Ann Rheum Dis* 41:612, 1982.
13. Beutner EH, Kumar V, Greenlee P: Basics in standardization and practical applications of immunofluorescent microscopy: Standardization of antinuclear antibody tests. In Aloisi R, Hyun J (Eds.): *Immunodiagnostics,* Alan R. Liss, New York, 1983, pp 49–70.
14. Bitterman PB, Crystal RG: Alveolar macrophages (AM) in idiopathic pulmonary fibrosis (IPF) and sarcoidosis are spontaneously secreting a growth factor causing human lung fibroblasts to replicate. *Clin Res* 49:443A, 1981.
15. Blaszczyk M, Beutner EH; Rogoziński T, et al: Substrate specificity of antinuclear antibodies in scleroderma. *J Invest Dermatol* 68:191, 1977.
16. Brentnall TJ, Kennally DA, Barnett AJ, et al: Antibodies to fibroblasts in scleroderma. *J Lab Clin Med* 1980.
17. Burnham TK: Antinuclear antibodies. A simplified classification of the nuclear immunofluorescent patterns. *Arch Dermatol* 114:1343, 1978.
18. Burnham TK, Bank PW: Antinuclear antibodies. I. Patterns of nuclear immunofluorescence. *J Invest Dermatol* 62:526, 1974.
19. Burnham TK, Fine G, Neblett TR: The immunofluorescent tumor imprint technique: II. The frequency of antinuclear factors in connective tissue diseases and dermatoses. *Ann Int Med* 65:9, 1966.
20. Burnham TK, Neblett TR, Fine G: The immunofluorescent tumor imprint technique. III. The diagnostic and prognostic significance of the "speckle" inducting antinuclear antibody. *Am J Clin Pathol* 50:683, 1968.
21. Burnham TK, Neblett TR, Fine G, et al: The immunofluorescent tumor imprint technique. *Arch Dermatol* 99:611, 1969.

22. Cathcart MK, Krakauer RS: Immunological enhancement of collagen accumulation in progressive systemic sclerosis (PSS). *Clin Immunol Immunopathol* 21:128, 1982.
23. Catoggio LJ, Bernstein RM, Black CM, et al: Serological markers in progressive systemic sclerosis: Clinical correlations. *Ann Rheum Dis* 42:23, 1983.
24. Chassagne J, Chollet Ph, Ferriere JP, et al: Correlation between active E-rosettes and antigens defined on peripheral lymphocytes by OTK 4 and OTK 8 monoclonal antibodies. *Immunol Lett* 4:335, 1982.
25. Chisarii FV, Edginton TS: Lymphocyte E rosette inhibitory factor: A regulatory serum lipoprotein *J Exp Med* 142:1092, 1975.
26. Chorzelski TP, Jablonska S, Beutner EH, et al: Anti-centromere antibody: An immunological marker of a subset of systemic scleroderma. *Br J Dermatol 113,* 381–389, 1985.
27. Claudy AL, Le Petit JC, Barthelemy H, et al: T-cell imbalance in progressive systemic sclerosis defined by monoclonal antibodies. *Arch Dermatol* 274:189, 1982.
28. Cohn ZA: The activation of mononuclear phagocytes: Fact, fancy and future. *J Immunol* 121:813, 1978.
29. Connolly SM, Winkelmann RK: Direct immunofluorescent findings in scleroderma syndromes. *Acta Dermatol Venereol* 61:29, 1981.
30. Cormane RH, Hamerlinck F, Nunzi E: Antibodies eluted from lymphoid cell membrane. *Ann Dermatol* 115:709, 1979.
31. Cunningham PH, Andrews BS, Davis JS: Immune complexes in progressive systemic sclerosis and mixed connective tissue disease. *J Rheumatol* 7:301, 1980.
32. Douvas AS, Achten M, Tan EM: Identification of a nuclear protein (Scl-70) as a unique target of human antinuclear antibodies in scleroderma. *J Biol Chem* 254:10514, 1979.
33. Fleischmajer R, Perlish JS:^{3}H-thymidine labeling of dermal endothelial cells in scleroderma. *J Invest Dermatol* 97::147, 1977.
34. Fleischmajer R, Perlish JS, Reeves JRT: Cellular infiltrates in scleroderma skin. *Arthritis Rheum* 20:975, 1977.
35. Fleischmajer R, Gay S, Meigel WN, et al: Collagen in the cellular and fibrotic stages of scleroderma. *Arthritis Rheum* 21:418, 1978.
36. Folkman J, Contran R: Relation of vascular proliferation to tumor growth. *Int Rev Exp Pathol* 16:207, 1976.
37. Friedrich W, O'Reilly RJ, Koziner B, et al: T-lymphocyte reconstitution in recipients of bone marrow transplants with and without GVHD: Imbalances of T-cell subpopulations having unique regulatory and cognitive functions. *Blood* 59:696, 1982.
38. Fritzler MJ, Kinsella TD, Garbutt E: The CREST syndrome. A distinct serologic entity with anticentromere antibodies. *Am J Med* 69:520, 1980.
39. Galoppin L, Saurat JH: In vitro study of the binding of antiribonucleoprotein antibodies to the nucleus of isolated living keratinocytes. *J Invest Dermatol* 76:264, 1981.
40. Garcia I, Wolbers R, Tan EM: Reactions between polyribonucleotides and low density lipoproteins in sera of patients with progressive systemic sclerosis. *J Immunol* 126:706, 1981.
41. Gerber MA: Immunohistochemical findings in the renal vascular lesions of progressive systemic sclerosis. *Human Pathol* 6:343, 1975.
42. Gilliam JN, Prystowski SD: Mixed connective tissue disease syndrome. Cutaneous manifestations of patients with epidermal nuclear staining and high titer serum antibody to ribonuclease-sensitive extractable nuclear antigen. *Arch Dermatol* 113:583, 1977.
43. Gliński W, Jablońska S: Subsets of progressive sclerosis with respect to experimental sensitization of patients to DNCB. Connective Tissue Diseases, Naples, Italy 5:14, 1986.
44. Gupta S, Malaviya AN, Rajagopalan P, et al: Subsets of human T lymphocytes: Imbalance of T cell populations in patients with progressive systemic sclerosis. *Clin Exp Immunol* 38:342, 1979.
45. Haustein UF: Das Gefässystem bei der progressiven Sklerodermie. *Dermatol Mschr* 162:721, 1976.
46. Heinzerling RH, Weyer R, Dziuba D, et al: Elevated levels of antibodies to polyuridilic acid detected and quantitated in systemic scleroderma patients by solid phase radioimmunoassay. *J Invest Dermatol* 75:224, 1980.

47. Horowitz DA, Garrett MA: Lymphocyte reactivity to mitogenes in subjects with SLE, RA and scleroderma. *Clin Exp Immunol* 27:92, 1977.
48. Hughes P, Holt S, Rowell NR: Leucocyte migration inhibition in progressive systemic sclerosis. *Br J Dermatol* 91:1, 1974.
49. Hughes P, Holt S, Rowell NR, et al: Thymus-dependent (T) lymphocyte deficiency in progressive systemic sclerosis. *Br J Dermatol* 95:469, 1976.
50. Hughes P, Holt S, Rowell NR, et al: The relationship of defective cell-mediated immunity to visceral disease in systemic sclerosis. *Clin Exp Immunol* 28:233, 1977.
51. Inoshita T, Whiteside TL, Rodnan GP, et al: Abnormalities of T lymphocyte subsets in patients with progressive systemic sclerosis (PSS, scleroderma). *J Lab Clin Med* 97:264, 1981.
52. Iwatsuki K, Tagami H, Imaizumi S, et al: The speckled epidermal nuclear immunofluorescence of mixed connective tissue disease seems to develop as an in vitro phenomenon. *Br J Dermatol* 107::653, 1982.
53. Izuno GT: Observation on in in vivo reaction of antinuclear antibodies with epidermal cells. *Br J Dermatol* 98:391, 1978.
54. Jabłońska S (Ed): *Scleroderma and Pseudoscleroderma.* Polish Medical Publishers, Warsaw, 1975.
55. Jablonska S, Rodnan GP: Localized scleroderma. In Rodnan GP (ed): *Clinics in Rheumatic Diseases.* Saunders, London, Philadelphia, Toronto, 1979.
56. Jabłońska S, Bubnow B, Lukasiak B: Acrosclerosis: A disease sui generis or a variety of diffuse scleroderma. *Br J Dermatol* 170:123, 1959.
57. Jabłońska S, Bubnow B, Lukasiak B: Ubergangsformen zwischen der Raynaud-schen Krankheit und der Sclerodermie. *Hautarzt* 6:278, 1960.
58. Jablonska S, Chorzelski T, Blaszczyk M: Role of autoimmunity (immunologic pheonomena in scleroderma). In Jablonska S (Ed): Scleroderma and Pseudoscleroderma. Polish Medical Publishers, Warsaw, 1975, pp. 15–35.
59. Jabłońska S, Chorzelski T, Maciejowska E: The scope and limitations of immunofluorescence method in the diagnosis of lupus erythematosus. *Br J Dermatol* 83:242, 1970.
60. Jaffee BD, Claman HN: Chronic graft versus host disease (GVHD) as a model for scleroderma. I. Description of model systems. *Cell Immunol* 77:1, 1983.
61. Jordon RE, Deheer D, Schroeter A, et al: Antinuclear antibodies. Their significance in scleroderma. *Proc Mayo Clin* 46:111, 1971.
62. Kahaleh MB, Osborn J, Le Roy EC: Increased factor (III)/von Willebrand factor antigen and von Willebrand factor activity in scleroderma and Raynaud's phenomenon. *Ann Intern Med* 94:482, 1981.
63. Kahaleh MB, Osborn J, LeRoy EC: Increased factor VIII/von Willebrand factor antigen and von Willebrand factor activity in scleroderma and Raynaud's phenomenon. *Ann Intern Med* 94::482, 1981.
64. Kahaleh MB, Sherar GK, LeRoy EC: Endothelial injury in scleroderma. *J Exp Med* 149:1326, 1979.
65. Kallenberg CGM, Pastoor GW, Wouda AA, et al: Antinuclear antibodies in patients with Raynaud's phenomenon: Clinical significance of anticentromere antibodies. *Ann Rheum Dis* 41:382, 1982.
66. Kallenberg CGM, de Jong MCJM, Walstra TM, et al: In vivo antinuclear antibodies (ANA) in biopsies of normal skin: Diagnostic significance and relation to serum ANA. *J Rheum* 10:733, 1983.
67. Kamiński MJ, Majewski S, Jabłońska S, et al: Lowered angiogeneic capability of peripheral blood lymphocytes in progressive systemic sclerosis (scleroderma). *J Invest Dermatol* 82:239, 1984.
68. Kay DM, Tuffanelli DL: Immunofluorescent technique in clinical diagnosis of cutaneous disease. *Ann Intern Med* 71:753, 1969.
69. Kelly RH, Scholl MA, Harvey VS, et al: Qualitative testing for circulating immune complexes by zone electrophoresis on agarose. *Clin Chem* 26:396, 1980.
70. Keystone EC, Lau C, Gladman DD, et al: Immunoregulatory T cell subpopulations in patients with scleroderma using monoclonal antibodies. *Clin Exp Immunol* 48:443, 1983.

71. Kleinsmith AM, Heinzerling RH, Burnham TK: Antinuclear antibodies as immunologic markers for a benign subset and different clinical characteristics of scleroderma. *Arch Dermatol* 118:882, 1982.
72. Kondo H, Rabin BS, Rodnan GP: Cutaneous antigen-stimulating lymphokine production by lymphocytes of patients with progressive systemic sclerosis (scleroderma). *J Clin Invest* 58:1388, 1976.
73. Krakauer RS, Sundeen J, Sauder DN, et al: Abnormalities of immunoregulation in progressive systemic sclerosis. Evidence for excess helper-cell function and altered B-cell function. *Arch Dermatol* 117:80, 1981.
74. Krawitt EL, Holdstock G, Bland JH, et al: Suppressor cell activity in progressive systemic sclerosis. *J Rheumatol* 9:263, 1982.
75. DeLustro F, LeRoy EC: Characterization of the release of human monocyte regulators of fibroblast proliferation. *J Reticuloendothel Soc* 31:295, 1982.
76. Mackel AM, DeLustro F, Harper FE, et al: Antibodies to collagen in scleroderma. *Arthritis Rheum* 25:522, 1982.
77. Maddison PJ, Mogavero H, Provost T, et al: The clinical significance of autoantibodies to a soluble cytoplasmic antigen in systemic lupus erythematosus and other connective tissue diseases. *J Rheumatol* 6:189, 1979.
78. Majewski S, Skopińska-Rozewska E, Jablonska S, et al: Modulatory effect of sera from scleroderma patients on the lymphocyte induced angiogenesis. *Arthritis Rheum* 28:1133, 1958.
79. Maricq HR: In vivo capillary microscopy for the clinician. *Arthritis Rheum* 21:173, 1978.
80. Maricq HR, LeRoy EC: Patterns of finger capillary abnormalities in connective tissue disease by "wide-field" microscopy. *Arthritis Rheum* 16:619, 1973.
81. Maricq HR, Spencer-Grean G, LeRoy EC: Skin capillary abnormalities as indicators of organ involvement in scleroderma (systemic sclerosis), Raynaud's syndrome and dermatomyositis. *Am J Med* 61:862, 1976.
82. Mattioli M, Reichlin M: Heterogeneity of RNA protein antigens reactive with sera of patients with systemic lupus erythematosus: Description of a cytoplasmic non-ribosomal antigen. *Arthritis Rheum* 17:421, 1974.
83. Mayes M, Cathcart M, Dustoor M: The role of immunoregulatory abnormalities in the immunopathogenesis of progressive systemic sclerosis. Proceedings of the Second International Conference on Progressive Systemic Sclerosis. Austin, Texas, October 20, 1982.
84. McCarty GA, Rico JR, Bembe ML, et al: Anticentromere antibody. Clinical correlations and association with favorable prognosis in patients with scleroderma variants. *Arthritis Rheum* 26:1, 1983.
85. McCarty GA, Valencia DW, Fritzler MJ et al: A unique antinuclear antibody staining only the mitotic-spindle apparatus. *N Engl J Med* 305:703, 1981.
86. Meffert H, Barthelmes H, Klug H, et al: Benziehungen zwischen morphologischen, immunologischen und klinischen Befunden bei progressiver Sklerodermie, dargestellt an der Muskulatur. *Dermatol Mschr* 161:556, 1975.
87. Moroi Y, Peebles C, Fritzier MF, et al: Complexity of antinuclear antibodies in scleroderma. *Arthritis Rheum* 22::640, 1979 (abstract).
88. Moroi Y, Peebles C, Fritzler MJ, et al: Autoantibody to centromere (kinetochore) in scleroderma sera. *Proc Natl Acad Sci* 77:1627, 1980.
89. Moroi Y, Murata I, Takeuchi A, et al: Human anticentriole autoantibody in patients with scleroderma and Raynaud's phenomenon. *Clin Immunol Immunopathol* 29:381, 1983.
90. Nishikawa T: Immunoglobulin deposition in the skin of localized scleroderma. Read at Maybashi Scleroderma Conference. October 1982.
91. Nishikawa T, Kurihara S, Sugiura A, et al: Localized scleroderma and PSS specific antibody to Og antigen. *Jpn J Dermatol* 91:859, 1981.
92. Northway JD, Tan EM: Differentiation of antinuclear antibodies giving speckled staining patterns in immunofluorescence. *Clin Immunol Immunopathol* 1:140, 1972.
93. Notman DD, Kurata N, Tan EM: Profile of antinuclear antibodies in systemic rheumatic diseases. *Ann Intern Med* 83:464, 1975.
94. O'Laughin S, Tappeiner G, Jordon RE: Circulating immune complexes in systemic scleroderma and generalized morphea. *Dermatologica* 160:25, 1980.

95. Osborn TG, Patel NJ, Ross GC, et al: Antinuclear antibody staining only centrioles in a patient with scleroderma. *N Engl J Med* 307:253, 1982.
96. Parker MD: Ribonucleoprotein antibodies: Frequency and clinical significance in systemic lupus erythematosus, scleroderma and mixed connective tissue disease. *J Lab Clin Med* 82:769, 1973.
97. Pietruszka M, Rabin BS: Abnormality of spontaneous lymphokine synthesis by lymphocytes of patients with connective tissue disorders. *Immunol Comm* 8:203, 1979.
98. Pisko E, Gallup K, Turner R, et al: Cardiopulmonary manifestations of progressive systemic sclerosis: Associations with circulating immune complexes and fluorescent antinuclear antibodies. *Arthritis Rheum* 22:518, 1979.
99. Prystowsky SD, Gilliam JN, Tuffanelli DL: Epidermal nuclear IgG deposition in clinically normal skin. *Arch Dermatol* 114::536, 1978.
100. LeRoy EC: Pathogenesis of scleroderma (Systemic sclerosis). *J Invest Dermatol* 79(Suppl i):87, 1982.
101. Reimer G, Huschka U, Keller J, et al: Immunofluorescence studies in progressive systemic sclerosis (scleroderma) and mixed connective tissue disease. *Br J Dermatol* 109:27, 1983.
102. Ritchie RF: Antinucleolar antibodies. Their frequency and diagnostic association. *N Engl J Med* 282:1174, 1970.
103. Rodnan GP: Progressive systemic sclerosis (scleroderma). In McCarty DJ (Ed): 9 *Arthritis and Allied Conditions,* ed. 9. Lea & Febiger, Philadelphia, 1979, pp 762–809.
104. Rodnan GP, Medsger TA, Buckingham RB: Progressive systemic sclerosis - CREST syndrome: Observations on natural history and late complications in 90 patients. *Arthritis Rheum* 23:423, 1975 (abstract).
105. Rowell NR, Scott DG: Immunohistological studies, with anti-connective tissue and anti-immunoglobulin antisera, of the skin in lupus erythematosus and scleroderma. *Br J Dermatol* 93:431, 1975.
106. Rutthorford R, Steffin K, Sexton J: Activated human mononuclear phyagocytes release a substance(s) that induces replication of quiescent human fibroblasts. *J Reticuloendothol Soc* 31:281, 1982.
107. Salem NP, Morse JH: Lymphocyte responses to mitogens in progressive systemic sclerosis. *Arthritis Rheum* 19:875, 1976.
108. Salerni R, Rodnan GP, Leon DF, et al: Pulmonary hypertension in the CREST syndrome variant of progressive systemic sclerosis (scleroderma). *Ann Intern Med* 86:394, 1977.
109. Schmidt JA, Mizel SB, Cohen D, et al: Interleukin I: A potential regulator of fibroblast proliferation. *J Immunol* 128:2177, 1982.
110. Scopelitis E, Biundo J, Jr, Alspaugh M: Anti-SS-A antibody and other antinuclear antibodies in systemic lupus erythematosus. *Arthritis Rheum* 23:287, 1980.
111. Segond P, Salliere D, Galanaud P, et al: Impaired primary in-vitro antibody response in progressive systemic sclerosis patients: Role of suppressor monocytes. *Clin Exp Immunol* 47:147, 1982.
112. Seibold JR, Rodnan GP, Medsger TA, et al: Circulating immune complexes in eosinophilic fasciitis. *Arthritis Rheum* 25:1180, 1982.
113. Sharp GC, Irvin WS, May CM, et al: Association of antibodies to ribonucleoprotein and Sm antigens with mixed connective-tissue disease, systemic lupus erythematosus and other rheumatic diseases. *N Engl J Med* 295:1149, 1976.
114. Shu S, Beutner EH: Studies on the apparent reactivity of ANA with viable cells. *Fed Proc* 35:512, 1976.
115. Shulman HM, Sale GE, Lerner KG, et al: Chronic cutaneous graft-versus-host disease in man. *Am J Pathol* 91:545, 1978.
116. Sidky YA, Auerbach R: Lymphocyte-induced angiogenesis: A quantitative and sensitive assay of the graft-vs-host reaction. *J Exp Med* 141:1084, 1975.
117. Simes MA, Johansson E, Rapola J: Scleroderma-like graft-versus-host disease as late consequences of bone-marrow grafting *Lancet* 2:831, 1977.
118. Sölling J, Sölling K, Jacobson KK: Circulating immune complexes in lupus erythematosus, scleroderma and dermatomyositis. *Acta Dermatol Venereol* 59:421, 1979.

119. Sönnichsen N, Brenke A, Barthelmes H, et al: Immunologische Befunde bei der progressiven Sklerodermie-diagnostische und nosologische Bedeutung. *Dermatol Mschr* 169:385, 1983.
120. Spielvogel RL, Goltz RW, Kersey JH: Scleroderma-like changes in chronic graft vs host disease. *Arch Dermatol* 113:1424, 1977.
121. Steen VD, Ziegler GL, Rodnan GP, et al: Clinical and laboratory associations of anticentromere antibody in patients with progressive systemic sclerosis. *Arthritis Rheum* 27:125, 1984.
122. Steffen C: Tissue antibodies in rheumatoid arthritis and other connective tissue diseases. *Ann Immunol* 1:47, 1969.
123. Stuart JM, Postlethweite AE, Káng AH: Evidences of cell-mediated immunity to collagen in progressive systemic sclerosis. *J Lab Clin Med* 88:601, 1976.
124. Subcommittee for Scleroderma Criteria of the American Rheumatism Association Diagnostic and Therapeutic Criteria Committee: Preliminary criteria for the classification of systemic sclerosis (scleroderma). *Arthritis Rheum* 23:581, 1980.
124[a] Swierczyńska Z, Woźniczko-Orłowska G, Rdułtowska H: A new method for the detection of circulating immune complexes by immunoelectrophoretic analysis. II. Studies on human pathological and normal sera. *Reumatologia* 17:279, 1979.
125. Takehara K, Moroi Y, Nakabayashi Y, et al: Antinuclear antibodies in localized scleroderma. *Arthritis Rheum* 26:612, 1983.
126. Tan EM, Rodnan GP, Garcia I, et al: Diversity of antinuclear antibodies in progressive systemic sclerosis. Anti-centromere antibody; Its relationship to CREST syndrome. *Arthritis Rheum* 23:617, 1980.
127. Thibierge G, Weissenbach RJ: Une forme de concretions calcaires sous-coutanées en relation avec la sclérodermie. *Bull Memr Soc Med Hôp* (*Paris*) 30:10, 1910.
128. Tsoi MS, Storb R, Jones E, et al: Deposition of IgM and complement at the dermo-epidermal junction in acute and chronic cutaneous graft-versus-host disease in man. *J Immunol* 120:1485, 1978.
129. Tuffanelli DL, McKeon F, Kleinsmith AM, et al: Anticentromere and anticentriole antibodies in the scleroderma spectrum. *Arch Dermatol* 119:560, 1983.
130. Villeneuve L: Role of adherent cells in graft-versus-host-induced suppression of the humoral immune response. *Scand J Immunol* 12:321, 1980.
131. Van Vloten WA, Scheffer E, Dooren LJ: Localized scleroderma-like lesions after bone marrow transplantation in man: A chronic graft versus host reaction. *Br J Dermatol* 96:337, 1977.
132. Wahl SM: Lymphocyte and macrophage derived fibroblast growth factors In Berk PD (Ed): *Myelofibrosis and the Biology of Connective Tissue,* Alan R. Liss, Inc., New York, 1983.
133. Wells VJ, Webb J, van Deventer M, et al: In vivo antinuclear antibodies in epithelial biopsies in SLE and other connective tissue diseases. *Clin Exp Immunol* 38:424, 1979.
134. Whitaker JN, Engel WK: Vascular deposits of immunoglobulin and complement in inflammatory myopathy. *Trans Am Neurol Assn* 96;24, 1971.
135. Williamson GG, Pennebaker J, Boyle JA: Clinical characteristics of patients with rheumatic disorders who possess antibodies against ribonucleoprotein particles. *Arthritis Rheum* 26:509, 1983.
136. Winkelmann RK: Pathogenesis and staging of scleroderma. *Acta Dermatol Venereol* 56:83, 1976.
137. Winkelmann RK, Carapeto FJ, Jordon RE: Direct immunofluorescence in the diagnosis of scleroderma syndromes. *Br J Dermatol* 96:231, 1977.
138. Winkelstein A, Rodnan GP, Heilman JD: Cellular immunity in progressive systemic sclerosis (scleroderma). *Ann Rheum Dis* 31:126, 1972.
139. Winterbauer RH: Multiple telangiectasia, Raynaud's phenomenon, sclerodactyly and subcutaneous calcinosis. A syndrome mimicking hereditary haemorrhagic telangiectasia. *Bull Johns Hopkins Hosp* 114:361, 1964.
140. Wright JK, Hughes P, Rowell NR: Spontaneous lymphocyte mediated (NK cell) cytotoxicity in systemic sclerosis. A comparison with antibody-dependent lymphocyte (K-cell) cytotoxicity. *Ann Rheum Dis* 41:409, 1982.
141. Zetter BR: Migration of capillary endothelial cells is stimulated by tumor-derived factors. *Nature* 285:41, 1980.

Section IV

OTHER DERMATOSES WITH SIGNIFICANT IMMUNOHISTOLOGIC FINDINGS

38
Wart Virus: Immunopathology

Stefania Jablonska
Maria Jarzabek-Chorzelska
Teresa Krainska
Tomasz Rogozinski

INTRODUCTION

Warts are epithelial tumors induced by human papillomavirus (HPV). They are, as a rule, self-limiting and regress spontaneously within 6 months to 2 years. Their regression is associated with immune responses of the host, and their persistence is generally associated with immune defects (11,12,20). Until recently, warts were presumed to be induced by a single type of HPV (30). The differences in their morphology were believed to depend mainly on the anatomic site of the lesions. The lack of a cell culture system allowing the propagation of wart viruses in vitro has impeded the characterization of the virus types present in clinically different cutaneous and mucosal lesions.

Papillomaviruses, which induce warts and papillomas in several animal species, proved to be highly host specific (20,26), so that animals are not suitable for studying HPVs. Recent studies with the use of molecular hybridization and restriction enzyme analysis have shown the existence of plurality—over 40 distinct HPV types inducing warts and wart-like lesions in humans. Preferential association of different virus types, with skin and mucosal lesions differing in morphology and location has been demonstrated (8,20,24,26).

There is also a growing body of evidence concerning the association of specific viruses with carcinomas. HPV-5 and HPV-8 genomes have been detected in cutaneous tumors of patients with epidermodysplasia verruciformis (12,14,21–23,27). Also, HPV-16 and HPV-18 genomes were found mainly in genital neoplasia and dysplastic lesions of the uterine cervix (6,10,37). Thus, HPVs differ in their biology. Some of them are associated with malignant neoplasia and seem to have an oncogenic potential.

HPV types cannot be differentiated in electron microscopy, (EM), since viral particles found in various warts do not differ in their structure and size. The type can be

Supported by grant PR6 of the National Polish Cancer Research Program.

determined by immunologic methods, if specific immune sera against the capsid protein antigens (i.e., virus-specific antisera) are available. However, at present, these are produced exclusively for experimental purposes.

SPECIFIC IMMUNE RESPONSES OF HPV-INDUCED LESIONS

Several techniques have been used for detecting circulating antibodies: immunodiffusion (28), complement fixation (1,7,9,28), radioimmunoassay (29), and immunofluorescence (IF) (17,33).

Since the studies were performed with the use of pooled wart virus and/or semipurified wart tissue antigens, the results are of limited value, and the procedures have to be repeated using characterized viral-specific antigens. Since viral particles in HPV-1 infection are much more abundant than in other cutaneous and mucosal lesions, the antigen for the first type-specific serologic study was prepared from plantar wart extract. With the use of purified HPV-1 virions, circulating antibodies to HPV-1 were found by a sensitive radioimmunoassay in 35% of nonselected adult individuals, and in about 50% of children between 5 to 15 years of age. Antibody activity paralleled a high incidence of infection with plantar warts in this age group (25). Our studies with the use of a less sensitive immunodiffusion technique revealed a lower incidence; that is, about 20% of HPV-1 infection in healthy adults (11). In further studies with the use of immunodiffusion, specific antibodies to HPV-2 were found in 25% of patients with common warts and in 12.5% of patients with persistent flat warts. There was no cross-reactivity; that is, specific anti-HPV-2 antibodies were not found in any patient with flat warts and vice versa (12).

The IF method allows the detection of capsid proteins in the nuclei of keratinized cells in the stratum granulosum and stratum corneum. Peroxidase-labeled immune sera may replace the IF procedure. Both the sensitivity and specificity of these two methods are comparable.

With the use of specific immune sera against purified virions of HPV-1, it is possible to visualize numerous large particles of viral antigen in the basophilic nuclei of keratinized cells of plantar warts (Fig. 1).

Using specific immune serum against purified HPV-2 virions, viral particles are detectable mainly in parakeratotic columns and in the upper keratinizing cells of common warts (Figs. 2 and 3). There is no cross-reactivity between these type specific immune sera. However, immune serum raised against purified virions of HPV-3, (i.e., virus-inducing flat warts in the general population and rare cases of epidermodysplasia verruciformis [EV]), does not reveal viral particles in all lesions of the flat wart type. This is due to the existence of HPV-3-related viruses, which were previously regarded as its subtypes. These viruses show less than 50% of sequence homology by cRNA-DNA hybridization experiments, and show different cleavage patterns in restriction enzyme analysis; they are therefore recognized as different types (24). Since HPVs are numbered according to the chronologic order of their identification, the new types were identified as HPV-10 and HPV-28.

Thus, HPV-3-type specific immune serum does not react with these related virus types, inducing flat warts or somewhat more elevated lesions, with a hyperkeratotic and proliferative surface; that is, with clinical features intermediate between the flat and common warts. The term transitional warts has recently been proposed for these lesions.

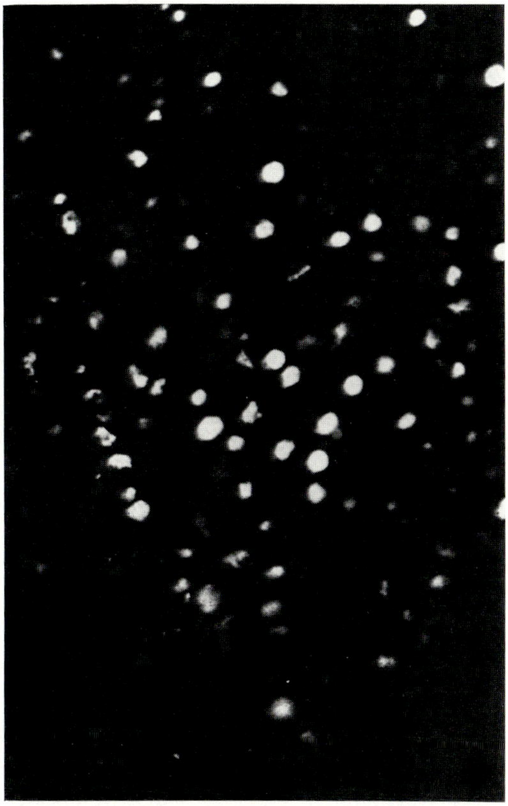

Figure 1. DIF staining with fluorescein-labeled guinea pig anti-HPV-1 immune serum. Protein concentration, 0.5 mg/ml; molar F/P ratio 2. Large viral HPV-1 antigens in the basophilic parakeratotic nuclei of a plantar wart (600×).

The HPV-3-related viruses have a cytopathogenic effect that is characteristic of HPV-3 type (vacuolated cells with small, heavily stained, somewhat pyknotic nuclei described as "bird's" eyes).

Since the immune sera against these new types are not available, IF is of limited value for identification of the causative viruses of flat warts. The IF method might be applied to detect EV-specific viruses in EV. A remarkable diversity of HPVs has been identified in EV: HPV-5, -8, -9, -12, -14, -15, -18, -19, -20 to -23, and others; and these viruses are EV specific (14,20–23,27). Some cases were shown to be associated with HPV-3 and HPV-10 (21,22). Patients infected with HPV-3 show flat wart-like lesions, a more protracted course, and less frequent malignant conversion. EV-specific viruses induce characteristic cutaneous changes; that is, reddish, brownish, or depigmented pityriasiform plaques, and very flat wart-like lesions. HPV-5 and HPV-8 were found in carcinomas associated with EV, and are therefore regarded as potentially oncogenic (22,23,27). Characteristically, several viruses could be identified from one patient, usually in different locations. Immune sera prepared from EV patients infected with nu-

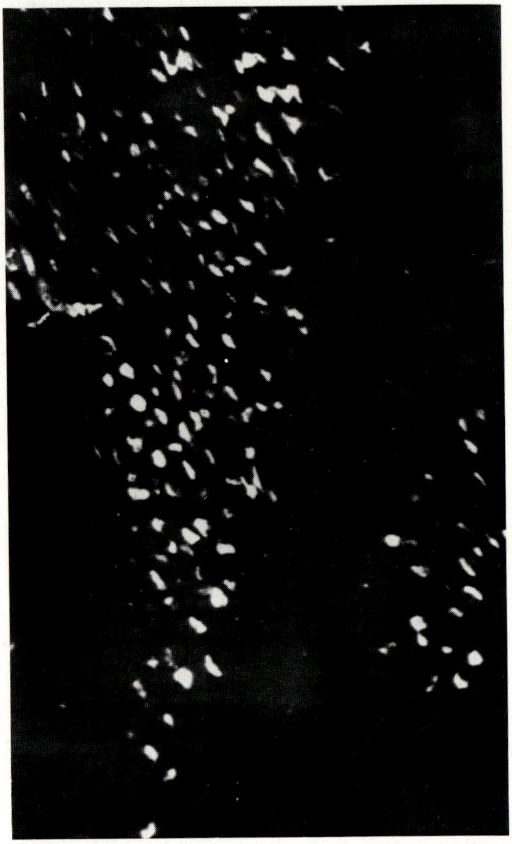

Figure 2. IIF test with guinea pig anti-HPV-2 immune serum at a dilution of 1:160, and fluorescein-labeled rabbit antiguinea pig IgG at a protein concentration of 0.5 mg/ml; molar F/P ratio 3. Viral particles appear in columnar arrangement within parakeratotic cells. Common wart (600×).

merous HPV types usually disclose the presence of EV-specific viruses, at least those that are closely related. In patients with mixed infections by non-EV-specific HPV-3 and EV-specific viruses, demonstration of such a double infection is possible by IF examination (Figs. 4 and 5), since there is no cross-reactivity between these virus types. Also, additional infections with HPV-1 or HPV-2 can be easily detected by IF. The complement-fixation IF technique, used for demonstration of the Epstein-Barr virus nuclear antigen (EBNA) (16,31), was also applied for detection of human papovavirus T antigens and HPVs in various warts and EV (3). This method is as specific as the indirect immunofluorescence (IIF) technique, and is superior to it in clarity of IF reading (i.e., no background or nonspecific staining) and with a somewhat higher sensitivity. If the concentration of viral particles is low, the routine IF method may not be sensitive enough. The IF complement-fixation test appears to be a more reliable method for detection of HPV types in cutaneous warts of different morphology.

Demonstration of specific virus types by IF is still not a routine procedure, because no specific immune sera against the main HPV types are commercially available.

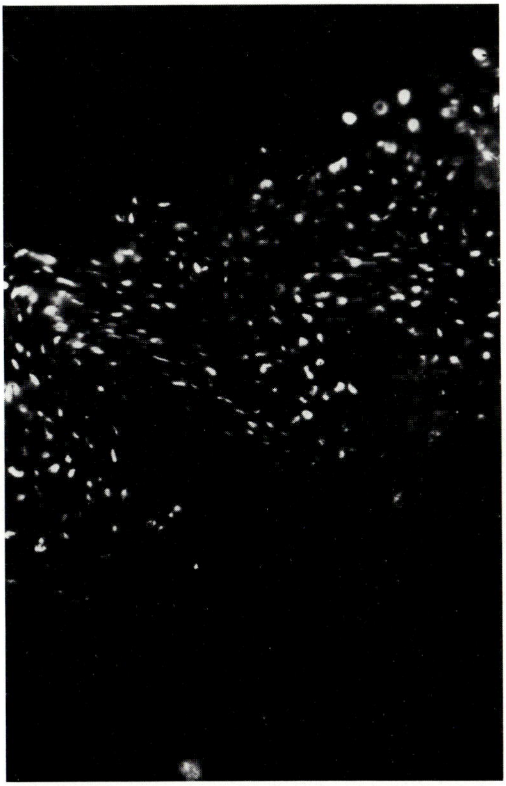

Figure 3. IIF test with guinea pig anti-HPV-3 immune serum at a dilution of 1:80, and the same fluorescein-labeled rabbit antiguinea pig IgG as in Figure 2. Viral antigens are present throughout the stratum corneum and granulosum. Flat wart (600×).

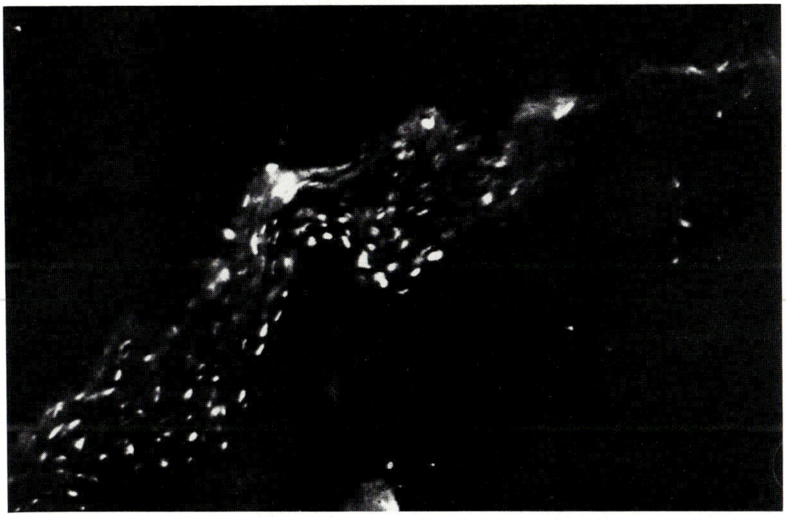

Figure 4. IIF test with guinea pig anti-HPV-3 immune serum at a dilution of 1:80, and the same fluorescein-labeled rabbit antiguinea pig IgG as in Figures 1 and 2. Epidermodysplasia verruciformis induced by HPV-3. Flat wart-like lesion (600×).

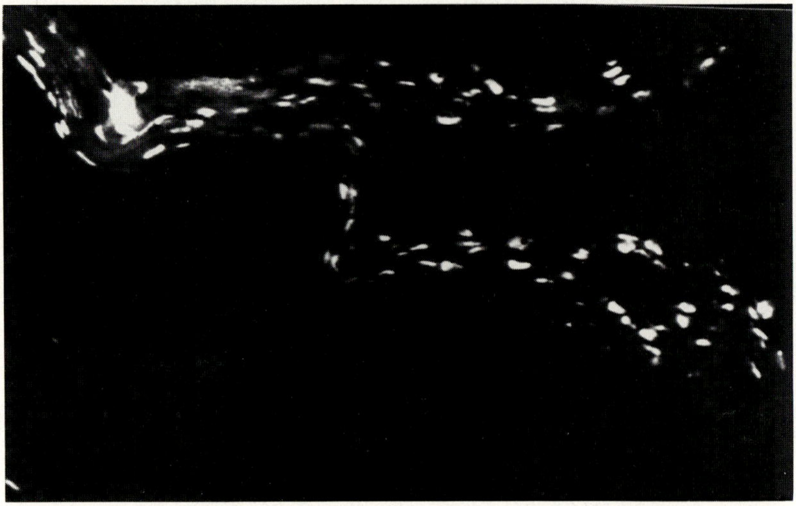

Figure 5. IIF test with guinea pig anti-HPV-5, -8, -9 immune serum at a dilution of 1:160, and the same fluorescein-labeled rabbit antiguinea pig IgG as in Figures 2 to 4. This immune serum detects viral antigens in the upper layers of a thinned epidermis in a patient found by molecular hybridization to be infected with HPV-5, -8, and other viruses. Epidermodysplasia verruciformis-red plaque (600×).

COMMON (GROUP-SPECIFIC) HPV ANTIGEN

Both IF and peroxidase-antiperoxidase (PAP) methods may be applied for detection of the papilloma virus (PV) common antigen in cutaneous and mucosal lesions. Its demonstration provides evidence for the presence of PV in a given lesion, without identification of virus type. The method is especially useful for the detection of as yet unidentified viruses, and for demonstration of HPV in lesions suspected of having a viral etiology. Since the immune serum is now commercially available,* these studies have a wide application.

IMMUNE SERUM AGAINST COMMON PAPILLOMA VIRUS ANTIGEN

Papilloma viruses (PV), despite their high specificity and noncross-reactive external capsidic antigens, were shown to share a common, genus-specific internal (structural) antigen (19). Antisera are prepared against purified viral particles disrupted with 1% sodium dodecyl sulfate (SDS). Since large quantities of virus are provided in HPV-1-induced infections (plantar warts) or experimentally induced bovine fibropapilloma (BPV-1), these two viruses are mainly used for preparing immune sera. The sera detect all PV in humans, cattle, Shope papilloma of rabbits, or other species. Common PV antigen may be demonstrated by IIF on frozen sections or by PAP on sections of formalin-fixed, paraffin-embedded tissues. In this way, specimens from

*Dako Corp., Santa Barbara, CA 93101. Code No. 521.

tumors of unknown origin, which have been stored in paraffin blocks, can be studied for presence of group-specific PV antigen. The PAP test with the use of SDS-disrupted viral particles is also applied for cytologic preparations. If paraffin blocks are not available, hematoxylin and eosin (H&E) stained sections or Papanicolau stained cytology preparations can be restained by PAP (13). In the PAP method, positive brownish staining is intranuclear, and confined, in cutaneous warts to keratinizing and parakeratotic cells (Fig. 6).

In the mucosal lesions, the staining is most pronounced in the nuclei of koilocytes and dyskeratocytes (15,18). Positive staining provides evidence for the presence of HPV. However, negative results occur in about half of the specimens of various cutaneous warts, and in oral and laryngeal papillomas (13).

PAP test for PV common antigen was reported to be positive in 7 of 15 patients with juvenile laryngeal papillomas, but negative in specimens from six patients with the adult form (2). Of special significance is the PAP test for gynecologic studies. Crum et al. (5) reported 75% positive results in cervical condylomata, whereas only 16% of lesions of atypical immature squamous metaplasia were positive; none of cervical in situ neoplasia (CIN) were positive. In another series of vulvar intraepithelial neoplasia, 4 of 68 specimens (6%) stained positively for PV common antigen, whereas only 1 of 35 (3%) aneuploid lesions was positive (4). There was also an inverse relationship between the presence of mitotic abnormalities and the expression of HPV antigen. The staining for PV was positive only in 23% of lesions with abnormal mitotic figures, which in a great majority were aneuploid (36).

Cervical dysplasias show a variable expression of HPV antigen. Positive results were reported in 30 to 40% of mild dysplasia, and in only about 20% of moderate dysplasias (13).

Immunoperoxidase staining for PV is a useful method for distinguishing benign from malignant vulvar and cervical neoplasias. Detection in some cases of PV antigen within aneuploid epithelium is evidence that HPV infection may progress into CIN (32).

Capsid protein production and virion assembly are readily detectable in condylomas and mild dysplasia, but not in CIN (4,32,36), since the epithelial maturation is required for virus assembly. Not infrequently, however, malignant lesions are found to contain specific HPV genomes, which can be characterized by molecular hybridization (22,37).

PV group-specific antigen could be detected in only 2 of 21 cases of bowenoid papulosis, and in 1 of 35 aneuploid lesions of vulvar intraepithelial neoplasia (4). A much more sensitive method of molecular hybridization permitted demonstration of a striking association of bowenoid papulosis with HPV-16 (6,10,37). HPV-16 and HPV-18 genomes were also found in other malignant lesions (6,10). The structural viral antigen is no longer expressed here, since its expression requires terminally differentiated keratinocytes.

Immunocytochemical methods for detection of group PV antigen are especially useful for differentiation between cervical condylomas and dysplasias. Positive results are suggestive of more benign lesions that are possibly contagious for a sexual partner, but with no immediate danger of malignant transformation. The method is simple and much more sensitive than EM, which is time consuming and does not easily disclose sparce viral particles. If cytologic or histologic preparations are positive for viral particles in EM, there is, as a rule, full agreement with cytochemical method for detection of group PV antigen.

Until specific antisera against HPV types are commercially available, PAP tests with immune sera against common structural antigens may be used for identification of PV associated with cutaneous or mucosal papillomas.

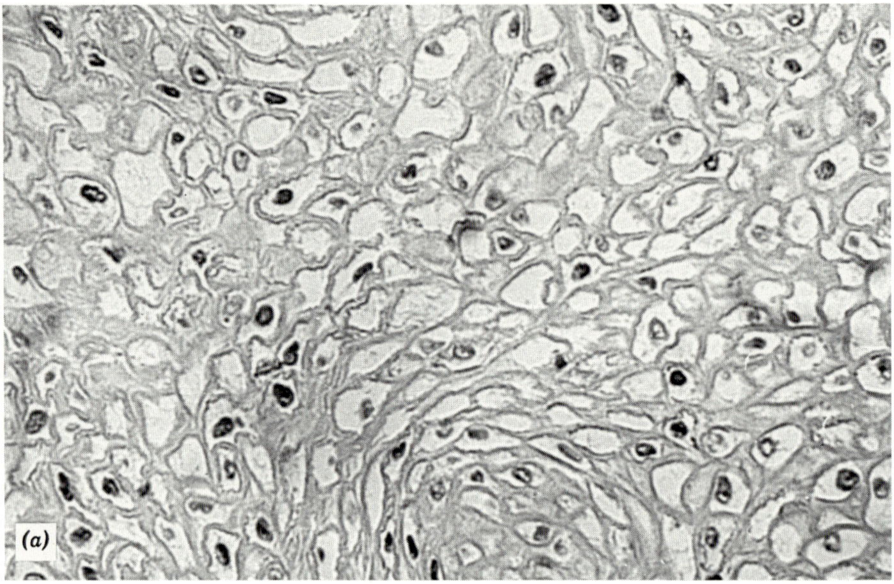

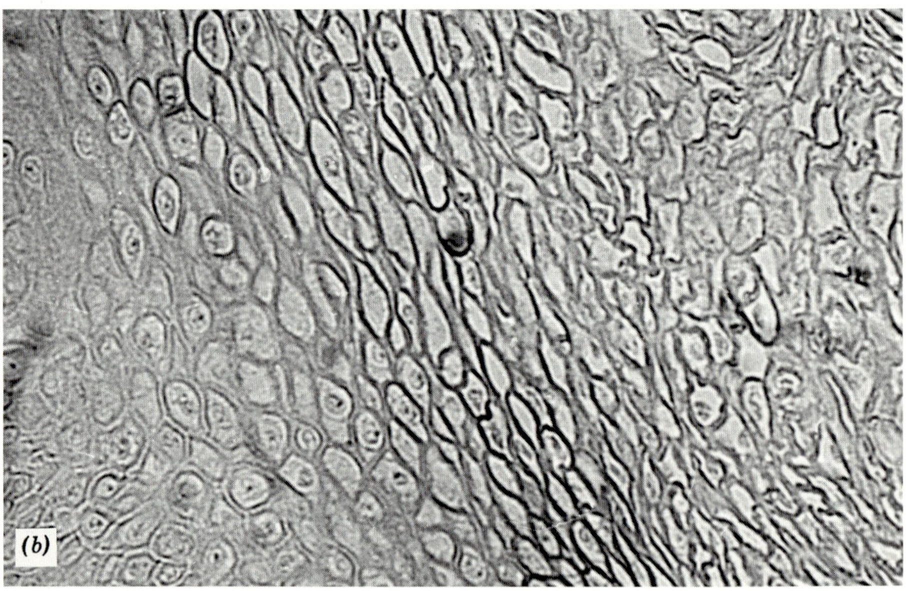

Figure 6. A. PAP staining with rabbit immune serum antidisrupted viral particles BPV-1 at a dilution of 1:25, goat antirabbit IgG in a dilution of 1:20, and rabbit PAP complexes in a dilution of 1:50. Viral antigens are seen as the brownish-stained nuclei of the koilocytes. Flat condyloma of the cervix uteri (600×). B. Control negative staining of the serial sections of the same specimen. Normal rabbit immune serum at a dilution of 1:25; goat antirabbit IgG and rabbit PAP complexes are at the same dilutions as in Figure 6A.

REGRESSING WARTS

Lymphocytes, macrophages, and Langerhans cells are associated with the regression of warts. Tagami et al. (34) believe that the attack of mononuclear cells is immunologically mediated, and is directed against the tumor cells transformed by virus (i.e., against wart tumor antigens). IF studies showed marginal IgM in parakeratotic nuclei; Tagami et al. considered this to be a specific reaction of antivirus antibody with the wart antigen (34). The role of cellular immunity is also suggested by the regression of flat warts, which suddenly become inflamed, edematous, and regress within a few weeks. With the degenerative changes in the epidermis and destruction of the proliferating rete ridges, the histologic features of the wart and the cytopathic effect are no longer recognizable as such.

Regression of common and plantar warts has not been studied in much detail. Besides invasion of inflammatory cells into the epidermis, there are perivascular infiltrates, hemorrhages, and thromboses. These features are suggestive of the role of specific humoral responses shown by IF (17) and other serologic methods (28,29) by use of immune sera against pooled wart antigens.

IMMUNE DEPOSITS IN THE STRATUM CORNEUM OF WARTS

Immune deposits in the stratum corneum (SC), although highly characteristic of psoriasis, may be encountered in various dermatoses, among others in HPV-induced tumors (Table 1).

Direct immunofluorescent (DIF) staining for in vivo-bound IgG, IgM, IgA, and complement (C3) was positive in a majority of the 47 warts studied. The pattern of apparent in vivo binding of SC antibodies characteristic of psoriasis was found in about one third of the specimens in both common warts and regressing flat warts in a similar frequency. Diffuse and focal diffuse staining, which can occur in various dermatoses, was also found in different types of warts.

IF staining in common warts may be similar to or identical with that found in

Table 1. Direct IF[a] in warts

Type of warts (no.)	*IF pattern*: Diffuse and *focal/diffuse nonpsoriatic pattern (no./%)*	*IF pattern*: *Focal psoriatic pattern (no./%)*
Plantar warts (4)	4(100)	0
Common warts (17)	6(35)	7(41)
Flat warts (4)	2(50)	1(25)
Regressing flat warts (22)	5(23)	7(32)
Total (47)	17(36)	15(32)

[a]IF tests for IgG, IgA, IgM, and complement C3.

psoriasis (35). Immune deposits are confined here to areas of parakeratotic columns harboring the virus. The presence of SC antibodies in these places could be a part of the repair mechanism (see Chap. 7), since replication of the virus is closely related to the terminal differentiation of keratinocytes; and also, the viral infection may induce changes in the structure and biology of keratin.

Regressing flat warts were not found to be associated with a significantly higher incidence of immune deposits. The histologic pattern of regressing warts has a close similarity to psoriasis; notably, papillomatosis and acanthosis with no discernible cytopathic effect, atrophy of the granular layer, and widespread parakeratosis. However, the basic difference consits of penetration of the activated mononuclear cells into the epidermis through the rete ridges, and not through the elongated papillae, as in psoriasis.

It is conceivable that lymphocytes and macrophages are activated by specific wart tissue-associated antigens located above the proliferating rete ridges; but this has yet to be documented experimentally for HPV. In psoriasis, inflammatory infiltrates penetrate into the SC through the "squirting papilla," and the formation of immune deposits starts above the papillae, becoming progressively more widespread throughout the entire SC. In verrucae, IF staining is usually focal and confined to the parakeratotic columns.

CONCLUSION

Immune deposition detected by IF in the SC (presumably SC antibodies) of some warts could be a secondary phenomenon; that is, a result of the presence of virus in the nuclei of keratinized cells, rather than a part of immune responses associated with human PV. It is also conceivable that the SC antibody binding may play a role in the regression of the warts via the autoimmune repair mechanism.

ACKNOWLEDGMENTS

We would like to thank Dr. G. Orth (Institut Pasteur) for the preparation of immune sera and for characterization of HPV types in the patients.

REFERENCES

1. Beth E, Cikes M, Giraldo G: Microfluorometric analysis of anti-complement and indirect immunofluorescence tests for human papovavirus (ICV and BKV) antigens. *Int J Cancer* 2:1–5, 1978.
2. Braun L, Kashima H, Eggleston J, et al: Demonstration of papillomavirus antigen in paraffin sections of laryngeal papillomas. *Laryngoscope* 92:640–643, 1982.
3. Chorzelski T, Jarząbek-Chorzelska M, Jablonska S, et al: An immunofluorescence complement-fixation test for detection of human papilloma viruses in various warts and wartlike lesions of epidermodysplasia verruciformis. *Arch Dermatol Res* 275:53–57, 1983.
4. Crum ChP, Braun LA, Shah KV, et al: Vulvar intraepithelial neoplasia: Correlation of nuclear DNA content and the presence of a human papilloma virus (HPV) structural antigen. *Cancer* 49:468–471, 1982.
5. Crum ChP, Egawa K, Yao SF, et al: Atypical immature metaplasia (AIM): A subset of human papilloma virus infection of the cervix. *Cancer* 51:2214–2219, 1983.

6. Durst M, Gissman L, Ikenberg H, et al: A papilloma-virus DNA from a cervical carcinoma and its prevalence in cancer biopsy samples from different geographic regions. *Proc Natl Acad Sci USA* 80:3812–3815, 1983.
7. Genner J: Verrucae vulgares II. Demonstration of a complement fixation reaction. *Acta Dermatol Venereol* 51:365–373, 1971.
8. Gissmann L, Pfister H, zur Hausen H: Human papilloma viruses (HPV): Characterization of four different isolates. *Virology* 76:569–580, 1977.
9. Hefton JM, Eisenger M: A quantitative micro-complement fixation method in studies of human wart viruses. *J Gen Virol* 38:179–182, 1977.
10. Ikenberg H, Gissmann L, Gross G, et al: Human papillomavirus type-16-related DNA in genital Bowen's disease and in bowenoid papulosis. *Int J Cancer* 32:563–565, 1983.
11. Jablonska S, Orth G, Gliński W, et al: Morphology and immunology of human warts and familial warts. In Bachmann PA (Ed): *Leukaemias, Lymphomas and Papillomas: Comparative Aspects*. Taylor and Francis, London, 1980, pp 107–131.
12. Jabłońska S, Orth G, Lutzner MA: Immunopathology of papilloma-virus-induced tumors in different tissues. *Springer Sem Immunopathol* 5:33–62, 1982.
13. Jensen AB, Lancaster WD, Hartmann DP, et al: Frequency and distribution of papillomavirus structural antigens in verrucae, multiple papillomas, and condylomata of the oral cavity. *Am J Pathol* 107:212–218, 1982.
14. Kremsdorf D, Jablonska S, Favre M, et al: Biochemical characterization of two types of human papillomaviruses associated with epidermodysplasia verruciformis. *J Virol* 43:436–447, 1982.
15. Kurman RJ, Sanz LE, Jenson AB, et al: Papillomavirus infection of the cervix: I. Correlation of histology with viral structural antigens and DNA sequences. *Int J Gynecol Pathol* 1:17–28, 1982.
16. Liabeuf A, Nelson RA Jr, Kourilsky FM: The detection of the Epstein-Barr virus (EBV) nuclear antigen (EBNA) by anticomplement immunofluorescence. Immunoglobulin class of antibodies and role of complement. *Int J Cancer* 15:533–556, 1975.
17. Matthews RS, Shirodaria PV: Study of regressing warts by immunofluorescence. *Lancet* 1:689–691, 1973.
18. Maisels A, Morin C, Casas-Cordero M: Human papillomavirus infection of the uterine cervix. *Int J Gynec. Pathol* 1:75–94, 1982.
19. Orth G, Breitburd F, Favre M: Evidence for antigenic determinants shared by the structural polypeptides of (Shope) rabbit papillomavirus and human papillomavirus type 1. *Virology* 91:243–255, 1978.
20. Orth G, Jablonska S, Breitburd F, et al: The human papillomaviruses. *Bull Cancer* (*Paris*) 65:151–164, 1978.
21. Orth G, Jablonska S, Favre M, et al: Characterization of two types of human papillomaviruses in lesions of epidermodysplasia verruciformis. *Proc Natl Acad Sci* 75:1537–1541, 1978.
22. Orth G, Favre M, Breitburd F, et al: Epidermodysplasia verruciformis: A model for the role of papillomaviruses in human cancer. In Essex M, Todaro G, van Hausen H (Eds): *Viruses in Naturally Occurring Cancers*. [Cold Spring Harbor Laboratory] New York, 1980, pp 259–282.
23. Ostrow RS, Bender M, Niimura M, et al: Human papillomavirus DNA in cutaneous primary and metastasized squamous cell carcinoma from patients with epidermodysplasia verruciformis. *Proc Natl Acad Sci USA* 79:1634–1638, 1982.
24. Ostrow R, Zachow KD, Watts S, et al: Characterization of two HPV-3 related papillomaviruses from common warts that are distinct clinically from flat warts or epidermodysplasia verruciformis. *J Invest Dermatol* 80:436–440, 1983.
25. Pfister H, zur Hausen H: Seroepidemiological studies of human papilloma virus (HPV-1) infections. *Int J Cancer* 21:161–165, 1978.
26. Pfister H, Gissmann L: Heterogeneity of human papilloma viruses. *Bull Cancer* 65:165–167, 1978.
27. Pfister H, Nurnberger F, Gissmann L, et al: Characterization of a human papillomavirus from epidermodysplasia verruciformis lesions of a patient from Upper-Volta. *Int J Cancer* 27: 645–650, 1981.

28. Pyrhonen S, Johansson E: Regression of warts: An immunological study. *Lancet* 1:592–595, 1975.
29. Pyrhonen S, Jablonska S, Obałek S, et al: Immune reactions in epidermodysplasia verruciformis. *Br J Dermatol* 102:247–254, 1980.
30. Rawson KEK, Mahy BWJ: Human papova (wart) virus. *Bacteriol Rev* 31:110–131, 1967.
31. Reedman BM, Klein G: Cellular localization of an Epstein-Barr virus (EBV)-associated complement-fixing antigen in producer and non-producer lymphoblastoid cell lines. *Int J Cancer* 11:499–520, 1973.
32. Reid R, Crum ChP, Herschman BR, et al: Genital warts and cervical neoplasia are linked by a spectrum of continuous morphologic and biologic change. *Cancer* 53:943–953, 1984.
33. Shirodaria PV, Matthews RS: An immunofluorescence study of warts. *Clin Exp Immunol* 21:329–338, 1975.
34. Tagami M, Ogushi M, Ofuji S: The phenomenon of spontaneous regression of numerous flat warts. *Cancer* 45:2557–2563, 1980.
35. Weiss VC, van den Brock H, Barrett S, et al: Immunopathology of psoriasis: A comparison with other parakeratotic lesions. *J Invest Dermatol* 78:256–260, 1982.
36. Winkler B, Crum ChP, Fujii T, et al: Koilocytotic lesions of the cervix. The relationship of mitotic abnormalities to the presence of papillomavirus antigens and nuclear DNA content. *Cancer* 53:1081–1087, 1984.
37. Zachow KR, Ostrow RS, Bender M; et al: Detection of human papillomavirus DNA in anogenital neoplasia. *Nature* 300:771–773, 1982.

39 Lichen Planus

Wilma Fowler Bergfeld

Rafael Valenzuela

Ernst H. Beutner

INTRODUCTION

Lichen planus (LP) is a papulosquamous disease of unknown etiology that involves the skin, mucous membranes, and nails. Clinically, it is characterized on skin by *violaceous* pruritic papules with superficial white lines: Wickham's striae (Fig. 1). LP is observed most frequently on the flexural areas of the body, but has also been observed in other areas including mucous membranes, scalp, genitalia, nail beds, and nail matrix. On the mucous membranes, the lesions present as white, lattice-like lines, as painful ulcerations, or as desquamative gingivitis.

Lichen planus presents as an acute, self-limiting disorder or a chronic recurrent disease, that affects men and women between 30 to 60 years of age. Common to both acute and chronic LP is an isomorphic, Koebner phenomena, which is a response of normal skin to trauma wherein LP is produced at the site of skin trauma.

Lichen planus-like lesions have been induced by a number of drugs that include gold (44) and other metals, streptomycin, tetracycline hydrochloride, para-aminosalicylic acid, antimalarial thiazide diuretics (57), penicillamine (51), hydrourea (33), fluorouracil (29), pyrithinol HCl (31), quindine (7), and photographic developing materials (47).

Even though LP is of unknown etiology, a literature review suggests a genetic predisposition, associated autoimmune diseases, and precipitating factors such as drugs. An attempt to demonstrate genetic predisposition was revealed in several reports of increased HLA frequencies; for example, HLA-A3 (53), HLA-B7 (36), and HLA-A28 (25), none of which have been statistically significant.

Other studies suggesting an autoimmune etiology of LP have reported that patients with LP have diminished peripheral IgA and IgM immunoglobulins, suggesting a B-cell deficiency (54). In contrast, immunohistochemistry studies of LP lesions demonstrate a predominantly T-cell infiltrate, with prominence of T-helper cells (3). LP has also been reported in association with diabetes (45), myasthenia gravis and thymoma (5), and biliary cirrhosis (24). Other interesting findings include reported overlap presentations with lupus erythematosus (LE) (32,48), bullous pemphigoid (BP) (34,55), psoriasis (39), and chronic graft-versus-host disease (GVHD) (49). All of these findings suggest an immunologic etiology of LP.

This work was supported, in part, by the IF Testing Service, Buffalo, NY.

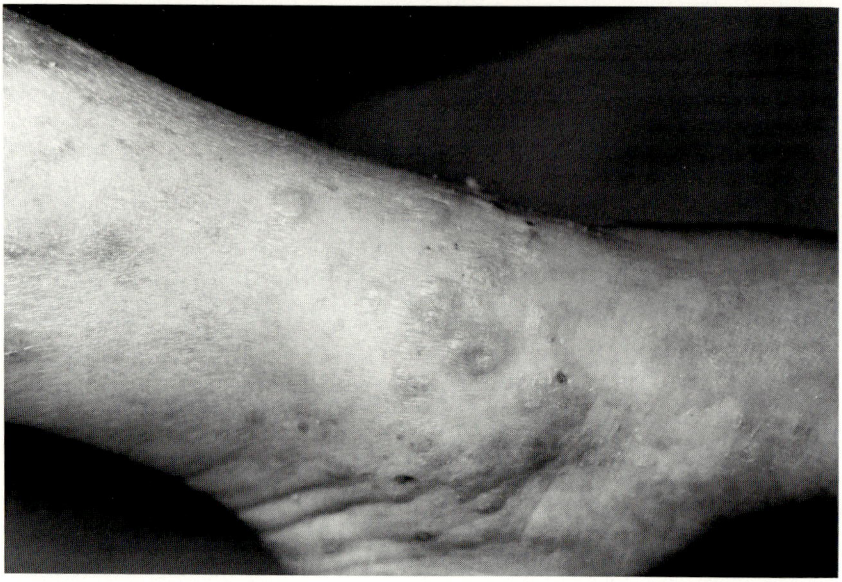

Figure 1. Typical violaceous papules of LP.

LIGHT MICROSCOPY

Characteristic histologic findings of LP include a lichenoid interface, chronic dermal infiltrate composed of lymphocytes, some macrophages, and (in the early lesions) diminished Langerhans cells. The epidermis may vary in thickness and demonstrate hyperkeratosis with acanthosis or atrophy. A striking hypergranulosis is usually present in all lesions. Basilar vacuolization, patchy and diffuse, can also be observed (Fig. 2). Subepidermal bullae are an occasional feature, and are especially observed in the atrophic LP lesions. Other features, including globular, homogeneous, eosinophilic, diastase-resistant, periodic acid Schiff (PAS) positive deposits (eosinophilic, hyaline, Sabouraud's bodies, and apoptotic cells) (6,21,22,36,40,56,59), are observed within the papillary dermis in small and large clumps (2); they may be observed within the adventitial dermis of telogen hair follicles (4,30). Other cells within the dermal infiltrate include melanophages and infrequent plasma cells. Acute inflammatory cells, eosinophils, and neutrophils are occasionally seen in very early lesions of LP. Exocytosis of lymphocytes in areas of focal epidermal spongiosis can also be observed in the more acute lesions.

IMMUNOHISTOCHEMISTRY AND IMMUNOFLUORESCENT PATTERNS

Immunohistochemistry reveals the dermal lichenoid infiltrate to be composed predominantly of T lymphocytes, especially T helper-inducer cells, which are OK T4+. There have also been reported increased numbers of OK T6+ Langerhans cells in older lesions (3,12,14,52).

The eosinophilic, homogeneous globules principally demonstrate deposits of immunoglobulin IgM; however, IgG and IgA with fibrin and complement can also be ob-

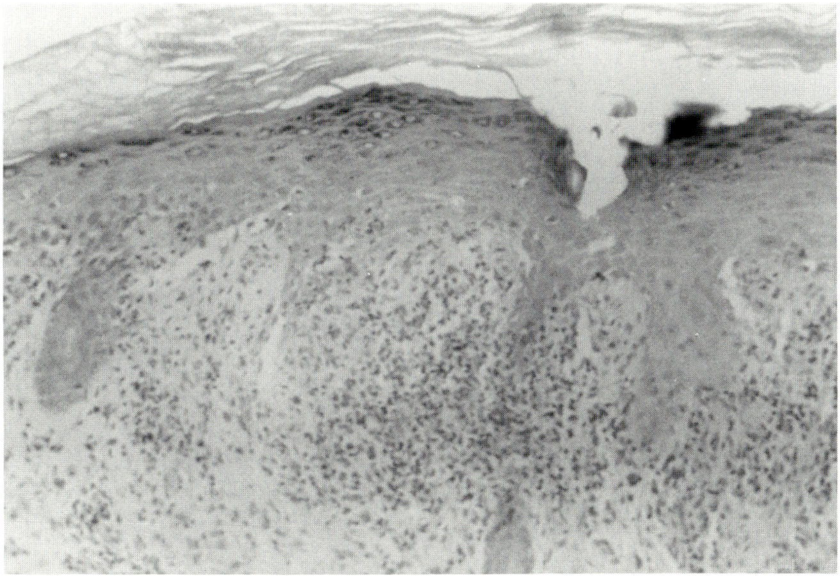

Figure 2. Lichenoid dermatitis with focal basilar vacuolization. The epidermis shows acanthosis, hypergranulosis, and hyperkertosis (H&E, 100×).

served (1,6,26). The globules cluster in groups of 10 or more, which may be helpful in differentiating LE from LP (31,57). The globules are round or oval, homogeneous, sharply marginated, and vary in size from 50 to 100 μ (Figs. 3 to 5). The oral lesions of LP may not contain the numerous papillary dermal globules; therefore, the histologic picture can be confused with LE. These globular deposits may be demonstrated in clinically uninvolved skin in 33 to 50% of all cases. Although most of the deposits are localized in the papillary dermis adjacent to the dermal-epidermal junction (DEJ), occasionally globular deposits can be found within the epidermis, the reticular dermis, and along hair follicles. In cases of alopecia (lichen planopilaris), globular deposits may be present in the external root sheath of hair follicles or just adjacent to the sheath within the adventitial dermis (30). In addition to globular deposits, a diffuse band of fibrin (1,6) has been shown along the DEJ and around follicular structures of active LP papules. Globular dermal deposits are usually not detected in lichen nitidus (58). The globular deposits of LP can also be demonstrated with different immunoperoxidase techniques (Fig. 6).

A diversity of immunofluorescent (IF) patterns are observed in desquamative gingivitis—a clinical condition that must be separated into its various clinical entities, including LP, LE, pemphigus, cicatricial pemphigoid, and psoriasis (23,35,41,50).

The presence of globular deposits of immunoglobulins and complement in the papillary dermis is not pathognomonic of LP. Similar deposits have been found in systemic lupus erythematosus (SLE), mixed connective tissue disease (MCTD), dermatomyositis, scleroderma, drug-induced LE, polymorphous light eruption, dermatitis herpetiformis (DH), bullous pemphigoid, pemphigus, porphyria cutanea tarda, erythema nodosum, drug eruption, eczema, lichen sclerosis et atrophicans, epidermolysis bullous simplex, erythema multiforme, granuloma annulare, neurodermatitis, Degos' malignant pustulo-

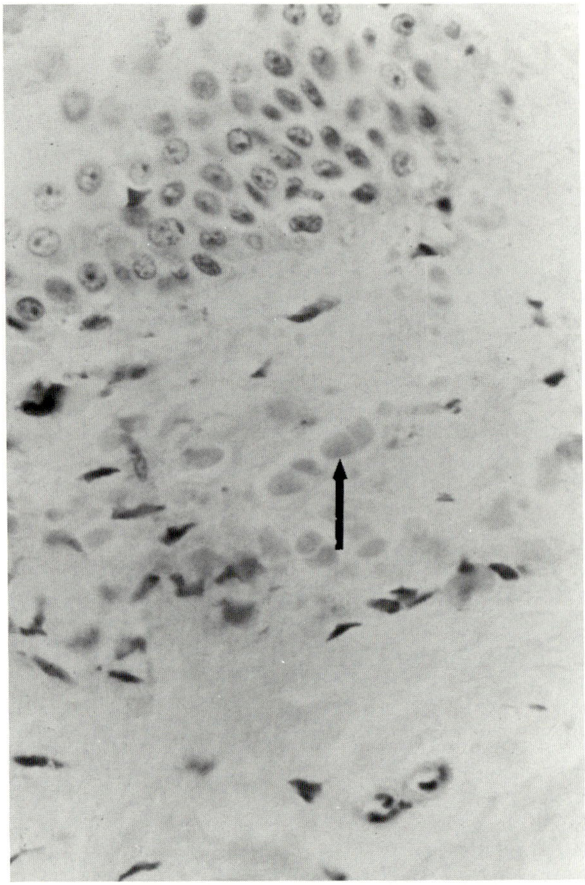

Figure 3. Globular hyaline bodies (arrow). These retain PAS positivity after diastase digestion, demonstrating a component of polysaccharides (PAS, 2244×). (Reprinted with permission from *Am J Clin Pathol* 79:486, 1983.)

sis, mycosis fungoides, pyoderma gangrenosum, poikiloderma congenitale (Rothman-Thomson syndrome), vasculitis, vitiligo, lichenoid eruptions of drug-versus-host reaction, and other dermatoses (1,22,40,56,57).

As indicated below, electron microscopic (EM) observations relate these globules to degenerated epithelial cells and apoptosis (20,27,38). Several immunologic studies indicate that the immunoglobulins in the globular deposits are physiologic autoantibodies that can bind in vivo to dead or altered epidermal cells (8). These antibodies (10), referred to variously as upper cytoplasmic or keratinocyte cytoplasm antibodies, are now recognized as being present in all normal sera (see Chap. 40). Other observations indicate that the stratum corneum (SC) antibodies seen by IF (9) are the same as the upper cytoplasmic antibodies (28; Chap. 40). The role of the apparent in vivo reactions of these antibodies with globular deposits appears to be to aid in the removal of degenerate epithelial cells (Chap. 7), quite possibly by apoptosis (8). In effect, the studies on the role of physiologic autoantibodies in normal repair mechanisms of the

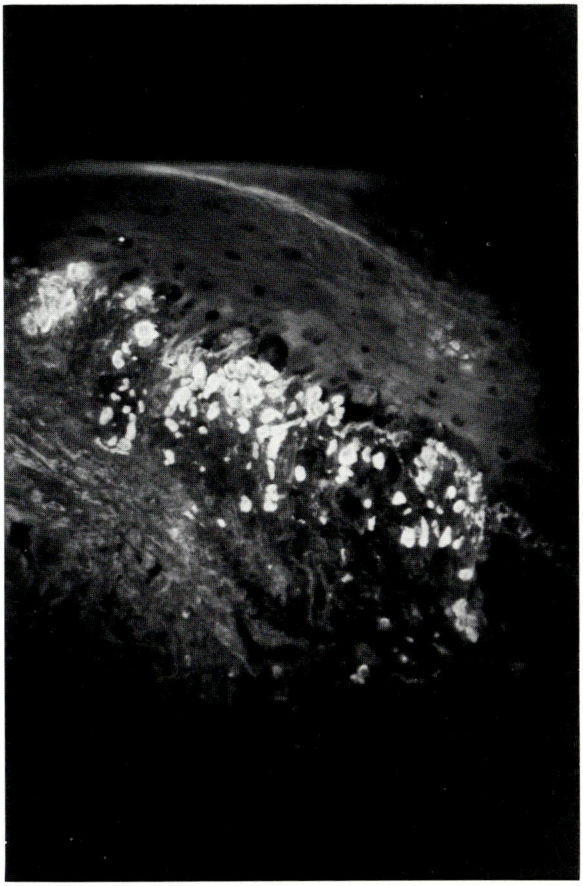

Figure 4. Focal, globular IF deposits in the papillary dermis. In this specimen from a patient with LP, the deposits are numerous (4+) and contain IgG, IgA, IgM, C3, and fibrinogen. They tend to cluster (DIF, 340×). (Reprinted with permission from *Am J Clin Pathol* 79:486, 1983.)

skin and the EM studies point to a similar conclusion. Such a mechanism for removal of epidermal cell remnants is also consistent with the above-mentioned finding of immunoglobulins bound to globular deposits in many diverse types of skin lesions. However, the globular deposits found in LP are not quite the same as those found in other dermatoses (as indicated in the next paragraph). These differences, together with the observation that LP lesions can be induced by skin injury (i.e., the Koebner phenomenon), suggest that the disease may be due to some abnormality in the repair of skin injury. If this is true, then LP may involve an autoantigen disturbance or a dysfunction of the autoimmune repair mechanisms (see Chap. 7) similar to those now implicated in the pathogenesis of psoriasis (see Chap. 42). Importantly, both LP and psoriasis can be induced by Koebnerizing. In light of these considerations, the differences in globular deposits seen in LP from those associated with other types of epidermal injury assumes special interest.

Certain features within the globulin deposits may be helpful in differentiating LP

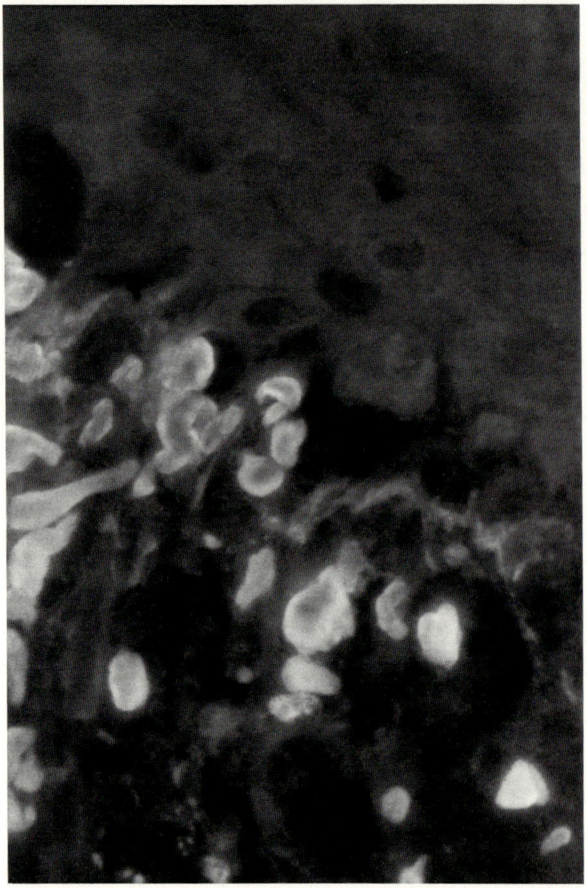

Figure 5. Specific fluorescence of large, spherical-to-oval dermal deposits at a higher magnification than in Figure 2. The deposits show considerable variation in size. Variation in the intensity of the fluorescence with different antisera is common; the IgM-containing deposits are usually the brightest. A pale brownish-yellow autofluorescence of the deposits may be observed in some sections, and indicates a negative fluorescence with the antiserum in question (DIF, 1360×). (Reprinted with permission from *Am J Clin Pathol* 79:486, 1983.)

from the other inflammatory dermatoses. In LP, the deposits are numerous (10^-), and demonstrate 3+ to 4+ IF. In addition, they tend to cluster in groups. They contain various immunoglobulins (IgM, IgG, and IgA), C3, and C5. Usually, in other dermatoses, the globular deposits are fewer and smaller (10−), IF is weaker (1+ to 2+), and they are located singularly along the DEJ rather than clustered. These globules contain mainly IgM immunoglobulin. Also, a more specific IF pattern, such as linear pattern of BP, may be seen in association with the globular deposits, thus making the diagnosis easier (17,35). Some patients with numerous globular deposits of immunoglobulins in skin lesions may initially be seen with overlapping clinical and histopathologic features, suggesting both LP and LE (32,48), BP (34,55), pemphigus, and psoriasis (39). In lichen amyloidosis, amyloid material contains immunoglobulin heavy chains, kappa and

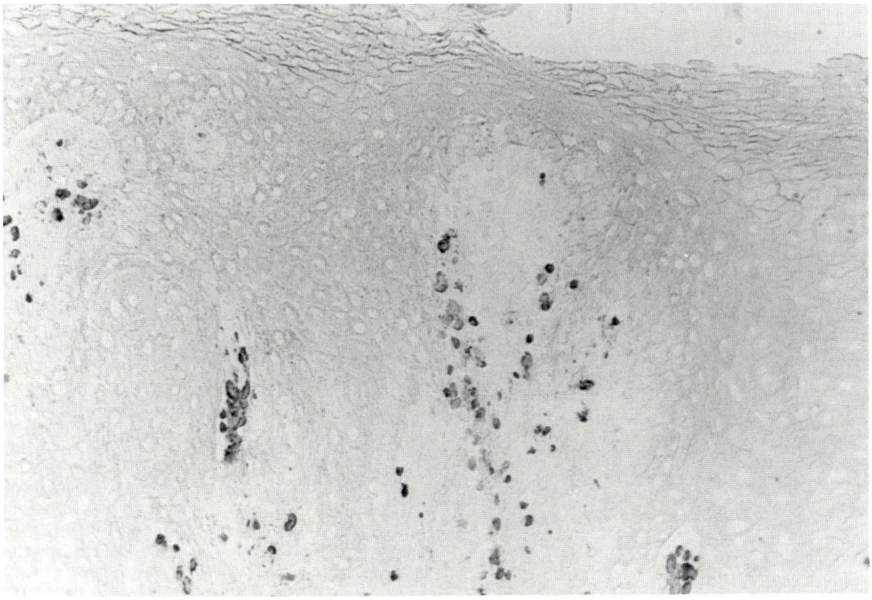

Figure 6. Globular, brown deposits of IgM in the papillary dermis of a case of LP. Clustering of the globules is evident (direct immunoperoxidase, 340×). (Reprinted with permission from *Am J Clin Pathol* 79:486, 1983.)

lambda light chains, C3, and C1q, and may exhibit a globular fluorescent appearance similar to that of the globular deposits (37). Globular deposits may also be seen in the presence of degenerated eosinophilic epidermal cells, apoptotic cells, and benign dermatoses, such as Mucha-Habermann disease (pityriasis lichenoides et varioliformis acuta) and sunburn erythema. In contrast, such globular fluorescent deposits are usually not detected in the eosinophilic cells of neoplastic conditions, such as actinic keratosis, Bowen's disease, and squamous cell carcinoma (19).

Attempts have been made to differentiate the overlapping cutaneous lesions by staining the disulfide bonds of the subepidermal hyaline bodies (SHB), which are globules with the fluorogenic maleimide derivative N-(7-dimethlyamino-4-methylcoumarinyl)-maleimide (DACM) (13,18). This procedure involved first blocking free sulfhydryl groups of the frozen tissue sections with 0.15 M N-ethyl maleimide at 37°C and pH 6.8. Next, disulfide linkages in the tissue were opened by incubating the sections with a solution of 40 mM dithiothreitol and 0.5 mM ethylenediamine tetracetic acid (EDTA) at 37°C and pH 6.8. The resulting sulfhydryl groups were stained with 0.1 mM DACM at room temperature and pH 6.8. DACM bound to tissue-SH groups is strongly fluorescent, with an absorption peak at 400 nm and an emission peak at 485 nm. For data analysis, two fluorescent patterns were recognized. Biopsy specimens with type I pattern contained moderate-to-many SHB, all of which showed strong DACM fluorescence. All other specimens were grouped as type II pattern, including those with few SHB regardless of DACM fluorescence intensity, and those with weak DACM fluorescence intensity regardless of the number of SHB. All four patients with LP showed a type I pattern. In contrast, 9 of 10 patients with LE had a type II pattern (Table 1). Although the total number of cases studied was small, the difference in disulfide group distribution between

Table 1.

Diagnosis	*DACM S-S staining pattern*[a] *I*	*II*
Lupus erythematosus	1	9
Lichen planus	4	0
Dermatomyositis	1	1
Bullous pemphigoid	0	2
Systemic vasculitis	0	1
Porphyria cutanea tarda	0	1
Rothmund-Thomson syndrome	1	0
Poikiloderma atrophicans vasculare	1	0
Lichenoid dermatosis	1	1

[a]Number of patients with each pattern. The patterns are defined in the text.
Reproduced with permission from *Am J Clin Pathol* 79:486–488, 1983.

LP and LE was significant by Fisher's exact test ($p = 0.01$). Since various dermastoses could demonstrate either pattern of DACM reactivity (Table 1), the technique may be useful when the differential diagnosis can be limited to lupus or LP by other clinicopathologic parameters.

Recently, an LP-specific antigen (LPSA) was demonstrated by double-layered indirect immunofluorescent (IIF) technique using either the patient's serum and autologous tissue or allogenic lesional tissue from other patients with LP. The LPSA was observed within the stratum spongiosum and stratum granulosum, but was absent in the SC, basal layer, basement membrane area, and dermis (Fig. 7) (2,42,43). Using IIF for identification of LPSA in lesional skin, Olsen reported LPSA in 80% (20/25) of patients with LP, compared to controls who demonstrated negative staining (0 of 36. patients). Using IIF for LPSA may be helpful in differentiating LP from other lichenoid dermatoses and overlapping syndromes (15,16). However, additional studies may be necessary to demonstrate conclusively the specificity of LPSA.

The common IIF studies for circulating intracellular and basement membrane autoantibodies invariably yield negative results in typical LP. However, positive direct IF (DIF) and IIF findings consistent with both LP and BP may be seen in the rare patient in whom these two diseases coexist (see also Chap. 8). Overlap diseases include LP and LE in which positive DIF and negative IIF findings are similar. Pemphigus vulgaris and LP have been reported together, but can be differentiated easily by different, positive DIF patterns, with pemphigus having positive intercellular IF of IgG by both DIF and IIF.

ELECTRON MICROSCOPY

Electron microscopy (EM) of dermal globular deposits of LP demonstrate an extracellular and electron-dense, nonmembrane-bound, finely granular material. These globules may also contain remnants of cytoplasmic organelles and other fibrillary substructures, probably cytokeratins. These fibrils measure 8 to 10 nm in diameter, tend to aggregate, and often show a whorled appearance similar to tonofibrils (Fig. 8). In contrast, the

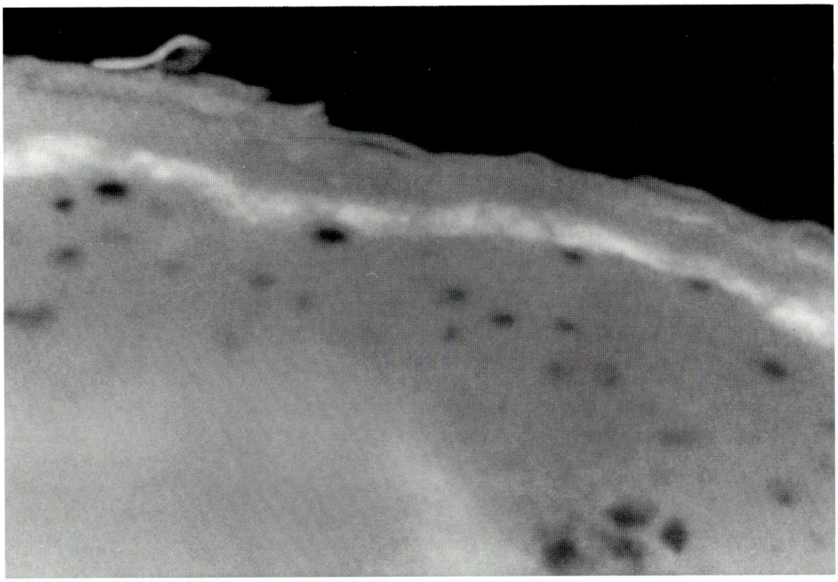

Figure 7. The positive, indirect autologous reaction of LP. Cryostat sections of lesional skin (perilesional if bullous) are incubated for 1 hour at 37°C with autologous serum diluted at 1:10, washed with PBS twice, and then incubated with fluorescein-conjugated rabbit antihuman IgG; counterstained with Evans blue (1% in PBS) (Original magnification, 400×). (The fluorescence is confined to the stratum granulosum. In this case, anti-IgA gave a similar reaction, but anti-IgM was negative. DIF for in vivo-bound immunoglobulins was negative. (Courtesy of Charles Camisa, M.D. and John C. Neff, M.D., Ohio State University, 1985.)

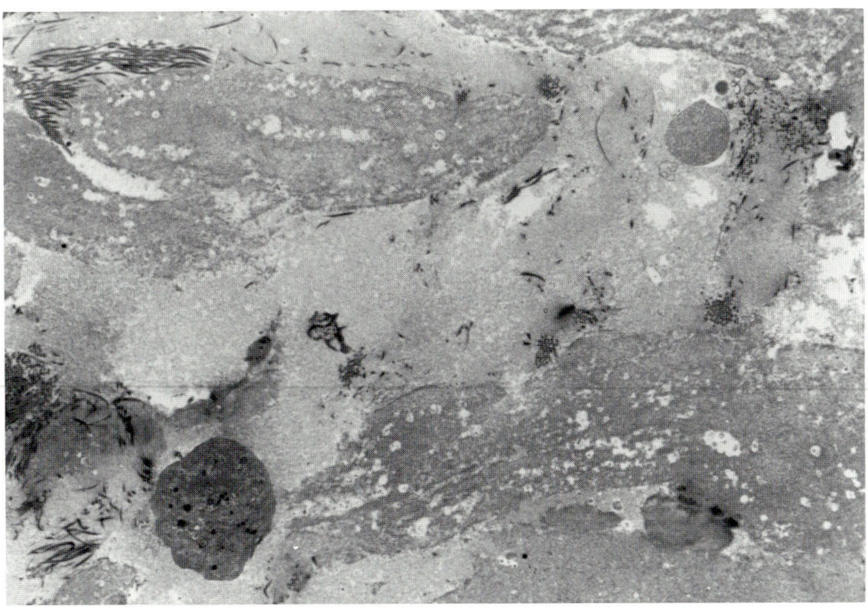

Figure 8. Extracellular globular deposits; same case as in Figure 4. Deposits are electron-dense and do not have a limiting membrane (uranyl acetate and lead citrate, 5685×). (Reprinted with permission from *Am J Clin Pathol* 79:486, 1983.)

amyloid fibrils do not aggregate, and measure 6 to 8 nm in diameter. These changes indicate that the dermal globules may be derived from degenerated epithelial cells (apoptosis) (20,27,38). Histochemical and EM findings suggest a dual origin for the globules of LP and LE.

SUMMARY

Although the exact pathogenesis of LP is unknown, the primary site of injury appears to be in the dividing epithelial cells, which may lose their regenerative capacity. Injured cells are replaced by the progressive migration from the periphery of the lesion, rather than by the act of mitotic division. The basement membrane of the lesion loses its anatomic integrity wherein antigens are released from the degenerating basalar epidermal cells, which appear to invoke a T-cell-mediated immune response as suggested by the predominantly T-cell lymphocytic dermal infiltrate with few macrophages and Langerhans cells (11,46).

Globular deposits of mixed immunoglobulins and complement are a consistent finding in lesions of LP. These globules primarily contain IgM and occasionally IgG and IgA. Complement is present in only about one-half the cases. Special staining with fluorogenic maleimide derivative to demonstrate disulfide bonding appears to be helpful in differentiating LP from LE. In addition, the presence of other IF patterns, such as the linear pattern seen in LE and absent in LP, is a second helpful pattern. In the overlap syndromes or the atypical LP patients, it may be necessary to employ IIF using the patient's serum and autologous lesional skin as a substrate to demonstrate intense staining of the stratum granulosum in patients with LP. This may identify a specific LP antigen within the stratum granulosum. It is also possible that LP may be shown to be an autoimmune disease related to a defect in cellular immunity, although this too remains to be proven. Several lines of evidence suggest that LP may be an autoantigen dysfunction involving over-reactions of physiologic autoantibodies. Clearly, further studies are needed to sort out the pathogenesis of LP.

REFERENCES

1. Abell E, Presbury DGC, Marks R, et al: The diagnostic significance of immunoglobulin and fibrin deposition in lichen planus. *Br J Dermatol* 93:17–24, 1975.
2. Abell E, Ramnarain D: Epidermal antigens in lichen planus. *Br J Dermatol* 92:631–636, 1975.
3. Alario A, Ortonne J-I, Schmitt D, et al: Lichen planus: Study with anti-human T lymphocyte antigen (anti-HTLA) serum on frozen sections. *Br J Dermatol* 98:601–604, 1978.
4. Anderson RL, Cullen SI: Pseudopelade of Brocq secondary to lichen planus. *Cutis* 17:916–918, 1976.
5. Aronson IK, SoHani K, Paik KI et al: Triad of lichen planus, myasthenia gravis and thymoma. *Arch Dermatol* 114:255–258, 1978.
6. Baart de la Faille-Kuyp, Baart de la Faille H: An immunofluorescence study of lichen planus. *Br J Dermatol* 90:365–371, 1974.
7. Berger TG, Aesody ST: Quinidine-reduced lichenoid photodermatitis. *Cutis* 29:595–600, 1982.
8. Beutner EH, Kumar V. Is the Ig bound to cytoid bodies antibody? *Int J Dermatol* 24:362–368, 1985.
9. Beutner EH, Jablonska S, Jarzabek-Chorzelska M, et al: Studies in immunodermatology. VI. IF studies of autoantibodies to the stratum corneum and of in vivo fixed IgG in stratum corneum of psoriatic scales. *Int Arch Allergy Appl. Immunol.* 48:301–323, 1975.

10. Beutner EH, Rhodes EL, Holborow EJ: Autoimmunity in chronic bullous skin diseases. Immunofluorescent staining of three types of antibodies to skin in sera of patients with pemphigus, bullous pemphigoid and in other human sera. *Clin Exp Immunol* 2:141–151, 1967.
11. Black MM: The pathogenesis of lichen planus. *Br J Dermatol* 86:302–305, 1972.
12. Bhan AK, Harrist TJ, Murphy GE, et al: T cell subsets and Langerhans cells in lichen planus: In situ characterization using monoclonal antibodies. *Br J Dermatol* 105:617–622, 1981.
13. Binkley W, Starsnic J, Valenzuela R, et al: A histochemical approach to the differentiation of lichen planus from lupus erythematosus. *Am J Clin Pathol* 79:486–488, 1983.
14. Bjerke JR, Krogh HK: Identification of mononuclear cells in situ in skin lesions of lichen planus. *Br J Dermatol* 98:605–610, 1978.
15. Camisa C, Neff GC, Olsen AG: Use of indirect immunofluorescence in lupus erythematosus/lichen planus overlap syndrome: An additional diagnostic clue. *J Am Acad Dermatol* 11:1050–1059, 1984.
16. Camisa C, Nesbitt LT Jr, Brantley JB: Lichen planus pemphigoides: Clinical and immunofluorescent findings in four cases. *J Am Acad Dermatol* 8:331–336, 1983.
17. Copeman PWM, Schroeter AL, Kierland RR: An unusual variant of lupus erythematosus of lichen planus. *Br J Dermatol* 83:269–272, 1970.
18. Danno K, Horio T: Sulphydryl and disulphide stainings of subepidermal hyaline bodies. *Br J Dermatol* 104:437–442, 1981.
19. Danno K, Imamura S, Horio T, et al: Benign and neoplastic eosinophilic staining cells: An immunofluorescence study. *Br J Dermatol* 102:155–160, 1980.
20. Ebner H, Gebhart W: Light and electron microscopic differentiation of amyloid and colloid or hyaline bodies. *Br J Dermatol* 92:637–645, 1975.
21. Fellner MJ: *Immunology of Skin Diseases.* Elsevier, New York, 1980, pp. 258–266.
22. Gogate P, Valenzuela R, Deodhar S, et al: Globular deposits of immunoglobulins and complement in the papillary dermis: Clinical significance. *Am J Clin Pathol* 73:512–517, 1980.
23. Goldstein BH, Katz SM: Immunofluorescent findings in oral bullous lichen planus. *J Oral Med* 34:8–12, 1979.
24. Graham-Bruron RA, Sarkany I, Sherlock S: Lichen planus and first degree biliary cirrhosis *Br J Dermatol* 106:699–703, 1982.
25. Halevy S, Zamir R, Gazit E, et al: HLA systems in relation to carbohydrate metabolism in lichen planus. *Br J Dermatol* 100:683–686, 1979.
26. Harrist TJ, Mihm MC: Cutaneous immunopathology: The diagnostic use of direct and indirect immunofluorescence techniques in dermatologic disease. *Hum Pathol* 10:625–653, 1979.
27. Hashimoto K: Apoptosis in lichen planus and several other dermatoses. *Acta Dermatol Venereol* 56:187–210, 1976.
28. Hintner H, Lawley TJ: Keratin intermediate filaments bear antigenic determinants for stratum corneum antibodies. *J Invest Dermatol* 82:491–495, 1984.
29. Horio T, Murai T, Ikai K: Photosensitivity due to a fluorouracil derivative. *Arch Dermatol* 114:1498–1800, 1978.
30. Horn R, Goethe D, Odom R, et al: Immunofluorescent findings and clinical overlap in two cases of folliculas lichen planus. *J Am Acad Dermatol* 7:203–207, 1982.
31. Ishibashi I, Hirano K, Nishiyamai Y: Photosensitive dermatitis due to pyritinol. *Arch Dermatol* 107:427–428, 1973.
32. Jamison TH, Cooper NM, Epstein WV: Lichen planus and discoid lupus erythematosus: Overlap syndrome associated with cryoglobulinemia and hypocomplementemia. *Arch Dermatol* 114:1039–1042, 1978.
33. Kennedy BJ, Smith LP, Goetz RW: Skin changes secondary to hydrourea therapy. *Arch Dermatol* 111:183–187, 1975.
34. Lang DG, Margo JC: Coexisting lichen planus and bullous pemphigus or lichen planus pemphigoides. *J Am Acad Dermatol* 9:133–140, 1983.
35. Laskaris G, Sklavounou A, Angelopoulos A: Direct immunofluorescence in oral lichen planus. *Oral Surg* 53:483–487, 1982.
36. Lowe J, Cudworth AG, Woodrow JC: HL-A antigens in lichen planus. *Br J Dermatol* 98:169–171, 1976.

37. MacDonald DM, Black MM, Ramnarain N: Immunofluorescence studies in primary localized cutaneous amyloidosis. *Br J Dermatol* 96:635–641, 1977.
38. Medenica M, Lorincz A: Lichen planus: An ultrastructural study. *Acta Dermatol Venereol* 57:55–62, 1977.
39. Menars N: Lichen planus occurring with PS. *Cutis* 16:105–107, 1975.
40. Michel B, Sy EK: Tissue-fixed immunoglobulins in lichen planus. In Beutner EH, Chorzelski TP, Bean SF, et al. (Eds): *Immunopathology of the Skin: Labeled Antibody Studies.* Dowden, Hutchinson, Ross, Stroudsburg, PA, 1973, pp 182–193.
41. Nisengard RJ, Alpert AM, Krestow V: Desquamative gingivitis: Immunologic findings. *J Periodontol* 49:27–32, 1978.
42. Olsen RG, du Plessis D, Barron C, et al: Lichen planus dermopathy: Demonstration of a lichen planus specific epidermal antigen in affected patients. *J Clin Lab Immunol* 10:103–106, 1983.
43. Olsen RG, du Plessis DP, Schultz EJ, et al: Indirect immunofluorescence-microscopy of lichen planus. *Br J Dermatol* 110:9–15, 1984.
44. Pennys MS, Acherman AB, Gottlieb NL: Gold dermatitis clinical and histopathologies study. *Arch Dermatol* 109:372–376, 1974.
45. Powel SM, Ellis JP, Ryan TJ, et al: Glucose tolerance in lichen planus. *Br J Dermatol* 91:73–75, 1974.
46. Presbury DGC, Marks R: The epidermal disorder in lichen planus: An in vitro study. *Br J Dermatol* 90:373–380, 1974.
47. Roed-Peterson J, Menne T: Allergic contact dermatitis and lichen planus from black and white photographic developing. *Cutis* 18:699–705, 1976.
48. Romero RW, Nesbitt LT, Reed RJ: Unusual variant of lupus erythematosus or lichen planus: Clinical, histopathologic, and immunofluorescence studies. *Arch Dermatol* 113:741–748, 1977.
49. Saurat JH, Gluckman E, Bussel A, et al: The lichen planus-like eruption after bone marrow transplant. *Br J Dermatol* 93:675–681, 1975.
50. Schiodt M, Holmstrup P, Dabelsteen E, et al: Deposits of immunoglobulins, complement, and fibrinogen in oral lupus erythematosus, lichen planus, and leukoplakia. *Oral Surg* 51:603–608, 1981.
51. Seehaefer JR, Rogers RS, Fleming CR, et al: Lichen planus-like lesion caused by penicillamine in first degree biliary cirrhoses. *Arch Dermatol* 117:140–142, 1981.
52. Shousha S, Svirbely J: Immunohistochemical study of lichen planus. *J Clin Pathol* 30:569–574, 1977.
53. Sodaify M, Vallium DI: Familial lichen planus: A case report. *Br J Dermatol* 98:579–581, 1978.
54. Stankler L: Deficiency of circulating IgA and IgM in adult patients with lichen planus. *Br J Dermatol* 93:25–27, 1975.
55. Stingl G, Holubar K: Coexistence of lichen planus and bullous pemphigoid. *Br J Dermatol* 93:313–320, 1975.
56. Ueki H: Hyaline bodies in subepidermal papillae: Immunohistochemical studies in several dermatoses. *Arch Dermatol* 100:610–617, 1969.
57. Valenzuela R, Bergfeld WF, Deodhar SD: *Lichen planus. Interpretation of Immunofluorescent Patterns in Skin Disease.* Am Soc Clin Pathologist Press, Chicago, 1984, pp 127–131.
58. Waisman M, Dundon BC, Michel B: Immunofluorescent studies in lichen nitidus. *Arch Dermatol* 107:200–203, 1973.
59. Weedon D: Civatte bodies and apoptosis. *Br J Dermatol* 91:357, 1974.

40
Keratinocyte Cytoplasmic Antibodies

Jean Hilaire Saurat
Liliane Didierjean

INTRODUCTION

The term keratinocyte cytoplasmic antibodies (KCAbs) applies to morphologically distinct patterns of epidermal cytoplasmic fluorescence seen with an indirect immunofluorescent technique (IIF) using human sera on epidermal substrates. The term KCAbs is preferable to *epidermal* cytoplasmic antibodies because keratinocytes appear to be the principal cell population with which these antibodies react. Whether or not some of these KCAbs also react with other epidermal cells, such as Langerhans cells, melanocytes, and/or Merkel cells, will not be considered in detail in this chapter. Some, if not all, KCAbs might be directed to keratin intermediate filament (KIF) proteins (24); it would therefore appear that at least these KIF/KCAbs are not directed to Langerhans cells and melanocytes.

To date, KCAbs have not been associated with any specific skin or systemic disease; and regardless of the target antigen within the keratinocyte, KCAbs have been considered to be formed in response to the liberation of epidermal antigens after epithelial injury or death. KCAbs have been most often characterized only by immunofluorescent (IF) patterns; however, it now appears that these patterns might represent a reaction to several unrelated antigens present in the cytoplasm of the keratinocytes. With the advent of more sophisticated techniques, the exact significance of KCAbs, in terms of target antigens and their possible link to pathologic states, might eventually be determined.

KERATINOCYTE CYTOPLASMIC ANTIBODIES: IMMUNOFLUORESCENT PATTERNS

The Three Basic Immunofluorescent Patterns: U-cyt, G-cyt, and B-cyt:

Beutner et al. (5) and Bystryn et al. (7) reported the occurrence of antibodies directed against antigens that are present in the cytoplasm of normal epidermal cells.

Burnham (6) outlined that two epidermal cytoplasmic IF patterns could be detected: 1) the *upper epidermal cytoplasmic* (called UEC, and subsequently U-cyt), in which the fluorescence was seen only in the upper and middle epidermis, with the basal cell layer

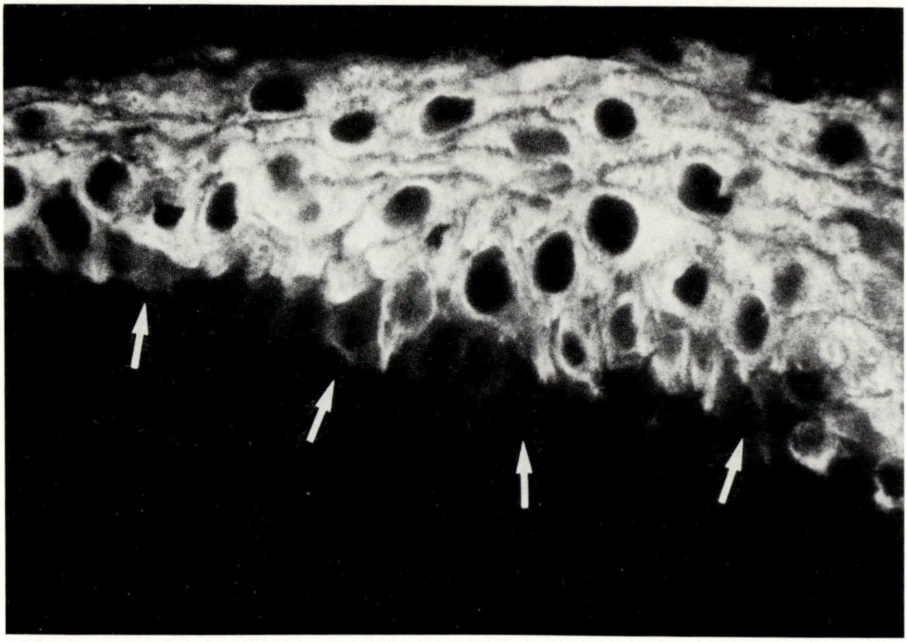

Figure 1. Indirect IF on human skin with a serum containing antibodies directed against upper cytoplasmic antigens. This is a U-cyt pattern (arrows show the basal membrane zone).

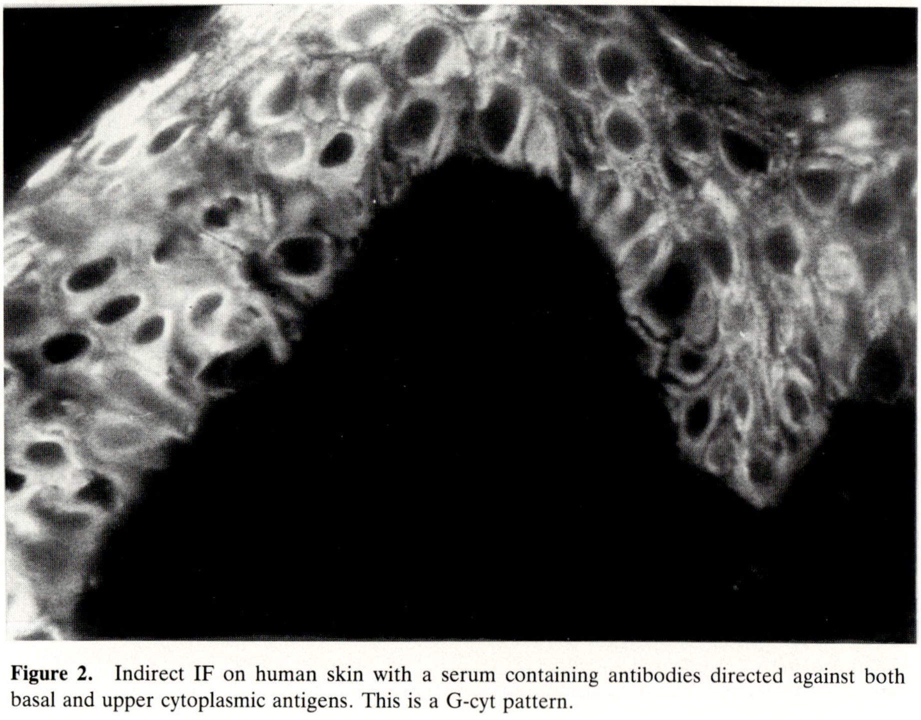

Figure 2. Indirect IF on human skin with a serum containing antibodies directed against both basal and upper cytoplasmic antigens. This is a G-cyt pattern.

being negative (Fig. 1); and 2) the *general epidermal cytoplasmic* (called GEC, and subsequently G-cyt), in which the entire epidermis fluoresced equally (Fig. 2). It was subsequently reported (1,27,54) that human sera could also contain antibodies that would react only with cytoplasmic components of the basal cell layer; the pattern observed with these "basal cell antibodies" was called BCL or B-cyt (Fig. 3).

For all three patterns, the criteria for positive reaction against epidermal cell cytoplasm were defined as follows: 1) fluorescence of epidermal cells that is distinctly brighter than that of dermal tissues; and 2) distinctly visible, nonfluorescing nuclei and interepidermal spaces in the epidermis.

Additional Patterns

The Focal B-cyt Pattern

Some sera are found to react only with some cells in the basal cell layer; this focal B-cyt staining contrasts with the regular B-cyt staining of the entire basal cell layer. This focal B-cyt pattern may represent at least two different kinds of reactions: 1) either a reaction of antibodies directed against melanocytes or Merkel cells (34,52), forming a pattern of scattered so-called "orphan cells"; or 2) an irregular basal cell staining with only about two-thirds of the basal cells being stained. That both the stained and unstained basal cells were keratinocytes had been shown by immunoelectron microscopy (IEM) (unpublished personal observations). This type of staining might represent the presence of antibodies directed against subsets of basal keratinocytes that express distinct cytoplas-

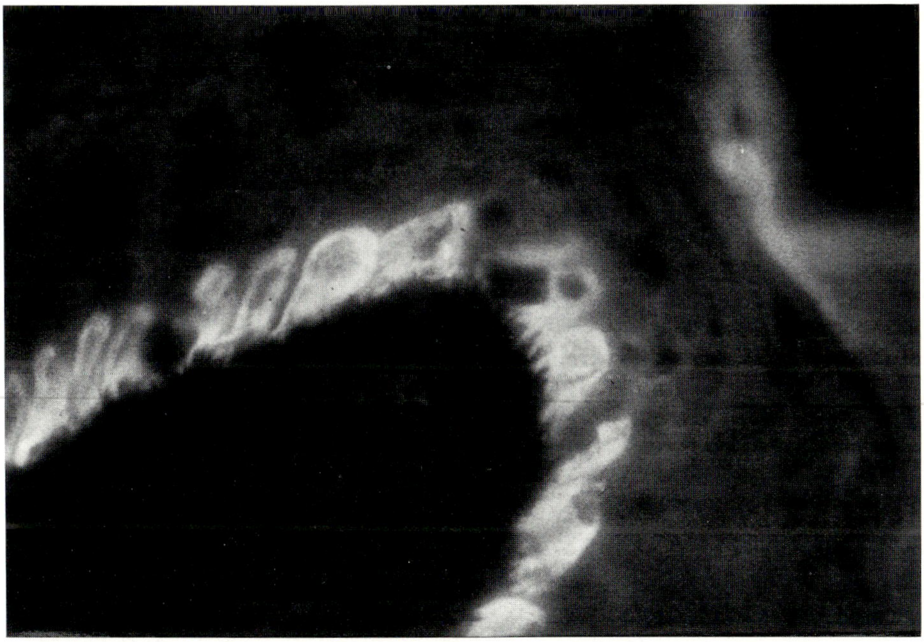

Figure 3. Indirect IF on human skin specimen with a serum containing antibodies directed against basal cell cytoplasmic antigens. This is a B-cyt pattern.

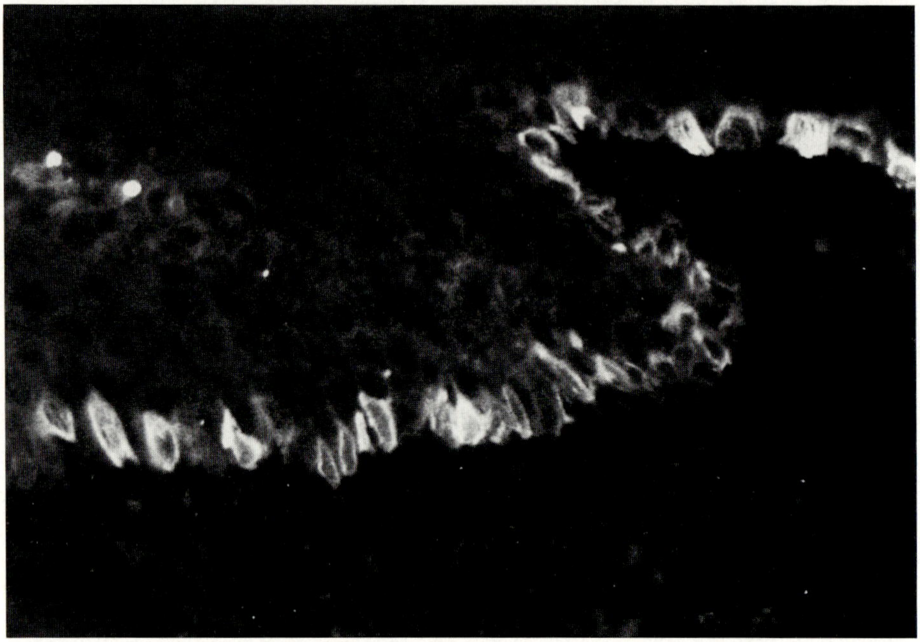

Figure 4. Indirect IF on the mucous side of a rabbit lip specimen. Not all of the basal cells are stained. This is a focal B-cyt pattern that might be related to the functional heterogeneity of the basal cells (see text).

mic antigens. Such a pattern was observed by our group (Fig. 4) and by van Joost (30). This is compatible with the concept of functional heterogeneity of basal cells (21).

The Outer Root Sheath of Hair B-cyt Pattern

Some human sera obtained from patients undergoing a bone marrow graft have been found to react with the basal cell layer of the outer root sheath of hair follicles, but not with the basal cell layer of the adjacent epidermis. The upper limit of this B-cyt outer root sheath pattern was situated at the orifice of the sebaceous gland canal (51) (Fig 5).

This suggested that basal cells below the sebaceous gland canal express antigen(s) distinct from those expressed by the epidermal basal cells.

This observation lends credence to the interpretation that KCAbs were reacting with differentiation antigens linked to the type of keratinocyte differentiation.

Patterns Linked to the Type of Keratinocyte Differentiation.

This was established by the study of staining patterns, observed with sera containing KCAbs, on several substrates involving a well-defined type of differentiation: orthokeratosis, parakeratosis, and mucosa (49,52).

Initial Findings: Human Skin (Orthokeratosis) and Rabbit Esophagus (Mucosa). When the sera were routinely studied by IIF on human skin (HS) and rabbit esophagus (RE) specimens, it was found that the staining patterns were different, depending upon the substrate used (43). For example, a single serum would react only with the basal cell layer when RE was used, and yet only with the upper layers when HS was the substrate.

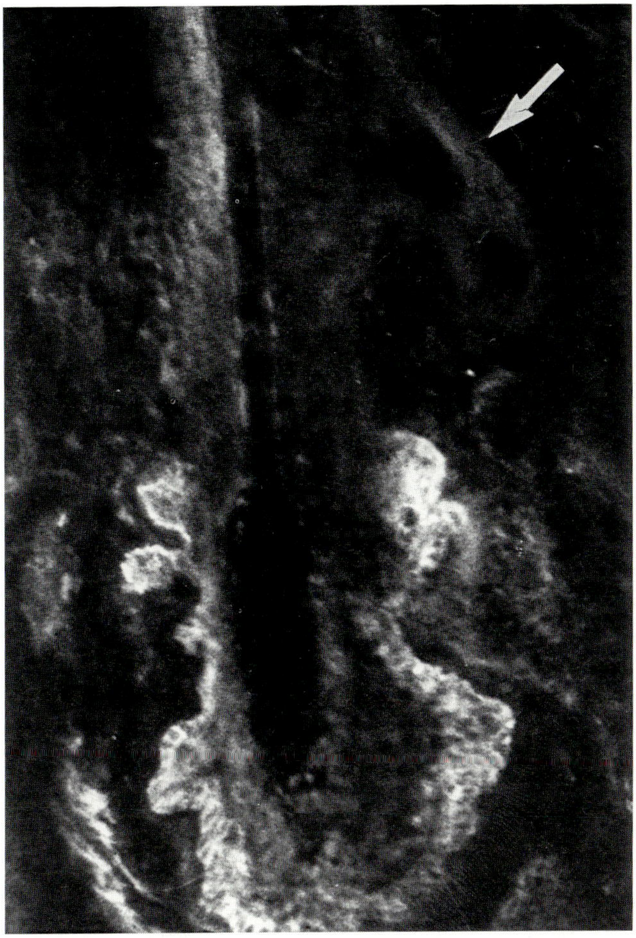

Figure 5. Indirect IF on human skin with a serum containing antibodies directed against antigens present in the basal cells of the outer root sheath of hair below the sebaceous gland. This is the ORS.B-cyt pattern (see text and Fig. 7 arrow showing the sebaceous gland). This serum did not react with the basal cells of the adjacent epidermis (Saurat and Didierjean [51]), but contained antibodies reacting with the arrector pili muscles.

The discrepancies between HS and RE reactivity could have been related either to species differences or to differentiation. This latter hypothesis was strongly supported by subsequent experiments performed on rabbit lip specimens.

THE RABBIT LIP MODEL. When the lower lip of a rabbit is cut sagitally, a specimen can be obtained that has areas of orthokeratosis (OK) with numerous hairs, areas of parakeratosis (PK), and areas of mucosa (M). The delineation between OK and PK, and then between PK and M, are both very well defined and constant from one animal to another. The advantages of such a specimen are twofold: first, it offers a single specimen with several types of keratinocyte differentiation (i.e., OK, PK, and M, plus the root sheath of hairs); second, there are sharply defined junctional zones in which the type of differentiation changes from OK to PK, and then from PK to M. This rabbit lip specimen was used as substrate for the study of distribution of the keratinocyte cytoplasmic staining obtained by IIF with well-defined sera containing KCAbs.

The two epidermal compartments, B-cyt and U-cyt, could be distinguished using rabbit lip specimens. More importantly, the staining of one compartment instead of the other depended on the *type* of differentiation. Sera were found to react only with the basal cell compartment on the mucosal side of the substrate, and then only with the upper compartment on the orthokeratotic side, and vice versa (Fig 6). There were *junctional zones* in which distribution of the staining changed: these were either at the junction between M and PK zones, or at the junction between PK and OK areas (47,48).

Therefore, the sera did not react identically all along the entire rabbit lip sections made through the junctional M, PK, and OK areas. This was not an artifact due to the sectioning of the substrates, as it was very reproducible. The same staining pattern was obtained with one serum on several sections from a single substrate, as well as on lip specimens from more than 100 rabbits. Furthermore, sera containing other types of antibodies, such as pemphigus antibodies, would react uniformly on the different parts of the substrates.

The distinct distribution of the staining was most probably due *to changes in antigenic properties of the substrate as it passed from mucosa to PK, and then to OK.*

This interpretation was supported by studies on species other than rabbit, including mouse tail epidermis, mouse, and guinea pig lip (52). These observations have both theoretic and practical interests: 1) they provide some information on the nature of the antigens to which KCAbs are directed (see later), and 2) they stress the need for several epidermal substrates for the detection of KCAb. Thus, if only OK human skin is used, KCAbs directed to PK or mucosal cytoplasmic antigens would not be detected (46).

Controls for the Specificity of Immunofluorescent Staining

Proper controls for verifying the specificity of the reaction producing these IF patterns should always be performed (48).

1. The FITC-labeled antihuman immunoglobulin serum should not contain naturally occurring antibodies to KIF. Rabbit sera often have such antibodies (38); checking reactivity of the labeled antiserum by omitting incubation with human serum to be studied is therefore necessary.
2. The FITC:protein ratio should not be too high, since it has been demonstrated that fluorescein readily binds to the cytoplasm of keratinocytes (12).
3. It should be necessary to demonstrate that the binding of human immunoglobulin(s) occurs via the Fab and not the Fc fragment, although the exact mechanism of such binding via Fc portion has not been established. By using Fab_2 fragments of human immunoglobulin prepared from sera containing KCAbs, we have demonstrated that the binding occurred via the Fab portion; therefore the IF pattern actually represented a true antigen-antibody reaction (20).

Immunoglobulin Class

In most cases in which this has been looked for, it was found that KCAbs were of the IgG class (4,28,29). A few cases were IgA (43), and IgM antibodies were seldom reported (6).

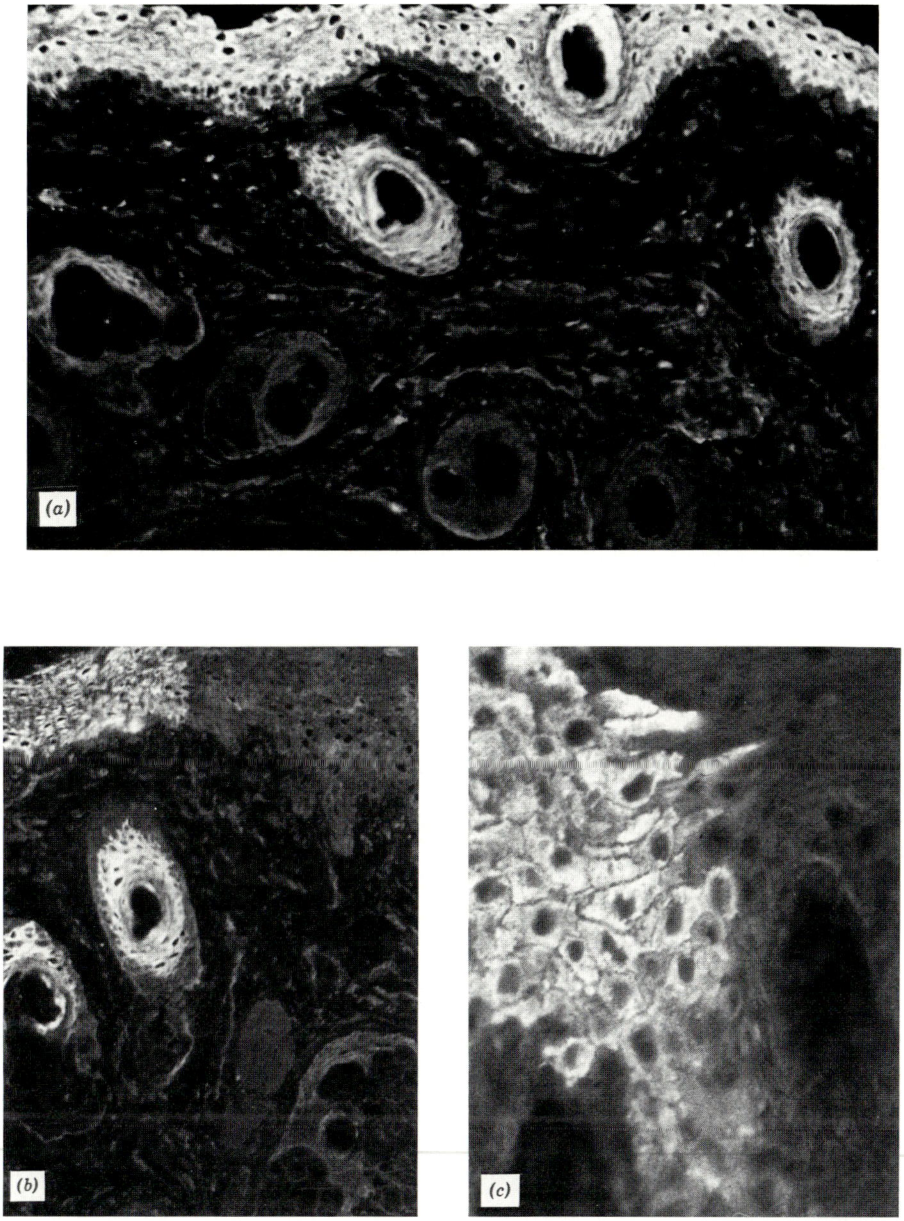

Figure 6. Indirect IF on a rabbit lip specimen with a serum containing antibodies directed to upper antigens of the orthokeratotic epithelia. This is a U-cyt.OK pattern (see text and Fig. 7). a. Pattern on the orthokeratotic side of the rabbit lip specimen. Note the U-cyt pattern. The hair follicles in the upper dermis are stained, whereas they are not in the deep dermis below the sebaceous glands. b. Pattern at the junction between the ortho- and parakeratotic sides. Note that the U-cyt pattern is no longer observed on the parakeratotic side. c. Again, a junction between the ortho- (positive U-cyt) and parakeratotic sides. This picture was obtained in a different rabbit, but with the same serum as in a and b.

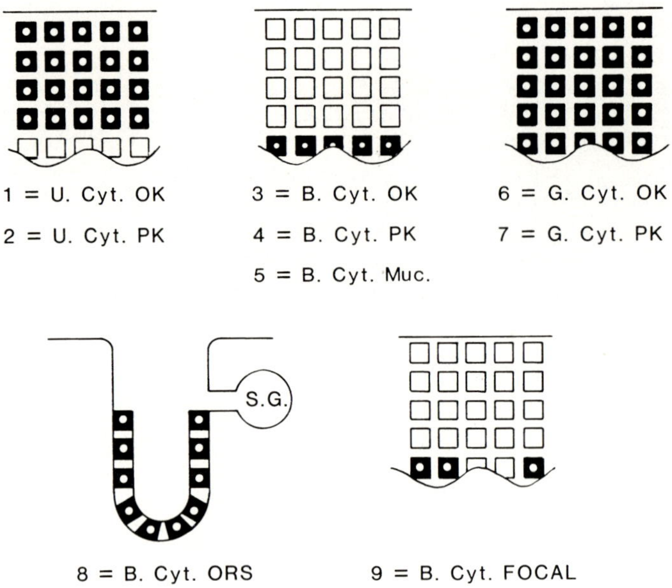

Figure 7. Schematic representation of the IF patterns observed with KCAbs.

ANTIGENS INVOLVED IN THE KERATINOCYTE CYTOPLASMIC IMMUNOFLUORESCENT PATTERNS

Keratin Intermediate Filament (KIF) Proteins

From the description of the different types of IF patterns obtained with KCAbs, and the link of these patterns with the type of keratinocyte differentiation, it would appear that if only one family of target antigens was involved, it should be a family of molecules tightly linked to the differentiation of keratinocytes. The major differentiation product of keratinocyte is keratin. Thus, keratin polypeptides would appear to be the best candidate. In fact, when animal antisera or monoclonal antibodies (MCA) raised against keratin polypeptides are studied by IIF on epidermal substrates, the IF patterns are very similar to that obtained with KCAbs; this is true at both cellular and tissue levels. At the cellular level, the IF pattern is usually not fibrillar in cryostat sections; it is rather homogeneous. Most important, at the tissue level, both U-cyt and B-cyt patterns may be observed. The U-cyt pattern is characteristic for the staining with antibodies directed against high molecular weight (67 and 63 kD) keratin polypeptides (60), whereas a B-cyt pattern has been observed with antibodies directed against low molecular weight (46 and 40 kD) keratin (57). Moreover, since it has been demonstrated that distribution of the different keratin polypeptides is not identical in OK, PK, and M epithelia (33,35,57), the patterns of KCAbs changing according to the type of substrate differentiation would also be explained, if KCAbs were indeed antikeratin antibodies.

In fact, Hintner, Steiner, and Lawley (24) recently reported that 12 sera giving U-cyt patterns on normal human skin all contained anti-KIF protein antibodies. This was demonstrated by the binding of the antibodies to transblotted KIF proteins on nitrocellulose sheets; the antibodies were mainly directed against high molecular weight (65, 63, and 61.5 kD) KIF proteins. Absorption of the sera with purified KIF removed U-cyt antibodies; absorbed U-cyt antibodies could be eluted from the same KIF preparation and shown to bind to U-cyt antigens by IIF. These data clearly demonstrated that KIF protein bore antigens to which U-cyt antibodies were directed.

It now remains to be established if *all* KCAbs are, in fact, antikeratin antibodies. Unless immunoblot analysis is systematically used for characterization of KCAbs, this issue will remain unresolved.

Presently, we can only analyze retrospectively the data published on several types of KCAbs patterns and review the evidences that are, or are not, compatible with an antikeratin immune reaction.

Retrospective Analysis of Data on KCAbs

Are previous observations compatible with the proposed anti-KIF nature of KCAbs?

Blocking Experiments, Immunodiffusion, and Immunoelectron Microscopy

Viac et al. (59,60) published two papers in which it was suggested that the cytoplasmic antigens defined by KCAbs appeared to be different from keratins. They reported the following: 1) Using a panel of sera with U-cyt-type KCAbs (IIF titers not given), they found that previous incubation of the substrate with a guinea pig antikeratin antiserum directed against 67-kD KIF protein did not prevent the binding of KCAbs; 2) KCAbs did not react by immunodiffusion test with purified stratum corneum (SC) keratin; 3) the IEM pattern obtained with KCAbs was not similar to that obtained with antikeratin antiserum, and, more precisely, there was no labeling of tonofilaments; they observed irregular deposits in the peripheral part of the cell cytoplasm; and 4) KCAbs did not react with thymic cells, as do keratin antibodies directed against the 67-, 55-, and 53-kD KIF proteins.

It might be that the discrepancy between the data reported by Hintner et al. (24) and Viac et al. (59,60) is due to differences in sensitivity of the methods used. It has been well established that the immunoblot technique is much more sensitive than immunodiffusion tests.

Organ Specificity of KCAbs

To our knowledge, a few attempts have been made at carefully analyzing the organ specificity of each serum containing KCAbs. Bystryn et al. (7) reported that KCAb-positive sera (U-cyt and G-cyt patterns) did not react with liver, kidney, and stomach. Van Joost (28) found that six sera with B-cyt antibodies (B-cyt Abs) did not react with stomach, thyroid, adrenal, and parotid glands, smooth and skeletal muscles, liver, and kidney. Bystryn (8) also found that three sera with B-cyt Abs did not react to rat liver, spleen, kidney, stomach, colon, and skeletal muscles, or to human kidney, liver, and spleen; one serum reacted to smooth muscle. Similarly, we (52) did not find any cytoplasmic staining when sera with B-cyt or U-cyt Abs were reacted with human liver, gall bladder, or bone marrow, and also rabbit brain, trachea, liver, colon, duodenum, pylorus, stomach, gall bladder, adrenal or thyroid glands, spleen, or aorta. Some sera with U-cyt Abs were found to react to the Hassall's corpuscules of rabbit thymus (14).

From these observations, it had been concluded that KCAbs were organ specific; that is, specific for stratified malpighian epithelia.

KIF proteins of 40, 46 and 52 kD have now been identified in a variety of simple epithelia, such as stomach, small intestine, kidney, and pancreas (57); therefore, it would seem that KCAbs in the studies previously mentioned were not KIF protein antibodies, since they did not react to these epithelia. However, it may well be that most of these KCAbs were, in fact, directed against KIF proteins over 52 kD, which according to the findings of Tseng et al. (57) are not expressed in simple epithelia. These data would then concord with the report of Hintner et al. (24), who found that U-cyt Ab mainly react with 65-, 63-, and 61.5-kD KIF proteins.

Regarding B-cyt antigens (B-Cyt Ags), the problem might be more complex. Tseng et al. (57) found that an MCA directed against 56-, 50-, and 40-kD KIF proteins selectively stained the basal cell layer of both epidermal and esophageal epithelium; since simple epithelia were found to express the 40-kD KIF protein, it might be extrapolated that KCAbs B-cyt Abs may well be KIF antibodies directed to KIF proteins of molecular weights between 56 to 50 kD.

Binding of KCAbs to Keratinocytes in Culture

It was hoped that in vitro studies would significantly increase our understanding of the nature of keratinocyte cytoplasmic antigens (KCAgs). The binding of U-cyt and B-cyt KCAbs has been studied in a human epidermal culture system by Didierjean et al. (15). In this system, epidermal cells migrate from a skin explant and form a stratified, keratinizing epithelium. It was found by IIF that B-cyt KCAbs reacted with cells in the basal layer of the reconstituted epithelium, whereas only upper level keratinocytes were stained with U-cyt KCAbs. This work demonstrated that: 1) KCAgs were found to be expressed in vitro, independent of any dermal influence; 2) localization in culture matched that found in vivo; and 3) KCAbs no longer bound to cultures older than 38 days.

These findings are compatible with the fact that KCAgs might be KIF proteins, although the loss of KCAbs binding after 38 days in culture is puzzling.

Faure et al. (18) studied the binding of KCAbs in a culture system in which keratinocytes were grown without feeder cells, dermal tissue, or collagen. They found that the expression of U-cyt Ags was markedly decreased. B-cyt antigens were not studied. These results are compatible with the fact that KC U-cyt Ags could be KIF proteins, since the high-molecular weight KIF proteins might not be synthetized in cell culture (25).

The Polymorphism of KCAgs

In their first report, Bystryn et al. (7) found that nine KCAbs sera did not react similarly to normal human skin obtained from four different donors. They later suggested (9) that there might be at least two different subgroups of U-cyt and G-cyt antigens that could be defined by serologic typing. One subgroup would be universally expressed in all individuals and demonstrated by the ability of a single serum to react to antigens present in all persons. The second subgroup would be common antigens expressed in some, but not all subjects. This was in accordance with our own previous results (43,44). We further demonstrated that such a polymorphism also exists for human B-cyt antigens (50) (Tables 1 and 2). In fact, the polymorphism, we observed was more pronounced than previously suggested, perhaps because the sera were obtained from bone marrow transplant patients. It appeared therefore that KCAbs could react to cytoplasmic antigens present in human keratinocytes, and that they might differ from person to person. Thus, it was tempting to speculate that these antigens were genetically determined alloantigens.

In fact, it has been reported by Ackermann-Schopf et al. (3), from the Terasaki group that U-cyt Ags might be HLA Ags. We clearly demonstrated that this was not the case (45) because: 1) although some human sera with HLA reactivity did react with a U-cyt pattern to normal human skin, there was, however, no correlation with the HLA typing of the skin used—furthermore, removal of HLA antibodies by absorption on platelets did not abolish U-cyt staining; and 2) the reaction of HLA-A and HLA-B

Table 1. Polymorphism of B-Cyt Antigens in Human Skin

B-cyt serum	Skin specimens from HLA identical persons								Additional normal human skin specimens (% of B-cyt reaction in 10–30 specimens)
	(1–1)	(2–2)	(3–3)	(4–4)	(5–5)	(6–6)	(7–7)	(8–8)	
I	− +	+ +	ND	ND	ND	ND	+ +	ND	ND
II	− −	+ −	− −	− −	− −	− −	− −	+ +	10
III	− −	− −	+ −	+ −	+ −	ND	ND	ND	ND
IV	− −	ND	− −	+ −	− −	ND	ND	+ −	26
V	− +	− −	− −	− −	− −	ND	+ −	ND	ND
VI	− −	− −	− −	− −	− −	+ +	ND	ND	ND
VII	− −	− +	+ −	− −	− −	ND	ND	ND	ND
VIII	− −	− +	− +	− −	+ +	ND	ND	ND	ND
IX	ND	ND	ND	ND	ND	+ −	+ +	− −	32
X	− −	+ −	− −	− −	− −	− −	− −	− −	17
XI	ND	− +	− +	− +	+ +	+ +	+ +	+ +	95
XII	ND	ND	+ +	+ −	+ +	ND	ND	+ +	83
XIII	ND	ND	+ +	+ +	+ +	− −	+ +	+ +	50
XIV	ND	ND	− −	− −	− +	− −	+ +	+ +	53

Polymorphism of B cyt antigens in human skin: Fourteen sera obtained from patients undergoing a bone marrow transplant were studied by IIF in frozen sections of human skin; serum dilution was 1:10, while the titers of B-cyt antibodies were greater or equal to 1:50. This table shows that B-cyt antigens may be different from person to person, but that this polymorphism is not related to the HLA antigens

Table 2. Polymorphism of U-Cyt Antigens in human skin

U-cyt serum	*Skin specimens from HLA identical persons*								*Additional normal human skin specimens (% of U-cyt staining reaction in 10–30 specimens)*
	(1–1)	*(2–2)*	*(3–3)*	*(4–4)*	*(5–5)*	*(6–6)*	*(7–7)*	*(8–8)*	
A	+ −	+ −	− −	− −	+ −	ND	ND	+ +	35
B	ND	ND	− −	+ −	− +	ND	ND	+ +	41
C	− +	ND	− +	− −	+ +	ND	ND	+ +	73
D	ND	ND	ND	ND	ND	+ −	+ +	+ +	100
E	+ ND	+ +	+ −	+ −	+ −	− +	− −	+ +	78
F	ND	− −	+ −	− −	− −	− −	− −	− +	5
G	ND	ND	+ +	− +	− −	− −	− +	+ +	25
H	ND	ND	− −	− −	− −	− −	+ +	+ +	30

Polymorphism of U-cyt antigens in human skin: Eight sera obtained from patients undergoing a bone marrow transplant were studied by IIF in frozen sections of human skin; serum dilution was 1:10, while the titers of U-cyt antibodies were greater or equal to 1:50. This table shows that U-cyt antigens may be different from person to person, but that this polymorphism is not related to the HLA antigens. See text for further discussion; +, positive U-cyt staining; −, no U-cyt staining; ND, not done. Parentheses indicate HLA-A and HLA-B identity and nonreactivity in MLR.

antisera to human skin was found to give a "pemphigus-like" pattern of staining (40,45). This has been largely confirmed since.

The significance of polymorphism of KCAgs remains unknown. An important issue would be to study whether this polymorphism is genetically determined. For this, extensive family studies would be necessary. We have performed a preliminary study, in this respect, in which a panel of KCAbs were reacted with skin specimens from the parents and relatives of patients undergoing a bone marrow transplantation. In all these subjects, the histocompatibility and other alloantigenic systems were analyzed. Unfortunately, we could not find strong evidence for any genetically determined polymorphism (Table 3).

At any rate, the polymorphism of KCAgs is difficult to interpret if it is assumed that all KCAbs are anti-KIF protein antibodies. At least two explanations could be given: 1) the polymorphism could be due to variable expression of KIF proteins within the epidermis from person to person, possibly in relation to the different sites from which the skin biopsy specimens were taken (a fact that has not been evaluated); and 2) not all KCAbs are anti-KIF antibodies.

Binding of KCAbs to Cutaneous Malignancies and Experimentally Modified or Pathologic Epidermis

Bystryn et al. (9) studied the binding of U-cyt, B-cyt, and G-cyt antibodies to basal cell and squamous cell carcinomas. In all cases, G-cyt antibodies reacted with the tumor tissues and adjacent normal skin; by contrast, the U-cyt and B-cyt antibodies did not react to the malignant lesions, whereas they reacted to the adjacent normal skin.

Didierjean et al. (16) studied the binding of U-cyt Abs specific for orthokeratotic scales (U-cyt OK), and of B-cyt Abs to the developing PK scales of newborn mouse tail epidermis. It was found that U-cyt OK reactivity progressively disappeared, while the natural switch from OK to PK occurred in the interfollicular areas of mouse tail

It was also demonstrated that KCAbs bind to psoriatic epidermis (10,49). B-cyt antibodies were found to bind to two or three basal layers; U-cyt OK antibodies were found to react to the PK psoriatic epidermis.

There are no observations in all of these cited studies suggesting that KCAbs might not be anti-KIF antibodies (33,35).

Conclusions

It appears, after reviewing the data published on KCAbs, that only the antigens involved in one of the three types of cytoplasmic IF patterns have been precisely characterized (24).

It was demonstrated, by the immunoblot technique, that the U-cyt KCAbs studied were anti-KIF antibodies. In light of present knowledge on the extremely variable subunit composition of KIF proteins and their variable distribution in epithelial tissues, most if not all previous observations made on U-cyt Abs would be compatible, with KCAbs being anti-KIF protein antibodies. Although this has not been demonstrated thus far, it seems reasonable to speculate that all of the other patterns described in the second section of this chapter might also reflect the binding of anti-KIF protein antibodies. It is, however, conceptually acceptable that some cytoplasmic IF patterns might be due to the binding of other antibodies directed against one of the numerous nonkeratinous proteins expressed in the cytoplasm of the keratinocytes.

It now appears that it is no longer acceptable to consider a simple IF picture as sufficient for defining KCAbs.

Table 3. The IF Staining Pattern of Sera From Patients with Bone Marrow Transplants

	Percentage of each pattern in a panel of 50 normal human skin specimens				*Patterns on Human skin specimens from related persons*						
					Family VA				*Family GU*		
KCAbs	*U-cyt*	*B-cyt*	*G-cyt*	*Neg.*	*Mother*	*Father*	*Son*[a]	*Daughter*[b]	*Mother*	*Father*	*Son*[b]
9	62	0	17	21	U-cyt	U-cyt	U-cyt	U-cyt	Neg.	U-cyt	U-cyt
28	4	88	0	8	B-cyt	B-cyt	B-cyt	B-cyt	B-cyt	B-cyt	G-cyt
110	0	21	26	53	G-cyt	G-cyt	B-cyt	U-cyt	Neg.	G-cyt	G-cyt
111	0	41	27	32	G-cyt	G-cyt	B-cyt	U-cyt	Neg.	G-cyt	G-cyt

[a]Donor of bone marrow graft.

[b]Recipient of a bone marrow graft. HLA-A and HLA-B are identical and nonreactive in MLR with donor of bone marrow graft.

Analysis of the IF patterns observed with 4 selected sera obtained from 3 patients undergoing a bone marrow transplant on: 1) a panel of 50 specimens of normal human skin, and 2) skin specimens obtained from the parents of two patients in which a bone marrow transplant was performed. These preliminary results, although showing some intrafamily differences (outlined), were not considered sufficient to pursue the search for the allogeneic nature of polymorphism of cytoplasmic antigens with the IF technique (see text). The families studied were from the bone marrow transplantation program of St. Louis Hospital, Paris (Prof E. Gluckman).

Each serum revealing such a pattern should be further characterized by the immunoblot technique performed with both keratin proteins and epidermal soluble proteins (see Table 4).

CLINICAL SIGNIFICANCE OF KCAbs

Occurrence of KCAbs in Skin Diseases

KCAbs in Normal People

KCAbs have been found in the serum of about 30% of normal people studied; the titers were usually low, and the patterns were mainly of the U-cyt and G-cyt type (1,7,41). It is interesting that Hintner et al. (24) found anti-KIF protein antibodies even in the sera of seven patients who were negative for U-cyt antibodies by IIF.

Skin Cancer

The incidence and titer of KCAbs appear to be greater in patients with basal and squamous cell carcinomas, as well as melanoma. (1,3,39). It was even suggested that the incidence and titers were greater when the patients had repeated relapses treated with cryosurgery (39). An increased incidence of KCAbs was also reported in patients with noncutaneous malignancies (3,39). The patterns were most often of the U-cyt and G-cyt type for all cutaneous and noncutaneous malignancies.

Burns

Thivolet and Beyvin (56) first reported the occurrence of B-cyt Abs in 13% of patients with burns. This was confirmed by several groups (2). The apparent greater occurrence of B-cyt Abs, as compared to U-cyt or G-cyt Abs, could be due to the fact that esophageal mucosa, which is not suitable for the detection of U-cyt Ab, have been used in most of these studies.

Bone Marrow-Transplanted Patients

KCAbs were found in 88% of patients undergoing a bone marrow transplant (41). Sequential analysis of 194 sera from 47 such patients demonstrated that there was no correlation with a graft-versus-host reaction (GVHR) (32,49). All types of patterns were observed in these studies, with the most frequent being type 5 (Fig. 7), in which KCAbs were directed against B-cyt on a rabbit lip mucosal side.

Drug Reactions

Van Joost (28) reported B-cyt Abs in 7 of 42 patients with a drug reaction. We (41,42) and others (8) have confirmed these observations. There was no correlation with either the clinical type of reaction or the drug responsible for it.

Bullous Dermatoses

KCAbs of the B-cyt type were found by Bystryn (8) in seven patients with pemphigus vulgaris (PV) and three with bullous pemphigoid (BP); the B-cyt antibodies appeared in patients who were improving at a time when pemphigus and BP antibodies were no longer detectable. Nishikawa et al. (37), via complement IF (in this technique, the serum to be tested is first incubated with the substrate, then with fresh serum containing complement, and finally with anti-C3 antiserum) were able to detect B-cyt Abs in 8 of 12 sera from patients with BP. Using a similar technique, we found B-cyt Abs in 5 of 16 patients with herpes gestationis (HG) (13) (Fig 8). Relevant to this might be the observation that when BP antibodies are used for the tracing of BP Ag in cultured keratinocytes, a cytoplasmic pattern may be observed (62). This pattern has been inter-

Table 4. IIF and Immunoblot Analysis of the Sera Obtained From Patients with Bone Marrow Transplants

		Rabbit lip	
		Orthokeratotic side	*Parakeratotic side*
KIF proteins			
Pattern as detected by SDS gel electrophoresis		66, 63, 61, 60, 56, 53, kD	64, 60, 57, 52, 49, kD
Serum with KC antibodies			
I. Staining pattern (IIF)		U-cyt	U-cyt
(Immunoblot analysis[a]	mainly 65, 63, 61.5 kD, serum dilution, 1:400)		
II. Staining pattern (IIF)		U-cyt	Negative
(Immunoblot analysis[a]	mainly 61.5 kD, serum dilution, 1:100)		
III. Staining pattern			
(Immunoblot analysis[a]	only weak staining of 55 kD KIF protein, serum dilution, 1:100)	B-cyt	B-cyt

[a]Molecular weight (kD) of KIF protein reactive with the particular serum (Dr. Hintner).

This table compares the staining patterns observed with three sera obtained from bone marrow transplant patients on rabbit lip specimens with: 1) the pattern of KIF proteins in the orthokeratotic and parakeratotic sides of the specimens, and 2) the immunoblot analysis of the three sera on human KIF proteins blotted on nitrocellulose sheets. The IF patterns were reproduced in more than 50 different rabbits. The immunoblot analysis was performed by Hintner et al. (24). It can be seen that although having similar anti-KIF protein antibodies, sera I and II did not react similarly on the parakeratotic side. Interestingly, serum III that did not react with upper cells did not contain detectable antibodies directed against 65, 63, and 61.5 kD KIF proteins. The staining pattern of serum II is illustrated in Figure 6.

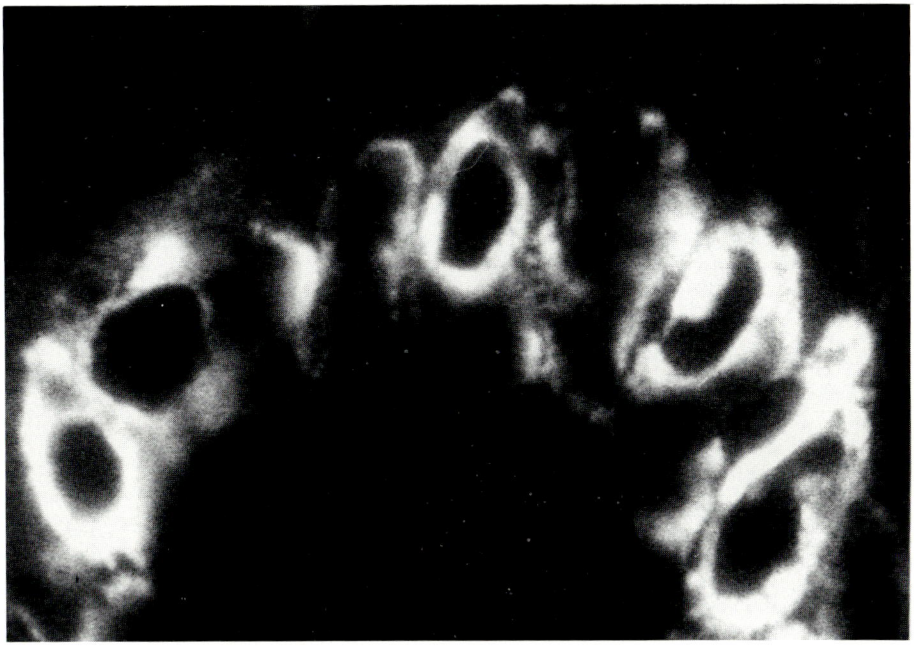

Figure 8. Basal cell antibodies detected by IIF (complement fixation) in a case of herpes gestationis (Didierjean and Saurat [13]).

preted as the retention of BP Ag within the cell; it is indeed well established that BP Ag is secreted by the basal keratinocyte (55,62).

Miscellaneous

KCAbs have also been reported in lichen planus (LP) (11,41), Darier disease (58), and various other dermatoses (43). Interestingly, an MCA with B-cyt activity was found in a patient with myeloma and a bullous dermatosis that could not be analyzed by electron microscopy (EM) (61); the precise antigenic specificity of this MCA could not be determined. We have found, in a patient with a chronic cold agglutinin disease (17), that the monoclonal cold agglutinin of Pr 1h specificity reacted with the cytoplasm of keratinocytes, giving either a B-cyt, U-cyt, or G-cyt pattern, depending on the OK, PK, or mucous differentiation of the substrate (53).

Comments on the Clinical Significance of KCAbs

KCAbs Are Not Disease Specific

It would appear that KCAbs do not seem to be associated with any specific skin disease. This is evident when no attempt has been made to correlate each of the nine patterns with clinical findings (described in the second section of this chapter (Fig 7)). It is difficult to attempt such a correlation because in most of the studies, only the three basic patterns (U-cyt, B-cyt, and G-cyt) were analyzed. From our experience with sera from patients undergoing a bone marrow transplant (31), in which the precise analysis and correlation of 194 KCAbs-positive sera were carried out, it appeared that no correlation could be found.

Therefore, unless future immunoblot analyses of KCAbs provide new insights in this respect, we consider that KCAbs are probably not disease specific.

KCAbs Do Not Seem to be Pathogenic

Although it was suggested that KCAbs could be cytotoxic to epidermal cells (3), this cannot be accepted without criticism because of the technique used. Most KCAbs are IgG; and in several instances, they have been found to fix complement (personal observations).

However, unlike most of the antibodies that have been found to react with skin structures and to have some clinical relevance, KCAbs seem to be directed against intracytoplasmic components. It is an immunologic dogma that unless specific membrane events take place, antibodies cannot cross the membrane of a living cell. To express a harmful effect (if any), KCAbs would have to reach their target and, therefore, have to cross the cell membrane. The first evidence that KCAbs were not likely to penetrate into keratinocytes came from the direct immunofluorescence (DIF) study of epidermis in bone marrow-grafted patients; we have studied 25 skin specimens from 13 patients, and we have never observed any epidermal binding of KCAbs in vivo. However, this study might be considered as incomplete because, for practical and ethical reasons, it was impossible to correlate the presence of circulating KCAbs with the absence of bound KCAbs at the same time in a sufficient number of patients (41).

Therefore, we performed in vitro experiments using trypsin-isolated keratinocytes from guinea pig ears. The cells were first incubated with various concentrations of several sera containing KCAbs; the staining was then done by FITC and peroxidase-labeled anti-IgG serum. No staining was demonstrated when the keratinocytes were living before incubation with KCAbs; a cytoplasmic staining was shown when the keratinocytes were altered (air dried) prior to exposure to KCAbs. Because the failure to demonstrate penetration of KCAbs into living keratinocytes might be related to technical problems, we have used anti-ribonucleoprotein (RNP) antibodies as controls. It is well established that some patients, most often those having so-called mixed connective tissue disease [MCTD], have in their serum high titers of anti-RNP antibodies; very frequently, the binding of such antibodies seems to occur in vivo, as shown by DIF of skin specimens. We could show that anti-RNP antibodies did seem to penetrate into living keratinocytes in an in vitro system similar to that used for the study of KCAbs; this might suggest that anti-RNP antibodies, because of the high titers or special biological properties, can reach their target even in living cells—a fact that could not be demonstrated for KCAbs (19).

KCAbs and the Physiologic Role of Autoantibodies

Besides their possible pathogenic role in some diseases, autoantibodies are now also considered to play a part in physiologic mechanisms—being transporters of metabolic or catabolic products, thus facilitating the cleansing of the organism by opsonization, which itself favors phagocytosis (22). The immunogenicity of self-Ag might be increased when, in physiologic conditions, they are not degraded by autolytic enzymes.

It would seem that this interpretation fits most of the available data concerning KCAbs. If most KCAbs are, in fact, anti-KIF protein antibodies, it is conceivable that since the natural route of elimination of KIF proteins is shedding with the corneocyte, any systemic absorption facilitated by any kind of skin injury would result in an increase of the natural production of KCAbs. This is the case with burns, cryosurgery for skin cancer, and so on. The incidence of KCAbs would even be increased if, together with the systemic release of KCAgs, a state of polyclonal B-cell activation exists; this would be the case for bone marrow-transplanted patients and, possibly, with some drug reactions.

If this interpretation is correct (presently, only supportive data are available), most KCAbs would appear only as a retrospective sign of epidermal injury.

SUMMARY

The term KCAbs was initially applied to morphologically distinct patterns of epidermal cytoplasmic fluorescence. It has been demonstrated that some KCAbs were directed against KIF proteins; it might also be that some KCAbs are directed against non-KIF proteins of keratinocytes, but the proof is currently lacking. KCAbs do not seem to be pathogenic and have not been associated with any specific skin disease. From present knowledge, it is presumed that KCAbs would rather appear as physiologic antibodies, formed after epidermal injury, for facilitating the cleansing of epidermal Ag not degraded by autolytic enzymes.

ACKNOWLEDGMENTS

This work was supported by grants from the Faculty of Medicine, University of Geneva. Ch. Wasung and C. Fonjallaz prepared the manuscript, Ph. Levy, MD, reviewed the English style and M. Pisteur made the illustrations. Dr. Hintner kindly performed the immunoblot analysis showed in Table 4.

NOTE ADDED IN PROOFS

Since this review has been written, two relevant papers have been published: K. Iwatsuki, et al. (*J. Invest. Dermatol.,* 87:179, 1986) studied sera containing KCAbs by immunoblotting, enzyme-linked immunosorbent assay and immunoelectron microscopy. By immunoblotting all the immunofluorescent positive KCAbs sera were found to bind to one or more keratin band and did not show any reactivity with epidermal Nonidet P-40 soluble proteins. U Cyt and G Cyt Abs were found to react with keratin proteins of 58-56 kD and 67-63 kD whereas B cyt Abs reacted strongly with 63 kD and slightly with 50 kD keratin proteins. In contrast to their previous reports (59, 60) the authors found that KC Abs reacted with tonofilaments in immunoelectron microscopy. They concluded that most though not all human KC Abs are directed against different keratin intermediate filaments proteins. Such findings confirm and extend the data reviewed page 666 of the present chapter. G. Grubauer et al. (*J. Invest. Dermatol.* 87:466, 1986) carefully studied the occurrence of apoptotic keratin bodies in the upper dermis of normal subjects. They showed that these bodies, that are constantly covered with immunoglobulins mainly IgM, were made of keratin intermediate filament proteins. Interestingly, this was associated with the presence in the serum of IgM antibodies reacting by immunoblotting with 51 and 58 kD keratin proteins, which are the constituents of keratin intermediate filaments of keratin bodies and basal keratinocytes. These findings are well in accordance with the concept of KC Abs/KIF Abs being naturally occurring antibodies as reviewed in page 676 of this chapter.

REFERENCES

1. Abel EA, Bystryn JC: Epidermal cytoplasmic antibodies: Incidence and type in normal persons and patients with melanoma. *J Invest Dermatol* 66:44, 1976.
2. Ablin RJ, Holder IA: Basal cell layer antibodies in patients with burns. *Arch Dermatol* 115:932, 1979.
3. Ackermann-Schopf C, Ackermann R, Terasaki PI, et al: Natural and acquired epidermal autoantibodies in man. *J Immunol* 112:2063, 1974.
4. Ackermann-Schopf CMA: Antibodies to basal epidermal cells in patients with basal or squamous cell carcinoma. *Arch Dermatol Res* 257:149, 1976.
5. Beutner EH, Rhodes El, Holborow EJ: Autoimmunity in chronic bullous diseases. *Clin Exp Imm* 2:141, 1967.
6. Burnham TK: Two epidermal cytoplasmic immunofluorescent patterns detected by indirect immunofluorescence. *J Invest Dermatol* 63:100, 1974.
7. Bystryn JC, Abel E, Weidman A: Antibodies against the cytoplasm of human epidermal cells. *Arch Dermatol* 108:241, 1973.
8. Bystryn JC: Clinical significance of basal cell layer antibodies. *Arch Dermatol* 113:1380, 1977.
9. Bystryn JC, Nash M, Robins P: Epidermal cytoplasmic antigens: II. Concurrent presence of antigens of different specificities in normal human skin. *J Invest Dermatol* 71:110, 1978.
10. Bystryn JC, Frances C: Cytoplasmic differentiation antigens of human epidermal cells. *Transplantation* 27:392, 1979.
11. Castells-Rodellas A, Castel T, Capdevila JM, et al: Immunofluorescencia del liquen plan. *Medicina Cutanea* 1:49, 1973.
12. Christophers E, Braun-Falco O: Fluorescein isothiocyanate as a stain for keratinizing epithelia. *Arch Dermatol Res* 241:199, 1971.
13. Didierjean L, Saurat JH: Herpes gestationis: Anticorps circulants contre les cellules basales dans cinq cas sur seize. *Ann Dermatol Venereol (Paris)* 107:1015, 1980.
14. Didierjean L, Saurat JH: Epidermis and thymus. Similar antigenic properties in Hassall's corpuscle and subsets of keratinocytes. *Clin Exp Dermatol* 5:395, 1980.
15. Didierjean L, Woodley DT, Regnier M, et al: Skin explant cultures: Expression of cytoplasmic differentiation antigens in outgrowth cells. *J Invest Dermatol* 76:38, 1981.
16. Didierjean L, Wrench R, Saurat JH: Expression of cytoplasmic antigens linked to orthokeratosis during the development of parakeratosis in newborn mouse tail epidermis. *Differentiation* 23:250, 1983.
17. Doutre MS, Beylot C, Conte Ph, et al: Les signes cutanés de la maladie des agglutinines froides. A propos d'un cas. *Ann Dermatol Venereol (Paris)* 105:541, 1978.
18. Faure M, Eisinger M, Bystryn JC: Decreased expression of epidermal cytoplasmic antigens in cultured human keratinocytes. *J Invest Dermat* 76:347, 1981.
19. Galoppin L, Saurat JH: In vitro study of the binding of antiribonucleoprotein antibodies to the nucleus of isolated living keratinocytes. *J Invest Dermatol* 76:264, 1981.
20. Galoppin L, Didierjean L, Saurat JH: Etude de la fixation des anticorps anticytoplasme des kératinocytes. Discussion du rôle du fragment Fc. *Ann Dermatol Veneréol (Paris)* 108:201, 1981.
21. Gelfant S: A new concept of tissue and tumor cell proliferation. *Cancer Res* 37:3845, 1977.
22. Grabar P: Autoantibodies and the physiological role of immunoglobulins. *Immunology Today* 4:337, 1983.
23. Hertz KC, Gazze LA, Kirkpatrick CH, et al: Autoimmune vitiligo. *N Engl J Med* 297:634, 1977.
24. Hintner H, Steinert P, Lawley TJ: Human upper epidermal cytoplasmic antibodies are directed against keratin intermediate filament proteins. *J Clin Invest* 71:1344, 1983.
25. Holbrook KA, Hennings H: Phenotypic expression of epidermal cells in vitro: A review. *J Invest Dermatol* 81(Suppl):11, 1983.
26. Houvanitz N, Nordlund JL, Lerner AB, et al: Antibodies to melanocytes. Occurrence in patients with vitiligo and chronic mucocutaneous candidiasis. *Arch Dermatol* 117:705, 1981.

27. Joost T van: IgG-class antibodies reactive with basal cells of human skin in certain dermatoses: An immunofluorescent study. Read before the 199th meeting of the Dutch Society of Dermatologists, Amsterdam October 4, 1973 (published as Society proceedings). *Ned Tijdschr Geneesk* 42:1616, 1974.
28. Joost T van: Incidence of circulating antibodies reactive with basal cells of skin in drug reactions. *Acta Dermatol Venereol* 54:183, 1974.
29. Joost T van, Asghar SS, Cormane RH: Skin reactions caused by phenylbutazone. *Arch Dermatol* 110:929, 1974.
30. Joost T van: Serum antibodies with affinity to the cytoplasm of epidermal basal cells. In Beutner EH, Chorzelski TP, Bean SF (Eds): *Immunopathology of the Skin,* ed. 2. Wiley, New York, 1979, p 476.
31. LeMarchand-Venencie F: Anticorps anti-cytoplasme des keratinocytes et greffe de moelle osseuse allogénique chez des patients aplasiques: Recherche de "correlations" avec d'autres paramètres immunologiques. MDr Thesis, Université Pet M Curie Paris 1980, p 36.
32. LeMarchand-Venencie F, Didierjean L, Gluckman E, et al: Anticorps anti-cytoplasme de Kératinocytes-sous-populations de keratinocytes, dysregulation immunitaire. *Ann Dermatol Venereol (Paris)* 108:187, 1981.
33. Loning T, Staquet MJ, Thivolet J, et al: Keratin polypeptides distribution in normal and diseased human epidermis and oral mucosa. Immunohistochemical study on unaltered epithelium and inflammatory, premalignant and malignant lesions. *Virchows Arch [Pathol Histol]* 388:273, 1980.
34. Merot Y, Didierjean L, Faucher F, et al: Antibodies to Merkel cells in human sera: Incidence and significance. *J Am Acad Dermatol* 11:568, 1984.
35. Moll R, Franke WW, Volc-Platzer B, et al: Different keratin polypeptides in epidermis and other epithelia of human skin: A specific cytokeratin of molecular weight 46,000 in epithelia of the pilosebaceous tract and basal cell epitheliomas. *J Cell Biol* 95:282, 1982.
36. Naughton GK, Eisinger M, Bystryn JC: Antibodies to normal human melanocytes in vitiligo. *J Exp Med* 158:246, 1983.
37. Nishikawa T, Kurihara S, Haraka T, et al: Binding of bullous pemphigoid antibodies to basal cells. *J Invest Dermatol* 74:389, 1980.
38. Osborn M, Franke WW, Weber K: Visualization of a system of filaments 7–10 nm thick in cultured cells of an epithelioid line (Pt K2) by immunofluorescence microscopy. *Proc Natl Acad Sci USA* 74:2490, 1977.
39. Paluch EP, Bloch KS: Antibodies to human epidermal cytoplasmic antigens: Incidence, patterns and titers, *J Invest Dermatol* 79:115, 1982.
40. Pujade-Lauraine MD, Saurat JH, Puissant A: Localisation des antigènes HLA sur l'épiderme humain. In E Panconesi (Ed): *Immunopathologica cutanea. Italian general review of Dermatology,* Firenze, 1977, p 38.
41. Saurat JH, Bonnetblanc JM, Gluckman E, et al: Skin antibodies in bone marrow transplanted patients. *Clin Exp Dermatol* 1:377, 1976.
42. Saurat JH, Puissant A, Tilles G, et al: 145 cas de toxidermies. Etude clinique, histologique et immunologique. *Ann Med Interne* 127:666, 1976.
43. Saurat JH, Gluckman E, Didierjean L, et al: Anticorps anti-cytoplasme des cellules de l'épiderme humain. *Ann Dermatol Venereol (Paris)* 104:121, 1977.
44. Saurat JH, Didierjean L, Gluckman E, et al: Studies on epidermal cytoplasmic antibodies. *J Invest Dermatol* 68:245, 1977.
45. Saurat JH, Gluckman E, Didierjean L, et al: Cytoplasmic and HLA antigens in the human epidermis. *Br J Dermatol* 96:603, 1977.
46. Saurat JH: Antibodies with affinity to the cytoplasm of keratinocytes. Importance of the substrates used for their detection. *Acta Dermatol Venerol* 58:378, 1978.
47. Saurat JH, Didierjean L, Gluckman E: Epidermal cytoplasmic antibodies distinguish orthokeratosis from parakeratosis and mucosa. *J Invest Dermatol* 70:233, 1978.
48. Saurat JH, Didierjean L, Beucher F, et al: Immunofluorescent tracing of cytoplasmic components involved in the keratinocyte differentiation. *Br J Dermatol* 98:155, 1978.

49. Saurat JH, Didierjean L, Galoppin L, et al: Antibodies with affinity to the cytoplasm of keratinocytes produced after bone marrow transplantation in man. A review. *Cut Immunopathol, INSERM* 80:77, 1978.
50. Saurat JH: Epidermal cytoplasmic antigens. *J Invest Dermatol* 72:194, 1979.
51. Saurat JH, Didierjean L: Antibodies to outer root sheath of hairs: Distinct antigenic properties of the basal cell layer of outer root sheath below the sebaceous gland canal. *Br J Dermatol* 102:419, 1980.
52. Saurat JH, Didierjean L, Gluckman E: New markers for keratinocyte differentiation. Antibodies with affinity to the cytoplasm of keratinocytes produced after bone marrow graft in humans, M. Paunieras (Ed): *Front Matrix Biol* KARGERI 9:36, 1981.
53. Saurat JH, Didierjean L, Habibi L: Pr antigens in the skin: Distinct localization linked to the stage and the type of keratinocyte differentiation. *Br J Dermatol* 105:25, 1981.
54. Shmunes E, Shu SY: Bullous disease of childhood. Report of a case demonstrating antibasal cell antibody. *Arch Dermatol* 113:325, 1977.
55. Stanley Jr, Hawley-Nelson P, Poirier M, et al: Detection of pemphigoid antigen, pemphigus antigen and keratin filaments by indirect immunofluorescence in cultured human epidermal cells. *J Invest Dermatol* 75:183, 1980.
56. Thivolet J, Beyvin AJ: Recherche par immunofluorescence d'autoanticorps sériques vis à vis des constituants de l'épiderme chez les brûlés. *Experientia* 24:945, 1968.
57. Tseng SCG, Jarvinen MJ, Nelson WG, et al: Correlation of specific keratins with different types of epithelial differentiation: Monoclonal antibody studies. *Cell* 30:361, 1982.
58. Vedtofte P, Joensen HD, Dabelsteen E, et al: Intercellular and circulating antibodies in patients with dyskeratosis follicularis, Darier's disease. *Acta Dermatol Venereol* (*Stockholm*) 58:51, 1978.
59. Viac J, Schmitt D, Staquet MJ, et al: Binding specificity of guinea pig antikeratin polypeptide sera on human keratinocytes: Comparison of their receptors with these of human epidermal cytoplasmic antibodies. *Acta Dermatol Venereol* (*Stockholm*) 60:189, 1980.
60. Viac J, Schmitt D, Reano A, et al: Expression of common cytoplasmic antigens by epithelial cells of thymus and epidermis. *Arch Dermatol Res* 274:113, 1982.
61. Vincendeau P, Claudy A, Thivolet J, et al: Bullous dermatosis and myeloma monoclonal anticytoplasmic antibody activity. *Arch Dermatol* 116:681, 1980.
62. Woodley DT, Didierjean L, Regnier M, et al: Bullous pemphigoid antigen synthesized in vitro by human epidermal cells. *J Invest Dermatol* 75:148, 1980. tested. See text for further discussion; +, positive B-cyt staining; −, no B-cyt staining; ND, not done. Parentheses indicate HLA-A and HLA-B identity and nonreactivity in MLR.

41
Nature and Function of Stratum Corneum/Keratinocyte Cytoplasm Autoantibodies and Their Antigens

Ernst H. Beutner
Vijay Kumar
Stefania Jablonska
Pamela C. Jones

INTRODUCTION

Autoantibodies to stratum corneum (SC) antigens (considered in this chapter) and to keratinocyte cytoplasm (KC) (reviewed in the preceding Chapter 40) can be detected in essentially all normal adult human sera, if appropriate methods are employed. These antibodies are classified as physiologic autoantibodies (Chap. 7). That is, they appear to trigger a normal autoimmune repair mechanism (ARM) (2,4–9,11,12). The key factor that distinguishes such physiologic forms of autoimmunity from pathologic ones is their inability to react in vivo with the normal, intact, self-antigens (Chap. 7). As indicated in Figure 1, reactions of such physiologic antibodies can occur only with altered self-antigens. Since one of the groups of SC antigens to which such physiologic autoantibodies are directed cross-react with KC antigens, we deal with the SC and KC systems together in this chapter.

BACKGROUND

Terasaki and Chamberlain in 1962 (55) found, in the course of their studies on "transplantation" that trypsinized suspensions of epidermal cells when incubated with fresh autologous sera of adult rabbits, rats, and guinea pigs induced cell lysis. This keratinocyte cytoplasmic antibody (KCAb) mediated lysis was complement-dependent. These studies were later extended by Ackermann-Schopf et al. (1).

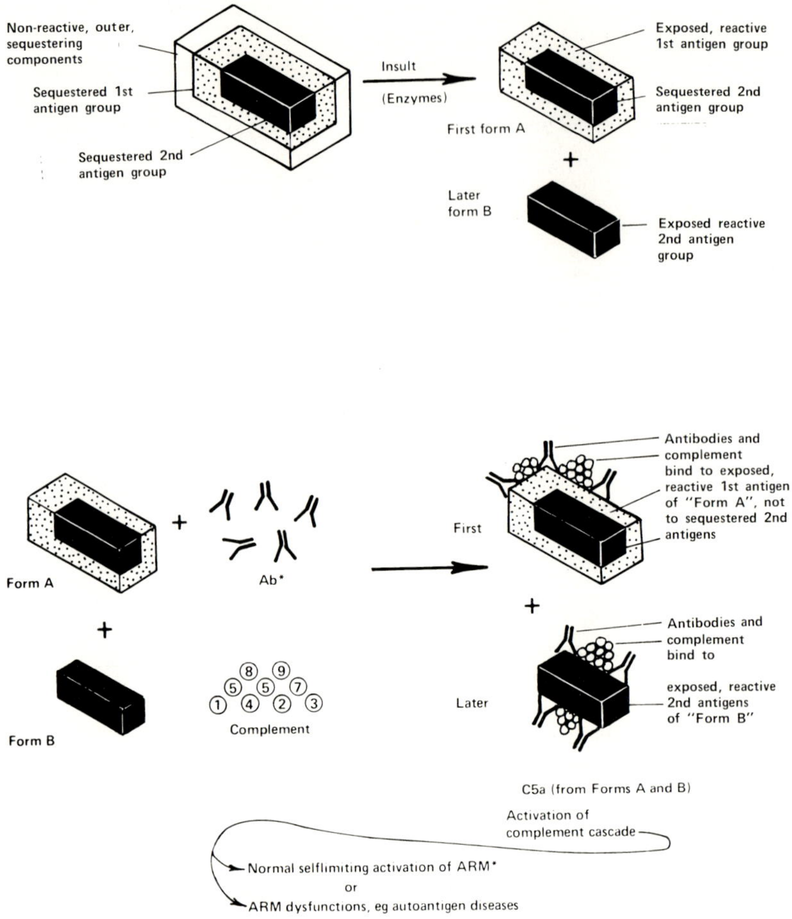

Figure 1. Diagram of molecular rearrangements of antigens for physiologic autoantibodies such as the SCAb-SCAg/KCAb-KCAg system. In vivo reactions of such physiologic autoantibodies trigger a cascade of reactions, including the unmasking of other self-antigens, the activation of the complement cascade, and other biologically active systems that implement the ARM. Normally, such an ARM is a self-limiting, healing mechanism. Dysfunctions of an ARM can cause diseases. We propose, for example, that healing defects may be due to such ARM dysfunctions.

Boyden, in 1964 (20), published a report on the demonstration of complement-fixing (CF) and tanned cell hemagglutinating antibodies in normal rabbit sera, using an aqueous extract of rabbit skin. The CF antigen served also as a coating agent for his tanned cell hemagglutinating method (19). These test systems gave positive reactions with all sera tested.

In 1964, Lehner (50) reported on antibodies to oral epithelial extracts by a passive hemagglutination. Parish et al. (54), in 1965, reported on antibodies detected by tissue culture methods in sera of patients with a certain form of eczema. However, in neither of these studies (50,54) were the antibodies found in all normal adult sera. In 1964, Tönder et al. (56), in their original work on the method of mixed agglutination on tissue sections, appear to have encountered a form of KCAb in normal sera.

Fisher (29), in 1965, reported on the demonstration of antibodies in the sera of 9 of 66 patients with various dermatoses, using a passive hemagglutination method with tanned red cells coated with aqueous extracts of callus. None of 20 normal control sera, however, gave such reactions. Beutner et al., in 1967 (15), reported the first immunofluorescence (IF) studies on human skin and guinea pig lip. They compared the intercellular (IC) antibodies found in 8 of 10 pemphigus cases and also the basement membrane zone (BMZ) antibodies found in two of three bullous pemphigoid (BP) cases, with the KCAb detected at 1:10 dilution in sera of 8 of 99 patients with diverse clinical conditions. Reactions in the horny layer were disregarded at that time since the authors prime concern were the distinctions of KCAb from pemphigus antibodies. The optical systems used at that time were less sensitive. Even with present optical systems, lower dilutions are needed to detect keratinocyte cytoplasmic/stratum corneum antibodies (KCAb/SCAb) in some sera. Krogh et al., in a series of papers, reported on SCAb in all normal human sera (39–46,56). They used: 1) the method of immune adherence to cryostat sections (43); 2) passive hemagglutination of fresh red cells coated with the water phase of a phenol water extract from a trypsin digest of callus (to detect what we now refer to as TR type SCAb) (41); and 3) other methods (45). In 1969 and 1970, Krogh also mentioned IF staining on the surface of "monolayers" of SC cells obtained with Scotch Tape (39,40) and suggested that the staining seen by indirect IF (IIF) of skin sections could be due to the same. Parish (53) questioned the existence of these universal autoantibodies. In 1975, Beutner et al. reported a "four-compartment" specificity test to demonstrate SCAb, using combinations of direct IF (DIF) and IIF and conjugates with and without antibodies (10). With this four-compartment test, they observed that particularly the stratum granulosum staining of the type reported by Krogh (40) could be due either to SCAb or to nonspecific staining associated with high fluorescein-to-protein (F/P) ratios of the conjugates. Using 1:10 dilutions of sera, they found SCAb in 20 of 24 adult sera, and noted that in the remaining four there was a questionable SCAb reaction. (The substage illuminators used then were less sensitive than the present epiillumination systems.) These SCAb were also found to fix complement in IF tests (7). Beutner et al., in 1981 (5), showed that the SCAb not only fail to react in vivo, but also do not react in organ culture explants. This serves to distinguish these antibodies from the pemphigus antibodies, which do react with their antigens in vivo and in organ cultures (28,52; Chaps. 8, 10, and 13). This affords the basis for classifying autoantibodies into physiologic and pathologic types (Chap. 7). The KCAb, on this basis, may also be classified as physiologic autoantibodies (11). Binder (16) and Binder et al. (17) demonstrated that the SCAb detected by IIF are directed against a different group of antigens (the trysin-sensitive [TS]-type SC antigens [SCAg]) than those detected by passive hemagglutination with the water phase antigen from the trypsin phenol water extraction, as described by Krogh et al. (42) (the trypsin-resistant [TR]-type SCAg). Those detected by IIF on normal skin sections are referred to here as TS type of SCAg or KCAg, while we refer to those detected by the previously mentioned passive hemagglutination method as the TR type of SCAg. Elution studies on psoriatic scales of Jablonska (36) and Kumar et al. (47), and the analytic studies on experimental scratches by Dabski (24), indicate that TR-type SCAg are the ones that commonly react in vivo.

Hintner et al. (34,35) suggested that KCAg and SCAg, as detected by IIF (i.e., TS type), appear to have antigenic determinants on keratin intermediate filament (KIF). They demonstrated by absorption and immunoblot methods that the KCAb producing the "upper cytoplasmic" staining are the same as the SCAb binding to the SC in IIF tests (see Figs. 2a to 2d). Hintner and Lawley (34) raised questions about the capacity of some sera to stain only the horny layer and others to react with cytoplasm of the

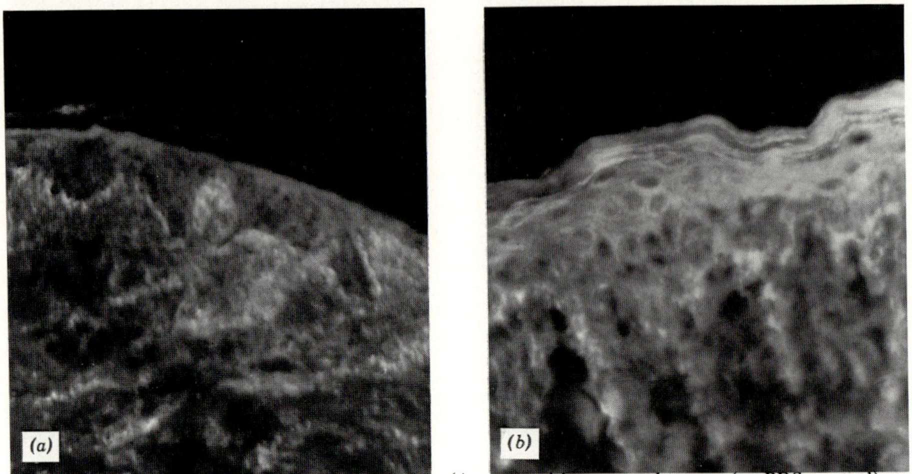

Figure 2. Normal human skin frozen section (4-μ test with a normal serum (or PBS control) and an antihuman IgG conjugate, with a molar F/P ratio of 2:7 and 4 U/ml diluted 1:16 to contain 1/4 unit and a normal human serum with a titer of SCAb/KCAb of 20 in IIF tests in skin. a. Skin section treated with pH 7.2 PBS and conjugate. Note lack of reaction in epidermis although the serum of the subject contains SCAb/KCAb (100×). b. Skin section treated with a normal human serum diluted 1:2.5 and conjugate. Note positive reaction in stratum corneum (SCAb) and in the stratum spinosum (KCAb) in other areas (200×). c. Same section as b. An area with positive reactions in the stratum corneum (SCAb) in some fields and in the stratum spinosum (KCAb) in most, but not all, fields (100×). d. Same section as b. An area with a positive upper cytoplasmic staining (KCAb), but almost no reaction in the stratum corneum (200×). e. Indirect IF stain of a frozen section of epidermal portion of monkey lip treated with a 1:2.5 dilution of another normal human serum and the same anti-human IgG conjugate as for a to d. Note staining of the stratum corneum, the upper layers of the stratum spinosum, and the basal cells. This serum contains both the SCAb/KCAb and the basal cell antibodies) (500×).

prickle cell layer, if the antibodies are directed to the same antigens. However, on re-examining the IF reactions (e.g., Fig. 2), it becomes more understandable. Goldsmith et al. (31) present evidence that the SCAg seen by IF staining is a soluble protein not associated with keratin, thus raising a question about the KIF nature of the antigen(s). The recent studies of Jones (37) suggests the TR-SCAg is localized to the cell envelope. It would be difficult to envisage keratin on the outside of the cell envelope, since its cellular location is cytoplasmic. Thus, there is a conflict still existing in these groups of studies, and until it is resolved, it is not yet appropriate to equate the TS-SCAg with KIF.

Kaneko et al. (38) demonstrated that the immune deposits in psoriatic scales contained not only IgA, but also the "S" or secretory component, and that dermal cells in lesions also contain the S piece, presumably due to the phagocytosis of immune complexes with S piece.

Immune complexes appear in the circulation in psoriasis (21,49); particularly immune complexes with IgA are elevated (32,49). It is noteworthy in this connection that IgA bound in vivo to psoriatic scales are equal to or greater than the bound IgG.

Allospecificity of SCAg was shown independently by Dabski et al. (26) and by Bystryn et al. (23). The first to recognize and characterize the sequestering factors to

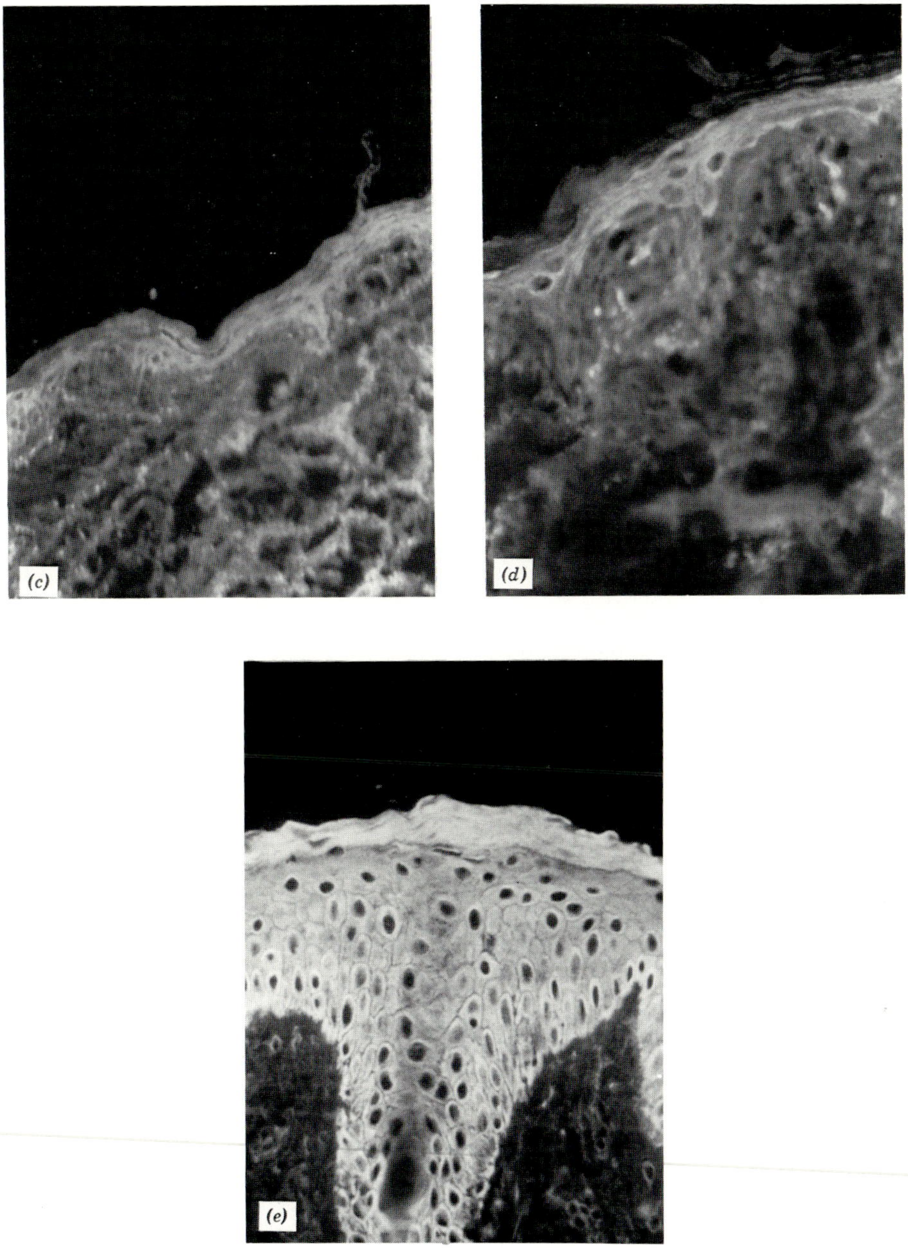

Figure 2 (continued)

SCAg detected by IF was Kumar et al. (48), and sequestering factor to the type KCAg was characterized by Beutner and Kumar (12) before it was shown that SCAg and KCAg may be the same. The relationship of the effects of proteases in these studies (48) to the SCAb-enhancing effects of proteases of polymorphonuclear leukocytes (PMN), reported by Dabski et al. (27), merits further study.

Studies of Lobitz and Buxman (51) on the IIF distribution of the substrate for bovine snout transglutaminase (as demonstrated with polyclonal rabbit antibodies induced by immunization) show that this substrate appears in the cytoplasm of keratinocytes and in the envelope of horny layer cells. This illustrates the general principle that antigens appearing in one layer of skin may be expected in others. Thus, while it has not been proven that the TR-type SCAg also occur in the prickle cell layer, it is doubtful that they form novel antigens.

A review of the background of the work on KCAb appears in the preceding Chapter 40.

METHODS FOR DETECTING STRATUM CORNEUM ANTIBODIES AND KERATINOCTYE CYTOPLASMIC ANTIBODIES

Details of methods for detecting SCAb are given in a book recently edited by Beutner (3). Some information on techniques also appears in Chapter 1 (IF methods) and in the preceding editions of this book (13,14). This section provides both brief overviews and some key data on methods in the sequence in which they were reported; notably: 1) complement fixation, 2) passive hemagglutination with tanned cells and fresh cells, 3) immune adherence, 4) IIF staining, and 5) immunoblot.

Complement Fixation

This classic method was used only by Boyden (20). Briefly, hemolytic complement fixation (CF) tests involve two steps. First, the reactions of either soluble or suspended particulate antigens with antibodies followed by the addition of quantitative amounts of complement in the form of fresh whole human serum. The amount of complement consumed by this first-step reaction of the antibodies is assayed by the second-step hemolytic system. This consists of sheep erythrocytes "sensitized with amboceptor"; that is, pretreated with a subagglutinating concentration of rabbit antibodies to sheep erythrocytes. The inhibition of lysis due to the consumption of complement in the first step of the reaction is a positive finding of CF antibodies if all of the controls give the expected reactions. Microtiter plates are used in more modern versions of CF tests (24). This classic method is gradually being superceded by other methods, which test for the presence of specific complement components (e.g., IF staining for C3) (7), rather than the consumption of total hemolytic complement.

Passive Hemagglutination with Tanned Red Blood Cells

This method, which was devised by Boyden (19) and refined by others (33), was used by Boyden (20), Fisher (29), and Lehner (50) for SCAb/KCAb studies. Either sheep or human group O red blood are usually employed. An example of a procedure with human group O cells is as follows: 1) Treat 4% cell suspension with 1:15,000 dilution of tannic acid (1:100 dilution in H_2O and 1:150 dilution in phosphate-buffered saline [PBS]) for 30 minutes at room temperature. 2) Wash 2% cell suspension three times in PBS and treat with antigen (approximately 1 mg protein/ml) for 30 minutes at room temperature. 3) Wash 2% cell suspension three times with 1:100 dilution of normal rabbit serum in PBS. And 4) place both coated and uncoated 2% suspensions in microtiter plates and add dilutions of sera made with 1:100 dilution of normal rabbit serum in

PBS, and read sedimentation patterns. This method, which detects protein antigens, may come back into use in future studies on SCAb/KCAb.

Passive Hemagglutination with Fresh Red Blood Cells

This technique, which was introduced into SCAb/KCAb studies by Krogh et al. (41,42), is regarded by immunologists as a method primarily for the detection of carbohydrate-type antigens. This method, which they described accurately (46) in the book on psoriasis (3), entails antigen preparation, red cell coating, and serologic testing. Most of the work reported by Krogh rests on a "trypsin-phenol/water" antigen prepared by 24-hour digestion of callus with Sigma* type IX trypsin followed by phenol water extraction. The water phase antigen is used to coat sheep erythrocytes (referred to here as TR-type SCAg). Also, the phenol phase of this extraction as well as the water phase of phenol water extraction of undigested lyophilized callus give small yields of reactive material. The antigenic specificities of these reagents, however, are distinct from those of the trypsin-phenol water reagent. This antigen, usually at a 0.25 to 1 mg/ml concentration, is incubated for 1 hour at 37°C, with 1% suspensions of sheep erythrocytes to sensitize them. The sensitized erythrocytes are washed in PBS and made up to a 0.5% suspension. For serologic tests, sera are absorbed with uncoated sheep erythrocytes and doubling dilutions are mixed with an equal amount of the sensitized red blood cells, in microtiter plates and then read for patterns.

Immune Adherence and Mixed Agglutination on Tissue Sections

Immune adherence, a complement-mediated method, was the first used in the SCAb studies of Krogh and Tönder (43) in 1968, but it has not been used by others since. Briefly, frozen sections of skin comparable to those used in IIF studies (see the following text) are placed on coverglasses fixed in 4% neutral-buffered formalin and dried. Fresh serum dilutions, which contain antibodies that bind to skin antigens and complement, are incubated for 20 minutes at 37°C. Secondly, the coverglasses are put on microtiter wells with human group O Rh-negative red blood cells, inverted 20 minutes, and then returned to allow unbound red blood cells to come off and read microscopically for immune adherence of the red blood cells to the fixed complement (56).

The mixed agglutination on the tissue section method, which was first described by Tönder et al. (56), was also used by Krogh and Tönder (46). Briefly, frozen sections of skin cut as for IF studies are treated with erythrocytes pre-sensitized to detect Ig or complement components or rheumatoid factor. This method has been used for studies of in vivo-bound immunoreactants.

Immunoblots

This method has been used by Hintner et al. (34,35) to characterize the TS-type SCAg/KCAg detected by standard IIF, but it has not been found to be as useful for studies of TR-type SCAg (37). Briefly, for immunoblots, solubilized antigens are electrophoresed in a polyacrylamide gel, the material is then transferred onto nitrocellulose paper, and the latter is pretreated with a nonreactive blocking agent (e.g., albumin) and treated with antisera (22,30). The binding of antibodies is commonly detected with ^{125}I-labeled

*Sigma Chemical Company, P.O. Box 14508, St. Louis, MO 63178.

protein A, although other methods can be used such as immunoenzyme staining with glucose oxidase labeled anti-IgG.

Immunofluorescence (IF)

The various forms of IF are now the most widely used techniques for studies of SCAb, KCAb, and their antigens. (for basics, see 3,13,14; and also Chap. 1).

The types of IF studies reported to date include the following:

1. Direct IF studies for localization of Ig, complement, fibrin, and other serum components in or on the skin, mucosa, or cells only give immunohistologic data in biopsy studies; but they can give data on antibody binding when used on explants or cells maintained in culture under controlled conditions. (See the next subsection on IF methods for studies on sequestering factors.)
2. Indirect IF tests may be performed for SCAb/KCAb on frozen sections (10,16), or with suspensions of keratinocytes (37).
3. Complement IF tests detect CF by SCAb (7); KCAb also, could be detected in this way. It can be performed as a two-step procedure with fresh serum as a source of both SCAb/KCAb and complement components.
4. Combinations of items 1 and 2 above afford the basis for the "four-compartment specificity test" (10). The first step is with diluent (PBS) or antiserum (e.g., with SCAb). The second step is with conjugate with or without antiglobulin antibody (see Fig. 1 in Chap. 42).
5. Indirect IF tests in the form of chessboard titrations with SCAb of the type shown in Table 1 illustrate the fact that high F/P ratios of conjugate give nonspecific staining of the stratum granulosum, while lower F/P ratios do not; for example, conjugates with molar F/P ratios of 2 or less give little or no nonspecific staining, while molar F/P ratios of 3 and up are progressively more troublesome in this respect.

Because of the importance of the sequestering protein(s) of SCAg and KCAg, the IF methods used in studying them merit a separate subsection.

IF Methods for Studies of Sequestering Factors of SCAg and KCAg

The differences between the DIF and IIF findings in studies of skin, mucosa, or callus from biopsy specimens, or explants cultured or maintained in media with or without SCAb/KCAb, provide test systems for characterization of the sequestering factors responsible for the H-self behavior of SCAg/KCAg. The combinations that have been used include the following:

1. Skin biopsy specimens incubated with known Ig class(es) and titers of SCAb and/or KCAb (see Fig. 1) (2,4,5,11).
   a) Direct IF for IgG, IgA, and IgM—*negative* in normal areas (*positive* at cut edges or at sites of lesions).
   b) Indirect IF for IgG, IgA, and/or IgM-class antibodies in the serum of the biopsy donor—*positive* for some.
   c) The difference(s) between the DIF and IIF finding are due to the sequestering of SCAg/KCAg.

2. Skin or mucosal explants cultured or maintained in media with or without SCAb or KCAb as normal fresh viable tissue (12,48).
   a) Direct IF (as for skin biopsy specimens above)—*negative* normally.
   b) Indirect IF (as for skin biopsy specimens above)—*positive* normally. Use same sera or Ig fractions, which are used for culturing explants.
   c) The differences are examined (as for biopsy specimens). The use of different methods for pretreating explants permits characterization of sequestering factors. Under those conditions, DIF can reveal antibody binding, since the media in which explants are maintained can be controlled; for example, by absorption of antibodies or the use of control media free of Ig or absorbed free of SCAb (16,18).

FORMATION OF STRATUM CORNEUM ANTIBODIES/KERATINOCYTE CYTOPLASMIC ANTIBODIES

SCAb/KCAb are formed during the first year of life (19,45,55). The same holds true for the formation of universal autoantibodies to the T antigens of red blood cells (Chap. 7). Importantly, it may well be true that *all universal physiologic autoantibodies form in the first year of life.*

Specifically, Terasaki and Chamberlain in 1962 (55) reported on the finding of CF KCAb in all adult sera of rabbits, rats, and guinea pigs, but not in sera of newborns. Similarly, Boyden (20), who demonstrated CF antibodies to skin extracts in all adult rabbit sera, found none in newborns or in 1- and 2-week-old rabbits, variable results with 3-week-old rabbits, and "normal" titers after 6 weeks with CF tests. Krogh and Tönder (46), using an immune adherence technique, found only the IgG-class antibodies at birth and during the first month. These presumably are of maternal origin. From the second to about the fourth month of life, increasing concentrations of IgM-class antibodies appear, and by about the sixth month, adult levels of IgG- and IgM-class SCAb appear. While Krogh and Tönder (45) suggest that these changes in titers reflect exogenous antigenic stimuli, such as microorganisms in normal flora, Boyden (20) advances the view that immunization results from injury to the skin. Until recently, there was little evidence to favor one view or another. The finding of cross-reactivity between species and some species specificity (45) for the producer's skin (23,26) favor the view that these antibodies form in response to self-antigen immunization by scratches or other forms of skin injury. The role of these antibodies in the repair of injury is discussed in Chap. 7 and elsewhere (2,4–9).

BASIC ROLES AND RELATIONSHIPS OF STRATUM CORNEUM ANTIBODIES/KERATINOCYTE CYTOPLASMIC ANTIBODIES, AND STRATUM CORNEUM ANTIGENS/KERATINOCYTE CYTOPLASMIC ANTIGENS

To gain a meaningful understanding of the nature of the normal reaction patterns of these SCAb/KCAb with their homologous self-antigens (SCAg or KCAg) both in vivo and in vitro, we need, at the outset, to consider three dimensions of the question and to integrate them. Notably, we need to consider: 1) the *functions* of the SCAb/KCAb reactions; 2) the antigenic *structures* to which these antibodies react, not merely at the

Table 1. Chessboard Titration of a Normal Human Serum and Low, Medium, and High F/P Ratio Conjugates on Monkey Skin

Sera	*Dilution*	*IIF*							*Comments*
SCAb	1/80	±	±	±	–	–	–		Tests of 1/1,
	1/40	±	±	±	–	–	–		1/2, 1/4, & 1/8
	1/20	w+	w+	w+	–	–	–		dilution of con-
	1/10	+	+	w+	w+	w+	±		jugate alone:
	1/5	+	+/++	+	+	w+	±		Saline controls
Abs SCAb[a]	1/5	±	±	±	–	–	±		yielded stratum
Saline		–	–	–	–	–	–		granulosum stain-
Dilution of the: C-433[b]		1/16	1/32	1/64	1/128	1/256	1/512		ing to a titer of
	U/ml	1/2	1/4	1/8	1/16	1/32	1/64		4 (16 μg F/ml).
	μg F/ml	2.1	1.0	0.52	0.26	0.13	0.06		
SCAb	1/80	±	±	–	–	–	–	–	This conjugate is
	1/40	w+	w+	–	–	–	–	–	of marginal use-
	1/20	+	w+	w+	w+	±	–	–	fulness for SCAb
	1/10	++	+	+	+	w+	±	–	detection, be-
	1/5	++	+/++	++	+	+	±	–	cause this use
Abs SCAb	1/5	w+	w+	±	±	–	–	–	dilution is close
Saline		±	±	–	–	–	–	–	to the NSS range.
Dilution of the: C-458[b]		1/32	1/64	1/128	1/256	1/512	1/1024	1/2048	
	U/ml	1/2	1/4	1/8	1/16	1/32	1/64	1/128	
	μg F/ml	2.2	1.1	0.55	0.27	0.14	0.07	0.03	
SCAb	1/80	++	+	w+	w+	±	±	–	Since this con-
	1/40	++	+/w+	w+	+/w+	±/w+	w+	–	jugate did not
	1/20	++	+	+	+/w+	w+	w+	–	give plateau
	1/10	++/+++	+	+	+/w+	+/w+	+/w+	–	titer, no use
	1/5	++/+++	++	+/++	+/w+	+	+/w+	–	dilution can be
Abs SCAb		++	+	+/w+	±	w+	±	–	selected.

Saline	++/+++	+/w+	w+	w+	±	−	−
Dilution of the: C-449[b]	1/32	1/64	1/128	1/256	1/512	1/1024	1/2048
U/ml	1/4	1/8	1/16	1/32	1/64	1/128	1/256
μg F/ml	4.7	2.3	1.2	0.6	0.3	0.15	0.07

[a]Abs SCAb: Serum absorbed free of SCAb by repeated absorptions with callus homogenate.
[b]The characteristics of these conjugates were as follows:

	C443	*C458*	*C449*
Primary conjugate property			
Molar F/P ratio	1.2	2.1	4.8
Findings of chessboard titrations			
Plateau titer range of SCAb	10–20	20	None (40)
Plateau endpoint (U/ml)	1/32 U/ml	1/32 U/ml	None (1/128)
NSS	None		
Threshold (μg F/ml)	8 mg/ml	0.55	0.15
Use dilution (2 to 3 dilutions before PEP)	1/4–1/8 U/ml	1/8 U/ml	None
Other conjugate properties			
Antibody (AB) in U/ml	8.0	16.0	8.0
in mg Ab/ml	2.0	4.3	3.5
mg Ab/U	0.25	0.28	0.43

histologic or cytologic level, but more importantly at the molecular levels; and 3) the biochemical features of the sequestering factor(s). The integration of these three dimensions provide us with an overview of the relationships of SCAb and KCAb with their SCAg and KCAg. The diagrams in Fig. 1 portray the types of relationships under consideration, and the following subsections provide overviews of the previously mentioned data. Fig. 2 depicts the IIF staining patterns of: 1) negative control (Fig. 2a), in which no in vivo reactions can be seen; 2) staining of both the SC (SCAb reaction) and stratum spinosum (KCAb reaction), which can be seen in some areas (Fig. 2b); 3) staining mostly of the SCAb form (Fig. 2c); and 4) upper cytoplasmic staining (KCAb) exclusively (Fig. 2d). The variation in the reaction patterns in Figures 2a to 2d may be due to the interference phenomenon or to the variation in antigenicity of the SCAg and KCAg in different areas. It seems probable that all sera can give both the SCAb and KCAb pattern, if tested on multiple skin samples. Repeated studies in this laboratory show that absorption of sera with SCAg in the form of ground callus removes the "KCAb" reaction pattern. Fig. 2e illustrates the appearance of the IF patterns obtained with the apparent coexistence of SCAb/KCAb with basal cell antibodies. The latter could be distinctly seen when the preparation was examined at different focal planes and in different areas.

Function of SCAb and KCAb

Physiologic autoantibodies such as SCAb and KCAb, as indicated in Fig. 1 and Chap. 7, can only react with injured or otherwise altered epidermis. They then undergo self-limiting in vivo reactions, which serve to activate physiologic repair mechanisms. These in vivo reactions, which occur when insults convert self-antigen from their normal nonreactive forms to forms that can undergo in vivo reactions with their physiologic autoantibodies, are apparently amplified by the conversions due to proteases of the tissue. Such conversions may appear to be mediated by endogenous hydrolytic enzymes, particularly of PMN. For example, the studies of Dabski et al. (27) demonstrate some of the effects of neutral serine proteases of PMN on SC antigens. In brief, in the SCAb-SCAg and KCAb-KCAg systems, conversion of antigens appears to be mediated by trauma (5,9,17,18), serine proteases (5,27,48), and certain other still unknown factors (see the following section on "Conversion of H-Self Forms of SCAg and KCAg to Reactive Forms" for details). When the converted reactive forms of hidden self-antigens undergo in vivo reactions with their homologous physiologic autoantibodies, they activate complement cascades and then kinins and chemotaxins, as well as other factors activated by immune complex formation (Chap. 5). While such ARM cascades are normally selflimiting, dysfunctions may occur; for example, "autoantigen" diseases such as Huebener, Thomsen, Friedenreich hemolytic anemia (Chap. 7), as suggested by Beutner et al. (2,4,6,8). Psoriasis may also be an autoantigen disease (see Chap. 42).

Divergent Observations on the Structures of SCAg and KCAg

Studies of the reactions of SCAg and KCAg at histologic and cytologic levels by conventional IIF methods yield results that are divergent with the findings that relate to the molecular architecture of these antigens. The molecular architecture portrayed in Figure 1 affords a more valid functional picture of the structures than the IF studies. Briefly, there are three discrepancies. The histologic structure of and sometimes even the tissue

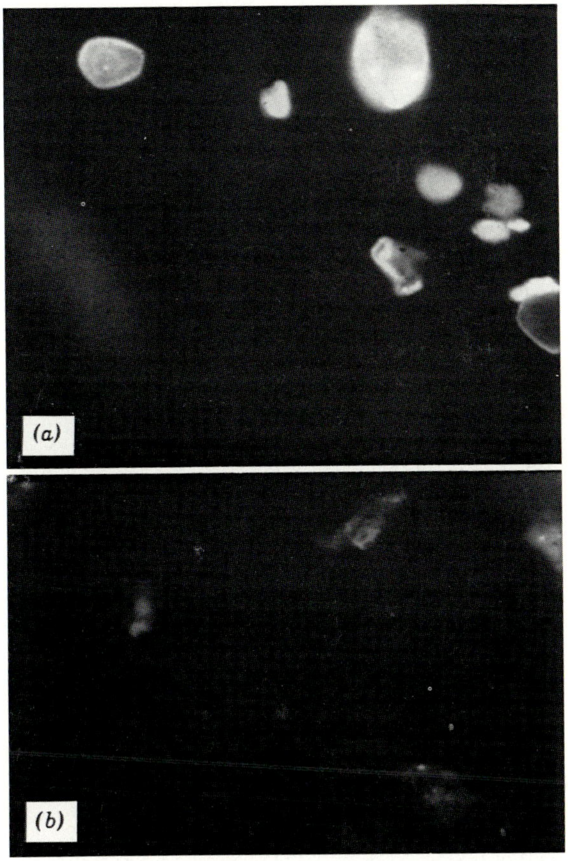

Figure 3. Samples of suspensions of viable, trypsinized monkey mucosal keratinocytes maintained in selected media for 2 hours, washed two times, resuspended in antihuman IgG conjugate for 30 minutes, washed three times, and then examined (500×). a. Keratinocytes maintained in a normal human serum. Note membrane IF. Dead cells also give cytoplasmic IF. b. Keratinocytes maintained in a calcium, magnesium-free buffer. This is a negative control.

specificity of SCAg and KCAg, as seen by IIF tests of frozen sections, appear to be quite distinct (see Figs. 2b, 2c, and 2d and Chap. 40). Yet, there is evidence to indicate that the upper cytoplamic and SC staining may be related to each other, and possibly to KIF antigenically; for example, as indicated above, absorption of sera with SCAg removes KCAb. Secondly, if we examine trypsinized keratinocytes by IIF, positive membrane IF is obtained with all normal sera tested (11). Also, dead cells give cytoplasmic staining (see Fig. 3). Similarly, suspensions of corneocyte give surface IF staining with normal sera (Fig. 4) and "basketweave" IIF patterns on sections (Fig. 2b here and Fig. 1 in Chap. 42). Yet, as indicated in Fig. 2a and in the "Introduction" section, these autoantibodies fail to react in vivo as demonstrated by DIF staining of normal skin biopsy specimens or of skin explants cultured in normal sera with SCAb and KCAb;—despite the apparent surface localization of the antigens. Finally, the SCAb detected by IIF tests of normal skin are distinct from those detected by passive hemagglutination (18). That is, despite the fact

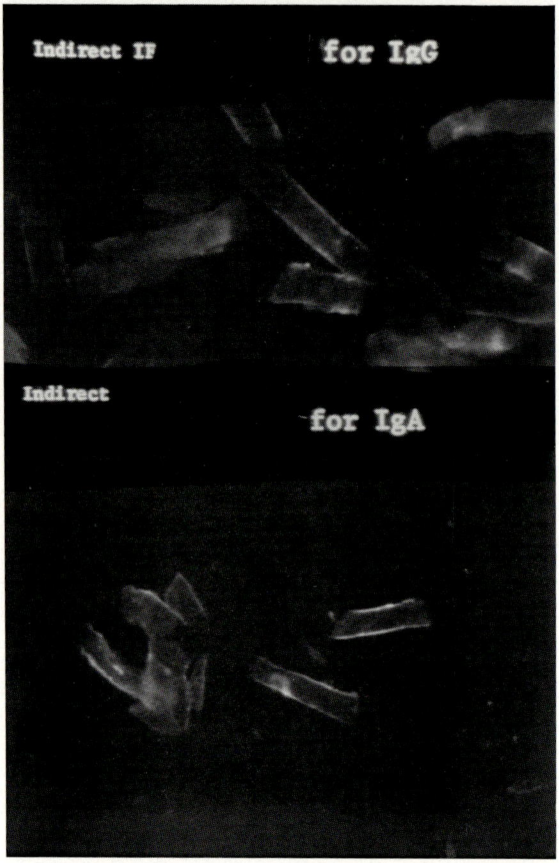

Figure 4. Suspension of scrapings from human callus treated with human serum for 30 minutes, washed three times, resuspended in antihuman IgG conjugate, washed three times, mounted with glycerol and coverglass, and examined. Note staining on surface of corneocytes (500×). Some sera contain SCAb of other Ig classes, but controls suspended in buffer alone give negative IF reactions.

that both kinds of antigen occur in the horny layer on the surface of corneocytes, they are unrelated antigenically or biochemically.

The diagram in Fig. 1 depicts the essential feature of the molecular architecture that fits all of these features of the SCAg-SCAb/KCAg-KCAb systems described with the previously mentioned discrepancies. Clearly, the histologic and cytologic localization cannot be used to interpret functions at molecular levels. The keypoint is that not only the SCAg and KCAg, but also *all other antigens that can react with all true physiologic autoantibodies, exist in a nonreactive form in freshly formed normal tissue.*

Characteristics of Sequestering Factors and SCAg/KCAg

From a functional viewpoint, the two tissue components associated with the antigens that play key roles in triggering these reaction sequences are: 1) the sequestering factors, and 2) the antigens themselves, as shown in Fig. 1.

In our present state of knowledge, the following statements seem justified.

1. Sequestering factors of SCAg and/or KCAg systems are sensitive to serine proteases. They are in the outermost component of the skin and stratified mucous membranes; that is, of keratinocytes and corneocytes.
2. Following initial trauma, the first antigens to convert to a reactive form are TS-type SCAg and/or KCAg (form A in Fig. 1). They can be detected by conventional IIF tests when the sequestering proteins are removed.
3. The antigens released by further serine proteases treatment are TR-type SCAg systems (form B in Fig. 1). These are detected by passive hemagglutination.
4. Reactions of the various forms of SCAg and KCAg occur in vivo; for example, at sites of trauma. These in vivo reactions appear to trigger ARM and the removal of the injured tissue.

Fig. 1 affords a realistic basis for studies of SCAb and KCAb reactions. These assume importance as normal clearing mechanisms (ARM) after skin and mucosal injury (e.g., 6,7,13,16). These appear to include normal ARM functions that manifest as sterile inflammation, apoptosis, and the formation of cytoid bodies (11), as well as dysfunctions of the ARM in diseases; most notably psoriasis (Chap. 42). Clearly, TR-type SCAg bind in vivo in virtually 100% of psoriatic scales, as indicated in Chap. 42. In addition, to the previously mentioned relationships, SCAb and/or KCAb have some allospecificity (23,26) (See the last section of this chapter which deals with specificity studies).

CONVERSION OF H-SELF FORMS OF STRATUM CORNEUM ANTIGEN AND KERATINOCYTE CYTOPLASMIC ANTIGENS TO REACTIVE FORMS

The previously mentioned IF methods for studies of sequestering factors of SCAg/KCAg systems afford the bases for identifying their in vivo behavior as H-self antigens and for characterizing the sequestering factors by tissue culture and other appropriate methods. These yield findings on stratified epithelial antigens comparable to those done on red blood cells in the past (Chap. 7).

Basic Observations on SCAg/KCAg in Skin and Mucosal Explants

Observations are considered, in this subsection, in a rational rather than a chronologic sequence. The most basic comparisons of DIF and IIF findings on SCAg/KCAg in skin explants and the conclusions we may draw from them are as follows:

1. Both in vivo and in normal skin or oral mucosal explants, the SCAb/KCAb complexes fail to react with homologous antigen in or on viable or normal intact epithelium, although the antigens can be detected by IIF in the same tissue (Fig. 1). Thus, studies of explants of skin afford a useful model system for studies of the sequestering factors.

2. Inversion of explants (SC down) brings about no changes in reactions of SCAg (or KCAg); that is, normal stratified epithelia fail to react (11,16). This raises doubts about the role of anatomic barriers as sequestering factors.

3. Comparisons of the behavior of SCAb/KCAb with that of pemphigus antibodies

(28,52; Chap. 13) and antiribonucleoprotein (anti-RNP) antibodies (Chap. 7), both in vivo and in organ culture explants of skin or mucous membranes, reveal that while the SCAb/KCAb fails to react, pathologic autoantibodies do react both in vivo and in cultures. For example: 1) The pemphigus antibodies do react at the surface of keratinocytes in vivo and in cultures of skin or mucosal explants under the same condition as KCAb of comparable titers; yet, KCAb fail to react. (b) The anti-RNP antibodies appear to bind to their nuclear antigens both in vivo and in organ and cell cultures (Chap. 7). These observations indicate that antibodies and other IgG can penetrate at least to the surface and apparently to the nucleus of the corneocytes, and that these histologic structures are not barriers to the reactions of SCAb/KCAb. The observations on the nuclear binding of anti-RNP nucleolar antibodies and certain other nuclear antibodies raise questions about the barrier functions of the cell and nuclear membranes. *Thus, at least for surface antigens and probably for other cellular antigens the barriers are at a molecular level as shown in Fig. 1—not at a histologic level.*

4. Trauma converts the horny layer (16–18) and the stratum spinosum, as well as callus (7), from nonreactive to reactive forms. For example, partial stripping of the horny layer converts the stripped surface from its normal nonreactive form to a form that reacts strongly with SCAb (48). Absorption studies with ground callus suggest that the antigen converted by cuts of the horny layer are TS-type SCAg (17,18). The findings that such conversions require time, e.g. 4 hours or more (48), and that they reach maxima in skin explants in 2 to 3 days (16), suggest that they may be mediated by endogenous or serum enzymes. Effects of exogenous enzyme on conversion are shown in Tables 2 and 3 and are discussed in the following text. The failure of trauma to convert TR-type SCAg to reactive forms may be due to the fact that they are sequestered by TS-type SCAg. Only the latter appears to be exposed by trauma (see below).

Table 2. Characterization of Sequestering Factors of the Antigens of the Stratum Corneum Autoantibodies

Tissue preparations examined	*Enzyme or other pretreatment*	*DIF (and IIF with autologous sera or sera used in cultures)*
Normal skin	None	Negative (IIF positive SCAb with autologous serum
Skin explants (in normal sera)	None	Negative (IIF positive for SCAb with serum used for culturing)
Skin explants (in normal sera) for 4 h)	Swabbed with:	
	1. trypsin	Surface positive
	2. chymotrypsin	Surface positive
	3. fibrinolysin	Surface positive
(same)	Stripped with Scotch tape	Surface positive
(same)	Scratched	Cut-edge positive
Callus	None	Cut-edge positive for GP-type SCAg; negative for CHO-type SCAg
Callus	Trypsin type IX digestion	Cut-edge variable, usually positive for CHO-type SCAg & negative for GP-type SCAg

Table 3. Characterization of the Sequestering Factors of the Antigens of Keratinocyte Cytoplasm Autoantibodies

Tissue preparations examined	*Enzyme pretreatment*	*DIF (and IIF) of autologous sera or sera used in cultures*
Normal skin or mucosal biopsy specimens	None	Negative (IIF positive for KCAb[a] in reaction with autologous serum)
Skin or mucosal explants cultured in normal serum of KCAb	None	Negative (IIF positive for KCAb in reaction in culturing serum)
Skin keratinocytes cultured in normal serum with KCAb	Trypsin digestion	Membrane of keratinocytes positive
Skin explant cultured in serum with pemphigus antibodies[a]	None	Membrane of keratinocytes positive, acantholysis (IIF positive for pemphigus antibodies)

[a]Test conditions and titers of one such autoreaction are shown in Figure 2. IIF titer of pemphigus antibodies of one reference serum used in replicate tests was 160.

Conversion of SCAg to Reactive Form

Direct IF and IIF examinations of skin biopsy specimens and explants with and without, respectively, enzyme pretreatment provide data on the H-self behavior of SCAg and on the nature of its sequestering factors. These findings, summarized in Table 2 excerpted from the studies of Kumar et al. (48), demonstrate that the factor sequestering the IF-reactive SCAg is sensitive to trypsin and other serine proteases. The biochemical nature of the antigens unmasked by these enzyme treatments remains to be determined.

Conversion of KCAg to Their Reactive Form

Direct IF and IIF examinations of skin or oral mucosal biopsy specimens; and of two types of tissue culture preparations of skin or mucous membranes cultured in normal sera containing KCAb, provide data on the H-self behavior of KCAg and on the nature of the sequestering factors (11) as indicated in Table 3. The keratinocytes in the biopsy specimens of neither normal skin or oral mucosa nor in normal skin or mucosal explants cultured 24 hours in normal sera (with KCAb or SCAb) yielded detectable DIF reactions. Yet, the antigen is present, at least on the surface, of the keratinocytes as revealed by membrane IF using an IIF staining of a suspension (Fig. 3). That is, tests with trypsinized keratinocyte suspensions reveal that all normal sera contain cytotoxic KCAb. The KCAb seen by IF staining of sections have been related to their cytotoxicity reactions (1,55) and to membrane IF. Figure 3 illustrates this type of membrane IF reaction. One fact that is evident from the observations in Table 3 is that while the membranes of keratinocytes react with pemphigus antibodies without trypsinization, reactions of normal sera occur only with trypsin-treated keratinocytes. Thus, the trypsin treatment removes or inactivates factor(s) that sequesters at least the surface components of the KCAg without killing the keratinocytes. Second, while the membrane IF due to both KCAb and the pemphigus antibodies entail membrane reactions, the IIF pattern of the two antigens is quite different. The pemphigus antibodies give essentially the same DIF and IIF patterns and kill the keratinocytes without the addition of complement. The KCAb, however, give divergent DIF and IIF patterns and require complement to kill keratinocytes.

BIOCHEMICAL NATURE OF SCAg AND SPECIFICITY OF SCAb

Biochemical Nature of SCAg

Hintner et al. (34,35) reported results of immunoblot and IF studies indicating that SCAg and KCAg are associated with KIF. However, observations of Goldsmith et al. (31) and Jones (37) raise some questions about this, as indicated previously. One possible interpretation is that TS-type and TR-type SCAg coprecipitate with KIF in the fractionation procedure. Interestingly, results of unpublished studies (S. Quitaishat and V. Kumar) on sera absorbed with TR type SCAg indicate that their SCAb are different from KIF antibodies as detected by immunoblot methods.

Extensive biochemical studies of Jones (37) on the composition and structure of TR-type SCAg provide several insights. Periodate treatment of TR-type SCAg, as well as hemagglutination inhibition of SCAb with glucosamine, yield partial inhibition. A part of the antigen appears to be a polypeptide of variable molecular size. Amino acid analysis of a highly active fraction reveals a composition similar to that of corneocyte envelopes. Absorption of sera with suspensions of purified corneocyte envelopes made by each of three methods removed all SCAb to TR-type SCAg. In brief, these and other findings indicate that these SCAb are directed to a heterogeneous group of epitopes on the corneocyte envelopes.

Biochemical Specificity of SCAb

The titers of SCAb in a given serum, vary depending on the method used to detect them. Indirect hemagglutination and IIF identify at least two, and probably many, independent antigen-antibody systems differing in their specificity for biochemical components of SC. Absorption of a serum with TR-type SCAg prepared according to the trypsin-phenol-water extraction method described by Krogh (51) significantly reduces or abolishes the titer of SCAb detectable by the indirect hemagglutination system, whereas titers of SCAb reactive in IIF remain unchanged. The opposite is true if crude preparations of ground callus are used for absorption. Pretreatment of the absorbing callus with proteolytic enzymes, such as trypsin or chemotrypsin, abolishes its affinity for SCAb detectable by IIF.

Direct IF tests with fluorescein-labeled antihuman IgG antibodies give negative results on frozen sections of normal human skin, but give positive reactions at 6-day-old monkey scratch sites (9). Indirect IF tests using antihuman IgG conjugate absorbed free of antibodies cross-reacting with monkey immunoglobulins, and normal human sera selectively absorbed with either TS- or TR-type antigen, provide an experimental model for studying SC antigens involved *in vivo* in immunologic reactions following traumatic insults to the epidermis; for example, scratching. Specifically, IIF tests with human sera absorbed with ground callus as a source of TS antigen render the reaction on normal skin negative, but have no effect on the IF titers at scratch sites. Conversely, sera absorbed free of antibodies to the TR antigens give significantly reduced titers at scratch sites, while titers on sections of normal skin remain unchanged (9). These findings indicate that: 1) 6-day-old scratch sites contain reactive, insoluble forms of TR-type antigen and monkey IgG bound to them; 2) antibodies to the TR antigen of monkey epidermis can be detected by both indirect hemagglutination and IIF; and 3) TR-type SC antigen is reactive *in vivo* with its corresponding SC antibodies as part of the ARM cascade. The same mechanism involving the TR antigen may be operating in the development of the early lesions of psoriasis, as indicated in Chapter 42.

Tissue-, Species-, and Allospecificities

Although the biochemical composition of SC antigens is not precisely known, it is established that while the indirect hemagglutination test detects IgM-class antibodies reacting with the TR or sequestered portion of the SC antigen, IIF identifies those IgG- or IgM-class antibodies that react with TS-type exposed portions of SCAg. It was shown that under certain conditions, the TR antigen can also be detected by IF (25). The question of tissue-, species-, and allospecificities of SCAb, however, has been investigated in several systems such as indirect hemagglutination, immune adherence, and IIF.

In the immune adherence test with normal human sera and skin sections, tissue specificity, but not species specificity, was shown (45). A similar lack of species specificity was demonstrated in SCAb of normal human and animal (rabbit and guinea pig) sera using the indirect hemagglutination test. In the latter system, however, some antibodies with activity against species-specific antigens can be detected in addition to the antibodies with specificity for common antigenic determinants on trypsin-phenol-water antigens (42).

The existence of allospecificity within the SC antibody-antigen system has long been suggested by observations in which marked discrepancies in SCAb titer of reference sera may exist between different laboratories and, even in one laboratory, if various skin substrates are used at different times.

Experiments in which human sera were selectively absorbed from SCAb reactive with ground callus from a single donor demonstrated that such absorptions remove antibodies reactive with some, but not all, skin substrates by IIF (26). The probability of removing all SCAb from a serum increases if a pool of callus from more donors is employed in absorptions. These results suggest the existence of antigenic dissimilarities between horny layers of human epidermis from different individuals. They also demonstrate the presence of allospecific SCAb in human sera. Since SCAb in human sera do not give significantly different titers on autologous skin substrates compared to homologous ones, they behave like both auto- and alloantibodies.

Further evidence for existence of allospecificity and for the presence of both species-specific and species-nonspecific TS-SCAg in human epidermis was gathered from recent experiments with blocking IF. In these studies, substrate specificities of monkey and human SCAb were compared by examining the capacity of the former to interfere with the reaction of the latter on the same epidermal substrate. A conjugate absorbed with monkey immunoglobulins, but still reactive with human immunoglobulins, was used to distinguish between IF reactions produced by human and monkey SCAb on tissue sections. The preincubation of frozen human skin sections with monkey sera containing SCAb blocked the reaction of human sera SCAb of some subjects in tests on some, but not all, skin specimens. These studies provided evidence that: 1) human SC contains several distinct antigenic determinants, some of which are common to monkey and human SCAb, while others are not; 2) human sera contain SCAb of nonidentical substrate specificities, since some are and others are not capable of reacting with SC antigens available after blocking; and 3) SCAb in most monkey sera react with human SC, but their corresponding SC antigens do not react with SCAb in all human sera.

REFERENCES

1. Ackermann-Schopf C, Ackermann R, Terasaki PI, et al: Natural and acquired epidermal autoantibodies in man. *J Immunol* 112:2063–2067, 1974.
2. Beutner EH: A unified concept of autoimmunity as visualized by immunofluorescence and as illustrated by contrasts between stratum corneum and pemphigus antibodies. In Knapp W, Holubar K, Wick G (Eds): *Proceedings of VIth International Conference on Immunofluorescence and Related Techniques.* Elsevier/North Holland, Amsterdam, 1978, pp 175–188.
3. Beutner EH (Ed): *Autoimmunity in Psoriasis.* CRC Press, Boca Raton, FL, 1982, 313 pp.
4. Beutner EH: Nature of autoimmunity: Unified concept and other theories as related to psoriasis. In Beutner EH (Ed): *Autoimmunity in Psoriasis.* CRC Press, Boca Raton, FL, 1982, pp 3–14.
5. Beutner EH, Binder WL, Jablonska S, et al: Nature of stratum corneum autoantibodies, antigens and antigen conversion and their role in healing and in psoriasis. In Marks R, Christophers E (Eds): *The Epidermis in Disease.* MTP Press, Lancaster, UK, 1981, pp 333–357.
6. Beutner EH, Chorzelski TP, Binder WL: Nature of autoimmunity: Pathologic versus physiologic responses and a unifying concept. In Beutner EH, Chorzelski TP, Bean SF (Eds): *Immunopathology of the Skin,* ed. 2. Wiley, New York, 1979, pp 147–180.
7. Beutner EH, Chorzelski TP, Jablonska S: Autoimmunity in psoriasis. I. Studies on the possible significance of the universal stratum corneum antibodies in the pathogenesis of psoriasis. In Farber EM, Cox AJ (Eds): *Psoriasis: Proceedings of the 2nd International Symposium.* Yorke Med. Books, New York, 1977, pp 63–72.
8. Beutner EH, Cunningham RK: Autoimmunity. In Stone J (Ed): *Dermatologic Immunology and Allergy.* CV Mosby, St Louis, 1985, pp 125–142.
9. Beutner EH, Dabski K, Jablonska S, et al: Stratum corneum antigens: Their role in psoriasis and in the autoimmune repair mechanisms. In Marks R, Plewig G (Eds): *Stratum Corneum.* Springer-Verlag, Heidelberg, 1983, pp 92–111.
10. Beutner EH, Jablonska S, Jarzabek-Chorzelska M, et al: Studies in immunodermatology. VI. IF studies of autoantibodies to the stratum corneum and of in vivo fixed IgG in stratum corneum of psoriatic scales. *Int Arch Allergy Appl Immunol* 48:301–323, 1975.
11. Beutner EH, Kumar V: Is the Ig bound to cytoid bodies? *Int J Dermatol* 24:362–368, 1985.
12. Beutner EH, Kumar V: Autoantibodies in health and disease: Classification of autoimmune response using universal stratified epithelial autoantibodies and other skin reactive autoantibodies as models. In Milgrom F, Abeyounis CJ, Albini B (Eds): *Antibodies: Protective, Destructive and Regulatory Role. Proceedings of 9th International Convocation on Immunology.* Karger, Basel, 1985 pp 158–163.
13. Beutner EH, Nisengard RJ: Defined immunofluorescence in clinical immunopathology. In Beutner EH, Chorzelski TP, Bean SF, Jordon RE (Eds): *Immunopathology of the Skin: Labeled Antibody Studies,* ed. 1. Dowden, Hutchinson, Ross, Stroudsburg, PA, 1973, pp 197–247.
14. Beutner EH, Nisengard RJ, Kumar V: Defined immunofluorescence: Basic concepts and their application to clinical immunodermatology. In Beutner EH, Chorzelski TP, Bean SF (Eds): *Immunopathology of the Skin,* ed. 2. Wiley, New York, 1979, pp 29–75.
15. Beutner EH, Rhodes EL, Holborow EJ: Autoimmunity in chronic bullous skin diseases. Immunofluorescent staining of three types of antibodies to skin in sera of patients with pemphigus, bullous pemphigoid and in other human sera. *Clin Exp Immunol* 2:141–151, 1967.
16. Binder WL: Studies on the role of the immune system in the pathogenesis of psoriasis. PhD Thesis, State University of New York at Buffalo, 1978, 164 pp.
17. Binder WL, Beutner EH, Jablonska S: Studies in immunodermatology. VIII. Immunofluorescence studies of stratum corneum antibodies. *Int Arch Allergy Appl Immunol* 61:407–416, 1980.
18. Binder WL, Beutner EH, Jablonska S: Immunofluorescence studies on stratum corneum antibodies. In Beutner EH (Ed): *Autoimmunity in Psoriasis.* CRC Press, Boca Raton, FL, 1982, pp 81–93.

19. Boyden S: The absorption of proteins on erythrocytes treated with tannic acid and the subsequent hemagglutination by anti-protein sera. *J Exp Med* 93:107–120, 1951.
20. Boyden S: Pathology. Autoimmunity and inflammation. *Nature* 201:200–201, 1964.
21. Braun-Falco O, Mannel C, Scherer R: Nachweis von zirkulierenden loeslichen Immunokorplexen im Sserum von Psoriatispatienten mit dem ^{125}J-Clq-Ablenkungs test. *Hautarzt* 28:658–660, 1977.
22. Burnette WN: "Western blotting". Electrophoretic transfer of proteins from sodium dodecyl sulfate-polyacrylamide gels to unmodified nitrocellulose and radiographic detection with antibody and radioiodinated proteins. *Analyt Biochem* 112:195–203, 1981.
23. Bystryn J-C: Natural stratum corneum antibodies and antigens. In Marks R, Plewig G (Eds): *Stratum Corneum.* Springer-Verlag, Heidelberg, 1983, pp 112–128.
24. Colombani J, D'Amaro J, Gabb BW, et al: International agreement on a microtechnique of platelet complement fixation. *Transplant Proc* 3:121–126, 1971.
25. Dabski K, Beutner EH, Jablonska S: Studies in immunodermatology. X. Detection of glycoprotein and carbohydrate type stratum corneum antigens by immunofluorescence. Conversion effects of enzymes and trauma. *Int Arch Allergy Appl Immunol* 71:200–209, 1983.
26. Dabski K, Beutner EH, Jablonska S: Studies in immunodermatology. XI. Demonstration of allospecificity of stratum corneum antibodies and antigens by indirect immunofluorescence. *Int Arch Allergy Appl Immunol* 71:210–213, 1983.
27. Dabski K, Glinski W, Beutner EH, et al: In vitro effects of enzymes of polymorphonuclear leucocytes on the antigenicity of stratum corneum. *Int Arch Allergy Appl Immunol* 77:287–291, 1985.
28. Deng J-S, Beutner EH, Shu S, et al: Pemphigus antibody action on skin explants. Kinetics and acantholytic changes and stability of antigens in tissue cultures of normal monkey skin explants. *Arch Dermatol* 113:923–926, 1977.
29. Fisher JP: Soluble substances of human stratum corneum. I. Immunochemical and immunological study. *J Invest Dermatol* 44:43–50, 1965.
30. Gershoni JM, Palade G: Protein blotting: Principles and applications. *Analyt Biochem* 131:1–15, 1983.
31. Goldsmith LA, Colbert M, McCoon P, et al: Characterization of a human stratum corneum antigen and its autoantibody. *J Invest Dermatol* 82:408, 1984 (abstract).
32. Hall RP, Peck G, Lawley TJ: Detection of IgA immune comlexes in patients with psoriasis. *J Invest Dermatol* 76:302–303, 1981 (abstract).
33. Herbert WJ: Passive hemagglutination with special reference to the tanned cell technique. In Weir DM (Ed): *Handbook of Experimental Immunology.* ed. 3, vol. 1. Blackwell Scientific Publ., Oxford, UK, 1978.
34. Hintner H, Lawley TJ: Keratin intermediate filaments bear antigenic determinants for stratum corneum antibodies. *J Invest Dermatol* 82:491–495, 1984.
35. Hintner H, Steinert PM, Lawley TJ: Human upper epidermal cytoplasmic antibodies are directed against keratin intermediate filament proteins. *J Clin Invest* 71:1344–1351, 1983.
36. Jablonska S, Beutner EH, Binder WL, et al: Immunopathology of psoriasis. *Arch Dermatol Res* 264:65–71, 1979.
37. Jones P: Immunopathology of psoriasis: Characterization of a stratum corneum antigen. PhD Thesis, State University of New York at Buffalo, 1985, 175 pp.
38. Kaneko F, Gushiken H, Kawagishi I, et al: Analysis of immunological response in psoriatic lesions: (1) Immunopathological studies on psoriatic lesions. *J Invest Dermatol* 75:436–439, 1980.
39. Krogh HK: Antibodies in human sera to stratum corneum. *Int Arch Allergy Appl Immunol* 36:415–426, 1969.
40. Krogh HK: The antigen involved in immune adherence with stratum corneum and human serum. *Int Arch Allergy Appl Immunol* 38:78–92, 1970.
41. Krogh HK, Maeland AJ, Tönder O: Indirect hemagglutination for demonstration of antibodies to stratum corneum of skin. *Int Arch Allergy Appl Immunol* 42:493–502, 1972.
42. Krogh HK, Maeland JA, Tönder O: Species specificity of skin antigens prepared by phenol water extraction. *Int Arch Allergy Appl Immunol* 47:839–849, 1974.

43. Krogh HK, Tönder O: Adherence of erythrocytes to stratum corneum of skin tissue sections. *Int Arch Allergy Appl Immunol* 34:170–180, 1968.

44. Krogh HK, Tönder O: Comparison of human stratum corneum, callus and psoriatic scales by means of serological methods. *Int Arch Allergy Appl Immunol* 53:434–440, 1977.

45. Krogh HK, Tönder O: Stratum corneum antigens and antibodies. In Beutner EH, Chorzelski TP, Bean SF (Eds): *Immunopathology of the Skin,* ed. 2. Wiley, New York, 1979, pp 413–425.

46. Krogh HK, Tönder O: Immune adherence and indirect hemagglutination tests for detection of stratum corneum antibodies. In Beutner EH (Ed): *Autoimmunity in Psoriasis.* CRC Press, Boca Raton, FL, 1982, pp 257–266.

47. Kumar V, Jones P, Beutner EH, et al: Immunofluorescence studies in psoriasis: Detection of antibodies to stratum corneum in psoriatic scales. In Beutner EH, Nisengard RJ, Albini B (Eds): *Defined Immunofluorescence and Related Cytochemical Methods. Ann NY Acad Sci* 420:361–368, 1983.

48. Kumar V, Rogozinski T, Beutner EH, et al: Studies in immunodermatology. IX. Effect of organic solvents and enzymes on the reactivity of stratum corneum antigens. *Int Arch Allergy Appl Immunol* 71:112–116, 1983.

49. Laurent MR, Ranayi GS, Shepherd P: Circulating immune complexes, serum immunoglobulins and acute phase proteins in psoriasis and psoriatic arthritis. *Ann Rheum Dis* 46:66–69, 1981.

50. Lehner T: Recurrent aphthous ulceration and autoimmunity. *Lancet* ii:1154–1155, 1964.

51. Lobitz CJ, Buxman MM: Characterization and localization of bovine epidermal transglutaminase substrate. *J Invest Dermatol* 78:150–154, 1982.

52. Michel B, Ko CS: Effect of pemphigus or bullous pemphigoid sera and leukocytes on normal human skin in organ culture. An in vitro model for the study of bullous diseases. *J Invest Dermatol* 62:541–542, 1974 (abstract).

53. Parish WE: General concepts of autosensitivity in disease. In Montagna W, Billingham RE: *Advances in Biology of Skin.* vol. 11. Appleton-Century-Crofts, New York, 1971, pp 233–282.

54. Parish WE, Rook AJ, Champion RH: A study of autoallergy in generalized eczema. *Br J Dermatol* 77:479–526, 1965.

55. Terasaki PI, Chamberlain CC: Destruction of epidermal cells in vitro by autologous serum from normal animals. *J Exp Med* 115:439–452, 1962.

56. Tönder O, Milgrom, F, Witebsky E: Mixed agglutination with tissue sections. *J Exp Med* 119:265–274, 1964.

42
Autoimmunity in Psoriasis

Ernst H. Beutner
Stefania Jablonska
Peter Hebborn
Vijay Kumar

INTRODUCTION

Psoriasis is a dermatosis mediated by genetic and environmental factors that is characterized clinically by inflammatory, scaling lesions and histologically first by a marked exocytosis of polymorphonuclear leukocytes (PMN), and later by acanthosis, a uniform papillomatosis, a marked parakeratosis, and a polymorphous perivascular infiltrate. The data summarized in this chapter indicate that psoriasis is characterized immunologically by a massive local Arthus reaction in the horny layer (3,34,46). Direct immunofluorescent (DIF) studies reveal strongly positive focal deposits of IgG, IgA, IgM, complement components, and fibrin in the stratum corneum (SC) (5,37). The immunoglobulin (Ig) deposits are due to the binding of the complement-fixing (CF) SC antibodies (SCAb) (33,49), which cause the just-mentioned localized Arthus-type reaction. These Arthus reactions are currently the only demonstrable antigen-specific, immunologic reactions that occur in vivo in virtually 100% of scales in patients with active psoriasis (3,34,46). The evidence for some roles which these Arthus reactions, in the horny layer of psoriatic lesions, play in inducing the subjacent epidermal hyperplasia is so compelling that it merits a reorientation of research on the mechanism of the disease (1). To stimulate more productive research in this field, we present in this chapter a "working hypothesis on the cause of psoriasis" (Table 1), which relates to this Arthus-type reaction. In effect, the basic thesis is that changes in the synthesis time of epidermal cells in patients with active psoriasis is secondary to the observed Arthus reaction in psoriatic scales and to the activation of PMN by it and lipoxygenase metabolites.

The present research on psoriasis focuses, to a large extent, on the synthesis time of epidermal cells (11,20,47) and fibroblasts (55) in psoriasis. Some findings in uninvolved psoriatic skin point to increased DNA turnover (11,20). However, Steigleder demonstrated that this DNA synthesis time is a function of the disease activity (59). His data can be summarized as follows:

This work was supported in part by the IF Testing Service and by the Polish Academy of Medicine.

Skin samples examined	*No.*	*Synthesis time ± SD*
Normal epidermis	35	6.9 ± 1.2
Uninvolved skin, no lesions elsewhere	10	6.7 ± 1.4
Uninvolved skin with lesions elsewhere	23	11.1 ± 1.2[a]
Pinpoint lesions	10	19.5 ± 1.4[a]
Psoriatic plaque	112	13.0 ± 1.4[a]

[a]Significant elevation ($p < 0.001$).

He concluded that synthesis time was "significantly prolonged in non-involved skin of patients but only if psoriatic lesions are present." Duell and Voorhees findings are at variances (20) with the data of Steigleder. The crucial studies, however, on the predictive value of any one of the diverse signs of hyperproliferative responses have not been done; that is, studies of responses of normal skin of children of couples with psoriasis who have no personal history of the disease with a view to predicting which offsprings will develop the disease in the future. In effect, it is not possible to determine if the DNA synthesis time, the Arthus-type reaction, or both or some other factors are primary events in the induction of psoriatic lesions. Either way, studies of the type reported by Krueger (48) on the transplantation of skin from psoriatics to nude mice and other studies on cell kinetics, as well as immunologic studies of the skin should, in the future, include controls of uninvolved skin from cases with both active and inactive psoriasis as was done by Steigleder (59).

ARTHUS TYPE REACTIONS IN PSORIATIC SCALES

The only documented in vivo reaction of autoantibodies that fix complement and that occur in all active psoriatic lesions are those of the universal SCAb. These reactions can

Table 1. Observed and Hypothetical Relationships Considered in Studies on the role of SCAb in the Etiology of Psoriasis

Observations	*Interpretation*	*Cause of psoriasis*
Genetic predisposition + Environmental factors: infections, etc.	Due to abnormal SCAg reactivity[a] Increased SCAg reactivity and PMN activation	Autoantigen disease, (i.e., a Self-perpetuating rather than self-limiting in vivo reactions of SCAb due to SCAg activation by PMN enzymes Complement activation (C5a)
Epidermal hyperplasia	Prolonged DNA synthesis time	Activated PMN release mitogens

[a]This abnormal SCAg reactivity is evident from the immunologic studies of psoriatic scales; but from the viewpoint of a genetic marker in the uninvolved skin from symptom-free subjects, it is a hypothetical SCAg abnormality. Therefore, this point is boxed and arrows to and from it are broken lines. Also, the "autoantigen disease" concept is boxed because this is also hypothetical.

be demonstrated in psoriatic scales by DIF (3,5,38) as well as by combinations of DIF and indirect immunofluorescence (IIF) examinations (Fig. 1a to 1f), and by elution studies (33,41,49) (see the next subsection). The SCAb, which are described in Chapter 41, occur in all normal adult sera. Previous studies in this laboratory (1,3) indicate that their normal function is probably to aid in the removal of injured skin components by triggering the autoimmune repair mechanism (ARM). Other types of autoantibodies reported in psoriasis do not entail in vivo reaction in psoriatic lesions. The increase in T-suppressor cells appears to be mediated by a soluble factor (25). None of the studies on T cells and Langerhans cells to date involve reactions with specific antigenic components of the skin. Also, kinetic studies of the latter show that changes in T-cell populations are events that occur late in the disease process (25). Thus, they are not considered here. This section provides a summary of the evidence for the in vivo reactions of SCAb in psoriatic scales, for their activation of complement, and for the release of chemotaxins since this clearly points to in situ Arthus reactions. Beutner's book on *Autoimmunity in Psoriasis* (1) provides a more detailed review of this field, including immunologic studies relating to T-suppressor and T-helper cell populations.

Direct IF Observations on Psoriatic Lesions and Identification of Reactants by Elution Studies.

The immunofluorescent (IF) demonstrations of IgG and complement binding to the SC antigen sites on psoriatic scales (5,37) serve to confirm and extend the previous studies by immune adherence and mixed agglutination on tissue sections (45). That is, IF studies reveal antigenic conversion to reactive forms, which is a phenomenon central to understanding these reactions. Basically, conjugates of goat Ig with fluorescein free of antibody serve as negative controls for comparable conjugates with antibodies to IgG or complement component C3 or to other immunoreactants for DIF studies of sections of psoriatic scales. Direct IF studies reveal binding of the immunoreactants in a baseketweave pattern (see Fig. 1d and 1f) in all psoriatic scales of active lesions. The failure to find such reactions in some biopsy specimens of typical psoriatic lesions is due to the loss of scales (see the following text). Thus, for some purposes, it is best to perform such studies with sections of scales. Indirect IF tests of psoriatic scales with normal human adult sera (all of which contain SCAb) frequently give more extensive basketweave patterns than DIF staining, thus suggesting that SC antigens are only partly saturated in vivo in such lesions.

The basic observations from DIF studies of psoriatic scales have been confirmed (19), but the interpretation that the observed basketweave pattern is due to in vivo binding of SCAb has been challenged by Kimura and Nishikawa (43). They initially reported, on the basis of their elution studies, that the observed Ig binding was nonspecific entrapment of serum proteins due to coagulation. However, they only examined sections eluted with pH 3.0 buffer, not the eluates for SCAb. By examining the eluates of psoriatic scales for two types of SCAb and IgG, Kumar et al. (49) were able to show that pH 2.0 (but not pH 3.0) eluates contain about 50-fold greater specific activity of SCAb than the pH 7.0 washing, as revealed by the indirect hemagglutination test for the antibodies to the trypsin-resistant (TR) SC antigen (Table 2). This affords direct evidence for the in vivo binding of this type of SCAb. Direct IF staining entails washing with pH 7.0 buffers; thus, only the residual IgG and other Ig is detected. Control elution studies on sections of eczema lesions and psoriatic lesions yield comparable results. Interestingly, most of the SCAb to the trypsin-sensitive (TS) type SC antigens

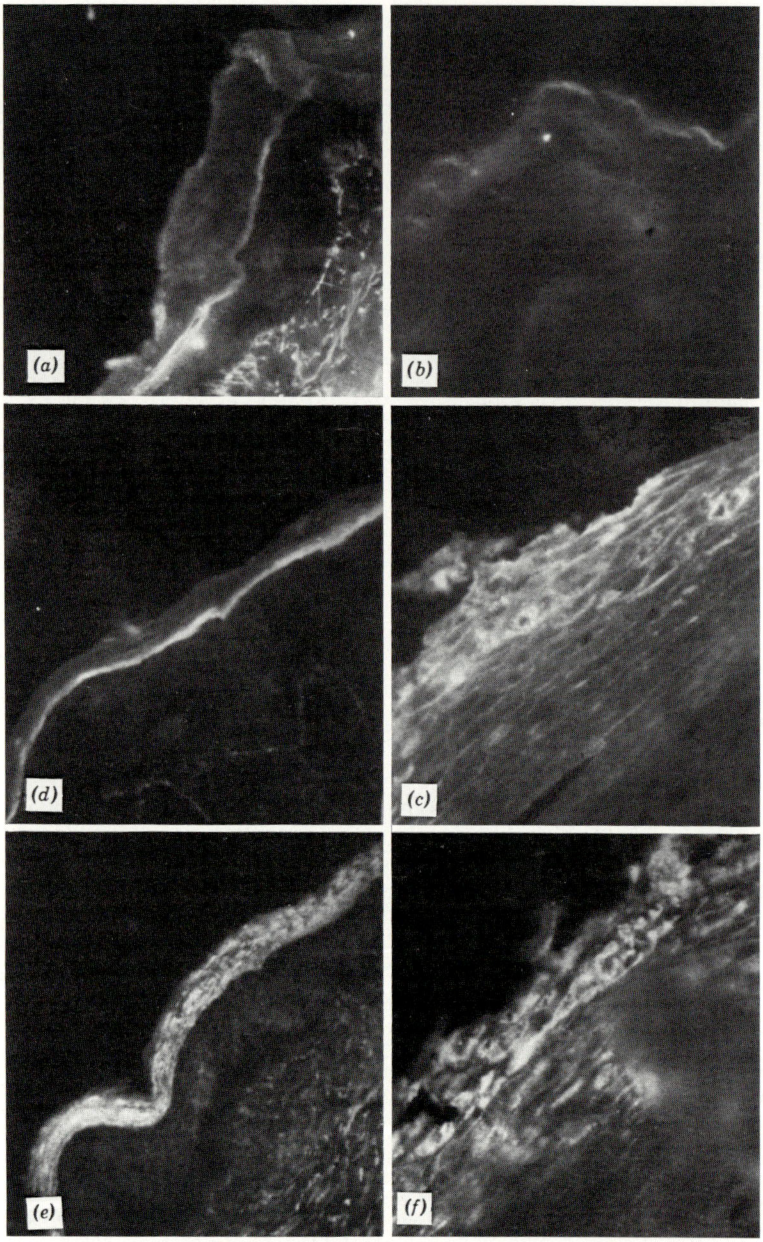

Figure 1. This six-part figure depicts the results obtained with the four-compartment test system with frozen sections of biopsy specimens of normal skin. (a) and (b) Normal skin (Fig. 1*a*) and psoriatic lesion (Fig. 1*b*) treated with labeled globulin free of anti-Ig antibody. The normal skin section was also pretreated with a normal serum containing SCAb. This has no effect. Note in Fig. 1*a*, the NSS of stratum granulosum. This layer is absent from the psoriatic lesions, as shown in Fig. 1*b*. Sections of some psoriasis lesions yield NSS of the nuclei in the parakeratotic stratum corneum. The weak line of staining seen in Fig. 1b was autofluorescence at the surface of the lesion (300x). (*c*) (*d*) Sections of normal skin (Fig. 1*c*) and of psoriatic lesion (Fig. 1*d*), which received DIF

Table 2. Elution Studies on Psoriatic Scales

	1	*2*	*3*	*4*	*5*	*Mean*
IgG eluted (mg/ml)						
pH 7.0[a]	0.51	0.94	0.54	0.78	0.41	0.63
pH 2.0[a]	0.028	0.078	0.048	0.097	0.014	0.049
Ratio: pH 7.0:2.0						13.1
Specific activity						
TR-SCAb titer/mg IgG						
pH 7.0[a]	2	—[b]	—	2	—	0.8
pH 2.0[a]	27	65	12	8	85	39
Ratio: pH 7.0:2.0						1:48.8

[a]Means of two separate elutions and assays of IgG and passive hemagglutination tests for SCAb.
[b]No detectable SCAb to the TR-SCAg.
From Jones (41).

were removed by pH 7.0 washings; 6 of 10 pH 7.0 washings were positive. SC antibodies to the TS antigen were present in the pH 2.0 eluates of only 1 of 10 cases examined. These findings indicate the following: 1) predominantly one type of SCAb do bind in vivo to psoriatic scales to produce Arthus reactions; and 2) usually only the TR-type SCAg is present in psoriatic scales. Other studies (44,49) now also point to the conclusion that SCAb do bind in vivo in psoriatic scales.

Frequency and Nature of Positive DIF Findings in Psoriatic Lesions

Direct IF finding of Ig, complement components, fibrin, and other serum proteins in the horny layer of psoriatic lesions need to be considered from two viewpoints: notably, findings with lesional biopsy specimens and observations on exfoliated psoriatic scales. Most studies to date deal with the former. Direct IF findings on biopsy specimens that have been reported over the past few years (1,3,5,9,32–37,39) show clearly that the typical positive reactions in SC occur with a significantly higher frequency in psoriatic lesions than in most other dermatoses studied to date. Table 3 summarizes some of these data. As indicated in Table 3, the frequency of IgG and C3 deposits in receding psoriatic lesions does not differ significantly from controls other than warts. However, the difference between the frequencies in active psoriatic lesions and most controls is a highly significant one. This difference becomes even more significant when we consider the differences between psoriatic scales and biopsy specimens.

---

staining for in vivo-bound IgG (Fig. 1*c*). Staining of the stratum granulosum on normal skin sections could not be distinguished clearly from the pattern obtained with the absorbed conjugate, although the intensity of the reaction tended to be stronger with the unabsorbed conjugate of the type used for this preparation (Fig. 1*d*) (150x). Note IC localization of IgG in the stratum corneum (300x). (*e*) and (*f*) Normal skin (Fig. 1*e*) and psoriatic lesion (Fig. 1*f*), which received IIF staining with SC antibodies (Fig. 1*e*). Note strongly positive IIF staining of SC. This stands in sharp contrast to the negative SC seen in Fig. 1*a* and 1*c* (150x). This may be compared with Fig. 1*f*. Since little difference could be detected between the DIF and IIF staining reactions, most if not all of the fluorescence seen in Fig. 1*f* was deemed to be due to the in vivo fixation of SC antibodies (300x). (Reprinted with permission from Beutner et al. [5], p. 301.)

Table 3. Frequency of Psoriatic Staining Pattern in Lesions of Psoriasis and Other Dermatoses as seen in Biopsy Specimens of Skin Lesions: DIF Reactions of SCAg Sites (Psoriatic Staining Patterns) in Skin Specimens

Clinical diagnosis	*No. of cases*	*Positive for IgG (% positive)*	*No. of cases*	*Positive for C3 (% positive)*
Active psoriasis	193	180 (93.3)	146	103 (70.5)
Receding psoriasis	18	5 (27.8)	15	0 (0)
Warts	20	13 (65)	20	12 (60)
Other controls[a]	89	17[b] (19.1)	89	8 (9.0)

Statistical analyses by chi square (x^2)
(x^2 > 10.83 is equivalent to P > 0.00005)

	For IgG	*For C3*
Active psoriasis vs. warts	x^2 = 17.02 *P > 0.0005*	x^2 = 0.00139 no difference[b]
Active psoriasis vs. other controls	x^2 = 159.10 *P* >>> 0. 00005	x^2 = 84.07 *P*>>>0.00005[a]
Active vs. receding psoriasis	x^2 = 64.35 *P* >> 0.00005	x^2 = 29.37 *P* > 0.00005
Receding psoriasis vs. other controls	No significant difference	No significant difference

[a]These included five cases with only a trace of IgG and two cases with only a trace of C3; cases with diffuse SC staining suggestive of extravasated plasma are included. The controls included lesional specimens from 56 cases of LE, 14 of eczema, 4 of seborrheic dermatitis, 4 of pityriasis rosea, and 11 miscellaneous cutaneous disorders.
[b]Significantly similar.
From Jablonska et al. (37) and unpublished data.

While 13 of 193 biopsy specimens from active psoriatic lesions gave negative IF findings (Table 3), virtually 100% of psoriatic scales yielded positive reactions. In effect, the occasional negative IF finding in biopsy specimens of psoriatic lesions appear to be due to the loss of the scale while obaining the specimen, or possibly in processing if they are loosely adherent. This may occur more commonly in receding lesions. Importantly, the finding of immune deposits in SC antigen sites in virtually all psoriatic scales indicates that in situ Arthus reactions occur in virtually 100% active psoriatic lesions.

Table 3 includes some previously unpublished data on DIF findings in warts that afforded the basis for our comments (32) on data of Weiss et al. (65). These authors reported that they found no significant difference between the frequency of immune deposits in psoriatic lesions (35 of 44 [80% positive]) and verruca vulgaris lesions (18 of 19 [95% positive]). They did not specify whether their biopsy specimens were from active psoriasis cases or whether they included significant amounts of scales. The data in Table 3 point to a higher frequency of IgG in psoriasis, but not of C3 deposits, in the cases examined. The contention of Weiss et al (65) is that Ig binding to psoriatic lesions is not a significant event. They do not address the finding that these Ig deposits in psoriatic scales are a sign of an Arthus reaction. In warts (regardless of their frequency of IF positivity), these reactions are triggered by infections of the horny layer with the human papilloma virus, and they probably serve as a defense mechanism—as they do against other superficial infectious agents (32; Chap. 38). Weiss et al., in their rebuttal

(66), cite as evidence for their interpretation on the lack of significance of the IF finding observations that relate to grafts of skin to nude mice (48). While the labeling index and the plasminogen activator levels of the latter are of interest, they do not relate to the patent Arthus reaction in psoriatic scales. However, the IF reactions in certain types of actinic keratosis mentioned by these investigators (65) and in certain other controls do merit mention.

The primary permeability barrier of the normal skin is the stratum granulosum (21,58). Since psoriatic lesions are characterized by the absence of a granular layer, the chemotactic factors and kinins from the complement cascade activated by the Arthus reaction in the horny layer may be expected to pass without a barrier into the stratum spinosum and corium. In effect, all control lesions with reactions in the SC antigen site, as seen by DIF reactions (e.g., warts and hyperkeratotic-type solar keratosis), need to be evaluated not only for the triggering factors, such as human papilloma virus, but also for the status of the granular layer to gain a better understanding of the effects of imune deposits in the horny layer.

Other observations on the immune deposits merit mention. First, they tend to be more widespread in psoriatic lesions than in other skin diseases. Secondly, preliminary observations indicate that the ratios of IgA to IgG in scales are equal or greater than 1 as judged by visual assessments. However, this does not always hold true for biopsy specimens. If this difference is confirmed in future studies, it would suggest that the IgG-class SCAb are degraded more rapidly than those of the IgA class. Thirdly, fibrin deposits are stronger and occur more frequently in fully developed spreading psoriatic plaques than they do in pinpoint lesions, as indicated by the following data (7).

Type of psoriasis	*No. of cases*	*No. with fibrin*		
		Positive	*Weak*	*Negative*
Pinpoint lesions	21	9	10	2
Peripherally spreading lesions	9	8	1	0

Dynamics of SC Antigen Degradation

Psoriasis appears to be a self-perpetuating form of the normally self-limiting reactions of the ARM (2), as indicated in Table 1. The triggering of the ARM depends on the changes in the reactivity of the SC antigens (see Chapter 41). That is, in normal nonreactive forms of the horny layer, the SC antigens are sequestered by TS material as indicated in Table 4. The same holds true for the keratinocyte cytoplasmic antigen (KCAg). Trauma quickly converts these antigens, which occur both as upper cytoplasmic (KCAg) and as SC antigens to reactive forms. They first appear as TS-type SC antigens. As these are degraded by proteolytic enzymes, TR-type SC antigens become reactive. These can be detected in tissue sediments and sections as insoluble TR-SCAg. Upon further degradation by proteolytic enzymes, these TR-SCAg are solubilized, and the remaining tissue seen in the section appears to be devoid of SCAg (Table 4).

Johannesson et al. (40) questioned the sequence of changes in psoriatic lesions on

Table 4. Stratum Corneum Antigen Involution: Reactivity at Selected Stages of Deterioration

State of skin	*Reactivity of SCAg and KCAg*	*IF with SCAb*
Normal unaltered	SCAg and KCAg sequestered by TS substance	Negative
Fresh trauma	TS-SCAg and KCAg convert to reactive form	Positive
Inflamed skin injury	TR-SCAg in insoluble form becomes active; TS-SCAg disappears	Positive
Receding lesion	TR-SCAg become solubilized, "disappears," or form soluble immune complexes	Negative

the basis of the observed localization of in vivo reactions of SCAb in psoriatic scales. That is, these investigators evaluated DIF localizations of immune deposits within the SC of psoriatic biopsy specimens by comparing them with the fluorochroming patterns of corneocytes staining. They observed that the IF reactions may be negative in the older, more superficial portions of the biopsy specimens and positive in the lower, more recently developed areas of the horny layer. From this, they concluded that the IF reactions are "secondary phenomena during the initiation of psoriatic lesions." These studies are based only on DIF tests for the immunologic studies. Thus, they fail to reveal the degraded TR-type SC antigens that become soluble and can no longer be detected by either IIF or DIF (Table 4). In effect, focal areas in psoriatic scales that do not bear in vivo-bound IgG may either have soluble SC antigen sites, which are lost in the IF staining procedures, or degraded nonreactive SC residues. The latter can be identified by appropriate IIF tests and by tests with scales soaked in SCAb containing sera and stained by DIF.

Evidence for the Fixation of Complement and the Release of Chemotaxins and Immune Complexes

The elution studies pointing to in vivo binding of SCAb in psoriatic scales, taken together with the observations that these SCAb fix complement in vitro and that DIF staining reveals in vivo-bound complement in sections of psoriatic scales, indicate that the bound SCAb fix complement in vivo. Direct evidence for this was provided by the studies of Tagami and Ofuji (60–64), which revealed that eluates of psoriatic scales are chemotactic and that purified fractions of the chemotactic components contain C5a and C3a. Finally, they showed that antisera to C5a abolish the chemotaxic activity of these eluates. Schöpf et al. (56) also found elevated levels of C3a, C3, and C4 in sera of patients with active psoriasis. Sera of psoriatic patients also increased chemotactic activity to casein, as shown by the extensive studies of Christopher et al. (16).

Immune complexes have been found in higher frequencies in sera of patients with active psoriasis (13,19). This does not relate to SCAb specifically. However, the titers of SCAb to the TR-soluble SC antigens drop during flares of psoriatic lesions (9,41) and return to their previous levels during remission. This indicates either that soluble forms of SC antigens are released from psoriatic scales into the circulation to form immune complexes or that SCAb to TR-SCAb are consumed by reactions in the horny layer, or both. The titers of SCAb to TS SC antigens do not fluctuate in the same way, possibly because reactions with them are transient minor components of the normal reaction sequence or because these SC antigens normally do not occur in soluble forms in vivo.

Other Studies of Autoimmunity in Psoriasis

Cormane et al. reported that eluates of white blood cells from psoriatic patients contain antibodies to nuclei of the stratum basale of the epidermis (17,18). The reactive antigen can be detected in frozen sections of normal epidermis by IIF tests with these eluates, but is absent from sections of psoriatic lesions. This suggests that these antibodies are directed toward a nuclear component that is altered to a nonreactive form in lesion formation. Absorption of eluates with psoriatic scales does not remove them, and there is no evidence of their in vivo reaction with the skin of patients. Cormane suggests that they are directed to nonhistone proteins of cell nuclei because of their specificity, and that they may have a regulatory role. The writers have seen such antibodies in normal sera. The previously mentioned absence of the antigen from psoriatic lesions suggest that the antibodies are a normal physiologic response to the tissue injury involved in lesion formation, and that they serve as ARM-triggering agents to aid in the removal of the injured tissue components.

While it seems clear that the antibodies to epidermal basal cell nuclei do not contribute to in vivo, in situ immune complex formation, it may be that some limited in vivo reactivity does occur with the cytoplasm of the upper stratum spinosum (6), as illustrated in Figure 1. If this is a true in vivo reaction of an autoantibody, it is obviously due to SCAb since they are the same as KC antibodies (KCAb); that is, the antibodies to the upper cytoplasmic antigens as shown by Hintner et al. (30,31) and confirmed in our laboratory (see Chap. 41).

ROLE OF POLYMORPHONUCLEAR LEUKOCYTES IN PSORIASIS

Jablonska et al. (14,15,34,35,39) together with Glinski et al. (26, 27) demonstrated that polymorphonuclear leukocytes (PMN) play key roles in responses to peritoneal dialysis as well as in the changes preceding the formation of psoriatic lesions, in Koebner reactions induced by scratches, and in those induced by stripping. (Interestingly, the apparent sequence of events, as they relate to the immunopathologic changes and prodromal histologic changes, differ somewhat in these two methods of inducing Koebner reactions as indicated in the next section). These observations concur with the classic hallmarks of the disease; notably, the Munro microabscesses and the "squirting papillae" that lead to their formation. That is, the pockets of PMN and leukoclastic debris in the horny layer make up the Munro microabscesses. The "squirting papillae" described by Pinkus and Mehregan (54) extrude PMN into the epidermis. As these PMN enter the horny layer, they lead to the formation of Munro microabscesses, which are well recognized as hallmarks of the histopathology of psoriasis. These events are, at least in part, induced by release of the powerful chemotactic activity of C5a from the in vivo reactions of SCAb in the horny layer as just described (56,64).

Effects of Peritoneal Dialysis on Psoriasis and on PMN

The key role of PMN in the induction of psoriatic lesions is best demonstrated by the therapeutic effects of peritoneal dialysis and leukopheresis (26,27). As shown in Table

Table 5. Relation Between Therapeutic Responses of 17 Cases of Severe Psoriasis to Peritoneal Dialysis and the Number of PMN removed

Responses of psoriasis to dialysis	*No. of psoriasis cases responding vs. no. of PMN × 10^9 removed by peritoneal dialysis*					
	1–5	*25–50*	*51–75*	*76–100*	*101–150*	*200–300*
Remission					1	2
Marked improvement			2	1	1	
Slight improvement		4	3			
No improvement	3					

From Glinski et al. (27).

Table 6. Relation of Koebner Reactions to DIF and Histologic Findings

No. of cases	*Extent of psoriatic type of IF deposits*	*Histologic changes of psoriasis*	*Development of positive Koebner reactions*	*Days after biopsy procedure*
2	Widespread	Yes	Yes	3
3	Focal	No	Yes	6–9
1	Focal	Yes	Yes	13
3	Focal	No	No	—
1	Focal	Yes	No	—

5, daily peritoneal dialysis for 3 to 4 weeks in patients with severe psoriasis yields significant treatment responses in 7 of 17 cases during the dialysis and in 8 of 16 cases two months after dialysis. As indicated in Table 5, these therapeutic responses were directly proportional to the number of PMN removed by the dialysis. The PMN removed from psoriatic patients also had significantly (four- to fivefold) elevated levels of neutral serine proteases in comparison to other patients. These investigators suggest that these enzymes activate the SC antigens in the horny layer of the skin, thereby contributing to the self-perpetuation of the lesions. The role of PMN in psoriasis is also demonstrated by analytic studies of the Koebner reaction, as summarized in Table 6 and the following subsections.

Koebner Reactions Induced by Scratch

Koebner reactions induced by scratch involve conversion of SC antigens of the cut edge of the horny layer from their normal nonreactive forms to forms reactive with SCAb to the TR types of SC antigens (3,4,7,8, Chap. 41) (see fresh trauma in Table 4). Reactions of SCAb at the cut edge of scratch sites adjacent to crusts (Fig. 2*a*) occur both in normal control subjects and in subjects with active untreated psoriasis in whom a Koebner phenomenon may be manifested. They occurred more frequently in the controls 2 to 3 days after scratching, but remained detectable for a longer period in patients

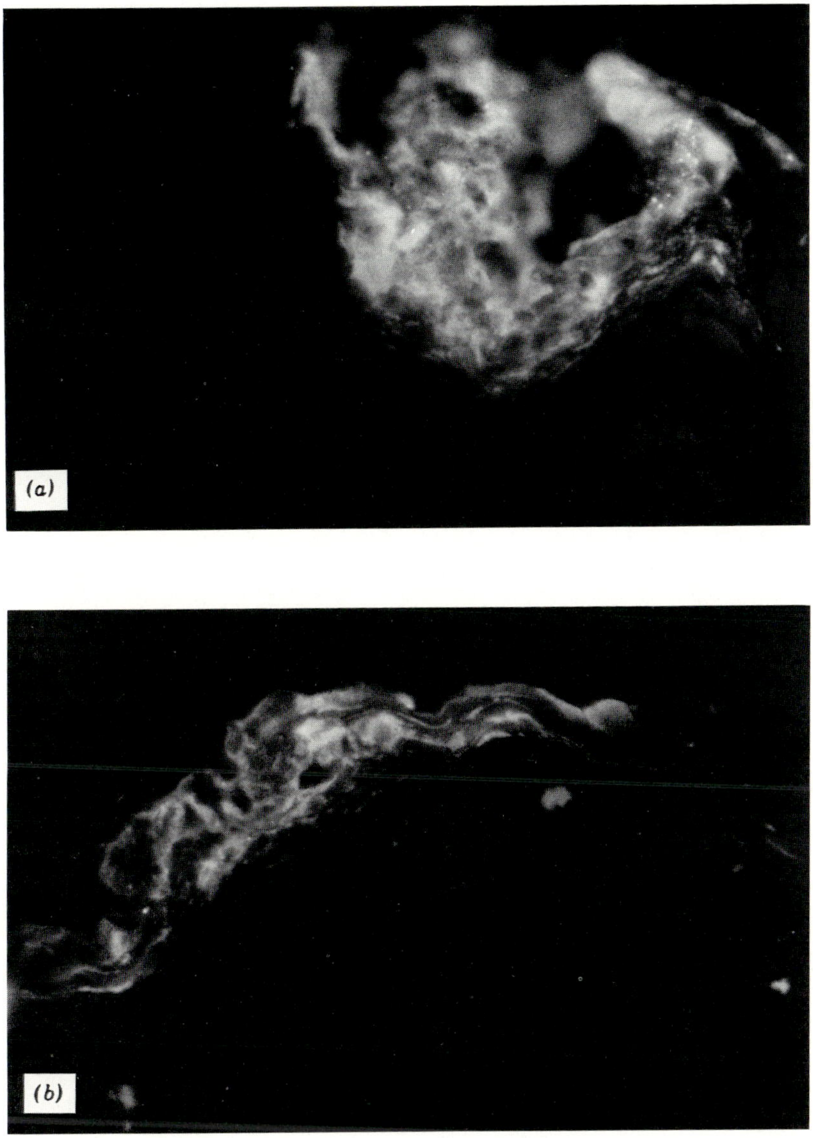

Figure 2.a Koebner phenomenon 72 hours after scratch; DIF staining for IgG. Diffuse staining of the crust and some immune deposits in the SCAg sites at the edge of the crust (IC staining visible at the lower right margin of stained crust). This IF pattern is the same in psoriatics and controls (300x). b. Koebner phenomenon 3 days after scratch in a patient with active psoriasis. This is an early development of the psoriatic IF pattern, as seen by direct staining for IgG. It is followed by the appearance of histologic features of psoriasis (300x). (Reprinted with permission from Jablonska et al. [35]).

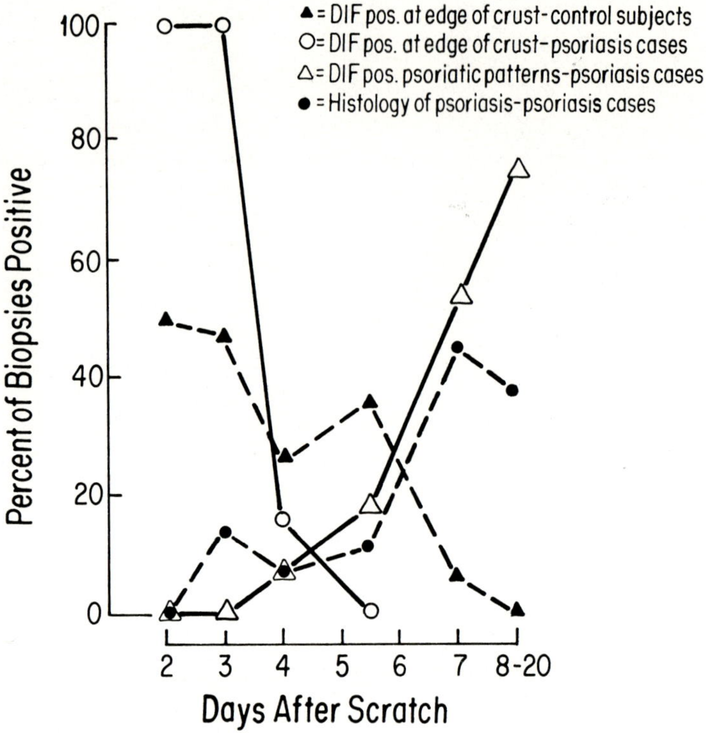

Figure 3. The data base of this graph is as follows:

Subjects tested	Days after scratch	*DIF*[a] at *edge of crust*		*DIF*[a] *of psoriatic type*		*Histology*[b] *of psoriasis*	
		Pos./Total	*% Pos.*	*Pos./Total*	*% Pos.*	*Pos./Total*	*% Pos.*
Psoriasis[c]	2	2/4	50	0/4	0	0/4	0
	3	7/15	47	0/17	0	1/7	14
	4	7/27	26	2/27	7	1/14	7
	5–6	12/33	36	6/33	18	2/17	12
	7	1/17	6	8/17	53	5/11	45
	8–20	0/16	0	12/16	75	1/3	33
Controls	2	4/4	100	0/4	0	0/4	0
	3	3/3	100	0/3	0	0/3	0
	4	1/6	16	0/6	0	0/1	0
	5	Since only normal skin was present at the scratch sites, no further biopsy specimens were taken from control subjects					

[a]Data from S. Jablonska, et al. (34).
[b]Data from S. Jablonska, et al. (35).
[c]Only untreated patients were included.

with active psoriasis. As shown by the studies of Jablonska et al. (34,35), the frequency of both the psoriatic type of DIF staining (Fig. 2*b*) (due to TR-type SCAb as shown above) and of psoriasiform type of histologic changes appeared as early as 3 to 4 days after scratching, and they increased in frequency up to at least the eighth day. As may be seen from kinetic studies (Fig. 3), the initial SCAb reactions at the edge of the crusts (Fig. 2a) are superseded in patients with active psoriasis by the psoriatic SCAb reaction patterns (Fig. 2b). These precede the appearance of Koebner reactions, as indicated by the data summarized in Table 6.

Koebner Reactions Induced by Stripping

Koebner reactions induced by partial stripping of the horny layer without oozing (39) induced the formation of minute red edematous papules randomly distributed in the stripped areas (Fig. 4). These minute lesions, referred to as prepinpoint papules (PPP) disappear within 3 to 4 days in patients with inactive psoriasis. In nonpsoriatic controls, erythema, and edema (but no frank PPP) were found. The frank PPP in stripped areas in patients with active untreated psoriasis go on to develop into both typical psoriatic

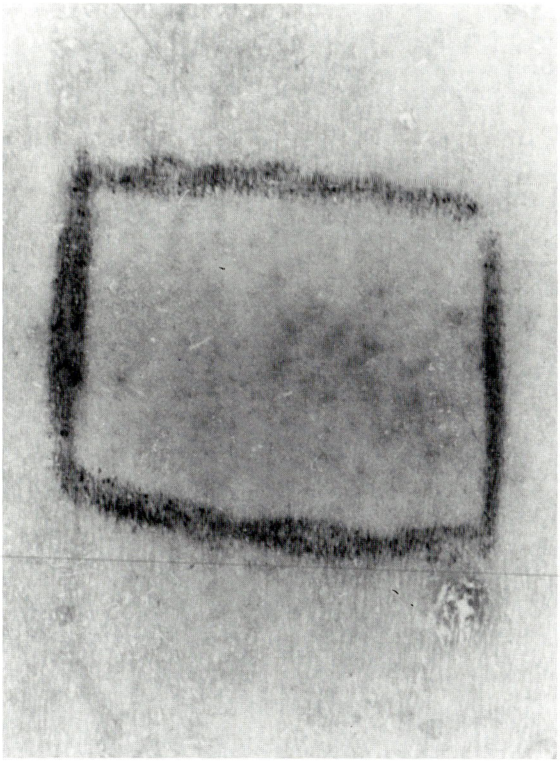

Figure 4. Small PPPs within stripped areas appeared more than 24 hours after stripping and lasted less than 24 hours. Note at least 15 PPPs distributed in clusters (in center and on right), and two singly (on left). Number of PPPs is unusually high and is related to very active disease. (Reprinted with permission from Jablonska et al. [39], p. 652.)

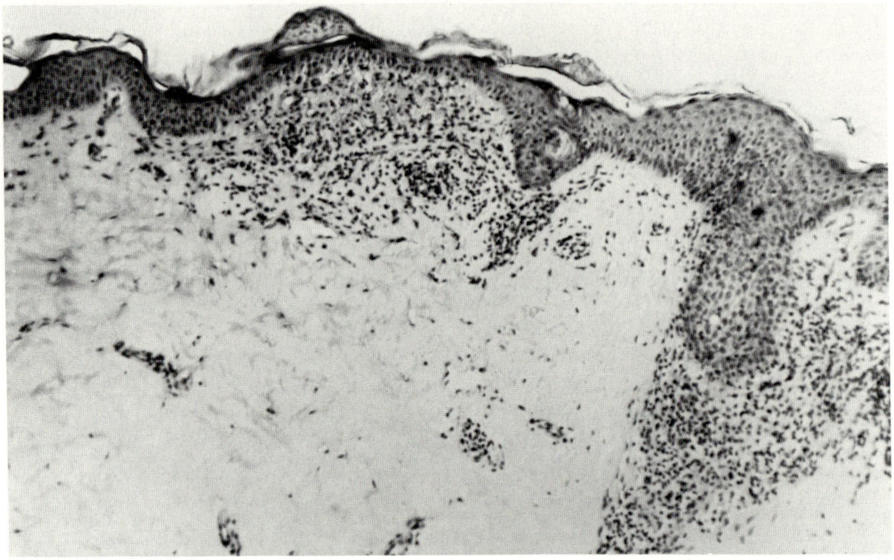

Figure 5. Specimen, taken 2 days after stripping, of PPPs that appeared less than 24 hours before the biopsy procedure. Note focal parakeratosis with accumulation of inflammatory cells, mainly PMNs, in SC. Stratum granulosum is thinned or absent; epidermis is thinned, edematous, and partly destroyed by penetrating inflammatory cells. Abundant infiltrates beneath epidermis contains numerous PMNs (H&E) (80x). (Reprinted with permission from Jablonska et al. [39], p. 652.)

pinpoint papules and full-blown psoriatic lesions. The PPP have characteristic histologic features with parakeratosis in the residual foci of the horny layer, with little or no stratum granulosum, and with massive penetration, predominantly of PMN into the thinning epidermis (Fig. 5). Immune deposits of IgG start to appear in the horny layer within 1 to 4 days (Fig. 6).

The dynamics of these changes are shown in Fig. 7. These indicate that the initial distinguishing changes observable by these methods are the continuation of massive exocytosis in patients with psoriasis and the rapid disappearance of PMN from controls within 2 to 3 days. Almost simultaneously, but shortly thereafter, a sharp increase in the frequency and extent of IgG binding to the horny layer is observed. In many of these cases, there is also an appearance, at least in some foci, of complement activation. In regenerated SC of PPP in the process of converting into psoriasis, there is also an increase of accumulation of PMN in SC.

Comparisons of Two Types of Koebner Reactions

The role of the horny layer in the induction of psoriatic lesions is also evident from earlier studies on the induction of the Koebner reaction to cuts made obliquely to the skin. Bizzozero (10) reported and Farber et al. (24) later confirmed that psoriatic lesions form only at the entrance points of a nearly horizontal cut of traumatizing instruments; that is, at the point of trauma to the SC. A role for PMN is evident from the characteristic exocytosis in psoriasis (38) and the formation of Munro microab-

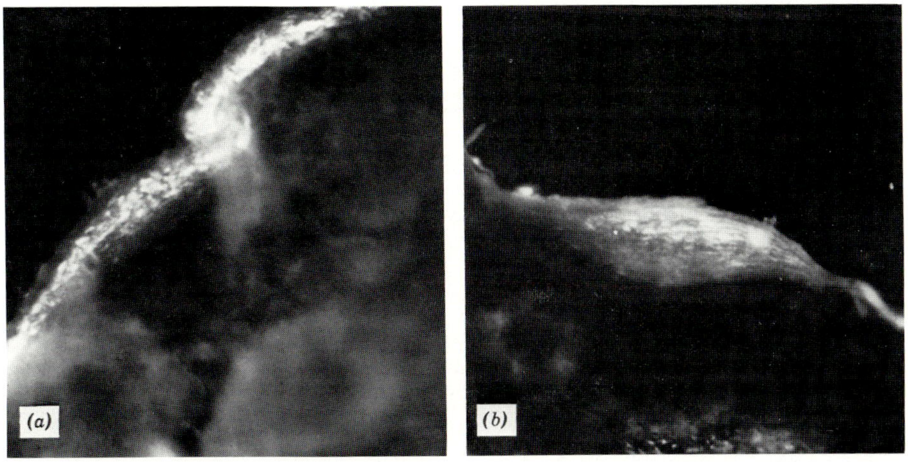

Figure 6. Direct IF tests of PPPs. (*a*) Specimen taken 72 hours after stripping. This papule had appeared less than 24 hours before the biopsy procedure. Note IgG staining patterns in SC of types associated with leukocytes (larger structures) and SCAg type seen in psoriasis (i.e., dots and dashes). Same findings appeared in IIF tests (original magnification 200x). (*b*) Specimen taken 8 days after stripping. This papule had appeared less than 24 hours before the biopsy procedure. Note focal area of typical linear psoriatic staining pattern, that is, IgG deposits on SCAg sites, presumably due to in vivo-bound SCAb. Histologically, slight acanthosis, but no other features of psoriasis, had developed (original magnification, 400x). (Reprinted with permission from Jablonska et al [39], p. 652.)

Table 7. Synopsis of Sequence of Histologic and Immunologic Changes Preceding the Induction of Psoriatic Lesions by the Koebner Reaction

Method of induction	*Prodromal events before psoriatic lesions develop*	*Earliest true psoriatic changes*
Scratches	SCAb bind at scratch site in controls and psoriatic patients	PMN penetrate into SC; massive Arthus reaction due to SCAb
Stripping	PMN accumulate in the corium and penetrate into epidermis in prepinpoint papules	SCAb seen in all lesions by DIF and elution studies

scesses. The immunologic and histologic studies on the two methods of inducing Koebner reactions afford some insights into the interactions of the horny layer with PMN.

The dynamics of a Koebner reaction induced by scratching, as shown graphically in Fig. 3, appear to differ somewhat from the sequence of changes depicted in Fig. 7. The basic difference, as indicated in Table 7, is that the binding of SCAb at the edge of the crust and its gradual extension to a psoriatic pattern appears to be an initial event in the Koebner reaction induced by scratches, while penetration of PMN into the epidermis

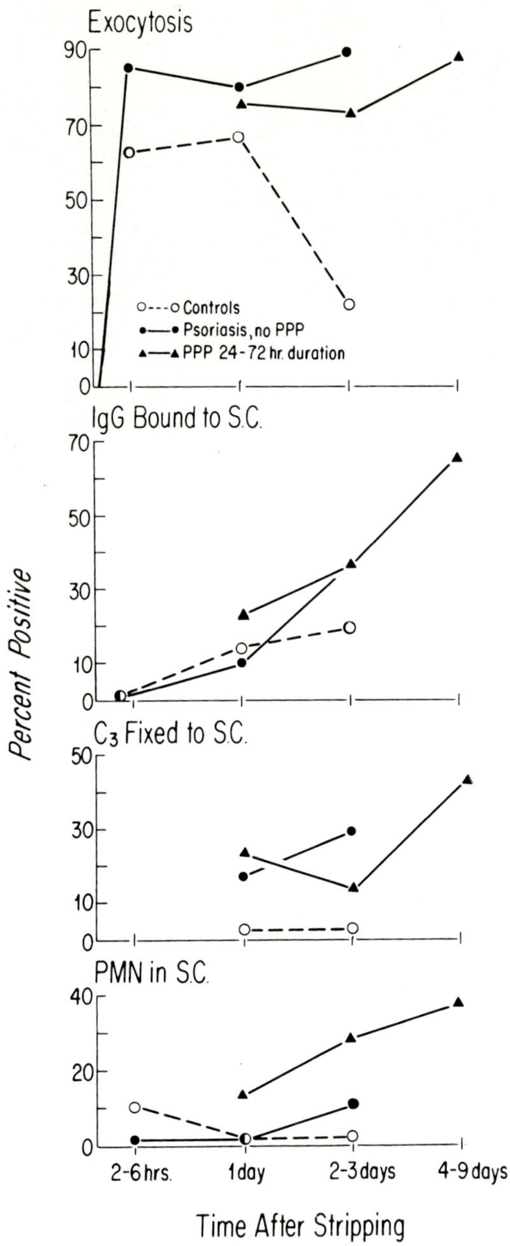
Exocytosis
90
70
50
30
10
0
o---o Controls
•—• Psoriasis, no PPP
▲—▲ PPP 24-72 hr. duration
IgG Bound to S.C.
70
50
30
10
0
Percent Positive
C3 Fixed to S.C.
50
30
10
0
PMN in S.C.
40
20
0
2-6 hrs.
1 day
2-3 days
4-9 days
Time After Stripping

Figure 7. (opposite) Kinetics of changes in frequencies of exocytosis, IgG bound to stratum corneum (SC), C3 component of complement fixed to SC and PMN in SC. The data base of the values plotted is as follows:

	Time (h or days)	Controls (Table 6)		Psoriasis No. of PPPs (Table 6)		PPPs (Table 5)	
		Pos./Total	*% Pos.*	*Pos./Total*	*% Pos.*	*Pos./Total*	*% Pos.*
A	1/2 h	2/2	—[a]	0/8	0		
Exocytosis	2–6 h	5/8	63	11/13	85		
	1 day	4/6	67	4/5	80		
	2–3 days	2/9	22	9/10	90	7/9	78
	4–9 days					19/23	83
B	2–6 h	0/10	0	0/22	0		
IgG bound	1 day	1/7	14	1/10	10		
to SC	2–3 days	2/10	20	7/19	37	2/9	22
	4–9 days					12/25	48
C	1 day	0/3	0	1/6	17		
C3 fixed	2–3 days	0/7	0	2/7	29	2/9	22
to SC	4–9 days					7/25	28
D	2–6 h	1/10	10	0/2	0		
PMN	1 day	0/6	0	0/5	0		
in SC	2–3 days	0/9	0	1/10	10	1/9	11
	4–9 days					7/22	32

[a]This value is not listed or plotted because the number of specimens is too small and because the number of PMN in the epidermis was minimal in each of the two cases.
Modified from Jablonska (39).

appears to precede the binding of SCAb in the Koebner reaction induced by stripping. In effect, it appears that the local Arthus reaction induced by the in situ binding of SCAb to the horny layer involves interactions of PMN with SC antigens, and that the sequence of events initiating this Arthus reaction may be somewhat variable.

We may postulate that, for example, a streptococcal infection activates PMN so highly that even trivial insults to SC antigens of the skin that cannot be detected by IF may trigger exocytosis and the formation of PPP. If these persist, they may, as reported by Jablonska et al. (39), convert into true psoriatic pinpoint papules. Alternatively, if the PMN are only moderately activated, then a frank scratch inducing a detectable reaction of SCAb may be needed to precipitate the development of psoriatic lesions. Either way, some interaction of PMN with SC antigens would be needed to induce the development of typical psoriasis.

MEDIATORS OF INFLAMMATION IN REPAIR AND PSORIASIS

Inflammation is a series of events following injury to tissues that is designed to remove the injurious stimulus, if persistent, and to culminate in repair of damaged tissues. The immunologic mechanisms mediated by the ARM (as described in Chap. 7) may fulfill these functions together with other mechanisms that mediate inflammation and presumably normal repair. Considerable effort has been expended in identifying mediators of the inflammatory process, including biogenic amines, oligopeptides, fatty acid derivatives, and more recently substances such as platelet activating factor, epidermal thymus activating factor, and interleukins (20). The relationships of these factors, particularly of metabolites of the cyclooxygenase and lipoxygenase pathway, merit attention.

Psoriasis has been studied extensively in this regard, and a significant elevation of lipoxygenase products of arachidonic acid metabolism has been described for lesional epidermis compared with uninvolved epidermis. Thus 12-hydroxyeicosatetraenoic acid (12-HETE) is elevated 80-fold in psoriatic epidermis (28) and 5-HETE derivatives; in particular, 5, 12, di-HETE, LTB_4 is elevated three- to sevenfold in psoriatic epidermis (12). Importance is attached to the elevation of leukotriene B4 (LTB_4) in psoriatic epidermis in view of the ability of this mediator to produce a persistent erythematous reaction in skin (associated with epidermopoiesis), a leukocyte infiltration in the dermis, and an appearance of microabscesses in the epidermis, all of which mimic some of the symptoms of psoriasis. The presence of an inhibitor of cyclooxygenase is found in lesional epidermis of psoriatic plaques (52,53), which may be similar in structure to 5, 8, 11-eicosatrienoic acid—a cyclooxygenase inhibitor produced in the skin of rodents suffering from essential fatty acid deficiency (57). Furthermore, compounds which strongly inhibit cyclooxygenase (e.g., indomethacin) exacerbate psoriasis (22,42).

In view of the fact that classic nonsteroidal anti-inflammatory agents have a common pharmacologic profile, which includes inhibition of the cyclooxygenase pathway of arachidonic acid metabolism, it is reasonable to equate ulcerogenic potential with inhibition of the major pathway for arachidonic acid metabolism in epithelial tissues, that is, prostaglandin synthesis. It is also reasonable to assume that prostaglandin synthesis, release, and action may be at least one of the primary chains of events in inducing inflammation and subsequent repair of damage locally to epithelial tissues of the gastrointestinal tract, and possibly of skin. Healing of thermal-induced burns of guinea pig skin was adversely affected by topical application of prostaglandin synthetase inhibitors: for example, indomethacin, piroxicam, tolmetin, and zomepirac (23).

The importance of prostaglandin synthesis as a primary event leading to repair of damage to skin is not clearly defined. However, circumstantial evidence exists to support this postulate. In psoriatic plaques, a natural inhibitor of prostaglandin synthesis exists (52). This is probably related to the inability of normal skin adjacent to a psoriatic plaque to produce an erythematous response to UVB irradiation (Woronov's ring) (53). Of greater importance is the observation that a potent inhibitor of prostaglandin synthesis, indomethacin, exacerbates psoriasis (42).

A recent study revealed that topically applied arachidonic acid may produce an amelioration of symptoms of psoriasis (29). This indicates that a prerequisite for healing of the lesion is an influx of PMN into the epidermis and, eventually, the SC overlying the plaque. The consequence of this is destruction and desquamation of the psoriatic SC leading to normalization of the epidermis and dermis.

The first point to emphasize is that the SC produced by and overlying a psoriatic plaque could be perpetuating the disease process. Evidence to support this is derived from the finding reviewed in this chapter on the massive focal Arthus reaction in the horny layer of virtually all scales from active psoriatic plaques, which are due to the activation of SC autoantigens (SCAg), the resultant in vivo reactions of SCAb, and the fixation of complement to these immune complexes (as described in the above section on "Arthus-type Reactions in Psoriatic Scales.")

It remains to be determined whether the immunologic mechanisms triggered by SCAb stimulate the lipoxygenase pathway, and thus the formation of such arachidonic acid metabolites as LTB_4, or whether the converse is true; or whether both of these mechanisms are secondary to some other initiating factors in repair and in psoriasis.

It is interesting to place in context the phenomenon of inflammation in the skin. Epithelial tissues, primarily epidermis and epithelium of the gastrointestinal tract, are the primary interfaces with the external environment. Consequently, these tissues are endowed with mechanisms to protect both themselves and, therefore, the body against insults from changes in the environment. Noxious stimuli produce an inflammatory response locally that is intended to result in healing and, therefore, survival of the tissue and the organism. It is interesting to note that epithelial tissue of the skin and gastrointestinal tract have the highest capability of all body tissues to metabolize arachidonic acid, particularly to cyclooxygenase derivatives of the prostaglandin series. It is reasonable to assume that continual mechanical or chemical insults to the gastrointestinal mucosa from daily ingestion of food are the causes of local trauma, as evidenced by a relatively constant level of occult blood loss under normal circumstances. Clearly, in most instances, such traumatic events culminate in healing of damaged tissues following a local inflammatory response.

In the same valence, the ARM (Chap. 7), which is triggered in the skin by the SCAb-KCAb complex (Chap. 41), is probably also triggered in the gastrointestinal mucosa by physiologic autoantibodies to the gut (50). Interestingly, these antibodies cross-react with a common antigen of enteric bacilli and of the colon of germ-free rats (50). They also react with kidney and liver of rats, mice, and humans (51,65). Low titers of antibodies to this common antigen occur in normal sera. It has been suggested that this cross-reaction of enteric bacilli with the gut antigen represents an adaptive mechanism of the bacteria to protect them against the normal defenses of the host. Such defenses may be examples of an ARM. Thus, it appears that such ARM cascades may accompany the body's capacity to metabolize arachidonic acid.

The abundant literature on the relationship of arachidonic acid and its metabolites to the skin (see Duell and Voorhees [20] for review) leaves no doubt that they play central roles as chemoattractants in inflammatory reactions of psoriasis. The evidence reviewed here and elsewhere (1) also leaves little doubt that the in vivo reactions of SC antibodies, which occur in virtually all scales of active psoriatic lesions, and their in situ fixation of complement regularly induce massive, local Arthus-type reactions that clearly play a role in the disease. The finding that topical applications of arachidonic acid induces temporary remission of psoriatic lesions (29) indicates that this agent and/or its chemotactic metabolites may aid in the removal of the immune complexes, as well as to induce lesion formation. The relationships between arachidonic acid metabolites and the Arthus reactions in the evaluation of psoriatic lesions clearly merits further study.

CONCLUSIONS

Fig. 8 depicts the type of relationships that are implicated by the working hypothesis shown in Table 1. These relationships were proposed prior to the performance of the previously mentioned studies on the use of arachidonic acid in the treatment of psoriasis. In effect, these latter findings afford supporting evidence for this interpretation.

If the interpretation in Fig. 8 is essentially correct, (i.e., if psoriasis is partly precipitated and perpetuated by an over-reaction of the ARM of the skin), then we can predict that it will be possible to find specific biochemical differences between normal control subjects and normal subjects with a history of psoriasis in terms of:

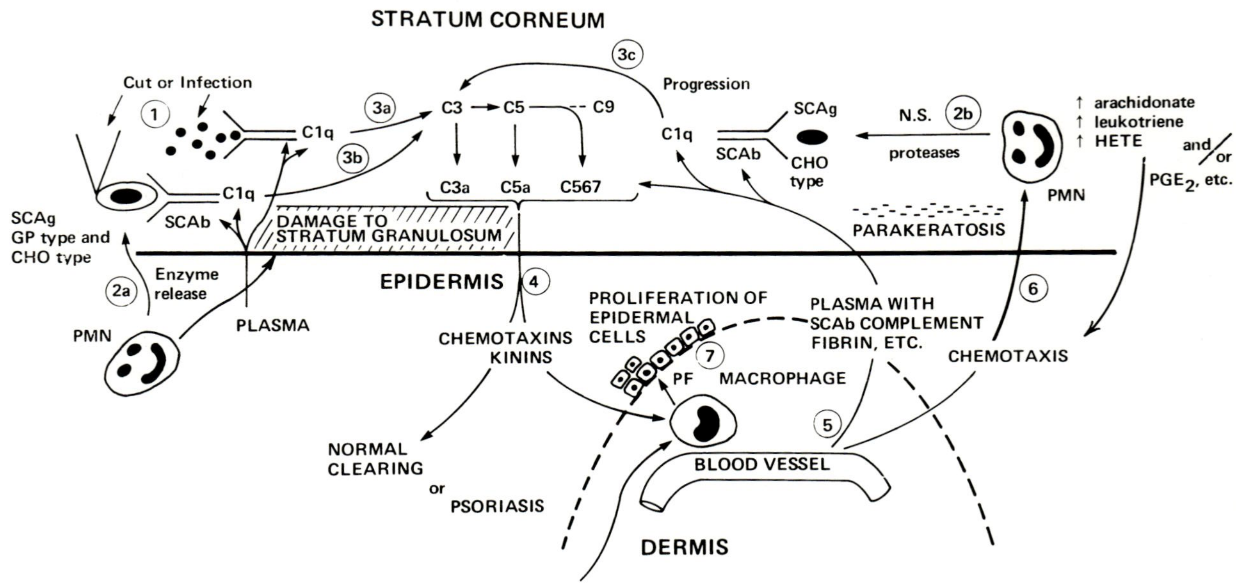

Figure 8. Postulated biological roles of SCAg-SCAb reactions. The following sequence of SCAg-SCAb-C and PMN reactions appears to play a self-limiting role in removal of damaged SC, and plays a self-perpetuating role in psoriasis: *1, 2*. Exogenous (1a, 1b) or endogenous (2a, 2b) damage to the SC activates PMN and unmasks SC antigens of the TS and TR types; antibodies (SCAb or antimicrobials) bind in SC and fix Clq there. *3*. The complement cascade releases C3a, C5a, and C567. *4*. These fragments acting as strong chemotoxins and kinins first activate PMN, and later macrophages. *5*. The kinin also promote release of more plasma proteins, including SCAb, C, and fibrin. *6*. The chemoattraction may be aided by arachidonic acid metabolites, including leukotrienes. The immune complexes in the SC attract more PMN into the epidermis. The PMN in the horny layer release neutral serine proteases, which can unmask more of the CHO-type SC antigen. The added SC antigen-SCAb-C complexes are also phagocytosed by PMN, which usually disrupt in the horny layer, although complexes with IgA-class SCAb may inhibit phagocytosis. *7*. Activation of inflammatory cells stimulate release of proliferative factor. (Reprinted with permission from Beutner et al. [4].)

1. The enzymes of their white blood cells, which convert SC antigens to the reactive forms;
2. Their SC antigens upon which these enzymes act; or
3. The specificities and/or titers of their SCAb.

If this prediction is proven by experimental studies, it will open a new sphere of research including such areas as the prediction of which individuals may develop psoriasis and how the disease can be prevented by overcoming the biochemical defect(s), as well as in areas related to mechanisms of the type depicted in Fig. 8.

REFERENCES

1. Beutner EH (Ed): *Autoimmunity in Psoriasis.* CRC Press, Boca Raton, FL, 1982, 313 pp.
2. Beutner EH: Nature of autoimmunity: Unified concept and other theories as related to psoriasis. In Beutner EH (Ed): *Autoimmunity in Psoriasis.* CRC Press, Boca Raton, FL, 1982, pp 3–14.
3. Beutner EH, Binder WL, Jablonska S, et al: Immunofluorescence findings on stratum corneum antibodies, antigens and their reactions in vitro and in vivo as related to repair and psoriasis. In Beutner EH (Ed): *Autoimmunity in Psoriasis.* CRC Press, Boca Raton, FL, 1982, pp 53–79.
4. Beutner EH, Dabski K, Jablonska S, et al: Stratum corneum antigens: Their role in psoriasis and in the autoimmune repair mechanisms. In Marks R, Plewig G (Eds): *Stratum Corneum.* Springer-Verlag, Heidelberg, 1983, pp 92–111.
5. Beutner EH, Jablonska S, Jarzabek-Chorzelska M, et al: Studies in immunodermatology. VI. IF studies of autoantibodies to the stratum corneum and of in vivo fixed IgG in stratum corneum of psoriatic scales. *Int Arch Allergy* 48:301–323, 1975.
6. Beutner EH, Kumar V: Autoantibodies in health and disease: Classification of autoimmune response using universal stratified epithelial autoantibodies and other skin reactive autoantibodies as models. In Milgrom F, Abeyounis CJ, Albini B (Eds): *Antibodies: Protective, Destructive and Regulatory Role. Proceedings of the 9th International Convocation on Immunology.* Karger, Basel, 1985 pp. 158–163.
7. Binder WL: Studies on the role of the immune system in the pathogenesis of psoriasis. PhD Thesis, State University of New York at Buffalo, 1978, 164 pp.
8. Binder WL, Beutner EH, Jablonska S: Studies in immunodermatology. VIII. Immunofluorescence studies of stratum corneum antibodies. *Int Arch Allergy* 61:407–416, 1980.
9. Binder WL, Beutner EH, Jablonska S: Immunofluorescence studies on stratum corneum antibodies. In Beutner EH (Ed): *Autoimmunity in Psoriasis.* CRC Press, Boca Raton, FL, 1982, pp 81–93.
10. Bizzozero E: Expériences sur le signe de Köbner dans le psoriasis. *Bull Soc Fr Derm Syph* 38:1047–1049, 1931.
11. Born W, Kalkoff KW: Die "gesunde" Haut des Psoriatikers im Tritium-Thymidin-Autoradiogramm. *Arch klin exp Derm* 234:125–132, 1969.
12. Brain S, Camp R, Dowd P, et al: Psoriasis and leukotriene B_4. *Lancet* ii:762–763, 1982.
13. Braun-Falco O, Scherer R: Immunoinflammatory phenomena in psoriasis. In Beutner EH (Ed): *Autoimmunity in Psoriasis.* CRC Press, Boca Raton, FL, 1982, pp 165–182.
14. Chowaniec O, Jablonska S, Beutner EH, et al: Earliest clinical and histological changes in psoriasis. *Dermatologica* 163:42–51, 1981.
15. Chowaniec O, Jablonska S: Pre-pinpoint papules. Changes preceding pinpoint lesions of psoriasis. *Acta Dermatol Venereol* 59:39–45, 1979.
16. Christophers E, Schröder JM, Langner A: Role of polymorphonuclear leukocyte chemotaxis in psoriasis. In Beutner E, (Ed): *Autoimmunity in Psoriasis.* CRC Press, Boca Raton, FL, 1982, pp 125–132.
17. Cormane RH: Immunopathology of psoriasis. *Arch Dermatol Res* 270:201–215, 1981.

18. Cormane RH, Hunyadi J, Hamerlinck F: The role of lymphoid cells and polymorphonuclear leukocytes in the pathogenesis of psoriasis. *J Dermatol* 3:247–259, 1976.
19. Diezel W, Meffert H, Metz D, et al: Psoriasis vulgaris—Abnahme der Serumimmunkomplexe nach Fotochematherapie. *Dermatol Monatschr* 165:10–12, 1979.
20. Duell EA, Voorhees JJ: Control of epidermal growth. In Goldsmith LA (Ed): *Biochemistry and Physiology of the Skin.* Oxford University Press, New York, 1983, pp 241–268.
21. Elias PM, Friend DS: The permeability barrier in mammalian epidermis. *J Cell Biol* 65:180–191, 1975.
22. Ellis CN, Fallon JD, Heezen JL, et al: Topical indomethacin exacerbates lesions of psoriasis. *Clin Res* 31:564A, 1983.
23. Fang C, Alexander JW, MacMillan BG, et al: Failure of topical prostaglandin inhibitors to improve wound healing following deep partial-thickness burns. *J Trauma* 23:300–304, 1983.
24. Farber EM, Roth RJ, Aschheim E, et al: Role of trauma in isomorphic response in psoriasis. *Arch Dermatol* 91:246–251, 1965.
25. Glinski W: Cellular factors in psoriasis and their interaction with humoral factors. In Beutner EH (Ed): *Autoimmunity in Psoriasis.* CRC Press, Boca Raton, FL, 1982, pp 205–218.
26. Glinski W, Jablonska S: Remission of psoriasis during peritoneal dialysis: A possible role of polymorphonuclear leucocytes (PMNL) and their neutral serine proteinases in the pathogenesis of the disease. In Beutner EH (Ed): *Autoimmunity in Psoriasis.* CRC Press, Boca Raton, FL, 1982, pp 219–232.
27. Glinski W, Jablonska S, Zarebska Z, et al: Role of blood-borne factors in psoriasis. In Marks R, Christophers E, (Eds): *The Epidermis in Disease.* MTP Press, Lancaster UK, 1981, pp 371–380.
28. Hammarstrom S, Hamberg M, Samuelsson B, et al: Increased concentration of nonsterified arachidonic acid, 12-L-hydroxy-5,8,10,14-eicosatetraenoic acid, prostaglandin E_2, and prostaglandin F_2 in epidermis of psoriasis. *Proc Natl Acad Sci USA* 72:5130–5134, 1975.
29. Hebborn P, Jablonska S, Beutner EH: Action of topically applied arachidonic acid on the skin of psoriatics and normal individuals. *Arch Dermatol,* 1987 (submitted).
30. Hintner H, Lawley TJ: Keratin intermediate filaments bear antigenic determinants for stratum corneum antibodies. *J Invest Dermatol* 82:491–495, 1984.
31. Hinter H, Steinert PM, Lawley TJ: Human upper epidermal cytoplasmic antibodies are directed against keratin intermediate filament proteins. *J Clin Invest* 71:1344–1351, 1983.
32. Jablonska S, Beutner EH: Report by Weiss VC, et al Immunopathology of Psoriasis. *J Invest Dermatol* 81:381, 1983 (letter to the editor).
33. Jablonska S, Beutner EH, Binder WL, et al: Immunopathology of psoriasis. *Arch Derm Res* 264:65–71, 1979.
34. Jablonska S, Beutner EH, Chorzelski TP, et al: IF studies of psoriatic scales and induced psoriatic lesions (Koebner phenomenon). In Beutner EH (Ed): *Autoimmunity in Psoriasis.* CRC Press, Boca Raton, FL, 1982, pp 93–110.
35. Jablonska S, Beutner EH, Jarzabek-Chorzelska M, et al: Clinical significance of autoimmunity in psoriasis. In Milgrom F, Albini B (Eds): *Immunopathology. Proceedings of the 6th International Convocation on Immunology.* Karger, Basel, 1979, pp 148–153.
36. Jablonska S, Chorzelski TP, Beutner EH, et al: Autoimmunity in psoriasis. Relation of disease activity and forms of psoriasis to immunofluorescence findings. *Arch Dermatol Res* 261:135–146, 1978.
37. Jablonska S, Chorzelski TP, Jarzabek-Chorzelska M, et al: Studies in immunodermatology. VII. Four compartment system studies of IgG in stratum corneum and of stratum corneum antigen in biopsies of psoriasis and control dermatoses. *Int Arch Allergy* 48:324–340, 1975.
38. Jablonska S, Chowaniec O, Maciejowska E: Histology of psoriasis: The role of polymorphonuclear neutrophiles. In Beutner EH (Ed): *Autoimmunity in Psoriasis.* CRC Press, Boca Raton, FL, 1982, pp 21–36.
39. Jablonska S, Chowaniec O, Beutner EH, et al: Stripping of the stratum corneum in patients with psoriasis. Production of prepinpoint papules and psoriatic lesions. *Arch Dermatol* 118:652–657, 1982.

40. Johannesson A, Hammar H, Sundquist KG: The deposition of immunoglobulins and complement in stratum corneum in microscopic lesions in patients with active psoriasis: The relationship to hyperproliferation. *Acta Dermatovenereol* 62:21–25, 1982.
41. Jones P: Immunopathology of psoriasis: Characterization of a stratum corneum antigen. PhD Thesis, State University of New York at Buffalo, 1985, 175 pp.
42. Katayama H, Kawada A: Exacerbation of psoriasis induced by indomethacin. *J Dermatol (Tokyo)* 8:323–337, 1981.
43. Kimura S, Nishikawa T: An immunohistochemical analysis of the deposited immunoglobulins and fibrinogen in parakeratotic psoriatic horny layer and pemphigus skin lesions. *Arch Dermatol Res* 261:55–62, 1978.
44. Kimura S, Nishikawa T: A further study on the deposition of plasma protein in psoriasis scale. *Arch Dermatol Res* 268:79–84, 1980.
45. Krogh HK, Tönder O: Antibodies in psoriatic scales. *Scand J Immunol* 2:45–51, 1973.
46. Krogh HK, Tönder O: Stratum corneum antigens and antibodies as revealed by immune adherence and indirect hemagglutination. In Beutner EH: *Autoimmunity in Psoriasis*. CRC Press, Boca Raton, Fl, 1982, pp 39–51.
47. Krueger GG, Bergstresser PR, Lowe NJ, et al: Psoriasis. *J Am Acad Dermatol* 11:937–947, 1984.
48. Krueger GG, Chambers DA, Shelby J: Involved and uninvolved skin from psoriatic subjects: Are they equally diseased? Assessment by skin transplanted to congenitally athymic (nude) mice. *J Clin Invest* 68:1548–1557, 1981.
49. Kumar V, Jones P, Beutner EH, et al: Immunofluorescence studies in psoriasis: Detection of antibodies to stratum corneum in psoriatic scales. In Beutner EH, Nisengard RJ, Albini B (Eds): Defined Immunofluorescence and Related Cytochemical Methods. *Ann NY Acad Sci* 420:361–368, 1983.
50. Lagercrantz R, Hammarstrom S, Perlmann P, et al: Immunological studies in ulcerative colitis. IV. Origin of autoantibodies. *J Exp Med* 128:1339–1352, 1968.
51. McDonald JC, Jacobbi LM, Johnson E: A heterophile system in human transplantation. V. Relationship of heterophile transplantation antigen and common antigen of enterobacteriaceae. *Transplantation* 21:141–148, 1976.
52. Penneys NS, Ziboh VA, Lord JT, et al: Inhibitors of prostaglandin synthesis in psoriatic plaque. *Nature* 254:351–352, 1975.
53. Penneys NS, Ziboh VA, Simon PS, et al: Pathogenesis of Woronoff ring in psoriasis. *Arch Dermatol* 112:955–957, 1976.
54. Pinkus H, Mehregan AH: The primary histologic lesion of seborrheic dermatitis and psoriasis. *J Invest Dermatol* 46:109–116, 1966.
55. Priestley GC, Adams LW, Oakley CA, et al: Proliferative responses of fibroblasts from psoriatic and normal skin to clobetasol proprionate. *Acta Dermatol Venerol* 63:393–396, 1983.
56. Schöpf E, Kapp A, Kownatzki H, et al: Involvement of the complement system in psoriasis—Levels of C3A, C5A, C3, C4 and C1INA. In *Proceedings of the 3rd International Symposium on the Treatment of Psoriasis and Psoriasis Arthritis*. 1984, p 84 (abstract).
57. Shier WT: Inhibition of prostaglandin synthesis by lysolecithin. *Biochem Biophys Res Comm* 78:1168–1174, 1977.
58. Squier CA, Hopps RM: A study of the permeability barrier in epidermis and oral epithelium using horseradish peroxidase as a tracer in vitro. *Br J Dermatol* 95:123–129, 1976.
59. Steigleder GK: Basic pathogenic aspects of psoriasis. In Farber EM, Cox AJ (Eds): *Psoriasis—Proceedings of the 3rd International Symposium*". Grune & Stratton, New York, 1982, pp 13–22.
60. Tagami H, Ofuji S: Leukotactic properties of soluble substances in psoriasis scale. *Br J Dermatol* 95:1–8, 1976.
61. Tagami H, Ofuji S: Demonstration of C3 cleavage product in leukotactic substances of scale extract from pustular psoriasis. *Br J Dermatol* 96:94–95, 1977.
62. Tagami H, Ofuji S: Characterization of a leukotactic factor derived from psoriatic scale. *Br J Dermatol* 97:509–518, 1977.

63. Tagami H, Ofuji S: A leukotactic factor in the stratum corneum of pustulosis palmaris et plantaris: A possible mechanism for the formation of intraepidermal sterile pustules. *Acta Dermatolvenereol* 58:401–405, 1978.
64. Tagami H, Ofuji S: Chemotactic factors in psoriatic scales. In Beutner EH (Eds): *Autoimmunity in Psoriasis*. CRC Press, Boca Raton, FL, 1982, pp 111–124.
65. Weiss VC, van den Broek H, Barrett S, et al: Immunopathology of psoriasis. A comparison with other parakeratotic lesions. *J Invest Dermatol* 78:256–260, 1982.
66. Weiss VC, van den Broek H, Barrett S, et al: Reply to letter to editor by Jablonska S, Beutner EH, on Immunopathology of psoriasis. *J Invest Dermatol* 81:381–382, 1983.

43
The Immunopathology of Graft-Versus-Host Disease

Patricia L. Myskowski
Bijan Safai

INTRODUCTION

Graft-versus-host disease (GVHD) is the consequence of immunocompetent lymphocytes reacting against an immunologically incompetent host. Such a reaction generally results in immunologic injuries in a number of organs. It is well recognized that certain conditions are needed in order for GVHD to develop. These include: 1) The presence of immunocompetent donor tissue; 2) host cells that differ sufficiently in their genetic make-up so that the host may be perceived as being foreign by the donor; and 3) an immunologically incompetent host that is thus incapable of rejecting the grafted tissue. Under such circumstances, a graft-versus-host reaction (GVHR) occurs in specific organs. This GVHR results in the development of specific clinical features, histopathologic findings, and immunologic changes, all constituting the entity of GVHD.

HISTORIC PERSPECTIVE

The first description of the clinicpathologic entity recognized later on as GVHD was reported by Murphy in 1916 (47). However, it was during the 1950s and 1960s that, through the use of experimental animal models, extensive work was done to describe the entity in a more comprehensive manner (4,67). It was shown that in animals with bone marrow failure induced by ionizing radiation, the administration of allogeneic spleen cells resulted in a fatal syndrome manifesting with diarrhea, wasting, and cutaneous lesions. Further experimental animal models of GVHD, such as runt disease and F1 hybrid disease, were then described. These observations and many others both expanded the knowledge of the pathophysiology of the syndrome and laid the groundwork for recognition of GVHD in humans. Mathe et al. (43) first observed the syndrome in humans in 1959, following bone marrow transplantation (BMT) in leukemic patients who had been pretreated with total body irradiation.

CLINICAL SETTINGS FOR DEVELOPMENT OF GRAFT-VERSUS-HOST DISEASE

GVHD may occur in the setting of congenital and iatrogenic immune deficiency states. In rare instances, GVHD has been seen in utero following maternofetal transfer of immunologically competent lymphocytes across the placental barrier in congenitally immunodeficient children (46). Similarly, GVHD has occurred following in utero transfusion of incompatible Rh blood (38,48,53). Rarely, it has occurred following the administration of nonirradiated blood products to immunosuppressed malignancy patients (14). However, the most common clinical setting in which GVHD occurs is as a consequence of allogeneic BMT.

Allogeneic BMT (i.e., when the donor and the patient are of the same species but of different genetic make-up) is the most frequently performed method of transplantation. It is usually done between siblings who are matched by HLA typing. Alternatively, syngeneic transplantation is performed when the donor and host are monozygotic twins, since the individuals are identical genetically. The most common indications for which BMT is performed include severe aplastic anemia and various hematologic malignancies; for example, acute lymphoblastic leukemia in second remission, acute nonlymphoblastic leukemia, and chronic myelogenous leukemia (52).

BMT has also been used in congenital immune deficiencies such as severe combined immune deficiency, Wiskott-Aldrich syndrome, and Chediak-Higashi syndrome, and it will probably prove to be a more frequently applied therapeutic modality in the future (52). With the increasing applications of BMT, and increasing survival of the transplant recipients, one can expect to see more instances of GVHD.

CLASSIFICATION

GVHD in humans is classified into acute and chronic forms. These two forms are defined by specific clinical, pathologic, and temporal parameters. Acute GVHD usually begins 5–47 days following BMT (25), most commonly between the fourth and fifth weeks after transplantation, but by definition within the first 100 days following BMT (25). Chronic GVHD has its onset more than 3 months, or 100 days, after transplantation (31).

CLINICAL FEATURES

Acute GVHD

The clinical and pathologic picture of acute GVHD may be expected to develop in up to 70% of patients who received successful allogeneic BMT (8,18,70,81). The primary targets of acute GVHR are the skin, mucous membranes, liver, and gastrointestinal tract (Table 1) (18).

The initial site of injury in acute GVHD is usually the skin. While the first cutaneous signs may be noted as early as 5 days after BMT, the time of onset is not related to the eventual severity of GVHD (31). The primary symptoms often include pruritus or a burning sensation of the skin. Initial signs are usually a faintly erythematous, blanching eruption. In an adult, the lesions may begin on the trunk or extremities; in children, the initial lesions are often on the face (29,44). The eruption may be evanescent or may

Table 1. Acute Graft-Versus-Host Disease

Frequency:	70% of allogeneic BMT recipients
Onset:	5–47 days after BMT (Always within first 100 days)
Targets	
Skin:	Morbilliform eruption with volar eruption
Gastrointestinal tract:	nausea diarrhea
Liver:	bile stasis hepatitis

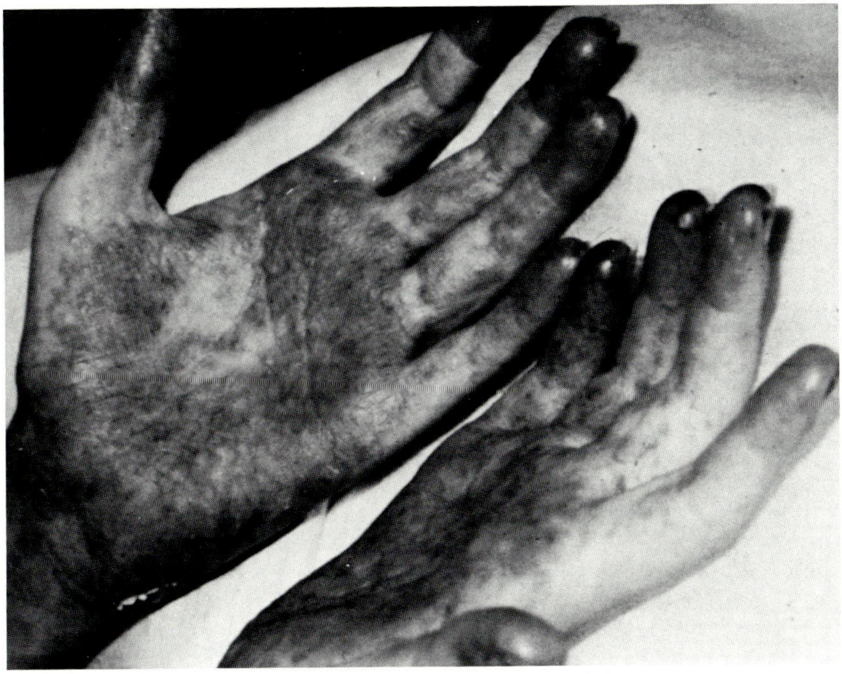

Figure 1. Palmar erythema in acute GVHD.

progress to present as a generalized erythroderma. Typical features include a morbilliform eruption simulating an allergic drug reaction (62) and marked erythema on the palms and soles (Fig. 1) (31). Less common features include a photosensitive distribution of the eruption, mucous membrane ulcerations, petechiae, bullae, and sloughing of the skin resembling toxic epidermal necrolysis (44,54,55).

Systemic features of acute GVHD often follow the skin findings. Systemic symptoms include fever, malaise, and myalgias. Gastrointestinal tract involvement is frequently observed, and is manifested by anorexia, nausea, and diarrhea. Hepatic dysfunction may reflect bile stasis or hepatitis. Thus, the usual triad of organ involvement in acute GVHD includes skin, gastrointestinal tract, and liver (18).

Chronic GVHD

This form of GVHD may occur as a result of a slow progression of the acute form, or it may develop de novo 3 or more months following BMT (Table 2). Chronic GVHD is observed in over 25% of BMT recipients; 80% of these cases have a history of acute GVHD (66). Skin involvement is virtually a universal feature of chronic GVHD (69). Cutaneous findings are often divided into early and late chronic GVHD (58–60). The typical features of early chronic GVHD include erythematous macules and papules, as well as buccal mucosa and scalp lesions, sometimes simulating lichen planus (LP) (59,62). Less common findings in early chronic GVHD include poikiloderma, alopecia, dystrophic nails, bullae, and discoid lupus erythematosus (DLE) like lesions (27,44,65).

The late form of chronic GVHD most often resembles scleroderma (Fig. 2) (31). Localized forms may resemble morphea, with peripheral extension into large areas of confluence and plaque formation (65,66,83). The trunk is the most frequently involved site in chronic GVHD, with extremities as the next most common site. Ulcerations and contractures may result from the sclerotic, bound-down skin.

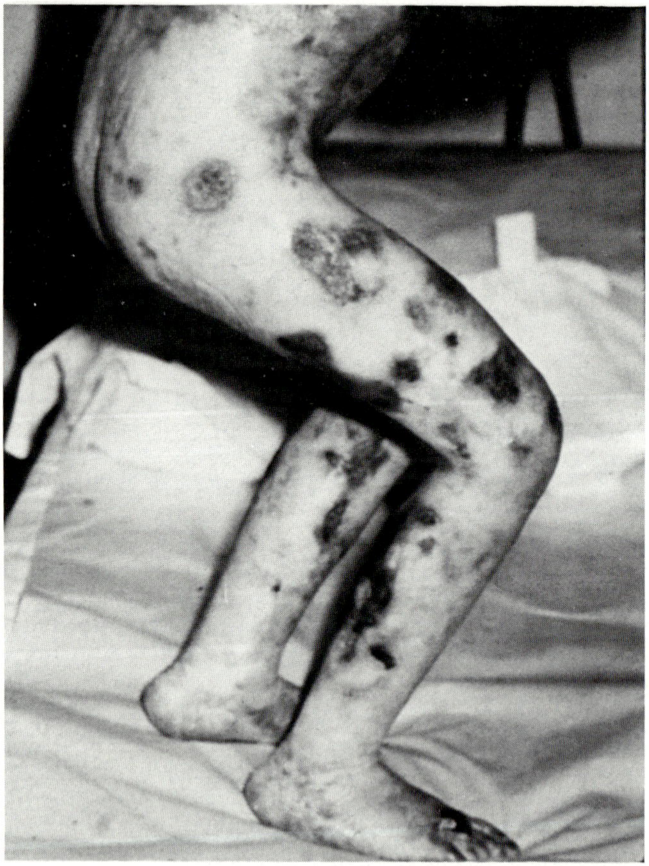

Figure 2. Sclerodermoid chronic GVHD with contractures.

Table 2. Chronic Graft-Versus-Host Disease

Frequency: 25% of allogeneic BMT recipients
Onset: 100 days or more after BMT
Targets
Skin: Lichenoid
Poikilodermatous
Sclerodermoid
Gastrointestinal tract: dysphagia
malabsorption
Pulmonary: fibrosis

Extracutaneous involvement is common in chronic GVHD, and resembles various autoimmune disorders (31,44). Ophthalmologic findings may mimic Sjögren's syndrome (66). Gastrointestinal involvement and pulmonary findings may resemble the changes of systemic scleroderma (44,65). Arthritis, circulating autoantibodies, and hematologic abnormalities are common findings that may also suggest rheumatologic disorders.

PROGNOSIS

The prognosis of acute GVHD appears to be directly related to the severity of reactions, and indirectly related to the complications of the immunosuppressive drugs used in its treatment (31). The mild form of acute GVHD may resolve spontaneously in approximately 15% of cases (25). Individuals with severe forms of the disorder, however, may face mortality rates up to 40%, with deaths resulting from end-organ failure and sepsis (9,86). The outcome of chronic GVHD is also related to the severity of disease. In the localized form, stabilization may occur, and some spontaneous softening of plaques has been observed (18,28). Generalized chronic GVHD may result in widespread contractures and ulcerations, as well as internal organ involvement, leading to bacterial sepsis and death.

HISTOPATHOLOGY

Light Microscopy

The earliest pathologic changes of acute GVHD occur in both the dermis and epidermis (Fig. 3) (28,88). General findings include sparse, perivascular lymphocytic infiltration in the upper and middle dermis, with mild edema of the papillary dermis (28). Epidermal changes consist of a vacuolar alteration at the dermal-epidermal junction, accompanied by sparse lymphocytic infiltrates, and epidermal cell necrosis. In its earliest lesions, acute GVHD may have a normal-appearing stratum corneum (SC); however, compact parakeratosis appears as the lesions become older. Within the epidermis, both keratinocytes and melanocytes show individual cell necrosis, and involvement may progress to the pilosebaceous unit (68). The essential finding of acute GVHD is satellite cell necrosis, which consists of individual necrotic keratinocytes surrounded by infiltrating lymphocytes within the epidermis (Fig. 4). Later changes involve both increasing edema of the papillary dermis, with some eosinophilic necrotic cells, and an admixture of the lymphocytic infiltrate with histiocytes and eosinophils (28).

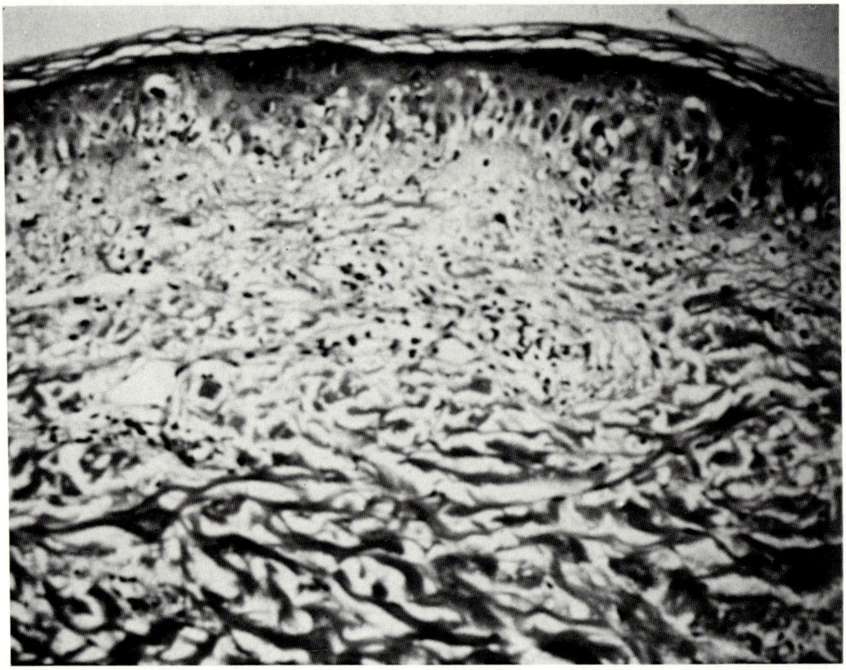

Figure 3. Acute GVHD. Sparse perivascular lymphocytic infiltrates. Vacuolization at dermal-epidermal junction (H&E stain).

Other patterns of acute GVHD may occur, especially as it enters a quiescent phase. Epidermal atrophy, sparse lymphocytic dermal infiltrate, and melanin and necrotic eosinophilic cells in the dermis may all be histologic findings of acute GVHD in a later, less active phase (28). Perhaps the most severe and rare histologic manifestation is a pattern similar to toxic epidermal necrolysis (28,34,54). In this form, necrosis within the epidermis and vacuolar changes at the dermal-epidermal junction result is subepidermal cleavage (28).

The histopathology of chronic GVHD may be divided into two patterns, lichenoid and sclerodermoid, which correspond to their clinical counterparts. Typical changes in lichenoid chronic GVHD include orthokeratosis and hyperkeratosis, hypergranulosis, and irregular acanthosis (18,58–60). Vacuolar alteration is usually evident at the dermal-epidermal junction; in addition, individual dyskeratotic keratinocytes may be present within the epidermis in a pattern mimicking the satellite cell necrosis of acute GVHD (Fig. 5) (62). The same histologic pattern may extend to adnexal structures (18,44). A lymphocytic infiltrate is usually present within the papillary dermis; it may be band-like, but is often more sparse and perivascular in distribution than true LP (18,62). This lichenoid phase of chronic GVHD usually occurs in the first year following BMT (61,65).

Chronic GVHD may then enter a poikilodermatous phase. Typical clinical and histologic findings of this stage include epidermal atrophy and telangiectasia (28,30,62). The sclerodermoid changes of late chronic GVHD often follow the lichenoid and poikilodermatous stages. In this last phase, the epidermis may show either atrophy or acanthosis,

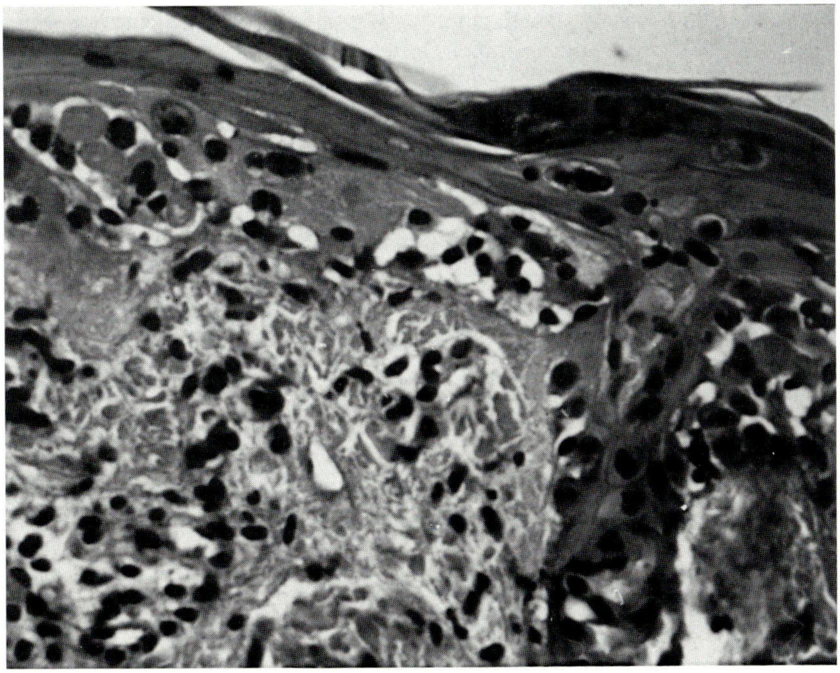

Figure 4. Acute GVHD. Vacuolar changes at dermal-epidermal junction, with necrotic keratinocytes surrounded by lymphocytes (H&E stain).

with diminution of the inflammatory process. There is progressive sclerosis of the dermis and subcutis, which may be similar to lupus profundus or scleroderma (Fig. 5) (28,30). Adnexal structures, including eccrine glands and hair follicles, also become involved by this progressive fibrotic process (28,65). A mixed cell infiltrate may also be found around vessels and adnexae (28). the dermal and subcutaneous changes of chronic sclerodermoid GVHD are most similar to those of scleroderma (18,28).

Electron Microscopy

Ultrastructural studies of acute and chronic GVHD have been confirmative of the light microscopic findings (12,13,57,87). The association of individual necrotic keratinocytes with lymphocytes within the epidermis in acute GVHD was first observed by Woodruff et al. in animal GVHD (87), and was later confirmed in humans (12). Ultrastructurally, epidermal damage appears to occur in three phases: 1) There is invasion of lymphocytes into the epidermis, with resulting acantholysis and formation of suprabasal clefts; 2) degeneration of epidermal cells occurs after their encounter with attacking lymphocytes; and 3) there is individual epidermal cell necrosis following surrounding of the degenerating keratinocyte by lymphocytes. This process appears to correlate well with the satellite cell necrosis of acute GVHD (57,81). Langerhans cells do not appear to be directly involved in this pathogenic process, although they are present (57).

Ultrastructural studies in chronic GVHD support the possible involvement of cell-mediated immune mechanisms in the pathogenesis of this disorder (22,32). Gallucci et

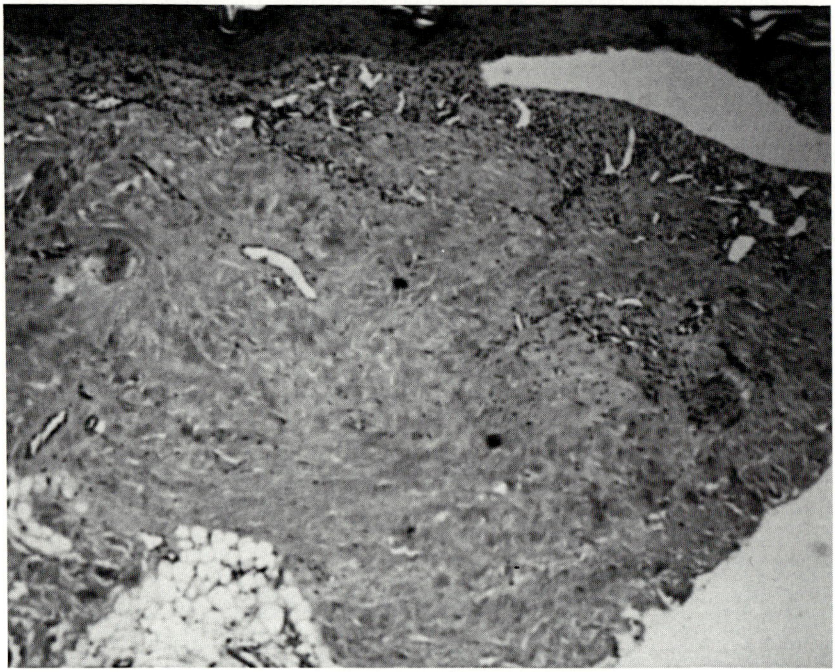

Figure 5. Chronic GVHD. Sclerodermoid changes. (H&E stain).

al. have described three types of epidermal injury in chronic GVHD. In the first type, prominent lymphocytic infiltration was present, but ultrastructural alterations of the keratinocytes were relatively minor. In the second type, acantholysis accompanied the prominent lymphocytic infiltrate, with subcellular injury being evident within most of the keratinocytes in the lower and middle epidermis. In the third type of injury, lymphocytic infiltration was sparse, but damage to keratinocytes was manifested by dilatation of organelles, followed by condensation and the formation of colloid bodies.(22) Lymphocytes and Langerhans cells also demonstrated evidence of subcellular damage. Changes in the basal lamina seemed to reflect the extent of injury to the basal cell layer (22). Janin-Mercier et al. have explored the relationship of the ultrastructural changes of chronic GVHD to those of LP and scleroderma (32). In lichenoid chronic GVHD, epidermal changes at the basal cell layer were similar to those of classic LP. However, lesions of chronic GVHD had certain features not found in LP: 1) Widening of the lamina lucida, and 2) satellite cell necrosis. The sclerodermoid type of chronic GVHD differed from classic scleroderma by the persistence of epidermal injury and by localization of active fibroblasts and collagen synthesis to the upper third of the dermis (32).

IMMUNOPATHOLOGY OF GRAFT-VERSUS-HOST DISEASE

The requirements for developing GVHR clearly demonstrate the immunogenetic basis of GVHD and the involvement of immunologic mechanisms in the pathogenesis of this disease. Although considerable advances have been made in this extremely complex phenomenon, the immunopathology of GVHD is not yet well defined. The problem is further compounded by the many controversial observations reported concerning both the immunopathology of GVHD and the different hypotheses presented by experts in the field. The following is a brief review of the large body of information available to date.

Circulating Abnormalities

Humoral Immune Mechanisms

It is well accepted that, in general, humoral immunity is less important than cellular immunity in the pathogenesis of GVHD, and that humoral immune alterations seen in GVHD are the epiphenomena of T-cell-mediated immune injuries.

Merritt et al. were the first to describe complement-dependent cytotoxic IgM antibodies against epithelial cell lines, but not lymphoid cells, in the sera of three recipients of HLA identical marrow (45). They reported that the onset of clinically evident GVHD coincided with the appearance of this antibody in the serum. In another series of studies, Saurat et al. demonstrated circulating specific antibodies against epidermal basal cells of the IgG type in two of four patients with chronic GVHD (58). Furthermore, these investigators used direct immunofluorescent (DIF) techniques to demonstrate IgG deposits in the skin of two of these four cases. Ullman et al. reported the presence of deposits of IgG, IgA, IgM, and C3 at the dermal-epidermal junction, and in blood vessel walls in one case of acute and one case of chronic GVHD (82). Tsoi et al. have reported a significant association between GVHD and deposits of IgM and C3 at the dermal-epidermal junction (Fig. 6) (74,79). They have demonstrated a consistent

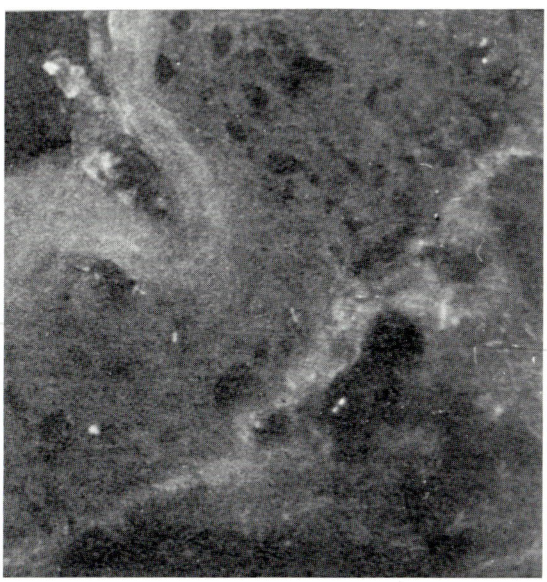

Figure 6. Chronic GVHD. Direct IF. Granular deposition of C3 at dermal-epidermal junction.

deposition of IgM in 86% of chronic GVHD cases, and of IgM deposits in 30% of those with acute GVHD. Only 11% of healthy bone marrow donors had a similar deposition of IgM. No IgM deposit was seen in the four recipients of syngeneic grafts. Furthermore, these investigators have observed C3 deposits in a less striking, but similar, pattern to that of IgM. It is unclear whether these antibodies are produced by the donor cells or by the recipient (79).

Cold autoantibodies and allolymphocytotoxic antibodies directed against non-HLA antigens on B and T lymphocytes have been reported in sera of 50% of BMT recipients (23,24). This is not a universal finding, and there have been reported cases of sustained engraftment without the presence of these antibodies (85).

Cellular Immune Mechanisms

It is believed that GVHD is initiated by cellular mechanisms. This includes development of alloreactive T lymphocytes capable of recognition of antigenic differences of the recipient, resulting in the development of lymphocyte-mediated injuries to the host target cell. However, the cell-mediated immunologic events causing the pathologic changes of GVHD are not yet well defined.

T-Lymphocytes and T-Cell Subsets. The number and percentage of T lymphocytes, determined by both E-Rosette and monoclonal anti-T-cell antibody methods, have been reported to be normal in patients with GVHD (16,56). However, early in the course of BMT, abnormally high numbers of immature T cells have been observed (11,17).

An imbalance of T-cell subsets has been reported by several different groups (1,20,56). It is reported that the ratio of T-suppressor to T-helper cells is reversed in both acute and chronic GVHD (1,11). The reversed ratio is demonstrated to return to normal in patients with an uncomplicated course, or in those with resolved GVHD (20). Other reports indicate that T-helper cells are depleted following BMT and remain low for over 2 years (1,19). In addition, suppressor-cytotoxic T cells are demonstrated to appear within 3 months after BMT, and to remain at normal or high levels for years (1).

Proliferative Response. In a mixed leukocyte culture assay (MLC), no evidence was observed of proliferation of lymphocytes of donor origin, from patients with or without acute GVHD, to cryopreserved pretransplant host cells (51,76). However, patients with chronic GVHD have been demonstrated to have more significant antihost responses than those without GVHD.

Natural Killer Activities. The possible role of natural killer cells in acute GVHD has been studied (15,37,39,40). It is reported that there is no correlation between the development of GVHD and the levels of natural killer (NK) activity against K562 target cells prior to BMT (37,39). However, normal NK activity against herpes simplex virus (HSV) type 1 infected fibroblasts, before BMT, has been shown to be predictive for the subsequent development of GVHD (39). The latter observation suggests that there are effector cells among the population of NK (HSV-1) effectors that could stimulate the transplanted marrow. In another series of experiments, Dokhelar et al. have shown a pretransplantation decrease in NK activity against K562 target cells that was restored after BMT (15). These investigators have reported a strong association between high NK levels and the development of acute GVHD during the first month post transplantation. These studies suggest that cells involved in GVHD might exert NK activity during some stage of their differentiation, or that NK cells may be involved in the development of acute GVHD (15).

CYTOTOXIC ACTIVITIES. Tsoi et al. have studied both specific cytotoxicity to host fibroblasts and the presence of serum-blocking activity for such cytotoxicity in GVHD (73,80). They have reported cytotoxicity during the first 2 months post-transplant in nearly 50% of tested patients with or without the presence of serum-blocking activity. The proportion of patients with cytotoxic activities decreased with time following grafting (80). After 1 year, 89% of the patients had neither serum-blocking nor cytotoxic activities, while the remaining 11% had both activities. These investigators have further suggested a correlation between the occurrence of acute GVHD and in vitro cytotoxicity to host fibroblasts by chimeric cells. No correlation was seen between the presence of serum-blocking factors and the development of acute GVHD in the early post-transplant phase (79).

IMMUNOREGULATION DEFECT. Nonspecific suppressor cell functions have also been studied in GVHD (75,78). This is done by measuring the ability of the patient's mononuclear cells to inhibit MLC reactivity of their bone marrow donors to various unrelated alloantigens. In this assay system, cells from 35 of 80 cases of chronic GVHD showed suppression, compared to 1 of 40 long-term BMT survivors without chronic GVHD (65). Suppressor effect was rarely seen in short-term BMT cases with or without acute GVHD (77). This nonspecific suppressor effect is said to be closely associated with clinical pictures of active chronic associated with clinical pictures of active chronic GVHD (21,77,80). Furthermore, presence of the suppressor effect is shown to be related to the development of late varicella-zoster infection (2). The cells responsible for the nonspecific suppressor activity are reported to be OKT8-positive T cells (80). In a series of experiments, it has been shown that the nonspecific suppressor activity could be abolished by either addition of helper factors or irradiation of the cells (50,75). These observations have been used to support a possible defect of helper-inducer function in patients with chronic GVHD. Several other studies have provided additional support for the presence of regulatory cell disorders in chronic GVHD (56,63).

B-CELL FUNCTION. Using pokeweed mitogen stimulation of polyclonal immunoglobulin (Ig) secretion, Lum et al. studied chronic GVHD and found T-suppressor cells that could suppress Ig synthesis, deficient T-helper cell activity, and B cells that were unable to secrete Ig despite of normal T-helper cells being present (41). Increased T-suppressor and decreased T-helper cell activity and defects in B-cell functions have all been observed in chronic GVHD, using similar assay systems (56,63). On the other hand, nonspecific T-suppressor cell activities, decreased T-helper cell function, and abnormal B-cell functions have not been observed in long-term stable BMT recipients without GVHD (49,63,75,77,78).

CUTANEOUS IMMUNOPATHOLOGY

The earliest work on local immune responses in acute GVHD centered upon the deposition of immunoglobulins in the skin. Tsoi et al. studied 88 recipients of allogeneic BMT by DIF methods. They noted that 39% (12 of 32) of patients with acute GVHD showed deposits of IgM at the dermal-epidermal junction. Deposits of C3 were also occasionally present, but were less specific. This group felt that the presence of IgM deposits was significantly associated with GHVD. No IgM deposition was seen in the skin of individuals receiving syngeneic grafts; and only 11% of healthy individuals, patients before transplantation and transplant recipients without GVHD, were found to have positive DIF findings (74). Ullman et al. noted depositions of IgG, IgM, IgA, and C3 at the dermal-epidermal junction and within blood vessel walls in a patient with acute GVHD (82). However, subsequent studies of immunoglobulin and complement deposition by DIF did not confirm the consistency of the findings (65). For example, Farmer et al. followed 22 patients with acute GVHD by examination of multiple sequential skin biopsy specimens. The specimens were examined by DIF techniques for the presence of immunoglobulin and complement. While C3 deposition was found at the dermal-epidermal junction in 41% of patients, immunoglobulins were absent in all of the patients with acute GVH who were examined. In addition, eight patients who did not develop clinical GVHD were found to have C3 deposition in the skin. The findings of immunoglobulin and complement deposition in skin biopsy specimens of patients with acute GVHD may therefore be nonspecific, and their clinical relevance has not yet been demonstrated (18).

Recent advances in the use of monoclonal antibodies (MCA) and immunohistochemical techniques have provided clues to the role of lymphocytes in the skin in acute GVHD (5,6,35,36). Beschorner et al. using immunoperoxidase methods with peroxidase-conjugated goat-antimouse IgG (Tago) and MCA from the Leu (Bectin-Dickinson) and Ortho (Orthoclone) series, demonstrated the presence of T cells and, specifically, T-nonhelper lymphocytes in skin biopsy specimens of acute GVHD. The lymphocytes were present within the epidermal infiltrate. NK cells and monocytes did not appear to participate in the epidermal injury (5,6). Lampert et al. studied nine patients who received BMT for aplastic anemia or leukemia, using indirect immunofluorescent (IIF) techniques (36). They used MCA which were coupled to fluorescein isothiocyanate or tetraethylrhodamine isothiocyanate. In four of their nine patients, a heavy infiltration by T lymphocytes was observed within the skin. In five of the nine patients, the lymphocytic infiltrate was moderate to minimal. In the four patients with dense lymphocytic infiltrates, more than 95% of the T lymphocytes were OKT8 positive and OKT4 negative. In addition, many of these cells invaded the basal layer and were in close apposition to keratinocytes in the epidermis. They felt that these findings confirmed a local role for T-suppressor/T-cytotoxic cells in the skin of acute GVHD. They noted that these findings, specifically the predominance of OKT8-positive cells, were similar to the lymphoid response seen in certain viral infections (e.g., cytomegalovirus and Epstein-Barr virus. They speculated that clinical or subclinical viral infections may possibly play a role as inciting factors in GVHD (35,36).

Recent interest has also centered upon the role of Langerhans cells and IA-staining cells in acute GVHD (3,10,33,35,42,64). Lampert et al. noted that in both rats and humans, Langerhans cells were lost in areas of maximal damage in acute GVHD, as determined by ATPase staining. However, Ia antigen staining was found on epidermal keratinocytes. These cells did not correspond to the Ia-positive, OKT6 positive, dendritic epidermal cells in humans (35). The finding of Ia-positive keratinocytes is not specific to acute GVHD, and may be present in other diseases with cellular immune dysfunction, such as LP (71) and mycosis fungoides (72). Studies of acute GVHD in the mouse have suggested that host keratinocytes may be synthesizing Ia in acute GVHD (10). Shearer and Levy have suggested that Ia synthesis by keratinocytes may result in "Ia-activated" immune suppression (64). However, the synthesis of Ia antigens by keratinocytes could represent a response to a cellular immune process, such as lymphokine (35). The Ia antigen does not appear to be passively acquired by the keratinocytes from other cells (10,35). The role of the Ia antigen in acute GVHD remains unclear, but further investigation of this phenomenon may help to explain the role of the skin as the major target organ in acute GVHD.

The earliest studies of immunologic processes in chronic GVHD centered upon the deposition of immunoglobulins and complement in the skin (74,79,82). Tsoi et al. found that 86% (12 of 14) of patients with chronic GVHD had marked deposition of IgM at the dermal-epidermal junction by DIF (74). They also found that C3 was frequently deposited at the dermal-epidermal junction in these patients. They noted that, in general, deposition of IgM and C3 was a far more consistent finding in chronic GVHD than in acute GVHD (Fig. 6) (74,79). Ullman et al. demonstrated the deposition of IgG, IgA, IgM, and C3 at both the dermal-epidermal junction and blood vessel walls in one patient with chronic GVHD (82). However, in studies of chronic GVHD in the rat radiation chimera, Beschorner et al. noted that some of the immunologic abnormalities found in spontaneously occurring GVHD, such as IgM deposition and circulating antinuclear antibodies (ANA), were not associated with the induced models of chronic GVHD and represented a paraphenomenon (7).

The use of immunohistochemical techniques and MCA has contributed further information about local immune responses in chronic GVHD (5,26,84). Gomes et al. studied skin biopsy specimens of three patients with a lichenoid form of chronic GVHD by IIF techniques. They noted the presence of a lymphocytic infiltrate in the dermis, which was primarily T cells; that is, OKT3+ cells. In addition, virtually all of the T lymphocytes were also OKT4− and OKT8+, thus identifying them as activated suppressor/cytotoxic lymphocytes. They also noted that Langerhans cells (OKT6+, HLA−DR+) were found in the epidermis, but could not be identified within the dermis (26). They felt that these studies supported the lack of Langerhans cells within the dermis, as previously demonstrated by EM (26,32). However, Beschorner et al. noted that many of the lymphocytes in the dermis in chronic GVHD were of the T-helper cell subset (5). Volc-Platzer et al. also found a dense lymphocytic infiltrate of helper/inducer cells within the dermis of lichenoid chronic GVHD by IIF techniques (84). They noted that Langerhans cells, as determined by HLA−DR+ and OKT6+ staining, were uniformly distributed within the epidermis. However, Ia staining, as determined by HLA−DR staining of keratinocytes, was present in the epidermis overlying the most dense lymphocytic dermal infiltrates (84). Recent work has also suggested that Langerhans cells in chronic GVHD are of donor origin (84). The heterogeneity of these findings is not easily explained. However, future studies may be expected to contribute to our understanding of local immune processes in chronic GVHD.

SUMMARY

Graft-versus-host disease (GVHD) is the consequence of immunocompetent donor lymphocytes reacting against a foreign, immunologically incompetent host. GVHD occurs in humans primarily in the settling of allogeneic BMT for hematologic disorders. In the acute form of the disease, the skin is the first target of injury. Acute GVHD appears to be initiated by cellular immune mechanisms, and T lymphocytes of the suppressor type appear to play a key role in the pathogenesis. The chronic form of the disease more closely resembles various autoimmune disorders. Both humoral and cellular immune abnormalities may be found in chronic GVHD. The deposition of IgM and complement in the skin, as well as the presence of circulating autoantibodies, support a role for humoral immunity. However, cellular immune dysfunction appears to be more important, with the persistent presence of increased circulatory suppressor cells and lymphocyte subset alterations in chronic GVHD. Further investigation is necessary to define the immune pathogenesis of acute and chronic GVHD, and to increase our understanding of this complex disorder.

REFERENCES

1. Atkinson K, Hansen JA, Storb R, et al: T cell subpopulations identified by monoclonal antibodies after bone marrow transplantation I. Helper-inducer and cytotoxic-suppressor subsets. *Blood* 59:1292, 1982.
2. Atkinson K, Farewell V, Storb R, et al: Analysis of late infections after human bone marrow transplantation role of genotypic non-identity between marrow donor and recipient and of non-specific suppressor cells in patients with chronic graft-versus-host disease. *Blood* 60:714, 1982.
3. Barclay AN, Mason DW: Induction of Ia antigen in rat epidermal cells and gut by immunological stimuli. *J Exp Med* 156:1665, 1982.
4. Barnes DWM, Loutit JF: Spleen protection: The cellular hypothesis. In Bacq ZM (ED): *Radiobiology Symposium.* Butterworth & Co, Ltd, London, 1954, pp 135.
5. Beschorner WE, Tutschka PJ, Santos GW: Chronic graft-versus-host disease in the rat radiation chimera. J Clinical features, hematology, histology and immunopathology in long term chimera transplantation. 33:393, 1981.
6. Beschorner WE, Constantino FA, Tutschka PJ, et al: Characterization of inflammatory cells of human skin with graft-versus-host disease (GVHD). *Exp Hematol* 6(Suppl):6, 1982 (abstract).
7. Beschorner WE, Tutschka PJ, Santos GW: Chronic graft-versus-host disease in the rat radiation chimera. *Transplantation* 35:224, 1983.
8. Blume KG, Beutler E, Bross KJ, et al: Bone marrow ablation and allogeneic marrow transplantation in acute leukemia. *N Engl J Med* 302:1041, 1980.
9. Bortin MM, Rimm AA, Rose WC, et al: Transplantation of hematopoietic and lymphoid cells in mice. *Transplantation* 21:331, 1976.
10. Breathnach SM, Katz SI: Ia antigen synthesis by keratinocytes and impaired Langerhans cell function in acute cutaneous graft-versus-host disease. *J Invest Dermatol* 80:314, 1983 (abstract).
11. Bruin HG, Astaldi A, Leupers T, et al: T lymphocyte characteristics in bone marrow transplanted patients. II. Analysis with monoclonal antibodies. *J Immunology* 127:244, 1981.
12. DeDobbeleer GD, Ledoux MH, Achten GA: Graft versus host reaction: An ultrastructural study. *Arch Dermatol* 111:158, 1975.
13. Dees JH, Charley MR, Sontheimer RD, et al: Sequential ultrastructural analysis of murine graft versus host skin disease (GVHD). *J Invest Dermatol* 80:379, 1983.
14. Dinsmore RE, Straus DJ, Pollack MS, et al: Fatal graft-vs-host disease following blood transfusion in Hodgkin's disease documented by HLA typing. *Blood* 55:831, 1980.
15. Dokhelar MC, Wiels J, Lipinski M, et al: Natural killer cell activity in human bone marrow recipients. *Transplantation* 31:61, 1981.
16. Elfenbein GJ, Anderson PN, Humphrey RL, et al: Immune system reconstitution following allogeneic bone marrow transplantation in man: A multiparameter analysis. *Transplant Proc* 8:641, 1976.
17. Elfenbein GJ, Bellis MB, Santos GW: Peanut agglutinin receptor bearing nonadherent mononuclear cells circulating in the blood after bone marrow transplantation in man. *Transplant Proc* 13:273, 1987.
18. Farmer ER, Hood AF: Graft-versus-host disease. in Fitzpatrick TB, Eisen AZ, Wolff K, et al. (Eds): *Update: Dermatology in General Medicine.* McGraw Hill, New York, 1983, p 28.
19. Fox R, McMillan R, Spruce W, et al: Analysis of T-lymphocytes after bone marrow transplantation using monoclonal antibodies. *Blood* 60:578, 1982.
20. Friedrich W, O'Reilly RJ, Koziner B, et al: T lymphocyte reconstitution in recipients of bone marrow transplants with and without GVHD: Imbalances of T cell subpopulations having unique regulatory and cognitive functions. *Blood* 59:696, 1982.
21. Gale RP, Opelz G, Mickey MR, et al: Immunodeficiency following allogeneic bone marrow transplantation. *Transplant Proc* 10:223, 1978.
22. Gallucci BB, Shulman HM, Sale GE, et al: The ultrastructure of the human epidermis in chronic graft versus host disease. *Am J Pathol* 95:643–672, 1979.
23. Gluckman E, Gluckman JC, Anderson E, et al: Lymphocytotoxic antibodies after bone marrow transplantation in aplastic anemia. *Transplantation* 29:471, 1980.

24. Gluckman E, Anderson E, Lepage V, et al: Non-HLA lymphocytotoxic antibodies during GVHD after bone marrow transplantation (BMT). *Transplant Proc* 9:761, 1977.
25. Glucksberg H, Storb R, Fefer A, et al: Clinical manifestations of graft vs. host disease in human recipients of marrow from HLA matched sibling donors. *Transplantation* 18:295, 1974.
26. Gomes MA, Schmitt DS, Souteyrand P, et al: Lichen planus and chronic graft-versus-host reaction. In situ identification of immunocompetent cell phenotypes. *J Cutaneous Pathol* 9:249, 1982.
27. Gratwhol AA, Moutsopoules HM, Chused TM, et al: Sjögren-type syndrome after allogeneic bone-marrow transplantation. *Ann Intern Med* 87:703, 1977.
28. Hansen JA, Woodruff JM, Good RA: The graft-vs-host reaction in man. In Safai B, Good RA (Eds): *Immunodermatology*. Plenum, New York, 1981, p 229.
29. Hathaway WE, Githins JH, Blackburn WR, et al: Aplastic anemia, histiocytosis and erythroderma in immunologically deficient children—probable runt disease. *N Engl J Med* 273:953, 1965.
30. Hood AF, Soter NA, Rappeport J, et al: Graft versus host reaction: Cutaneous manifestations following bone marrow transplantation. *Arch Dermatol* 113:1087, 1977.
31. James WD, Odom RB: Graft-vs-host disease. *Arch Dermatol* 119:183, 1983.
32. Janin-Mercier A, Saurat JH, Bourges M, et al: The lichen planus like and sclerotic phases of the graft versus host disease in man: An ultra structural study of six cases. *Acta Dermatol Venereol (Stockh)* 61:187, 1981.
33. Krueger GG, Emam M, Roberts LK, et al: Ia expression by murine epdermis in vivo without evidence of skin disease. *J Invest Dermatol* 80:315, 1983 (abstract).
34. Krueger GRF. Graft-vs-host disease and toxic epidermal necrolysis. *Lancet* 1:268, 1973.
35. Lampert IA, Suitters AJ, Janossy G, et al: Lymphoid infiltrates in skin in graft-versus-host disease. *Lancet* 2:1352, 1981.
36. Lampert IA, Janossy G, Suitters AJ, et al: Immunological analysis of the skin in graft versus host disease. *Clin Exp Immunol* 50:123, 1982.
37. Livnat S, Seigneuret M, Storb R, et al: Analysis of cytotoxic effector cell function in patients with leukemia or aplastic anemia before and after marrow transplantation. *J Immunol* 124:481, 1980.
38. Loke YW: *Immunology and Immunopathology of the Human Foetal Maternal Interaction.* Elsevier, Amsterdam, 1978, p 108.
39. Lopez C, Sorell M, Kirkpatrick D, et al: Association between pre-transplant natural kill and graft-versus-host disease after stem-cell transplantation. *Lancet* 2:1103, 1979.
40. Lopez C, Kirkpatrick D, Livant S, et al: Natural killer cells in bone marrow transplantation. *Lancet* II:1025, 1980.
41. Lum LG, Seigneuret MC, Storb RF, et al: In vitro regulation of immunoglobulin synthesis after marrow transplantation I. T-cell and B-cell deficiencies in patients with and without chronic graft-versus-host disease. *Blood* 58:431, 1981.
42. Mason DW, Dallman M, Barclay AN: Graft versus host disease induces the expression of Ia antigens in epidermal cells and gut epithelium in the rat. *Nature* 293:150, 1981.
43. Mathe G, Bernard J, Schwarzenberg L, et al: Essai de traitement de sujets atteints de leucemie aigue en remission par irradiation totale suivie de transfusion de moelle osseuse homologue. *Rev Fr Etudes Clin Biol* 4:675, 1959.
44. Matsuoka L: Graft-vs-host disease. *J Am Acad Dermatol* 5:595, 1981.
45. Merritt CB, Mann DL, Rogentine GN Jr: Cytotoxic antibody for epithelial cells in human graft versus host disease. *Nature* 232:638, 1971.
46. Morhenn VB, Maibach HI: Graft-vs-host reaction in a newborn. *Acta Dermatol Venereol* 54:133, 1974.
47. Murphy JB: The effect of adult chicken grafts on the chicken embryo. *J Exp Med* 24:1, 1916.
48. Naiman JL, Punnet HH, Lischner HW, et al: Possible graft-versus-host reaction after intrauterine transfusion. *N Engl J Med* 281:697 1969.
49. Neely JE, Neely AN, Kersey JH: Immunodeficiency following human marrow transplantation in vitro studies. *Transplant Proc* 10:229, 1978.
50. Okado M, Klimpel GR, Kuppers RC, et al: The differentiation of cytotoxic T cells in vitro. I.

Amplifying factor(s) in the primary response is Lyt 1+ cell dependent. *J Immunol* 120:2527, 1979.
51. Opelz G, Gale RP, and the UCLA Bone Marrow Transplant Team: Absence of specific mixed leukocyte culture reactivity during graft-versus-host disease and following bone marrow transplant rejection. *Transplantation* 22:474, 1976.
52. O'Reilly RJ: Allogenic bone marrow transplantation: Current status and future directions. *Blood* 62:941, 1983.
53. Parkmann R, Mosier D, Umansky I, et al: Graft versus host disease after intrauterine and exchange transfusion for hemolytic disease of the newborn. *New Engl J Med* 290:359, 1974.
54. Peck GL, Herzig GP, Elias PM: Toxic epidermal necrolysis in a patient with graft versus host reaction. *Arch Dermatol* 101:561, 1972.
55. Peck GL, Elias PM, Graw RG Jr: Graft-versus-host reaction and toxic epidermal necrolysis. *Lancet* II:1151, 1972.
56. Reinherz EL, Parkman R, Rappeport J: Aberrations of suppressor T cells in human graft versus host disease *N Engl J Med* 300:1061, 1979.
57. Rozman C, Mascaro JM, Granema A, et al: Ultrastructural findings in acute and chronic graft-vs-host reaction. *J Cutaneous Pathol* 7:354, 1980.
58. Saurat JH, Gluckman E, Bussel A, et al: The lichen-planus-like eruption after bone marrow transplantation. *Br J Dermatol* 93:675, 1975.
59. Saurat JH, Gluckman E: Lichen planus like eruption after bone marrow transplantation: A manifestation of the graft versus host disease. *Clin Exp Dermatol* 2:335, 1977.
60. Saurat JH, Gluckman E: Lichen planus eruption: A marker for chronic graft versus host reaction. *Br Med J* 2:1480, 1977.
61. Saurat JH, Gluckman E: Graft versus host reaction. *Arch Dermatol* 114:801, 1978.
62. Saurat JH: Cutaneous manifestations of graft-versus-host disease. *Int J Dermatol* 20d:249, 1981.
63. Saxon R, McIntyre RE, Stevens RH, et al: Lymphocyte dysfunction in chronic graft versus-host disease. *Blood* 58:746, 1981.
64. Shearer GM, Levy RB. Graft-vs-host-associated immune suppression is activated by recognition of allogenic murine 1-A antigens. *J Exp Med* 157:936, 1983.
65. Shulman HM, Sale GE, Lerner KG, et al: Chronic cutaneous graft-versus-host disease in man. *Am J Pathol* 91:545, 1978.
66. Shulman HM, Sullivan KM, Weiden PL, et al: Chronic graft-versus-host syndrome in man: A long term clinicopathologic study of 20 Seattle patients *Am J Med* 69:204, 1980.
67. Simonsen M: Graft versus host reactions. Their natural history and applicability as tools of research. *Progr Allergy* 6:349, 1962.
68. Slavin RE, Santos GW: The graft versus host reaction in man after bone marrow transplantation: Pathology pathogenesis, clinical features and implication. *Clin Immunol Immunopathol* 1:472–498, 1973.
69. Sullivan KM, Shulman HM, Storb R, et al: Chronic graft-versus-host disease in 52 patients: Adverse natural course and successful treatment with combination immunosuppression. *Blood* 57:267, 1981.
70. Thomas ED, Storb R, Clift RA, et al: Bone marrow transplantation. *N Engl J Med* 292:832, 1975.
71. Tjernlund UM: Ia like antigens in lichen planus. *Acta Dermatol Venereol* 60:309, 1980.
72. Tjernlund UM: Epidermal expression of HLA-DR antigen in Mycosis fungoides. *Arch Dermatol Res* 261:81, 1978 1980.
73. Tsoi MS, Storb R, Weiden PL, et al: Studies on cellular inhibition and serum-blocking factors in 28 human patients given marrow grafts from HLA identical siblings *J Immunol* 118:1979, 1977.
74. Tsoi MS, Storb R, Jones E, et al: Deposition of IgM and complement at the dermo-epidermal junction in acute and chronic graft versus host disease in man. *J Immunol* 120:1485, 1978.
75. Tsoi MS, Storb R, Weiden P, et al: Sequential studies of cell inhibition of host fibroblasts in 51 patients given HLA identical marrow grafts. *J Immunol* 129:239, 1982.
76. Tsoi MS, Storb R, Dobbs S, et al: Cell-mediated immunity to non-HLA antigens of the host

by donor lymphocytes in patients with chronic graft-versus-host disease. *J Immunol* 125:2258, 1980.

77. Tsoi MS, Storb R, Dobbs S, et al: Suppressor cells in patients with HLA identical marrow grafts. In Gale RP, Fox CF (Eds): *Biology of bone Marrow Transplantation.* Academic Press, New York, 1980, p 119.
78. Tsoi MS, Storb R, Dobbs S, et al: Specific suppressor cells in graft-host tolerance of HLA-identical marrow transplantation. *Nature* 292:355, 1981.
79. Tsoi WT, Storb R, Jones E, et al: Deposition of IgM and complement at the dermo-epidermal junction in acute and chronic graft versus host disease in man. *J Immunol* 120:1485, 1978.
80. Tsoi MS: Immunological mechanisms of graft-versus-host disease in man. *Transplantation* 33:459, 1982.
81. Tutschka PJ, Bortin MM: Graft versus host disease. *Transplant Pro* 8:1267, 1981.
82. Ullman S, Spielvogel RL, Kersey JH, et al: Immunoglobulins and complement in skin in graft versus host disease. *Ann Intern Med* 85:205, 1976 (letter to the editor).
83. Van Vloten WA, Scheffer E, Dooren LJ: Localized scleroderma-like lesions after bone marrow transplantation in man. *Br J Dermatol* 96:337, 1977.
84. Volc-Platzer B, Stingl G, Wolff K, et al: Cytogenetic identification of allogeneic epidermal Langerhans cells in a bone marrow graft recipient. *N Engl J Med* 310:1123, 1984.
85. Warren RP, Storb R, Weiden PL, et al: Immunologic monitoring of marrow graft recipients following transplantation from HLA-identical siblings. *Transplant Proc* 10:535, 1978.
86. Weiden PL, Storb R, Tsoi MS, et al: Infusion of donor lymphocytes into stable canine radiation chimeras: Implications for mechanism of transplantation tolerance. *J Immunol* 116:1212, 1976.
87. Woodruff JM, Butcher WI, Hellerstein LJ: Early secondary disease in the rhesus monkey. II. Electron microscopy of changes in mucous membranes and external epithelia as demonstrated in the tongue and lip. *Lab Invest* 27:85, 1972.
88. Woodruff JM, Hansen JA, Good RA, et al: The pathology of the graft versus host reaction (GVHR) in adults receiving bone marrow transplants. *Transplant Proc* 8:675, 1976.

44 Immunopathology of Blood Vessels

Immunopathologic studies of skin reveal immune deposits in vessels in certain vasculitides. Specifically, immunofluorescent studies of biopsy specimens, particularly of lesional skin, reveal highly characteristic reaction patterns. The first part of this chapter affords a review of the relevant findings in vasculitides. While such immune deposits in vessels occur primarily in lesional skin, some may also occur in clinically normal skin. One striking example of this, which is reported in the second part of this chapter, occurs in viral hepatitis. This latter finding is so characteristic that the finding of typical granular complement and IgM deposits in the vessels of normal skin merits the suggestions that viral hepatitis be considered in the differential diagnosis.

IMMUNOPATHOLOGY OF VASCULITIS

Vijay Kumar

Ernst H. Beutner

Tadeusz P. Chorzelski

INTRODUCTION

Vasculitis may be defined as a clinical syndrome that, on pathologic examination, shows destructive and inflammatory changes in the blood vessels. Vasculitis presents a polymorphic picture depending upon vessel size, rate and degree of damage, and the repair mechanism of the tissue (5,7,8,21,25,26). Vasculitis may be classified based upon clinical presentation, pathologic findings, and laboratory findings, as indicated in the following three subsections.

Clinical Presentation

The separate names that have evolved for vasculitic syndromes imply that unique clinical patterns exist (5,7,21,25). Clinical manifestations of vasculitis may be separated into two groups: Cutaneous and systemic. Palpable purpura is the hallmark and most diagnostic feature of cutaneous vasculitis. Other cutaneous features are urticaria, petechiae, papules, plaques, nodules, bullae, and necrotic ulcerations. In the absence of palpable purpura, clinical diagnosis is extremely difficult, and only pathologic examination may provide the confirmation.

Cutaneous lesions are most predominant on dependent parts; that is, lower parts of the legs and ankles, and also on forearms and hands. The course in any single individual is unpredictable. There may be only one episode, or the disease may be recurrent for months or years. The more chronic cases may be due to the presence of circulating immune complexes (CIC).

Since vessels are obviously found in all organs of the body, it follows that all organs could potentially be involved. Systemic involvement in necrotizing vasculitis is quite common. Arthritis occurs in about one-quarter of these patients and arthralgia in about one-third (8,11). Infiltration lesions in the lungs, sometimes diffuse and sometimes nodular, are seen in about 30% of patients. Vasculitis of the kidneys is frequent and poses the most serious threat to the patient. In the studies of Winkelmann (24) and McCombs (12), about 40% of their patients had renal involvement. Gastrointestinal involvement is especially prominent in Henoch-Schonlein purpura. The bleeding may be so severe as to require a blood transfusion. Neurologic involvement, presenting as headache, diplopia, and dysphagia, has been found to occur in about 25 to 30% of cases. Other organs may be involved, but less frequently.

Pathologic Findings

The size of the vessel involved and the evidence of the inflammatory response have been used as the basis for classification. Most vasculitides can be classified into two broad categories based upon the histologic appearance: 1) Lymphocytic, and 2) necrotizing. Excellent reviews of the histopathology of vasculitis appear in standard texts (5,7,25).

Laboratory Findings

Based upon the laboratory findings, various vasculitides have been classified as hypergammaglobulinemic, cryoglobulinemic, hypocomplementemic, immune complex vasculitis, etc. (21,26). This chapter affords a review of the key findings.

LABORATORY STUDIES

Laboratory studies that have been found to be useful include blood, urine, and skin studies. *Blood* studies should include leukocyte and platelet count, erythrocyte sedimentation rate (ESR), cryoglobulins, antinuclear antibodies (ANA), rheumatoid factor, complement levels, coagulation and fibrinolysis, and hepatitis-associated antigen. *Urinalysis* studies of proteinuria, creatine clearance, casts, and hematuria are very important to detect possible renal involvement. In patients with persistent proteinuria or abnormal renal sediment, a renal biopsy procedure may be necessary. *Skin* biopsy studies are very important, and may be the only unequivocal tests for diagnosis and classification. Both routine histologic examination (H&E) and immunologic studies should be performed (Table 1).

Table 1. Diagnostic Criteria of Vasculitis

Histologic			Immunologic
Major	1. Cellular infiltration		1. Immune deposits of Ig (most commonly, IgM and IgG) and complement in blood vessels
	2. Fibrin deposits		2. Fibrin deposits in and around vessels
	3. Necrosis		
Minor	1. Endothelial swelling		
	2. Extravasation of erythrocytes		
	3. Thrombosis in the lumen		

The histologic criteria for diagnosis are divided into major and minor. For the diagnosis of vasculitis, two of the three major criteria should be fulfilled (21). Characteristically, cellular infiltrate is seen within the vessel wall. The infiltrate may be polymorphonuclear leukocytes (PMN) that may undergo fragmentation (leukocytoclasia), lymphocytes or monocytes, or monocytes and histiocytes. From the practical standpoint, this picture is variable. This variability stems not only from the severity of the reaction, but is also dependent on the time at which the biopsy specimen is obtained (9,16,18). Rarely is no cellular infiltrate seen.

IMMUNOFLUORESCENT STUDIES

Direct immunofluorescent (DIF) studies of the skin biopsy specimen may be very helpful in confirming the diagnosis of vasculitis. It is of particular diagnostic value when routine histology is not revealing. The immunofluorescent (IF) studies may be positive in over 80% of such cases (15). In our laboratory, we studied 42 chronic hepatitis patients with no skin lesions and found a relatively high frequency of IgM (79%) and C3 (38%) in normal skin biopsy specimens (see Part II of this chapter).

The age of the biopsy specimen obtained for DIF studies is very important. Older lesions may show neither typical histopathologic characteristics of vasculitis nor the presence of immunoglobulins or complement. If early lesions (<18 hours) are not available for IF studies, a possible approach is reproduction of the lesion by local injection of histamine to cause vasodilatation and fixation of immune complexes, as described by Braverman and Yen (2). Such an experimental lesion may be produced by an intradermal injection of 50 μl of a 0.1 mg/ml of histamine solution. The biopsy examination of the specimen should be performed at about 3 to 4 hours post procedure from an area of histamine injection. Direct IF studies of these specimens should be positive for immunoglobulins or complement in patients with vasculitis. Since the immune deposits in blood vessels are transitory and may be negative in older lesions, the type of studies discussed above formed the basis for a study of both kinetics of the appearance of immune reactants and inflammatory changes at known times (9). As summarized in Table 2, the studies of Sams et al. (17) demonstrate that initial deposition of immunoglobulins and complement is followed by infiltration of inflammatory cells, followed by diapedesis of erythrocytes. These changes are accompanied by the development of clinically palpable purpuric lesions. These studies also indicate why biopsy specimens of spontaneous lesions for IF studies often show negative results; that is, they were too old at the time of the procedure and immune reactants had been phagocytosed.

Table 2. Immune Mechanism in Histamine-induced Lesions of Vasculitis Patients

Time of biopsy after histamine injection (h)	*DIF studies for C3*	*Histopathology*
1	+	No inflammatory cells
4	+	Mononuclear cells, some PMN
8	±	Predominantly PMN
24	−	Predominantly PMN

Note: Clinical lesions appeared 8 hours after injection of histamine.

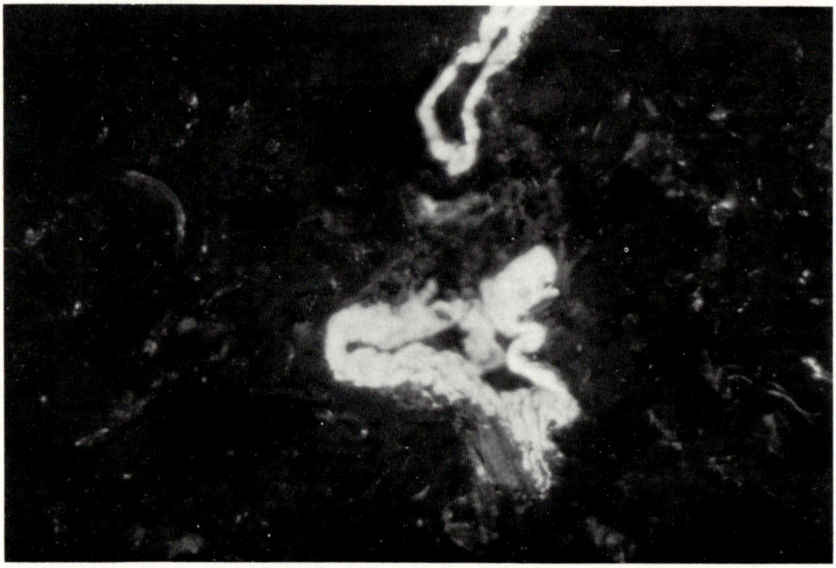

Figure 1. Direct IF studies of a lesional biopsy specimen from a patient with vasculitis that is positive for IgM and also for other immunoglobulins (220x).

Direct IF studies of lesional skin biopsy specimens from patients with necrotizing and non-necrotizing vasculitis showed that vascular deposits of immunoglobulins and complement C3 can be detected both in necrotizing and non-necrotizing types of vasculitis (Fig. 1). However, the number of positive results were lower in non-necrotizing vasculitis (55%), compared to necrotizing vasculitis (80%) (22). As shown in Table 3, the incidence of this positivity may not only vary for different immunoglobulins or complement, but may also vary from report to report (10,15,17,19). This may be due to the fact that skin biopsy specimens might have been taken from lesions of different ages. Normal skin biopsy specimens from normal individuals, as reported by Schroeter et al., were negative for immune deposits (19). However, IF studies of normal skin from vasculitis patients without skin lesions yielded 27% positivity (15).

Table 4 lists the incidence of immunoglobulins and complement in various forms of

Table 3. IF in Vasculitis

	IgG	*IgA*	*IgM*	*Fibrin*	*Complement*	*Reference*
Normal	0/3	0/2	0/2	0/2	0/2	Schroeter et al. (19)
Lesional	15/26	0/18	8/18	11/13	6/7	
	3/22	1/22	NR	2/22	6/22	Handel et al. (10)
	NR	4/13	4/13	5/13	9/13	Sams et al. (17)
	NR	NR	≈50/100	NR	≈50/100	Planuphak et al. (15)

NR-not reported.

Table 4. IF Findings in Selected Forms of Vasculitis

	IgG	*IgA*	*IgM*	*Fibrin*	*Complement*	*References*
Henoch-Schonlein purpura	(8)/8	8/8	(8)/8	NA	(8)/8	Baart de la Faille-Kuyper (1)
Hypocomplementemic vasculitis	NR	1/4	1/4	NA	1/4	McDuffie (13)
Mixed cryoglobulinemia	5/6	5/6	3/6	6/6	6/6	Cream (3)
Vasculitis associated with rheumatic diseases	10/12	NR	NR	11/12	9/12	Tuffanelli and Kay (23)

NR-not reported.

vasculitis. IF studies in Henoch-Schonlein purpura, a special type of leukocytoclastic vasculitis, show immunoglobulin and complement in cutaneous blood vessels. IgA is the most predominant of all the immunoglobulins (1). The reason that vascular deposits of IgA occur so often in Henoch-Schonlein purpura may be related to the upper respiratory infections that often precede this type of vasculitis.

Immunoglobulins and C3 are present in the blood vessels of specimens taken from early lesions of hypocomplementemic vasculitis, which is another variant of leukocytoclastic vasculitis (13). In mixed cryoglobulinemia, a third distinctive type of leukocytoclastic vasculitis, immune deposits containing C3, has been demonstrated (3,4). The immune deposits in blood vessels are of the same class(es) as the circulating cryoprecipitins. Thus, the detection of circulating cryoprecipitins is essential for the diagnosis of cryoglobulinemic vasculitis. Most mixed cryoglobulins contain IgG and IgM, and the IgM component has rheumatoid factor activity. Vasculitis associated with connective tissue diseases such as systemic lupus erythematosus (SLE) and rheumatoid arthritis (RA), has deposits of IgG, IgM, and C3 in both lesional and normal skin biopsy specimens (23). In polyarteritis nodosa, immunoglobulins and complement are again detected in a majority of cases (6). In approximately 30% of patients with polyarteritis nodosa, hepatitis B surface antigen (HBsAg) has been detected both in blood and vessel walls. In livido vasculitis, the immune deposits in blood vessels are predominantly or exclusively of the IgM type and have a smooth or homogeneous morphology (20). The diagnostic significance of the IF studies has been summarized in Table 4.

Etiology

Etiologic or predisposing factors involved in vasculitis are infections, drugs, foreign proteins, chemicals, and various collagen diseases. In addition, various other factors, such as food additives (salicylates, sodium benzoate), physical factors (gravitational), cold, trauma, insect bites, and chronic and malignant diseases, are predisposing facors for vasculitis.

Pathomechanism

Some potential mechanisms involved in vasculitis are described in the following subsections.

Microbial Agents

Microbial agents have long been recognized as agents of vasculitis. These microorganisms could invoke inflammatory reactions by several mechanisms. Gram-negative bacteria, by releasing endotoxins, could activate the alternate pathway of complement. Bacteria could release chemotactic factors. Bacterial, rickettsial, tuberculous, fungal, and viral organisms could act as antigens and could cause humoral and/or cellular immune reactions leading to an inflammatory response. Parish presented direct evidence for the role of streptococci in some cases of vasculitis (14).

Immune Complexes

There is compelling evidence that vasculitis is an immune complex disease. Tappeiner et al. correlated the presence of CIC with immune deposits in blood vessels (22). They studied 34 patients with various forms of vasculitis (22 with necrotizing, 17 with and 5 without systemic involvement, and 12 with non-necrotizing vasculitis). They found elevated Clq-binding ability in 13 of 17 patients with necrotizing vasculitis with systemic involvement, and in one of five patients without systemic involvement. The immune complexes were found in only 1 of 12 cases of non-necrotizing vasculitis. In these patients, vascular deposits of immunoglobulins and/or of complement were present in 18 of 19 cases of necrotizing vasculitis with high levels of immune complexes in circulation.

Immune complexes seen to play a significant role in the pathogenesis of vasculitis (16–18,22). Antigen-antibody complexes in antigen excess may develop in soluble immune complexes that escape the clearing mechanism of the reticuloendothelial system and, thus, circulate in blood. Upon lodging against lamina propria of blood vessels, they induce an inflammatory response predominantly via the activation of the complement sequence. Vasoactive amine may also be playing a significant role in lodging the immune complexes in blood vessels. Vasoactive amines induce vascular permeability, which allows immune complexes to cross the blood vessels and induce inflammation.

There are several mechanisms that result in local vasodilatation. In areas of increased turbulence, such as bifurcation of blood vessels, platelets aggregate and release vasoactive amines, or immune complexes upon binding to platelets can also induce the release of vasoactive amines. In addition, antigenic challenge to the host may result in the production of IgE antibodies. These antibodies, upon binding to circulating basophils and mast cells, result in the release of vasoactive amines, and they also cause platelet aggregation resulting in additional release of vasoactive amines. Once immune complexes are deposited in blood vessels, they result in the elaboration of chemotactic factors C3a, C5a, and C567. PMN are attracted to the site and release lysosomal enzymes, elastase, and collagenase, which cause tissue destruction, hemmorhage, and inflammation.

Practical Considerations Relating to DIF Findings

Most DIF studies of vasculitis are performed with biopsy specimens of lesional skin. Studies of muscle or other tissues usually are not as revealing and are of questionable value. While IF studies of lesion skin can give useful information, tests of normal skin usually yield negative findings even in well-characterized cases of vasculitis. Also, serum tests for tissue-specific antibodies are essentially of no value in studies of vasculitis. The indicated IF studies and the most characteristic finding in the major vasculitides are summarized in Table 5.

IF bands along the dermal-epidermal junction usually do not occur in vasculitis. Some false-positive reactions may appear. Also, the IF band may occur in erythematous or uninvolved skin in overlap cases with SLE (19).

In cutaneous vasculitis, the biopsy specimen should be taken from early lesions. If fresh lesions are not available, the local injection of histamine, as described by Braverman and Yen (2), is indicated. Specifically, 0.05 ml of a histamine solution containing 0.1 to 1.0 mg/ml is injected intradermally. A deep 3- to 5-mm biopsy incision is made in the center of the injection area in 3 to 4 hours. In such specimens, findings usually include deposits of IgG, IgM, IgA, complement, and fibrin or fibrinogen in and around blood vessels. However, the results are not always positive. In older lesions and in atrophie blanche, vascular and perivascular deposits of fibrin alone may be the only finding by the DIF method.

SUMMARY

Immunologic studies of early lesional or normal skin biopsy specimens are an important adjunct to histologic studies in confirming the diagnosis of vasculitis. Approximately

Table 5. Summary of Diagnostic Significance of Biopsy Findings in Vascular Diseases

Diseases	*Biopsy Findings by DIF in Lesional Skin*	*Serum Findings*	*Relevance of Findings*
Allergic (leukocytoclastic) vasculitis[a]	Mainly IgM and C in vessel walls in fresh lesions	No specific antibodies	
Henoch-Schonlein purpura[a]	Mostly IgA in vessel walls in fresh lesions	No specific antibodies	DIF suggestive of immunologic pathogenesis, but not diagnostic itself in most cases
Essential mixed cryoglobulinemia	IgG, other Ig, and C in vessel walls in fresh lesions	Cryoglobulins	
Polyarteritis nodosa	IgG and C in walls of medium (cutaneous & subcutaneous) vessel is rare; mainly IgM and C in vessel walls	No specific antibodies	
Necrotizing vasculitis	C mostly; sometimes IgM, IgA, & F in lumen of vessels	No specific antibodies	
Atrophie blanche		No specific antibodies	

[a]For reliable IF studies, skin biopsy specimens must be obtained either of very early lesions or 3 to 4 hours after intradermal injection of 0.05 ml of a histamine solution containing 0.1 to 1.0 mg/ml into the normal skin, according to the method of Braverman and Yen (2).

30% of skin specimens of patients with known systemic and cutaneous vasculitis show no skin pathology; and in 80% of these patients, IF studies of the presence of immunoglobulins or complement are positive. Immunologic studies are of help in understanding the pathogenesis of disease, which in turn helps in patient management and treatment by: 1) removal of an offending antigen; 2) treatment of an underlying disease; and 3) treatment directed at the primary vasculitic process by prevention of deposition of CIC by modulation of the immune response, or by suppression of inflammatory response.

REFERENCES

1. Baart de la Faille-Kuyper EM, Kater L, Kooiker CJ, et al: IgA deposits in cutaneous blood vessel walls and mesangium in Henoch-Schonlein syndrome. *Lancet* I:892–893, 1973.
2. Braverman IM, Yen A: Demonstration of immune complexes in spontaneous and histamine-induced lesions and in normal skin of patients with leukocytoclastic angiitis. *J Invest Dermatol* 64:105–112, 1975.
3. Cream JJ: Immunofluorescent studies of the skin in cryoglobulinemic vasculitis. *Br J Dermatol* 84:48–53, 1971.
4. Cream JJ: Immune complex disease and mixed cryoglobulinemia. In Beutner EH, Chorzelski TP, Bean SF, Jordan RE (Eds): *Immunopathology of the Skin: Labeled Antibody Studies*, ed. 1. Dowden, Hutchinson, Ross, Stroudsburg, PA, 1973, pp 137–152.
5. Cupps TR, Fauci AS: *The Vasculitides.* Saunders, Philadelphia, 1981, 221 pp.
6. Diaz-Perez JL, Winkelmann RK: Cutaneous periarteritis nodusa. A study of 33 cases. In Wolff K, Winkelmann RK (Eds): *Vasculitis.* Saunders, Philadelphia, 1980, pp 273–284.
7. Fauci AS: *Vasculitis* In Parker LW (Ed): *Clinical Immunology.* Saunders, Philadelphia, 1980, pp 473–519.
8. Gilliam JN, Smiley D: Cutaneous necrotizing vasculitis and related disorders. *Ann Allergy* 37:328–339, 1976.
9. Gower RG, Sams WM Jr, Thorne EG, et al: Leukocytoclastic vasculitis. Sequential appearance of immunoreactants and cellular change in serial biopsies. *J Invest Dermatol* 69:477–484, 1977.
10. Handel DW, Roenigk HH, Shainoff J, et al: Necrotizing vasculitis. Etiologic aspects of immunology and coagulopathy. *Arch Dermatol* 111:846–852, 1975.
11. McCluskey RT, Fienberg R: Vasculitis in primary vasculitides, granulomatoses and connective tissue diseases. *Human Pathol* 14:305–315, 1983.
12. McCombs RP: Systemic "allergic" vasculitis. JAMA 194:1059–1064, 1965.
13. McDuffie FC, Sams WM Jr, Maldonado JE, et al: Hypocomplementemia with cutaneous vasculitis and arthritis. *Mayo Clin Proc* 48:340–348, 1973.
14. Parish WE: Cutaneous vasculitis. The occurrence of complexes of bacterial antigens with antibody and of abnormalities associated with chronic inflammation. In Beutner EH, Chorzelski TP, Bean SF, Jordan RE (Eds): *Immunopathology of the Skin: Labeled Antibody Studies,* ed. 1. Dowden, Hutchinson, Ross, Stroudsburg, PA, 1973, pp 153–169.
15. Planuphak P, Kohler PF, Stanford RE, et al: Value of skin biopsy in vasculitis. *Clin Res* 26:123A, 1978 (abstract).
16. Sams WM Jr: Leukocytoclastic vasculitis. In Beutner EH, Chorzelski TP, Bean SF (Eds): *Immunopathology of the Skin,* ed. 2. Wiley, New York, 1979, pp 463–471.
17. Sams WM Jr, Claman H, Kohler PF, et al: Human necrotizing vasculitis: Immunoglobulins and complement in vessel walls of cutaneous lesions and normal skin. *J Invest Dermatol* 64:441–445, 1975.
18. Sams WM Jr, Thorne EG, Small P, et al: Leukocytoclastic vasculitis. *Arch Dermatol* 112:219–226, 1976.
19. Schroeter AL, Copeman PWM, Jordon RE, et al: Immunofluorescence of cutaneous vasculitis associated with systemic disease. *Arch Dermatol* 104:254–259, 1971.

20. Schroeter AL, Diaz-Perez JL, Winkelmann RK, et al: Livedo vasculitis. (The vasculitis of atrophie blanche). *Arch Dermatol* 111:188–193, 1975.
21. Sibbald RG, Roberts JT, Rosenthal D: Cutaneous vasculitis. *CMA J* 118:142–150, 1978.
22. Tappeiner G, Jordon RE, Wolff K: Circulating immune complexes in necrotizing vasculitis. In Wolff K, Winkelmann RK (Eds): *Vasculitis,* Saunders, Philadelphia, 1980, pp 68–75.
23. Tuffanelli DL, Kay DM: Morphological and immunological studies of necrotizing vasculitis in systemic lupus erythematosus. *Clin Res* 17:278, 1969 (abstract).
24. Winkelmann RK, Ditto WB: Cutaneous and visceral syndrome of necrotizing or "allergic" angitis: A study of 38 cases. *Medicine* 43:59–89, 1964.
25. Wolfe K, Winkelmann RK: *Vasculitis.* Saunders, Philadelphia, 1980, 338 pp.
26. Zvaifler NJ: Vasculitides: Classification and pathogenesis. *Austr NZ J Med* 8(Suppl):134–138, 1978.

STUDIES ON CLINICALLY NORMAL SKIN IN CHRONIC HEPATITIS

Jerzy Januszkiewicz

Tadeusz P. Chorzelski

INTRODUCTION

Most immunofluorescent (IF) studies of skin in patients with chronic hepatitis deal with examinations of skin lesions, and not with normal skin (6–8,10). Various types of skin lesions associated with hepatitis B (HB) infection have been reported; notably urticaria, palpable purpura of the Henoch-Schonlein type, erythema multiforme, lichen planus (LP)-like dermatitis, and polyarteritis nodosa. Since some of the dermatologic syndromes may be accompanied by hypocomplemententemia, leukocytoclastic vasculitis with immunoglobulins (Ig), and/or complement deposits as well as HB surface antigen (HBsAg) deposits in the perivascular distribution (3,6,8), it is believed that immune complexes may account for skin manifestations (6). In two cases of viral HB, HBsAg, Clq, and C3 deposits were found in the small superficial blood vessels, but not Ig. Normal skin gave negative results (7). In another case, IgM and C3 vascular deposits were found in clinically normal skin, which histologically showed, however, lymphocytic perivascular infiltrate (8). In 1977, we studied a case of chronic active hepatitis (CAH) with skin rash to exclude systemic lupus erythematosus (SLE). In both lesional and normal skin, we found IgM and C3 deposits in papillary vessels. Since the findings were not consistent with a diagnosis of SLE, it prompted us to study normal skin of patients with CAH without skin lesions for immune deposits.

IMMUNOFLUORESCENT FINDINGS OF NORMAL SKIN IN CHRONIC HEPATITIS

On the basis of our preliminary findings, we undertook a study of normal skin of chronic hepatitis patients. In the period 1979 to 1982, we examined 42 patients with chronic hepatitis, 37 with CAH-type B, 2 with type non-A/non-B, and 3 with protracted (over 1 year duration) HB. The classification of De Groote et al. (4) was applied. In the

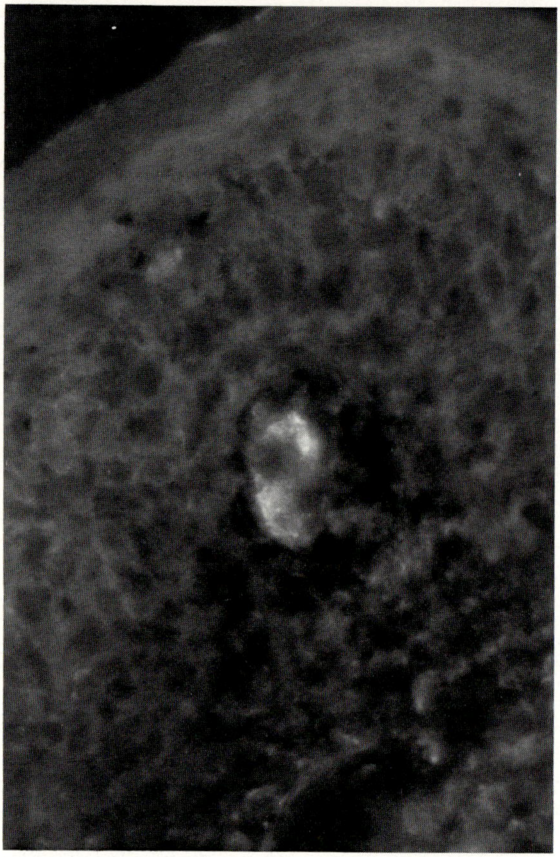

Figure 1. Direct IF tests for IgM in a 4-μ section of a normal skin biopsy specimen from a patient with chronic active hepatitis. The patient was positive for HBsAg. Note IgM deposits in the lumen of a blood vessel (200x).

Table 1. IF Deposits in Superficial Vessels of Normal Skin in Chronic Hepatitis

Group	*No. of cases*	*No. of cases with immune deposits*			
		IgA	*IgG*	*IgM*	*C3*
Protracted hepatitis type B	3	0	0	2	1
Chronic active hepatitis B	37	3	7	30	14
Chronic active hepatitis non-A/non-B	2	0	0	1	1
Total	42	3	7	33	16
Percentage		7.1	16.7	78.6	38.1

Table 2. IF Deposits in the Dermal-Epidermal Junction of Normal Skin in Chronic Hepatitis

Forms of hepatitis	*No. of cases*	*No. of cases with immune deposits*			
		IgA	*IgG*	*IgM*	*C3*
Protracted hepatitis B	3	0	0	0	1
Chronic active hepatitis B	37	1	5	0	10
Chronic active hepatitis non-A/non-B	2	0	1	0	1
Total	42	1	6	0	12
Percentage		2.4	14.3	0	28.6

monitoring of patients' liver morphology, clinical, biochemical, and immunologic studies were used.

The standard skin biopsy specimen was obtained from the dorsal area of the hand, between the thumb and the forefinger. The routine histology and the IF methods according to Beutner et al. (1), with IgG, IgA, IgM, and C3 conjugates, were used.

In our 15 consecutive cases of CAH-type B, we found no abnormalities in routine histology of clinically normal skin. Therefore, we discontinued further histologic examinations. In contrast, the immunologic examinations of the clinically normal skin revealed a high frequency of IgM (Fig. 1) and C3 deposits in superficial capillaries (Table 1).

The finding of IgM in skin vessels seems to be a characteristic of hepatitis, as it was present in 78.6% of cases. In 16 of 33 cases characterized by IgM in vessels, the C3 was also present. Three cases with negative IF findings on repeated biopsy examinations showed IgM deposits in the just-described distribution.

In none of 58 biopsy specimens of clinically normal skin was IgM found in the dermal-epidermal junction (Table 2).

SUMMARY OF IMMUNOFLUORESCENT FINDINGS IN NORMAL SKIN IN CHRONIC HEPATITIS

While IgM deposits in normal skin capillaries are characteristic of chronic hepatitis, this is not a disease-specific finding. IgM and C3 deposits in capillaries in the papillary dermis occur in rheumatoid arthritis (2,5). These deposits, which according to Rapaport et al. (9) are related to circulating immune complexes, occur in a significantly lower frequency than in chronic hepatitis.

From the practical point of view, the detection of IgM in superficial blood vessels of normal skin in problem cases strongly suggests chronic hepatitis. Indeed, three cases were referred to us with a tentative diagnosis of collagen disease in which IgM was found in perivascular distribution. A final diagnosis of CAH was eventually confirmed in each of these three cases.

REFERENCES

1. Beutner EH, Chorzelski TP, Jordon RE: *Autosensitization in Pemphigus and Bullous Pemphigoid.* Charles C Thomas, Springfield, IL, 1970, 194 pp.

2. Conn DL, Schroeter AL, Michel B: Cutaneous vessel deposits in rheumatoid arthritis. *Arthritis Rheum* 19:15, 1976.
3. Dienstag JL, Rhodes AR, Ehan AK, et al: Urticaria associated with acute viral hepatitis type studies of pathogenesis. *Ann Intern Med* 1:34, 1978.
4. De Groote J: Classification of chronic hepatitis. *Ann Clin Res* 8:130, 1976.
5. Ma ASP, Soltani K, Bristol LA, et al: Cutaneous immunofluorescence studies in adult rheumatoid arthritis in sun-exposed and non-sun-exposed areas. *Int J Dermatol* 23:269, 1984.
6. McElgunn PSY: Dermatologic manifestations of hepatitis B virus infection. *J Am Acad Dermatol* 8:539, 1983.
7. Neumann HAM, Berretty PJM, Reinders Folmer SCC, et al: Hepatitis B surface antigen deposition in the blood vessel walls of urticarial lesions in acute hepatitis B. *Br J Dermatol* 104:383, 1981.
8. Popp JW Jr, Harrist TJ, Dienstag JL, et al: Cutaneous vasculitis associated with acute and chronic hepatitis. *Arch Intern Med* 141:623, 1981.
9. Rapaport JR, Kozin F, Mackel SE: Cutaneous vascular immunofluorescence in rheumatoid arthritis: Correlation with circulating immune complexes and vasculitis. *Am J Med* 68:325, 1980.
10. Weiss TD, Tsai CC, Baldassare AR, et al: Skin lesions in viral hepatitis. Histologic and immunofluorescent findings. *Am J Med* 64:269, 1978.

Index